The Textbook of Peritoneal Dialysis

Edited by

Ram Gokal
Department of Renal Medicine, Manchester Royal Infirmary, Manchester, United Kingdom

and

Karl D. Nolph
Division of Nephrology, Department of Internal Medicine, School of Medicine, University of Missouri,
Health Sciences Center and Dalton Cardiovascular Research Center, Columbia, Missouri,
United States of America

Kluwer Academic Publishers

Dordrecht / Boston / London

Library of Congress Cataloging-in-Publication Data

```
The Textbook of peritoneal dialysis / edited by Ram Gokal & Karl D.
  Nolph. -- 1st ed.
      p.   cm.
   Includes index.
   ISBN 0-7923-2661-X (HB : alk. paper)
   1. Peritoneal dialysis.   I. Gokal, R.   II. Nolph, Karl D.
   [DNLM: 1. Peritoneal Dialysis.  2. Peritoneum--physiology.
  3. Peritoneum--drug effects.   WJ 378 T355 1994]
  RC901.7.P48T46 1994
  617.4'61059--dc20
  DNLM/DLC
  for Library of Congress                                93-40474
```

ISBN 0-7923-2661-X

Published by Kluwer Academic Publishers,
P.O. Box 17, 3300 AA Dordrecht, The Netherlands.

Kluwer Academic Publishers incorporates
the publishing programmes of
D. Reidel, Martinus Nijhoff, Dr W. Junk and MTP Press.

Sold and distributed in the U.S.A. and Canada
by Kluwer Academic Publishers,
101 Philip Drive, Norwell, MA 02061, U.S.A.

In all other countries, sold and distributed
by Kluwer Academic Publishers Group,
P.O. Box 322, 3300 AH Dordrecht, The Netherlands.

Printed on acid-free paper

All Rights Reserved
© 1994 Kluwer Academic Publishers
No part of the material protected by this copyright notice may be reproduced or utilized in any form or by any means, electronic or mechanical, including photocopying, recording or by any information storage and retrieval system, without written permission from the copyright owner.

Printed in the Netherlands

nka RN

The Textbook of P

1st Edition

(Combining *Continuous Ambulatory Peritoneal Dialysis*, 2nd ed. and *Peritoneal Dialysis*, 4th ed.)

Table of Contents

Foreword   vii
B. H. Scribner

Preface   ix
R. Gokal and K. D. Nolph

List of Contributors   xi

1. Historical developments and overview of peritoneal dialysis   1
   Ram Gokal and Karl D. Nolph

2. Ultrastructure and pathology of the peritoneum in peritoneal dialysis   17
   James W. Dobbie

3. The peritoneal microcirculation in peritoneal dialysis   45
   Randall White, Ronald Korthius and D. Neil Granger

4. Peritoneal physiology-transport of solutes   69
   Bengt Rippe and Raymond Theodorus Krediet

5. Peritoneal lymphatics   115
   Robert A. Mactier and Ramesh Khanna

6. Ultrafiltration in peritoneal dialysis   135
   John K. Leypoldt and Chandra D. Mistry

7. Pharmacologic alterations of peritoneal transport rates and pharmacokinetics of the peritoneum   161
   Przemyslaw Hirszel, Norbert Lameire and Marc Bogaert

8. CAPD systems and solutions   233
   Mariano Feriani, Giuseppe LaGreca, Frank L. Kriger and James F. Winchester

9. Peritoneal dialysis access and exit site care   271
   Zbylut J. Twardowski and Ramesh Khanna

10. Placement, repair, and removal of chronic peritoneal catheters   315
    Stephen R. Ash and W. Kirt Nichols

11. Organization of the peritoneal dialysis program – the nurses' role   335
    L. Uttley and B. Prowant

12. Continuous ambulatory peritoneal dialysis   357
    J. W. Moncrief, R. P. Popovich, N. V. Dombros, G. E. Digenis and D. G. Oreopoulos

13. Automated peritoneal dialysis — 399
    Jose A. Diaz-Buxo and Wadi N. Suki

14. Adequacy of peritoneal dialysis — 419
    Prakash Keshaviah

15. Nutritional requirements of peritoneal dialysis patients — 443
    Bengt Lindholm and Jonas Bergström

16. Peritonitis — 473
    William F. Keane and Stephen I. Vas

17. Host defence and effects of solutions on peritoneal cells — 503
    Gerald A. Coles, Sharon L. Lewis and John D. Williams

18. Calcium, phosphate and renal osteodystrophy — 529
    Alastair J. Hutchison and Ram Gokal

19. Noninfectious complications of peritoneal dialysis — 555
    Joanne M. Bargman

20. Peritoneal dialysis in children — 591
    Steven R. Alexander, J. Williamson Balfe and Elizabeth Harvey

21. Peritoneal dialysis in diabetic end-stage renal disease — 639
    Ramesh Khanna

22. Peritoneal dialysis in the elderly patient — 661
    Allen R. Nissenson

23. Quality of life — 679
    Ram Gokal

24. Outcome of peritoneal dialysis: comparative studies — 699
    Rosario Maiorca and Giovanni C. Cancarini

25. Registry results — 735
    Karl D. Nolph

26. The use of peritoneal dialysis in special situations — 751
    Sarah S. Prichard and Joanne M. Bargman

27. Intraperitoneal chemotherapy — 769
    Michael F. Flessner and Robert L. Dedrick

Index — 791

Foreword

In May 1992 a landmark article entitled "Survival as an Index of Adequacy of Dialysis" was published by Charra et al. [1]. Although it was based only on hemodialysis results, I believe it has important implications for peritoneal dialysis as well.

The importance of this article is that their patient survival data are superior to any previously reported. The authors clearly recognized the pitfalls inherent in comparing survival data among various series. They employed sophisticated statistical methods to reduce these pitfalls to a minimum and were careful to draw conclusions only when the survival data were clearly superior to data reported by others for a similar sub-group of patients.

Using old fashioned Kiil dialysis, each of the 445 patients received 24 hours of long slow dialysis a week. Since the average KT/V was 1.67, under dialysis, which has been shown to adversely effect mortality [2], was eliminated as a variable in this study. Similarly, the adverse effects of protein malnutrition [3] were eliminated as a variable since protein intake was generous as indicated by an average protein catabolic rate of 1.43 grams/kg/day and an average serum albumin of 4.1 grams/100 ml. Thus the authors were able to concentrate on the two other controllable variables that can effect patient survival namely *smoking* and *hypertension*, and to conclude that their superior survival rate was due entirely to adequate control of blood pressure. This conclusion was made even more explicit in a recent editorial by Charra [4]. He also offered further documentation to the principle, long adhered to by our group [5], that the only way to control blood pressure among dialysis patients is to normalize the volume of the extracellular space while phasing out antihypertensive medications. Dialysis patients are resistant to antihypertensive medications unless the extracellular space is normalized. At the same time, because they cause vascular instability during ultrafiltration, these drugs make it virtually impossible to gain control of blood pressure by using ultrafiltration to normalize the size of the extracellular space. These drugs should be withdrawn slowly at the initiation of dialysis therapy as the extracellular space is normalized by aggressive ultrafiltration.

Despite the fact that hypertension was first implicated back in 1978 by Haire and Sherrard [6] as a high risk factor for premature mortality among the dialysis population, I believe that far too little attention is paid to its control in the day to day administration of renal replacement therapy. (I use the term *renal replacement therapy* to include the pre-dialysis management of the patient, as well a treatment by both dialysis and transplantation). Also, I agree with Charra's suggestion that the definition of adequacy of dialysis should be expanded to include adequate control of blood pressure [4].

I believe that many of the points discussed above have important implications for the future of peritoneal dialysis. Since this mode of therapy has only been in widespread use for a little over a decade, it will be some time before long term survival can be used to judge adequacy. Nevertheless, it is important to begin now to initiate the proper studies including patient registries that will one day delineate what effect if any the time spent being maintained on peritoneal dialysis has on patient survival [7].

In the meantime it is essential to monitor carefully in each patient on peritoneal dialysis the four *controllable* variables known to affect patient survival. These are: the dose of peritoneal dialysis, adequate protein intake, avoidance of smoking and control of blood pressure.

As to the first two variables, dose of peritoneal dialysis and protein intake, it is important to develop similar methods to follow them [7], and to express the results in terms that the patient himself can readily understand.

Referring to the above discussion by Charra regarding blood pressure control, it seems to me that CAPD should offer the ideal mode of dialytic therapy to control blood pressure without drugs, since removal of extracellular fluid is both constant and easily adjusted as compared to hemodialysis with its inherent wide swings in extracellular volume. A recent publication presents data consistent with this idea [8].

In line with Charra's opinion [4] that control of blood pressure is the variable most often neglected in the care of patients on renal replacement therapy, the subject of blood pressure control received almost no mention in an otherwise excellent scientific meeting which compared overall results of hemodialysis and peritoneal dialysis [9].

Belding H. Scribner M.D.
Seattle, Washington
March, 1993

References

1. Charra B, Calemard E, Ruffet M, Chazot C, Terrat JC, Vanel T, Laurent G. Survival as an index of adequacy of dialysis. Kidney Int 1992; 41: 1286-91.
2. Held JH, Levin NW, Bovbjerg RR, Pauly MV, Diamond LH. Mortality and duration of dialysis treatment. JAMA 1991; 265: 871-5.
3. Lowrie EG, Lew NL. Death risk in hemodialysis patients: the predictive value of commonly measured variables and an evaluation of death rate differences between facilities. Am J Kidney Dis 1990; 15: 458-82.
4. Charra B. Does empirical long slow dialysis result in better survival? Proc ASAIO (in press).
5. Scribner BH. Kidney Int (editorial) 1992; 41: 1286.
6. Haire HM, Sherrard DJ, Scardapane D, Curtis FK, Brunzell JD. Smoking hypertension and mortality in a maintenance dialysis population. Cardiovasc Med 1978; 3: 1163-7.
7. Keshaviah P. Urea kinetic and middle molecule approaches to assessing adequacy of hemodialysis and CAPD. Kidney Int 1993; 43 (suppl 40): S28-38.
8. Saldanha LF, Weiler E, Gonick HC. Effect of continuous ambulatory peritoneal dialysis on blood pressure control. Am J Kidney Dis 1993; 21: 184-8.
9. Nolph KD, Henderson LW. Options in renal therapy. Kidney Int Supplement 40, Feb 1993.

Preface
Textbook of Peritoneal Dialysis

In 1986, the first edition of *Continuous Ambulatory Peritoneal Dialysis*, edited by R. Gokal, was published. In 1989, the third edition of *Peritoneal Dialysis*, edited by K. D. Nolph, was published. Rather than edit new editions of each of these books separately, we have decided to combine our efforts to edit this single book which is called *The Textbook of Peritoneal Dialysis*.

Peritoneal dialysis represents an internal technique for blood purification. In this dialyzer, the blood path, the membrane and the dialysate compartment are provided by nature. Interest in and utilization of peritoneal dialysis has been stimulated by the developments of chronic peritoneal catheters, automated cycling equipment, manipulations of transport, experiences with continuous ambulatory peritoneal dialysis, experiences with peritoneal dialysis using cyclers, decreases in peritonitis rates with new connection approaches and better definitions of adequate peritoneal dialysis. New advances in our understanding of the physiology of peritoneal dialysis (including the role of peritoneal lymphatics) and peritoneal dialysis kinetics are examples of the dynamic nature of the field.

Publications related to peritoneal dialysis usually exceed 400 annually. *Peritoneal Dialysis International*, the official journal of the International Society for Peritoneal Dialysis, is a journal solely devoted to peritoneal dialysis experiences and development. The Sixth Congress of the International Society for Peritoneal Dialysis was held in Thessaloniki, Greece, in 1992. The next meeting of this international society will be held in Stockholm, Sweden, in 1995. The 13th Annual Peritoneal Dialysis Conference was held in San Diego, California, in 1993 and attracted 2,500 participants from 40 countries. At this time, more than 70,000 patients are estimated to be maintained on chronic peritoneal dialysis worldwide.

This book is meant to provide an overview of the state of the art of peritoneal dialysis. Many clinicians are making extensive commitments to peritoneal dialysis. Nephrologists, anatomists, physiologists, pharmacologists, biomedical engineers, and even physicists are involved in studies to better understand peritoneal dialysis. The complexities of peritoneal dialysis and the peritoneal membrane are becoming apparent. Studies of peritoneal dialysis increase understanding of the anatomy and physiology of biological membranes and the factors influencing the paths for movement of solutes across the microcirculation and related structures. Peritoneal dialysis provides a "window" to the visceral microcirculation in animals and in humans.

Peritoneal dialysis may be useful to treat problems other than renal failure. Beneficial effects in the treatment of dysproteinemia, psoriases, hypothermia and metabolic problems have been reported. The intraperitoneal administration of chemotherapeutic agents draws upon and contributes to our understanding of peritoneal dialysis. This book contains a chapter dealing with the concepts of intraperitoneal chemotherapy.

The editors feel fortunate to have been involved in peritoneal dialysis research and development for over 50 years of combined experience. New ideas and new developments have been an almost daily occurrence. Yet, our understanding of this dialysis system is still in its infancy. The authors of the chapters in this book have been actively investigating and writing about their respective topics for many years. Most are individuals with whom we have had the good fortune to have had frequent contacts. Many coauthors of chapters have somewhat different opinions, and yet, they have made an effort to combine their thoughts in a single chapter.

As in our previous books, each chapter is an extensive review of a given topic. We have not edited out all overlap between chapters since we feel the reader benefits by exposure to slightly different perspectives of complex material, and this allows each author to deal with all issues that relate to his respective topics.

We hope that this book will serve as a reference text for all those with more than a casual interest in peritoneal dialysis.

August 1993
Ram Gokal
Karl D. Nolph

List of Contributors

Stephen R. Alexander
University of Texas
Health Science Center
Dept. of Clinical Pediatric Nephrology
523 Harry Hines Blvd.
Dallas, TX 75235–9063
U.S.A.

Stephen R. Ash
Ash Medical Systems, Inc.
2701 B. Kent Avenue
West Lafayette, IN 47906
U.S.A.

J. Williamson Balfe
The Hospital for Sick Children
555 University Avenue
Toronto, Ontario M5G 1X8
Canada

Joanne M. Bargman
Division of Nephrology
Dept. of Medicine, ECW 7-034
Toronto Western Hospital
399 Bathurst St.
Toronto, Ontario M5T 2S8
Canada

Jonas L. Bergstrom
Department of Renal Medicine
K 56, Huddinge University Hospital
Karolinska Institute
S-141 86 Huddinge
Sweden

Marc Bogaert
Heymans Institute of Pharmacology
University of Gent Medical School
Gent, Belgium

Giovanni C. Cancarini
Department of Nephrology – Spedali Civili
Pizzo Ospedale, 1
Brescia
Italy 25125

Gerald A. Coles
Institute of Nephrology
Cardiff Royal Infirmary
Newport Road
Cardiff, Wales CF2 1SZ
United Kingdom

Robert Dedrick
1633 Warner Ave.
McLean, VA 22101
U.S.A.

Jose A. Diaz-Buxo
Metrolina Kidney Center
928 Baxter Street
Charlotte, NC 28204
U.S.A.

George E. Digenis
48 Dekelia Street
Aharnes, Attika
Greece 13671

James W. Dobbie
Baxter R & D Europe, S.C.
Parc Industriel
Rue du Progrès, 7
1400 Nivelles
Belgium

Nicholas V. Dombros
Karolov Diehl 13
54623 Thessaloniki
Greece

Mariano Ferriani
Department of Nephrology
St. Bortolo Hospital
36100 Vicenza
Italy

Michael F. Flessner
Box 675, Nephrology Unit
Department of Medicine
University of Rochester
601 Elmwood Ave.
Rochester, NY 14642
U.S.A.

Ram Gokal
Department of Renal Medicine
Manchester Royal Infirmary
Oxford Road
Manchester, England M13 9WL
United Kingdom

D. Neil Granger
Dept. of Physiology and Biophysics
Louisiana State University Medical Center
1501 Kings Highway
P.O. Box 33932
Shreveport, LA 71130–3932
U.S.A.

Elizabeth Harvey
The Hospital for Sick Children
555 University Avenue
Toronto, Ontario M5G 1X8
Canada

Przemyslaw Hirszel
Professor of Medicine
Department of Medicine
Nephrology Division
Uniformed Services University
of the Health Sciences
4301 Jones Bridge Road
Bethesda, MD 20814
U.S.A.

Alistair J. Hutchison
Dept. of Renal Medicine
Manchester Royal Infirmary
Oxford Road
Manchester, England M13 9WL
United Kingdom

William F. Keane
Professor of Medicine
University of Minnesota School of Medicine
Hennepin County Medical Center
701 Park Avenue
Minneapolis, MN 55415
U.S.A.

Prakash Keshaviah
Baxter Clinical Engineering Laboratory
825 S. 8th Street – Suite 722
Minneapolis, MN 55404
U.S.A.

Ramesh Khanna
Division of Nephrology
MA 436 Health Sciences Center
University of Missouri
Columbia, MO 65212
U.S.A.

Ronald Korthius
Dept. of Physiology and Biophysics
Louisiana State University Medical Center
1501 Kings Highway
P.O. Box 33932
Shreveport, LA 71130–3932
U.S.A.

Raymond T. Krediet
Renal Unit
Academic Medical Center
Meibergdreef 9
Amsterdam 1105 AZ
The Netherlands

Frank L. Kriger
Division of Nephrology
Georgetown University School of Medicine
3800 Reservoir Road, N.W.
Washington, DC 20007–2113
U.S.A.

Giuseppe LaGreca
Department of Nephrology
St. Bartolo Hospital
Via Rodolfi
36100 Vicenza
Italy

LIST OF CONTRIBUTORS

Norbert Lameire
Professor of Medicine
Afdeling Nefrologie
Universitair Ziekenhuis
De Pintelaan 185
B-9000 Gent
Belgium

Sharon Lewis
University of New Mexico
BRF 321 – Dept of Pathology
Albuquerque, NM 87131–5301
U.S.A.

John K. Leypoldt
Research Service
VA Medical Center and Departments
of Internal Medicine
and Bioengineering
VA Medical Center (11H)
500 Foothill Boulevard
Salt Lake City, UT 84148
U.S.A.

Bengt Lindholm
Department of Renal Medicine
K 56, Huddinge University Hospital
Karolinska Institute
S-141 86 Huddinge
Sweden

Robert A. Mactier
Consultant Physician
Renal Unit
Stobhill General Hospital
Glasgow, Scotland, G21 3UW
United Kingdom

Rosario Maiorca
Spedali Civili, Brescia
Piazza Spedali Civili 1
25125 Brescia
Italy

Chandra D. Mistry
Institute of Nehprology
Cardiff Royal Infirmary
Newport Road
Cardiff CF2 1SZ
Wales
United Kingdom

Jack W. Moncrief
Moncrief Popovich Research Institute
4211 Medical Parkway
Austin, TX 78765
U.S.A.

W. Kirt Nichols
Department of Surgery
University of Missouri
NW301 Health Sciences Center
1 Hospital Drive
Columbia, MO 65212
U.S.A.

Allen R. Nissenson
UCLA School of Medicine
Department of Medicine
Director, Dialysis Program
Los Angeles, CA 90024
U.S.A.

Karl D. Nolph
Division of Nephrology
MA 436 Health Sciences Center
University of Missouri
Columbia, MO 65212
U.S.A.

Dimitrios G. Oreopoulos
Division of Nephrology
Department of Medicine
Toronto Western Hospital
399 Bathurst St.
Toronto, Ontario M5T 2S8
Canada

Robert P. Popovich
Moncrief Popovich Research Institute
4211 Medical Parkway
Austin, TX 78765
U.S.A.

Sarah Prichard
Royal Victoria Hospital
Room A417
687 Pine Avenue West
Montreal, Quebec H3A 1A1
Canada

Barbara Prowant
Division of Nephrology
MA 436 Health Sciences Center
University of Missouri
Columbia, MO 65212
U.S.A.

Bengt Rippe
Department of Nephrology
University Hospital of Lund
S-221 85 Lund
Sweden

Jacques Rottembourg
Dept. of Nephrology
Groupe Hospitalier de la Pitie-Salpetriere
47–83 Blvd. de l'Hopital
75651 Paris, Cedex 13
France

Belding H. Scribner
University of Washington
Division of Kidney Diseases
Room 11
Seattle, WA 98195
U.S.A.

Wadi N. Suki
Department of Medicine
Baylor College of Medicine
6550 Fannin, Suite 1275
Houston, TX 77030
U.S.A.

Zbylut J. Twardowski
Division of Nephrology
MA 436 Health Sciences Center
University of Missouri
Columbia, MO 65212
U.S.A.

Linda Uttley
Department of Renal Medicine
Manchester Royal Infirmary
Oxford Road
Manchester, England M13 9WL
United Kingdom

Stephen I. Vas
Dept. of Medical Microbiology
Toronto Western Hospital
399 Bathurst Street
Toronto, Ontario M5T 2S8
Canada

Randall White
Division of Nephrology
Dept. of Medicine
Louisiana State University Medical Center
1501 Kings Highway
P.O. Box 33932
Shreveport, LA 71130–3932
U.S.A.

John D. Williams
Institute of Nephrology
Cardiff Royal Infirmary
Newport Road
Cardiff, Wales CF2 1SZ
United Kingdom

James F. Winchester
Professor of Medicine
Division of Nephrology
Georgetown University School of Medicine
Room 2212
3800 Reservoir Road, N.W.
Washington, DC 20007–2113
U.S.A.

1 Historical developments and overview of peritoneal dialysis

RAM GOKAL AND KARL NOLPH

1. Historical review of peritoneal dialysis — 1
   1.1. Early studies of peritoneal anatomy — 1
   1.2. Invention of peritoneal lavage — 1
   1.3. Early studies of peritoneal physiology (1877–1923) — 2
   1.4. Early experiences of PD in uraemia (1923–1960) — 2
   1.5. Methods, techniques and PD fluids — 3
2. Intermittent chronic peritoneal dialysis (1960 onwards) — 4
   2.1 Indwelling catheters — 4
3. Continuous ambulatory peritoneal dialysis — 5
   3.1 Growth of CAPD worldwide — 6
   3.2 Evolution of CAPD technique — 6
4. Automated peritoneal dialysis — 8
5. Recent developments and areas of research — 9
   5.1. Adequacy of dialysis — 10
   5.2. Nutrition — 10
   5.3. Peritoneal membrane — 10
6. Patient selection — 10
   6.1. Indications for CAPD — 11
   6.2. Contraindications — 11
      6.2.1. Other relative contraindications — 11
References — 12

Peritoneal Dialysis (PD) has now become an established form of renal replacement therapy. Its use throughout the world is increasing (see Chapter 25) and has provided a means of managing some patients who would otherwise have been denied treatment because haemodialysis was inappropriate, failed or unavailable. The current state of art has been a combination of painstaking efforts, dedication and ingenuity on the part of several innovative pioneers in this field over the last two centuries. This chapter describes these historical developments leading up to PD as it is practised today. This chapter also gives an overview of the state of the art of peritoneal dialysis, details of most aspects being given in the relevant chapters that follow.

1. Historical review of peritoneal dialysis

1.1. Early studies of peritoneal anatomy

Probably the first observers of the peritoneal cavity were the early morticians in Egypt, who delicately prepared the remains of influential Egyptians to ensure that the body would remain "uncorrupted" for eternity [1]. Cunningham [2] reports that "the Egyptians recorded in the Ebers papyrus, written about 3000 BC, the peritoneal cavity to be a definite entity in which the viscera were somehow suspended". In conjunction with these anatomical studies these Egyptians also attempted to treat impaired renal function by inducing diarrhoea with the use of purgatives or forced diuresis using beer. They were thus aware of oedema and understood the effects of diuresis. In Greek times, Galan, a Physician, made detailed descriptions of the abdomen whilst treating injuries of gladiators. He provided precise details of the peritoneal cavity and peritoneum [1]. Even though gradually, over the centuries, the peritoneal structure became more clearly defined, its functioning and role better understood, it has remained an enigma and enchanted physiologists, surgeons and gynecologists. More recently nephrologists joined this band of investigators.

1.2. Invention of peritoneal lavage

The concept of peritoneal lavage goes back over 150 years when it served a purpose totally different from removal of toxins. Christopher Warrick, a Surgeon from Truro in England, presented his findings about a new – rather drastic method of treating recurrent ascites [3]. He managed a female patient aged 50 with severe ascites by infusing a mixture of one half bristol water and one half claret into the peritoneal cavity after draining the ascites. She miraculously recovered from the ensuing syncope and pain and underwent two further such "exchanges". It is interesting to note that Warrick felt that this was "ascitic lymph" and was looking for a method whereby the "ruptured lymphatics must close their mouths".

The idea of peritoneal lavage came from a clergyman, Reverend Stephen Hales, who happened to be present at the presentation of Warrick at the Royal Society of Medicine. Reverend Hales felt pity for the old lady and wrote a letter to the Secretary of the Royal Society suggesting a more gentle modification of Warrick's methods [4]. His technique entailed introducing two trochars, one on each side of the abdomen allowing the "liquor" to flow in and out of the abdomen. This first description of peritoneal lavage was essentially identical to the continuous peritoneal lavage later to be used for the treatment of uraemia.

1.3. Early studies of peritoneal physiology (1877–1923)

Not much is known of the fate of lavage in managing recurrent ascites. The next publication on experimental peritoneal lavage was published more than 130 years later in the late 19th century by Wegner, a German investigator [5]. He found that hypertonic solutions of sugar, salt or glycerine increased in volume when injected into the peritoneal cavity of a dog. Starling and Tubby in 1884 showed that hypertonic intraperitoneal solutions would increase whilst hypotonic solutions would decrease in volume [6]. They studied the absorption of such substances as indigo, carmine, methyline blue from the peritoneal cavity and concluded that the solute exchange was primarily between solutions and blood; the exchange with lymph was negligible. Cunningham in 1920 showed the complete absorption of a 10% dextrose solution from the rat peritoneal cavity in about 12 hours and concluded that most of the absorption could be explained on the basis of the "known physical laws of osmosis and diffusion" [7]. Similar results were obtained by Clark who further showed that absorption was temperature related; it increased by elevating the temperature of the solution or applying heat to the abdominal wall [8].

Spurred on by these interesting physiological studies and the report of Abel in 1913 on "vivi" diffusion (haemodialysis) in animals [9], Putnam published his work in dogs, characterising the peritoneum as a dialysing membrane [10]. His studies were extensive, looking at fluid removal (ultrafiltration) and exchange of various solutes and varying intervals of dwell time. He concluded that "under certain circumstances, fluids in the peritoneal cavity can come into an apparently complete osmotic equilibrium with the plasma", and that the "speed of diffusion of different molecules through the peritoneum appeared to vary with their respective sizes". He also pointed out that "changes in volume reflected the osmotic forces at work". This work as well as that of others [7, 8] presented convincing evidence that the peritoneal membrane was permeable in two directions in a similar way to the pigs bladder membrane or a membrane of non biological material like parchment invitro, a phenomenon first described by Graham in 1861 who also coined the word dialysis [11]. These studies on transfer of colloids and crystalloids in a bidirectional manner across the peritoneal membrane were fundamental in establishing the principles of solute transport and ultrafiltration which are still true to this day. These studies were further amplified by Engel who showed that the clearance of solute was proportional to the molecular size and solution pH, and high flow rate maximized the transfer of solutes which also depended on peritoneal surface area and blood flow [12].

Further progress and practical application of this acquired knowledge was relatively slow. However, two paediatricians Blackfan and Maxey did utilize the peritoneal cavity for the administration of fluids to dehydrated children [13].

1.4. Early experiences of PD in uraemia (1923–1960)

Ganter, a German clinical investigator, is traditionally credited with the first attempts to utilise PD in a human being [14]. Initially he performed a series of experimental PD in rabbits and guinea pigs made uraemic by ureteric ligation. Utilising 2–4 hour exchanges there was almost complete equilibration of non protein nitrogen in dialysate with that in the blood. There appeared to be some clinical improvement in the animal. Ganter used this technique to treat a uraemic woman suffering from obstructive uropathy from uterine cancer. He introduced 1.5 litres of salt solution through a needle in the peritoneal cavity. There was transient improvement in symptoms when the solution was removed but the patient subsequently died. From his experience with the use of peritoneal dialysis he was able to elicit several features upon which he based his recommendation: the use of 1–1.5 litres per exchange with close monitoring of the equilibration time; the use of hypertonic solutions with an anaesthetic to minimise pain; and continuous lavage for cases of poisoning but a dwell phase between exchanges for uraemia. He postulated that with improvements this procedure could become an innovative and useful form of renal care.

A number of other reports subsequently confirmed the usefulness of peritoneal dialysis in uraemia. Heusser and Werder performed peritoneal dialysis in three patients with acute renal failure from mercury poisoning [15], as did Balazc and Rosenak [16] and Wear et al. [17]. In all these reports outcome was very poor related to poor removal of urea. Rhodes et al. [18] treated two uraemic patients with chronic renal failure with peritoneal dialysis using for the first time intermittent methods as first described in his experimental animals with a single catheter and a dwell period of about 15 minutes.

During the second world war, thousands of cases of acute renal failure died of uraemia. Soon afterwards Fine, Frank and Seligman from Boston produced their landmark paper on the successful use of PD in acute renal failure [19]. Their investigations were based on sound scientific evidence on the effects of peritoneal lavage. Odel et al. reviewed the literature between 1923 and 1948 and reported that 101 patients had received peritoneal dialysis over this period. Of these 63 had reversible causes, 32 irreversible and in 2 the diagnosis was uncertain [20]. There was recovery in 32 of the cases with reversible causes; death in 40 cases was predominantly related to uraemina, pulmonary oedema and peritonitis. Derot et al. reported the first successful experience in acute renal failure with 9 out of 10 survivors [21]. Following the work of Grollman et al. [22] who demonstrated the use of intermittent peritoneal dialysis in nephrectomised dogs, Legrain and Merrill [23] used this form of dialysis in three patients. In one of them three procedures were performed in a 2 week period. They stressed frequent dialysis, dietary salt and protein restrictions and avoidance of infection.

1.5. Methods, techniques and PD fluids

Over this period, up to 1950, the methods and techniques involved ingenious improvisation. Catheters were made from tubings available on the ward and included gall bladder trocars [17] rubber catheters, whistle tip catheters and stainless steel sump drains [19]. In the early fifties, polyvinylchloride [21, 23] and polyethylene plastic tubes [22] were employed to gain peritoneal access but were troubled with kinking and blockage. Maxwell et al. [24] described a nylon catheter with small perforations and a curved distal end. This catheter became commercially available and widely used subsequently.

The techniques varied from continuous flow (two catheters used) [19, 21, 23] or intermittent (one catheter with tip in pelvis) [12, 24, 25]. The former technique was bedevilled by fluid leakage and the risk of peritonitis was later avoided.

The fluid composition varied considerably from normal saline to 5% Dextrose. In retrospect the complications and undesirable side effects were readily explained by the unsuitable composition of different dialysis fluids. Odel et al. [20] in their literature review, also assessed the electrolyte composition and found that hyperchloraemic metabolic acidosis was a frequently observed side effect with the Lock-Ringer and modified Tyrode solutions and normal saline. High dialysis fluid sodium concentrations were used and Reid et al. [26] who performed the first PD in England in 1946 used twice normal saline. Peripheral and pulmonary oedema and hypertension often accompanied peritoneal dialysis in the fifties; soon a low dialysate sodium and appropriate amounts of bicarbonate (or acetate/lactate) were incorporated as a routine to avoid these complications. Bicarbonate in PD fluids ranged from 26 mmol/l, [27] to 35–40 [25]. The bicarbonate was soon replaced by lactate when commercial fluid became available in 1959. Since dextrose (up to 7 gm/100 ml) was being used to induce ultrafiltration this created a problem during the sterilisation process. Caramalisation of glucose had to be avoided during the sterilisation and in addition solutions containing both calcium and bicarbonate could not be stored because of precipitation of calcium carbonate. In the late fifties intermittent peritoneal dialysis became a relatively safe and standardised procedure in particular related to the work of Doolan et al. [28] and Maxwell and colleagues [29] who developed the hanging bottle peritoneal dialysis using commercially prepared rinsing fluids.

These changes and improvements, though important, did not allow the use of peritoneal dialysis on a longterm basis for the management of patients in endstage renal failure. Further advances were primarily related to catheter improvements which made longterm therapy possible.

2. Intermittent chronic peritoneal dialysis (1960 onwards)

The successful application of intermittent peritoneal dialysis to acute renal failure, led to the use of repeated peritoneal dialysis in patients with terminal end stage renal failure at a time when a similar venture was being tried with intermittent haemodialysis. The first such patient was treated in early 1960 by Rubin and Doolan at the US Naval Hospital in Oakland, California, by what later became known as "periodic" peritoneal dialysis. This patient survived for six months [29]. Just from the single case experience it became obvious that the major problem lay with adequate and safe peritoneal access.

In the early sixties various devices were tried to achieve easy and frequent access into the peritoneal cavity. In Seattle, Boen and colleagues tried the Seattle Teflon and silicone rubber tubes [30]. Boen and colleagues [31] attempted repeated peritoneal irrigation in four patients with endstage renal failure utilising a plastic conduit for repeated insertion of the catheter. They had little success: a number of technical problems necessitated revision or removal of the conduits within two weeks to four months. Boen and colleagues [32], developed the repeated puncture technique with automatic cycling machines. Initially 20 litre pyrex carboys were tried to be replaced by even larger bottles with volumes of 45 litres. The improved cycling machine facilitated uninterrupted cycling without breaking the continuity of the closed sterile fluid administration circuit. It also enabled complete freedom between dialysis sessions and this technique could be adapted for home use. Tenckhoff et al. [33], carried this out in a patient for three years entailing 380 catheter punctures with a low peritonitis rate. However, this procedure could not be used on a large scale as it was too time consuming. Overall, this early experience was indeed discouraging. The main problem being peritonitis from infection along the channel of the indwelling devices and from manually changing bottles. Repeated episodes of peritonitis were often followed by the development of adhesions with partial and more extensive obliteration of the peritoneal cavity, decreasing the dialysis efficiency. Most patients died within a few months. Peritoneal dialysis was utilised as a "holding procedure" for patients waiting for a place in a chronic haemodialysis programme or while waiting for vascular access to mature. In an editorial in *The Lancet* [34], it was stated that "peritoneal dialysis is obviously no silver bullet for renal failure but in suitable cases it is a good leaden bullet, which is more commonly fired".

2.1. Indwelling catheters

A major advance was brought about in gaining peritoneal access by Palmer et al. [35] with further advances made by Gutch [36] and McDonald et al. [37], who all utilised silicone rubber catheters, which incorporated perforations at the distal end and a triflanged step or a teflon velour skirt for seating the tube in the deep fascia and pertioneum. However, it was not until Tenckhoff's design of the indwelling silicone rubber catheter which had two dacron cuffs that intermittent peritoneal dialysis became accepted as a longterm therapy for renal failure patients [38]. This catheter or its subsequent modifications became accepted as the only practical access device. The original Tenckhoff catheter was basically a modification of the curled Palmer catheter [35]. It was inserted either surgically through a mini laporotomy or with local anaesthesia and the aid of a special Trocar at the bedside. Using automated machines and this catheter a large experience was built up in the Seattle area [39]. Tenckhoff and colleagues in this report related the experience of 12,000 peritoneal dialysis sessions in 69 patients who were mostly at home. By 1977, in the Seattle area 161 patients had been on peritoneal dialysis, many of them for over four years and a few for eight years [40]. Similar experience, was reported by Oreopoulous in 1975 [41] and subsequently by centres in Europe [42, 43]. Longterm therapy beyond four years was not often achieved with a cumulative technique survival of 27% for three years in the Seattle group of patients [44]. Inadequate dialysis was one reason for conversion to haemodialysis as was repeated peritonitis. Enhancement of peritoneal dialysis efficiency was attempted in various ways; the influence of dialysis fluid flow and exchange volumes, effect of temperature, optimisation of dwell time, increase of solute transfer by convection, and utilisation of pharmacological methods were all tried without too much success [45]. For these reasons, haemodialysis remained the cornerstone of dialysis therapy and for peritoneal dialysis to challenge this position, a major rethink was necessary. This came about in the mid seventies.

3. Continuous ambulatory peritoneal dialysis

The concept of CAPD had its origin in Austen, Texas, USA, when in 1975 Dr. R. Popovich and Dr. J. Moncrief were discussing ways to dialyse a patient who could not receive haemodialysis or intermittent peritoneal dialysis. This "brainstorming" session induced Dr. Popovich, a biomedical engineer with knowledge of membrane kinetics, to theorise the use of long dwell cycles to achieve adequate removal of uraemic waste products to sustain life. Based on mathematical calculations, which suggested that adequate control could be achieved on five daily exchanges of 2 ltr, 7 days a week, Moncrief tried this in a patient and found that the results matched the theoretical ones. Ironically, the first description and account of the clinical experiences was not accepted for presentation at the American Society for Artifical Internal Organs (Fig. 1) [46]. It was initially called a "portable/wearable equilibrium dialysis techniques". This group described the theoretical mass transfer characteristics for this procedure.

Popovich demonstrated that a double pool model is valid for a low dialysis clearance system, such as the equilibration dialysis he described. The accumulation of the metabolites in the body would be equal to the rate of generation minus the rate of residual renal clearance, minus the overall dialysate clearance (diffusive and convective). Popovich postulated that the accumulation term being a time derivitive of total mass of the metabolite in the system, should equal zero if the dialysis treatment is continuous and the concentrations and volumes remain constant. Working on an accepted urea generation rate [47] and a desired steady state BUN level (0.8 gm/1) he estimated that over a 24 hour day, the daily clearance requirements equalled about 10 litres of dialysis fluid exchanged. The theory therefore predicted that a patient will maintain a steady BUN level of about 80 mg/dl, if 10 ltr of PD fluids are allowed to equilibrate with body fluids on a daily basis. This indeed was borne out in the clinical experiences, described in three patients [48].

A major cooperative study was begun in 1977 supported by the National Institute of Health. These included clinical studies at the Austin Diagnostic clinic, Texas (Dr. Moncrief), at the University of Missouri (Dr. K. Nolph), with the biomedical engineering support of the University of Texas (Dr. Popovich). This joint experience in 9 patients (duration of CAPD 5–26 weeks) was described in 1978 [49] and the name of the technique was changed to Continuous Ambulatory Peritoneal Dialysis (CAPD).

The main advantages of this new technique were good steady state biochemical control, more liberal dietary and fluid intakes than haemodialysis, improvement in anaemia and wellbeing of the patients and freedom from machines which allowed patients to travel long distances. However, these studies utilised peritoneal dialysis solutions in bottles. Connections and disconnections of tubing and bottles to the Tenckhoff catheter were required with each exchange and chances of contamination were high. Hence, not only was the technique cumbersome and time consuming, but was complicated by a high incidence of peritonitis (1 episode/10 patient weeks).

THE DEFINITION OF A NOVEL PORTABLE/WEARABLE EQUILIBRIUM PERITONEAL DIALYSIS TECHNIQUE.
Robert P. Popovitch, Jack W. Moncrief, Jonathan F. Decherd, John B. Bomar* and W. Keith Pyle.'
Depts. Chem. Engr. and Biomed Engr., The Univ. of Texas and Austin Diag. Clin., Austin, Texas.

An analysis will be presented which predicts that acceptable blood metabolite levels will result if 10 liters of dialysate per day are allowed to continuously equilibrate with body fluids. Accordingly, a portable/wearable dialysis procedure based upon equilibrium-intermittent peritoneal dialysis has been defined. Two liters of standard hypertonic dialysate fluid are infused peritoneally via a Tenckhoff catheter and allowed to equilibrate 5 hours while the patient conducts his normal activities. The dialysate is then drained and replaced with the procedure being repeated five times per day.

In a preliminary clinical study metabolite equilibration between blood and dialysate was achieved for BUN and creatinine but not for vitamin B-12. Steady state metabolite levels for BUN and creatinine were 40 and 9.5 mg% respectively. The patient was maintained 5 months with the new procedure with excellent clinical results followed by a successful transplant.

It is concluded that a new portable/wearable dialysis procedure has been defined. The technique does not require blood access and results in steady, low blood metabolite levels: middle molecule removal greatly exceeds that of conventional techniques.

Figure 1. The abstract of the first description of CAPD by the pioneers Dr Popovich and Dr Moncrief as it appeared in the abstract book of the American Society of Artificial Organs Meeting of 1976 [46].

In September 1977, Dr. Oreopoulos started his first patient on CAPD using a novel modification of the above technique with PD fluid in polyvinylchloride (PVC) bags. Following instillation of the fluid, the plastic bag, still connected to the administration set, was rolled up and carried under clothing without much difficulty. After a dwell period of (4–8h) the fluid was allowed to drain into the same bag under the "force of gravity" without disconnecting the tube from the Tenckhoff catheter [50]. The technique details were first presented in January 1978, at the 11th Annual Contractors Conference of the Artifical Kidney programme, Institutes of Arthritis, Metabolism, Digestive Disease in Bethesda, USA. The Oreopoulos modification made CAPD easier to perform and decreased (but did not eliminate) the rather high incidence of peritonitis when using bottled PD fluid (1 episode/10 patient weeks, to 1 episode/8 patient months). This represented a major advance and the use of CAPD increased in an explosive way. By June 1980, 115 patients were managed on CAPD at the Toronto Western Hospital [51].

In September 1978, the Food and Drug Administration approved sale of peritoneal dialysis solution in plastic bags in the United States; this led to many centres developing CAPD Programmes [52]. Another major step in the growth of CAPD in the USA was the announcement by the Health Care Financing Administration (Medicare) in October 1979, that CAPD was reimbursable and an accepted alternative to chronic haemodialysis. The growth therefore, has been exponential. By July 1980 over 1700 patients were treated in 190 centres [53].

3.1. Growth of CAPD worldwide

The growth in the United States was mirrored in other leading Western Nations with rapid increasing numbers in Canada [51], Europe [54–58] and Australia [59]. All these reports related to certain advantages of CAPD over IPD and Haemodialysis, but the technique was still compromised by the high rate of peritonitis and catheter related problems. These reviews were substantiated by individual centre experiences in the UK and Canada [60, 61] and proved beyond any doubt that maintenance of good dialysis and well being could be achieved over several years on CAPD treatment.

Over the ensuing years there has been a steady increase in the number of patient on peritoneal dialysis worldwide and industrial sources report that this number worldwide was 76,000 patients at the end of 1992. Also over the years the percentage increase of patients on an annual basis has been much higher on peritoneal dialysis as compared to haemodialysis and for the difference 1991/92 this was 16% increase for peritoneal dialysis as compared to 9% for haemodialysis (Table 1).

3.2. Evolution of CAPD technique

The CAPD technique, as eventually proposed by Popovich and Moncrief, entailed four exchanges of 21 volumes, using a combination of three 1.36% glucose and one 3.8% glucose to produce a ten litre dialysate volume over a 24 hour period. This necessitated 4–8 hour dwell period adjusted to fit into the patients daily routine. The initial use of glass bottles resulted in an unacceptable peritonitis rate [49] but with the introduction of the PVC bags there was a dramatic improvement [50].

The basic CAPD system, which to this day remains unchanged, consists of the PVC bag containing 0.5–3 litres of peritoneal dialysis fluid, a transfer set and a Tenckhoff catheter (Fig. 2). The connection between the bag and transfer set is broken four times a day, and the exchange procedure transferring the set from the spent bag to the new bag has to be performed using a strict non-touch technique. Various devices (connectors) have been developed to minimise the risk of contamination and given rise to the science of "connectology". However, this site remains the major source of contamination and peritonitis [62]. "Initially spike" connectors, at Site 1 and 2 (Fig. 2), led to accidental

Table 1. Global Dialysis Patients by Region Data show actual number of patients on either haemodialysis or peritoneal dialysis at end of 1992 and the % increase in comparison with 1991 numbers.

	Hemodialysis		Peritoneal dialysis	
	1992 (000s)	'91–'92 %Δ	1992 (000s)	'91–'92 %Δ
U.S.	132.0	9.0%	27.2	13.5%
Europe	108.0	3.8%	18.0	14.7%
Japan	110.0	5.3%	7.0	14.8%
Canada	4.5	12.2%	2.8	16.7%
Latin America	32.1	14.6%	13.6	20.4%
Far East	31.6	12.9%	7.7	22.2%
Rest of world	37.0	9.8%	3.6	12.5%
	455.2	9%	79.9	16%

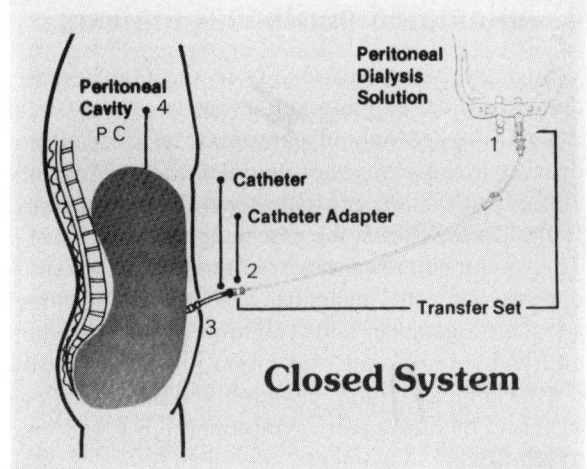

Figure 2. The CAPD System: 1, Denotes connection between transfer set and PD fluid bag. This connection is broken 3–4 times a day to effect exchanges. 2, Connection between Tenckhoff catheter and transfer set, incorporating a titanium connector. This connection is undone every 6 months for transfer set changes. 3, Exit site. 4, Peritoneal cavity (PC). (Reproduced with permission – Baxter).

catheter and bag disconnections. In addition, bag leaks and fluid leaks from defective materials used in the manufacture of connectors [63] plagued the procedure and maintained a high peritonitis rate. The connection between Tenckhoff catheter and transfer set (Site 2) was improved substantially by the introduction of a luer-locking titanium peritoneal catheter adaptor in 1979 [52]. This led to a further reduction in the peritonitis rate. From the initially weekly transfer set changes advocated by Oreopoulos [50], monthly set changes were introduced in 1979 [64]. Improvements in transfer set material has led to set changes being performed at roughly six monthly intervals.

An inherent problem with this technique is that having made a connection of transfer set to a new bag, fluid is instilled into the peritoneal cavity. If the exchange procedure has led to a contamination of the connector, the micro-organisms will pass with the fluid into the peritoneal cavity. The Italian Y set connector system utilising the closed double bag, overcomes this inherent problem [65, 66]. Buoncristiani and colleagues [65] were the first to use this system which includes two bags, one containing the peritoneal dialysis fluid while the other is empty. They are connected by a Y tubing with a sterile capped needle. After the connections are made the dialysate from the peritoneal cavity is drained into the empty bag followed by drainage of fresh fluid from the other bag into the peritoneal cavity. The two bag system is then disconnected and the Y piece is filled with chlorhexidine. This system had two major advantages: any contamination at the time of the connection was "washed out" and in addition it enabled the patient to be bag free at all times, between the exchanges. This is the principle of "flush before fill" (Fig. 3). Use of the system has

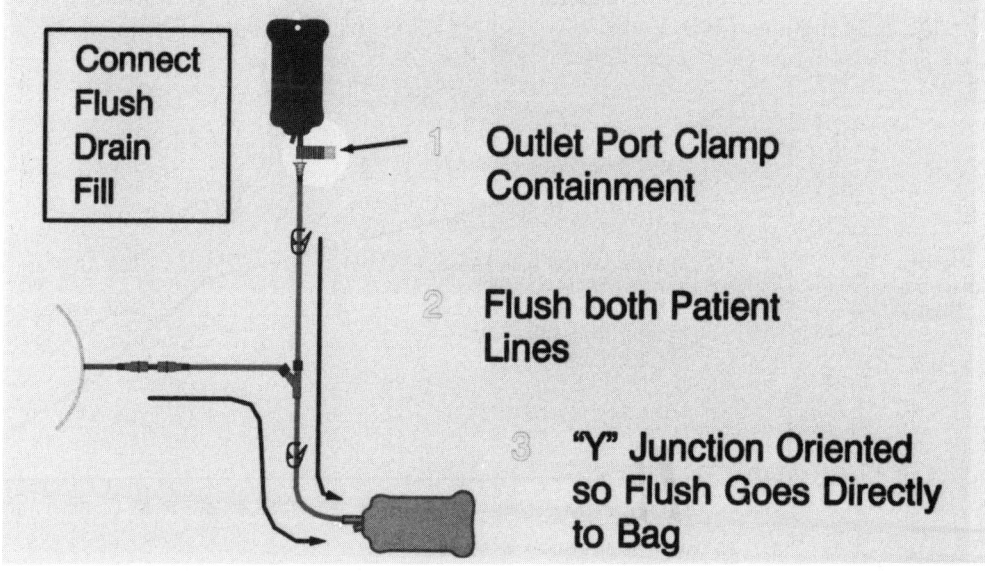

Figure 3. The disconnect system. This diagramatically shows the effective "Flush before Fill" principle, entailing the four steps, Connect, flush, Drain and Fill. The particular system shown describes the actual technique (Step 1–3) and does not utilise a disinfectant in the line after the twin bag is "disconnected".

resulted in low peritonitis rates and in a controlled randomised trial peritonitis rates were halved as compared to the standard system [67]. Initially, other than in Italy, the use of the system was limited but in the late eighties there has been a dramatic increase in its use and now there is a whole range of disconnect systems that are available. [68], which have substantially reduced the peritonitis rate. Thus disconnect/Y systems are now accepted as the normal and the use is increasing [59]. The effects of all these technical changes with the introduction of the new systems and connector devices has had, over the years, a dramatic impact on the peritonitis rate (Fig. 4). It is now generally accepted that with the use of disconnect systems a peritonitis rate of an episode every two years should be possible and this has been verified in several individual centre reports. In addition the impact of the disconnect system on CAPD results is also significant [70, 71].

The development of techniques of CAPD has brought with it the realisation that though CAPD is simple, the procedure does require motivation, discipline, compliance and a certain degree of technical skill. The early literature emphasised the need to have an organised programme for training and an adequate nursing staff to fulfil the teaching aims [72, 73]. This of course still applies today and where this has not been possible (as in some countries like the UK) where the use of CAPD has expanded rapidly the high dropout and peritonitis rates may be related to limited facilities and staff especially in the early eighties [74].

4. Automated peritoneal dialysis

Whilst the growth of CAPD in the eighties was dramatic, the use of intermittent modes of peritoneal dialysis lagged behind considerably. Intermittent dialysis therapy in 1986 provided dialysis for only 700 out of 90,000 endstage renal disease patients. In the United States, the percentage was 0.7% [75]. The major disadvantages compared to haemodialysis were the inadequacy of dialysis, minimal adequate clearances and symptoms of thirst, sodium and water imbalance and blood pressure control. CAPD compared more favourably to haemodialysis in terms of clearances, symptomatology and also pyschosocial adjustments.

However, there was a resurgence of interest in automated peritoneal dialysis (APD) with the introduction of continuous cyclic peritoneal dialysis (CCPD) described by Nakagawa et al. [76] in 1981. CCPD is based on the concept of continuous equilibration dialysis initially proposed by Moncrief and Popovich but incorporates the automation provided by a cycler [77]. CCPD uses multiple short, nocturnal exchanges, while the patient is connected to the cycler and a long diurnal exchange with the patient ambulatory. Thus, it is a virtual reversal of the CAPD schedule. The primary objective of CCPD is to provide automated, continuous peritoneal dialysis in a convenient manner, freeing the daytime hours from all procedures. The secondary goal is to reduce the rate of peritonitis. After over a decade and a half of experience of CCPD it is felt that the original goals have been

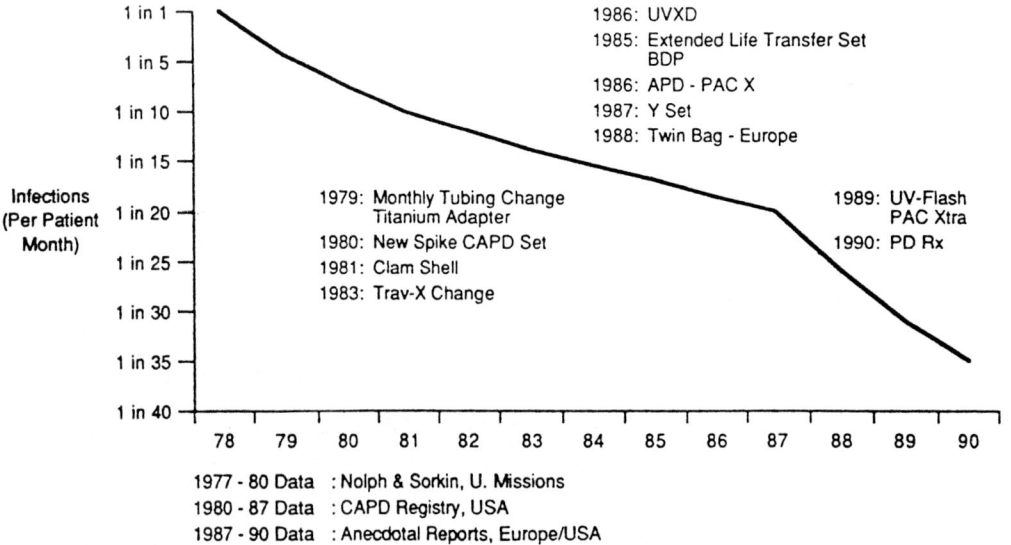

Figure 4. The improvement in peritonitis rate with time in relationship to various developments in technology. With the disconnect system an overall peritonitis rate in excess of an episode every 24 months should be possible [68].

fulfilled. CCPD has been of particular benefit to those patients in need of assistance with the procedure due to their poor muscular coordination, blindness and generalised weakness and patients who are unable to perform manual dialysis exchanges. Thus, the interest of CCPD for the very young, the elderly, and the diabetic patient has been substantial. Growth of CCPD has been monitored, with about 10% of the dialysis population undertaking this treatment in the mid eighties.

Another variant of intermittent dialysis therapy was the development of nightly peritoneal dialysis (NPD). This is performed every night and may be considered as CCPD without longdwell daytime exchanges. NPD performed with an intermittent flow technique is called nightly intermittent peritoneal dialysis (NIPD) and was utilised to a small extent by Twardowski [75]. It was used mainly in patients with recurrent abdominal leaks and hernias, bladder prolapse, rapid glucose absorption resulting in poor ultrafiltration on CAPD, abdominal discomfort, chronic hypertension and patient preference. In 1985 Scribner postulated "some form of nightly peritoneal dialysis (NPD), may prove as the best compromise of all forms of peritoneal dialysis" [78]. However, because of reduced dialysis time compared to CAPD or CCPD, the main problem was to achieve adequate clearances. The efficiency of peritoneal dialysis is dependent upon peritoneal transport characteristics in individual patients and the measurement of this was established in a simplified procedure called a peritoneal equilibration test (PET), first indicated by Twardowski in 1987 [79].

The curves that were obtained over a four hour dwell of 2.27% glucose solution discriminated patients into four categories of low, low average, high average and high peritoneal transport rates based on measurements of glucose and creatinine in dialysate and bloods. Using this test one could prognosticate and prescribe the preferred dialysis regime. This ability to tailor dialysis has certainly popularised automated peritoneal dialysis which is now the fastest growing peritoneal dialysis modality in percentage terms.

Other intermittent dialysis techniques have been introduced to try to maximize the efficiency of the dialysis. One such technique is tidal peritoneal dialysis (TPD). Here, after an initial flow into the peritoneal cavity, only a portion of the dialysate is drained and replaced by fresh dialysis fluid, leaving the majority of dialysate in constant contact with the peritoneal membrane until the end of the dialysis session when the fluid is drained as completely as possible [75]. TPD is approximately 20% more efficient than NIPD with a dialysis flow of 3.5 litre per hour.

The introduction of APD has certainly meant that patients on peritoneal dialysis can be maintained longer on this technique and it also means that psychoscocial factors and patient preference can be more readily accommodated such that therapy can be adjusted depending upon clinical situations, changes in peritoneal membrane characteristics, and loss of residual renal function. Dialysis adequacy can be better maintained as can the nutritional status.

5. Recent developments and areas of research

In the early eighties several innovations were introduced to improve dialysis outcome and decrease morbidity. Buoncristiani introduced the so called "combined peritoneal dialysis" in which they proposed two different schedules so as to omit exchanges during the day time [80]. In a similar vein Forbes *et al.* [81], outlined three 2 litre exchanges daily irrespective of patient size and residual renal function and found no significant difference in biochemical parameters although there was a rise in haemoglobin values. This manoeuvre proved cheaper and more acceptable but there was the real danger that some patients may well be under dialysed on this regime or require a high number of hypertonic exchanges, which potentially could be detrimental to the peritoneum. It was apparent even at those early stages of dialysis, that the prescription was virtually dependent on age, dietary intake, size of the patient, and residual renal function and regimes needed to be individually tailored to the patients requirements.

In order to achieve adequate dialysis and also decrease the exchanges it was necessary to increase instillation volumes. Several workers attempted this with instillation of 2.5–3 litre exchanges [82, 83]. The major determinant of patient tolerance of large volumes appeared to be the respiratory vital capacity which was significantly low in patients not able to tolerate the 2.5 litres. All these initial studies were directed at improving the efficiency and adequacy of dialysis as well as trying to minimize the inconvenience to patients and so was borne an entirely new area of study of adequacy of dialysis.

5.1. Adequacy of dialysis

The term adequacy usually implies sufficiency for a specific requirement. In so far as it applies to dialysis it has been defined clinically as the amount of dialysis which results in the absence of symptoms and signs of uraemia, and needs to be linked with clinical outcomes associated with a particular dialysis prescription or "dose". It is clear that clinical outcomes will be determined by factors other than dialysis dose for example comorbid conditions and age.

The estimation of dialysis dose mostly derives from the National Cooperative dialysis study, (NCDS), which demonstrated the importance of removal of small molecular weight substances for haemodialysis patients treated with cellulosic membranes and led to the development of the KT/V urea removal index [84, 85]. The KT/V urea for standard CAPD measurement has been calculated [86]. Other indices have also been proposed: the dialysis index described by Teehan *et al.* [87] and weekly creatinine clearance [88]. While these guidelines of adequacy markers are useful and appear reasonable they need to be linked with outcome. There are two studies addressing dialysis adequacy and clinical outcome [89, 90]. However, controversy persists as to what constitutes an adequate dialysis dose for PD and prospective studies are awaited.

That adequacy of dialysis is important is not in question nor is the realization that the residual renal function plays an important role in adding to the dialysis prescription; when this declines as it does with time, the patient may then become inadequately dialysed.

5.2. Nutrition

It has always been recognized that protein energy malnutrition and wasting are present in a significant proportion of dialysis patients. In a recent study in CAPD patients, mild to moderate malnutrition was present in 40% of patients and severe malnutrition 8% [92]. Contributing factors are increased protein requirements and low supply of energy and protein in relation to the needs. Anorexia with low protein and energy intakes results from a variety of factors of which underdialysis with insufficient control of uraemia, and continuous dialysate protein losses which are enhanced considerably during episodes of peritonitis are important. Underlialysis may well be a causative factor in the malnourished state in some patients. Lindsay proposes that nutrition will not be improved unless dialysis is increased [93]; this may be done by increasing the number of daily exchanges or the exchange volumes or converting to high flow and/or daily long hour APD. Recognition that metabolic acidosis is a catabolic factor has led to the practise of correcting this by oral sodium bicarbonate, or an increase in the PD fluid lactate. That nutrition has a bearing on outcome is now well recognized [94] as is the link between nutrition and adequacy of dialysis [95].

5.3. Peritoneal membrane

An area of major research and advance has been in our understanding of peritoneal morphology, its physiological functions and the role that the cellular components play in host defence [96, 97]. These are important aspects as are the fluid transport characteristics across the peritoneum [98] and lymphatic absorption [99], all of which will be discussed in subsequent chapters. Other areas of development include: study of more physiological peritoneal dialysis solutions [100] and improved osmotic agents [101], better catheter designs and placement techniques [102] and a better understanding of the mineral metabolism in peritoneal dialysis [103]. All these advances have certainly had an impact on the quality of life that is imparted to the patient [104].

6. Patient selection

The availability of peritoneal dialysis makes a renal centre more flexible in managing a patient in endstage renal failure. In spite of nearly fifteen years of experience with CAPD there is as yet no "profile" of a perfect CAPD patient. Selection, therefore, becomes a process of assessing a multitude of factors, some of which are stated in Table 2.

For new patients, essential factors are motivation, physical and mental capabilities of carrying out the procedure, and some insight into symptoms of uraemia and low key scientific knowledge of dialysis for renal failure. A desire to be independent and attain home dialysis is important. Certain categories of patients may have major difficulties in undergoing other types of dialysis. These are the "high risk" patient population like diabetics and those with severe cerebro and cardiovascular disease, in whom there may well be little option but to treat on CAPD.

6.1. Indications for CAPD

For patients already on haemodialysis or IPD, CAPD is indicated for problems such as vascular access, excessive weight gain between dialysis, severe hypertension, postdialysis disequilibration and severe anaemia. It may also be indicated for those in certain (hospital) dialysis patients showing a desire to undertake home dialysis.

For new patients, about to commence dialysis therapy, the factors in Table 2 need to be assessed carefully. However, certain diseases may be preferentially managed by CAPD. Diabetics may be a group in whom CAPD may be an absolute indication as would those in whom HD would be hazardous. Patients awaiting a kidney transplant can be safely maintained on CAPD and this is even more important for children in whom CAPD would be preferred therapy prior to transplantation.

6.2. Contraindications

An inappropriate peritoneal cavity from adhesions, secondary to previous operations or systemic inflammatory disease is the only absolute contradiction to CAPD. According to Moncrief & Popovich poor clearance can be detected in advance by instilling 2 liter of PD fluid via an acute catheter and measuring the creatinine concentration in the dialysate and blood after 6 hours [105]. If this ratio is < 40% failure of CAPD is likely. Adhesions may also lead to poor inflow and drainage. In general, previous abdominal surgery is not a contraindication to CAPD.

Table 2. Factors influencing choice of CAPD in new patients starting dialysis.

Medical Factors	Psychosocial fractors
Age	Patient preference
Ischaemic heart disease	motivation
Diabetes mellitus	Compliance
Ease of transplantation	Family support
Extensive abdominal surgery	Distance from centre
Blindness	Occupation
Severe pulmonary disease	Concern with blody image
Peripheral vascular disease	Travel
Lumbar disc problems	
Extensive diverticulitis	

6.2.1. Other relative contraindications are

1. Recurrent chronic backache with pre-existing disc disease. This may be aggravated by the exaggerated lordosis associated with the constant presence of fluid in the peritoneal cavity.
2. Abdominal hernias. These may well have to be repaired before CAPD is started.
3. The presence of colostomy, ileostomy, nephrostomy and ileal conduit may increase the risk of peritonitis; unless absolutely necessary these patients are better managed on HD.
4. Progressive neurological diseases, movement disorders and severe arthritis make CAPD impossible to perform. In such cases a spouse or relative may be able to carry out the exchanges.
5. Severe psychological and social problems. A co-operative and compliant patient is essential for independent home dialysis. Patients who are psychic, belligerent, or uncooperative are unlikely to succeed in this form of therapy and may be better managed on hospital/in centre HD.
6. Immunosuppressive drugs. Patients receiving these may have poor healing of catheter and exit sites. There is no evidence that these patients are more prone to peritonitis.
7. Chronic obstructive airways disease patients may not be able to tolerate 2 litres of fluid because of an impaired vital capacity; this is however relatively uncommon.
8. Severe diverticular disease of the colon in the elderly may be associated with repeated Gram negative peritonitis or perforation, which has a high mortality.
9. "Profile" of the patient prone to develop peritonitis. Although there is no absolute data available on this, it has been noted that patients with repeated attacks of peritonitis are less motivated, more depressed and often have suffered major life crises. Stegman and Berger [106] found that when host, agent and environmental factors are controlled, age (younger patients), low patient motivation and minimal social support were significant risk factors for peritonitis.
10. Hepatitis B antigenaemia (HBsAg). For units that do not routinely dialyze these patients this may be an absolute contraindication because of the risk to staff and other patients within the

unit. However, CAPD may be carried out in designated hepatitis units where the staff have been vaccinated or in departments or a hospital for infectious diseases. It is important to remember that the dialysate is HBsAg positive and needs to be treated with 1% hypochlorite before discarding.

Patient selection will remain a problem where the various treatment modalities are not integrated. The important point to remember is that renal units should be able to provide all the therapies and be prepared to adjust treatment according to the patients' needs or justified desire.

References

1. McBride P. Taking the first steps in the development of Peritoneal Dialysis. Perit Dial Bull 1982; 2: 100–2.
2. Cunningham RS. The physiology of the serous membranes. Physiol Rev 1926; 6: 242–56.
3. Warrick C. An improvement of the practice of tapping, whereby that operation instead of relief of symptoms, becomes an absolute cure for acsites, exemplified in the case of Jane Roman. Philosophy Trans Royal Society 1744; 43: 12–9.
4. Hale S. A method of conveying liquors into the abdomen during the operation of tapping. Philosophical Trans Royal Soc 1744; 43: 20–1.
5. Chirurgische Bemerkungen uber die Peritonealhohle, mit besonderer Berucksichtigung der ovariotome. Arch fur Klin Cher 1877; 20: 51.
6. Starling EH, Tubby AH. The influence of mechanical factors on lymph production. J. Physiol 1894; 16: 140–8.
7. Cunningham RS. The effect of dextrose upon the peritoneal mesothelium. Am J Physiol 1920; 53: 458–88.
8. Clark AJ. Absorption from the Peritoneal Cavity. J Pharmacol Exper Therap 1921; 16: 415–22.
9. Abel JJ, Rowntree LG, Turner BB. Removal of diffusible substances from the circulating blood of living animals by dialysis. J Exper Therap 1913; 5: 275–316.
10. Putnam J. The living peritoneum as a dialysing membrane. Am J Physiol 1923; 63: 548–65.
11. Graham T. Liquid diffusion applied to analysis. Philosoph Trans Royal Soc 1861; 151: 183.
12. Engel D. Beitrage permeabilitas problem: Entgeft ungsstudien mettils des Lebendin peritoneums als "Dialysator". Z Gesarite Ex Med 1927; 55: 544–601.
13. Blackfan KD, Maxey KF. The intraperitoneal injection of saline solution. Am J Dis Child 1918; 2: 1257–65.
14. Ganter G. Uber die Beseitigung giftiger Stoffe aus dem Blute durch Dialse. Muench Med Wochenschr 1923; 70: 1478–80.
15. Heusser H, Werder H. Untersuchungen uber Peritonealdialyse. Bruns Beitr Klin Chir 1927; 141: 38–49.
16. Balazc J, Rosenaks S. Zur behandlung der sublimatanurie durch Peritoneal Dialse. Wein Klin Wochenschr 1934; 47: 851–4.
17. Wear JB, Sisk IR, Trinkle AJ. Peritoneal lavage in the treatment of uraemia. J Urol 1938; 39: 53–62.
18. Rhoads JE. Peritoneal lavage in the treatment of renal insufficiency. Am J of Med Sc 1938; 39: 53–62.
19. Fine JH, Frank HA, Seligman AM. The treatment of acute renal failure by peritoneal irrigation. Ann Surg 1946; 124: 857–75.
20. Odel HM, Ferris DO, Power H. Peritoneal lavage as an effective means of extra-renal excretion. Am J Med 1950; 9: 63–77.
21. Derot M, Tanzet P, Roussillion J, Bernier JJ. La dialyse peritoneal dans le traitement de l'ureme aigue. J Urol 1949; 55: 113–21.
22. Grollman A, Turner LB, McLean JA. Intermittent peritoneal lavage in nephrectomised dogs and its application to the human being. Arch Int Med 1951; 87: 379–90.
23. Legrain M, Merrill JP. Short term continuous transperitoneal dialysis. New Engl J Med 1953; 248: 125–9.
24. Maxwell MH, Rockney RE, Kleman CR, Twiss MR. Peritoneal Dialysis. JAMA 1959; 170: 917–24.
25. Boen ST. Kinetics of peritoneal Dialysis. Medicine 1961; 40: 243–87.
26. Reid R, Penfold JB, Jones RN. Anuria treated by renal encapsulation and peritoneal dialysis. Lancet 1946; 2: 749–51.
27. Abbot WE, Shea P. The treatment of temporary renal insufficiency by peritoneal lavage. Am J Medi Sc 1946; 211: 312–9.
28. Doolan PD, Murphy WP, Wiggins RA, Carter NW, Cooper WC, Watten RH, Alphen EL. An evaluation of intermittent peritoneal lavage. Am J Med 1959; 26: 831–44.
29. Drukker W. History of Peritoneal Dialysis. In: Maher JF (ed), Replacement of Renal Function by Dialysis. Kluwer Academic Publishers, Dordrecht 1989; pp 476–515.
30. Boen ST, Milman AS, Dillard DH, Scribner BH. Periodic peritoneal dialysis in the management of chronic uremia. Trans Am Soc Artif Int Organs 1962; 8: 256–62.
31. Merrill JP, Sabbaga E, Henderson L, Welzant W, Crane C. The use of an inlying plastic conduit for chronic peritoneal irrigation. Trans Am Soc Artif Int Organs 1962; 8: 256–62.
32. Boen ST, Mion C, Curtis F, Shilipetar G. Periodic peritoneal dialysis using the repeated puncture technique and an automatic cycling machine. Trans Am Soc Artif Organs 1964; 10: 409–13.
33. Tenckhoff H, Shillipetar G, Boen ST. One year's experience with home peritoneal dialysis. Tran Am Soc Artif Unt Organs 1965; 11: 11–4.
34. Editorial. Intermittent Peritoneal Lavage. Lancet 1959; 2: 551–2.
35. Palmer RA, Quinton WE, Gray JF. Prolonged peri-

toneal dialysis for chronic renal failure. Lancet 1964; 1: 700–2.
36. Gutch CF. Peritoneal Dialysis. Trans Am Soc Artif Int Organs 1964; 10: 406–7.
37. McDonald HP, Gerber N, Mishra D, Woln L, Peng B, Waterhouse K. Subcutaneous Dacron and Teflon cloth adjuncts for silastic AV shunts and peritoneal dialysis catheters. Trans Am Soc Artif Int Organs 1968; 14: 176–80.
38. Tenckhoff H, Schechter H. A bacteriologically safe peritoneal access device. Trans Am Soc Artif Int Organs 1973; 10: 363–70.
39. Tenckhoff H, Blagg C, Curtis HF, Hickman RO. Chronic peritoneal dialysis. Proc EDTA 1973; 10: 363–70.
40. Tenckhoff H. Advantages and shortcomings of peritoneal dialysis. Seminar Uro Nephrologie Hopital Pitie 1977; pp 107–18.
41. Oreopoulos DG. Home peritoneal dialysis. Proc EDTA 1975; 12: 139–42.
42. Buoncristiani V. Clinical results of long term peritoneal dialysis. Proc EDTA 1975; 12: 145–8.
43. Heal MR, England AG, Goldsmith HJ. Four years experience with indwelling silastic cannulae for long term peritoneal dialysis. Brit Med J 1975; 2: 596–600.
44. Ahmed S, Gallagher N, Shen F. Intermittent peritoneal dialysis: status reassessed. Trans Am Soc Artif Int Organs 1979; 25: 86–8.
45. Gutman RA. Towards enhancement of peritoneal clearances. Dial Transplant 1979; 8: 1072–6.
46. Popovich RP, Moncrief JW, Decherd JF, Bomar JB, Pyle WK. The definition of A novel portable/wearable equilibrium dialysis technique. Abstact. Trans Am Soc Artif Int Organs 1976; 5: 64.
47. Gotch FA, Sargeant JA, Keen M, Lam M, Prowitt M, Grasy M. Solute kinetics in intermittent dialysis therapy. 9th Annual Contractors Conference. Artificial Kidney Chronic Uremia Prog (NIAMDO) 1976; 9: 98–101.
48. Popovich RP, Moncrief JW, Dechert JF, Pyle WK, Morris S, Lindley JD. Clinical developments of the low dialysis clearance hypothesis via equilibium peritoneal dialysis. Proc Annual Contractors Conf. Artif Kidney-Chronic Uremia Prog (NIAMDO) 1977; 10: 123–5.
49. Popovich RP, Moncrief JW, Nolph KD, Ghods AJ, Twardowski Z, Pyle WK. Continuous Ambulatory Peritoneal Dialysis. Ann Int Med 1978; 88: 449–56.
50. Oreopoulos DG, Robson M, Izatt S, Clayton S, de Veber GA. A simple and safe technique for CAPD. Trans Am Soc Artif Int Organs 1978; 24: 484–9.
51. Oreopoulos DG, Khanna R, Williams P, Dombros N, Carmichael D. Efficacy of and clinical experience with CAPD in Canada. In: Aktins R, Thomson N, Farrell PC (eds), Peritoneal Dialysis. Churchill Livingstone, Edinburgh 1981; pp 114–25.
52. Nolph KD. Continuous Ambulatory Peritoneal Dialysis. Am J Nephrol 1981; 1: 1–10.
53. Moncrief JW, Popovich PR. Efficiency and clinical experience with CAPD in the USA. In: Atkins R, Thomson N, Farrell PC (eds), Peritoneal Dialysis. Churchill Livingstone, Edinburgh 1981; pp 165–70.
54. Lamiere N, De Paepe M, Van Holder R, Verbanck J, Ringoir S. Experience with CAPD in Belgium. In: Atkins R, Thomson N, Farrell PC (eds), Peritoneal Dialysis. Churchill Livingstone, Edinburgh. 1981; pp 104–13.
55. Mion C, Slingeneyer A, Canard B. CAPD in France: results of a national survey and two years experience at one centre. In: Atkins R, Thomson N, Farrell PC (eds), Peritoneal Dialysis. Churchill Livingstone, Edinburgh 1981; pp 126–35.
56. La Greca G, Biasioli S, Chiaramonte S, Fabris A, Feriani M, Pisani E, Ronco C. Italian clinical experience of CAPD. In: Atkins R, Thomson N, Farrell PC (eds), Peritoneal Dialysis. Churchill Livingstone, Edinburgh 1981; pp 136–8.
57. Gokal R, Ward MK. Clinical experience with CAPD in the United Kingdom. In: Atkins R, Thomson N, Farrell PC (eds), Peritoneal Dialysis. Churchill Livingstone, Edinburgh 1981; pp 162–4.
58. Lindholm B, Alverstrand A, Furst P, Trandeus A, Bergstrom J. Efficiency and clinical experience of CAPD – Stockholm, Sweden. In: Atkins R, Thomson N, Farrell PC (eds), Peritoneal Dialysis. Churchill Livingstone, Edinburgh 1981; pp 147–61.
59. Thomson N, Atkins R, Hooke D, Maydom B, Scott D. Long term clinical experience with CAPD in Australia. In: Atkins R, Thomson N, Farrell PC (eds), Peritoneal Dialysis. Churchill Livingstone, Edinburgh 1981; pp 93–103.
60. Gokal R, McHugh M, Fryer R, Ward MK, Kerr DNS. CAPD: one year's experience in a UK dialysis unit. Brit Med J 1980; 281: 474–7.
61. Fenton SSA, Cattram DC, Allen AF, Rutledge P, Ampil M, Dodson J, Locking H, Smith SD, Wilson DR. Initial experience with CAPD, Artif Organ 1979; 3: 206–9.
62. Gokal R. Peritonitis in CAPD. Antimicrobial Chemotherap 1982; 9: 417–22.
63. Gokal R, Manos J, Mallick NP. Defects in CAPD equipment. Lancet 1982; 2: 382, 671.
64. Oreopoulos DG, Khanna R, Williams P, Vas SI. Continuous Ambulatory Peritoneal Dialysis Nephron 1982; 30: 292–303.
65. Buoncristiani V, Bianchi P, Cozzari M. A new safe simple connection system for CAPD. Int J Nehrol Urol Androl 1980; 1: 50–3.
66. Bazzato G, Coli U, Landini S. CAPD without wearing a bag: complete freedom of patient and significant reduction of peritonitis. Proc EDTA 1980; 17: 266–75.
67. Maiorca R, Cantaluppi A, Cancarini GC, Scalamonga A, Broccoli R, Graziani G, Brasa S, Ponticelli C. Prospective controlled trial of a Y-connector and disinfectant to prevent peritonitis in CAPD. Lancet 1983; 2: 642–4.
68. Viglino G, Cantaluppi A, Gandolfo C, Peluso F, Cavalli PL. Y-set evolution. In: La Greca G, Ronco C, Feriani M, Chiaramonte S, Conz P (eds),

Peritoneal Dialysis. Wichtig Editore, Milan 1991; pp 281–93.
69. Buoncristiani V. The Y-set with disinfectant is here to stay. Perit Dial Int 1989; 9: 149–50.
70. Maiorca R, Cancarini GC, Comerini C, Monili L. Morbidity and mortality of CAPD and Haemodialysis. Kidney Int 1993; 43 (suppl 40): S4–15.
71. Maiorca R, Cancarini GC, Comerini C, Monili L, Brunori G. The impact of the Y-system and low peritonitis rate on CAPD results. In: Hatano M (ed), Nephrology. Springer Verlag, Tokyo 1991; pp 1592–601.
72. Clayton S, Finer C, Quinton C, Jabaz O, Clark S, Kelman B, Oreopoulos DG. Training patients for CAPD at Toronto Western Hospital. In: Legrain M (ed), Continuous Ambulatory Peritoneal Dialysis. Excerpta Medica, Amsterdam 1980; pp 162–6.
73. Oreopoulos DG. Requirements for the organisation of a CAPD programme. Nephron 1979; 24: 261–3.
74. Gokal R, Marsh FP. Survey of CAPD in the United Kingdom, 1982. Perit Dial Bull 1984; 4: 261–3.
75. Twardowski ZJ. New approaches to Intermittent Peritoneal Dialysis therapies. In: Nolph KD (ed), Peritoneal Dialysis. Kluwer Academic Publishers, Dordrecht 1989; pp 133–51.
76. Nakayawa D, Price C, Stinebraugh B, Suki W. Continuous cyclic peritoneal dialysis: a viable option in the treatment of chronic renal failure. Trans Am Soc Artif Intern Organs 1981; 27: 55–7.
77. Diaz-Buxo JA, Walker PJ, Farmer CD. Continuous Cyclic Peritoneal Dialysis – A preliminary report. Artif Organs 1981; 5: 157–62.
78. Scribner BH. Forward to 2nd Edition. In: Nolph KD (ed), Peritoneal Dialysis. Martinus Nijhoff Publishers, Dordrecht 1985; pp XI–XII.
79. Twardowski Z, Nolph KD, Prowant BF, Ryan LP, Moore HL, Nielson MP. Peritoneal equilibration test. Perit Dial Bull 1987; 7: 138–47.
80. Buoncristiani V, Cozarri M, Carobi C, Quintaliana G, Barbarossa D, Di Paolo N. Combined Peritoneal Dialysis. Proc EDTA 1980; 17: 328–32.
81. Forbes AMW, Reed VL, Goldsmith HJ. The adequacy of six litre daily CAPD. Proc EDTA 1980; 17: 276–81.
82. Twardowski Z, Nolph KD, Prowant BF, Moore HC. Efficiency of high volume low frequency CAPD. Trans Am Soc Artif Int Organs 1983; 29: 53–7.
83. Kim D, Khanna R, Wu G, Clayton S, Oreopoulos DG. Continuous Ambulatory Peritoneal Dialysis with three-litre exchanges: a prospective study. Perit Dial Bull 1984; 4: 82–5.
84. Gotch F, Sargent JA. A mechanistic analysis of the National Cooperative Dialysis Study (NCDS). Kidney Int 1985; 28: 526–34.
85. Lowrie EG, Laird NM, Parker TF, Sargent JA. Effect of the haemodialysis prescription on patient morbidity. Report from the NCDS. N Engl J Med 1981; 305: 1176–81.
86. Keshaviah PK, Nolph KD, Van Stone JC. The peak concentration hypothesis: Perit Dial Int 1987; 9: 257–60.
87. Teehan B, Schleifer CR, Sigler MH, Gilgour GS. A quantitative approach to the CAPD prescription. Perit Dial Bull 1985; 5: 152–6.
88. Twardowski Z, Nolph KD. Peritoneal Dialysis: how much is enough? Semin Dial 1988; 1: 75–6.
89. Blake PG, Sombolos K, Abraham G, Weissgarten J, Pemberton R, Chu GL, Oreopoulos DG. Lack of correlation between urea kinetic indeces and clinical outcomes in CAPD patients. Kidney Int 1991; 39: 700–6.
90. Keshaviah P, Nolph KD, Prowant B, Moore H, Ponferrada L, Van Stone J, Twardowski ZJ, Khanna R. Defining adequacy of CAPD with urea kinetics. Adv Perit Dial 1990; 6: 173–7.
91. Churchill DN. Adequacy of Peritoneal Dialysis and other outcome related risk factors: a critical appraisal. Semin Dial 1992; 5: 142–6.
92. Young GA, Kopple JD, Lindholm B, Vonesh EF, De Vecchi A, Scalamogna A, Castelnova C, Oreopoulos DG, Anderson GH, Bergstrom J, Dichiro J, Gentile D, Nissenson A, Sahkrani L, Brownjohn A, Nolph KD, Prowant BF, Algrim CE, Martis L, Serkes K. Nutritional assessment of CAPD patients: an International Study. Am J Kidney Dis 1991; 7: 462–71.
93. Lindsay RM, Spanner E, Heidenheim PR, LeFebvre JM, Hodsman A, Baird J, Allison MEM. Which comes first, Kt/V or PCR – Chicken or Egg? Kidney Int 1992 (suppl 38); 42: S32–6.
94. Teehan BP, Scheifer CR, Brown JM, Sigler MH, Raimondo J. Urea kinetic analysis and clinical outcome on CAPD. A five year longitudinal study. Adv Perit Dial 1991; 6: 181–5.
95. Bergstrom J, Lindholm B. Nutrition and adequacy of dialysis. Kidney Int 1993 (suppl 40); 43: S39–50.
96. Dobbie J, Lloyd JK, Gall CA. Categorisation of ultrastructural changes in peritoneal mesothelium, stroma and bloods vessels in uremia and CAPD patients. Adv Perit Dial 1990; 6: 3–12.
97. Lamperi S, Carozzi S. Immunologic defences in CAPD. Blood Purif 1989; 7: 126–43.
98. Mistry C, Mallick NP, Gokal R. Ultrafiltration with an isosmotic solution during long peritoneal dialysis exchanges. Lancet 1987; 2: 178–82.
99. Mactier R, Khanna R. Peritoneal cavity lymphatics. In: Nolph KD (ed), Peritoneal Dialysis. Kluwer Academic Publishers, Dordrecht 1989; pp 48–66.
100. Hutchison A, Gokal R. Improved solutions for peritoneal dialysis: Physiological calcium solutions, osmotic agents and buffers. Kidnet Int 1992; 42 (suppl 38): S153–9.
101. Gokal R. Osmotic agents in Peritoneal Dialysis. In: Coles G, Davies M, Williams J (eds), CAPD: Host defence, Nutrition and Ultrafiltration. Karger, Basel 1990; pp 126–33.
102. Gokal R, Ash SR, Helfrich GB, Holmes CJ, Joffe P, Nichols K, Oreopoulos DG, Riella M, Slingerneyer A, Twardowski Z, Vas Sl. Peritoneal catheters and exit site practices: towards optimum peritoneal access. Perit Dial Int 1993; 13: 29–39.
103. Coburn J. Mineral metabolism and renal bone

disease: effect of CAPD versus haemodialysis. Kidney Int 1992: 42 (suppl 38): S92–100.
104. Gokal R. Quality of life in patients undergoing renal replacement therapy. Kidney Int 1992; 42 (suppl 38): S23–7.
105. Moncrief J, Popovich R. CAPD worldwide experience. In: Nolph KD (ed), Peritoneal Dialysis. Martinus Nijhoff, Hauge 1981; pp 178–212.
106. Stegman MR, Berger AM. Peritonitis among CAPD patients: Host agent and/or environment? Perit Dial Bull 1984; 4: 206–8.

2 Ultrastructure and pathology of the peritoneum in peritoneal dialysis

JAMES W. DOBBIE

1. Collection and processing of peritoneal tissue for morphological examination — 18
2. Recognition of artefact — 18
3. Distribution of type of biopsy — 18
   3.1. Change of modality — 19
   3.2. Surgical opertions while on CAPD — 19
   3.3. Catheter-related problems — 19
   3.4. Deterioration in dialysis performance of the peritoneum — 19
   3.5. Peritonitis — 19
   3.6. Repeat biopsies — 19
4. Role of a peritoneal biopsy registry in monitoring the effects of peritoneal dialysis — 20
5. Morphology of the normal peritoneum — 20
   5.1. Mesothelium — 20
      5.1.1. Surface features — 20
      5.1.2. Cell junctions — 20
      5.1.3. Nuclei — 20
      5.1.4. Organelles — 20
      5.1.5. Mesothelial cytoskeleton — 21
      5.1.6. Lamellar bodies — 22
   5.2. Submesothelial stroma — 25
6. Comparative morphology and physiology of serous cavities — 26
7. Morpho-functional correlates — 27
8. Pathological peritoneum — 28
   8.1. Uremic peritoneum — 28
9. Peritoneum in CAPD — 31
   9.1. Mesothelium — 31
      9.1.1. Surface topography — 31
      9.1.2. Nuclei — 32
      9.1.3. Organelles and cytosol — 32
      9.1.4. Peritonitis — 33
      9.1.5. Recovery from peritonitis — 33
10. Basement membrane reduplication — 35
    10.1. Non-enzymatic glycosylation of structural protein — 36
11. Peritoneal fibrosing syndromes in peritoneal dialysis — 37
12. Macroscopic appearance and histopathology of peritoneal fibrosis — 37
    12.1. Peritoneal opacification — 37
    12.2. "Tanned" peritoneum syndrome — 37
    12.3. Mural fibrosis — 37
    12.4. Sclerosing encapsulating peritonitis (SEP) — 38
13. Morphological insights into the pathogenesis of peritoneal fibrosis in CAPD — 39
    13.1. Failure of remesothelialization — 40
    13.2. Cellular desert — 40
    13.3. Fibrin exudation — 40
14. The pathogenesis of uncontrolled fibrous dysplasia of the peritoneum — 41
    14.1. Characterizing mesothelial stem cells — 41
    14.2. Proliferation of stem cells and fibrogenesis — 41
    14.3. Growth factors and the control of stem cells — 41
    14.4. Entrapment of mesothelial stem cells — 42
15. Durability of peritoneum in CAPD — 42
References — 42

Following the first histological description by Von Recklinghausen in 1863 of the endothelioid covering of the peritoneum [1], the limited resolution of the light microscope prevented any deeper probing of the structure of the thin cellular monolayer we now call the mesothelium. Thus it is not surprising that little interest was shown in the barely visible lining of the peritoneum until the inception of CAPD in the late 1970s stimulated a natural curiosity in the morphological determinants of peritoneal dialysis and a concern over the possible pathological consequences of continual immersion in dialysate. It was therefore as recent as 1981 before the first electron micrographs of human mesothelium were published [2]. In the succeeding years there has been a quickening of interest in peritoneal ultrastructure, both in regard to a furthering of our understanding of what structures are interposed between the capillary bed and the dialysate, as well as a developing awareness of changes associated with the process of dialysis. In the last decade there has been a significant increase in our knowledge of the fine structure of the peritoneum which has in turn been responsible for new insights into the molecular biology of this neglected structure. A tissue which was previously thought to consist of a simple, leaky, cellular monolayer mounted on a non-descript thin backing of loose areolar connective tissue, has been shown to possess highly conserved and complex functions designed to provide the most successful, lubricated, "non stick" surfaces yet identified in the natural world [3].

1. Collection and processing of peritoneal tissue for morphological examination

Peritoneum is a delicate tissue and requires care and common sense in its collection at surgical operation [4]. If one is to have any confidence in obtaining mesothelium which is free from artefactual damage and in which observed ultrastructural changes may be reasonably attributed to pathological processes, the biopsy must be taken as soon as the peritoneum is opened. If on the other hand a biopsy is taken just prior to closure of the peritoneum, an unquantifiable number of artefacts may have been created during the procedure. Mesothelium dries very quickly on exposure to air; it reacts topically to blood and plasmatic exudates oozing from the wound edge, while even mild abrasion from the surgeon's gloves or more rough treatment from retractors may induce ultrastructural changes [5, 6]. The ideal sample is an ellipse (18 mm × 3 mm) of parietal peritoneum from the anterior abdominal wall obtained from the edge of the freshly opened peritoneum. If a catheter is present, the biopsy should be taken as far from the peritoneal exit site as is practically possible.

Most ultrastructural information has been derived from biopsies of parietal peritoneum obtained at routine abdominal operations in normal controls and during surgical insertion, removal or replacement of the catheter in patients on CAPD [5, 6]. With the exception of variation in microvillous density there would appear to be no readily identifiable ultrastructural difference between visceral and parietal mesothelium. Likewise there does not appear to be any striking differences between mesothelium from different species, or from different serous cavities. A legitimate concern that morphological changes seen in a small biopsy from the anterior abdominal wall cannot be truly representative of what is happening throughout the entire peritoneum is not supported by our experience. Where biopsies have been available from several sites (visceral and parietal), they show that the histopathological changes associated with the dialysis process have a diffuse, global, peritoneal expression. That this be so is but common pathological sense, since to the best of our knowledge, all peritoneal surfaces are equally exposed to the dialysis process. Likewise there is every indication that peritonitis in CAPD is a diffuse phenomenon, where the constant filling of the abdomen with several liters of dialysate prevents the fibrinous adhesive loculation of the peritoneum which is the natural course of events in surgical peritonitis.

Thus by virtue of its accessibility and the representative nature of its mesothelium, the parietal peritoneum of the anterior abdominal wall has been the site of choice for biopsies in studying the reaction of peritoneum to the process of peritoneal dialysis [5, 6].

2. Recognition of artefact

Denudation of mesothelium and surface coating with fibrin may falsely suggest peritonitis. Where the tissue also exhibits widespread stromal insudation with RBCs, crimping of collagen bundles and mild perivascular cuffing of capillaries with leukocytes, then surgical trauma is the likeliest explanation of the findings. Additional findings which assist in differentiating peritonitis from trauma is the detection of active or necrotic mesenchymal cells (macrophages, fibroblasts and possible mesothelial stem cells) which are indicative of a more chronic process than can possibly develop within a 30 minute time frame. Infiltration of stroma by acute inflammatory cells is an unreliable indicator of an infective process since biopsies of antibiotic-treated peritonitis may show only scanty infiltrate.

Stratified layers of surface fibrin with necrotic debris and deep stromal insudation with bands of fibrin in the presence of damaged collagen are strong indicators of peritonitis.

Necrotic, partially detached, edematous or fragmented mesothelium may be due to drying artefact, inappropriate use of solutions (e.g. saline) or scuffing injury.

3. Distribution of type of biopsy

The number and nature of the situations in which biopsies are collected are directly related to events which occur in the course of a patient's treatment on peritoneal dialysis. Thus there is an automatic bias in the nature of the specimens collected, since they can only be obtained when an "event" results in surgical access to the peritoneum. This bias however is not necessarily disadvantageous, since most of the events represent possible pathological states of the peritoneum in which we seek to obtain further histopathological enlightenment [5, 6].

Of the 700 biopsies received by the International Peritoneal Biopsy Registry, approximately one third of them is from uremic patients at the time of first insertion of the catheter. These samples serve as non-dialysate exposed controls being representative of uremic peritoneum, distinct from normal human peritoneum. The circumstances during CAPD therapy which offer an opportunity to biopsy the peritoneum can be categorized as follows [5].

3.1. Change of modality

a) *Change to hemodialysis.* Samples obtained from patients who were changed to hemodialysis for social causes or medical causes other than peritoneal problems or increasing uremia, provide an insight into the interval appearances of peritoneum during stable peritoneal dialysis.

b) *Renal transplantation.* Biopsies are often obtained at catheter removal at varying time intervals following cessation of CAPD therapy after successful renal transplantation. Such specimens are extremely informative in documenting the presence or absence of restorative morphological changes which may occur in the weeks and months after peritoneal dialysis stops.

3.2. Surgical operations while on CAPD

A not inconsiderable number of biopsies are supplied by elective surgical procedures which may occur at random throughout a patient's time on CAPD. Hernia repairs represent the most common surgical procedure, but operations elsewhere in the abdominal cavity do provide generous samples of visceral and parietal peritoneum concomitantly, whereby we can ascertain whether parietal peritoneal changes fairly represent what is happening diffusely throughout the peritoneum.

3.3. Catheter-related problems

Catheter migration from the pelvis or omental blockage, leakage, tunnel and exit site infections frequently give rise to surgical removal of the catheter and an opportunity for peritoneal biopsy. In most instances the patient and his peritoneum have been quietly attempting to proceed with normal dialysis and therefore most samples in this category are similar to those found in 1(a). Specimens obtained in such circumstances also serve to document extension of inflammation from the catheter tract into the peritoneum.

3.4. Deterioration in dialysis performance of the peritoneum

In these instances peritoneal tissue may be obtained either through catheter removal when the patient is deliberately transferred to another modality, or an elective surgical biopsy is taken in order to determine if there is a morphological explanation for the deterioration in dialysis performance. We therefore receive biopsies from patients in clinical situations in which our most pressing task is to establish what histopathological counterpart correlates with the clinical syndrome. Thus access to peritoneal samples in patients who are causing clinical concern, either through loss of ultrafiltration capacity or through decreased permeability and poor biochemical control of uremia, does provide extremely important biopsies.

3.5. Peritonitis

Catheters are usually only removed in cases of severe or persistent peritonitis, in most instances as a direct consequence of the pathogenicity of the infecting organisms which are most commonly either *Staphylococcus aureus*, *Pseudomonas aeruginosa* or fungal infections. Thus biopsies obtained under these circumstances represent the most severe and possibly damaging forms of peritoneal inflammation. From many of these patients a second biopsy may be obtained together with a visual description of the peritoneum when the surgeon replaces the catheter some three to four weeks later. Such biopsies have been extremely instructive in following the rate of resolution, extent of fibrogenesis and remesotheliatization of the inflamed peritoneum [5].

3.6. Repeat biopsies

The advantage of taking a biopsy on initial catheter emplacement pays dividends on subsequent occasions when events give rise to opportunities for sampling the peritoneum. With the passage of time the International Peritoneal Biopsy Registry has accumulated a series of biopsies from individual patients which have been instructive in documenting progressive alterations in structure when they occur.

4. Role of a peritoneal biopsy registry in monitoring the effects of peritoneal dialysis

In the 1960s and 1970s the creation of biopsy registries (adrenal, ovarian, testicular tumor, jejunum, kidney, etc.) was instrumental in advancing histological classification and interpretation of many complex pathological conditions. Biopsy registries accumulated large pools of tissue sections, allowing panels of histopathologists the opportunity to jointly examine hundreds or thousands of examples of specific pathologies that they might otherwise see only in small numbers in a professional lifetime. The acknowledged beneficial findings of such registries with regard to the unmasking of patterns of sequential histopathological change, quantification of lesions, and insights into etiology have likewise been attained by the International Peritoneal Biopsy Registry which began in an informal manner in Glasgow Royal Infirmary in 1978.

The introduction of several liters of a hypertonic, hypo-oncotic electrolyte solution possibly contaminated by plasticizers, trace elements, particulates of diverse origins into a patient's peritoneal cavity every day for five, ten or fifteen years non-stop, is an unnatural act which requires extremely careful monitoring [5, 6]. In this respect examination of peritoneal biopsies is the ultimate in quality assurance. Mesothelial loss, metaplasia, hyperplasia or neoplasia, fibroneogenesis, cellular infiltrates of the peritoneum in peritoneal dialysis patients as in pathologies of other body surfaces, must ultimately be examined by histological, immunocytochemical and/or electron microscopical techniques in order to determine beyond reasonable doubt the nature and prognosis of the acquired lesions. Thus as the composition of dialysate evolves and the dialysate pathway is exposed to new materials, a continual monitoring of peritoneal reaction is mandatory.

5. Morphology of the normal peritoneum

5.1. Mesothelium

5.1.1. *Surface features*

Normal mesothelial cells are flat or discoid in cross section. Silverstained en face preparations of peritoneum display the mesothelium as a mosaic of polygonal cells which are all of similar size. Cells have 4–7 borders. Normal mesothelium is covered by a thick mantle of microvilli which are 2–3 µ in length and 0.08 µ in diameter (Figs. 1, 2) [7–9]. Most samples of peritoneum exhibit an even distribution of microvilli over the cell surface, but patterns of either marginal or central ratification are observed. Most cells bear a single motile cilium (Fig. 2) [7–9]. Other surface features which may be observed on scanning electron microscopy are small, spherical globules 0.5–1 µ in diameter, entangled in the microvilli (Fig. 3). These are lamellar bodies, packets of phospholipid lubricant released from the underlying mesothelium by exocytotic extrusion. Both inner and outer cell surfaces exhibit a profusion of micropinocytotic vesicles which appear as pits when viewed in scanning electron microscopy [7–9].

5.1.2. *Cell junctions*

Seen in cross section, the cell junctions of mesothelial cells, slope, overlapping in the manner of roof tiles. Tight junctions are present in the outermost part of the junctional complex, deep to which desmosomes are encountered. At the basal region of the complex, adjacent cells are interlocked with interdigitating processes (Figs. 2, 4) [7–9].

5.1.3. *Nuclei*

Mesothelial cell nuclei occupy a central position within the cell, being oval or cigar-shaped in sectional profile (Fig. 5) [8]. Adjacent to the inner nuclear membrane there is a band of medium electron density, known as the nuclear fibrous lamina. This specialisation is found in nuclei of cells which undergo significant alterations in shape and volume (e.g., muscle cells). The nuclei show peripheral margination of chromatin and a preponderance of euchromatin over heterochromatin. Two prominent nucleoli are commonly encountered (Fig. 5) [8].

5.1.4. *Organelles*

The rough endoplasmic reticulum (RER) is prominent, exhibiting ribosome-studded cisternae scattered throughout the cytosol (Figs. 2, 4) [7–9]. A well-developed Golgi apparatus consisting of stacks of flattened, curvilinear sacs and associated vesicles is found in a juxtanuclear position facing the peritoneal surface (Fig. 2) [7–9]. Mesothelial cells are well-endowed with mitochondria, possessing a complement not inferior to that of the distal renal tubular epithelium (Fig. 2). They exhibit circular or elongated profiles in section while the cristae are lamellar in type. Their matrix, which is of moderate

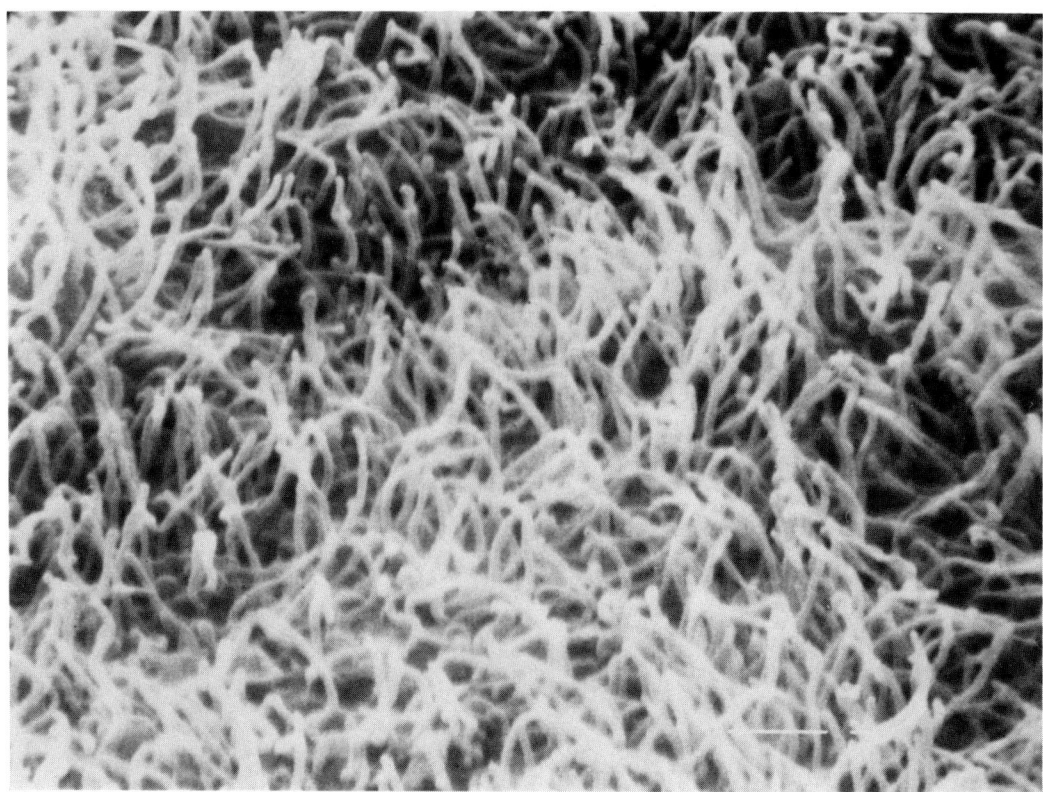

Figure 1. A scanning electron micrograph of mesothelial surface of a biopsy of parietal peritoneum from a normal non-uremic individual displaying the profuse carpet of microvilli. Magnification ×14,000.

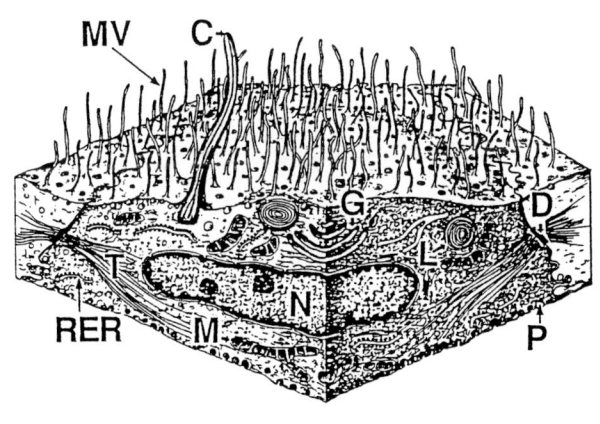

Figure 2. Diagrammatic representation of a normal mesothelial cell based on data obtained from reconstructions of serial electron micrographs. The configuration of the cell, its surface topography and its organelle composition are displayed. Cilium, C: micropinocytotic vesicles, P; lamellar body, L; Golgi apparatus, G; mitochondrion, M; desmosome, D; tonofibrils, T; rough endoplasmic reticulum, RER; nucleus, N.

electron density, contains prominent matricial dense granules [7–9].

5.1.5. *Mesothelial cytoskeleton*

Immunocytochemical staining of the mesothelial cytoskeleton has in the last few years provided totally new information on the tissue origin of mesothelium, its manner of regeneration and a facility for determining its maturity in culture. *In vivo* injury and loss of surface mesothelium stimulates the proliferation of multipotential subserosal cells. These exhibit the ultrastructural features of myofibroblasts but co-express low molecular weight cytokeratin and vimentin (Fig. 6) [11]. As these cells migrate upwards to re-establish surface mesothelium, they acquire high molecular weight cytokeratin and lose vimentin. cultured mesothelial cells usually express low molecular weight cytokeratin and vimentin. Moreover it has been shown that during rapid growth in culture, human mesothelium shows reversible loss of cytokeratins and increase in vimentin. In non-dividing cells, vimentin synthesis decreases [12]. The important role of the immunocytochemical characterization

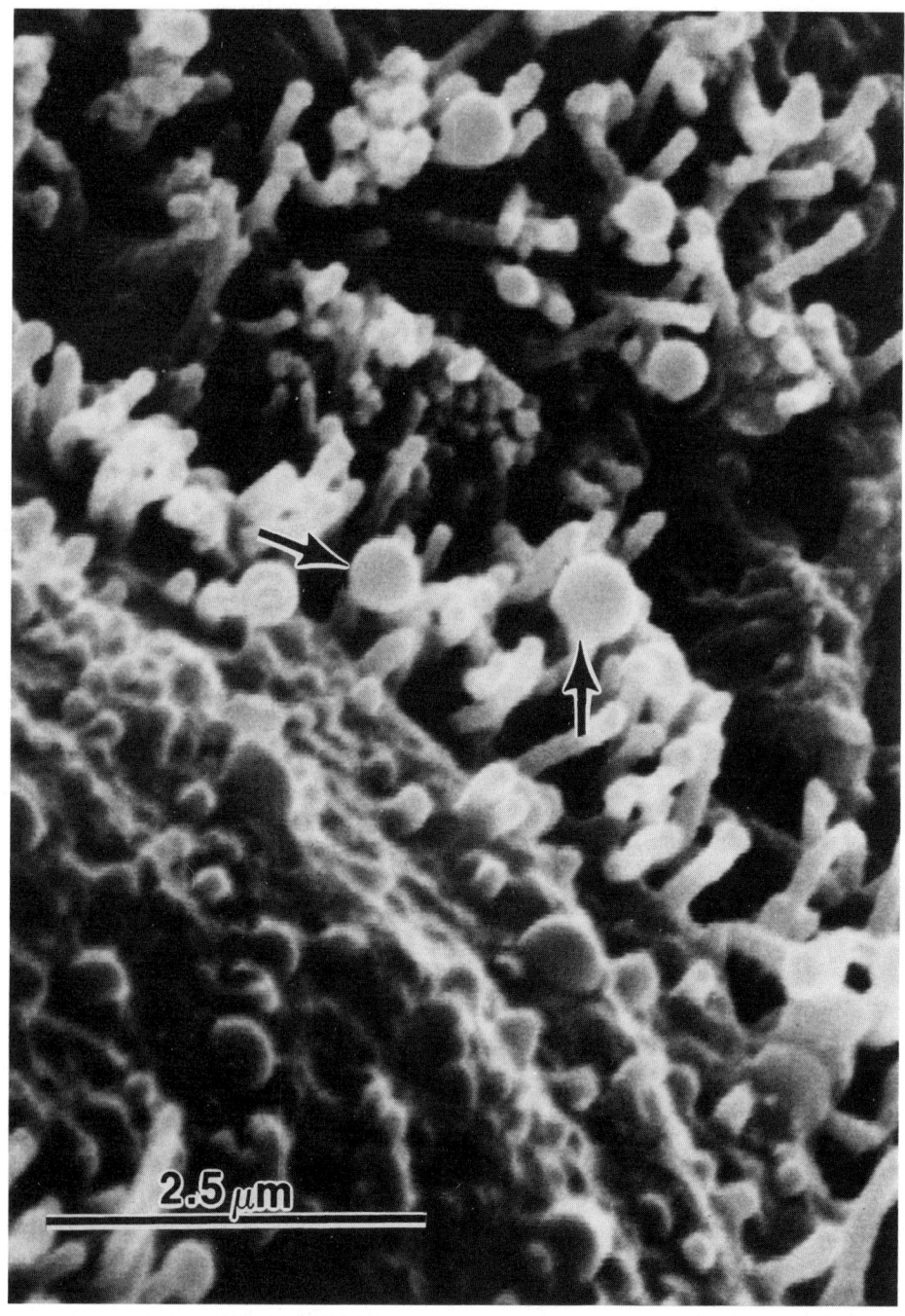

Figure 3. Scanning electron micrograph of a peritoneal biopsy from a non-uremic patient showing several spherical lamellar bodies (arrows) lying on the surface among microvilli. Magnification ×21,600.

of the cytoskeleton as a marker for mesothelial maturity, *in vivo* and *in vitro*, is summarized in Fig. 6.

5.1.6. *Lamellar bodies*

Investigations carried out in 1987 into the source of phosphatidylcholine (PC) in peritoneal dialysate effluent revealed that transparent mesentery in rat synthesized as much PC as pulmonary alveolar tissue in an *in vitro* system [13]. This prompted an investigation which compared the ultrastructural organisation of mesothelium and type II pneumocytes, the known secretory source of alveolar surfactant. Electron microscopic examination of

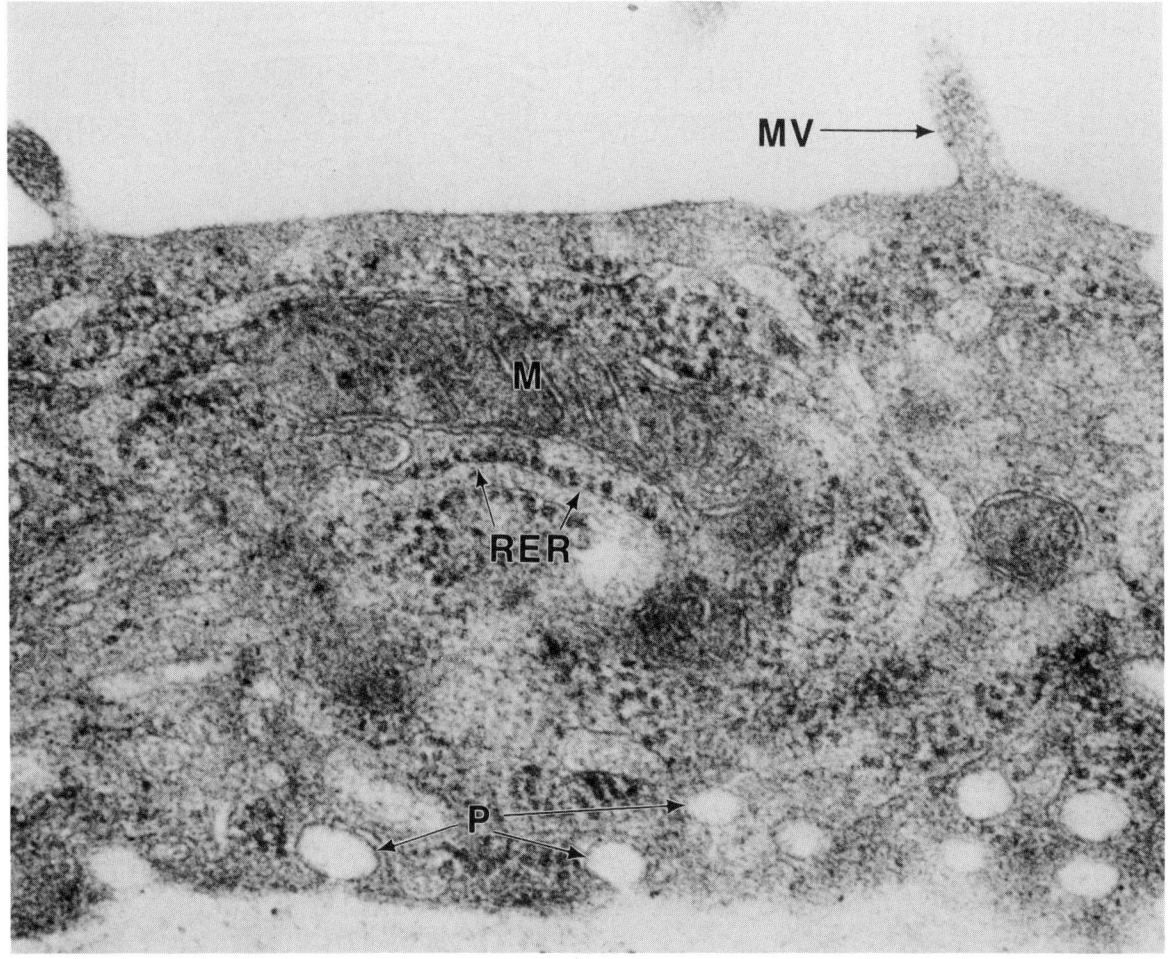

Figure 4. Transmission electron micrograph of mesothelial cell from a biopsy of parietal peritoneum of a non-uremic patient displaying ultrastructural detail of cytoplasm. Microvilli, MV; mitochondria, M; rough endoplasmic reticulum, RER; micropinocytotic vesicles, P. Magnification ×140,000.

tissue fixed and processed for embedding in standard resins showed hitherto unsuspected similarities in the fine structure of mesothelium and type II pneumocytes [14]. Both cells bear microvilli on their lumenal surface and possess similarly structured intercellular junctional complexes. Both cell types contain prominent endoplasmic reticulum, well-developed Golgi regions and an abundance of mitochondria. Numerous micropinocytotic vesicles line both surfaces of each cell type. A distinctive feature shared by both mesothelium and type II pneumocytes is the presence of prominent cytoplasmic lipid inclusions. Under certain pathological conditions both cells exhibit lanceolate clefts representing intracytoplasmic crystals of cholesterol [14].

In the light of such unexpected ultrastructural concordance [14], it was obvious that the next step in establishing if there was homology between the two cell types was the application of specific techniques of electron microscopic preparation developed for the study of type II pneumocytes. The highly structured cytoplasmic inclusions in type II pneumocytes had eluded recognition until the early 1970s because their lipid contents are readily extracted by the organic solvents used in conventional tissue processing for electron microscopy [15]. Following the discovery that tannic acid fixation and the use of polar dehydrants in tissue processing showed a complex lamellar substructure within these inclusions [16, 17], the role of these so-called lamellar bodies in the storage and secretion of pulmonary surfactant was rapidly elucidated. A recent study in which these techniques were

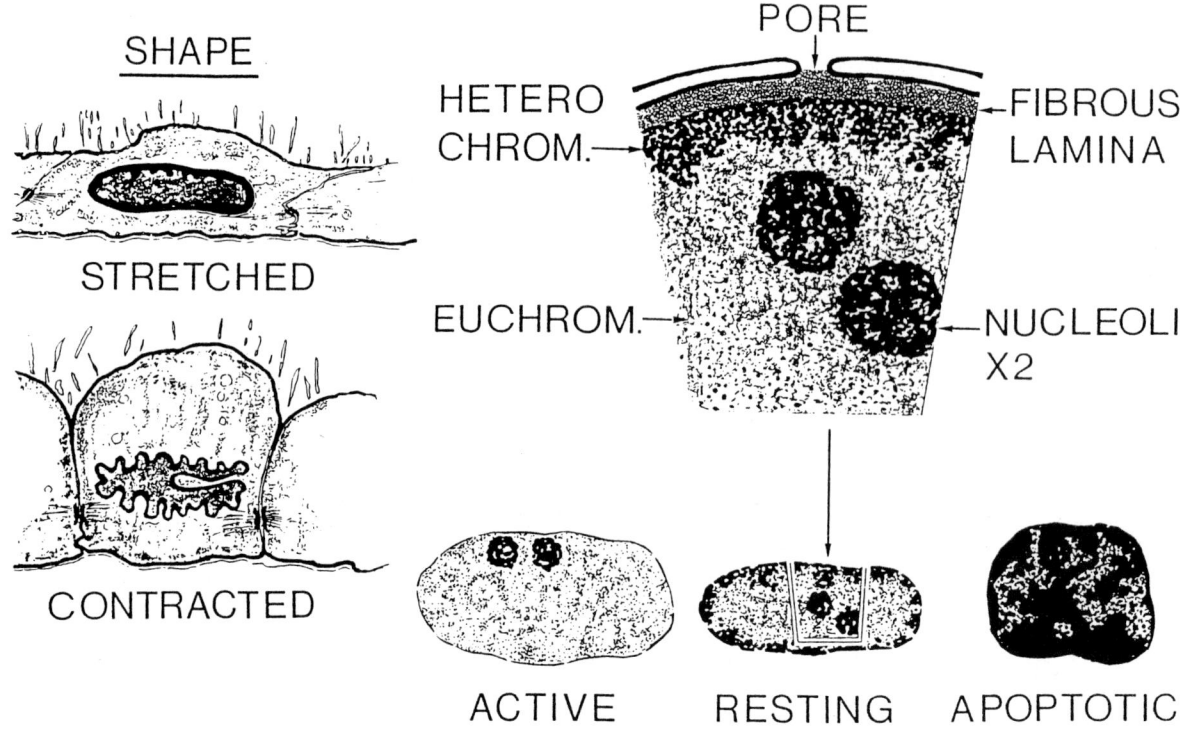

Figure 5. Diagrammatic summary of mesothelial cell nuclear profiles. In stretched cells, the nucleus assumes a cigar-shaped outline. In contracted cells, the nucleus may be highly convoluted with cytoplasmic invaginations. The nucleus possesses a fibrous lamina interposed between the inner nuclear membrane and the thin band of marginated heterochromatin. Euchromatin generally predominates over heterochromatin. Two nucleoli are commonly encountered.

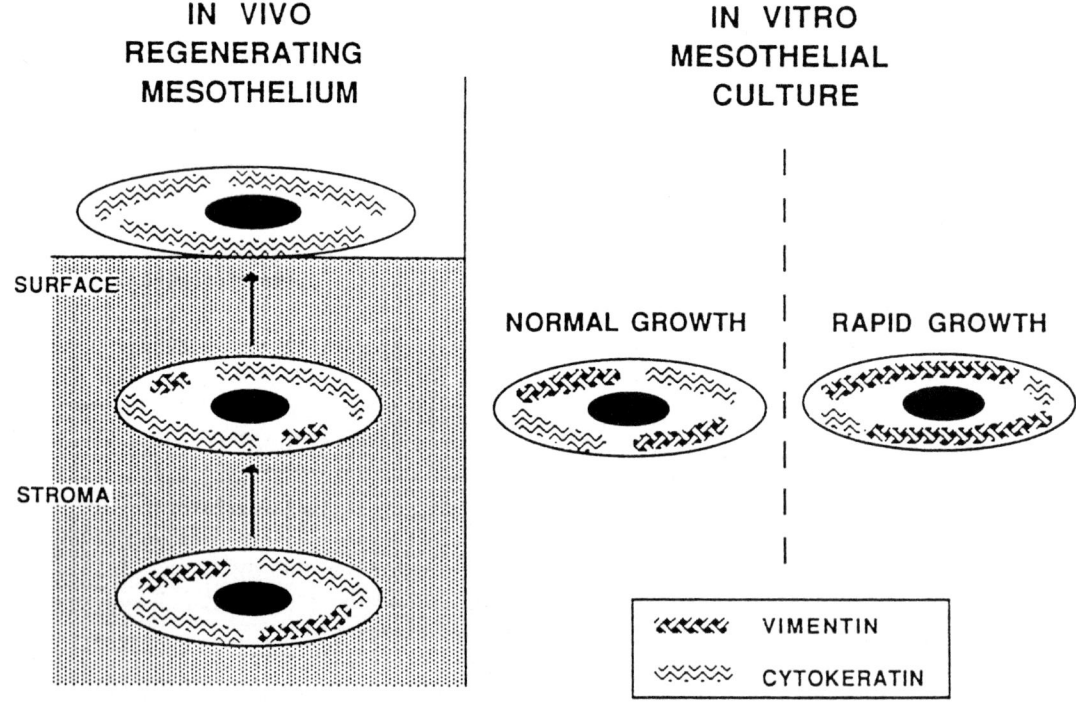

Figure 6. Diagrammatic summary of the distinctive cytoskeletal markers which serve to distinguish the state of maturity of mesothelial cells *in vivo* and *in vitro*.

applied directly to peritoneal tissue likewise unmasked the existence of lamellar bodies in parietal and visceral mesothelium in humans, monkeys, rabbits and mice [18]. The bodies, which were up to 1.5 μ in diameter, exhibited repeating patterns of alternate electron dense lamellae and electron lucent zones (Figs. 7, 8). Arranged in concentric or parallel planar series, the lamellar structure and periodicity was found to be the same as that encountered in the type II pneumocytes of the same species processed for microscopy by the same techniques. Lamellar profiles were also identified in the endoplasmic reticulum and the Golgi complex of mesothelial cells as first described in type II pneumocytes. Similarly, exocytotic extrusion of lamellar bodies from the apical portion of the mesothelial cell and the presence of lamellar bodies on the cell surface in a manner identical to that found in type II pneumocytes was also observed (Figs. 8, 9). These findings have provided evidence that a process of specialized biosynthesis and secretion of phospholipids similar to that established for type II pneumocytes also occurs in mesothelial cells.

5.2. Submesothelial stroma

Mesothelium rests on a thin but readily visible basement membrane (Fig. 10) [7–9]. In both parietal and visceral sites the stroma consists of a layer of areolar tissue, some 1–2 mm in thickness which is composed of oriented bundles of collagen fibers set in a matrix of ground substance of moderate electron density [7–9]. At a variable distance from the surface, a retiform elastic lamina is present in both visceral and parietal peritoneum (Fig. 10) [7–9]. The collagenous and elastic elements achieve varying degrees of structural organisation and

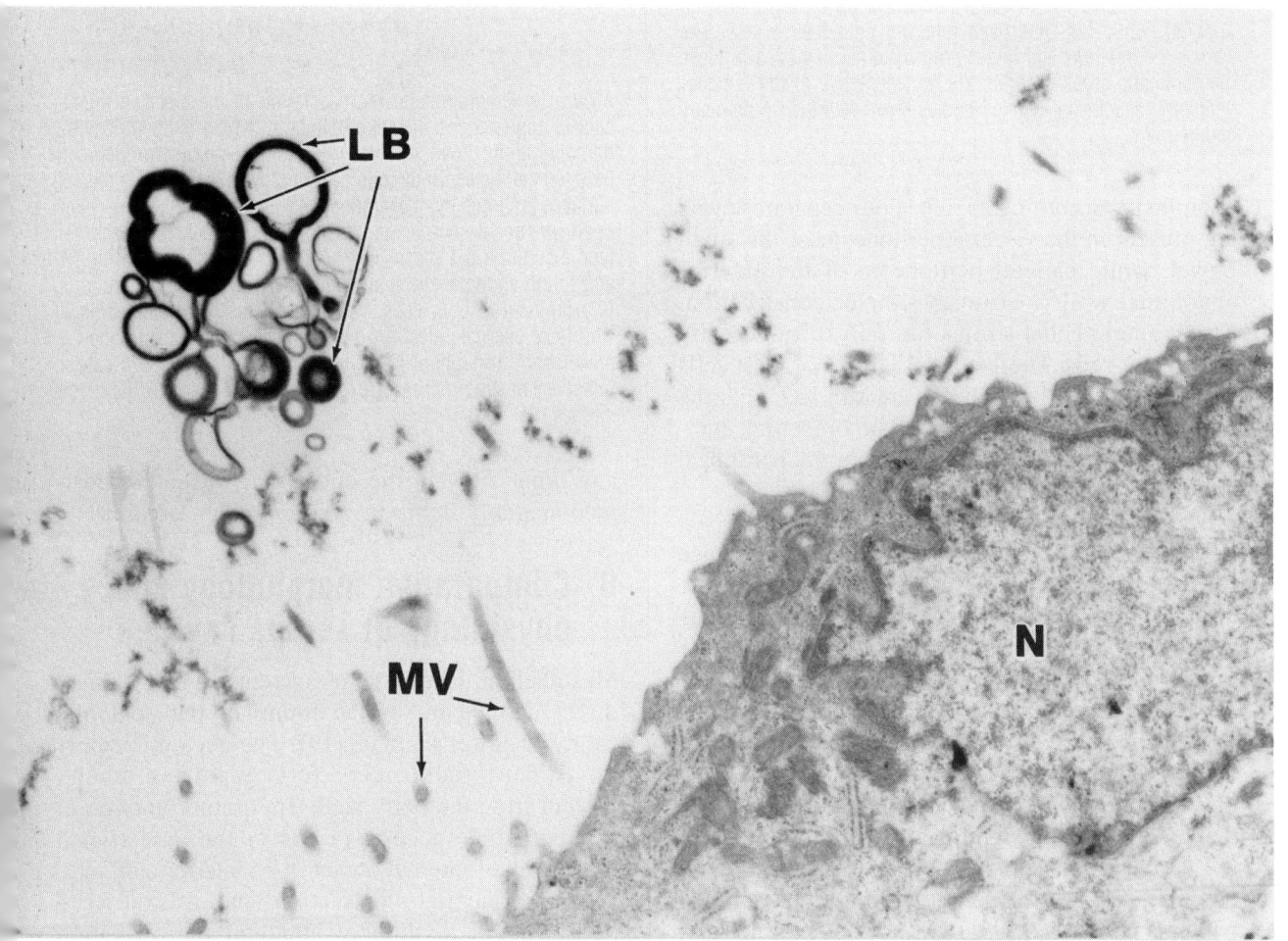

Figure 7. Transmission electron micrograph of biopsy of parietal peritoneum from a non-uremic patient at elective abdominal surgery. A cluster of unravelling lamellar bodies (LB) are present at the outer edge of the microvillous layer (MV). Nucleus, N. Magnification x23,100.

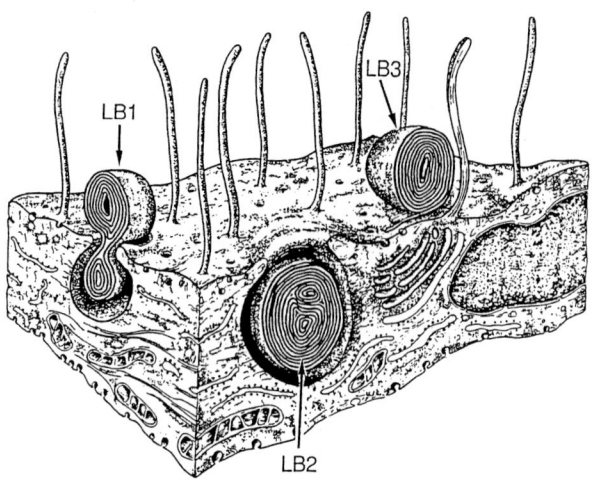

Figure 8. Diagrammatic representation, based on serial sections of human parietal mesothelium illustrating the form and disposition of lamellar structures. LB2 is a fully formed body contained in a vesicle which is developing an opening to the cell surface. LB1 is in the process of exocytotic extrusion through such an opening, while LB3 has been released onto the surface. The whorls, bifurcations and finger print patterns displayed in these diagrammatic cross-sections are representative of the lamellar geometry mesothelial-derived bodies share with their pulmonary counterparts.

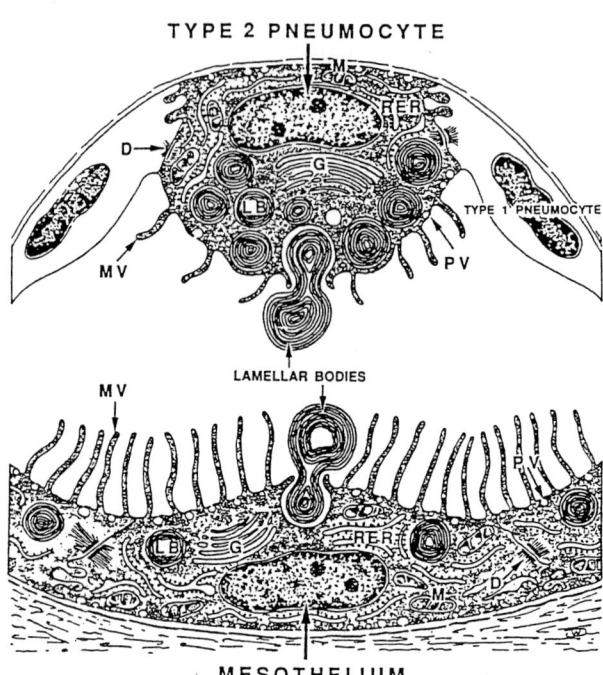

Figure 9. Diagrammatic representation of the electron microscopic appearances of mesothelium and type II pneumocytes, demonstrating close similarity of ultrastructural arrangements between cell types. Both cells bear microvilli (MV), while the cell surfaces are lined by micropinocytotic vesicles (PV). Well-developed junctional complexes contain desmosomes (D). Each cell type exhibits a cytoplasm well endowed with mitochondria (M) and rough endoplasmic reticulum (RR). The Golgi apparatus (G) is prominent in both cells. Lamellar bodies (LB), consisting of whorls of alternate electron-dense and electron-lucent lamellae, are present throughout the cytoplasm in both cells and can be observed in the process of exocytotic extrusion from the apical surface.

complexity according to site. Four separate layers are present in the visceral peritoneum of the small bowel, while parietal peritoneum of the anterior abdominal wall is of much simpler construction. The submesothelial stroma has only a low density of resident cells. These consist largely of mast cells and fibroblasts. Macrophages are rare and, with the exception of the milk spots in the omentum, lymphoreticular tissue is not found in normal peritoneal stroma [7–9].

The peritoneum is not a highly vascularised tissue, the capillary bed lying at some little distance from the mesothelium. In the adventitial matrix around larger vessels are cells with long tenuous processes which encircle the vessel. These have the typical morphology of veil cells, perivascular cells distinct from pericytes which have been described in other parts of the body. These are believed to belong to the dendritic cell family.

Under stimulus of the inflammatory response there is a rapid and significant apparent increase in the vascular bed. This is most probably due, as in other tissues, to the opening up of a capillary bed which is normally shut down and is not readily discernible on histological examination. The most vascular region of the peritoneum is that which covers the liver. The stroma is no thicker than at any other site but the underlying vascular bed is incomparably richer than at any other location.

6. Comparative morphology and physiology of serous cavities

Mesothelium is a tissue of ancient lineage, being a direct descendant of the lining of the coelomic cavity of lower animals [19]. The coelomic cavity in its most rudimentary form separates tubular viscera from the body wall. The prime function of this potential space is to permit the unrestricted movement of internal organs, e.g., intermittent, integrated sequential contraction and relaxation – peristalsis, or rhythmic contraction and relaxation of strictures – ventricular beating [19]. This space is also used in annelid worms for effecting locomotion and is the precursor for synovial lined joints.

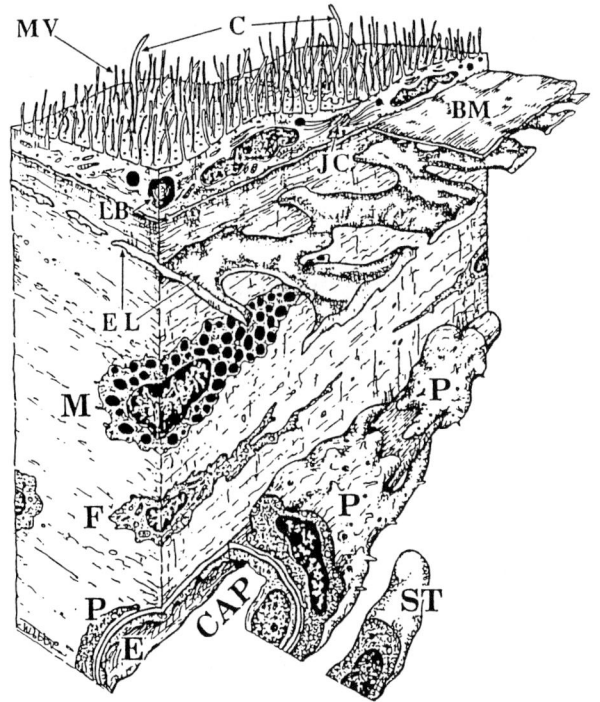

Figure 10. Diagrammatic representation of the morphology of normal peritoneum showing the spatial relationships between component parts. Microvilli, MV; cilium, C; junctional complex, JC; lamellar body, LB; elastic lamina, EL; mast cell, M; fibroblast, F; pericyte, P; endothelium, E; capillary, CAP; basement membrane, BM.

In order to subserve all of these related functions the cavity has from an early stage developed the property of self-lubrication [19]. It would appear that the ability of the cavity to maintain non-stick surfaces with very low coefficients of friction is an example of a highly conserved evolutionary development. As species have evolved, the cavity has been used successively as a convenient conduit for fluids distributing oxygen, nutriments, cells, waste products and reproduction [19].

The evolutionary history of the coelomic cavity as a conduit for external voiding of waste products is particularly pertinent in view of the success of peritoneal dialysis. In 1982 a study in fish [20] showed that salmonids excreted peritoneal fluid through abdominal pores (peritoneal canals). This investigation brought to the attention of the zoological world previous research on the function of the peritoneal cavity as an accessory excretory organ in vertebrates. Indeed, there exists an interesting reciprocal and compensating correlation between the presence or absence of abdominal pores and the method of waste excretion in elasmobranch fish, *Ganoidei, Dipnoi* and *Teleostei* species, amphibia, certain *Chelonia* and *Crocodilia*. In species where nephrostomes drain the peritoneal cavity into mesonephric ducts there are no abdominal pores. Conversely, in animals where abdominal pores are present, nephrostomes are absent (Fig. 11) [20]. In installing an artificial abdominal pore (peritoneal catheter) it could be argued that the process of peritoneal dialysis in man recapitulates the accessory excretory function of the peritoneal cavity in lower vertebrates [19].

No striking differences have been observed between a variety of mammalian species with respect to the ultrastructure of the mesothelium. Piscine mesothelium, however, does not bear microvilli but possesses motile cilia [19].

7. Morpho-functional correlates

The role of the mesothelium in peritoneal dialysis must be viewed in the context of its normal function in normal mammals. There seems little doubt that

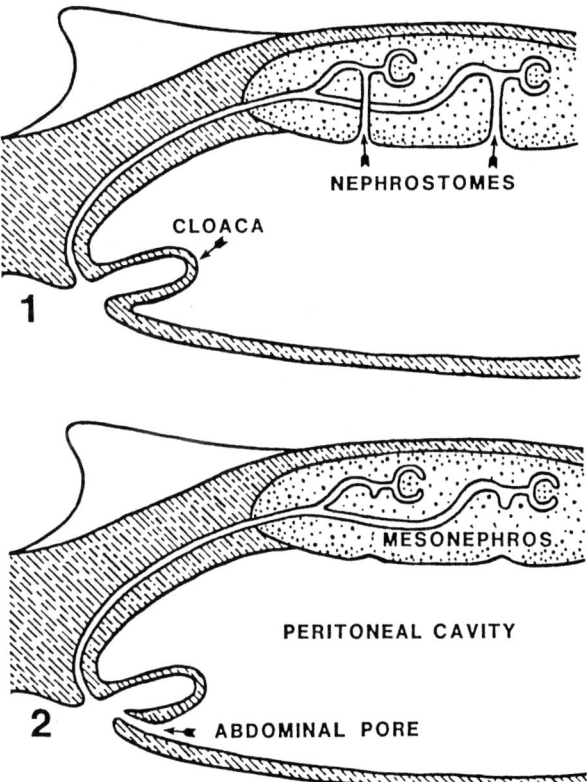

Figure 11. The two different forms of peritoneal drainage found in fish. In some species peritoneal drainage is effected through nephrostomes which join mesonephric tubules (1). In other species drainage is achieved through abdominal pores (2). Thus there is a reciprocal relationship between these structures; where abdominal pores are present, nephrostomes are absent.

the primary function of mesothelium, as it is throughout the animal kingdom, is the provision of a non-adhesive surface which permits unrestricted mobility for the viscera it subtends (Fig. 12) [18]. In this regard the ultrastructural organisation of the cells demonstrates its role as a resilient lining cell which has well-developed secretory capabilities. Although the surface microvilli are profuse, they do not attain the high density found in tissues where the structural requirements are a very large surface area for adsorptive transport [18]. It is therefore believed that mesothelial microvilli exist as a device to lower friction between opposing surfaces when they are coated with lubricant secretions (Fig. 12) [10, 13, 14, 18].

With respect to mesothelial sub-cellular organisation, organelle content betrays a secretory function [7–9]. This secretory capability is devoted to producing lubricants (phospholipids and glycosaminoglycans) and agents which suppress adhesion (prostacyclin and tissue plasminogen activators) (Fig. 12) [18]. The structure of the cell junctions is responsible for two main functional attributes; the occurrence of tight junctions determines the volume and composition of transmembrane fluid transport, while the structure and frequency of desmosomes determines the mechanical strength of the lining membrane. Transmembrane fluid transport and mesothelial secretion are directly related in that the peritoneal transudate is the solvent or carrier solution for the secreted surfactant lubricant [18].

8. Pathological peritoneum

8.1. Uremic peritoneum

The low resolution of light microscopic examination of the thin mesothelial monolayer has in the past one hundred years failed to reveal a single cytoplasmic lesion. This deficiency has recently been rectified by transmission electron microscopy which has uncovered highly distinctive ultrastructural abnormalities exclusively in human uremic mesothelium. Dobbie et al. [9] have detected paracrystalline intracytoplasmic inclusions in the mesothelium of over one third of the biopsies obtained from uraemic patients at catheter insertion, prior to the initiation of CAPD (Figs. 13, 14). The exclusiveness of this uremic association is con-

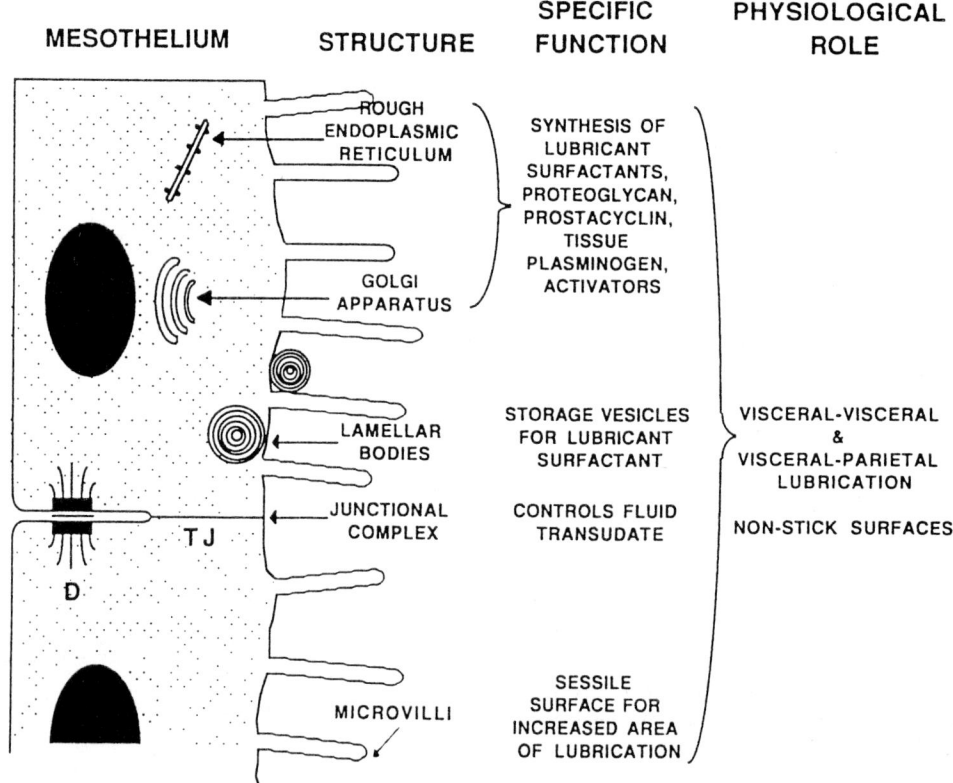

Figure 12. Diagrammatic summary of the important subcellular structures and organelles which together subserve the prime functions of normal mesothelium. Desmosome, D; tight junction, TJ.

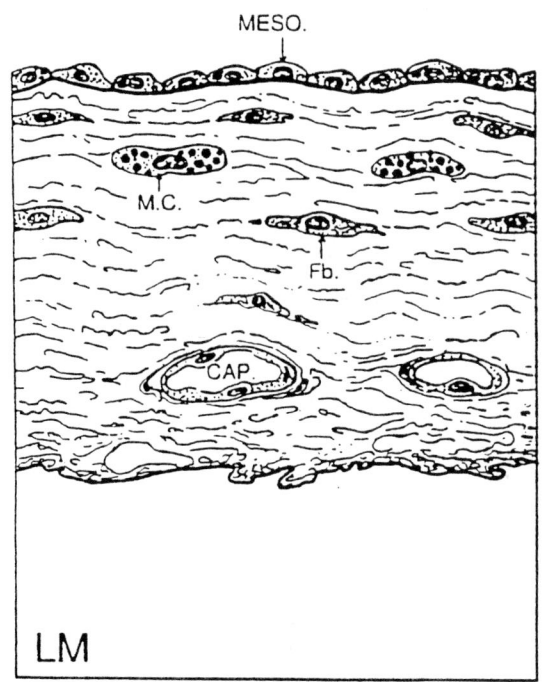
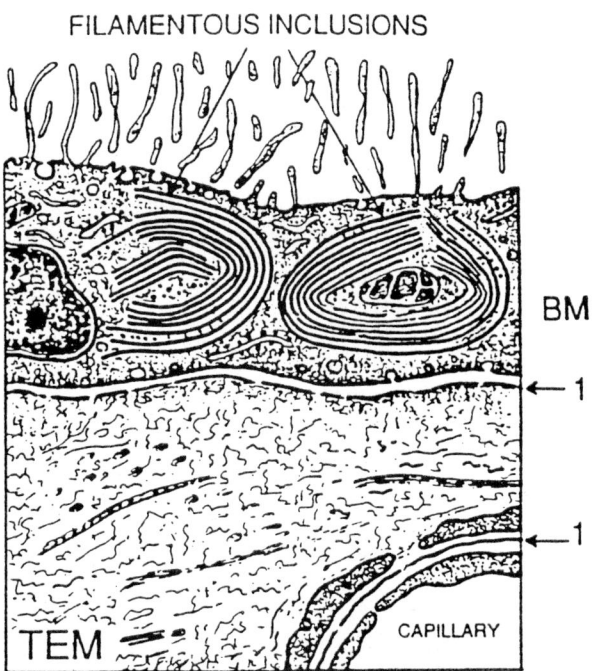

Figure 13. Diagrammatic summary of morphological findings in peritoneal biopsies from uremic (non-dialysed) patients. Light microscopic examination (LM) reveals no abnormality as compared to normal controls. Transmission electron microscopy (TEM) in 36% of uremic biopsies shows intracytoplasmic filamentous inclusions in mesothelial cells. Mesothelium, MESO; mast cell, MC; fibroblast, Fb; capillary, CAP; basement membrane, BM (1).

firmed by their failure to detect either *in vivo* or *in vitro*, the lesion in normal human and animal mesothelium [20].

The initial process in the formation of the inclusion is the appearance of a single, densely osmiophilic filament within the cisterna of the RER [9]. Accumulation of multiple filaments arranged in parallel arrays with a regular periodicity is observed in association with sacular dilatations of the cisternae which usually contain electron dense granular material. These appearances strongly suggest retention of locally synthesized molecules within the RER which then proceed to crystalline assemblage and deposition. Where the filaments are profuse, the inclusions burst from the confines of the RER to lie free in the cytosol. These filaments may constitute structures of considerable dimension which result in distortion of the affected cells. The preference of the filaments for assuming straight or gently curvilinear profiles implies a certain rigidity, an impression supported by the observations that large accumulations cause angular deformations of inner and outer cell membranes. Where this is observed, the cells exhibit signs of active detachment from the basement membrane.

The end result of this process is illustrated by the appearance in these biopsies of numerous detached cells replete with bundles of inclusions, many of which have cascaded out of ruptured cell membranes to lie scattered on the peritoneal surface. Thus, defoliation of mesothelium would appear to be the pathological consequence of this cytological inclusion disorder [9].

Non-infective pericarditis [21], pleuritis [22] and ascites [23] have been accepted as significant uremic manifestations of renal failure since their original description by Richard Bright in 1836 [24]. Since then there has been no advance in our understanding of the etiology of uremic serositis and any literature on the subject is confined to speculation on possible serosal irritation caused by the retention of unidentified nitrogenous waste products. Although we do not as yet possess any information on either the nature of the inclusions or the factors involved in the causation, the exfoliative mesothelial lesion which results therefrom would appear to be an extremely important histopathological and etiologic candidate for the initiation of the exudative serositis so characteristic of the uremic state.

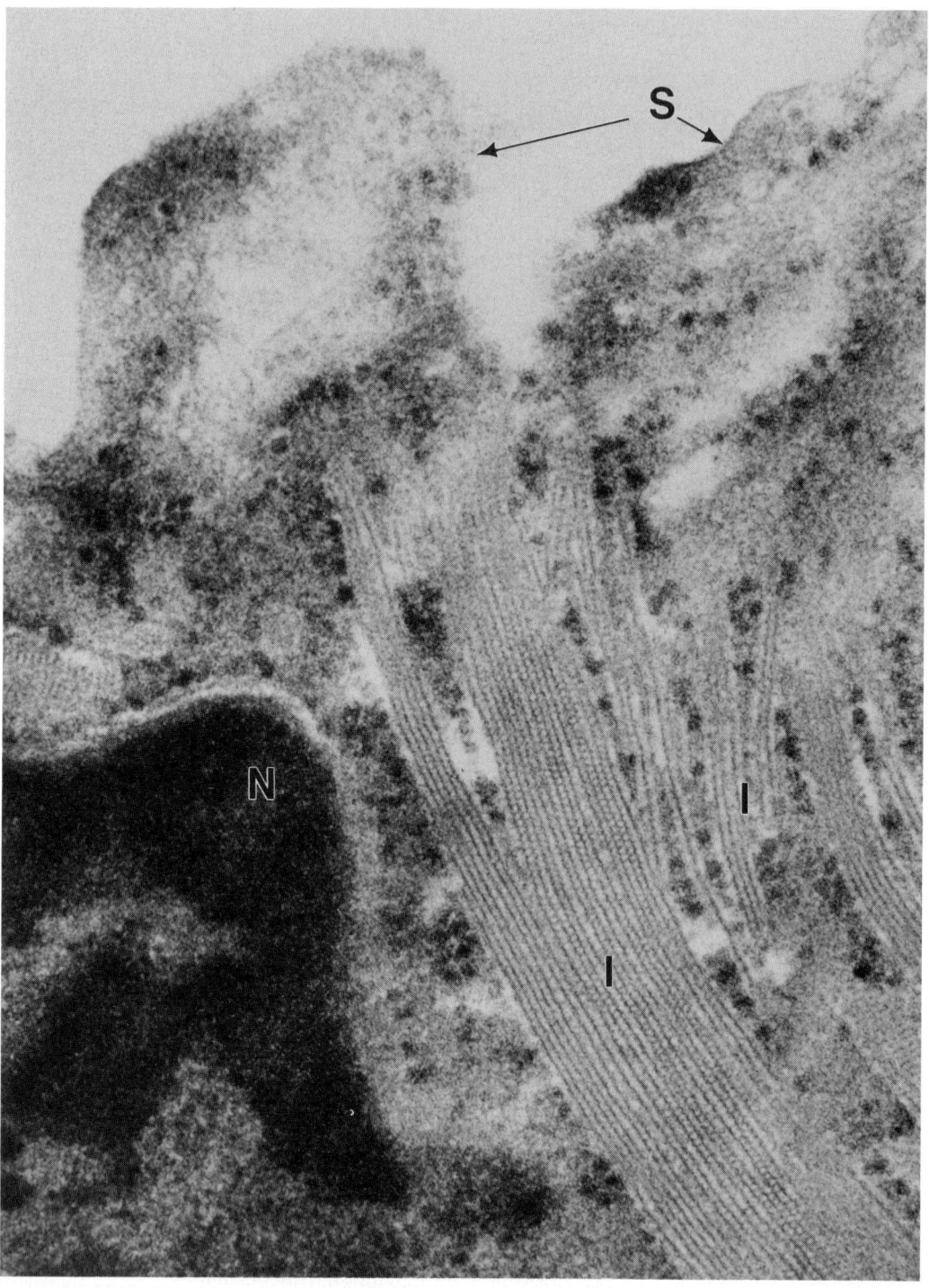

Figure 14. Transmission electron micrograph of peritoneal biopsy of uremic patient prior to onset of peritoneal dialysis. Rod-like structures arranged in parallel bundles are found free in the mesothelial cytosol exhibiting the appearance of paracrystalline cytoplasmic inclusion (I). Surface, S; nucleus, N. Magnification ×180,000.

9. Peritoneum in CAPD

9.1. Mesothelium

9.1.1. Surface topography

Observations made on scanning electron microscopy provide a tantalizing indication that mesothelium subjected to the process of continuing dialysis may undergo reactive changes in response to the new environment [9]. This would appear to consist of a reactive proliferation of mesothelium giving an increased number of cells per unit area. In this respect, mesothelium would simply be following an innate response shown by all epithelial surfaces to the continued presence of an irritant. If the existence of this phenomenon could be established through accurate measurement it might have significant bearing on our concepts of peritoneal permeability and mass transfer. Increased density of cells means increased length of the cellular junctions. The equations relating cell number to junctional length and mesothelial permeability might provide important new insights regarding the inter-patient variability of peritoneal permeability. Unfortunately randomly collected and variably processed biopsies received by the International Peritoneal Biopsy Registry do not readily lend themselves to accurate morphometry.

Scanning electron microscopy also shows a diminution in density of microvillous projections with continued exposure to dialysate (Fig. 15) [8, 9]. As with cell numbers, morphometric analysis of density changes in microvillous cover is yet to be performed. Likewise, the density of surface micropinocytotic vesicles is reduced in biopsies from patients on CAPD. Research on other tissues has shown a connection between microvillous density and numbers of surface vesicles. In normal circumstances mesothelial microvilli contain a considerable reserve of cell membrane. Under certain conditions this reserve can be rapidly converted to vesicles. This conversion can be seen in active cells, as in mesothelial cell culture [9]. In CAPD patients the diminution of microvillous density may be the

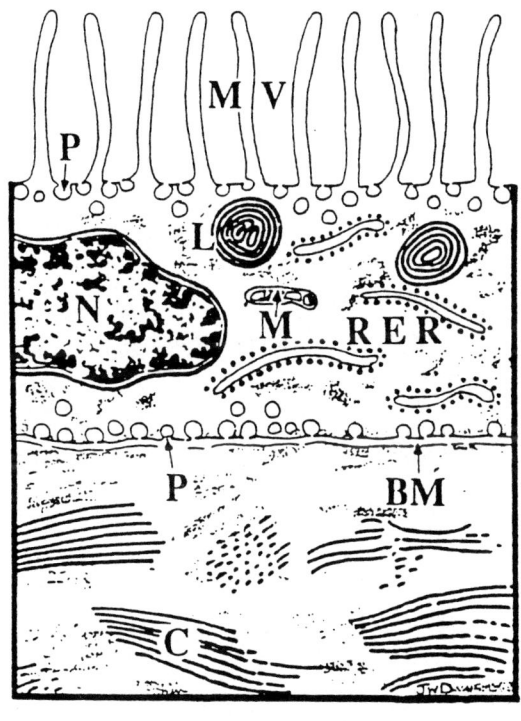
NORMAL MESOTHELIUM

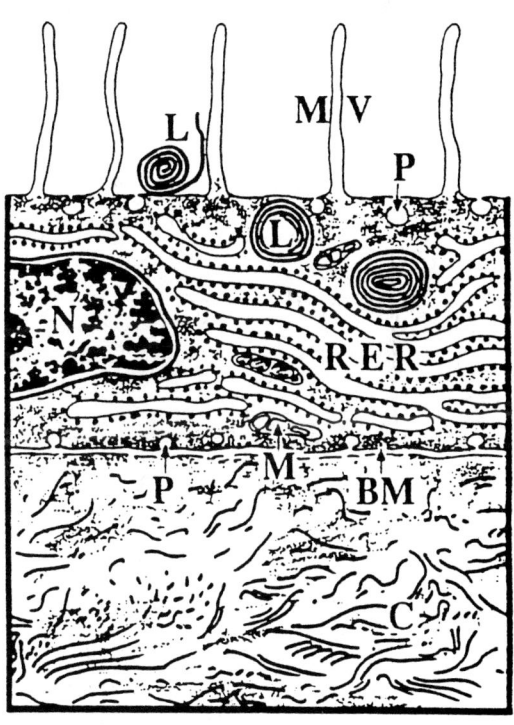
MESOTHELIUM AFTER CAPD

Figure 15. Diagrammatic representation of the ultrastructure of the mesothelium and subjacent serosal stroma in normal individuals and CAPD patients as determined by electron microscopic examination of peritoneal biopsies. The most striking differences are found in the decrease in numbers of mesothelial microvilli (MV) and micropinocytotic vesicles (P), and the hyperplasia of the RER in biopsies from CAPD patients as opposed to the findings in normal controls. There are also differences in the submesothelium in CAPD patients where variations in texture of ground substance and disposition of collagen fibres (C) may be observed. Lamellar bodies, L; mitochondria, M; nucleus, N; basement membrane, BM.

cause of the decreased numbers of micropinocytotic vesicles. Whatever the nature of the cause or the effect it seems likely that these changes in surface topography of mesothelium in CAPD signifies a reduction in cell membrane reserve.

Abnormal surface protuberances is a further category of topographical alterations encountered in biopsies from CAPD patients [9]. These variously shaped projections, termed blisters and blebs, are known from work in other tissues to represent focal damage to the structural integrity of the cell membrane and its underlying cytoskeleton, whereby cytosol and organelle herniate through weak points in the structure. Since these appearances may also be observed in uremic mesothelium, it is as yet unclear whether these abnormalities represent evidence of continuing in vivo cell damage or whether they have been induced by handling during collection.

9.1.2. Nuclei

An alteration in nuclear profile occurs in inflamed mesothelium in biopsies from CAPD patients. Concomitant with cuboidal transformation of the cell shape, the nucleus assumes a circular outline while the ratio of euchromatin to heterochromatin increases (Fig. 16) [8]. Intranuclear inclusions called perichromatin granules have been observed in the regenerating mesothelium found in biopsies from CAPD patients [25]. Consisting of spherical, highly electron dense granules (300–350 Å in diameter) and surrounded by a prominent electron-lucent halo, the inclusions must probably represent intranuclear ribosomes. Their appearance is such however, that they can easily be confused with virus particles.

9.1.3. Organelles and cytosol

In stable CAPD patients with normally functioning peritoneum there is a variety of ultrastructural changes which are relatively minor with respect to their deviation from the appearances encountered in mesothelium of normal controls.

A characteristic feature of mesothelium in patients who have been treated with CAPD is the hyperplasia of the RER (Fig. 15) [7–9]. These

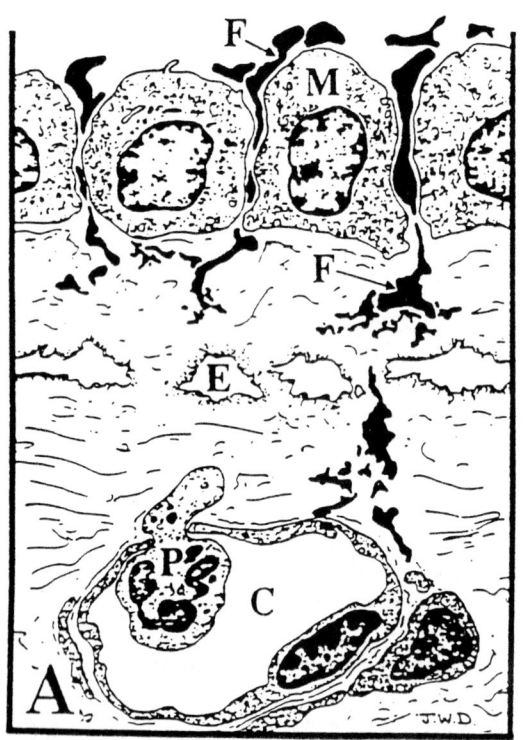
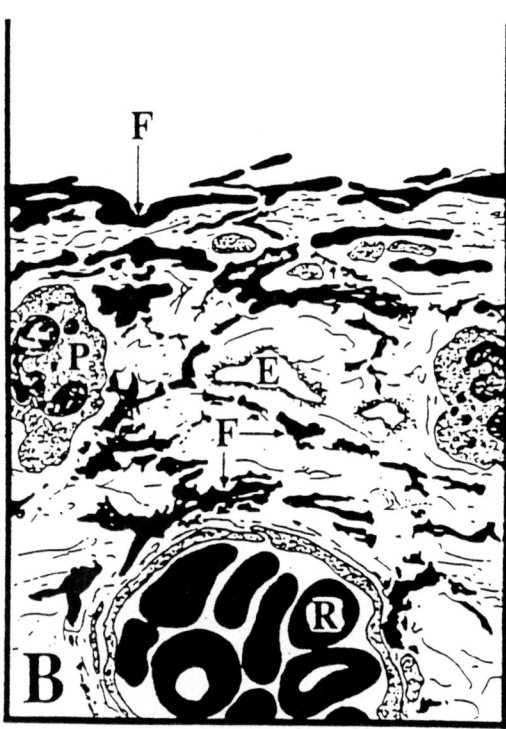

Figure 16. Diagrammatic representation of the essential ultrastructural changes encountered in biopsies of human peritoneum during peritonitis. In the early stages of inflammation (A), there is exudation of fibrin (F) which appears in the submesothelial tissue between and on the surface of mesothelial cells (M). Migration of polymorphs (P) from the superficial capillaries occurs. In advance peritonitis (B), there is loss of mesothelium; fibrin covers the surface and insudates the submesothelium in stratified layers. Dilated capillaries are packed with red blood cells (R). In interpreting these biopsies, identification and location of the elastic lamina (E) is important in judging the degree of thickening due to accretion of fibrin or granulation tissue or even loss of tissue due to necrosis.

findings may be part of the tissue's adaptive response to constant removal of secretory products in the effluent dialysate. Biopsies from some patients on CAPD may show degenerative changes in the RER as part of a generalized process of cell damage or toxicity. These findings may be part of the tissue's adaptive response to constant removal of secretory products in the effluent dialysate. Biopsies from some patients on CAPD may show degenerative changes in the RER as part of a generalized process of cell damage or toxicity. These lesions are evidenced by variable cisternal dilatation and vesiculation with disaggregation of the polyribosomes [9].

Degenerative changes in mitochondria may be observed in peritoneal biopsies from patients on CAPD, particularly in the presence of signs of inflammation. The most common pathological changes are those of mitochondrial pyknosis and intracristal swelling. The latter phenomenon, which is also referred to as condensed configuration is due to influx of water into the outer chamber of the mitochondrion. Extensive mitochondrial swelling in association with marked endoplasmic dilatation together represent the ultrastructural appearance of cloudy swelling [8]. We have observed variation in size and number of matriceal dense granules in the mitochrondria in biopsies from patients on CAPD. Since it is known that these granules are the site of accumulation of divalent cations, and that they are prominent in tissues involved in the transport of solutes and water, a study of their variation in size and density in CAPD patients with respect to normal controls would be an important exercise, particularly in regard to the unphysiologically high calcium levels in normal dialysate.

9.1.4. *Peritonitis*
The majority of biopsies obtained from patients with active or recent peritoneal inflammation were those in which the infection had been of such severity as to require removal of the catheter [9]. Thus there is a high incidence of cases where the causative organism was either *Staphylococcus aureus, Pseudomonas aeruginosa* or fungi. Most biopsies in this category show grossly damaged or denuded mesothelium. Stratified variegated layers of surface fibrin suggest successive episodes of deposition. Deep in the edematous stroma there may be lozenges of insudated fibrin (Figs. 16, 17). Acute or chronic inflammatory infiltrate is usually sparse while organisms are but rarely observed [9]. This probably reflects the fact that the patients had been heavily dosed with antibiotics and that active infection of the membrane had ceased. There, persistent exudative response in the absence of signs of pus-forming bacterial inflammation in these biopsies may however indicate that permeation of the peritoneal cavity by exo- or endotoxins from surviving colonies of organisms in or around the catheter continues to cause a 'scalded membrane' and is the explanation why catheter removal is usually attended by clinical signs of peritoneal healing.

9.1.5. *Recovery from peritonitis*
Random biopsies from CAPD patients may unexpectedly show a peritoneum denuded of mesothelium, together with stromal changes indicative of a chronic non-healing process (Fig. 18) [9]. The history usually reveals a recent, often severe, episode of peritonitis some one to three months previously. To all clinical appearances the patient had made a good recovery, but enquiry invariably reveals problems with ultrafiltration. The histological appearances of these biopsies closely resemble those seen in the persistent exudative lesions found in biopsies from patients whose catheters were removed because of 'unresolving inflammation' following severe peritonitis [9].

A striking histopathological feature of biopsies where remesothelialization has failed to occur is the conversion of the stroma to a 'cellular desert' (Fig. 18) [9]. Pale hyalinised fibrous tissue with abnormal horizontal banding of collagen exhibits large featureless tracts completely devoid of any cell content. The deepest edge of the stroma and the occasional blood vessel may show focal aggregates of chronic inflammatory cells. On examination of such specimens it is obvious that there is no sign of recruitment of cells which might be construed as mesothelial stem cells. Neither does the naked stroma show any evidence of repopulation of the surface by mesothelial reseeding (Fig. 18).

Examination of such specimens suggests three likely explanations for the pathogenesis of this striking lesion [9, 26]. It is eminently possible that due to the severity of the last episode of peritonitis the stromal mesenchymal reserve was damaged beyond recovery. Conversely, continued permeation of the peritoneal cavity by bacterial toxins from an infected catheter might in itself prevent healing. The third and likeliest explanation is that the continuing effect of a hostile environment has inhibited or destroyed the recuperative ability of stromal mesenchymal cells to heal the peritoneum after the last

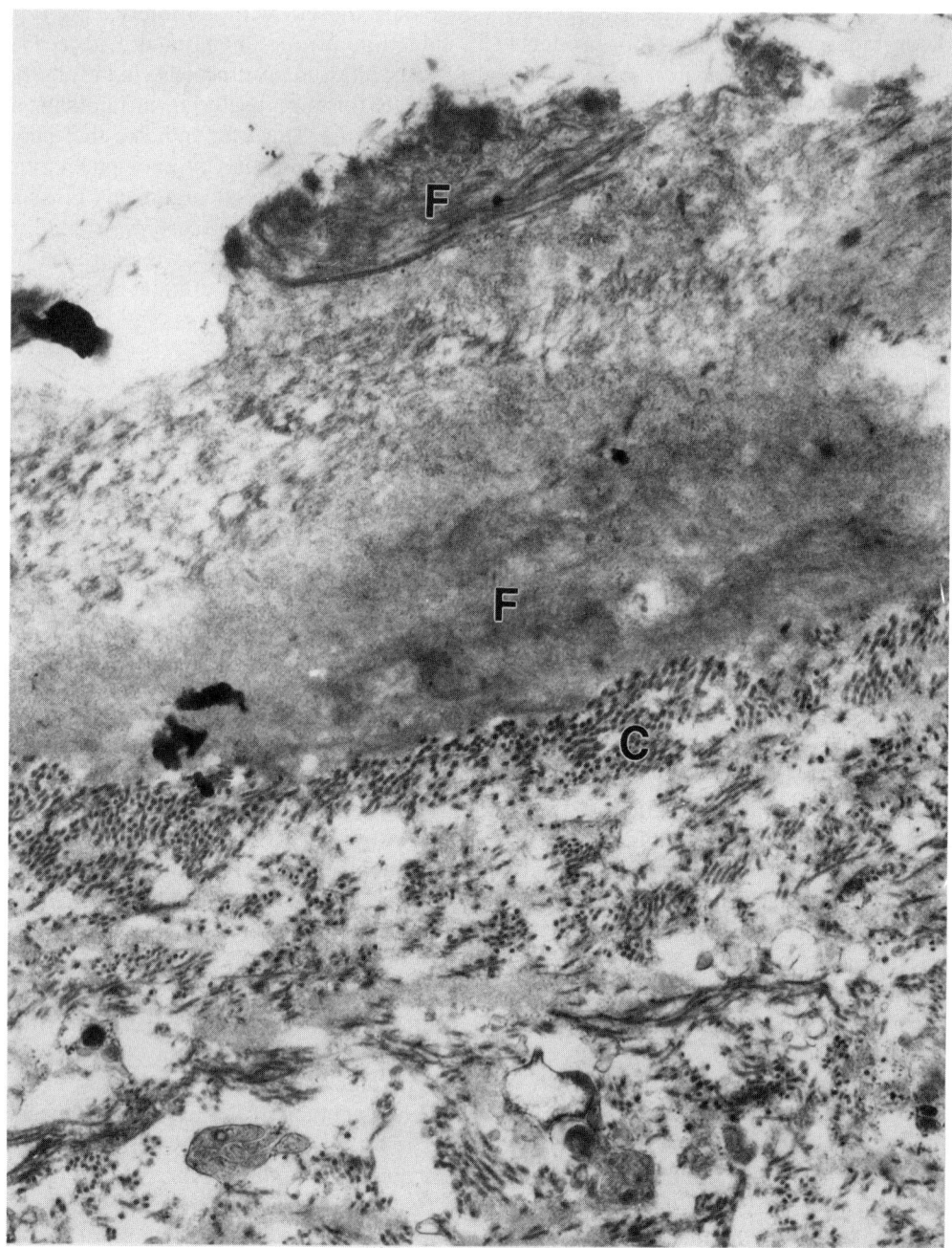

Figure 17. Transmission electron micrograph of biopsy of CAPD patient with active peritonitis. Mesothelium is missing from the surface which is covered by stratified layers of fibrin (F) which abut on edematous stromal collagen (C). Magnification ×73,000.

episode of peritonitis. Collateral evidence linking the pathogenesis of stromal diabetiform lesions to hyperglycemic damage incurred during peritonitis tends to support the theory that continued use of hypertonic glucose during and after peritoneal inflammation perpetuates the stromal cellular desert and frustrates remesothelialization (vide infra) [9, 26].

This distinct entity represents the most severe type of lesion associated with peritoneal dialysis. Information derived from a limited number of serial biopsies strongly supports the concept that this syndrome is the precursor of peritoneal fibrosis and sclerosing peritonitis [9, 10, 26].

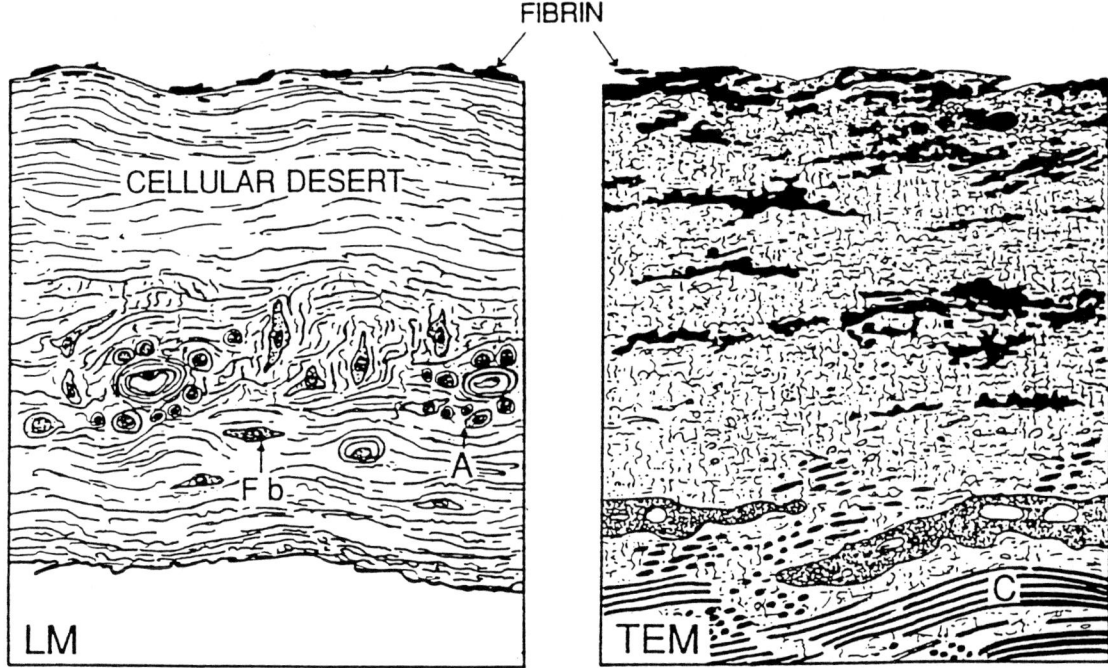

Figure 18. Diagrammatic representation of morphological findings found in random biopsies of patients on CAPD one to three months after an episode of peritonitis in which remesothelialization has not taken place in the area sampled. The outer zone of the stroma consists of acellular, variably hyalinised collagen. The surface is sparingly flecked with fibrin. Light microscopy, LM: fibroblast, Fb; aggregates of chronic inflammatory cells, A; transmission electron microscopy, TEM; collagen, C.

10. Basement membrane reduplication

Significant morphological alterations may be encountered in the basement membrane of mesothelium and stromal blood vessels of non-diabetic patients treated with peritoneal dialysis (Fig. 19) [9, 10, 26–28]. At both sites the lesions present as thickening and diabetiform reduplication of the membrane. The presence of pericyte debris in the walls of the blood vessels implies increased cell death and turnover.

Basement membrane changes of this nature in association with pericyte pathology is in fact pathognomonic of diabetic angiopathy. In direct contrast, other non-diabetic patients who had been successfully treated with CAPD for many years show either minimal or no alterations in the morphology of their peritoneal basement membranes [9].

In pursuit of possible etiologic factors which might account for the presence or absence of diabetiform basement membrane pathology in these non-diabetic patients, a cohort of 14 biopsies was identified which showed no or minimal alterations in basement membrane morphology. Review of historical data revealed that these biopsies belonged to patients on CAPD for 1–7 years who had either no history of peritonitis (33%) or had experienced one or two episodes (67%). Biopsies from 26 patients showing significant basement membrane pathology were characterized by a history of multiple episodes [3–6] of peritonitis, many of which had been severe. Thus by comparing the opposite ends of the spectrum of basement membrane and pericyte morphology we can discern that pathological change would appear to be linked to incidence and severity of peritonitis [9].

A similar association between increasing episodes of peritonitis and basement membrane pathology is encountered in biopsies from diabetic patients on CAPD. As is the case in non-diabetic patients, uremic diabetics unexposed to dialysis do not show reduplication of the mesothelial basement membrane, although they exhibit vascular pathology [5]. It is noteworthy that the most extreme cases of angiopathy, evident on light microscopic examination, and in which there is vessel calcification, obliteration and adventitial proliferation of smooth muscle, are encountered in the biopsies of diabetic patients with a history of multiple and severe episodes of peritonitis.

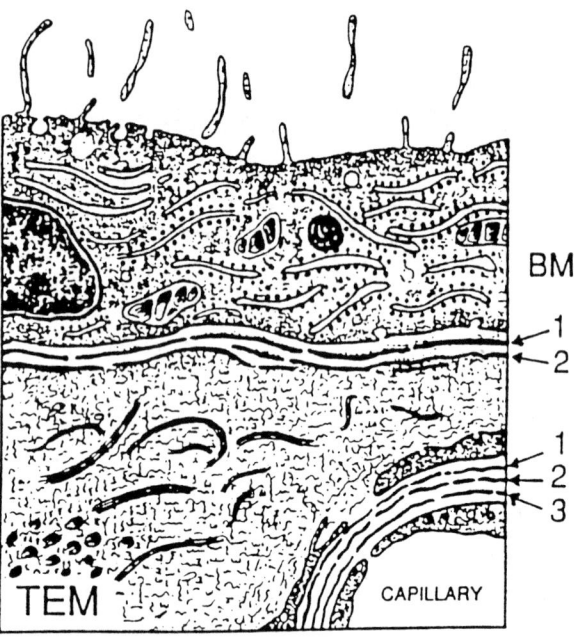

Figure 19. Diagrammatic representation of ultrastructural changes which may be encountered in biopsies of patients (diabetic and non-diabetic) after exposure to CAPD for many months (6–60). Reduplication of the mesothelial basement membrane may be seen, usually in patients with a history of frequent and/or severe peritonitis, independent of their diabetic status. Reduplication of the basement membrane in capillaries may also be encountered but is usually most pronounced in diabetic patients.

10.1. Non-enzymatic glycosylation of structural protein

The apparent association between incidence and severity of peritonitis and the diabetiform stromal pathology encountered in biopsies of non-diabetic patients who had been exposed to glucose-based dialysis offers significant clues as to the possible etiology. In CAPD during any dwell period there is a decay in glucose concentration through loss of glucose by diffusion across mesothelium to the peritoneal vascular bed. It is well recognized that during and for some time after peritonitis there may be a marked increase in peritoneal permeability to glucose. The loss of mesothelium observed in biopsies from such patients underscores the importance of its role as a barrier to rapid stromal ingress of glucose during normal circumstances. These findings are further supported by the fact that patients whose biopsies show failure to remesothelialize after peritonitis exhibit loss of ultrafiltration.

Thus in patients who have lost their mesothelium, naked stroma may be exposed to glucose concentrations 10–40 times greater than that found in normal serum.

In recent years considerable *in vitro* research into the non-enzymatic glycosylation of protein has established the etiologic importance of diabetic hyperglycemia in inducing pathological changes in basement membranes, matrix ground substance and long-lived collagen. It has been demonstrated that the process occurs as a direct chemical reaction between sugars and primary amino groups in the protein [29]. The reaction is initiated when glucose reacts with the e-amino group of the lysine residues in proteins. The condensation product, an aldosylamine, undergoes an Amadori rearrangement to form 1-deoxy-fructosyl adduct. Whereas these initial reactions are reversible, a series of further reactions of the Amadori products gives rise to advanced glycosylation end products (AGE) which are irreversible. AGE continue to accumulate indefinitely and are responsible for accelerated diabetic aging of mesenchymal structures. *In vitro* studies have shown that the rate of protein cross linkage was markedly dependent on glucose concentration in the range of 5–25 mmol/L which represents the range of blood glucose concentration from normoglycemia to severe diabetic hyperglycemia. Moreover, it has been demonstrated that glycosylated proteins continue to generate polymeric products 2–3 weeks after removal of free glucose from the reactants [30].

It is therefore not surprising that there would appear to be an association between diabetiform stromal pathology and peritonitis, a situation where the stroma is exposed to glucose concentrations 10 times greater than that experienced in the most severe episodes of diabetic hyperglycemia [10]. This concept of pathogenesis is strongly supported by the observation that non-diabetic patients without history of peritonitis may show no stromal pathology. If this were not so, and mesothelium did not protect stromal mesenchyme and vessels from hyperglycemia, then CAPD would not now be with us as an established long-term therapeutic option as all patients presumably would develop 'peritoneal diabetes' [9]. The probable verity of such a pathogenetic mechanism as explanation for the diabetiform lesions is also strongly supported by the histological findings in biopsies from patients who have sustained long periods of mesothelial denudation [9]. Here the advanced degenerative changes in the stroma typified by acellular hyalinized collagen are precisely the findings one might predict if naked stroma was immersed in a 214 mmolar solution of glucose for 2–3 months.

11. Peritoneal fibrosing syndromes in peritoneal dialysis

In safeguarding the motility of hollow viscera evolution has endowed the peritoneum with a remarkable ability to heal by total resolution any inflammatory exudate, on most occasions leaving the cavity in its pristine pre-morbid condition [31]. Even chronic inflammation may resolve with minimal local residual damage. Such is the vital nature of maintaining a mobile alimentary tube that in man and animals, diffuse or widespread chronic peritoneal inflammation resulting in a global fibrous dysplasia is a most unusual and uncharacteristic peritoneal reaction. Until recently, diffuse obliteration of the peritoneal cavity by fibrosis was only encountered in specific conditions such as tuberculosis, talc granulomata, and practolol peritonitis. Whereas for the last century surgeons have confronted the problem of highly localised fibrous adhesions, the development of continuous ambulatory peritoneal dialysis (CAPD) has been associated with the appearance of a new form of iatrogenic fibrosis which is remarkable both for the aggressiveness of its fibroneogenesis and the global nature of its peritoneal involvement [26].

12. Macroscopic appearance and histopathology of peritoneal fibrosis

In both degree and distribution, CAPD-associated fibrosis of the peritoneum covers a wide spectrum, from simple opacification of the normally transparent serosa, through to the formation of new fibrous sheaths and plaques. Based on examination of biopsies collected by the Peritoneal Biopsy Registry, a categorization of the histological appearances has been made of fibrosing syndromes (Fig. 20) [26].

12.1. Peritoneal opacification

Most surgeons with any experience of observing the peritoneum in patients treated by CAPD describe a diffuse opacification as the hallmark of this therapy. Those with extensive experience in examining the peritoneum of CAPD patients speak of local accentuation of this phenomenon, particularly in relation to the distal end of the catheter, the pelvis and paracolic gutters [26].

As far as I am aware, no designed studies have been carried out in order to correlate degree of opacification with microscopic appearances. The only information on this score which may be relevant is our observation that the immediate submesothelial tissue in CAPD patients can exhibit disorganisation of the normally oriented collagen fibers and expansion of the matrix ground substance [8]. Additional ultrastructural findings peculiar to patients on CAPD which may also contribute to the opacification process, is the pheonomenon of mesothelial basement membrane thickening and reduplication [9, 10, 26].

12.2. "Tanned" peritoneum syndrome

Experience accumulated over the last fourteen years in the International Peritoneal Biopsy Registry, has culminated in the recognition of a phenomenon known as a "tanned" peritoneum [26]. At operation in this condition, CAPD patients are found to have a peritoneum (both visceral and parietal) which is dry, wrinkled and light brown in color. The peritoneum thus exhibits a thickened leathery appearance implying as it were, that the membrane has been "tanned" in situ. In our experience this syndrome is most often encountered in patients maintained on CAPD for a considerable number of years. Biopsies obtained from patients with these macroscopic appearances on light microscopy show that the outer portion of the peritoneum has been replaced by an acellular rind of hyalinized collagen (the cellular desert) (Figs. 18, 21) [9, 26]. The mesothelium is absent. A sparse infiltrate of mononuclear cells may be found in the underlying tissues. Sclerotic changes in the stromal vessels are usually prominent. Scanning electron microscopy of the surface shows collagen fibers, fibrin, the occasional erythrocyte and cellular debris. Transmission electron microscopy reveals occasional surface flecks of fibrin and degenerate collagen fibers.

12.3. Mural fibrosis

Following the formation of the condensed superficial layer of hyalinized fibrous tissue produced by tanning of the peritoneum, an aggressive process of fibrosis may subsequently develop in the underlying serosa (Fig. 20) [26]. Capped by the impervious layer of altered collagen, the hyperplastic fibrous tissue is constrained and deflected inwards to invade the outer longitudinal muscle layer which

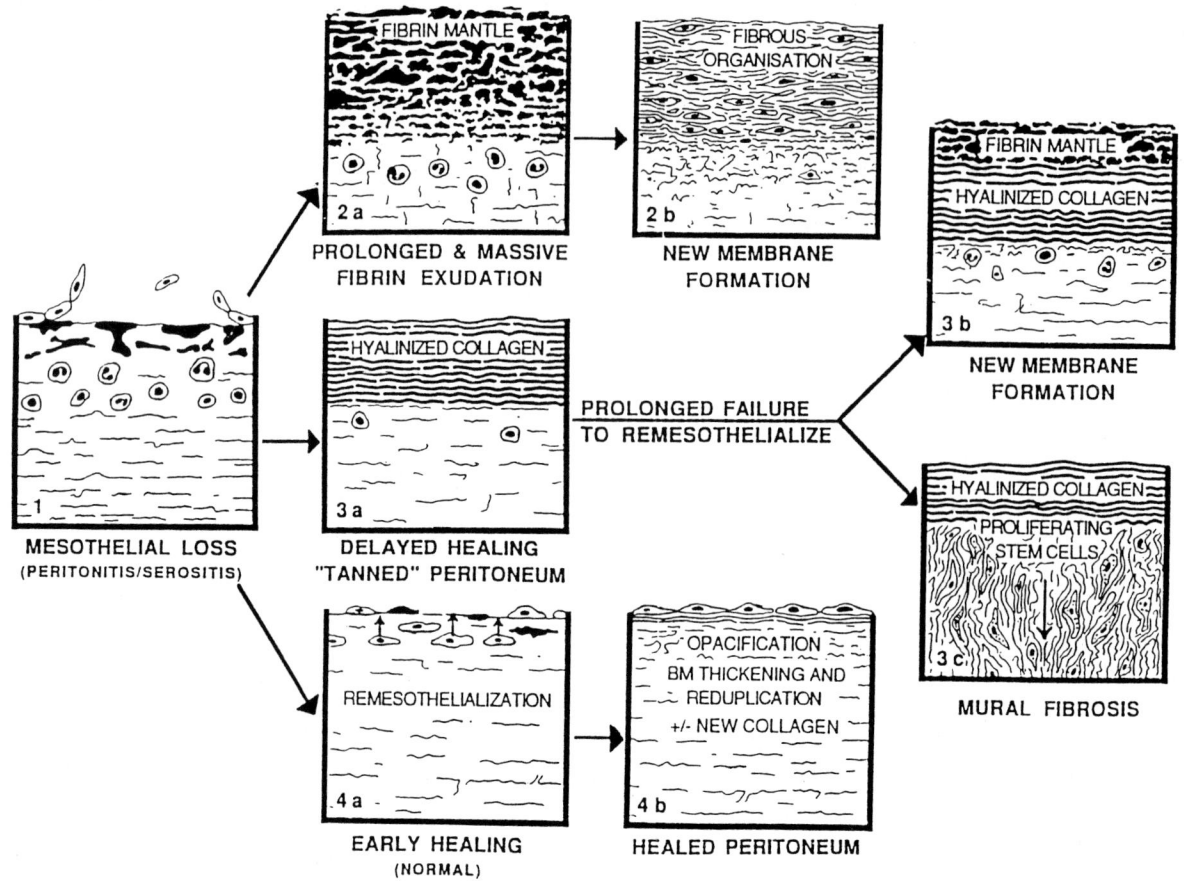

Figure 20. Flow diagram of possible sequelae to peritonitis in which there is mesothelial loss followed by either early or delayed resolution. In early healing (4a and 4b) with prompt remesothelialization, residual damage may be minimal and the only evidence of the event can be detected in some patients as opacification, basement membrane (BM) changes, and minimal new collagen formation. Delayed healing is characterized by a "tanned" peritoneum, manifesting as a superficial band of hyalinized collagen (3a). This may proceed to fibrin mantle superimposition and eventually to new membrane formation (3b) or to exuberant underlying fibroneogenesis with invasion of bowel wall (3c). Prolonged or massive fibrin exudation (2a) can lead *ab initio* to new membrane formation (2b). Based on histological interpretation of peritoneal biopsies (random and serial).

may be obliterated along with the myenteric plexus. Thus our histological assessment of the rare cases of this syndrome collected by the International Peritoneal Biopsy Registry strongly favors the interpretation that mural fibrosis represents a pathological progression of the tanned peritoneum syndrome. Macroscopically the peritoneum presents similar appearances to that found in tanned peritoneum, but the bowel is stiffened and apparently thickened. Although the patient presents with symptoms of bowel obstruction at operation, adhesions may be conspicuously absent, and in the pure syndrome an encapsulating membrane is never found. Histological examination reveals that there is no true thickening of the peritoneum and that the stiffness is due to fibrotic replacement of the outer bowel wall. This entity was first described clinically and histologically in association with peritoneal dialysis by Hauglustaine *et al.* [32, 33].

12.4. *Sclerosing encapsulating peritonitis (SEP)*

This is the most frequently used and familiar term applied to the process of peritoneal fibrosis found in association with peritoneal dialysis [31, 34–41]. Unfortunately SEP is used indiscriminately in the literature for any form of intra-abdominal pathology which apparently thickens the peritoneum. "Sclerosing" implies progressive formation of dense collagenous tissue. "Encapsulating" refers to the cocooning of the small bowel by a sheath of new fibrous tissue, while "peritonitis" acknowledges the histological reality that this new tissue is invariably permeated by a mononuclear inflammatory infiltrate. SEP is the end-stage of an intra-abdominal

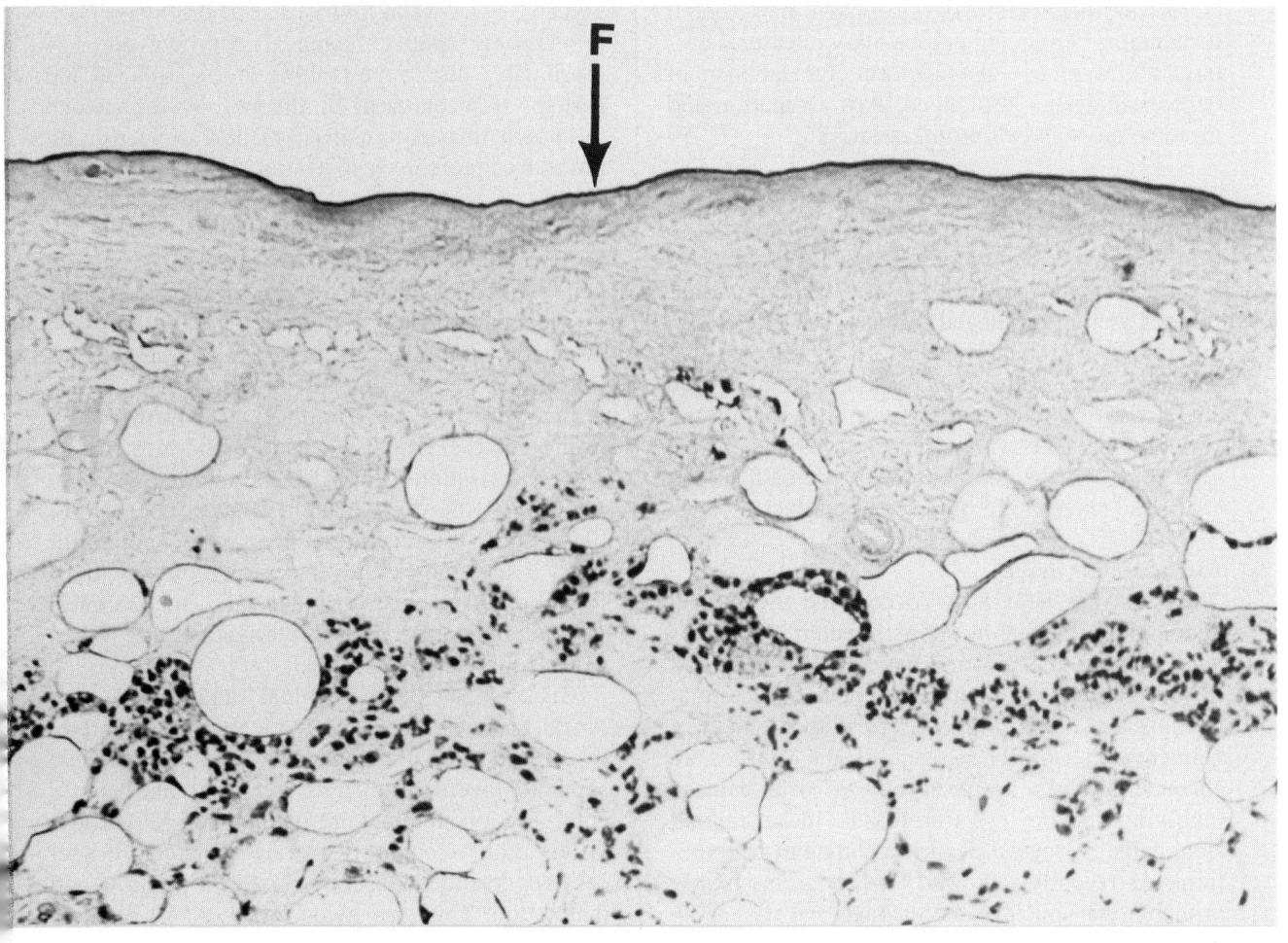

Figure 21. Biopsy of parietal peritoneum of patient who had been on CAPD for 137 months and who developed generalised small bowel obstruction. At operation the parietal and visceral peritoneum was dry and wrinkled and uniformly light brown in color. There were few adhesions. Histological examination of biopsies of both visceral and parietal peritoneum showed the characteristic appearances of "tanned peritoneum". Mesothelium was extensively missing. The surface was covered in places with a thin layer of fibrin apparent in this photomicrograph as a thin black line (F). The superficial collagen was virtually acellular – the cellular desert. In the deeper layers, chronic inflammatory infiltrate was present. Stained by Lendrum's MSB trichrome. Magnification ×400.

inflammatory process resulting in the formation of sheets of new fibrous tissue which cover, bind and constrict the viscera, thereby compromising the motility of the bowel [26, 31]. At operation or autopsy the principle finding is a thickened, leathery, fibro-connective sheath of marbled appearance which envelopes the small intestine [34–41]. Although the bulk of the encapsulating sheath lies anteriorly, septae dip between bowel loops to involve the mesentery. Plaques of variable size may affect stomach, spleen, liver, gall bladder and pelvic organs. Parietal involvement with or without adhesions to the visceral mass is not uncommon.

The histopathology of the sclerotic tissue from different cases invariably reveals dense fibrous tissue permeated with a chronic inflammatory infiltrate of variable density (Fig. 20). Special stains show either traces or widespread insudation of fibrin. Electron microscopy confirms at higher resolution the basic histological findings and shows that mesothelium is generally absent from the surface of the new fibrous tissue. When found, mesothelium is cuboidal rather than endothelioid in form [8].

13. Morphological insights into the pathogenesis of peritoneal fibrosis in CAPD

It is our considered opinion that the following constitute the key pathogenetic factors in dialysis-associated peritoneal fibrosis – extensive mesothelial denudation, continuing intracavitary release of bacterial toxins, glucose derangement of metabolism of peritoneal stroma, prolonged fibrin exudation and mesothelial stem cell proliferation [26].

13.1. *Failure of remesothelialization*

Following severe peritonitis there is ample evidence from serial and random biopsies that there may be a failure in the healing process whereby remesothelialization is delayed for many weeks or even months [9]. Although the factors involved in this process are not known with absolute certainty, the characteristic features of the histopathology strongly implicate two mechanisms, namely, hyperglycemic damage to the naked stroma [9] and continued exposure to organismal products.

13.2. *Cellular desert*

This term has been used to describe the typical histological findings in the peritoneum of patients where remesothelialization has failed to occur. At this stage the peritoneum is lined by acellular hyalinized collagen (Figs. 18, 21). Rather than there being evidence of fibroneogenesis, the biopsies are characterized by widespread cellular loss or damage involving leukocytes, fibroblasts, mesenchymal stem cells, pericytes, dendritic cells and endothelium. As recently reviewed [26], it seems highly probable that much of the damage and its persistence may be attributable to the effect of prolonged exposure to very high tissue levels of dextrose. If healing with remesothelialization occurs after such an episode, the effect of the glucose damage is permanently etched in the tissue in the form of thickening and reduplication of basement membranes, matrix and collagen abnormalities. It has been argued that this process entails a diabetiform mechanism involving non-enzymatic glycosylation of structural elements resulting in accelerated aging of long-lived collagen [9, 10]. The histological appearances of a scalded peritoneum without demonstrable pus-forming organisms are also compatible with unremitting exposure to bacterial exotoxins or even endotoxins, presumably derived from catheter biofilm or vegetations.

This histological appearance correlates with the "tanned" peritoneum where the cavity is lined by a rind of "tanned" collagen (Fig. 21). Macroscopically the surface is dry, wrinkled and brown in color. The dryness is presumably due to the loss of mesothelium and its secretory potential (phospholipid lubricant, prostacycline and glycosoaminoglycans). The wrinkling is due to the hyalinized, prematurely aged collagen. The brown color is presumably due to the tanning of the collagen and perhaps is accentuated by the yellow color which is known to occur in the Amadori condensation process of protein glycosylation.

13.3. *Fibrin exudation*

Fibrin continues to exude slowly from this deadened membrane, presumably at a rate which is balanced by clearance through daily dialysate washing and evacuation (Fig. 20). At this stage anything which disturbs the balance of fibrin exudation and removal in favor of fibrin accretion leads to a further stage in the process. In our experience and also that of others, cessation of CAPD is the most potent initiator of this further step. However it is most likely that slow accretion over many months or years is inevitable. With the formation of a stratified fibrin mantle on top of the hyalinized peritoneal stromal remnants, neovascularization and fibrogenesis inevitably ensue [26].

Histological, "archeological" analysis of peritoneal biopsies from these patients shows distinctive stratification of the thickened peritoneum where separate layers of different cellular and matrix configuration are piled one on the other [26]. These observations eloquently narrate a history of successive episodes of new mantle formation and maturation. Thus this evidence speaks of a quasi-geological process of continuing events where episodes of fibrin deposition are followed by periods of low fibrin exudation or rapid fibrin removal (Fig. 20). These findings correlate well with the known phenomenon of episodic rise and fall of fibrin content of dialysate effluent.

Clinical observations confirm pathological findings that the development of a thick fibrin exudate can occur rapidly and fibroneogenesis spreads throughout the recently formed fibrin mantle. In many instances this new tissue is pseudo-neoplastic, and in this respect is most probably analogous to the invasive pannus of rheumatoid arthritis which penetrates soft tissue, cartilage and bone [26].

The role of proliferating mesothelial stem cells in aggressive fibroneogenesis is now discussed in depth.

14. The pathogenesis of uncontrolled fibrous dysplasia of the peritoneum

At a certain stage following acute or chronic peritoneal injury, an aggressive fibroblastic reaction can occur. Evidence drawn from many sources now allows us to focus attention on the importance of uncontrolled proliferation of mesenchymal stem cells as a key factor in the production of excess fibroconnective tissue. Only recently has the mesenchymal stem cell responsible for regeneration of mesothelium been identified and investigated [11]. Its role in a variety of pathological conditions associated with peritoneal dialysis has been reviewed by Dobbie [9].

14.1. *Characterizing mesothelial stem cells*

Brunschwig and Robbins [42], who observed that repair of the peritoneal surface occurs simultaneously and rapidly over the whole of the denuded area, maintained that mesothelium arose from subjacent connective tissue cells which migrated to the surface and underwent metaplasia. Subsequent experimental studies by Raftery [43] strongly supported this concept of regeneration from mesenchymal stem cells and cast serious doubt on earlier theories of mesothelial reimplantation and macrophage transformation. Bolen *et al.* [11] in extending the experimental studies of Raftery, provided a much clearer understanding of mesothelial regeneration. Their investigations demonstrated a striking proliferation of stromal cells which the authors have designated subserosal multipotential cells, following the loss of surface mesothelium. Although these cells possess ultrastructural features of myofibroblasts, they also exhibit from an early stage the immunocytochemical markers of epithelia. Thus the active subserosal multipotential cells show peripherally arranged myofilaments, focal investment by basal lamina, abundant rough endoplasmic reticulum and occasional wavy 10 nm filaments. Immunocytochemical studies demonstrate the presence of low-molecular-weight, cytokeratins, co-expression of vimentin and absence of desmin. These cells are thus distinct from connective tissue myofibroblasts which show only vimentin. As the cells rise through the stroma to cover the denuded surface, they progressively acquire higher-molecular-weight, cytokeratins and lose vimentin. These findings derived from experimental studies are compatible with our ultrastructural observations in human peritoneal biopsies which show active remesothelialization [45].

14.2. *Proliferation of stem cells and fibrogenesis*

In investigating a case of idiopathic SEP, Lee [45] brought this new-found knowledge to bear on the pathogenesis of uncontrolled serosal fibrogenesis. Immunocytochemical staining of the fibroconnective tissue in this patient demonstrated reactivity for cytokeratin (AE 1/AE 3, Hybritech) and vimentin (Enzo Biochem). These findings therefore identified the proliferating spindle-shaped cells in the connective tissue as multipotential subserosal cells (mesothelial stem cells) and not fibroblasts as the cells responsible for the fibrous dysplasia in this case of SEP.

We have shown that mesothelial cells in culture have the same immunocytochemical markers as stem cells (co-expression of cytokeratins and vimentin) [46]. Renvall and his colleagues have also demonstrated that mesothelial cells in culture produce collagen and connective tissue matrix molecules [47–49]. Drawing together all of this information from these separate studies, it is therefore likely that Lee's contention that the multipotential subserosal stem cells immunocytochemically identified as the predominant cell in his case of sclerosing peritonitis, is indeed responsible for the overgrowth of fibroconnective tissue.

14.3. *Growth factors and the control of stem cells*

Regulatory growth factors for mesothelial cells in culture and stem cells *in vivo* were reviewed by Dobbie [10], where the proliferative response of mesothelium to transforming growth factor-β-1 (TGF-β-1) was highlighted. An important linkage in the pathological response of serosal tissues was recently furnished by the studies of Lafyatis *et al.* [50] who showed that synoviocytes in culture secrete TGF-β-1. They further observed in rheumatoid synovium that TGF-β-1 secretion may function as part of an autocrine (self-stimulating) system whereby it regulates synoviocyte phenotype, determining whether cell growth inhibition and collagenase secretion, or conversely cell growth promotion and collagen synthesis, results. They therefore suggested that this factor may be one of the important agents in promoting and sustaining the exuberant fibroblastic reaction seen in rheumatoid joints and tendons. That many factors may be involved in this process is further supported by the work of Melnyk *et al.* [51] who have shown that synoviocytes synthesize, bind and respond to basic fibroblast growth factor (βFGF). Also working with rheumatoid synovium they have shown that βFGF, a 146-amino acid protein of molecular weight of 16,000 appears to function in a similar autocrine loop in promoting hyperplasic invasive fibrous tissue.

14.4. Entrapment of mesothelial stem cells

Following the identification of the phenomenon of tanned peritoneum, there arose in our minds a concern that this dense acellular band of consolidated collagen might represent an insurmountable barrier to the upward migration of mesothelial stem cells which would be thus prevented from reaching the surface and effecting remesothelialization (Fig. 20) [26]. When eventually we had the opportunity to examine specimens of small bowel serosa from patients with mural fibrosis, we observed proliferating fibrous tissue lying beneath and presumably trapped by the zone of hyalinized collagen. A plausible explanation therefore for the pathogenesis of aggressive fibrogenesis in these cases is that the mesothelial stem cells, prevented from rising to the surface where attainment of polarity would induce maturity, continue to proliferate, lay down collagen and extend inwards (Fig. 20). It is possible that, trapped in this situation, they are continually subjected to uninhibited autocrine, paracrine or cytocrine stimulation. It follows that this process may suitably account for the existence of fibrous plaques in all serosal surfaces, e.g. as in the pleura and sugar icing on the spleen.

Thus a critical review of all of this diverse but related data on serosal tissue strongly implies that the development of excessive reactive peritoneal fibrosis most probably arises from the unrestrained stimulation of mesenchymal stem cells. It is probable that this stimulation is of an autocrine nature.

15. Durability of peritoneum on CAPD

In conclusion, experience gained over 15 years of examining peritoneal histology from normal controls, uremic individuals and CAPD patients leads us to believe that the peritoneum is a tough and resilient membrane. If this had not been so it is doubtful that peritoneal dialysis in general and CAPD in particular would have developed into the life-maintaining therapy which now sustains so many patients worldwide.

Evidence from the International Peritoneal Biopsy Registry supports the clinical impression that peritonitis due to *staphylococcus epidermidis* does not result in significant pathological sequelae, even in patients with multiple episodes. However, the greatest threat to the durability of the peritoneum as a dialysing membrane would appear to be from the effect of severe peritonitis which fails to resolve quickly and completely. As the cohort of patients who have been on CAPD for a long time span (10 years) increases in size, the International Peritoneal Biopsy Registry increasingly recognises the existence of a syndrome of a dry, brown (tanned) peritoneum, which is not associated with a history of frequent or severe peritonitis. Although there is strong indication that the histologically demonstrable changes in the peritoneal collagen in this condition are due to glycosylation, much work is required before the true case and nature of those changes are understood.

References

1. Von Recklinghausen F. Zur fettresorption. Virchows Arch. Path. Anat. 26: 172 (1863).
2. Dobbie JW, Zaki MA, Wilson LS. Ultrastructural studies on the peritoneum with special reference to chronic ambulatory dialysis. Scott Med J 1981; 26: 213–23.
3. Dobbie JW. Morpho-functional correlations in human mesothelium. In: La Greca G, Ronco C, Feriani M, Chiaramonte S, Conz P (eds), Peritoneal Dialysis. Proceedings of Fourth International Course on Peritoneal Dialysis, Vicenza, Italy 1991; pp 33–9.
4. Dobbie JW, Zaki MA. The ultrastructure of the parietal peritoneum in normal and uremic man and in patients on CAPD. In: Mahrer JF, Winchester JF (eds), Frontiers in Peritoneal Dialysis. Field, Rich & Associates, Inc., New York, 1986; pp 3–10.
5. Dobbie JW. Monitoring peritoneal histopathology in peritoneal dialysis: Dial Transplant 1989; 18: 319–35.
6. Dobbie JW. The peritoneal biopsy registory: A watchdog for peritoneal dialysis. Seminars in Dial 1992; 5: 20–3.
7. Dobbie JW. The morphology of the peritoneum. In: Khanna R, Nolph KD, Prowant B, Twardowski ZJ, Oreopoulos DG (eds), Advances in Continuous Ambulatory Peritoneal Dialysis. Peritoneal Dialysis Bulletin, Inc., Toronto, 1985; pp 3–6.
8. Dobbie JW. Morphology of the peritoneum in CAPD. Blood Purification 1989; 7: 74–85.
9. Dobbie JW, Lloyd JK, Gall CA. Categorization of ultrastructural changes in peritoneal mesothelium, stroma and blood vessels in uremia and CAPD patients. In: Khanna R, Nolph KD, Prowant B (eds), Advances in Continuous Ambulatory Peritoneal Dialysis; University of Toronto Press, Toronto 1990; pp 3–12.

10. Dobbie JW. New concepts in molecular biology and ultrastructural pathology of the periotoneum: their significance for peritoneal dialysis. Am J Kid Dis 1990; 15: 97–109.
11. Bolen JW, Hammer SP, McNutt MA. Serosal tissue: Reactive tissue as a model for understanding mesotheliomas. Ultrastruct Path 1987; 11: 251–62.
12. Connell MD, Rheinwald JG. Regulation of the cytoskeleton in mesothelial cells. Reversible loss of keratin and increase in vimentin during rapid growth in culture. Cell 1983; 34: 245–53.
13. Dobbie JW, Pavlina T, Lloyd J et al. Phosphatidylcholine synthesis by peritoneal mesothelium: its implication for peritoneal dialysis. Am J Kid Dis 1988; 12: 31–6.
14. Dobbie JW. Ultrastructural similarities between mesothelium and type II pneumocytes and their relevance to phospholipid surfactant production by the peritoneum. In: Khanna R, Nolph KD, Prowant B (eds), Advances in Continuous Ambulatory Peritoneal Dialysis. University of Toronto Press, Toronto 1988, pp 32–41.
15. Stratton CJ. Multi-lamellar body formation in mammalian lung: An ultrastructural study utilising three lipid-retention procedures. J Ultrastruct Res 1975; 52: 309–20.
16. Futaesaki Y, Mizukira, Nakamura H. A new fixation method using tannic acid for electron microscopy and some observations of biological specimens. J Histochem Cytochem 1972; 4: 155–7.
17. Kalina M, Pease DC. The preservation of ultrastructure in saturated phosphatidylcholine by tannic acid in model systems and Type II pneumocytes. J Cell Biol 1977; 74: 726–41.
18. Dobbie JW, Lloyd JK. Meothelium secretes lamellar bodies in a similar manner to Type II pneumocyte secretion of surfactant. Perit Dial Int 1989; 9: 215–9.
19. Dobbie JW. From philosopher to fish: The comparative anatomy of the peritoneal cavity as an excretory organ and its significance for peritoneal dialysis in man. Perit Dial Int. 1988; 8: 3–6.
20. George CJ, Ellis AE, Bruno DW. On the remembrance of the abdominal pores in rainbow trout Salmo gairdneri Richardson, and other salmonid spp. J Fish Biol 1982; 21: 643–7.
21. Rutsky EA, Rostand SG. Treatment of uremic pericarditis and pericardial effusion. Am J Kid Dis 1987; 10: 2–8.
22. Maher JF. Uremic pleurities. Am J Kid Dis 1987; 10: 19–22.
23. Gluck Z, Nolph KD. Ascites associated with End-Stage Renal Disease. Am J Kid Dis 1987; 10: 9–18.
24. Bright R. Tabular view of the morbid appearances in 100 cases connected with albuminous urine: With observations. Guys Hosp Rep 1836; 1: 380–400.
25. Dobbie JW, Henderson I, Wilson LS. New evidence on the pathogenesis of sclerosing encapsulating peritonitis (SEP) obtained from serial biopsies. In: Khanna R, Nolph KD, Prowant B et al. (eds), Advances in Continuous Ambulatory Peritoneal Dialysis. Peritoneal Dialysis Bulletin, Inc, Toronto 1987; pp 138–49.
26. Dobbie JW. Pathogenesis of peritoneal fibrosing syndromes (sclerosing peritonitis) in peritoneal dialysis. Perit Dial Int 1992; 12: 14–27.
27. Gotloib L, Bar Sella P, Shostak A. Reduplicated basal lamina of small venules and mesothelium of human parietal peritoneum: Ultrastructural changes of reduplicated peritoneal basal membrane. Perit Dial Bull 1985; 5: 212–5.
28. Di Paolo N, Sacchi G. Peritoneal vascular changes in continuous ambulatory peritoneal dialysis: An in vivo model for the study of diabetic microangiopathy. Perit Dial Int 1989; 9: 41–5.
29. Eble AS, Thorpe SR, Baynes JW. Non-enzymatic glycosylation and glucose dependent cross-linking of protein. J Biol Chem 1983; 258: 9406–12.
30. Vlassara H, Brownlee M, Cerami A. High affinity receptor mediated uptake and degradation of glucose-modified proteins: A potential mechanism for the removal of senescent macromolecules. Proc Natl Acad Sci USA 1958; 82: 5588–92.
31. Dobbie JW. Pathology of the peritoneum. In: Bengmark S (ed), The peritoneum and peritoneal access. Wright, London 1989; pp 42–52.
32. Hauglustaine D, Monballyu J, van Meerbeek J et al. Report of sclerotic alterations of the peritoneum in patients on CAPD. Lancet 1983: 734.
33. Hauglustaine D, van Meerbeek J, Montballyu J et al. Sclerosing peritonitis with mural bowel fibrosis in a patient on long-term CAPD. Clin Nephrol 1984; 22: 158–62.
34. Gandhi VC, Humayan HM, Ing TS et al. Sclerotic thickening of the peritoneal membrane in maintenance peritoneal dialysis patients. Arch Intern Med 1980; 140: 1201–3.
35. Slingeneyer A, Mion C, Mourad G et al. Progressive sclerosing peritonitis: A late and severe complication of maintenance peritoneal dialysis. Trans Am Soc Artif Intern Organs 1983; 29: 633–8.
36. Ing TS, Daugirdas JT, Gandhi VC, Leehey DJ. Sclerosing peritonitis after peritoneal dialysis. Lancet 1983; 2: 1080.
37. Ing TS, Daugirdas JT, Gandhi VC. Peritoneal sclerosis in peritoneal dialysis patients. Am J Nephrol 1984; 4: 173–6.
38. Mion C, Slingeneyer A. Sclerosing peritonitis. What is it? Perit Dial – Proc 2nd Internat Course. Proc 1986: 215–22.
39. Novello AC, Port KF. Sclerosing encapsulating peritonitis. Intern J Artif Organs 1986; 9(6): 393–6.
40. Pusateri R, Ross r, Marshall R, et al. Sclerosing encapsulating peritonitis: Report of a case with small bowel obstruction managed by a long term home parenteral hyperalimentation, and a review of literature. Am J Kidney Dis 1986; 13(1): 56–60.
41. Korzets A, Korsets Z, Peer G et al. Sclerosing peritonitis – possible early diagnosis by computerized tomography of the abdomen. Am J Nephrol 1988; 8: 143–6.
42. Brunschwig A, Robbins GF. Regeneration of peritoneum: experimental observations and clinical experience in radical resections of intra-abdominal cancer. Fifteenth Cong Soc Int Chir Lisbonne, 1953, Bruxelles, Hennde Smedt, 1954; pp 756–65.

43. Raftery AT. Regeneration of parietal and visceral peritoneum: an electron microscopical study. J Anat 1973; 115: 375–92.
44. Dobbie JW, Henderson I, Wilson L. New evidence on the pathogenesis of sclerosing encapsulating peritonitis (SEP) obtained from serial biopsies. In: Khanna R, Nolph KD, Porwant B et al. (eds), Advances in continuous ambulatory peritoneal dialysis. Peritoneal Dialysis Bulletin Inc, Toronto 1987; 3: 138–49.
45. Lee RG. Scelrosing peritonitis. Dig Dis Sci 1989; 34: 1473–6.
46. Hjelle JT, Golinska BT, Waters DC et al. Isolation and propagation in vitro of peritoneal mesothelial cells. Perit Dial Inter 1989; 9: 341–7.
47. Renvall S. Peritoneal metabolism and intra-abdominal adhesion formation during experimental peritonitis. Thesis. Acta Chir Scand (suppl) 1980: 503.
48. Aalto M, Kulonen E, Penttinen R, Renvall S. Collagen synthesis in cultured mesothelial cells. Acta Chir Scand 1981; 147: 1–?.
49. Renvall S, Lehto M, Penttinen R. Development of peritoneal fribrosis occurs under the mesothelial layer. J Surg Res 1987; 43: 407–12.
50. Lafyatis R, Thompson NL, Remmers EF et al. Transforming growth factor-B production by synovial tissues from rheumatoid patients and streptococcal cell wall arthritic rats. J Immunol 1989; 143: 1142–8.
51. Melnyk VO, Shipley GD, Sternfeld MD et al. Synoviocytes synthesize, bind and respond to basic fibroblast growth factor. Arth Rheum 1990; 33: 493–500.

3 The peritoneal microcirculation in peritoneal dialysis

RANDALL WHITE, RONALD KORTHUIS AND D. NEIL GRANGER

1. Introduction 45
2. Anatomy of the peritoneum and the peritoneal microcirculation 45
　2.1. Definition and structure of the visceral and parietal peritoneum 45
　2.2. Blood supply to the peritoneum 46
　2.3. Peritoneal microvascular network 46
　2.4. Peritoneal microvascular ultrastructure 47
3. Physiologic modulation of the peritoneal microcirculation 50
　3.1. The peritoneal microvasculature in transport model 51
　3.2. Blood flow in relation to peritoneal dialysis 52
　3.3 The effects of vasoactive agents on the peritoneal microcirculation 54
　3.4. The effects of peritoneal dialysis on the peritoneal microcirculation 56
4. The peritoneal microcirculation in inflammation 58
　4.1. General principles of leukocyte-endothelial interactions 58
　4.2. Inflammatory mediators and the microcirculation 60
　4.3. The inflammatory process in peritoneal dialysis 62
5. Summary 62
References 63

1. Introduction

The peritoneal microcirculation provides the framework for the physiological interactions between the systemic vasculature and the peritoneal cavity. In peritoneal dialysis, these dynamic interactions are of paramount importance in maintaining effective dialysis. The peritoneal microcirculation participates in numerous physiologic functions including solute transfer and exchange, regulation of fluid dynamics and ultrafiltration, delivery of nutrients and hormones, delivery of leukocytes to areas of inflammation, gas exchange, and distribution of drugs. Knowledge of the dynamics of the peritoneal microcirculation in relation to peritoneal dialysis provides a basis for the rational use of drugs and other manipulations to increase the efficiency of peritoneal dialysis. In addition, studies of the peritoneal microcirculation provide investigators a unique window through which many basic microcirculatory processes may be explored. The focus of this chapter will be to review the available information regarding peritoneal microcirculatory function in relation to peritoneal dialysis by examining the following areas: (1) the functional anatomy of the peritoneal microcirculation, (2) the physiologic factors modifying the peritoneal microcirculation and (3) the role of the peritoneal microcirculation in inflammation.

2. Anatomy of the peritoneum and the peritoneal microcirculation

2.1. Definition and structure of the visceral and parietal peritoneum

The peritoneum is a large, intricately arranged serous membrane which lines the abdominal wall (parietal peritoneum) and visceral organs of the abdominal cavity (visceral peritoneum). The peritoneal cavity is the potential space between the parietal and visceral layers of the peritoneum [1]. The peritoneal cavity is lined by a layer of mesothelial cells encasing tissue perfused with circulatory and lymphatic vessels [2]. Normally, the peritoneal cavity contains less than 100 ml of fluid but can accommodate a 20 fold increase without patient discomfort [3]. Specialized regions, the omenta and mesenteries, are double-layer folds of peritoneum which connect certain viscera to the posterior abdominal wall or to each other. For example, the greater omentum extends from the greater curvature of the stomach to attach to the inferior border of the transverse colon. Specific double-layered peritoneal folds attach solid viscera to the abdominal wall (e.g. the falciform ligament of the liver). Lying between the liver and diaphragm is the subphrenic space which is bound by two layers of peritoneum. This area is of particular importance in view of the generous and specialized lymphatic drainage associated with the undersurface of the diaphragm [4].

The total surface area of the peritoneum in adults approximates the surface area of the skin (1–2 m^2) [5]. However, the effective surface area of the peritoneal membrane is probably well below 1m^2 and may be further reduced as a result of adhesion formation secondary to infections or prior abdominal surgery [6, 7]. The visceral peritoneum accounts for approximately 90% of the total peritoneal membrane surface area, while the parietal peritoneum accounts for only 10% [8]. Considering that the majority of the surface area is composed of visceral peritoneum, one might intuitively suspect that the contribution of the visceral peritoneum to total peritoneal membrane exchange would predominate over that contribution made by the parietal peritoneum. However, eviscerated rats exhibit only slight reductions in peritoneal absorption rates for urea, creatinine, glucose and inulin relative to control animals. In other studies using a similar evisceration model, the parietal peritoneum accounts for 56–59% of ultrafiltration and absorbs 75–77% of intraperitoneally instilled glucose [9]. These results suggest that the contribution of the visceral peritoneum to peritoneal exchange is much less than would be predicted from the relative surface area of the parietal and visceral peritoneum (10% vs. 90% of the total peritoneal membrane area). However, this interpretation is complicated by the possibility that evisceration results in improved contact between the dialysate and the remaining peritoneal membrane [10]. Nevertheless, the aforementioned studies in eviscerated rats strongly indicate that the relative contribution of the visceral and parietal peritoneum in peritoneal dialysis may not necessarily correlate to the anatomic surface area.

2.2. Blood supply to the peritoneum

The vascular and lymphatic systems supplying the peritoneal membrane and intraperitoneal organs constitute a complex and efficient system for fluid and solute exchange in the peritoneal cavity. This exchange system is composed of three separate but interdependent components: (1) the blood circulation to the visceral peritoneum, (2) the blood circulation to the parietal peritoneum, and (3) the lymphatic circulation of the parietal and visceral peritoneum. Physiologic, pharmacologic, and pathologic modifications of the transport properties of these components can dramatically influence the efficiency of peritoneal dialysis.

The arterial blood supply to the visceral peritoneum and intraperitoneal organs arises from the celiac, superior mesenteric and inferior mesenteric arteries. The arterial blood supply to the parietal peritoneum and underlying musculature arises from the circumflex, iliac, lumbar, intercostal, and epigastric arteries. The veins draining the visceral peritoneum and intraperitoneal organs empty into the portal vein, while the venous system of the parietal peritoneum empties into the systemic veins.

A potentially important consequence of this venous vascular arrangement is that drugs and other solutes which are absorbed primarily across the visceral peritoneum are subject to hepatic metabolism. For example, pharmacologic studies have shown intraperitoneal administration of compounds such as atropine, caffeine, glucose, glycine and progesterone are absorbed primarily by the visceral peritoneum and are subject to first pass metabolism by the liver [11]. In addition, the effects of some intraperitoneally administered vasoactive drugs may be modified by the liver through hepatic metabolism [12].

2.3. Peritoneal microvascular network

The large vessels supplying the peritoneal cavity function primarily as conduits to supply blood to the visceral organs. As the large vessels course through the mesentery they divide and reflect over the bowel surface forming capillary beds which presumably can participate in transperitoneal fluid and solute exchange [3]. Nearly fifty years ago, Chambers and Zweifach described the topography of the mesenteric circulation [13]. The typical mesenteric microcirculatory network is composed of arterioles, terminal arterioles, precapillary sphincters, arterio-venous anastomoses, thoroughfare channels, capillaries and venules (Fig. 1) [14]. Blood flows into the capillary system through arterioles and exits through venules. Arterioles and thoroughfare channels modulate blood flow into the network, while precapillary sphincters regulate blood flow to single capillaries. Arterio-venous anastomoses can divert blood flow from arterioles directly into venules, thereby bypassing the capillary networks. The flow through a capillary network can be extremely variable with individual capillary flow starting, stopping, and sometimes reversing direction [15, 16].

The architecture of the peritoneal microvascula-

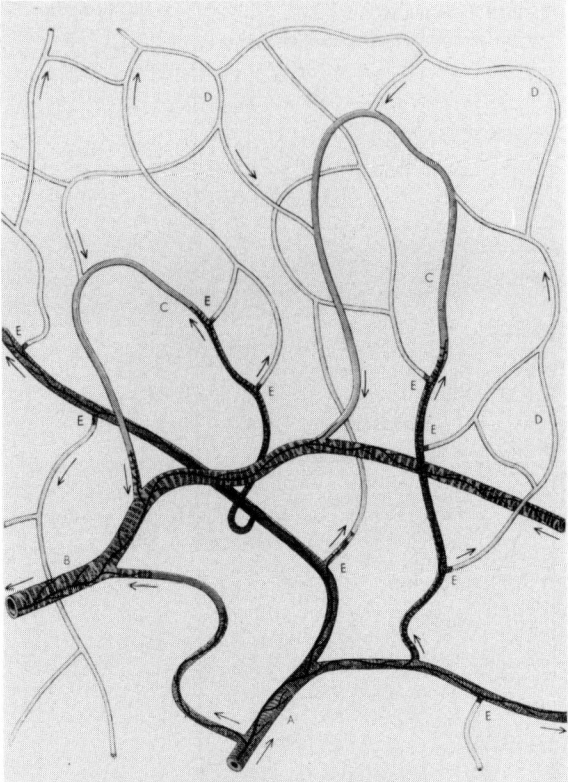

Figure 1. Structural elements of a typical mesenteric microcirculatory bed. A = arteriole, B = venule, C = thoroughfare channel, D = capillary, E = precapillary sphincter, (B W Zweifach: The microcirculation of the blood. Scientific American January: 54–60, 1959). © 1959 by Scientific American, Inc. All rights reserved.

ture has been previously reviewed by Miller [17]. In general, the microvascular architecture of the parietal peritoneum may be represented by that supplying the cremaster muscle, as this muscle extends from the abdominal wall musculature [17]. The visceral microvasculature may be directly visualized on the mesenteric surface in such areas as the cecum. Features of the cremasteric microvasculature include the absence of short artery to vein anastomoses and the formation of arteriolar and venular arcades from which capillaries may arise [17–19]. In the visceral mesentery, abundant arterial and venular arcades are present which may function to equalize flow and ensure perfusion during bowel compression [17].

The hemodynamic pressure profiles of the microvasculature are illustrated in Fig. 2. Under normal conditions, the microvasculature appears to be in a slightly vasoconstricted state. Since the greatest slope for microvascular pressure change occurs in the arterioles 8 to 40 µm in diameter, these vessels account for the bulk of the vascular resistance exhibited by the mesenteric circulation. Figure 2 also illustrates the pressure changes associated with vasoconstriction and vasodilation and the typical microvessel size gradations for arterioles, capillaries and venules [20].

2.4. Peritoneal microvascular ultrastructure

Terminal arterioles may participate in the exchange process since they have a discontinuous muscle layer. As a consequence, portions of these vessels are lined only by endothelium and basement membrane. However, the relative contribution to overall peritoneal transport is minimal since the surface area and permeability of these vessels are much less than in the capillaries and postcapillary venules. Peritoneal solute transfer occurs primarily across capillaries and postcapillary venules [21, 22]. There are three types of capillary endothelium present in the peritoneum: (1) continuous endothelium as in the mesenteric vessels, (2) fenestrated endothelium as in the intestinal villi and (3) discontinuous endothelium as found in the liver sinusoids [17]. Since mesenteric capillaries represent the dominant vessel involved in peritoneal exchange, emphasis will be placed on the mesenteric capillary.

Structurally, the endothelial cells which line the continuous capillary are joined by tight junctions. Cytoplasmic vesicles may exist in the capillary which can function to transport solutes. These vesicles may fuse and form open channels through the endothelium [20]. The endothelial surface is lined by a glycocalyx which produces an electronegative surface charge along the luminal surface. This surface charge may act as a physiologic barrier for anionic proteins [23].

Permeability of the mesenteric microcirculation has been measured using estimates of the osmotic reflection coefficient (σ) for total protein. The osmotic reflection coefficient describes the degree of macromolecule selectivity exhibited by the microvascular barrier and determines the effectiveness of an oncotic pressure gradient across the capillary membrane for a particular solute. An osmotic reflection coefficient of zero would imply a freely permeable membrane, while an osmotic reflection coefficient of one would indicate that the solute is impermeable and would generate 100% of its potential osmotic pressure [24].

Studies of capillary osmotic reflection coefficients in the peritoneum indicate that the σ values

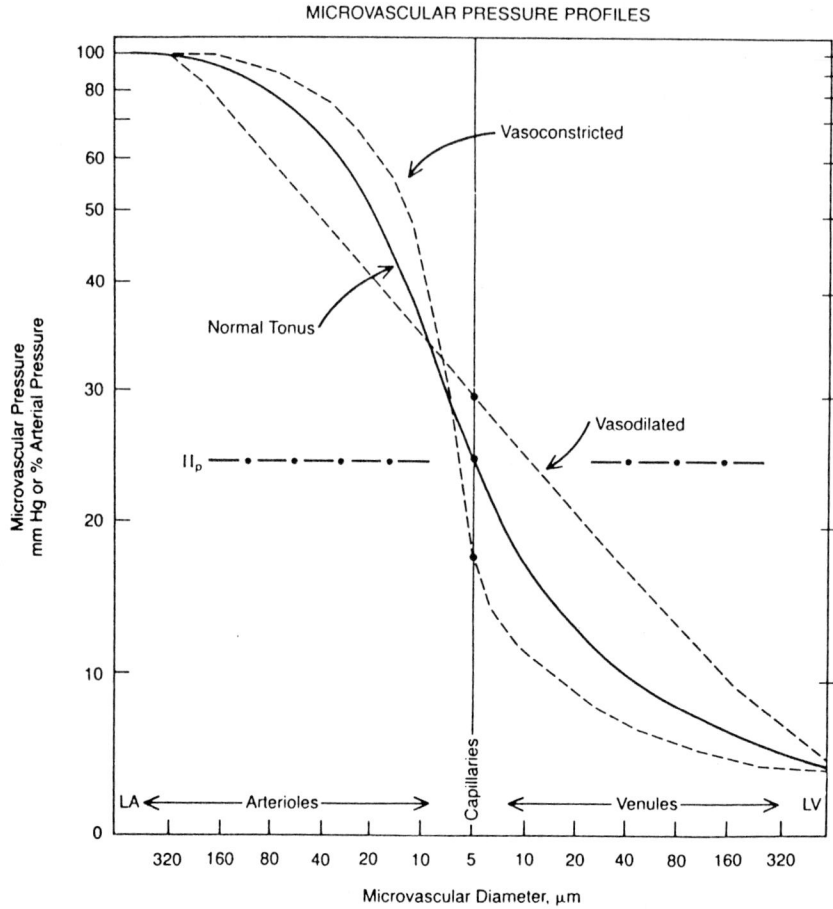

Figure 2. Microvascular pressure profiles as related to microvascular diameter. Normal vascular tone is in a state of partial vasoconstriction (solid line). The dotted lines represent changes in microvascular pressure which occur with vasoconstriction and vasodilation. (Renkin EM: Microcirculation and Exchange. In: Patton HD, Fuchs AF, Hille B, Scher AM, Steiner R (eds), Textbook of Physiology, Philadelphia, W. B. Saunders, pp 860–878, 1989).

of the peritoneal membrane are comparable to those reported for the continuous capillary beds of other organs [22, 24–27]. The reflection coefficients for sodium chloride (MW 58), urea (MW 61), sucrose (MW 342), raffinose (MW 504), and vitamin B_{12} (MW 1354) range between 0.02–0.20 in the frog mesentery and rabbit, cat, and human peritoneum [28–34]. The reflection coefficients for myoglobin (21Å radius), albumin (36Å radius), Dextran 118 (61Å radius) and Dextran 242 (90Å radius) are 0.35, 0.82, 0.99 and 1.00, respectively [31, 33]. These studies indicate that there is a strong correlation between σ and molecular size. Thus, the peritoneal capillary membrane is not freely permeable to solutes but is a highly selective barrier with restrictive properties similar to those reported for other continuous capillary beds.

The peritoneal capillary has the ability to regulate solute exchange in such a manner as to allow the transport of relatively small molecules such as urea while restricting the movement of macromolecules such as albumin. There appears to be a differential in permeability to solutes in the proximal portion of the capillary as compared to the distal end of the capillary. The proximal portion provides ultrafiltration with low solute permeability while the distal portion is more permeable to larger solutes. Indeed, intravital fluorescence microscopy of mesenteric capillaries have shown the rapid passage of small solutes with MW 389–3400 occurs along the entire length of most capillaries with a majority of the leakage occurring in the venous capillaries and venules. In addition, large molecular weight solutes such as dextrans (MW 19000) exhibit localized leakage in the venular end of the microcirculation [36]. These findings suggest that peritoneal capillaries contain populations of small and large 'pores' which allow solute transport.

Recently, Rippe and Stelin have proposed a three pore model of permselectivity which provides an ultrastructural framework to explain the restrictive properties and functional characteristics of the peritoneal capillaries. In this model there are three population of pores: (1) a large number of transcellular pores 4–5 Å radius, (2) a large number of small pores 40–50 Å radius, and (3) a small number of large pores 200–300 Å radius, as illustrated by Flessner in Fig. 3 [37–40]. This theory predicts that under conditions simulating peritoneal dialysis, approximately 40% of the total ultrafiltrate is obtained through the transcellular path and would therefore be solute free. The transcellular ultrafiltration would be primarily driven by osmotic pressure differentials from the large glucose gradient across the peritoneal membrane. Most of the small solutes would be transported through small pores by diffusion and convection, while relatively large proteins and macromolecules would be transported through large pores primarily under the influence of hydrostatic forces. Capillary hydrostatic pressures are in the range of 18 mm Hg, while interstitial hydrostatic pressures are in the range of 0.4 to 0.5 mm Hg [40, 41]. Thus, across large pores, where hydrostatic pressure is the predominant force, there appears to be a unidirectional convective force from the capillary to the interstitium. Large molecules such as proteins leave the capillaries under the influence of this hydrostatic force, and their return to the blood compartment would primarily be under the influence of the lymphatic system [40].

The exact anatomic structures which correlate with the different pores are not known with certainty [20]. The structural correlates of the small pores may be the intercellular junctions, while large pores may be represented by vesicles or chains of vesicles. In addition, there may exist subsets of large pores which are static and account for solute fluxes under normal physiological conditions and a subset of large pores which are normally quiescent but can react to certain stimuli such as inflammation resulting in increased permeability [23].

Another interesting concept to consider is whether or not individual pore populations may have differential responses to certain modulators of

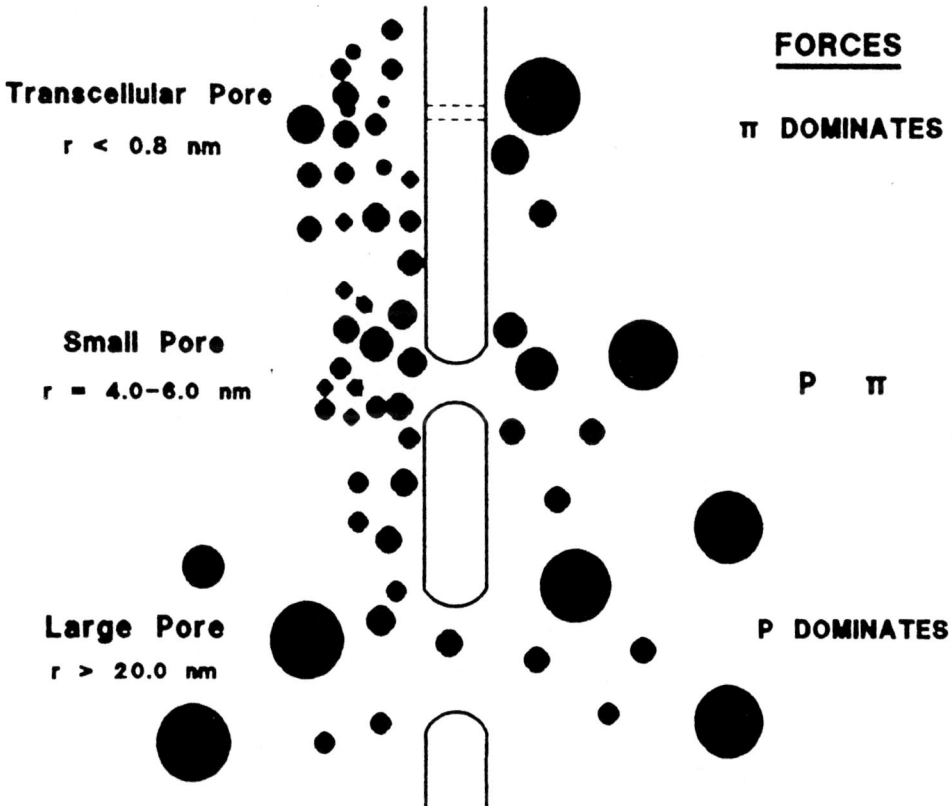

Figure 3. Hypothetical three-pore capillary membrane which illustrates the governing forces across each pore. The pore radius is given under each pore name. The forces are: P, hydrostatic pressure, Π, osmotic pressure. Large circles represent protein; small circles represent small solutes. (Flessner MF: Peritoneal Transport Physiology: Insights from basic research. © J Am Soc Nephrol 2:122–135, 1991).

permeability. For example, Harper *et al.* have shown that in intestinal capillaries, neurotension (a tridecapeptide present in intestinal mucosal N cells) can preferentially increase large pore size [42], while the predominant effect of hypoxia is to increase small pore radius [42a].

The basement membrane functions as a substratum which acts as a solid support to anchor cells and limits the domain of connective tissue, thus producing distinct cellular compartments [43]. With the exception of large molecules such as plasma proteins, the basement membrane appears to be freely permeable to most solutes [44–48]. This concept is supported by the fact that the restrictive properties of the intestinal capillaries to endogenous macromolecules are similar to the capillaries found in the mesentery, skin and skeletal muscle, despite the fact that numerous large fenestrations are present in the intestinal capillary endothelium [49]. It has also been shown that colloidal carbon penetrates the intercellular clefts of continuous capillaries after exposure to histamine, but the transport of the colloidal carbon into the interstitial space is impeded at the basement membrane [50, 51]. These observations suggest that the basement membrane or interstitial gel matrix constitute an important component of the barrier to the blood-to-lymph transport of macromolecules. In addition, the proteoglycans in the basement membrane and interstitial gel matrix create a strong electrostatic barrier that retards the movement of anionic solutes [52]. These findings suggest that although the basement membrane is permeable to small solutes, it may provide a significant transport barrier for macromolecules under conditions of endothelial contraction and/or injury.

In summary, peritoneal microvascular ultrastructure provides a framework to explain the restrictive properties and functional characteristics of microvascular transport. The ability of the microvascular wall to preferentially regulate solute exchange from the capillary to the interstitium is closely associated with these ultrastructural characteristics. Transport properties may be modeled by a three pore system of permselectivity based on solute size and the number and types of pores. The rate of filtration of fluids and solutes is governed by the differences in oncotic and hydrostatic pressures. Increases in permeability have been linked to preferential effects on small versus large pore populations. Finally, the basement membrane appears to be freely permeable to small solutes but restricts the transport of macromolecules.

3. Physiologic modulation of the peritoneal microcirculation

Transport across the microvascular wall is the initial process involved in solute and fluid exchange from the systemic vasculature to the peritoneal cavity. In the above section, structural properties of the microcirculation were described and related to its functional characteristics. In this section, the emphasis will be focused on the physiologic principles involved in the manipulation of the microcirculation during peritoneal dialysis. At the microcirculatory level, the physiologic variables which may affect transport and peritoneal dialysis efficiency include changes in:

1. peritoneal capillary blood flow,
2. microvascular permeability,
3. capillary surface area (perfused capillary density);
4. capillary hydrostatic pressure;
5. ultrafiltration.

These variables may be affected by drugs, peritoneal dialysis fluid, hormones, neurotransmitters, ions, local metabolic demands, certain pathophysiologic processes (e.g., vasculitis), inflammation, and procedural variables involved in peritoneal dialysis.

The concept of clearance provides a useful index to assess efficiency of peritoneal dialysis. Clearance represents the volume of plasma cleared of a substance per unit time. It is a measure of the rate at which solutes move from the blood to the peritoneal cavity. The peritoneal clearance may be calculated by the following equations:

$$C(\text{ml/min}) = (D_i/P_i) \times (V_D/T)$$

C : Clearance
D_i : Dialysate solute concentration
P_i : Plasma solute concentration
V_D : Drainage volume
T : Time of exchange

Many of the physiologic effects of certain substances in peritoneal dialysis are related to alterations in clearance. As will be seen, numerous vasoactive substances can alter clearance through changes in blood flow, in capillary permeability and microvascular surface area.

3.1. The peritoneal microvasculature in transport model

Although a detailed description of peritoneal transport processes will be provided in chapter 4, the role of the peritoneal micro-vasculature in transport models will be described to emphasize the critical importance of the microcirculation in peritoneal solute exchange and fluid movement. The transport of solutes and water from the capillary lumen to the peritoneal cavity occurs across several physiologic and anatomic barriers, summarized by Nolph et al. [53]. These barriers include (Fig. 4):

R_1: a stagnant fluid layer within the peritoneal capillary,
R_2: the capillary endothelium,
R_3: the capillary basement membrane,
R_4: the interstitium,
R_5: the mesothelium,
R_6: the stagnant fluid films within the peritoneal cavity.

According to this model, three of the major resistance barriers reside at the level of the capillary wall (i.e., $R_1 - R_3$). The capillary endothelium, (R_2), appears to be the most important area of resistance for larger solutes. Vasoactive agents appear to alter R_2 primarily by modulating perfused capillary density and permeability. R_1, which is the resistance attributable to a stagnant fluid layer within the peritoneal capillary, is thought to have minor effects with high capillary flow rates [53]. The characteristics of the capillary basement membrane, R_3, were described in the previous section. Factors that may alter peritoneal resistance to solute movement in this model are summarized in Table 1. This conceptualization provides an important visual model of the transport process, and facilitates understanding how modifications of microcirculatory transport resistance properties may affect clearance and peritoneal dialysis efficiency.

Flessner et al. have developed a mathematical description of peritoneal transport. According to this model, capillaries are uniformly distributed in the tissue space surrounding the peritoneal cavity but are separated by varying distances from the dialysate (Fig. 5). Transacapillary transport of solutes are described in terms of tissue diffusion, convection, capillary membrane transport and lymphatic transport [54–56]. This model allows for the prediction of solute concentration gradients within the tissue space in relation to the peritoneal capillary. It emphasizes that solute concentration profiles allow for a quantitative measure of the depth of tissue involved in transport and for the

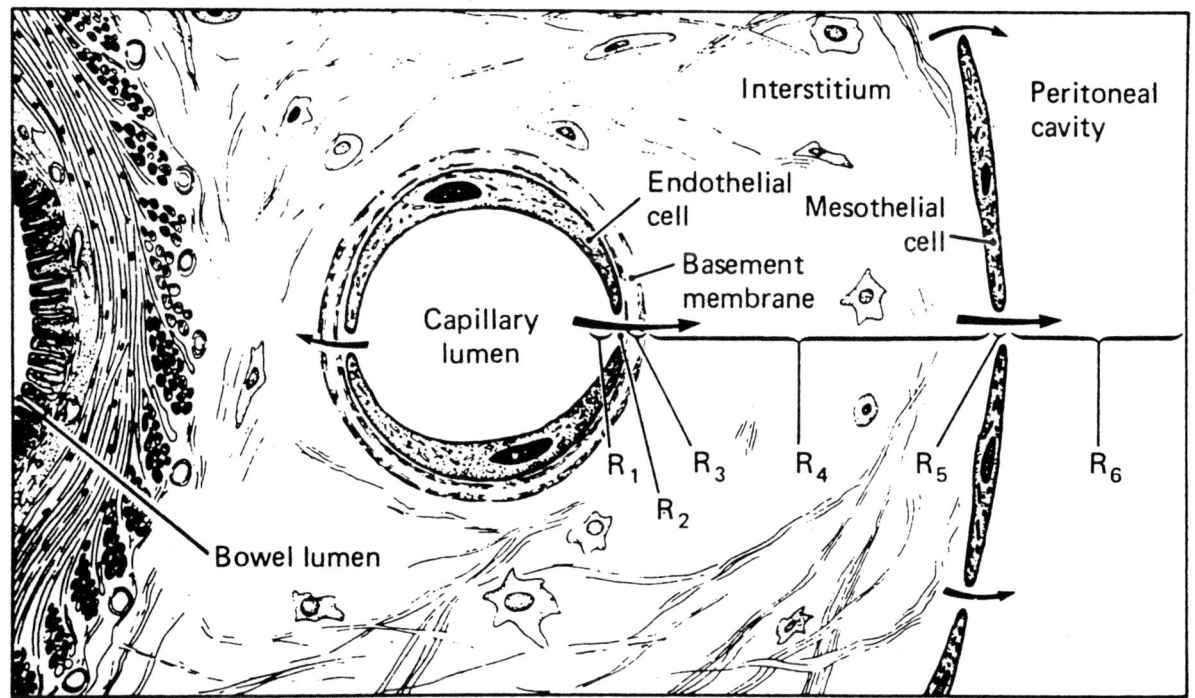

Figure 4. Diagramatic representation of resistance to solute passage from peritoneal capillaries to dialysate (Nolph KD, Miller F, Rubin J, Popovich R: New directions in peritoneal dialysis concepts and applications. Used with permission from Kidney Int 18: S111–S116, 1980).

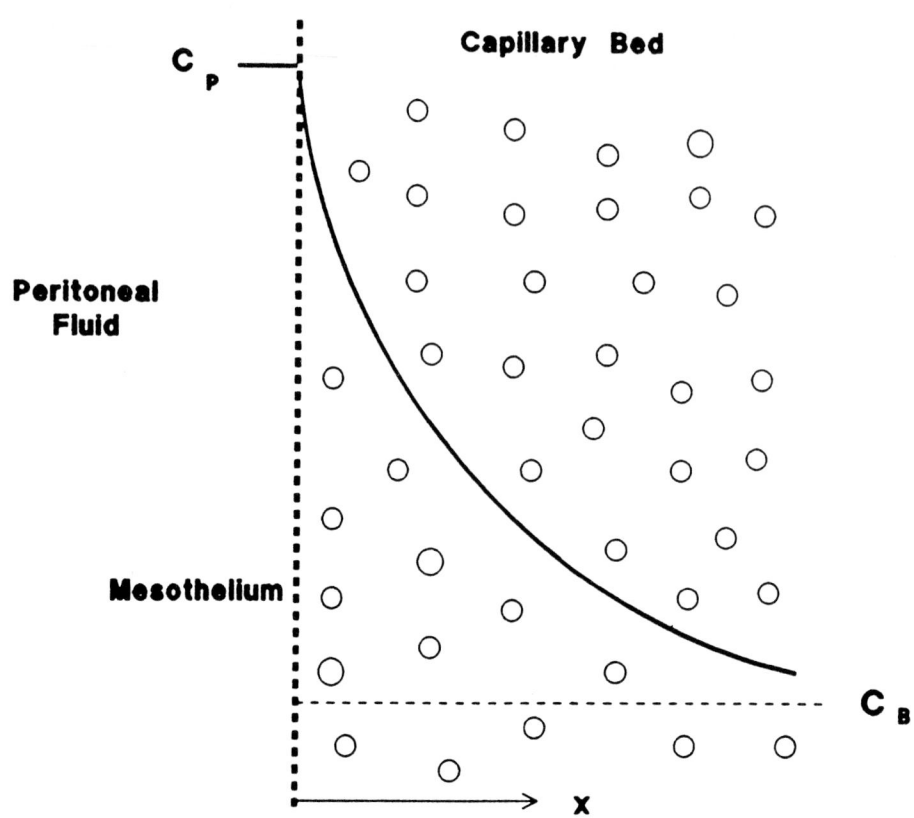

Figure 5. Distributed model concept in which transport in the peritoneal cavity-to-blood direction occurs as diffusion and convection across the mesothelium, through the tissue space, and into blood capillaries which are distributed throughout the tissue space. "x" is the distance into the tissue from the peritoneal surface. The small circles represent capillaries in the tissue space. C_P is the concentration of a substance in the peritoneal cavity. C_B is the concentration of a substance in the blood. (Flessner MF: Peritoneal transport physiology: Insights from basic research. © J Am Soc Nephrol 2: 122–135, 1991).

Table 1. Factors that may alter peritoneal resistances to solute movement (modified from Nolph KD, Miller F, Rubin J, Popovich R. New directions in peritoneal dialysis concepts and applications. Kidney Int 1980; 18: S111–S116).

Resistance	Potential modulators of resistance
R_1 (Stagnant fluid layer in the capillary)	Capillary flow rate, turbulence, blood viscosity
R_2 (Capillary endothelium)	Vasodilation, changes in capillary permeability, capillary recruitment
R_3 (Capillary basement membrane)	Thickening of the basement membrane?
R_4 (Peritoneal interstitum)	Inaccessible stagnant fluid, variations in the hydration status of the interstitum
R_5 (Mesothelium)	Drugs, dialysis fluid, inflammation
R_6 (Stagnant fluid layer in the peritoneal cavity)	Rapid cycling

differentiation of the dominant transport process occurring based on tissue type. For example, this model predicts that the predominant mode of small solute transport in the viscera is diffusion to a depth of 400–600 μm from the serosal surface. Mathematical modeling of small solute transport suggests that the mechanisms of transport are identical in both directions.

3.2. Blood flow in relation to peritoneal dialysis

Approximately 25% of the cardiac output is directed to the splanchnic vascular bed in normal, resting individuals [57]. Excluding the parietal peritoneum, the total abdominal splanchic blood flow usually exceeds 1200 ml/min at rest [58]. The precise blood flow available to peritoneal capillaries which participate in solute exchange during peritoneal dialysis is unknown. Due to the heterogeneous nature of peritoneal tissue and its vasculature, there is currently no direct method to precisely measure the effective blood flow in the peritoneal capillary bed. Much of the blood flow is routed to the abdominal viscera supplying areas which contribute minimally to solute exchange [52]. Indirect measures of effective peritoneal blood flow have been made using inert gas (H_2, X_e) washout techniques. Estimates of peritoneal blood flow range between 2.5 ml and 6.2 ml/min per kg body weight in rabbits to 7.5 ml/min × 100 g body weight in rats [59, 60]. In rats, splanchnic blood flow accounts for 91% of the effective peritoneal perfusion with superior mesenteric blood flow alone accounting for 89% of peritoneal perfusion [60]. In man, carbon dioxide diffusion techniques estimate peritoneal blood flow ranging between 68 and 82 ml/min, or approximately 1–2 ml/min per kg body weight [61].

When considering effective capillary blood flow, an important question arises. Is the effective blood flow adequate to deliver solutes and fluid such that solute clearance and ultrafiltration are not primarily blood flow limited? Nolph et al. have presented indirect evidence that maximum clearance is not primarily blood flow limited [61]. This evidence relies on the interpretation of urea clearance data under conditions of decreased mesenteric blood flow or vasodilation as well as data derived from kinetic modeling.

Maximum urea clearances obtained with rapid cycling and predicted clearances at infinite dialysis flow are in the range of 30–40 ml/min. If urea clearances were blood flow limited, a severe restriction in mesenteric blood flow would be expected to reduce urea clearance. However, the results of studies in dogs subjected to circulatory shock have shown that urea clearances remain at 74% of control values despite a 38% reduction in mean arterial pressure [62]. In rabbits, urea clearances are affected when blood flow is reduced to 20% of normal [59, 63]. These findings demonstrate that despite marked reductions in mesenteric blood flow, only modest decreases in urea clearance occur, suggesting that urea clearance is not primarily blood flow limited.

As noted above, estimates of effective capillary blood flow have been made using gas diffusion techniques and range between 68–82 ml/min. Thus, peritoneal clearances of carbon dioxide are approximately two to three times the maximum urea clearance. Using the ratio of urea clearance to peritoneal blood flow, Aune predicted that a doubling in blood flow would produce less than a 10% increase in urea clearance [59]. These observations suggest that blood flow does not limit the delivery of urea to the microcirculation for exchange. However, results obtained using gas diffusion techniques should be viewed with caution since they are based on the assumption that peritoneal gas clearance is equal to effective blood flow. Model analysis predicts that peritoneal gas clearance is equal to apparent peritoneal surface area (A) multiplied by the square root of the product of gas diffusivity (D) and tissue blood perfusion (q):

Peritoneal gas clearance = $A\ (Dq)^{1/2}$.

Thus, without precise knowledge of all these parameters (data does not exist for "D"), the true blood flow cannot be calculated exactly by gas clearance [40, 64].

Another approach to evaluate whether clearance is blood flow limited is to consider the effects of intraperitoneal vasodilators on solute clearance. If blood flow limitations are present, proportionally greater increases in clearance of small solutes such as urea should occur when compared to increases in clearance of large solutes. Since urea clearances are increased by only 20% with intraperitoneal vasodilators, it appears that the clearance of small solutes such as urea are not primarily blood flow limited [52, 61, 65–70].

Kinetic models of peritoneal dialysis and simulations using hollow fiber dialyzers also yield results which are consistent with the concept that blood flow becomes limiting for small solute exchange only when the blood flow is less than 50 ml/min [52]. However, peritoneal blood flow easily exceeds this model-derived value under most conditions (e.g., in the presence of vasoactive peritoneal dialysis solutions, the blood flow may exceed 100 ml/min). Taken together, the bulk of the evidence suggests that clearance of solutes such as urea is not blood flow limited.

Finally, to evaluate whether ultrafiltration may be limited by effective peritoneal blood flow (EPBF), Grzegorzewska et al. studied the effects of ultrafiltration and effective peritoneal blood flow during peritoneal dialysis in the rat [71]. When maximum net ultrafiltration rate (NUFR) was obtained with hypertonic solutions, EPBF was approximately five times greater than NUFR, and under isosmotic conditions, EPBF exceeded NUFR by fifty-seven times. They conclude that since there is a great difference between EPBF and NUFR, it is unlikely that normal EPBF significantly limits NUFR during peritoneal dialysis.

In summary, the effective capillary blood flow in peritoneal tissue has not been precisely measured. Using gas diffusion techniques in man, the effective peritoneal capillary blood flow is estimated to be 68–82 ml/min. Several lines of evidence indicate that ultrafiltration and the clearance of solutes such as urea are not blood flow limited. Newer techniques which allow precise evaluation of gas diffusivity in tissue may help to further define the exact relationship between peritoneal gas clearance and effective capillary blood flow.

3.3. The effects of vasoactive agents on the peritoneal microcirculation

Numerous endogenous and exogenous vasoactive agents have been shown to modify blood flow in the peritoneal microcirculation. For example, a wide variety of drugs, hormones, neurotransmitters and mediators of inflammation alter mesenteric vascular resistance. Peritoneal dialysis solutions also exhibit vasoactive properties. In addition to altering blood flow, many of these agents can also simultaneously affect perfused capillary density and microvascular permeability.

Based on a review of the literature, two generalizations concerning vasoactive agents in the splanchnic circulation may be proposed. The first is that vasodilators in the splanchnic circulation generally enhance peritoneal clearances while vasoconstrictors decrease peritoneal clearances [72]. The second generalization is that vasodilators increase the capillary filtration coefficient and the number of perfused capillaries; while, vasoconstrictors reduce the capillary filtration coefficient and the number of perfused capillaries (alterations in capillary filtration coefficients may reflect changes in perfused capillary density and permeability) [24, 52, 65, 68]. While no broad generalization regarding the relationship between vasoactive agents and permeability may be made, it should be noted that many vasodilators also act to increase microvascular permeability [24]. As with most generalizations there are some exceptions. Many of these exceptions will be noted in the following discussion.

The effect of a particular vasoactive agent on capillary blood flow, perfused capillary density and capillary permeability combine to determine the final physiological effect a particular agent has on microvascular exchange. For example, bradykinin, glucagon, histamine and neurotensin increase both blood flow and permeability [42, 73–75]. Secretin and cholecystokinin infusions increase blood flow but do not alter microvascular permeability to macromolecules [76]. This example demonstrates the lack of an absolute relationship between blood flow and alterations in vascular permeability [24]. Despite the lack of effect of secretin and cholecystokinin on macromolecular permeability, these agents increase the capillary filtration coefficient. The latter observation suggests that changes in capillary surface area secondary to capillary recruitment primarily account for the ability of these agents to increase peritoneal clearances. In contrast, adenosine exhibits vasodilator properties but reduces the intestinal capillary filtration coefficient presumably by redistributing flow from mucosal capillaries to less permeable capillaries of the intestinal muscle layer [24, 77]. Aminophylline increases intestinal blood flow but does not alter peritoneal clearances [78–80].

Vasoactive agents may also demonstrate dose dependent effects on the microcirculation. Glucagon and serotonin generally increase the capillary filtration coefficient; however, certain doses of these agents decrease the capillary filtration coefficient [24, 81]. Epinephrine may also exhibit dose dependent effects due to differential alpha and beta adrenergic stimulation [24, 82].

Histamine increases microvascular permeability in the rat stomach, an effect that is inhibited by H_1 receptor blockade. Histamine also increases permeability in the rat mesentery. However, this effect appears to be mediated by H_2 receptors. In the intestine, H_1-receptors are primarily responsible for the initial vasodilation occurring with histamine while H_2-receptors account for the changes in permeability [24, 75]. Therefore, effects on certain receptor populations are important in determining physiologic actions and may be tissue specific.

Another important consideration is the route of administration of a particular substance. Glucagon increases clearances when given intravenously, but requires a very high dosage to influence clearance when given via the intraperitoneal route [83]. Thus, in addition to dose dependent effects and receptor specificity, the route of administration may be additional parameters which determine the physiologic action of an individual pharmacological agent.

Thus, there are no absolute relationships relating alterations in blood flow to changes in permeability and clearance, but the net effect an agent has on blood flow, perfused capillary density, and permeability determine the agent's physiologic consequences in the microvasculature. In addition, the effect of a particular agent on peritoneal blood flow, microvascular surface area, and permeability is affected by the agent's dose, route of administration, and receptor specificity.

With regard to the various factors that modify peritoneal exchange in the clinical setting, perhaps the most important parameter is clearance. Table 2 catalogues many substances which affect clearance

Table 2. Drugs and hormones which modify peritoneal clearance (modified from references 72 and 84).

Agents that increase clearance

Albumin [85–89]
Aminoproprionate [90]
Anthranilic acid [91, 92]
Arachidonic acid [93]
Bradykinin [94]
Calcium channel blockers [95]
Cetyl trimethyl NH_4Cl [96]
Cholecystokinin [97]
Cytochalasin D [98]
Desferrioxamine [99–101]
Dialysate alkalinization [102, 103]
Diazoxide [12]
Dioctyl sodium sulfosuccinate [104, 105]
Dipyridamole [106]
Dopamine [107, 108]
Edentate calcium disodium [109]
Ethacrynic acid [110]
Furosemide [110, 111]
Glucagon [113–116]
Histamine [117, 118]
Hydralazine [119]
Hypertonic glucose [120, 121]
Indomethacin [119]
Insulin [122]
Isoproterenol [123–126]
Lipid in dialysate [127]
Nitroprusside [12, 120, 128–130]
N-myristyl alanine [91]
Procaine hydrochloride [131]
Prostaglandin A1 [132, 133]
Prostaglandin E1 [132, 133]
Prostaglandin E2 [132, 133]
Phentolamine [134]
Protamine [135]
Puromycin [136]
Salicylate [107, 119]
Secretin [97]
Serotonin [107]
Streptokinase [107]
Tris hydroxymethl aminomethane (THAM) [114, 119]

Agents that decrease clearance

Calcium [114]
Dopamine [138]Norepinephrine [139]
Prostaglandin F2 [132]
Vasopressin [107, 108]

in peritoneal dialysis. Most vasoactive agents produce changes in clearance ranging from 15–65%. Nitroprusside and isoproterenol are perhaps the most extensively studied vasodilators in peritoneal dialysis. Nitroprusside and isoproterenol are among the most effective agents which augment peritoneal clearances [12, 120, 128–130, 140–144]. Nitroprusside increases the clearance of urea, creatinine, inulin, and protein in a dose-dependent fashion. Small solute clearance appears to be most affected at lower doses, while large solute clearances are significantly increased at higher doses [145]. The maximum effect of intraperitoneally administered nitroprusside appears to occur after three to five consecutive exchanges with the drug, and the effects of nitroprusside are reversed when the drug is removed from the dialysis fluid. With nitroprusside, mass transfer coefficients increase proportionately more for inulin than for urea suggesting that alterations in permeability occur with exposure to the drug [130]. In addition, nitroprusside enhances the leakage of fluorescein-tagged albumin across the mesenteric microvessels [17, 146]. Studies of the effects of vasodilators and peritoneal dialysis solutions on small arteries (70 μm) and small veins (140 μm) in the rat cecum demonstrate that peritoneal dialysis solutions dilate both arteries and veins. While subsequent addition of nitroprusside produces no further arterial vasodilation, a significant increase in venular diameter occurs [147]. This experimental evidence suggests that a primary site of action of nitroprusside during peritoneal dialysis resides at the venule, both in terms of the blood flow response and the increase in permeability.

Intraperitoneal nitroprusside has been used in certain clinical situations. Patients with vascular diseases such as scleroderma may experience decreased clearances during peritoneal dialysis. Addition of nitroprusside to the dialysis fluid appears to improve clearance in such patients [140]. A possible major disadvantage for the clinical use of nitroprusside is the potential for systemic vasodilation. However, some studies indicate the peripheral vasodilation effects are limited with appropriate intraperitoneal dosing [130].

Isoproterenol administered intraperitoneally accelerates peritoneal transport. The route of administration is important in determining its effects on clearance. Intravenous isoproterenol increases superior mesenteric blood flow by 88% but does not alter peritoneal clearances of creatinine and inulin. In contrast, intraperitoneally administered isoproterenol increases superior mesenteric blood flow and increases solute clearance. The clinical use of isoproterenol is hindered by its potential cardiac stimulatory actions [141].

Intraperitoneal administration of the calcium channel blockers verapamil and diltiazem has been shown to increase the clearance of urea in animal models. Verapamil increases urea dialysate to plasma ratios by 16 to 44%, while diltiazem increases the ratio by 25%. With both verapamil and diltiazem, the dialysate protein concentration does not increase, suggesting that no significant alterations in permeability occur with intraperitoneal exposure to these drugs. In addition, these drugs show no effect on peritoneal ultrafiltration [95]. However, other investigators have found intraperitoneally instilled verapamil does appear to increase permeability and ultrafiltration [152].

3.4. The effects of peritoneal dialysis on the peritoneal microcirculation

Routine peritoneal dialysis can markedly affect the mesenteric microcirculation. For example, topical application of dialysis fluid to arterioles in the rat cecum or cremaster muscle produces a transient vasoconstriction lasting one to four minutes followed by a sustained vasodilation [17, 66, 147–149]. Since standard peritoneal dialysis solutions have a high osmolality as a result of elevated glucose concentrations (calculated osmolality of 346 mosmol/L for 1.5% Dianeal to 485 mosmols/L for 4.25% Dianeal), a low pH, (pH of 4–6.5 for Dianeal), and contain an acetate or lactate buffer system, it is logical to postulate that these alterations may contribute to the vasoactive properties of peritoneal dialysis solutions. Indeed, superfusion of mesentery with a hypertonic solution containing glucose produces submaximal arteriolar vasodilation. Isosmolar acetate or lactate solutions also produce submaximal arteriolar vasodilation. The combination of hyperosmolality and acetate or lactate produces maximal arteriolar vasodilation. Although maximal arteriolar vasodilation is achieved with peritoneal dialysis solutions, maximum mesenteric venular vasodilatation does not occur. In the presence of peritoneal dialysis solutions, the addition of nitroprusside produces significant increases in venular diameter [147].

In an analogous fashion, vasodilation occurs following intravascular infusions of hyperosmolar solutions. Local infusion of hypertonic glucose or sodium chloride solutions into the superior mesenteric artery of the cat produces a marked reduction in intestinal vascular resistance. Glucose produces a 2.70% decrease in vascular resistance per 1% increase in osmolality while sodium chloride produces a 4.87% decrease in vascular resistance per 1% increase in osmolality. For glucose, the reduction in vascular resistance was maintained throughout the infusion period while the response to sodium chloride waned with time [150].

Granger et al. have measured superior mesenteric and peritoneal blood flow during intraperitoneal administration of a commercial dialysis solution (Dianeal) in anesthetized cats. The dialysis fluid significantly increased blood flow to the mesentery, omentum, intestinal serosa and parietal peritoneum; however, significant alterations in blood flow were not present in the major abdominal organs including the liver, stomach, intestine, pancreas and spleen. This selective vasodilation presumably results from decreased diffusion distance of the fluid to the tissue in the microvasculature of the "thin" tissues [151]. If blood flow per unit tissue in the cat and man are similar, then extrapolation of this data to man suggests that total peritoneal blood flow in man may exceed 100 ml/min during dialysis [72].

It is unlikely that the low pH of peritoneal dialysis solutions accounts for their vasoactive properties since adjustment of pH to 7.0–7.4 does not alter the vasodilator response in the rat cremaster muscle [66]. Furthermore, clearances of urea, creatinine, inulin and protein are not altered with adjustments in pH.

Ultrafiltration occurs in peritoneal dialysis when there is net fluid filtration into the peritoneum. The increased osmolality of hypertonic, glucose containing peritoneal dialysis solutions creates an osmotic gradient which favors fluid movement from the vascular compartment to the peritoneal cavity [153, 154]. In the rabbit, 1.5% glucose containing peritoneal dialysis fluid produces an ultrafiltration rate of 3.0 ml/min/m^2 and increases by approximately 1.7 ml/min/m^2 for each 1% increase in glucose concentration [137, 155]. The intraperitoneal glucose concentration decreases with time resulting in decreased osmolality and reduced ultrafiltration. Eventually, osmotic equilibrium is obtained and at this point it would seem reasonable to assume intraperitoneal volume would be maximized. However, peritoneal lymphatic absorption can significantly influence estimations of ultrafiltration rates. Lymphatic absorption produces a net ultrafiltration rate significantly below the true transcapillary filtration rate. Therefore, peak intraperitoneal volume does not coincide with osmotic equilibrium but occurs when the transcapillary ultrafiltration rate equals the lymphatic absorption rate (Fig. 6) [156].

At equilibrium, the absorption of fluid between the peritoneal cavity and the capillary is described by Starling's equation.

$$J_v = L_P A\ (\Delta P - \sigma \Delta \Pi) - J_L$$

J_v : Fluid flow from the peritoneum to the plasma
$(L_P A)$: Peritoneal membrane filtration coefficient
ΔP : Effective hydrostatic pressure gradient between capillaries and peritoneal cavity
σ : Osmotic reflection coefficient
$\Delta \Pi$: Effective colloid pressure gradient between the capillaries and peritoneal cavity
J_L : Lymph flow from the peritoneal cavity

When crystalloids are allowed to equilibrate, the rate of fluid absorption across the peritoneal membrane (J_v) is –0.9 to 1.1 ml/min [157, 158]. The peritoneal membrane filtration coefficient ($L_P A$) is calculated to be approximately 0.1 min^{-1} mm Hg^{-1}. This value is similar to 0.12 ml min^{-1} mm Hg^{-1} obtained for the cat peritoneum [33, 159]. Comparisons of the ratios of hydraulic conductivity and potassium permeability in skeletal muscle and mesentery are similar. This suggests that the molecular and structural characteristics responsible for the resistance to water and solute movement across capillaries in these tissues are similar [72, 160].

In summary, it appears that hyperosmolality and the presence of acetate or lactate buffers contribute to the vasodilation of mesenteric arterioles induced by peritoneal dialysis solutions. A number of substances alter vascular tone in the mesenteric microcirculation including nitroprusside and isoproterenol. In the presence of peritoneal dialysis solutions, the addition of nitroprusside produces no additional mesenteric arteriolar dilation but a significant increase in mesenteric venular dilation does occur. In animals, intraperitoneal administration of peritoneal dialysis fluid demonstrates tissue selective vasodilator responses. The rate of ultrafiltration from the vasculature to the peritoneal cavity may be affected by lymphatic absorption with peak intraperitoneal volume occurring when the transcapillary ultrafiltration rate equals the lymphatic absorption rate.

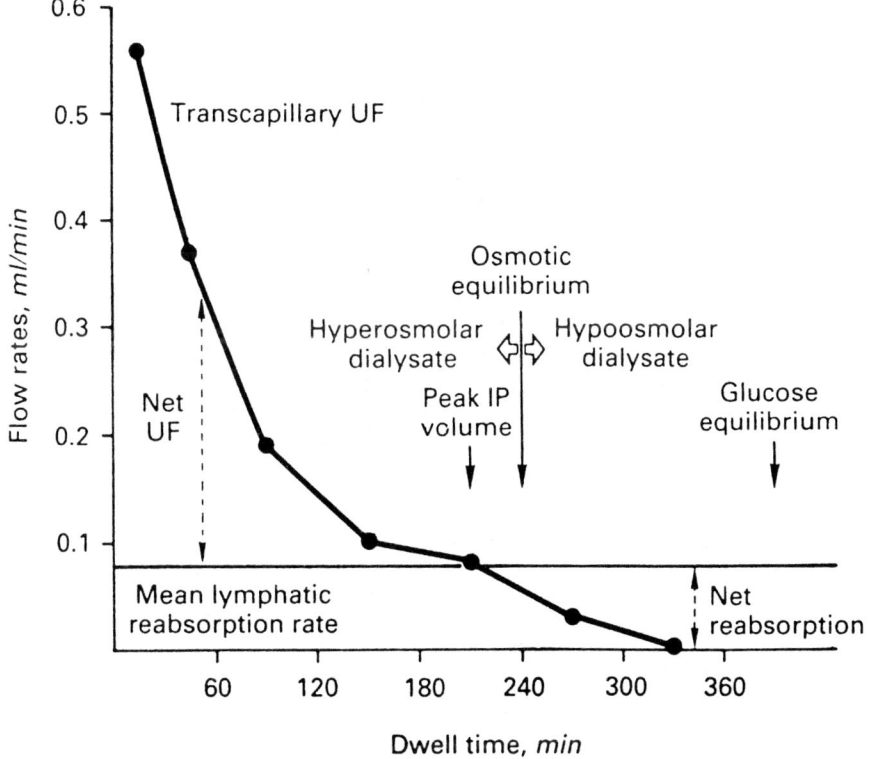

Figure 6. Effect of dwell time on mean transcapillary ultrafiltration. Note that peak intraperitoneal volume occurs when transcapillary ultrafiltration rate equals the lymphatic absorption rate (Nolph KD, Mactier R, Khanna R, Twardowski ZJ, Moore H, McGary T. The kinetics of ultrafiltration during peritoneal dialysis. Used with permission from Kid Int 1987; 32: 219–226).

4. The peritoneal microcirculation in inflammation

4.1. General principles of leukocyte-endothelial interactions

A fascinating and emerging area of investigation with relevance to the field of peritoneal dialysis is the role of the microcirculation in inflammation. An important facet of this work is the interaction of leukocytes with the vascular endothelium during inflammation. Leukocyte migration from the microcirculation to the peritoneal cavity in inflammatory states such as peritonitis begins with the initial interaction between the leukocyte and the endothelial cells lining the vascular wall. The leukocyte cell count in the peritoneal dialysis effluent may increase rapidly during an infectious process. This rapid rise in the number of peritoneal leukocytes is dependent on factors that govern the initial adhesive interaction between leukocytes and the venular endothelium. Furthermore, many of the mediators produced in the inflammatory process can affect microvascular permeability and vascular tone. This section will focus on the basic physiologic interactions involved in leukocyte adherence and migration and describe how these interactions are regulated. The influence of the inflammatory process in peritoneal dialysis will also be addressed.

The attachment and subsequent migration of leukocytes from the vascular to the extravascular compartment involves numerous steps which occur in a sequential fashion. Leukocyte adhesion is localized primarily to postcapillary venules [161–164]. In order for a leukocyte to establish an adhesive interaction with the endothelium, it must first be displaced from the center stream to the vessel wall. This appears to be related to microvascular network topography and radial dispersive forces. As the blood vessel diameter increases from the capillary to the postcapillary venules, the more flexible erythrocytes begin to pass the leukocytes and deflect them toward the vessel wall [165]. Once displaced to the vessel wall, the leukocyte can begin to adhere. Adhesion begins as a rolling movement along the postcapillary endothelium. As the inflammatory process proceeds, the number of rolling neutrophils increases and the velocity of the rolling decreases. This exposes the leukocyte to low concentrations of chemotactic agents released from parenchymal cells and/or the endothelium. Leukocyte activation allows the establishment of firm (stationary) adhesive interactions (Fig. 7). As noted below, the firmly adherent leukocyte may

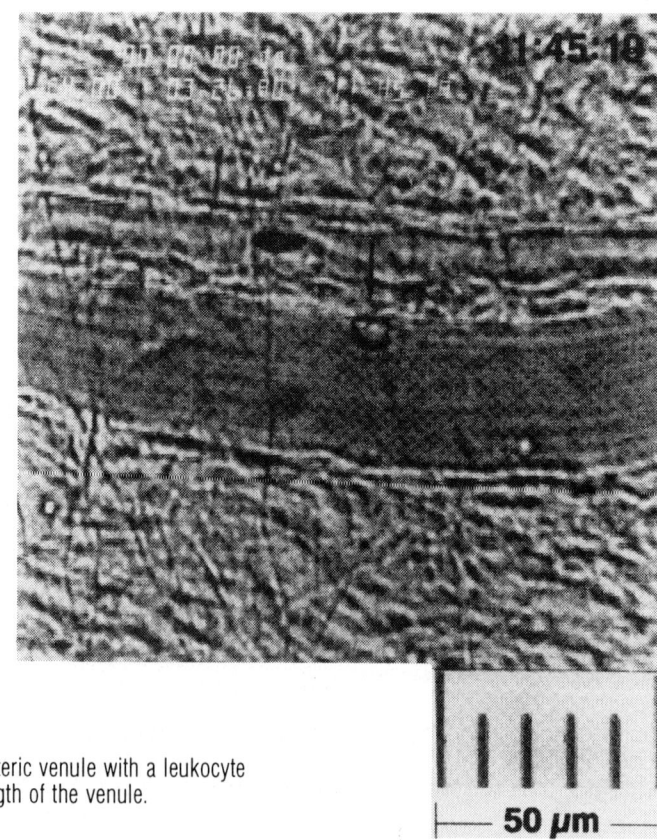

Figure 7. Panel A: A mesenteric venule with a leukocyte (arrow) rolling along the length of the venule.

B.

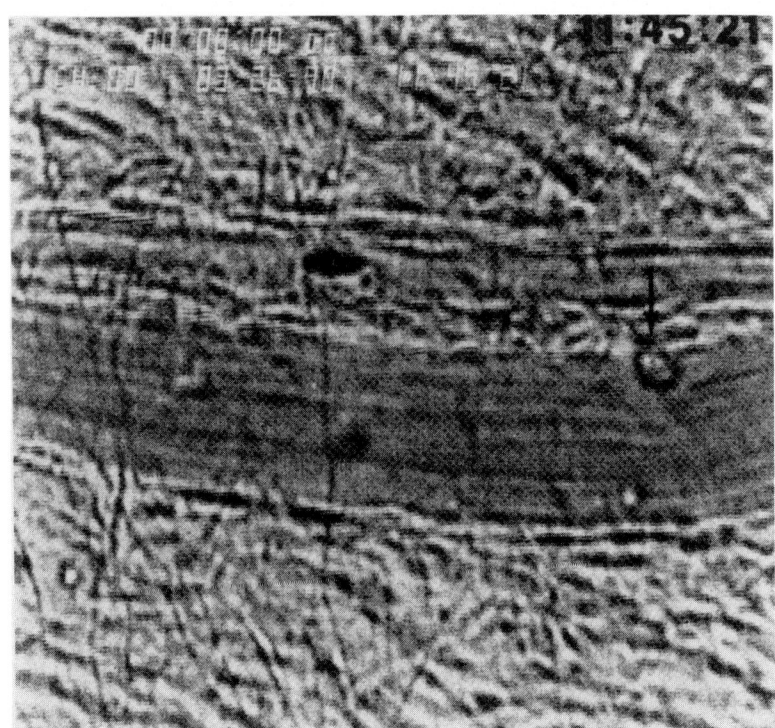

C.

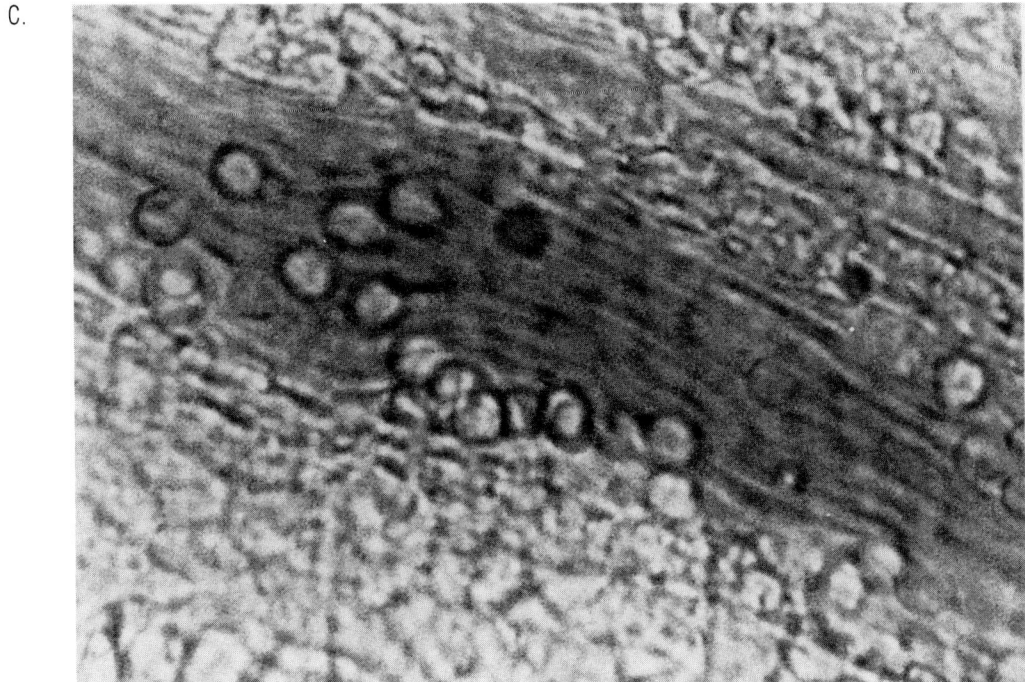

Fig. 7. Panel B: This micrograph was taken two seconds after the micrograph depicted in Panel A to demonstrate that the leukocyte moved approximately 40 μm downstream in the venule. Panel C: A mesenteric venule during 2 ng/min platelet activiting factor (PAF) infusion. Note the numerous white blood cells adhering to the endothelial wall after PAF infusion. (Kubes P, Suzuki M, Granger DN: Modulation of PAF – induced leukocyte adherence and increased microvascular permeability. Am J Physiol 259: G858–G864, 1990).

then migrate across the endothelial barrier and enter the interstitium [166].

The adhesive interaction between the leukocyte and the endothelium is mediated by a complex, highly coordinated, dynamic interplay between adhesion glycoproteins expressed on the surface of both the leukocyte and the endothelium. Each of these glycoproteins belong to one of three main families: the integrins, superimmunoglobulins, and selectins. The integrins are heterodimers composed of a common beta subunit (CD18) and a specific alpha subunit (CD11a, CD11b or CD11c). These subunits combine to form the intergrins CD11a/CD18(LFA-1), CD11b/CD18 (Mac-1, MO1 or CR3) and CD11c/CD18 (p150, 90). The superimmunoglobulin family is represented by intercellular adhesion molecules known as ICAMs. The selectins are represented by L-selectin (LAM-1), E-selectin (ELAM-1), and P-selectin (GMP-140). The integrins and L-selectin are expressed on the surface of neutrophils. ICAM-1 is present on endothelial cells and its expression may be increased by endotoxin and cytokines such as interleukin-1 and tumor necrosis factor (IL-1 and TNF). Cytokines can also activate endothelial cells to express E-selectin. P-selectin is present on platelets and vascular endothelial cells (Table 3) [166–172].

The sequence of events involved in neutrophil adherence and migration to sites of inflammation requires coordination of the adhesive interactions between the neutrophil and vascular endothelium (Fig. 8). The initial leukocyte rolling appears to involve interactions between L-selectin on the neutrophil and E-selectin and P-selectin on the vascular endothelium. This interaction allows for the upregulation of CD11b/CD18 which can bind to ICAM-1 and strengthen neutrophil adhesion. L-selectin is then downregulated (shed) from the cell surface. The firmly adherent neutrophil may then migrate across the vessel wall by a process that is dependent on CD11a/CD18 (LFA-1), CD11b/CD18(Mac-1), and ICAM-1 [166–173].

4.2. Inflammatory mediators and the microcirculation

The physiologic interaction between the neutrophil and the endothelium may be influenced by several factors. Intravital videomicroscopic approaches have provided a wealth of information regarding the influence of intravascular hydrodynamic dispersal forces [161, 173, 174], leukocyte capillary plugging [175–177], electrostatic charge [178], and chemical mediators on leukocyte-endothelial cell interactions during inflammation. The following discussion will focus primarily on information concerning the chemical mediators of these adhesive interactions including platelet activating factor (PAF), arachidonic acid metabolites, complement and reactive oxygen species.

Platelet activating factor (PAF), arachidonic acid metabolites and certain components of complement have been shown to increase microvascular permeability [179–181]. Platelet activating factor is formed by a variety of cells including endothelial cells, neutrophils, macrophages and platelets. The effects of PAF on vascular tone may vary from vasodilation at low concentrations to vasoconstriction at higher concentrations. In addition to the vascular effects, PAF may cause mesenteric ischemia, interstitial edema, hemoconcentration, increased microvascular permeability as well as

Table 3. Leukocyte adhesion receptor families.

Family	Localization	Counter-receptor	Function
Integrins CD11a/CD18 CD11b/CD18 CD11c/CD18	Leukocytes	ICAM-1 ICAM-2	Adherence Emigration
Super-immunoglobulins ICAM-1 ICAM-2	Endothelial Cells	CD11a, CD11b, CD11c	Adherence Emigration
Selectins L-selectin P-selectin E-selectin	Leukocytes Endothelial cells	? SIALYL LEWIS X SIALYL LEWIS X	Rolling

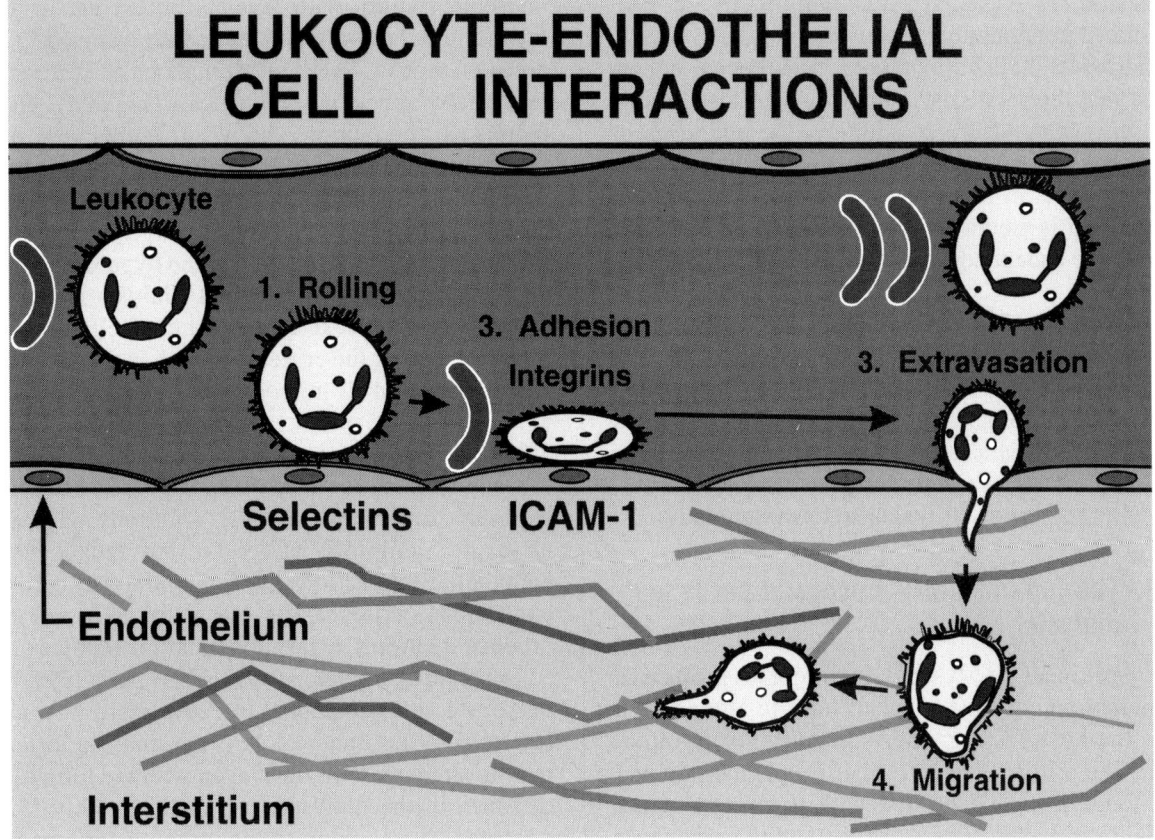

Figure 8. The sequence of events involved in leukocyte adherence and migration to sites of inflammation requires coordination of the adhesive interactions between the leukocyte and vascular endothelium. (1) The initial leukocyte rolling appears to involve interactions between L-selectin on the neutrophil and E-selectin and P-selectin on the vascular endothelium. (2) This interaction allows for the upregulation of the leukocyte integrin CD11b/CD18 which can bind to ICAM-1 and strengthen neutrophil adhesion. (3) The firmly adherent leukocyte may then extravasate by a process that is dependent on CD11a/CD18, CD11b/CD18, and ICAM-1. (4) The leukocyte may then migrate into the interstitial tissue. (Figure courtesy of Kristine Bienvenu).

increased leukocyte adherence in post capillary venules. Interestingly, adherent leukocytes appear to mediate PAF-induced vascular leakage. This observation is supported by experimental evidence which demonstrates that pretreatment with monoclonal antibodies directed against the common beta subunit of CD11/CD18 largely prevents the increased vascular protein leakage caused by intraarterial infusion of PAF [183].

The arachidonic acid metabolite leukotriene B4 (LTB4) has been shown to increase microvascular protein efflux in the presence of a transvascular chemotactic gradient [181]. However, Kubes *et al.* have shown that in the cat mesentery, local intraarterial infusion of either LTB4 or PAF promotes leukocyte adherence, but only PAF alters microvascular permeability. This indicates that leukocyte adhesion alone does not always result in increased microvascular permeability, but leukocyte adhesion in the presence of an appropriate chemotactic stimulus may alter microvascular permeability. When LTB4 and PAF are infused simultaneously, LTB4 causes a further increase in microvascular permeability than is observed with PAF alone. While PAF *per se*, may increase microvascular permeability in the presence of adherent leukocytes, it may also serve as a "priming agent" that sensitizes neutrophils to other stimuli such as LTB4 [184]. The complement factor C5a can increase macromolecular permeability in postcapillary venules. Neutropenia attenuates C5a-induced increases in microvascular permeability [185].

Reactive oxygen metabolites such as superoxide and hydrogen peroxide may be produced by neutrophils and endothelial cells [186–188]. Reactive oxygen metabolites have been shown to increase neutrophil adherence in postcapillary venules [189]. Hydrogen peroxide appears to promote leukocyte adhesion to vascular endothelium by a PAF mediated upregulation or activation of CD11/CD18. Superoxide induced increases in leukocyte adherence may be related to inactivation of nitric oxide by superoxide [190]. In addition, the inhibition of nitric oxide production by the vascular endothelium can produce an increase in microvascular protein efflux that is mediated by leukocyte dependent and leukocyte independent mechanisms in the mesentery [191].

Mesothelial cell monolayers have also been shown to express adhesion molecules [192]. C5a has been shown to increase leukocyte adherence and migration through the mesothelial monolayers. Thus, it appears that both the microvascular endothelium and mesothelium can actively participate in the peritoneal response to inflammation.

4.3. The inflammatory process in peritoneal dialysis

In peritoneal dialysis, a patient's protective immunologic defense mechanisms are altered such that the host has a greater susceptibility to infection. The primary protective barriers of the skin and peritoneum are penetrated with a foreign object providing easier access for potential pathogenic organisms. These patients may experience depressed immunologic function secondary to uremia and may have underlying medical illnesses such as diabetes mellitus.

It appears that peritoneal dialysis solutions, *per se*, have a negative impact on host defenses. The activity of peripheral blood leukocytes as measured by chemiluminescence, phagocytosis and bacterial killing is suppressed by peritoneal dialysis solutions. This suppression is believed to be secondary to such factors as the solution's high osmolality and low pH [193]. It has also been shown that peritoneal dialysis solutions can decrease peritoneal macrophage function by decreasing the cell's phagocytic activity and respiratory burst [194]. The requirement for frequent exchanges may dilute the intraperitoneal immunoglobin concentrations, thus rendering the patient more susceptible to infection [195]. Many of these observations are dependent on alterations in leukocyte function. The microcirculation plays a critical role in this process as it delivers these cells to the interstitial environment and peritoneal cavity.

To form a complete picture of the normal immunologic process during peritoneal dialysis, there must be integration of events occurring in the microcirculation with events occurring in the interstitium, mesothelium and peritoneal cavity. As noted previously, cytokines stimulate the expression of certain adhesion molecules. This may elicit increased interactions between leukocytes and microvascular endothelium. The cells would then be able to respond to the inflammatory challenge. However, the picture is complicated by a nonphysiologic environment created by the hyperosmolality and low pH of the peritoneal dialysis fluids. It appears that at least acutely, these cells may be inhibited during the critical time when the potential for introduction of microorganisms is the greatest [196]. Whether or not peritoneal dialysis fluids affect leuckocyte – endothelial interaction is under investigation. Preliminary data suggests that acute exposure to peritoneal dialysis solutions may have an acute inhibitory effect on the leukocyte – endothelial interactions [197]. In contrast, chronic exposure to peritoneal dialysis solutions appears to produce a chronic local inflammation [196].

In pathophysiologic states such as peritonitis, the leukocyte cell count may increase rapidly from a few cells to thousands of cells per mm^3. In inflammation an increase in fibrinogen with the formation of fibrin in the dialysate can occur quickly [52]. As noted above, many of the inflammatory mediators can alter permeability. An intriguing question is whether some of the basic microcirculatory processes involved in inflammation can account for clinical observations such as alterations in solute clearance and decreased ultrafiltration capacity commonly associated with peritonitis.

5. Summary

In summary, interactions between the leukocyte and the vascular endothelium appear to play an important role in a number of pathophysiologic processes associated with inflammation. Elucidation of the mechanisms involved in producing the well-described alterations in microvascular permeability, vascular tone and leukocyte adherence that accompany peritonitis have important clinical implications for the patient on peritoneal dialysis. Although the relative contribution of adhesion molecules and inflammatory mediators to peritoneal inflammation remains undefined, it is hoped that this discussion will stimulate research in this intriguing and clinically relevant area.

References

1. Williams PL, Warwick R (eds) Grays Textbook of Anatomy. Philadelphia: W. B. Saunders 1980; pp 1319–89.
2. Baron MA. Structure of the intestinal peritoneum in man. AM J Anat 1941; 69: 439–96.
3. Nolph KD, Twardowski Z. The Peritoneal Dialysis System. In: Nolph KD (ed), Peritoneal Dialysis. Martinus Nijhoff, Boston 1985; pp 23–50.
4. Mactier RA, Khanna R, Twardowski ZJ, Nolph KD. Role of peritoneal cavity lymphatic absorption in peritoneal dialysis. Kid Int 1987; 32: 165–72.
5. Verger C. Peritoneal Ultrastructure. In: KD Nolph (ed) Peritoneal Dialysis. Martinus Nijhoff, Boston 1985; pp 95–113.
6. Henderson LW. The problem of peritoneal membrane area and permeability. Kidney Int 1973; 3: 409–10.
7. Mion CM, Boen ST. Analysis of factors responsible for the formation of adhesions during chronic peritoneal dialysis. Am J Med Sci 250: 675–9.
8. Knapowski J, Feder E, Simon M, Zabel M. Evaluation of the participation of parietal peritoneum in dialysis: physiological morphological and pharmacological data. Proc Eur Dial Trans Assoc 1979; 16: 155–64.
9. Rubin J, Jones Q, Andrew M. An analysis of ultrafiltration during acute peritoneal dialysis in rats. Am J Med Sci 1989; 298: 383–9.
10. Rubin J, Jones Q, Planch A, Stanek K. Systems of membranes involved in peritoneal dialysis. J Lab Clin Invest 1987; 110: 448–53.
11. Lukus G, Brindle SD, Greengard P. The Route of Absorption of Intraperitoneally Administered Compounds. J Pharm Exp Ther 1971; 178: 562–6.
12. Nolph KD, Ghods AJ, Stone JV, Brown PA. The effects of intraperitoneally vasodilators on peritoneal clearances. Trans Am Soc Artif Inter Organs 1976; 22: 586–94.
13. Chambers R, Zweifach BW. Topography and function of the mesenteric capillary circulation. Am J Anat 1944; 75: 173–205.
14. Zweifach BW. The microcirculation of the blood. Scientific America, January 1959; pp 54–60.
15. Richardson DR. Basic circulatory physiology. Little, Brown and Co., Boston 1976; pp 101–36.
16. Johnson PC, Wayland H. Regulation of blood flow in single capillaries. Am J Physiol 1967; 212: 1405–15.
17. Miller FN. The peritoneal microcirculation. In: Nolph (ed), Peritoneal Dialysis. Martinus Nijhoff, Boston 1985; 51–93.
18. Buez S. An open Cremaster muscle preparation for the study of blood vessels by in vivo microscopy. Microvas Res 1973; 5: 384–94.
19. Smuje L, Zweifach BW, Intaglietta M. Micropressure and capillary filtration coefficients in single vessels of the cremaster muscle in the rat. Microvas Res 1970; 2: 96–110.
20. Renkin EM. Microcirculation and Exchange. In: Patton HD, Fuchs AF, Hille B, Scher AM, Steiner R (eds), Textbook of Physiology. W. B. Saunders, Philadelphia 1989; 860–78.
21. Chambers R, Zwiefach BW. Functional activity of the blood capillary bed, with special reference to visceral tissue. Ann NY Acad Sci 1946; 46: 683–94.
22. Taylor AE, Granger DN. Exchange of macromolecules across the circulation. In: Renkin EM, Michel CC (eds), Handbook of Physiology, Microcirculation Section, Chapter 11. American Physiological Society, Baltimore 1984; pp 467–520.
23. Gotloib L, Shostak A. The functional anatomy of the peritoneum as dialyzing membrane. In: Stein JH, Twardowski ZJ, Nolph KD, Khanna R (eds), Contemporary Issues in Nephrology Peritoneal Dialysis. Churchill Livingstone, New York 1990; pp 1–27.
24. Harper SL, Bohlen, HG, Granger DN. Vasoactive agents and the mesenteric microcirculation. Am J Physiol 1985; 249: G309–15.
25. Diana JN, Laughlin MH. Effect of ischemia on capillary pressure and equivalent pore radius in capillaries of the isolated dog hind limb. Cir Res 1974; 35: 77–101.
26. Korthuis RJ, Granger DN. Peritoneal Dialysis: An analysis of factors which influence peritoneal mass transport. In: Stigmark B (ed), Peritoneum and Peritoneal Access. John Wiley and Sons, London 1988; pp 24–41.
27. Rippe B, Haraldson B. Capillary permeability in rat hindquarters as determined by estimations of capillary reflection coefficients. Acta Physiol Scand 1986; 127: 289–303.
28. Aune S. Transperitoneal Exchange. IV. The effect of transperitoneal fluid transport on the transfer of solutes. Scand J Gastroent 1970; 5: 241–52.
29. Curry FE, Mason JC, Michel CC. Osmotic reflection coefficients of capillary walls to low molecular weight hydrophilic solutes measured in single perfused capillaries of the frog mesentery. J Physiol 1976; 261: 319–36.
30. Michel CC. Reflection coefficients in single capillaries compared with results from whole organs. Bibl Anat 1977; 15: 172–6.
31. Michel CC. Filtration coefficients and osmotic reflection coefficients of the walls of single frog mesenteric capillaries. J Physiol 1980; 309: 341–55.
32. Pyle WK, Moncrief JW, Popovich RP. Peritoneal transport evaluation in CAPD. In: Moncrief JW, Popovich RP (eds), Proc 2nd Int Symp on CAPD. Masson, New York 1981; pp 35–9.
33. Rippe B, Perry MA and Granger DN. Permselectivity of the peritoneal membrane. Microvasc Res 1985; 29: 89–102.
34. Rippe B, Stelin G, Ahlmen J. Basal permeability of the peritoneal membrane during continuous ambulatory peritoneal dialysis (CAPD). In: Advances in Peritoneal Dialysis. Proc. of the 2nd International Symposium in Peritoneal Dialysis, Excerpta Medica, Amsterdam 1981; pp 5–9.
35. Nolph KD, Miller FN, Pyle WK, Popovich RP,

Sorkin MI. An hypothesis to explain the ultrafiltration characteristics of peritoneal dialysis. Kid Int 1981; 20: 543–8.
36. Nakamura Y, Watalnd H. Macromolecular transport in the cat mesentery. Microvasc Res 1975; 9: 1–21.
37. Rippe B, Stelin G. Simulations of peritoneal solute transport during CAPD. Application of two pore formalism. Kid Int 1989; 35: 1234–44.
38. Stelin G, Rippe B. A phenomenologic interpretation of the variation in dialysate volume with dwell time in CAPD. Kid Int 1990; 38: 465–72.
39. Rippe B, Simonsen O, Stelin G. Clinical implications of a three-pore model of peritoneal transport. In: Khanna R, Nolph KD, Prowant BF, Twardowski ZJ, Oreopoulos D (eds), Advances in Peritoneal Dialysis 1991, Vol 7, Peritoneal Dialysis Bulletin 1991; pp 3–9.
40. Flessner MF. Peritoneal transport physiology: insights from basic research. J Am Soc Nephrol 1991; 2: 122–35.
41. Hargens AR, Cologne JB, Menninger FJ, Hogan JS, Tucker BJ, Peters RM. Normal transcapillary pressures in human skeletal muscle and subcutaneous tissue. Microvas Res 1981; 22: 177–89.
42. Harper SL, Barrowman JA, Kvietys PR, Granger DN. Effect of neurotensin on intestinal capillary permeability and blood flow. Am J Physiol 1984; 10: G161–6.
42a. Perry MA, Shepherd AP, Kvietys PR, Granger DN. Effect of hypoxia on feline intestinal capillary permeability. Am J Physiol 1985; 248: G272–6.
43. Bernfield M. Introduction. In: Porter R et al. (eds), Basement Membranes and Cell Movement. Ciba Foundation Symposium 108. Pitman, London 1984; pp 1–5.
44. Clementi F, Palade GE. Intestinal capillaries. I. Permeability to peroxidases and ferritin. J Cell Biol 1969; 41: 33–58.
45. Fox JR, Wayland H. Interstitial diffusion of macromolecules in the rat mesentery. Microvas Res 1979; 18: 255–74.
46. Johansson BR. Permeability of muscle capillaries to interstitially microinjected ferritin. Microvas Res 1978; 16: 362–8.
47. Laurent TC: Interaction between proteins and glycosaminoglycans. Fed Proc 1977; 36: 24–7.
48. Watson PD, Grodin FS. An analysis of the effects of the interstitial matrix on plasma-lymphtransport. Microvas Res 1978; pp 16–41.
49. Granger DN, Taylor AE. Permeability of intestinal capillaries to endogenous macromolecules. Am J Physiol 1980; 238: H457–64.
50. Majno G. Ultrastructure of the vascular membrane. In: Handbook of Physiology-Circulation, Section 2, vol. 3, Williams and Wilkins, Baltimore 1965; pp 2293–376.
51. Majno G, Palade GE. Studies on inflammation. I. The effect of histamine and serotonin on vascular permeability: an electron microscopic study. J Biophys Biochem Cytol 1961; 11: 571–606.
52. Nolph KD. Peritoneal Anatomy and Transport Physiology. In: Maher JF: Replacement of Renal Function by Dialysis [3rd ed]. Kluwer Academic Publishers, Boston 1989; 516–36.
53. Nolph KD, Miller F, Rubin J, Popovich R. New directions in peritoneal dialysis concepts and applications. Kidney Int 1980; 18: S111–6.
54. Flessner MF, Dedrick RL, Schultz JS. A distributed model of peritoneal-plasma transport: theoretical considerations. Am J Physiol 1984; 246: R597–607.
55. Flessner MF, Dedrick RL, Schultz JS. A distributed model of peritoneal-plasma transport: analysis of experimental data in the rat. Am J Physiol 1985; 248: F413–24.
56. Flessner MF, Fenstermacher JD, Dedrick RL, Blasberg RG. A distributed model of peritoneal-plasma transport: tissue concentration gradients. Am J Physiol 1985; 248: F425–35.
57. Stephenson RB. Microcirculation and Exchange. In: Patton HD, Fuchs AF, Hille B, Scher AM, Steiner R (eds), Textbook of Physiology. W. B. Saunders, Philadelphia 1989; pp 911–23.
58. Wade OL, Combes B, Childes AW, Wheeler HO, Dournand D, Bradley SE. The effect of exercise on the splanchnic blood flow and splanchnic blood volume in normal man. Clin Sci 1956; 15: 457.
59. Aune S. Transperitoneal exchange II. Peritoneal blood flow estimated by hydrogen gas clearance. Scand J Gastroent 1970; 5: 99–104.
60. Bulkey GB. Washout of intraperitoneal Xenon: effective peritoneal perfusion as an estimation of peritoneal blood flow. In: Granger DN, Bulkey GB (eds), Measurement of Blood Flow: Application to the splanchnic circulation. Williams and Wilkins, Baltimore 1981; pp 441–53.
61. Nolph KD, Popovich RP, Ghods AJ, Twardowski Z. Determinants of low clearances of small solutes during peritoneal dialysis. Kid Int 1978; 13: 117–23.
62. Erb RW, Greene JA Jr., Weller JM. Peritoneal dialysis during hemorrhagic shock. J Appl Physiol 1967; 22: 131–5.
63. Texter E, Clinton JR. Small intestinal blood flow. Am J Dig Dis 1963; 8: 587–613.
64. Dedrick RL, Flessner MF, Collins JM. Schultz JS. Is the peritoneum a membrane. ASAIO J 1989; 5: 1–8.
65. Miller FN, Nolph KD, Harris PD, Rubin J, Wiegman DL, Joshua IG. Effects of peritoneal dialysis solutions on human clearances and rat arterioles. Trans Am Soc Artif Intern Organs 1978; 24: 131–2.
66. Miller FN, Nolph KD, Harris PD, Rubin J, Wiegman DL, Joshua IG, Twardowski ZJ, Ghods AJ. Microvascular and clinical effects of altered peritoneal dialysis solutions. Kid Int 1979; 15: 630–9.
67. Nolph KD. Effects of intraperitoneal vasodilators on peritoneal clearances. Dial Transpl 1978; 7: 812.
68. Nolph KD, Ghods AJ, Brown PA, Twardowski ZJ. Effects of intraperitoneal nitroprusside on peritoneal clearances with variations in dose, frequency of administration, and dwell times. Nephron 1979; 24: 114–20.

69. Nolph KD, Ghods AJ, Van Stone J, Brown PA. The effects of intraperitoneal vasodilators on peritoneal clearances. Trans Am Soc Artif Intern Organs 1976; 22: 586.
70. Nolph KD, Ghods AJ, Brown PA, Miller FN, Harris P, Pyle K, Popovich R. Effects of nitroprusside on peritoneal mass transfer coefficients and microvascular physiology. Trans Am Soc Artif Intern Organs 1977; 23: 210–8.
71. Grzegorzewska AE, Moore HL, Nolph KD, Chen TW. Ultrafiltration and effective peritoneal blood flow during peritoneal dialysis in the rat. Kid Int 1991; 39: 608–17.
72. Korthuis RJ, Granger DN. Role of the Peritoneal Microcirculation in Peritoneal Dialysis: In: Nolph KD (ed), Peritoneal Dialysis (3rd ed), Kluwer Academic Publishers, Boston, 1989.
73. Granger DN. Richardson PDI, Taylor AE. The effects of isoprenaline and bradykinnin on capillary filtration in the cat small intestine. Br J Pharm 1979; 67: 361–6.
74. Granger DN, Kvietys PR, Wilborn WH, Mortillaro NA, Taylor AE. Mechanisms of glucagon-induced intestinal secretion. Am J physiol 1980; 239: G30–8.
75. Mortillaro NA, Granger DN, Kvietys PR, Rutili G, Taylor AE. Effects of histamine and histamine antagonists on intestinal capillary permeability. Am J Pysiol 1981; 240: G381–6.
76. Granger DN, Perry MA, Kvietys PR, Taylor AE. Permeability of intestinal capillaries: effects of fat absorption and gastrointestinal hormones. Am J Physiol 1982; 242: G194–201.
77. Granger DN, Valleau, JD, Parker RE, Lane RS, Taylor AE. Effects of adenosine on intestinal hemodynamics, oxygen delivery and capillary fluid exchange. Am J Physiol 1978; 235: H707–19.
78. Granger DN, Richardson PDI, Kvietys PR, Mortillaro NA. Intestinal blood flow. Gastroenterology 1980; 78: 837–63.
79. Chou CC, Kvietys PR. Physiological and pharmacological alterations in gastrointestinal blood flow. In: Granger DN, Bulkley GB (eds), Measurement of Blood Flow: Applications to the Splanchnic Circulation. Williams and Wilkins, Baltimore 1981; pp 477–509.
80. Maher JF, Cassetts M, Shea C, Hohnadel DC. Peritoneal dialysis in rabbits. A study of transperitoneal theophylline flux and peritoneal permeability. Nephron 1978; 20: 18–23.
81. Richardson PDI. the effects of glucagon and pentagastrin on capillary filtration coefficient in innervated jejunum of the anesthetized cat. Br J Pharm 1975; 54: 255.
82. Richardson PDI. Pharmacology of intestinal blood flow and oxygen uptake. In: Shepherd AP, Granger DN (eds), Physiology of Intestinal Circulation. Raven, New York 1984; pp 393–402.
83. Hirszel P, Maher JF, LeGrow W. Increased peritoneal mass transport with glucagon acting at the vascular surface. Trans Am Soc Artif Intern Organs 1978; 24: 136–8.
84. Nolph KD. Peritoneal dialysis. In: Brenner BM, Rector FC, Jr. (eds), The Kidney, vol 2. WB Saunders, Philadelphia, pp 1847–1906.
85. Campion DS, North JDK. Effect of protein binding of barbiturates on their rate of removal during peritoneal dialysis. J Lab Clin Med 1965; 66: 549–63.
87. Cole DEC, Lirenman DS. Role of albumin enriched peritoneal dialysate in acute copper poisoning. J Pediatr 1978; 92: 955–77.
88. Etteldorf JN, Dobbins WT, Summit RL, Rainwater WT, Fischer RI. Intermittent peritoneal dialysis using 5% albumin in the treatment of salicylate intoxication in children. J Pediatr 1961; 58: 226–36.
89. Schultz JC, Crouder DG, Medart WS. Excretion studies in ethylchlorovynol (placidil) intoxication. Arch Intern Med 1966; 117: 409–11.
90. El-Bassiouni EA, Mattocks AM. Acceleration of peritoneal dialysis with minimal N-myristyl-B-aminopropionate. J Pharm Sci 1973; 62: 1314–6.
91. Kudla RM, ElBassiouni EA, Mattocks AM. Accelerated peritoneal dialysis of barbiturates, and salicylate. J Pharm Sci 1971; 60: 1065–7.
92. Mattocks AM. Accelerate removal of salicylate by additives in peritoneal dialysis fluid. J Pharm Sci 1969; 58: 595–8.
93. Hirszel P, Lasrich M, Maher JF. Arachidonic acid increases peritoneal clearances. Trans Am Soc Artif Intern Organs 1981; 27: 61–3.
94. Maher JF, Hirszel P, Lasrich M. Effects of gastrointestinal harmones on transport by peritoneal dialysis. Kid Int 1979; 16: 130–6.
95. Lal SM, Nolph KD, Moore HS, Khanna R. Calcium channel blockers enhance urea transport without increasing protein loss. Clin Res 1986; 34: 40.
96. Penzotti SC, Mattocks MA. Acceleration of peritoneal dialysis by surface-acting agents. J Pharm Sci 1968; 57: 1192–5.
97. Maher JF, Hirszel P, Lasrich M. Effects of gastrointestinal hormones on transport by peritoneal dialysis. Kid Int 1979; 16: 130–6.
98. Hirszel P, Dodge K, Maher JF. Acceleration of peritoneal transport by cytochalasin D. Uremia Invest 1984; 8(2): 85.
99. Covey TJ. Ferrous sulfate poisoning: a review, case summaries and therapeutic regimen. J Pediatr 1964; 64: 218–26.
100. Stanbaugh GH Jr, Homes AW, Gillit D. Iron chelation therapy in CAPD: A new effective treatment for iron overload disease in ESRD patients. Perit Dial Bull 1983; 3: 99–103.
101. Williams P, Khanna R, Crapper McLachlan DR. Enhancement of aluminium removal by desferrioxamine in a patient on continuous ambulatory peritoneal dialysis with dementia. Perit Dial Bull 1981; pp 73–7.
102. Knochel JP, Clayton E, Smith WL, Barry KG. Intraperitoneal THAM: An effective method to enhance phenobarbital removal during peritoneal dialysis. J Lab Clin Med 1964; 64: 257–68.
103. Knochel JP. Mason AD. Effect of alkalinization on peritoneal diffusion of uric acid. Am J Physiol 1966; 210: 1160–4.

104. Penzotti SC, Mattocks MA. Acceleration of peritoneal dialysis by surface-acting agents. J Pharm Sci 1968; 57: 1192–5.
105. Mattocks AM, Penzotti SC. Acceleration of peritoneal dialysis with minimum amounts of dioctyl sodium sulfosuccinate. J Pharm Sci 1972; 61: 475–6.
106. Maher JF, Hirszel P, Abraham JE. The effect of dipyridamole on peritoneal mass transport. Trans Am Soc Artif Intern Organs 1977; 23: 219–223.
107. Hare HG, Valtin J, Gosselin RE. Effects of drugs on peritoneal dialysis in the dog. J Pharmacol Exp Ther 1964; 145: 122–9.
108. Shear L, Harvey JD, Barry KG. Peritoneal sodium transport: enhancement by pharmacologic and physical agents. J Lab Clin Med 1966; 67: 181–8.
109. Mehbod H. Treatment of lead intoxication. Combined use of peritoneal dialysis and edentate calcium disodium. JAMA 1967; 201: 972–4.
110. Maher JF, Hohnadel DC, Shea C, SiSanzo F, Cassetts M. Effects of intraperitoneal diuretics on solute transport during hypertonic dialysis. Clin Nephrol 1977; 7: 96–100.
111. Grzegorzewska A. Baczyk K. Furosemide-induced increase in urinary and peritoneal excretion of uric acid during peritoneal dialysis in patients with chronic uremia. Artific Organs 1982; 6: 220–4.
113. Maher JF, Hirszel P, Lasrich M. Effects of gastrointestinal hormones on transport by peritoneal dialysis. Kid Int 1979; 16: 130–6.
114. Nolph KD, Ghods AJ, Brown P, Van Stone JC. Factors affecting peritoneal dialysis efficiency. Dial Transpl 1977; 6: 52–6.
115. Felt J, Richard C, McCaffrey C, Lefy M. Peritoneal clearance of creatinine and inulin during dialysis in dogs. Effect of splanchnic vasodilators. Kid Int 1979; 16: 459–69.
116. Hirszel P, Maher JF, Legrow W. Increased peritoneal mass transport with glucagon acting at the vascular surface. Trans Am Soc Artif Organs 1978; 24: 136–8.
117. Rasio EA. Metabolic control of permeability in isolated mesentery. Am J Physiol 1974; 226: 962–8.
118. Brown EA, Kliger AS, Goffinet J, Finkelstein FO. Effect of hypertonic dialysate and vasodilators on peritoneal dialysis clearances in rats. Kid Int 1978; 13: 271–7.
119. Granger DN, Richardson PDI, Kvietys PR, Mortillaro NA. Intestinal blood flow. Gastroenterology 1980; 78: 837–63.
120. DeSanto NG, Capodicasa G, Capasso G. Development of means to augment peritoneal urea clearances: the synergic effects of combining high dialysate temperature and high dialysate flow rates with dextrose and nitroprusside. Artif Organs 1981; 5: 409–14.
121. Henderson LW, Nolph KD. Altered permeability of the peritoneal membrane after using hypertonic peritoneal dialysis fluid. J Clin Invest 1969; 48: 992–1001.
122. Rasio EA. Metabolic control of permeability in isolated mesentery. Am J physiol 1974; 226: 962–8.
123. Nolph KD, Ghods AJ, Van Stone J, Brown PA. The effects of intraperitoneal vasodilators on peritoneal clearances. Trans Am Soc Artif Intern Organs 1976; 22: 586–94.
124. Brown ST, Aheran DJ, Nolph KD. Reduced peritoneal clearances in scleroderma increased by intraperitoneal isoproterenol. Ann Intern Med 1973; 78: 891–7.
125. Maher JF, Shea C, Cassetta M, Hohnadel DC. Isoproternol enhancement of peritoneal permeability. J Dial 1977; 1: 319–31.
126. Nolph KD, Miller L, Husted FC, Hirszel P. Peritoneal clearances in scleroderma and diabetes mellitus. Effects of intraperitoneal isoproterenol. Int Urol Nephrol 1976; 8: 154–61.
127. Shinaberger JH, Shear L, Clayton LE. Dialysis of intoxication with lipid soluble drugs: enhancement of glutethimide extraction with lipid dialysate. Trans Am Soc Artif Organs 1965; 11: 173–7.
128. Miller FN, Nolph KD, Harris PD. Effects of peritoneal dialysis solutions on human clearances and rat arterioles. Trans Am Soc Artif Intern Organs 1978; 24: 131–2.
129. Nolph KD. Effects of intraperitoneal vasodilators on peritoneal clearances. Dial Transpl 1978; 7: 812.
130. Nolph KD, Ghods AJ, Brown PA, Twardowski ZJ. Effects of intraperitoneal nitroprusside on peritoneal clearances with variations in dose, frequency of administration, and dwell times. Nephron 1979; 24: 114–20.
131. Breborowicz A, Knapowski J. Augmentation of peritoneal dialysis clearances with procaine. Kid Int 1984; 26: 392–6.
132. Maher JF, Hirszel P, Lasrich M. Modulation of peritoneal transport rates by prostaglandins. Adv Prostaglandin Thromboxame Res 1980; 7: 695–700.
133. Hirszel P, Larisch M, Maher JF. Peritoneal transport rates and inhibition of prostaglandin synthetase by mefenamic acid. Abstr Am Soc Artif Intern Organs 1980; 9: 48.
134. Parker HR, Schroeder JP, Henderson LW. Influence of dopamine and Regitine on peritoneal dialysis in unanesthetized dogs. Abstracts Am Soc Artif Int Organs 1978; 7: 43.
135. Alavi N, Lianos E, Andres G. Effect of protamine on the permeability and structure of rat peritoneum. Kidney Int 1982; 21: 44–53.
136. Avasthi PS. Effects of aminonucleoside on rat blood peritoneal barrier permeability. J Lab Clin Med 1979; 94: 295–302.
137. Maher JF, Hirszel P, Lasrich M. An experimental model for study of pharmacologic and hormonal influences on peritoneal dialysis. Contr Nephrol 1979; 17: 131–8.
138. Gutman RA, Nixon WP, McRae RL, Spencer HW. Effect of intraperitoneal and intravenous vasoactive amines on peritoneal dialysis: Study in anephric dogs. Trans Am Soc Artif Intern Organs 1976; 22: 570–3.
139. Hirszel P, Larisch M, Maher JF. Divergent effects of catecholamines on peritoneal mass transport.

Trans Am Soc Artif Intern Organs 1979; 25: 110–3.
140. Brown ST, Aheran DJ, Nolh KD. Reduced peritoneal clearances in scleroderma increased by intraperitoneal isoproterenol. Ann Intern Med 1973; 78: 891–7.
141. Maher JF, Shea C, Cassetta M, Hohnadel DC. Isoproternol enhancement of peritoneal permeability. J Dial 1977; 1: 319–31.
142. Nolph KD, Miller L, Husted FC, Hirszel P. Peritoneal clearances in scleroderma and diabetes mellitus. Effects of intraperitoneal isoproterenol. Int Urol Nephrol 1976; 8: 154–61.
143. Hirszel P, Maher JF, Chamberlin M. Augmented peritoneal mass transport with intraperitoneal nitroprusside. J Dial 1978; 2: 131.
144. Raja RM, Kramer MS, Rosenbaum JL. Enhanced clearance with intraperitoneal nitroprusside in high flow recirculation peritoneal dialysis. Trans Am Soc Artif Int Organs 1978; 24: 133–5.
145. Nolph KD, Rubin J, Wiegman DL, Harris PD, Miller FN. Peritoneal clearances with three types of commercially available peritoneal dialysis solutions. Nephron 1979; 24: 35–40.
146. Miller FN, Joshua IG, Anderson GL. Quantitation of vasodilator – induced macromolecular leakage by in vivo fluorescent microscopy. Microvas Res 1982; 24: 56–7.
147. Miller FN, Nolph KD, Joshua IG, Rubin J. Effects of vasodilators and peritoneal dialysis solution on the microcirculation of the rat cecum. Proc Soc Expt Biol Med 1979; 161: 605–8.
148. Miller FN, Nolph KD, Joshua IG, Weigman DL, Harrid PD, Anderson DB. Hyperosmolality, acetate and lactate: Dilatory factors during peritoneal dialysis. Kid Int 1981; 20: 397–402.
149. Miller FN, Joshua JG, Harris PD, Weigman DL, Jauchem JR. Peritoneal dialysis solutions and the microcirculation. Contr Nephrol 1977; 17: 51–8.
150. Levine SE, Granger DN, Brace RA, Taylor AE. Effect of hyperosmolality on vascular resistance and lymph flow in the cat ileum. Am J Physiol 1978; 234: H14–20.
151. Granger DN, Ulrich M, Perry MA, Kvietys PR. Peritoneal dialysis solutions and splanchnic blood flow. Clin Exp Pharmacol Physiol 1984; 11: 473–83.
152. Vargemezis V, Pasadakis P, Thodis E. Effect of a calcium antagonist (verapamil) in the permeability of the peritoneal membrane in patients on continuous ambulatory peritoneal dialysis. Blood Purif 1989; 7: 309–13.
153. Rubin J, Nolph KD, Popovich RP, Moncrief JW, Prowant B. Drainage volume during continuous ambulatory peritoneal dialysis. Am Soc Artif Int Org 1979; 22: 54–60.
154. Twardowski ZJ, Khanna R, Nolph KD. Osmotic agents and ultrafiltration in peritoneal dialysis. Nephron 1986; 42: 93–101.
155. Maher JF. Peritoneal transport rates: mechanisms, limitation and methods for augmentation. Kid Int 1980; 18: S117–21.
156. Nolph KD, Mactier R, Khanna R, Twardowski ZJ, Moore H, McGary T. The kinetics of ultrafiltration during peritoneal dialysis. Kid Int 1987; 32: 219–26.
157. Pyle WK, Moncrief JW, Popovich RP. Peritoneal transport evaluation in CAPD. In: Moncrief JW, Popovich RP (eds), Proc 2nd Int Symp on CAPD, Masson, New York 1981; pp 35–9.
158. Pyle WK, Popovich RP, Moncrief JW. Mass transfer in peritoneal dialysis. In: Advances in peritoneal dialysis: Proc of the 2nd international symp on peritoneal dialysis. Excerpta Medica, Amsterdam 1981; pp 41–9.
159. Rippe B, Stelin G, Ahlmen J. Lymph flow from the peritoneal cavity in CAPD patients. In: Frontiers in Peritoneal Dialysis. Field, Rich and Associates, New York 1986; 24–30.
160. Curry FE, Frokjaer-Jensen J. Water flow across the walls of single muscle capillaries in the frog, rana pipiens. J Physiol 1984; 350: 293–307.
161. Atherton A, Born GVR. Relationship between the velocity of rolling granulocytes and that of blood flow in venules. J Physiol 1973; 233: 157–65.
162. Granger DN, Benoit JN, Suzuki M, Grisham MB. Leukocyte adherence to venular endothelium during ischemia-reperfusion. Am J Physiol 1989; 257: G683–8.
163. Perry MA, Granger DN. Role of CD11/CD18 in shear rate-dependent leukocyte-endothelial cell interactions in cat mesenteric venules. J Clin Invest 1991; 87: 1798–804.
164. Ley K, Gaehtyens P. Endothelial, not hemodynamic differences are responsible for preferential leukocyte rolling in rat mesenteric venules. Circ Res 1991; 69: 1034–41.
165. Schmid-Schonbein GW, Usami S, Skalak R, Chien S. The interaction of leukocytes and erythrocytes in capillary and post capillary vessels. Microvas Res 1980; 19: 45–70.
166. Bienvenu K, Hernandez L, Granger DN. Leukocyte Adhesion and Emigration in inflammation. Ann New York Acad Sci 1992; 664: 388–99.
167. Tonneson MG. Neutrophil-endothelial cell interactions: mechanisms of neutrophil adherence to vascular endothelium. J Invest Dermatol 1989; 93: 535–85.
168. Kishimoto TK, Jutila MA, Bery EL, Butcher EC. Neutrophil Mac-1 and MEL-14 adhesion proteins are inversely regulated by chemotactic factors. Science 1989; 245: 1238–41.
169. Bevilagua MP. Strengelin S, Gimbrone MA, Seed B. Endothelial leukocyte adhesion molecule 1: an inducible receptor for neutrophils related to complement regulatory proteins and lectins. Science 1989; 243: 1160–5.
170. McEver RP. Selectins: Novel adhesion receptors that mediate leukocyte adhesion during inflammation. Thromb Haem 1991; 65: 223–8.
171. Smith GW. Molecular determinants of neutrophil-endothelial cell adherence reactions. Am J Respir Cell Molec Biol 1990; 2: 487–99.
172. Springer T, Anderson DC, Rosenthal, Rothelein R. Leukocyte Adhesion Molecules. Springer-Verlag New York, 1989.

173. Kishimoto TK. A dynamic model for neutrophil localization to inflammatory sites. J NIH Res 1991; 3: 75–7.
174. House SD, Lipowsky JJ. Leukocyte-endothelium adhesion: microhemodynamics in mesentery of the cat. Microvas. Res. 1987; 34: 363–79.
175. Engler RL, Schmid-Schonbein, Pavelec RS. Leukocyte capillary plugging in myocardial ischemia and reperfusion in the dog. Am J Pathol 1983; III: 98–111.
176. Worthen GS, Schwab B, Elson EL, Downey OP. Cellular mechanics of stimulated neutrophils: stiffening of cells induces retention in pores in vitro and lung capillaries in vivo. Science 1989; 245: 183–6.
177. Carden DL, Smith JK, Korthuis RJ. Neutrophil-mediated microvascular dysfunction in postischemic canine skeletal muscle: role of granulocyte adherence. Circ Res 1990; 66: 1436–44.
178. Harlan JM. Leukocyte-endothelial cell interactions. Blood 1985; 65: 513–25.
179. Leter AM. Significance of lipid mediators in shock states. Circ Shock 1989; 37: 3–12.
180. Bjork J, Lindbom L, Gerdin B, Smedegard G, Arfors KE, Benveniste J. PAF-acether [platelet-activating factor] increases microvascular permeability and affects endothelium-granulocyte interactions in microvascular beds. Acta Physiol Scand 1983; 119: 305–8.
181. Dahlen SE, Bjork J, Hedqvist P, Arfors KE, Hammarstrom S, Lindgren JA, Samuelsson B. Leukotrienes promote plasma leakage and leukocyte adhesion in postcapillary venules: In vivo effects with relevance to the acute inflammatory response. Proc Natl Acad Sci USA 1981; 78: 3887–91.
182. Braquet P, Touqui L, Shen TV, Vargafting BB. Perspectives in platelet activating factor research. Pharmacol Rev 1987; 39: 97–145.
183. Kubes P, Suzuki M, Granger DN. Platelet activating factor – induced microvascular dysfunction: role of adherent leukocytes. Am J Physiol 1990; 258: G158–63.
184. Kubes P, Grisham MB, Barrowman JA, Gaginella T, Granger DN. Leukocyte – induced protein leakage in cat mesentery. Am J Physiol 1991; 261: H1872–9.
185. Bjork J. Hagli TE, Smedegard G. Microvascular effects of anaphylatoxin C3a and C5a. J Immunol 1985; 134: 1115–9.
186. Weiss S. Oxygen, ischemia and inflammation. Acta Physiol Scand 1986; 126 (supp 584): 9–38.
187. Weiss SJ. Tissue destruction by neutrophils. NEJM 1989; 320: 365–76.
188. Reilly PM, Schiller HJ, Bulkley GB. Pharmacological approach to tissue injury by free radicals and other reactive oxygen metabolites. Am J Surg 1991; 161: 488–503.
189. Suzuki M, Asako H, Kubes P, Jennings S, Grisham MB, Granger DN. Neutrophil derived oxidants promote leukocyte adherence in postcapillary venules. Microvasc Res 1991; 42: 125–38.
190. Kubes P, Suzuki M, Granger DN. Modulation of PAF – induced leukocyte adherence and increased microvascular permeability. Am J Physiol 1990; 259: G858–64.
191. Kubes P, Suzuki M, Granger DN. Modulation of PAF – induced leukocyte adherence and increased microvascular permeability. Am J Physiol 1990; 259: G858–64.
192. Zeillemaker AM, Hoynck van Papendrecht AAGM, Roos D, Leguit P. Neutrophil adherence and migration through human mesothelial monolayers (abstract). Peritoneal Dial Int 1993; 13 (supp 1): s30.
193. Duwe AK, Vas SI, Weatherhead JW. Effects of the composition of peritoneal dialysis fluid on chemiluminescence, phagocytosis, and bactericidal activity in vitro. Infection and Immunity 1981; 33: 130–5.
194. H van Bronswijk, Verbrugh HA, Heezius HCJM, J van der Meulen, Oe PL, Verhoef J. Dialysis fluids and local host resistance in patients on continuous ambulatory peritoneal dialysis. Eur J Clin Microbiol Infect Dis 1988; 7: 368–73.
195. Verbrugh HA, Keane WF, Hoidal JR, Freiberg MR, Elliott GR, Peterson PK. Peritoneal macrophages and opsonins: antibacterial defense in patients undergoing chronic peritoneal dialysis. J. of Infectious Diseases 1983; 6: 1018–29.
196. Lewis S, Holmes C. Host defense mechanisms in the peritoneal cavity of continuous ambulatory peritoneal dialysis patients. Peritoneal Dialysis Int 1991; 11: 14–21.
197. White R, Work J, Korthius R. The effect of a hypertonic peritoneal dialysis solution on leukocyte adhesion to postcapillary venules in the rat mesentery (abstract). FASEB J 1993; A343: 1985.

4 Peritoneal physiology-transport of solutes

BENGT RIPPE AND RAYMOND THEODORUS KREDIET

1. Introduction 69
2. The peritoneum as a dialysis membrane 70
  2.1. The surface area of the peritoneal membrane 70
  2.2. Functional characteristics of the capillary endothelium 71
  2.3. The peritoneal interstitium 74
  2.4. The peritoneal lymphatic system 75
  2.5. The mesothelium 75
3. Physiology of solute transport during peritoneal dialysis 76
  3.1. Membrane models vs. distributed models 76
  3.2. Diffusive transport 76
  3.3. Diffusive and convective transport 77
  3.4. Determination of PS (MTAC) 78
  3.5. Transperitoneal ultrafiltration and osmosis (convection) 79
  3.6. Restricted diffusion 80
  3.7. Restricted convection and theory for the reflection coefficient 81
  3.8. Role of electric charge 81
4. Parameters of solute transport from the blood to the peritoneal cavity 82
  4.1. D/P ratios 82
  4.2. Peritoneal clearance 83
  4.3. Obtaining transport parameters in patients 84
5. Interpretation of peritoneal PS (MTAC) or clearance values 85
  5.1. Solute MTAC (PS) and clearance as related to solute molecular weight 85
  5.2. Three-pore model 86
  5.3. A three-pore (capillary) membrane series-coupled with an interstitial diffusion resistance 90
  5.4. Conditions of increased capillary permeability 92
  5.5. Electrolyte transport 92
  5.6. Individual characterization of surface area and intrinsic permeability 92
6. Solute transport from the peritoneal cavity 95
  6.1. Low molecular weight solutes 95
  6.2. Macromolecules 96
7. The regulation of surface area and permeability 97
8. Peritoneal permeability in system diseases 100
  8.1. Uremia 100
  8.2. Diabetes mellitus 100
  8.3. Systemic lupus erythematosus 100
  8.4. Systemic sclerosis 100
  8.5. Amyloidosis and paraproteinemia 100
9. Solute transport during peritonitis 101
  9.1. Low molecular weight solutes 101
  9.2. Macromolecules 101
  9.3. Sclerosing encapsulating peritonitis 102
10. Solute transport during long-duration peritonitis dialysis 102
Acknowledgements 104
References 104

1. Introduction

The peritoneal cavity, which lodges the abdominal viscera, represents the largest serosal cavity in the body. Functionally it may be regarded as a large continuous interstitial space. It is lined by a thin, translucent membrane, the peritoneum, which covers the inner surface of the abdominal wall (parietal peritoneum) and the majority of visceral organs (visceral peritoneum) and which forms omenta. The lining structure of the peritoneal cavity is usually denoted the 'peritoneal membrane'. Because of its relatively large surface area (1-2 m^2 in adults) [1], its high dregree of capillarization and relatively high blood flow, it can be rather effectively utilized as an endogenous dialysis membrane to remove uremic toxins and water from the body fluids of patients with end-stage renal disease during peritoneal dialysis (PD). The peritoneal cavity is also suitable as a portal entry for various drugs and hormones administered intraperitoneally (i.p.). In peritonitis (during PD), for example, antibiotics can be given i.p. for systemic use, because of the high transport capacity of the peritoneal membrane.

In this treatise we will discuss the basic mechanisms underlying the transport of small solutes, macromolecules and fluid between the blood capillaries and the peritoneal cavity. These rather complex processes involve peritoneal transport pathways arranged in parallel and in series, i.e. mainly the capillary walls coupled in series with the interstitium. The presence of a rather large peritoneal interstitium with a relative sparsity of lymph vessels, causes among other things an asymmetry in bidirectional transport of macromolecules between the blood and the peritoneal cavity. This will be discussed at some length. We will also discuss peritoneal exchange in various pathophysiological and disease states.

2. The peritoneum as a dialysis membrane

What we commonly denote 'the peritoneal membrane' is a complex structure comprising at least three sequential anatomical layers: (1) The peritoneal and mesenteric capillary walls with their surrounding basement membranes, (2) the interstitium and (3) the highly permeable mesothelium. Of these barriers we will mainly focus on the capillary walls, which serve as a major exchange barrier between the blood and the interstitium. At first, however, we will consider the peritoneal membrane exchange surface area and what portions of the peritoneum take part in the transperitoneal exchange.

2.1. The surface area of the peritoneal membrane

During peritoneal dialysis the surface area of the peritoneal exchange vessels, i.e. the capillaries (diameter 5–6 µm) and the so-called postcapillary venules (diameter 7–20 µm) mainly determine the peritoneal exchange capacity when there is no blood flow limitation of exchange. Somehow the *capillary* surface area should be related to the *total* surface of the peritoneal membrane. Only a few measurements of this parameter have been performed previously, the first measurements being published by Wegener [2]. Putiloff [3], who assessed the parietal and visceral peritoneal surface area of an infant (weight 2.9 kg) and an adult (70 kg) post mortem, found that the peritoneal surface area per unit body weight was about two-fold larger in the infant than in the adult (522 cm^2/kg and 284 cm^2/kg, respectively). More recent measurement [1] have essentially confirmed these results, although the total surface area per kg body weight was found to be lower. In adults an average value of 1.04 m^2 was determined. Esperanca and Collins [1] found that only 10 per cent of the total surface area was parietal, whereas 90 per cent was either visceral, omental or hepatic. The same results were obtained in a recent study by Rubin *et al.* [4], who pointed out that the peritoneal surface area in man seems to correspond to only 40–50 per cent of the body surface area. In the same study the peritoneal surface area of Sprague-Dawley rats was also measured. The rats were shown to have a higher peritoneal surface area than predicted from their body surface area, i.e., from scaling their body surface area (from man) using (body weight)$^{0.67}$.

It should be pointed out that it is the *functional*, not the anatomical, peritoneal surface area that is of importance in peritoneal exchange. The functional surface area relates to the capillary density and to the spatial arrangements of capillaries in the peritoneal interstitium. Removing the visceral peritoneum in animal experiments has been shown to just minimally reduce the glucose absorption rate from the peritoneal cavity [5]. Furthermore, Rubin *et al.* have demonstrated that the absorption of urea, creatinine and inulin decreases only slightly, if at all, following evisceration [6]. The situation may be different in other species. Bell *et al.* [7] found considerably lower values for the transport rates of creatinine and para-aminohippuric acid in eviscerated rabbits than those in intact animals reported by the same group [8]. In a recent study Fox *et al.* showed that this reduction in transport rate could be prevented by the application of circumferential abdominal compression [9]. The contribution of the visceral peritoneum to solute transport in humans is not known, but effective peritoneal dialysis has been described in an infant with acute renal failure after virtually complete resection of the small intestine [10]. It may therefore be that the effective (functional) capillary surface area is actually much higher in the parietal peritoneum than in the visceral, i.e. the density of capillaries (and postcapillary venules) that can exchange with the peritoneal surface is much higher in the parietal than in the visceral peritoneum.

The functional surface area of the peritoneal membrane cannot be measured directly, only the functional cross sectional exchange pore area divided by the effective diffusion path length ($A_0/\Delta x$) (see below). This parameter is in the order of ~25,000 cm in PD as measured for the whole series-coupled capillary-interstitial barrier [11, 12]. Let us assume that the Δx in the expression $A_0/\Delta x$ is actually referring only to the capillary wall thickness (and much less to the thickness of the whole peritoneal membrane). Then, for a capillary wall thickness of 0.4 µm (see below) one would calculate an A_0 (i.e., an 'unrestricted' cross sectional pore area) of ~1cm^2, when setting $A_0/\Delta x$ at 25,000 cm. This pore area corresponds to an approximately total *capillary* wall surface area which is 10^3 times larger [13]. In turn, this corresponds to the anatomical capillary surface area that is found in 10 g (10 cm^3 of skeletal muscle [14, 15]. Let us assume that the total peritoneal surface area is 1 m^2 in adults and that 10 per cent of the total surface area is parietal, the visceral portion being of little importance for total exchange. If the capillary density in the tissue underlying the mesothelium would be the same as in muscle, then the thickness of such a tissue having a surface area of 1000 cm^2 would need to be 100 μm (corresponding to 10 cm^3 of tissue) to account for the exchange seen in CAPD, provided that there are no diffusion resistances in the interstitium. As we will discuss later, however, the interstitium is not freely permeable to solutes. The transport resistance in the interstitium is at least 10-fold higher than that in a pure water solution. The overall $A_0/\Delta x$ measured for the entire peritoneal membrane may thus be considerably lower than the *capillary* $A_0/\Delta x$ (see below). Therefore, a considerably *larger* portion of the peritoneal (parietal) tissue than that having a thickness of 0–100 μm must normally take part in peritoneal exchange [16].

2.2. Functional characteristics of the capillary endothelium

Of the three major anatomical structures that a solute has to pass on its way between the blood and peritoneal cavity, the continuous capillary endothelium and the interstitium represent the most important functional barriers. The capillary membrane restricts solute exchange to less than 0.1 per cent of the total capillary wall surface area (small pores, see below). Furthermore, solutes larger than glucose are restricted in their transport across the permeable pathways ('pores') in the capillary wall, although the interstitium will markedly modify the degree of restricted diffusion of small solutes across the capillary-interstitial barrier.

The microvascular exchange vessels comprise both true capillaries (diameter 5–6 μm) and so-called postcapillary venules (diameter 7–20 μm). Electron microscopy of microvessels has revealed that the two distinct types of capillary endothelium exists: 'continuous' and 'fenestrated'. Continuous capillaries are found in skin, muscle, lung and connective tissue, such as in the peritoneal membrane. In continuous capillary walls, endothelial cells form a continuous layer, surrounded by a basement membrane (Fig. 1a). Although the cells are considerably flattened, the luminal and abluminal endothelial plasmalemmal membranes (cell membranes) are always separated by a thin layer of cytoplasm. The plasmalemma is enwrapped in a negatively charged 'slimy' layer, the so-called glycocalyx. The cytoplasm is rich in mitochondria, rough and smooth endoplasmatic reticulum, Golgi apparatus and other organelles. The dominating cytoplasmic feature is, however, a large number of endoplasmic vesicles ('plasmalemmal vesicles'). Recent electron microscopic studies using ultrathin serial sectioning, have shown that the majority of these structures, usually envisioned as 'free vesicles' in routine electron microscopy, actually represent parts of complex invaginations from either the luminal or abluminal endothelial surface. Only one per cent are truly *free* vesicles [17, 18]. Occasionally, channels may be formed by random confluences of vesicles or invaginations [18], but such channels are extremely rare, and even considered to be absent in *true* capillaries [19].

The endothelial plasmalemma (cell membrane) is permeable to lipid soluble species (such as O_2 and CO_2) and to some extent also to water [20–22] through ultra-small pores (radius 2–4Å). These ultra-small pores may be specialized (water) channels, probably represented by certain 28 kD intramembrane proteins [23]. The major transcapillary exchange route for water and for small solutes is, however, through the clefts between endothelial cells, commonly denoted 'small pores', with a functional 'equivalent' radius of 40–55Å [for review see 14, 22, 24]. The interendothelial cleft is for most of its length 150–200Å wide. On separate points between the luminal and abluminal surface, the cleft is narrowed and the outer leaflets of the adjacent cell membranes here seem to fuse. The three-dimensional cleft structure has recently been revealed by serial section electron microscopy [25]. Membrane fusions were demonstrated to show branching irregular strands on the junctional surface of the endothelial cell, occasionally interrupted by discontinuities (Fig. 1b). These discontinuities are approximately 60–80Å wide. Water and small solutes up to the size of albumin are able to pass between these junctional strands and via their small discontinuities, whereas solutes larger than ~50Å in radius apparently are excluded from this paracellular pathway.

How macromolecules pass the endothelium has been a matter of much controversy over the last few decades [26]. Ever since the discovery of plasmalemmal vesicles in endothelium, vesicles have been postulated to take part in the bulk transport of large solutes across the endothelial barrier

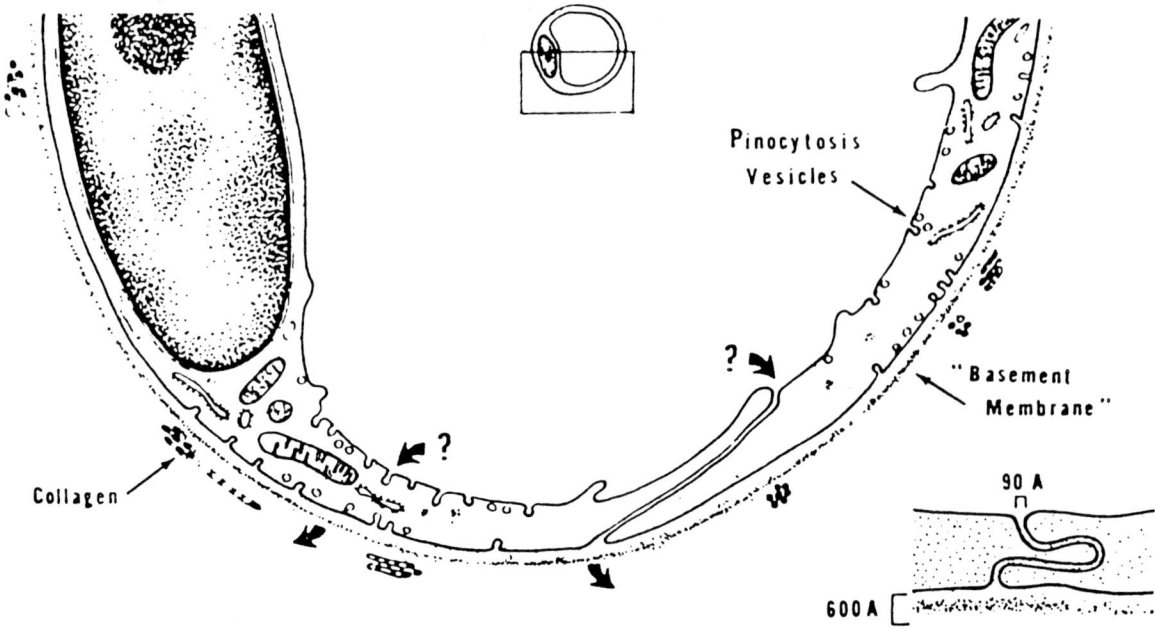

Figure 1a. Schematic drawing of a continuous capillary wall [from 14].

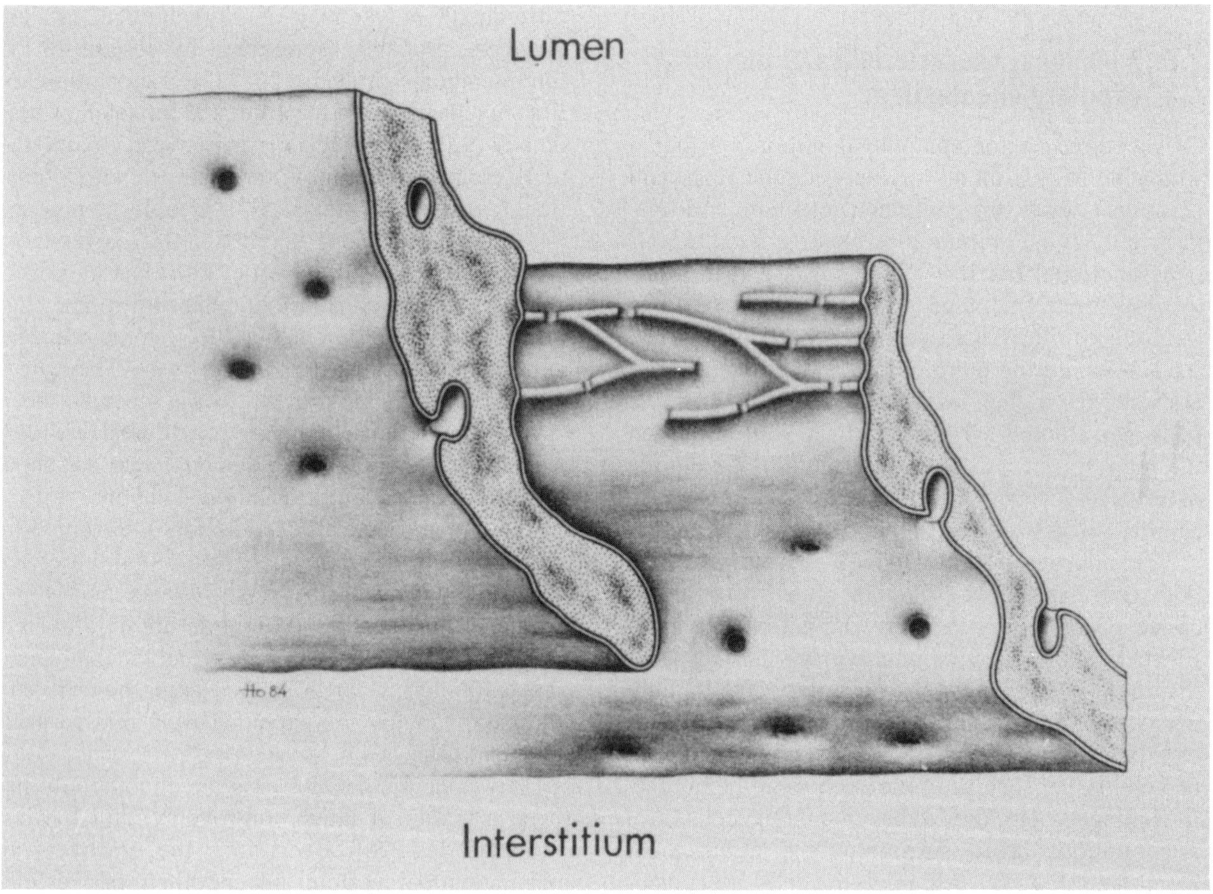

Figure 1b. A three-dimensional reconstruction of an interendothelial slit (cleft) in continuous endothelium [from 25].

by 'cytopempsis' or 'transcytosis' [27–29]. However, according to several recent studies transcytosis may not significantly contribute to the overall transport of macromolecules between blood and tissue [26, 30–32]. Actually, the bulk of evidence seems to favour passive transport of macromolecules across so-called large pores with a radius of ~250Å [33]. these large pores are probably modified interendothelial clefts and constitute only one part per 30,000 of the small pores.

The evidence in support of large pore transport is based on physiological studies of the sieving characteristics of the blood-interstitial barrier and the blood-lymph barrier performed in a variety of microvascular beds [24, 30–35]. Although it is generally assumed that the transport of macromolecules occurs through a 'large pore system', it is still under debate whether convection or diffusion is the main mechanism during peritoneal dialysis. If large pores exist, then the mechanism of protein transport should be convection directed from blood to the peritoneal cavity [24, 30–35]. However, a study using peritoneal dialysis with protein containing dialysate has suggested diffusion as a major mechanism for transperitoneal protein transport [36].

In summary, the bulk of experimental evidence favours the existence of at least two different exchange pathways across the capillary wall; one transcellular (or ultra-small pore) pathway available for water exchange, but excluding solutes, and another paracellular pathway available for fluid and for small solutes up to the size of albumin. In addition, there seems to be a pathway available for macromolecules being > 50 Å in radius, probably represented by specialized paracellular pores ('gaps') with a large radius, or alternatively, by channels formed by fused plasmalemmal vesicles. This three-pore model of capillary permeability is illustrated in Fig. 2. Crystalloid osmosis (such as induced by small solutes) is very effective across the water-exclusive pores. Across small pores,

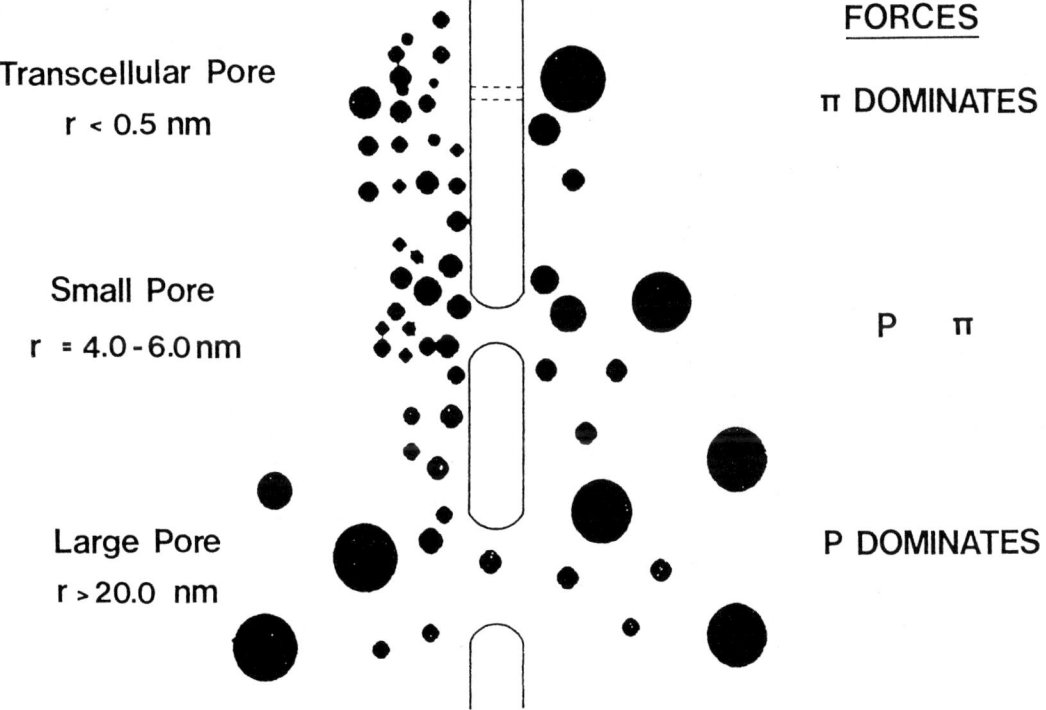

Figure 2. The three-pore model of capillary permselectivity [from 16]. The 'small pores' (interendothelial slits) is the dominant transcapillary pathway for small water soluble solutes and water. Across these pores the so-called Starling equilibrium (the balance between hydrostatic and colloid osmotic pressures) is established, where hydrostatic pressure (ΔP) usually slightly outweights the effective colloid osmotic pressure ($\alpha_{prot} \Delta\pi_{prot}$). Normally around 40–50 per cent of the total transcapillary ultrafiltration rate (lymph flow) occurs through large pores, where hydrostatic pressure dominates over the effective colloid osmotic pressure gradient, which is here very low. Approximately 85–90 per cent of the ultrafiltration coefficient (L_pS) is accounted for by small pores, and 5–10 per cent by large pores. In addition a few per cent of the total UF coefficient is accounted for by transcellular pores having a radius less than 5Å. Crystalloid osmotic gradients are very efficient through these pores. However, they normally play an insignificant role in transcapillary exchange, because normally there are just negligible differences in crystalloid osmotic pressure between plasma and the interstitium.

colloid osmotic and hydrostatic pressures are in balance (cf. Starling equilibrium), where however, the hydrostatic pressure normally slightly outweighs the effective colloid osmotic pressure gradient, causing some net fluid filtration from blood to tissue. Across the large pores colloid osmotic forces are of negligible significance in comparison to hydrostatic pressure gradients, and in these pores there is normally always (slight) filtration from blood to tissue. If there is no *net* UF, there will be recirculation of fluid from large pores (filtering plasma from blood to tissue) to small pores (absorbing essentially protein free fluid from tissue to blood).

2.3. The peritoneal interstitium

The interstitium is usually envisioned as a two-phase system [37–39] of gel and sol, the two phases being in equilibrium with each other. The colloid-rich phase consists of mucopolysacharides, mostly (mobile) hyaluronan and (fixed) proteoglycans (the combination of glycosaminoglycan and protein). The free fluid phase is interspaced between areas of the colloid-rich phase. Water and small solutes may easily enter the colloid-rich phase, whereas macromolecules are partly 'excluded' from this compartment. The total exclusion of albumin in skin, for example, is approximately 50 per cent, but decreases with increasing tissue hydration [39].

Recent studies of the interstitium in transilluminated mesentery demonstrate a remarkably high degree of inhomogeneity of the interstitium [40]. Some regions appeared to be practically devoid of plasma proteins, while other regions contained 'tunnels' of interstitial fluid having a protein concentration of about two thirds of that of plasma. The overall concentration of plasma proteins in the (mesenteric) interstitium was calculated to be ~10 g/l, but corrected for the concentration in the 'available' space, it was as high as 40 g/l, or more than half of the plasma protein concentration. The bulk of data available thus indicates that the interstitium may be regarded as a gel, penetrated by more or less continuous channels of free fluid. Such a gel may act as a gel chromatographic column [41]. Here, smaller macromolecules would have longer transit times across the tissue ('column') than larger, reflecting a larger volume of distribution of the smaller than the larger macromolecules.

The physiology of the interstitial space was recently reviewed in general terms [39] and also with special reference to the peritoneum [16].

Flessner pointed out that the interstitial effective diffusivity of solutes is at least one order of magnitude lower than in free solution, mostly due to the tortuosity of the free fluid phase and solute interactions with the colloid rich phase [43]. He also argued very convincingly against the impact of 'unstirred' or 'stagnant' fluid layers on total transport resistance, because the solute diffusivity in the tissue space is much lower than that in stagnant fluid layers. It could be calculated that only ~1 µm of interstitial depth would have the same impact as a 300 µm thick layer of 'stagnant fluid'. The interendothelial cleft in the capillary wall may be regarded as part of the interstitium as well, where diffusion is affected by volume exclusion, tortuosity, etc. Such effects are, however, incorporated into the 'equivalent pore' concept (see below).

For a full description of transperitoneal transport *both* the capillary wall and the interstitium must be taken into account (see below). Flessner et al. [43–46] have assessed experimentally (and by computer simulation) solute concentration profiles in the interstitium, of visceral and parietal peritoneum and the underlying tissue in muscle and visceral and parietal peritoneum and the underlying tissue in muscle and visceral organs, respectively, as a function of distance from the serosal surface. The measurements (and calculations) were performed for solute transport in the direction from plasma to the interstitium or *vice versa*. There is a fundamental difference in tissue solute concentration profiles depending on the direction of driving forces. For peritoneal-to-blood transport, rather steep solute concentration gradients build up in visceral organs from the peritoneal surface down to a depth of 700–800 µm from the serosal surface. In parietal organs the steepest portion of the tissue concentration vs. depth profile curve is established during the first 100–200 µm of tissue depth (below the serosal surface), after which tissue concentration profiles are rather flat. This may indicate that convection plays an important role in parietal tissue transport in the peritoneal-to-blood direction. With regard to the transport from the plasma to the peritoneal cavity, very flat tissue concentration curves are obtained throughout the interstitium except near the serosal surface. Concerning tissue concentration profiles for macromolecules, there are even greater differences between visceral and parietal organs than outlined here. At 120 minutes after the i.p. injection of bovine serum albumin (BSA) in the rat, tracer albumin had distributed at a concentration identical to that in the peritoneal cavity throughout a tissue depth of 1,000 μm from the serosal surface in parietal muscles and the diaphragm. In small intestine and liver there was, however, a rather significant drop in concentration as a function of 'depth' of the tissue from the serosal surface. A tissue concentration as high as the peritoneal concentration implies that tracer is actually concentrated several times in the free tissue fluid spaces, as compared to the concentration in free dialysate. convective transport of fluid and colloid tracer causing a concentration-hyperpolarization effect may explain this phenomenon. This may occur if the fluid accompanying the tracer albumin is taken up by the capillaries, due to colloid osmosis (see below) and if tracer albumin is left in regions of the interstitial tissue, which are only slowly exchanging with the capillaries and the peritoneal cavity.

The compliance of the interstitial space is bimodal [39]. The interstitial pressure is normally thought to be slightly negative [47]. In the negative pressure range, the compliance of the interstitium is low. However, during PD, the peritoneal cavity pressure is positive, which may also hold for the interstitial hydrostatic pressure. In this situation there is a high compliance of the interstitial space [39]. Thus, the peritoneal tissue can sustain edema formation without the hydrostatic pressure rising significantly. In the positive pressure range, the interstitium of the peritoneal 'membrane' (tissue) may therefore act as a variable depot of fluid, which can increase its volume considerably for moderate changes in tissue pressure.

In summary, the interstitium may be regarded as a two-phase system of gel and sol, where free fluid channels permeate the more colloid rich phase in a complex fashion. Macromolecules are restricted to a much smaller interstitial volume than smaller molecules, due to the mechanism of 'exclusion'. The tissue diffusivity of solutes is smaller than in free fluid, mainly due to tortuosity effects and solute interactions with the colloid rich phase. Interstitial transport of small solutes is dominated by diffusion, while convective forces appear to be of importance in parietal tissues and dominate the transport of macromolecules. The capillary wall determines the amount of solute transported to the interstitium. for a full description of transperitoneal transport *both* interstitial transport barriers and capillary wall resistances should be taken into account. Finally, the interstitium has a high compliance. This implies that large amounts of fluid can accumulate in the peritoneal interstitium without large elevations in interstitial hydrostatic pressure, and that small pressure gradients directed from the peritoneal cavity to the interstitium can effectively move large amounts of fluid into the interstitial compartment.

2.4. The peritoneal lymphatic system

The lymphatic drainage of the peritoneal cavity occurs primarily via lymphatic vessels located in the subdiaphragmatic peritoneum [47, 48]. Absorption by lymphatic capillaries within the interstitium of the mesentery, omentum and the rest of the visceral and peritoneal peritoneum only contributes a relatively minor proportion to the total peritoneal lymphatic drainage. In the subdiaphragmatic region terminal lymphatic lacunae are separated from the peritoneal cavity only by thin mesothelial cells. Between these cells there are 'gaps' (so-called von Recklinghausen's stomata), through which particles up to the size of erythrocytes seem to be able to enter the subdiaphragmatic lymphatic system, to be further transported via retrosternal lymphatics and the right lymphatic duct to the blood [48, 49]. Lymphatic absorption implies bulk drainage of fluid and macromolecules into the blood, which is size independent [50]. The matter of magnitude of the absorption of intraperitoneally administered macromolecules into the lymphatic system and into the peritoneal tissue is controversial. Daugirdas *et al.* [51] administered radio-labelled serum albumin (RISA) dissolved in 1.5 to 2 liters normal saline in nine patients with chronic renal failure. they found that 17% of it had disappeared after seven hours, but that only 24% of the absorbed amount could be recovered in the plasma. Similar results were obtained in ten CAPD patients using 1.36 per cent glucose dialysate [52]. Hence, the rate of elimination of colloids from the peritoneal cavity is about four to five times higher [53–55] than the appearance rate of colloids in the systemic circulation [51, 52, 56, 57]. This is further discussed in Chapter 5.

2.5. The mesothelium

The mesothelium reduces the friction between the visceral organs by continually secreting lubricant and by providing the peritoneum with a smooth surface. It appears as a continuous layer of flattened, elongated cells. The mesothelial cell thickness ranges between 0.6 and 2 μm. The luminal aspect of the mesothelial cell plasmalemma has numerous cytoplasmic extensions, so-called microvilli, the distribution of which varies, or may be even absent [58]. The plasmalemma of mesothelial cells shows (like that of the endothelial cells) a negatively charged glycocalyx. Similar to endothelial cells the cytoplasm is rich in intracellular organelles, and also in plasmalemmal vesicles. There is good evidence that the latter represent just invaginations from the cell surface, enhancing the cell surface area, and that they do not take part in transcytosis [19]. In the cytoplasm there are also numerous so-called lamellar bodies (Weibel-Palade bodies) containing phospholipid surfactant that can be released by exocytosis. The excretion of phospholipid surfactant appears similar to that seen in type II pneumocytes [58].

As we recently reviewed [16] the mesothelium seems to offer very little resistance to transport of small and large solutes across the peritoneal membrane. Especially *in vitro* measurements of transport across mesentric tissue have given extremely high values of mesothelial permeabilities [59, 60]. Studies on protein absorption from the peritoneal cavity to the peritoneal tissue have demonstrated that protein is absorbed at the same rate as water and that there are hardly no concentration gradients across the mesothelial layer [45, 46]. Indeed, in physiological studies of capillary permeability of single mesenteric microvessels, the mesothelium has not been regarded as a significant transport barrier between the superfusate medium and the capillaries in the mesentery [13, 21, 61].

3. Physiology of solute transport during peritoneal dialysis

3.1. Membrane models vs. distributed models

The peritoneum is a complex structure having parallel exchange pathways as well as transport resistances coupled in series. To adequately model the transport processes determining solute and fluid exchange between the blood and the peritoneal cavity, all pathways and resistances have to be taken into account. The combination of a distributed exchange model [16, 43, 44] and a parallel pathway model would be ideal to describe peritoneal exchange [62]. In this treatise, however, we will use a (modified) 'membrane concept' because of its simplicity. Such an approach may be reasonably accurate to model the blood-to-peritoneal transport.

However, when modelling peritoneal-to-blood exchange the simple membrane model is inadequate, and a distributed model would be far more accurate.

In membrane models of peritoneal exchange a single membrane is assumed to separate two well-mixed pools, the blood compartment and the peritoneal cavity compartment, respectively. The solute concentration in the blood compartment is usually assumed to stay constant over the dwell time. The mathematics describing the exchange through a single membrane is simple and straight-forward and can be easily handled on an ordinary pocket computer. Distributed model approaches are far more complicated and require much more data power for their application [43, 44, 62]. Applying the single membrane model one usually models permeability characteristics in terms of sizes and relative numbers of 'equivalent pores' and also of parameters linked to the membrane surface area and permeability [63]. According to the membrane concept the peritoneal dialysis system is compared with an artificial membrane having cylindrical, fluid filled pores, penetrating the membrane at right angles. Equivalent pores can be of several different discrete radii and relative frequencies. The equivalent pore concept has been particularly useful in capillary physiology, where it has been employed to describe the three main pathways available for the passage of solutes and water across the capillary membrane, i.e. the water-exclusive ultra-small pores (radius 2–4Å), the interendothelial slits, i.e., the regular 'small pores' (radius 40–55Å) and the 'large pores' (radius 200–300Å) [22, 24, 26, 31–35, 63].

3.2. Diffusive transport

Transport of solutes between the blood and the peritoneal cavity follows two major principles: diffusion and convection. *Diffusive transport* through a membrane is driven by the difference in solute concentration on either side of the membrane and occurs in the direction of the electrochemical (concentration) gradient. If solute transport is unrestricted (free), the rate of solute transfer (J_s) is proportional to the driving concentration gradient, ΔC, the solute's diffusion constant (D), to the surface area available for diffusion (A) and inversely proportional to the diffusion distance (μx) according to Fick's first law of diffusion:[1]

---

[1] The terminology used in this section is in principle that recommended by the American Physiological Society [64].

$$J_s = \frac{D}{\Delta x} \cdot A\Delta C. \qquad (1a)$$

The diffusion constant is inversely proportional to the solute radius. This follows from the definition of D:

$$D = \frac{RT}{6\pi \cdot N \cdot a_e \cdot \eta} = \frac{k}{a_e} \qquad (2)$$

where a_e refers to the solute radius and RT is the product of the gas constant and the temperature in degrees Kelvin and N is Avagadro's number, while η is water viscosity (here set to 0.007 dyn·sec·cm^{-2}). Thus, D is inversely proportional to A_e, the proportionality constant (k) being $3.3 \cdot 10^{-5}$ at 37°C. For glucose, having a solute radius of 3.67Å, $D = 9 \cdot 10^{-6}$ (cm^2·sec^{-1}), while albumin (radius 35.5Å) has a diffusion coefficient of $9.3 \cdot 10^{-7}$ cm^2·sec^{-1} at 37°C.

The ratio of the solute's diffusion constant to the effective diffusion distance is named permeability (P). The product of permeability and surface area is usually denoted 'permeability surface area product' (PS), or in conjunction with dialysis, 'mass transfer area coefficient' (MTAC). If the uphill solute concentration is denoted C_B and the downhill concentration denoted C_D, then according to Fick's first law of diffusion we have:

$$J_s = \frac{D}{\Delta x} A (C_B - C_D) = PS (C_B - C_D). \qquad (1b)$$

3.3. Diffusion and convective transport

Solute can also be moved by *convective* forces. The magnitude of solute *convection* is determined by the rate of ultrafiltration (UF) occurring through the permeable membrane pathways (J_v), the average solute concentration existing in the membrane during UF ($\overline{C}$) and the solute sieving coefficient (S). The sieving coefficient is defined as the downhill concentration divided by the uphill concentration at the prevailing UF rate when diffusion is negligible. In iso-porous membranes the sieving coefficient equals $(1 - \sigma)$, where σ is the so-called reflection coefficient of the membrane.[2] The combination of diffusion and convection can be described by so-called phenomenological equations [65] as:

$$J_s = PS (C_B - C_D) + J_v \overline{C} S \qquad (3a)$$

or

$$J_s = PS (C_B - C_D) + J_v \overline{C} (1 - \sigma). \qquad (3b)$$

$\overline{C}$ varies in a non-linear fashion with the rate of UF. For highly diffusive solutes, especially when the rate of UF is not extremely high, $\overline{C}$ equals $(C_B+C_D)/2$. Then equation 2 can be written as:

$$J_s = PS (C_B - C_D) + J_v \frac{(C_B - C_D)}{2} S. \qquad (3c)$$

For the peritoneal membrane equation 3c is valid for all solutes up to the size of approximately inulin (mol. radius 14 Å) at least when 1.36 per cent or 2.25 per cent glucose solutions are used as dialysis fluids. Integration of equation 3b across the membrane between the boundary conditions C_B and C_D yields the following eq:

$$J_s = J_V (1 - \sigma) \frac{C_B - C_D e^{-Pe}}{1 - e^{-Pe}} \qquad (4)$$

where Pe = $[J_v(1 - \sigma)]/PS$, i.e., here Pe represents a modified 'Peclet number', which expresses the ratio of convective to diffusive transport. Equation 4 is known as the familiar non-linear global convection-diffusion equation, and in the form written above, as the Patlak equation [66]. In this equation the diffusion component (PS) approaches zero when the rate of UF (J_v) is high, because then the term e^{-Pe} approaches zero. This occurs already for $Pe > 3$ and then equation 4 can be written as:

$$J_s = C_B J_v (1 - \sigma). \qquad (5)$$

Pe may exceed 3 also when PS values are low (as for macromolecules) at moderate or low rates of UF, and then equation 5 is again valid.

Furthermore, for the special condition of C_D being zero equation 4 can be reduced to:

$$J_s = \frac{C_B J_v (1 - \sigma)}{1 - e^{-Pe}}. \qquad (6a)$$

Here, J_s represents the so-called *unidirectional* solute transport, as will be mentioned further below. Note that when $J_v = 0$ (or approaches 0) equation 6

---

[2] σ denotes the fraction of the *ideal* solute osmotic pressure gradient (exerted across a semipermeable membrane), which is operative across a leaky membrane. σ equals 1 for semipermeable membrane from which the molecule is totally reflected and σ equals zero if the membrane is freely permeable to solute.

is identical to equation 1b. If both sides of equation 6 are divided by C_B, we obtain the unidirectional solute *clearance*:

$$Cl = \frac{J_v(1-\sigma)}{1-e^{-Pe}}. \tag{6b}$$

The unidirectional solute clearance approaches the mass transfer area coefficient of the membrane when J_v approaches zero.

3.4. Determination of PS (MTAC)

For small solutes equation 3c can be used with high accuracy to assess the mass transfer area coefficient in CAPD, provided that the solute mass transfer per unit time (J_s) as well as the solute sieving coefficient (S) are known. The solute mass transfer across the peritoneal membrane can be directly determined from the peritoneal solute concentrations and the dialysate volumes sequentially determined as a function of dwell time (t) from:

$$J_s = \frac{V_2 C_{D2} - V_1 C_{D1}}{(t_2 - t_1)} \tag{7}$$

where V_1 and V_2 and C_{D1} and C_{D2} are the dialysate volumes and dialysate solute concentrations prevailing at time t_1 and time t_2, respectively. If mass transfer occurs by diffusion alone, then PS can be directly measured using equation 1b. The blood concentration of solute (C_B) as assessed under the period of investigation, is usually regarded to remain constant during the period. Inserting equation 7 in equation 1b and rearranging yields:

$$PS = \frac{V_2 C_{D2} - V_1 C_{D1}}{(t_2 - t_1)(C_B - \overline{C_D})} \tag{8}$$

where $\overline{C_D}$ is the average concentration of solute in the dialysate during time $(t_1 - t_2)$. $\overline{C_D}$ can be determined as the arithmetic mean of C_{D1} and C_{D2}, i.e. $[(C_{D1}+C_{D2})/2]$, or more correctly, as the mean value of a saturation curve of the type $C = C_{max}(1 - e^{-kt})$, yielding:

$$\overline{C} = C_B - \frac{C_{D1} - C_{D2}}{\ln\left[\frac{C_B - C_{D1}}{C_B - C_{D2}}\right]}. \tag{9}$$

Inserting this expression for $\overline{C_D}$ (eq 9) into equation 8 and setting the mean i.p. volume ($\overline{V}$) identical to the arithmetic mean of V_1 and V_2 yields:

$$PS = \frac{V_1 + V_2}{2(t_2 - t_1)} \cdot \ln \frac{(C_B - C_{D1})}{(C_B - C_{D2})}$$
$$= \frac{\overline{V}}{t_2 - t_1} \ln \frac{(C_B - C_{D1})}{(C_B - C_{D2})}. \tag{10}$$

This is the classical formula of Henderson and Nolph [67]. It was also used by Garred *et al.* [68] for assessing PS (MTAC) from intraperitoneal solute saturation curves during CAPD under conditions of no net UF.

The situation is more complicated during UF. For small solutes PS can be modelled with high accuracy from equation 3c. Replacing C_D by $\overline{C}_D$ and rearranging equation 3 yields:

$$PS = \frac{J_s - J_V \frac{(C_B - \overline{C}_D)}{2} \cdot S}{C_B - \overline{C}_D}. \tag{11}$$

Here J_s is defined by equation 7 and $\overline{C}_D$ has been defined above (eq 9).

More correctly the mass transfer area coefficient (PS) can be solved directly from equation 4 yielding:

$$PS = J_V(1-\sigma)/\ln\left[\frac{J_s - J_{V_s}(1-\sigma)\,\overline{C}_D}{J_s - J_{V_s}(1-\sigma)\,C_B}\right]. \tag{12}$$

where J_{V_s} denotes the fluid flow occurring through small pores (see below).

The difference between equation 11 and 12 regarding modelling results for *small* solutes under conditions of PD is less than 1 per cent.

Eqs 12 and 4 can be considered to be identical to the equations applied by Pyle and Popovich [69, 70, 71] for evaluating mass transfer area coefficients from the rate of solute transfer through the peritoneal membrane.

For conditions of net UF Garred *et al.* [68] suggested that PS can be approximately modelled by:

$$PS = \frac{\overline{V}}{(t_2 - t_1)} \ln\left[\frac{V_1(C_B - C_{D1})}{V_2(C_B - C_{D2})}\right]. \tag{13}$$

which is equivalent to:

$$PS = \frac{J_s - J_V C_B}{C_B - \overline{C}_D}. \tag{14}$$

However, equation 13 and equation 14 greatly underestimate PS for transport as measured in the blood-to-peritoneal direction and overestimate PS for transport in the peritoneal-to-blood direction. This becomes evident when equation 14 is compared with equation 11. This is because Garred et al. assumed S to be = 1 and $\bar{C} = C_B$. The maximal underestimation of transport occurs when $\bar{C}_D$ is zero, or close to zero during net convection. Then transport may be underestimated by $J_V[1 - (S/2)]$.

In none of the above equations has lymphatic absorption of solutes from the peritoneal cavity been taken into account. Uptake of solutes by peritoneal cavity lymphatics is a non-restrictive process [16, 50, 56], and according to equation 3c, the mass transfer of *small* solutes from the blood to the peritoneal cavity will become

$$J_s = PS(C_B - \bar{C}_D) + (J_V + L) \frac{C_B + \bar{C}_D}{2} S - \bar{C}_D \cdot L \quad (15)$$

For peritoneal to blood transport we have:

$$J_s = PS(\bar{C}_D - C_B) - (J_V + L) \frac{C_B + \bar{C}_D}{2} S + \bar{C}_D \cdot L \quad (16)$$

where L is the convective (non-restrictive) fluid flow directed from the peritoneal cavity to the interstitium or to the blood and $(J_v + L)$ is the *total* fluid transfer from the blood to the peritoneal cavity, whereas J_v is the net fluid transfer. Note that equation 7 has to be modified to:

$$\frac{(V_2 + L \cdot t_2)C_{D2} - (V_1 + L \cdot t_1)C_{D1}}{t_2 - t_1} \quad (17)$$

to account for lymphatic transport occurring during the period of measurement ($t_1 - t_2$). Furthermore equations 15 and 16 can be rearranged in a fashion similar to equation 11 to yield *PS* values corrected for lymphatic uptake of solutes from the peritoneal cavity.

All the equations described above are valid for homoporous membranes. The situation is more complicated if the membrane is not homoporous. In heteroporous membranes great discrepancies may for example exist between $(1 - \sigma)$ and S. Actually, this a key feature of the three-pore model recently described by Rippe et al. [63], as will be further discussed below.

Excellent reviews have been published on the various models for assessing transperitoneal transport [72–74]. Many membrane models are highly sophisticated to an extent that is far beyond the quality of input data. However, the simple linear equation 11 (in combination with equation 9) can be used with high accuracy for assessing small solute PS (MTAC) during CAPD under most circumstances.

3.5. Transperitoneal ultrafiltration and osmosis (convection)

The rate of net convection (J_V) across the peritoneal membrane is determined by the membrane ultrafiltration coefficient (L_PS) and the balance between the hydrostatic, colloid osmotic and crystalloid osmotic pressures acting across the peritoneal membrane, as well as by the lymph flow from the peritoneal cavity. The net volume flow across the membrane (J_V) can then be described by [65]:

$$J_V = L_P S(\Delta P - \sigma_{\text{prot}} \Delta \pi_{\text{prot}} - \sum_{i=1}^{n} \sigma_i \Delta \pi_i) - L. \quad (18)$$

Here ΔP represents the mean hydrostatic pressure difference prevailing between the blood capillaries and the peritoneal cavity (being of the order of 8–15 mm Hg during PD), $\Delta \pi_{\text{prot}}$ is the colloid osmotic pressure difference caused by the plasma proteins (usually ~25 mm Hg), whereas σ_{prot} represents the average reflection coefficient for total proteins across the peritoneum (~0.9) [63]. The third term in parenthesis denotes the sum of all 'effective' crystalloid osmotic gradients acting across the peritoneal membrane, where that for glucose usually dominates. Finally, L represents the lymph flow from the peritoneal cavity to the blood.

$\Delta \pi_i$ is defined by:

$$\Delta \pi_i = P T \Delta C_i \quad (19)$$

according to van 't Hoff's law, where RT (defined above) equals 19.3 mm Hg per mmol/L of solute concentration difference (ΔC_i) across the membrane. The *effective* osmotic gradient is determined by the product of the osmotic solute reflection coefficient and $\Delta \pi_i$. Osmotic small solute reflection coefficients in the peritoneal membrane are probably very low as discussed recently by Stelin and Rippe [75]. In animal studies values of 0.02 to 0.03 have been found [76, 77]. These values can be calculated to correspond to 0.04 and 0.05, respectively, if the impact of "ultrasmall" pores (see below) on σ is accounted for. Low values of peritoneal small solute reflection coefficients (of the order of 0.05–0.15) have also been employed by other authors to simulate alterations in i.p. fluid volume during CAPD [78, 79]. An average value of 0.05 was recently calculated [80] in CAPD patients. Indeed, if the permeability of the peritoneal membrane can be characterized by 'equivalent pores' of radius ~50Å, then the σ for glucose should be in the order of or less than 0.05 (see below).

Attempts have been made to solve equation 18 analytically. For example, Stelin and Rippe [75] made the simplifying assumption that the third term in the parenthesis of equation 18 would be mainly determined by glucose. Furthermore, the glucose concentration was assumed to decrease with a single exponential over time. Then a very simplistic analytical solution of equation 16 was obtained [75]. More explicit solutions of equation 18 have recently been derived by Vonesh et al. [81]. Although this derivation yields essentially the same results as that by Stelin and Rippe, the equations are in some aspects fundamentally different. In the solution by Vonesh et al. $L_P S$ is one order of magnitude lower, and σ_i one order of magnitude higher than in the former analysis. Since $L_P S$ and σ_i are multiplicatively linked, the net modelling results are, however, essentially the same, except that Vonesh et al. had to assume a highly inflated lymph flow parameter to fit experimental data to the model [82]. Stelin and Rippe [75] used a heteroporous concept, where ultra-small pores account for a very large fraction of fluid transport during crystalloid osmosis [63], whereas Vonesh et al. [81] applied the conventional transport theory according to Pyle and Popovich [69, 70, 71], essentially assuming an isoporous membrane, where $(1 - \sigma) = S$. According to the heteroporous membrane concept, however, there is a large discrepancy between S and $(1 - \sigma)$. The heteroporous concept has been used with good accuracy to *numerically* integrate equation 18 (using a PC) under simulated conditions of normal and altered peritoneal transport [12]. A heteroporous transport concept is necessary if one wants to predict with reasonable accuracy the UF profiles produced when high molecular weight solutes are used as osmotic agents in CAPD [82, 83].

3.6. Restricted diffusion

So far we have discussed the kind of diffusion and convection occurring in free solution, so-called *free* diffusion/convection. Solute transport by diffusion can, however, be *restricted* because of solute interactions with, for example, pores or other permeable pathways existing in a membrane. In a membrane having pores of a radius that is similar to, or even very much larger than that of the solute, transport is restricted by the pore passage. First, the molecule has to hit the pore cross-sectional entrance area. Second, there are interactions of the solute with the pore walls by frictional forces. If the total cross sectional pore surface area is denoted by A_0 and if transport is restricted, then the apparent pore surface area (A) will become smaller than the total cross-sectional pore area by the restriction factor A/A_0. Inserting the restriction factor into the PS term of equation 1 yields:

$$PS = \frac{D \cdot A}{\Delta x} = \frac{D \cdot A_0}{\Delta x} \frac{A}{A_0}. \quad (20)$$

In the right part of equation 20 we thus have the solute's diffusion constant (D), a restriction factor (A/A_0) and also the entity $A_0/\Delta x$. The latter parameter represents the total unrestricted pore area (A_0) over unit diffusion path length (in cm). Since Δx is usually difficult to estimate for biological membranes, A_0 may be hard to calculate exactly. Therefore $A_0/\Delta x$ is the surface area linked parameter that can usually be determined in studies on permeability of biological membranes. Note that the dimension of $A_0/\Delta x$ is cm and not cm².

The degree of diffusion restriction occurring in a membrane with cylindrical pores, i.e., A/A_0, is dependent on the solute radius (a_e) over pore radius (r_p), here denoted λ, as can be described by [84]:

$$\frac{A}{A_0} = \frac{(1-\lambda)^{9/2}}{1 - 0.3956\lambda + 1.0616\lambda^2}. \quad (21)$$

Glucose has a diffusion coefficient which is approximately 10 times higher than that for albumin. If both the passage of glucose and albumin across the peritoneal membrane occurred by free diffusion, then the ratio of free diffusion of glucose to that of albumin, would be of the order of 10. However, since albumin has a peritoneal clearance of approximately 0.1 ml/min and the mass transfer area of glucose usually of the order of 10 ml/min, there is a marked *restriction* of peritoneal albumin transport in the peritoneal membrane. To be able to use equation 21 one may have to convert solute molecular weight to solute radius. Theoretically the solute radius should be related to the solute mass (volume) by the cubic root of the latter. In practise, however, a_e seems to be proportional to $(MW)^{0.4}$

(where MW stands for molecular weight) instead of $(MW)^{0.33}$[63].[3] Thus, if solute transport is reduced by *more* than $(MW)^{-0.4}$ as molecular weight increases, then transport occurs by restricted diffusion.

3.7. Restricted convection and theory for the reflection coefficient

As discussed above the permeable pathways of the peritoneal membrane seem to be much larger than the radius of most small solutes. Therefore the peritoneal membrane is far from being semipermeable. If the peritoneal membrane were completely semipermeable, then the reflection coefficient would be unity for all solutes. The initial osmotic force for a 1.36% (76 mmol/L) glucose solution would then be of the order of 70 × 19.3 = 1,350 mm Hg according to equation 1! However, if the peritoneal membrane had equivalent pores of radius ~50Å, then only a very small fraction of the total osmotic force would be exerted across the membrane. This fraction is described by the osmotic reflection coefficient (σ) of the solute in the membrane. the reflection coefficient for a solute in a certain membrane is governed by the ratio solute radius to the 'equivalent pore' radius. Denoting this ratio by λ we have [according to 84]:

$$1 - \sigma = \frac{(1-\lambda)^2[2-(1-\lambda)^2](1-\lambda/3)}{1-\lambda/3+2/3\lambda^2}. \quad (22)$$

For a 50 Å 'equivalent' pore σ for glucose is thus only 0.024, whereas the reflection coefficient for albumin would be ~0.89. Note also that $(1-\sigma)$ is the coupling coefficient between solute flux and volume flow for solutes that have very low diffusion capacities such as macromolecules [cf. IgG (mol radius = 54 Å) and larger solutes]. The peritoneal passage of solutes larger than albumin can thus be modelled by equation 5 [31–34]. J_V then refers to the *large pore* volume flow, denoted J_{VL}.

3.8. Role of electric charge

Both the endothelial and mesothelial cell have a high density of negative charges on their surface. The capillary wall charge markedly seems to affect the transport of negatively charged macromolecules between blood and tissue [85–88]. It was recently shown that the negative capillary wall charge can be modulated by the highly negatively charged acute phase reactant orosmucoid [89, 90]. However, lymphatic flux analyses in intestinal and pulmonary capillary beds have indicated that the lymph-to-plasma concentration ratio at high lymph flows (primarily a measure of capillary permeability) for cationic macromolecules may be lower than that for neutral anionic ones. This is opposite to results reported using other techniques. Parker *et al.* studied the effects of molecular charge on macromolecular transport within the pulmonary circulation and suggested that the electro-chemical properties of the interstitium may be of equal importance as those of the capillary walls [91, 92]. The data were consistent with the hypothesis that the negatively charged interstitial colloid-rich phase behaved as a cation exchange column, facilitating the transport of negatively charged solutes through the tissue and retarding that of catonic macromolecules. Cationic molecules may even bind to the interstitial matrix. Actually, in a recent study Leypoldt and Henderson [93] found that the transport of positively charged dextrans (DEAE Dextran) was less than that for both neutral and negatively charged dextran sulphates.

At present it seems clear, however, that at least the capillary walls are negatively charged. Since peritoneal transport is affected by *both* the properties of the capillary wall *and* the interstitium, the overall effect of the peritoneum on solute transport with respect to charge can be highly variable. Actually, Krediet *et al.* found no effect of charge on transport of dextrans from blood to the peritoneal cavity [94]. Differently charged isoforms of IgG showed nearly identical peritoneal clearances [95]. However, since IgG penetrates the capillary wall through the 'large pore equivalent', where charge effects are small, this does not contradict the notion of the peritoneal membrane as a charge selective barrier. In a recent study intraperitoneal administration of protamine sulphate has been reported to increase the permeability to inulin [96] and to proteins [97]. Whether these changes are due to an opening of large pores by protamine (i.e., due to a general increase in capillary permeability) [98], or to selective charge effects, cannot be determined presently. It was recently proposed that mesothelial negative fixed charges may be lost during peritonitis (inflammation) [99]. Inflammation, however, implies opening of capillary large pores, and because large pores show little charge restric-

---

[3] Rippe & Stein [63] used the formula $a_e = 0.465 \cdot (Mw)^{0.39}$ to approximately model a_e vs Mw.

tion, the mentioned findings are also consistent with an increased solute flux through unselective pores in the peritoneal membrane.

Munck et al. [100] suggested that transport restriction due to equal solute and membrane charges can be modelled by simply increasing the solute radius a_e by one so-called Debye-length (l_D), which is 8Å at normal ionic strength of the medium. Furthermore, the pore radius (r_p) should be decreased by 1 l_D. The modified soluted radius to pore radius ratio (λ^*) then becomes $(a_e+l_D)(r_p-l_D)$. The authors [100] found a surprisingly good agreement between data and theory using this modified solute-to-pore radius to model reflection coefficients of albumin across artificial membranes containing track etched-pores (of radius 220Å). Rippe and Haraldsson recently used this model for predicting the negative charge effects in capillaries of rat hindquarters and for the glomerular barrier [31, 32]. The consequence of incorporating charge in the calculations of peritoneal transport is that albumin, which is negatively charged at normal pH, will be more severely restricted than predicted by the *uncharged* pore radius. The coupling of albumin flux to fluid flow will be considerably less than predicted by e.g., 45–50Å equivalent (uncharged) pores. Actually, albumin can be predicted to be completely restricted in 50Å pores if the Munck model is utilized. Determining the equivalent pore radius in continuous capillaries usually yields values in the order of 40–45Å [22, 24, 33, 34], by not taking charge interactions into account. However, these pore radii may correspond to ~55–60Å when *uncharged*. Pores of those radii will offer almost no restriction to small solute diffusion, but will markedly restrict the transport of negatively charged macromolecules.

4. Parameters of solute transport from the blood to the peritoneal cavity

4.1. D/P ratios

The peritoneal equilibration test (PET) [101] is a simple and feasible technique that can be used to estimate the transport properties of the peritoneal membrane. It is semi-quantitative and actually does not yield direct measures of PS (MTAC) for the peritoneal membrane. The method to determine PS (MTAC) from PET data was discussed above (section 3). Using the PET the dialysate to plasma concentration ratio (D/P) of urea and creatinine can be obtained in a standardized way. Also the ratio between the dialysate glucose concentration at the end of the dwell and that after inflow (D/D_0) is calculated. In addition the drained volume after four hours is assessed.

It has been claimed that D/P ratios show rather high reproducibility in the same patient. In contrast, PS (MTAC) values have an intra-individual coefficient of variation of about 15% [103]. The difference is probably caused by the lower sensitivity of the D/P ratio after four hours to detect alterations in membrane characteristics, because these D/P ratios often approach equilibrium at the end of the dwell. Yet, good correlations have been reported between PS (MTAC) and D/P ratios [103, 104]. This is illustrated in Fig. 3. The largest deviations are found in patients with very low and very high PS (MTAC) values.

The baseline peritoneal equilibration test has been proved to have a good prognostic value. Patients with high peritoneal transport rates ('high transporters') rapidly dissipate their glucose concentration gradients during the dwell and therefore have poor UF on standard CAPD. In long dwell exchanges their solute removal will therefore be less efficient than in patients with an average transport capacity. The best candidates for standard CAPD (8–9 L of dialysis solution/24 h in adults) are patients with a high-average peritoneal transport capacity, whereas most patients with low-average peritoneal transport can be maintained on standard dose CAPD provided that they have a reasonable residual renal function (2–3 ml/min).

In Fig. 4a and b we have analyzed D/P ratios for creatinine (Fig. 4a) and D/D_0 values for glucose (Fig. 4b) obtained by Twardowski et al. [101], using their published values of *average D/P* and (D/D_0) vs time curves and of D/P (and D/D_0) vs time relationships being +1 SD above and 1 SD below the mean. We have used equation 11 as modified by lymphatic flow (eq 15) and also equation 12 (the Pyle-Popovich model) to calculate PS sequentially during the dwell. Since the i.p. dialysate volume vs time curve was not known, we used an arbitrary function describing the i.p. volume vs time relationship:

$$V_t = V_0 + a_1(1 - e^{-kt}) - a_2 \qquad (23)$$

where V_t represents the i.p. dialysate volume as a function of t. V_0 is the dialysate volume at time zero and a_1, a_2 and k are some arbitrary coefficients that

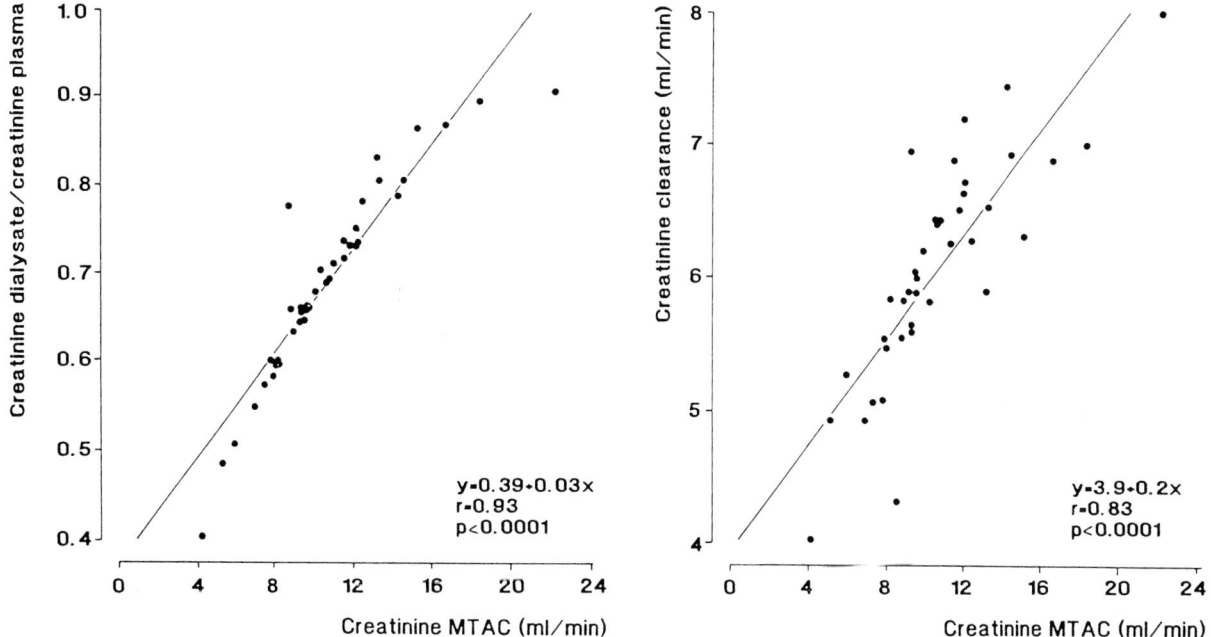

Figure 3. Relationship between creatinine D/P vs creatinine MTC (left panel) and creatinine clearance vs creatinine MTC (right panel) from the study of Struijk *et al.* [103].

determine the change occurring in V_t over dwell time. The parameters, a_1, a_2 and k were fitted to the average drain volume vs time data published by Twardowski *et al.* obtained in PET [101]. V_0 was set at 2,350 (ml), k at 0.013, a_1 at 570 (ml) and a_2 at 1.25 (ml/min). The data given in the figure were obtained using the Pyle-Popovich (P&P) model setting S for glucose and creatinine at 0.55. The P&P model actually yielded the same results as the recently published three-pore model of peritoneal exchange [63] where $S \sim 1$ in 'small pores', but where the UF rate through small pores (J_{Vs}) is ~55 per cent of the total rate of UF (J_{Vnet}). The lymphatic drainage from the peritoneal cavity was (initially) set at 0.3 ml/min.

As can be seen from the figures there is an initially enhanced PS (MTAC) for glucose and creatinine, at least during the first 60 min of the dwell. For both curves, the tendency of an initial increase in PS is blunted, however, if the rate of lymphatic absorption is increased form 0.3 to 1.5 ml/min (data in parenthesis). Furthermore, if a non-linear regression analysis is employed to assess both PS and S values for the *whole* dwell period using the Pyle-Popovich model, then abnormally inflated S-values ($S > 1$) for the blood-to-peritoneal transport, and negative S-values ($S < 0$) for the peritoneal-to-blood transport, respectively, will result [73, 74]. This indicates an initially enhanced solute transport when the UF-rate is high. the initial rapid dissipation of the glucose gradient may be due to initial rapid glucose equilibration with the large peritoneal tissue interstitium or may be the result of initial vasodilation (induced by hyperosmolality, lactate and low pH) and recruitment of capillary surface area, as was recently discussed at some length elsewhere [12, 74, 105].

4.2. Peritoneal clearance

Clearance represents the mass transfer per unit of time divided by the plasma concentration of solute. It is a valuable parameter if one wants to assess the efficiency of peritoneal dialysis and it can easily be obtained from individual drained *D/P* values multiplied by the corresponding drain volumes and divided by the total dwell time. Furthermore, determination of peritoneal clearances for solutes that are only slowly accumulating in the peritoneal cavity over time, such as proteins, seems to be the most appropriate way of measuring their transport capacities across the peritoneal membrane. It should be realized that both diffusive and convective transport are included when peritoneal clearances are calculated. Since convection should dominate over diffusion as transport mode for large solutes, the PS (MTAC) which is a diffusive parameter, is not appropriate for assessing the transport of solutes

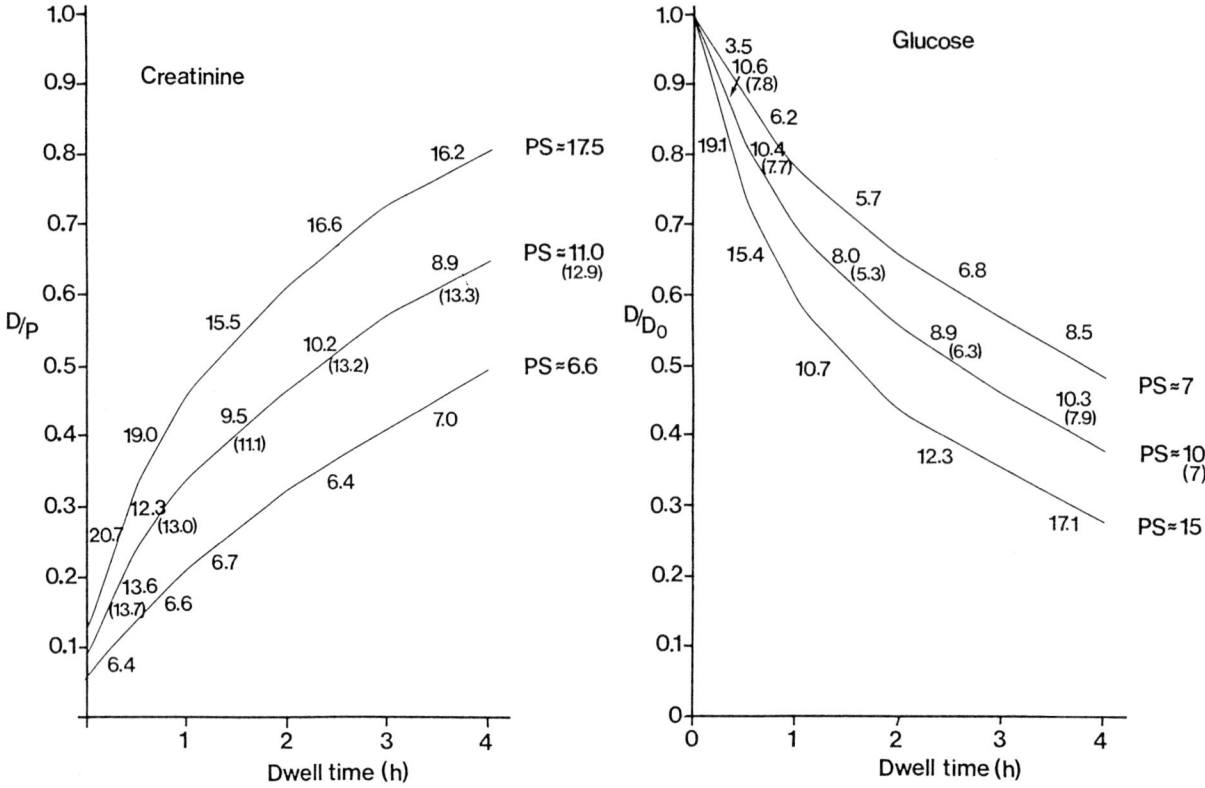

Figure 4. Dialysate to plasma creatinine concentration ratios (D/P) and dialysate to "initial" glucose concentration ratios vs. dwell time in a population studied by Twardowski *et al.* [101] using the peritoneal equilibration test (PET) as introduced by these authors. PS values calculated sequentially according to equation 12 setting $S = 0.55$ for both glucose and creatinine are shown in the figure. These were identical to those obtained using equation 15 and the three-pore model of peritoneal exchange setting $L = 0.3$. The modelling results using equation 15 setting $L = 1.5$ is shown in parenthesis. Note, when setting S at a fixed value, then the MTAC values (PS values) are higher during the first 60 min than afterwards. Assuming a high rate of non-selective transfer of tracer to the interstitium and to the lymph ('lymphatic absorption') partly blunts this pattern.

that are larger than approximately inulin. Only at absolute zero UF rate it would be theoretically possible to obtain macromolecular PS values for an ideally isoporous membrane. However, if the membrane is heteroporous, such conditions may hardly be created, because then fluid recirculation between small and large pores will occur at zero *net* convection [30, 31, 32]. Therefore, it is more appropriate to estimate the plasma clearance than the apparent PS (MTAC) for large solutes in the peritoneal membrane.

4.3. Obtaining transport parameters in patients

The PET (peritoneal equilibration test) is the most widely used assessment of peritoneal transport capacity for low molecular weight solutes. It should be realized, however, that although the obtained *D/P* ratio of creatinine reflects mainly diffusive transport, it also includes some convective transport. The D/D_0 ratio for glucose represents mainly diffusive transport, but it is also dependent on the initial dissipation of the glucose gradient within the interstitial compartment and on lymphatic absorption. The effect of convection can be minimized by using dialysate with a low glucose concentration. In a recent study by Davies *et al.* [124] the reproducibility of the PET test appeared good on the short term. When it was repeated with an interval exceeding three months in 28 patients, mainly to investigate an apparent clinical change, 61% of the test showed *D/P* values for creatinine exceeding the 95% confidence limit of the normal variability.

Using the laboratory determinations that are normally done during a PET, MTAC values of various low molecular weight solutes can easily be calculated [102]. The drainage volume (V_2), the intraperitoneal solute concentration at drainage time and a blood solute concentration (C_B) have to be determined. For urea and creatinine, the following equation can be used:

$$PS = \frac{V_2}{t} \ln \frac{V_1 C_B}{V_2(C_B - C_{D2})}. \qquad (24)$$

For lactate and glucose:

$$PS = \frac{V_2}{t} \ln \left[\frac{V_1}{V_2} \frac{(C_B - C_{D1})}{(C_B - C_{D2})} \right]. \qquad (13b)$$

With these formulas, values close to the 'average' PS values given in Fig. 4a and b are obtained.

These calculations can be improved by expressing the plasma solute concentration per volume of plasma water [106]. A theoretically justified correction for convective transport can be obtained setting the mean intraperitoneal membrane concentration at the arithmetic mean of C_B and C_D, i.e., according to the Pyle and Popovich model, by setting $F = 0.5$ using dialysate with a low glucose concentration. For dialysate with a high glucose concentration F may be set at 0.67, implying that C is close to the plasma concentration [73]. However, this modification seems to have little or no significant effect on the calculation of MTAC values obtained during a dwell using glucose 1.36% or glucose 3.85% [107].

Another way of overcoming the problem of separating diffusion from convection is to analyze transport of small solutes at relative 'isovolemia', i.e., during a time period when the i.p. dialysate volume remains more or less constant. In this situation, transport evaluation can be made according to eq 10 and the problems using equations 13 and 14 can be avoided [73, 74, 105, 108]. One major disadvantage of determining MTAC at isovolemic conditions is, however, that small solute concentrations are then relatively close to their equilibrium values, and that the relative changes in solute concentrations will be relatively small, enhancing the uncertainty of measurements.

Another approach to estimate the MTAC is the assessment of peritoneal clearances of different solutes during relatively short dwell times. It can easily be done by multiplying the *D/P* ratio with the drained volume, divided by the dwell time. This was the conventional technique during intermittent peritoneal dialysis, and has also been employed by Rubin *et al.* in CAPD patients [109]. Although this may seem attractive, it has a number of disadvantages. First, the contribution of the time of inflow and drainage is relatively large compared to the dialysis time, making it difficult to establish the precise dwell time. The second problem is the contribution of convective transport, leading to an inflated estimate of the MTAC. Another cause for overestimation of the MTAC is the finding that the PS during the first hour of a CAPD dwell is significantly higher than during the subsequent hours (see also Fig. 4) [11, 105, 108, 110, 117].

For accurate calculations of transport parameters the residual volume should also be taken into account, especially since this parameter can show marked intra and inter-patient variations, even when the drainage of the peritoneal cavity has been performed in a standardized way [55]. The residual volume after drainage of a (test) bag, used for the calculation of MTAC or D/P ratio, can easily be determined by adding a specific volume (V_x) of fresh solution intraperitoneally, followed by immediate draining. By comparing the concentration of solutes in this rinsing bag and comparing them to those in the drained (test) bag, the residual volume (V_r) can be calculated by: $V_r = V_x \times [C_2/C_1 - C_2)]$, in which C_1 represents the concentration in the (test) bag and C_2 that in the rinsing bag. In a comparison between various endogenous solutes present in drained dialysate and intraperitoneally administered inulin and dextran 70, a good correlation was found between the residual volume determined with the two exogenous solutes [111]. All endogenous low molecular weight solutes and proteins overestimated the residual volume, probably due to mass transport during the procedure. After correction for mass transport, albumin appeared the most useful endogenous marker for the estimation of the residual volume.

5. Interpretation of peritoneal PS (MTAC) or clearance values

5.1. Solute MTAC (PS) and clearance as related to solute molecular weight

Solutes of the size of inulin and smaller are almost completely *non-restricted* in their passage through the peritoneal membrane. The situation mimics that which applies for transcapillary transport. For over two decades it has been discussed whether restricted diffusion does or does not occur across continuous capillary walls [112]. We now know, that the degree of restricted diffusion for solutes is hard to determine from physiological measurements of small solute PS values. This is due to methodological problems that usually lead to progressive underestimation of PS values for small solutes as molecular size decreases [22]. Therefore capillary PS measurements usually indicate non-restricted capillary diffusion of small solutes. In whole-organ vascular beds, small solute PS values are underestimated due to heterogeneity of plasma flow and capillary morphology and due to flow limitation of solute delivery to the tissue. To avoid flow-limitation in a perfectly homogenous tissue, plasma flow should exceed the capillary solute PS by at least a factor three or four. For the peritoneal membrane, the blood flow in the peritoneum should be at least 100 ml/min for a PS of urea of 20–25 ml/min to allow correct estimations of urea diffusion capacity. Although literature data seem to be consistent with blood flows of this magnitude (see below), at least urea seems to be on the border of being flow-limited. The impact of a distributed capillary bed on solute transport, and most importantly, interstitial diffusion resistances in the peritoneal tissue, is similar to that of blood flow limitation and heterogeneity as will be demonstrated below. All these factors reduce clearances (or MTACs) of *small* solutes proportionally more than they affect the transport of larger solutes, and the effects are amplified progressively with decreasing molecular size.

Hence, there are a number of factors that make transport across the peritoneal membrane of small solutes apparently non-restricted. The transport of larger solutes, however, such as β_2-microglobulin, myoglobin and albumin, appears to be clearly restricted, i.e., the clearances are reduced more with increasing molecular size than in proportion to the free diffusion coefficients. In Fig. 5 peritoneal mass transfer area coefficients, obtained from a number of different laboratories for small and intermediate-size solutes [55, 68–70, 73, 74, 102, 105, 106, 108, 113–120] and for large solutes [94, 107, 110, 121–123], have been plotted vs molecular weight (MW) on a log-log scale. As discussed above, free diffusion of any solute should decrease linearly in this log-log diagram with approximately $(MW)^{-0.4}$. Values of the exponent larger than 0.4 indicate *restricted* diffusion.

In Fig. 5, three power functions relating MW to measured peritoneal clearances are plotted, namely that by Pyle and Popovich: $333.6 \, (MW)^{-0.561}$ [69, 70], that by Lasrich et al.: $121.8 \, (MW)^{-0.442}$ [123] and that by Krediet et al.: $59 \, (MW)^{-0.34}$ [115]. The power function by Pyle and Popovich and that by Lasrich et al. indicate restricted diffusion, while that of Krediet et al. has a slope which is actually *less* than that characterizing free diffusion. These power functions seem to work satisfactorily for small solutes up to the size of inulin. However, as seen from the figure, they all *overestimate* the β_2-microglobulin clearance. Above all, they overestimate clearances of macromolecules by approximately one order of magnitude. This is because they do not comprise any theory to describe restricted diffusion (and convection). In Fig. 5 equations 2, 20 and 21 have been employed to model restricted diffusion in a membrane having equivalent cylindrical pores of radius 50, 60 and 72Å, respectively (solid lines), when $A_o/\Delta x$ was set at 45,000 cm, as fitting to the experimental data of Rippe et al. [113] and those by Pyle and Popovich [69, 70]. Note that in this very simplistic analysis, the influence of convection (UF) is not taken into account. Furthermore, 'large pore' transport of macromolecules is not considered when modelling the small pore radius. Therefore, the best fit of theory to the experimental data of Rippe et al. [113; filled squares], and those of Pyle and Popovich [69, open circles] occurred for a small pore radius of 72Å. This value is an overestimate, since transport of solutes occurs by both convection and diffusion and, most likely, through a heteroporous capillary membrane (see below).

Whilst small solutes seem to be non-restricted across the peritoneal membrane, this more or less also seems to hold for solutes larger than albumin. This may, however, be fortuitous. If solutes larger than albumin are permeating across *pores* larger than 200Å in radius, then there should be no diffusion in these pores. However, if transport occurs by transcytosis, diffusion is a major transport mode for macromolecules. Assuming macromolecular transport through large pores, then the Pe-numbers (for large solutes) through these pathways can be shown to always exceed 3, and transport is *completely convective* in nature [24, 32–35]. If convection dominates large solute transport, then clearances of solutes > 50Å in radius may be modelled as just the product of the rate of UF occurring through large pores (J_{VL}) and the large pore sieving coefficient of the solute ($1 - \sigma_L$) (eq 5).

5.2. Three-pore model

Rippe et al. [63, 113] claimed that peritoneal transport may be approximately modelled in the same way as transport across the peritoneal microvessels. This implies that there would be a 'bimodal' selec-

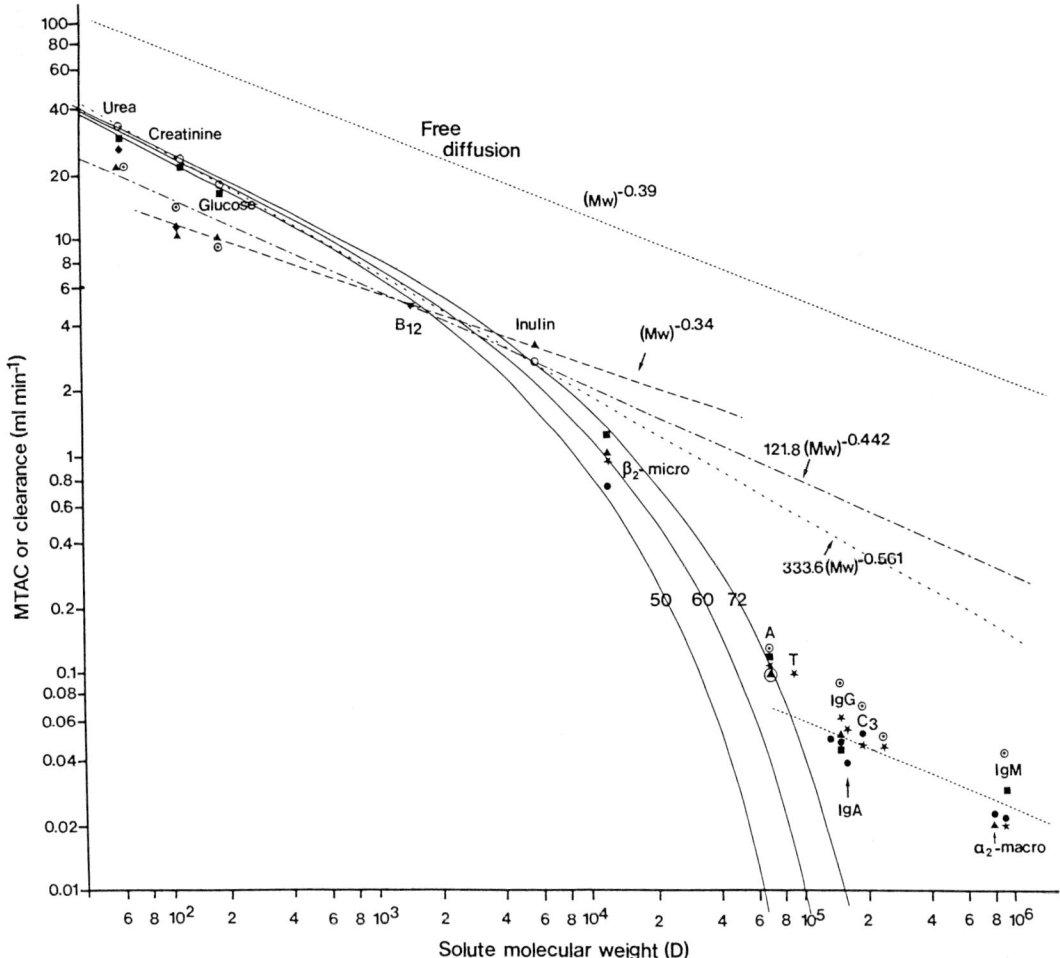

Figure 5. Selected literature data of mass transfer area coefficients (PS) or clearance plotted vs molecular weight. The data are plotted on a log-log scale where power functions of MTAC vs molecular weight become linear. Open circles: data from Pyle and Popovich [69, 70]; Filled triangles: *average* data from the laboratory of Krediet and Struijk [94, 102, 107, 114–118, 123]; Filled squares: data from Rippe *et al.* [63, 113]; Dotted circles: data from Kagan *et al.* [110]; Stars: data from Blumencrantz *et al.* [121]; Filled triangles, pointing down: Garred *et al.* [68]; Filled diamond(s); average data from Lindholm, Waniewski, Heimbürger *et al.* [73, 74, 106, 108, 119]. Note that the MTAC values calculated for conditions of intermittent peritoneal dialysis or during the *early* phase of the dwell are relatively high [69, 70, 113], whereas small solute PS values obtained for the long (4–6 h) dwells are usually much lower. Solutes up to the size of inulin seem to be more or less unrestricted in their transport across the peritoneal membrane, whereas solutes larger than inulin are markedly restricted in their transport. Three power functions describing the transport of small solutes are shown in the figure. All these functions are inadequate in describing the degree of diffusional restriction across the peritoneal membrane. Therefore, solid lines indicating the 'restricted diffusion' in membranes containing 50Å, 60Å and 72Å 'equivalent' pores, respectively, are depicted in the figure. Note that for the data of Rippe *et al.* [113] and those of the Pyle and Popovich [69, 70] the situation can be described by the existence of 72Å equivalent pores for solutes up to the size of albumin and assuming an $A_0/\Delta x$ of 45,000 cm. This is when convective transport and transport through large pores are not included in the analysis [cf. 113].

tivity of the peritoneal membrane with respect to solute transfer, i.e., an apparent restriction across capillary walls of transport of intermediate size solutes, buy a nearly unrestricted transport of the largest solutes. Furthermore, fluid transfer may be modelled to occur, not only through protein-selective (small) pores and unselective (large) pores, but also through water-exclusive [20–22] pathways across the endothelial (and mesothelial) cells.

Although capillary transport appears to occur via at least three permeable pathways, *solute* transport may with little error be modelled using a simple two-pore model. If macromolecules, the clearances of which are depicted in Fig. 5, are assumed to pass through the peritoneal membrane through porous pathways, then the mode of transfer is probably convection, as discussed above. It is then possible to fit data for solutes larger than albumin to a function defined by equation 5, namely to $J_{VL}(1 - \sigma_L)$. If at least two large solute clearances (for $a_e > 50\text{Å}$) are known, then one can solve this equation for J_{VL} and σ_L and can thereby estimate the large pore radius (according to equation 22). Having determined the large pore radius and large pore volume flow, the ultrafiltration rate through small pores can now be determined for the two-pore model. In the next step the 'unidirectional small pore solute clearances' for solutes < 50Å in radius, can be obtained by subtracting their large pore solute clearances (eq 5) from their total (measured) clearances, by inserting the resulting clearance value into equation 6. Small pore reflection coefficients and small pore PS values are modelled according to equations 20 and 21, respectively. Using an iterative procedure the $A_0/\Delta x$ and the small pore radius (r_s) are varied to obtain the best fit of experimental data to the model. The fractional pore area occupied by large pores in relation to the small pore area can be obtained according to Poiseuille's law by:

$$\frac{A_L}{A_s} = \frac{\alpha_L}{1 - \alpha_L} \left(\frac{r_s}{r_L}\right)^2 \quad (25a)$$

when α_L denotes the fraction of $L_P S$ accounted for by large pores (5–10 per cent). Furthermore, the large to small pore number ratio can be obtained by:

$$\frac{n_L}{n_s} = \frac{\alpha_L}{1 - \alpha_L} \left(\frac{r_s}{r_L}\right)^4. \quad (25b)$$

Figure 6 shows the original analysis of the data by Rippe et al. [113] employing these principles, as modelled for a net filtration rate of 1 ml/min. Adaptation of experimental data from (seven) patients to the two-pore theory was made using a non-linear least squares regression analysis. The analysis yielded a small pore radius (r_s) of 47 ± 1.02Å (±SE) and a large pore radius of 305 ± 41Å and a non-restricted pore area over unit diffusion path length ($A_0/\Delta x$) of 45,000 ± 2,300 cm. The large pore volume flow became 0.0523 ± 0.006 ml/min, whereas the fractional UF coefficient accounted for by large pores (α_L) was estimated to be ~0.06. A_L/A_s was calculated to be $2.3 \cdot 10^{-3}$ and n_L/n_s to 1/12,500. When comparing these data with the majority of the literature data (cf. Fig. 5), clearances for β_2-microglobulin, albumin, IgG and IgM conform to literature data, whereas small solute clearance data are consistently higher. This is probably due to the fact that the measurements were performed within the first 40 min of the dwell (see above). Readjustment, from 45,000 to 27,000 cm [12], which is more consistent with the 'average' PS value during 4–6 h dwells, only slightly affects the data for β_2-microglobulin and larger solutes, but has a vast impact on the small solute clearances (and PS values).

The two-pore model cannot account for the fact that small solute sieving coefficients are in the range of 0.5–0.6. Thus, a strict two-pore model would predict small solute sieving coefficients of the order of 0.95–1.0, not 0.5–0.6! However, taking into account the water conductance across endothelial cells, recognised by capillary physiologists for many years [20], small solute sieving coefficients of the order of 0.5 are indeed possible. Rippe and Stelin [63] showed that if only 1.5–2 per cent of the total hydraulic conductance is accounted for by transcellular pores, exclusive for water, but rejecting solutes, then approximately one half of the peritoneal fluid filtration will occur through these pathways for large glucose osmotic pressure gradients. Actually, heteroporosity of this kind was suggested already by Nolph et al. [125] as a cause of the marked small solute sieving during peritoneal dialysis. The total fluid filtration occurring across such a heteroporous peritoneal membrane is obtained by summing up the partial small pore flow, the large pore flow, and the transcellular UF flow and the lymph flow:

$$J_{V\text{net}} = J_{Vs} + J_{Vc} + J_{VL} - L \quad (26)$$

where J_{Vc} approximately equals $0.55 \cdot J_{V\text{net}}$ [63]. The total (lumped sum) osmotic reflection coefficient is obtained by:

$$\sigma = \alpha_s \sigma_s + \alpha_L \sigma_L + \alpha_c \cdot 1 \quad (27)$$

where α denotes the fraction of $L_P S$ accounted for by small pores (α_s), large pores (α_L) or transcellular pores (α_c). Thus $\alpha_s + \alpha_L + \alpha_c = 1$.

The total (unidirectional) clearance is obtained by:

$$Cl = Cl_L + Cl_s \quad (28)$$

where J_{Vs} instead of $J_{V\text{net}}$ is used to model Cl_s. Cl_L is modelled in the same way as for the two-pore model. The sieving coefficient for the three-pore membrane is modelled by:

$$S = \frac{Cl_L + Cl_s}{J_{V\text{net}} + L}. \quad (29)$$

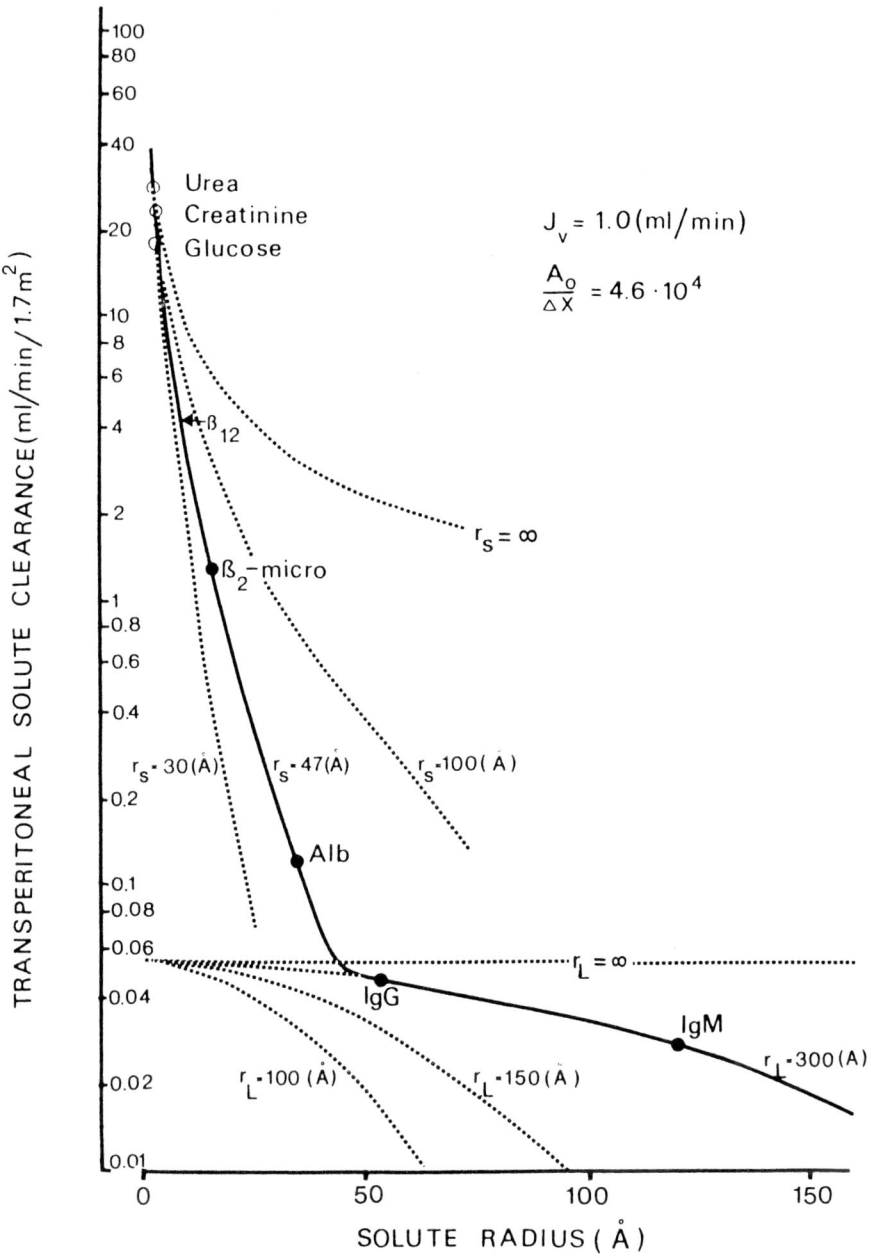

Figure 6. Semilogarithmic plot of transperitoneal unidirectional clearances vs molecular radius together with data from the study of Rippe *et al.* [113] using the two-pore theory of transmembrane transport. Solid line is simulated for a small pore radius of 47Å and the large pore radius of 300Å and a pore area over unit diffusion path length ($A_o/\Delta x$) of 45,000 when the total blood-to-peritoneal filtration rate is set at 1 ml · min^{-1} 1.73 M^2 body surface area.

To model peritoneal transport of small solutes one can also use the *net* fluid filtration rate ($J_{V_{net}}$), but then in conjunction with a sieving coefficient (S) of the order of 0.5–0.6 (cf. Pyle-Popovich model). Both models yield the same modelling results. However, when modelling osmosis and macromolecular transport, the three-pore model is superior to conventional models in accuracy [82, 83].

The data of Rippe *et al.* [113], as analysed according to the two-pore model, were further remodelled by Rippe and Stelin [63] using the three-pore concept with essentially similar results as using the two-pore model. Actually, the small pore radius increased to slightly above 50Å using the three-pore model. However, there is evidence that this value may be too high. A small pore radius much larger than 43–45Å, implies that the coupling of albumin flux to the rate of UF would be very pronounced. Albumin transport is, however, just moderately elevated during increased UF [107], such as during the initial portion of hypertonic dwells.

5.3. A three-pore (capillary) membrane series-coupled with an interstitial diffusion resistance

To fully understand the mechanisms of peritoneal exchange one has to model fluid and solute transport across *both* the capillary wall and the interstitial compartment. The capillary wall is highly permeable to small solutes, whereas the interstitium, due to the rather large diffusion distances, may offer a considerable diffusion impedance for small solutes. As solute size increases, the *capillary* wall diffusion resistance will increase progressively relative to the interstitial transport resistance and determine the rate of solute transfer for intermediate and large solutes. Hence, the impact of interstitial diffusion resistances will be relatively small for large solutes. In Fig. 7 the data depicted in Fig. 5 are shown together with predictions by the three-pore model for total net fluid filtration rate of 1 ml/min. the small pore volume flow J_{V_S} is set at 0.54 ml/min, the large pore volume flow is set at 0.06 ml/min and the transcellular volume flow at 0.60 ml/min. Curve A represents the curve fit by the three-pore model using the same modelling technique as in Fig. 6 [63] (r_L = 250Å), but $A_o/\Delta x$ is set here at 27,000 cm instead of at 45,000 cm and α_L is set at 0.09. Curves B and C are modelled using $A_o/\Delta x$ = 270,000 cm and assuming that the interstitial PS for urea is as low as 16 ml/min. The interstitial PS (PS_{int}) is assumed to decrease with increasing molecular radius just in proportion to the free solute diffusion coefficient, whereas the *capillary* permeability surface area product (PS_{cap}) is modelled as in Fig. 6 using equation 2, 20 and 21. The total peritoneal transport resistance (PS_{tot}) is then obtained by:

$$\frac{1}{PS_{tot}} = \frac{1}{PS_{cap}} + \frac{1}{PS_{int}}. \tag{30}$$

Modelling clearance data according to this technique yields a nearly *unrestricted* diffusion for solutes of radius less than inulin, followed by a sharp decline in clearance with increasing solute radius up to the size of albumin. An analysis of the kind described here was performed already in the early eighties by Smeby and Wideröe et al. [78, 79]. In those studies the interstitial transport resistance was attributed to 'unstirred layers'.

A relatively good fit of data to the model can be obtained for a pore radius of 47Å (Curve C), but the fit is reasonably good also for a small pore radius of 43Å (Curve B), for which the coupling of albumin flux to fluid flow (UF rate) is more realistic than for 47Å small pores [107]. The most interesting consequence of this very simplistic analysis of a three-pore membrane with a series-coupled interstitial diffusion resistance, is that the $A_0/\Delta x$ for the capillary wall will become much more realistic than previous estimates calculated for the whole peritoneal membrane. Actually, according to Poiseuille's law, it is now possible to calculate an ultrafiltration coefficient (LPS) using the *capillary* $A_0/\Delta x$ from:

$$L_P S = \frac{n_s \cdot \pi \; r_s^4}{\Delta x} \frac{60 \cdot 1320}{8\eta}$$
$$= \frac{A_0}{\Delta x} \frac{r_s^2}{8\eta} \frac{60 \cdot 1320}{8\eta} \tag{31}$$

where η has been defined above and where 60 is used to convert sec to min and 1320 converts dynes/cm^2 to mm Hg. Inserting $A_0/\Delta x$ = 270,000 (cm) and small pore radius of 47Å (47 · 10^{-8} cm) yields and $L_P S$ of 0.084 ml·min^{-1}·mm Hg^{-1}. Setting r_s = 43 (Å) yields a value of $L_P S$ of 0.07 ml·min^{-1}·mm Hg^{-1}. Both these values are very close to those estimated for the human peritoneal membrane [75]. The estimated $A_0/\Delta x$ for the capillary walls is thus in close accordance with the peritoneal UF coefficient. The latter parameter should (according to Poiseuille's law) be determined nearly entirely by the *capillary* wall and very little by the interstitium.

In summary, the peritoneal barrier exchange characteristics may be rather adequately described using a three-pore model of membrane permeability. Solute transport can be simulated as occurring through a membrane having a large number of small pores of radius 40–50Å, and a small number of large pores of radius 200–300Å. Furthermore, there seems to be an abundancy of transcellular pores of radius 2–4Å allowing substantial osmosis of fluid, but rejecting solute transport. Solute sieving during high rates of osmotic fluid flow (UF) may be explained by dilution of the dialysate, by water free of solutes passing through these pathways. Molecules larger than ~50Å seem to pass the peritoneal membrane mainly by unidirectional

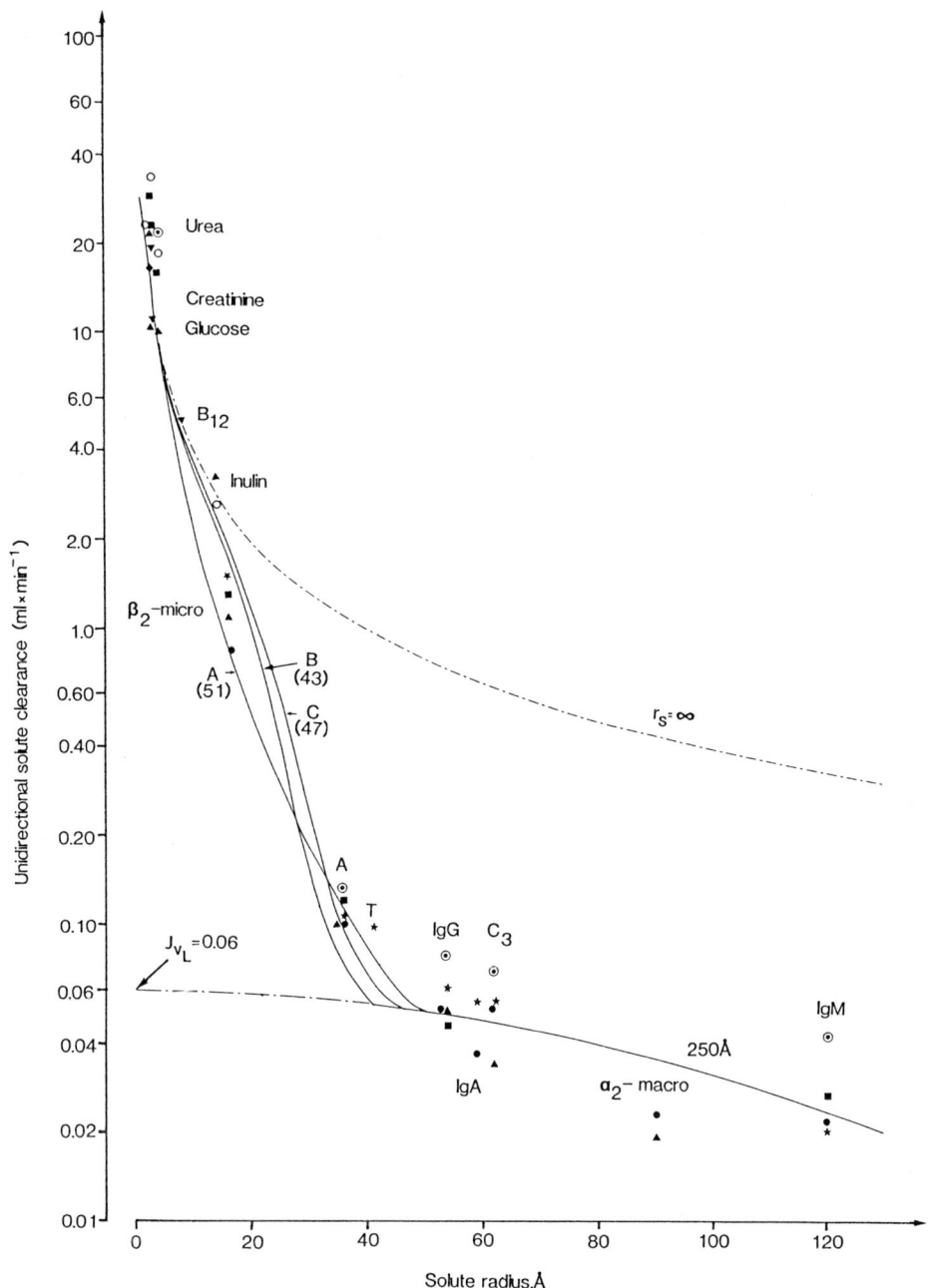

Figure 7. Semilogarithmic plot of unidirectional solute clearance employing either the simple three-pore theory where $A_0/\Delta x$ is set at 27,000 cm (curve A) or a three-pore membrane having $A_0/\Delta x$ = 270,000 with a series-coupled interstitial compartment where PS for urea is set at 16 ml/min. The latter simulation is shown for a small pore radius of 43Å (curve B) and 47Å (curve C). The symbols are identical to those in Figure 5. Note that the parallel pathway model with a series-coupled resistance yields essentially no diffusional restriction of solutes up to the size of inulin, and then a sharp decline in clearance as molecular size increases. The transfer of IgG, C3, α_2-macroglobulin and IgM are modelled to occur through large pores of radius 250Å through which the rate of UF (unaffected by the rate of *net* UF) is 0.06 ml/min. Free diffusion is depicted by a hatched line ($r_s = \infty$).

convection from the blood to the peritoneal cavity in these models. The role of diffusion remains controversial at present. The interstitium markedly modified transport across the peritoneal membrane. Interstitial diffusion resistances tend to make transport of small solutes (up to the size of inulin) nearly *unrestricted*, whereas larger solutes are restricted in their peritoneal transport. Excluding interstitial transport resistances from transport simulations leads to marked underestimations of the effective capillary cross-sectional pore area available for diffusion. Concerning the absorption of macromolecules from the peritoneal cavity, this seems to occur by non-size selective drainage via lymphatic absorption, and also most likely, due to transport into peritoneal tissues bordering the peritoneal cavity.

5.4. Conditions of increased capillary permeability

During peritonitis (inflammation) one can expect blood flow to the peritoneal tissue and the number of perfused capillaries to increase. Thus, there is recruitment of vascular surface area. Probably there are also increases in the hydrostatic capillary pressure. Furthermore, inflammation usually implies opening of large gaps in post-capillary venules. The impact of such alterations would be to increase small solute clearances in proportion to the degree of capillary recruitment (the increase in effective capillary surface area) and also to markedly increase clearances of large molecules (mostly albumin and larger solutes). Actually, the relationship in Fig. 7 depicting large solute transfer (the large pore curve) will move 'upwards'. This will be reflected by a decrease in the ratio of small solute diffusion capacity to large solute diffusion capacity, i.e., in diffusion terms, as a decreased degree of 'restricted diffusion'. In reality this change in 'restricted diffusion' reflects leakage of large solutes and fluid out from the blood capillaries via large pores. Opening of large pores in the peritoneal membrane will not markedly affect the UF profile *per se* [12]. However, recruitment of capillaries as occurring during peritonitis will cause a left-ward displacement of the i.p. dialysis volume vs time curve and a reduction of peak height of the curve.

5.5. Electrolyte transport

In the original three-pore model it was assumed that urea and sodium chloride had approximately the same PS. Rippe *et al.* [12] modelled sodium transfer across the peritoneal membrane using a *unidirectional* clearance concept (eq 6b) instead of employing the bi-directional clearance formula (eq 4). This automatically deflated sodium transport across the peritoneal membrane. Sodium chloride therefore showed marked sieving across the peritoneum, as desired. However, correcting the modelling approach by employing equation 4 instead of equation 6b, the degree of NaCl sieving was markedly reduced to the extent that it did not fit with experimental data [74, 120]. The PS for NaCl had to be deflated down to ~5–7 ml/min to make the model fit the data [82]. Indeed, Heimbürger *et al.* [105] and Waniewski *et al.* [120] have found PS values for Na of the order of 5 ml/min. This is less than 50% of the value predicted by the three-pore model. Low PS values have also been presented for other extracellular cations such as Ca but *not* for (intracellular) potassium [74, 120] and phosphate [110].

Both Na and Ca, that are extracellular, are thus moving through the peritoneum at much lower rates than predicted from their diffusion coefficients. The reason for this is not known. One explanation for the retardation of extracellular cations across the peritoneal tissue may be found in the fact that interstitium is highly negatively charged. The interstitial gel contains a high number of polyelectrolyte chains with negatively charged groups distributed along them. These fixed negative charges are counter-balanced by (mobile) cationic ions. Mobile ions would interact with these ions in a way that retards the transport of mobile ions across the interstitium [126]. It should be noted, however, that the low PS values obtained for sodium in humans have not been reported in animal studies [127], where the impact of completely sodium-free i.p. glucose solutions on sodium transport from blood to peritoneum has been studied. Further research is needed to clarify the mechanisms underlying electrolyte transport across the peritoneal capillary-interstitial barrier.

5.6. Individual characterization of surface area and intrinsic permeability

The magnitude of solute transport across the peritoneum is determined by membrane and solute properties. The transport ability of the peritoneal membrane is governed by both its surface area and its intrinsic permeability, i.e., the resistance the membrane offers to the diffusion and convection of solutes.

As has been pointed out in the section on the surface area of the peritoneal membrane, the functional or effective surface area is smaller than its anatomic equivalent, and can be regarded as the pore area available for transport divided by the effective diffusive path length. The capillary wall is probably the most important size selective restriction barrier to solute transport as stated previously in this chapter, but the other layers may also contribute [128, 129], as discussed earlier. Experiments using topically or intraperitoneally administered vasoactive solutes, such as isoproterenol and nitroprusside have made it likely that the number of perfused capillaries is the most important determinant of the effective peritoneal surface area [130–133]. Under normal conditions only 25% of the peritoneal capillaries is perfused [132]. The presence of dialysate in the peritoneal cavity has been found to increase splanchnic blood flow in cats as measured by microspheres [134]. It suggests that the effective peritoneal surface area is not constant, but may be influenced by splanchnic blood flow and splanchnic blood volume [135].

As the effective surface area is not a static property of the peritoneum, but a dynamic one, that can change depending on the number of perfused capillaries, or depending on changes in the interstitium and mesothelial cell barrier, a functional characterization is necessary. This can be achieved by taking the MTAC of a solute whose transport is only dependent on the surface area of the membrane, and not on its intrinsic permeability. Changes in the MTAC of such a solute are caused by changes in the effective peritoneal surface area.

The relationship between parameters of solute transport and solute molecular weight can be described by power functions as has been pointed out in the section on restricted diffusion and in Fig. 5. In fact, this is one of the starting points of the described three pore model. This model, especially with an added interstitial resistance is however a complex mode of assessing changes in effective surface area and permeability in individual patients. Therefore, a more simple way was developed, that allows assessment of these membrane properties in individual patients [123].

When the free diffusion coefficient of urea, glucose and inulin are plotted against their molecular weights on a double logarithmic scale, the slope of the correlation coefficient (the power) was −0.46. [115, 116]. This implies that values exceeding this power indicate restricted diffusion. This power holds only for solutes smaller than sucrose. Most values reported for the power relationship between MTAC and molecular weight are within the order of magnitude of −0.46 (see section: Solute MTAC (PS) and clearance as related to solute molecular weight [115, 116, 124, 136]). Therefore, the figures found for low molecular weight solutes give no indication for a size-selective restriction barrier during peritoneal dialysis, but are more in favour for a transport process, similar to free diffusion in water. It implies that the effective peritoneal surface area, defined as the number of perfused capillaries and the mainly size independent resistances exerted by the interstitium and the mesothelium, is the only membrane characteristic that influences the MTAC of a low molecular weight solute. Consequently, the MTAC of such a solute, e.g., creatinine can be used as a functional measurement of the effective peritoneal surface area. Changes in the MTAC of creatinine in individual patients reflect changes in their effective surface area.

A power relationship between peritoneal clearances and molecular weights has also been established for the transport of serum proteins from the blood to the dialysate, both during intermittent peritoneal dialysis [137] and CAPD [123]. However, the slope of the regression line is much steeper than that obtained when the free diffusion coefficients of these proteins were plotted against molecular weights. Therefore an additional barrier to the transport of macromolecules must be present in the peritoneal membrane, i.e., the intrinsic permeability. The size-dependence of transport of proteins (at least up to the size of α_2-macroglobulin) reveals the intrinsic permeability properties of the peritoneal membrane. A similar size selective restricted transport has also been found in CAPD patients for non-protein macromolecules, such as neutral dextran fractions with diffusion radii ranging from 30 to 90 Å [94], but not for smaller fractions, up to 20 Å in rabbits [138].

Molecular size is not the only determinant of transport velocity. Also the shape, and in some instances the charge of a molecule can have an effect. This is very evident for non-protein macromolecules, such as dextrans. Based on the equation: radius = 3.05 MW$^{-0.47}$ [139] as derived from the data of Granath and Kvist [140], it can be calculated that a dextran fraction with a diffusion radius identical to that of β_2-microglobulin (MW 11,800) has a molecular weight of 4,600. For α_2-macroglobulin (MW 820,000) the molecular weight of the corresponding dextran fraction is only 176,000 [141]. Therefore, the establishment of relationships between MTACs (low molecular weight solutes) or clearances (macromolecules) and the free diffusion coefficients in water of these solutes is a more rational approach. A power relationship was found for peritoneal protein clearances and their free diffusion coefficients in water [142]. The exponent of the equation was called the restriction coefficient. This clinical parameter of restricted transport, that can be determined in individual patients by plotting MTAC values of low molecular weight solutes, and also clearances of macromolecules, against the free diffusion coefficients in water of these solutes on a double logarithmic scale, should not be confused with the terms restriction factor and reflection coefficient. As pointed out in the section on restricted diffusion, the restriction factor (A/A_0) is the ratio between the apparent pore surface area and the total cross sectional pore surface area. To estimate this factor used in membrane physiology, assumptions have to be made on the size of the small pores. The reflection coefficient (see transperitoneal ultrafiltration and osmosis section) is a determinant of the effective osmotic pressure a solute can exert over a pore.

A restriction coefficient that equals 1.0 means a linear relationship between clearances and free diffusion coefficients, so no hindrance by the restriction barrier. In this situation the effective peritoneal surface area is the only membrane characteristic that determines solute transport. A restriction coefficient higher than 1.0 means size-selectivity restricted transperitoneal transport. This implies that the restriction coefficient can be used as a clinical measurement of the intrinsic peritoneal permeability. The higher the restriction coefficient, the lower the permeability to solute transport. The use of the restriction coefficient has been validated both for serum proteins and neutral dextrans [143, 144]. In another study (Fig. 8) the mean value of the restriction coefficient was 1.24 for low molecular weight solutes and 2.37 for serum proteins, which is again consistent with a process of mainly free diffusion for low molecular weight solutes and restricted transport for macromolecules [107].

In Table 1, a summary is given of the relationship between the parameters of solute transport and the permeability characteristics of the peritoneal membrane. The effective peritoneal surface area can be characterized by the MTAC of creatinine or, when this is not possible because of very long dwell

Table 1. The relationship between membrane characteristics and parameters of solute transport.

	Effective peritoneal surface area	Intrinsic peritoneal permeability
MTAC of low molecular weight solutes	+	−
Clearance of macromolecules	+	+
Restriction coefficient	−	+

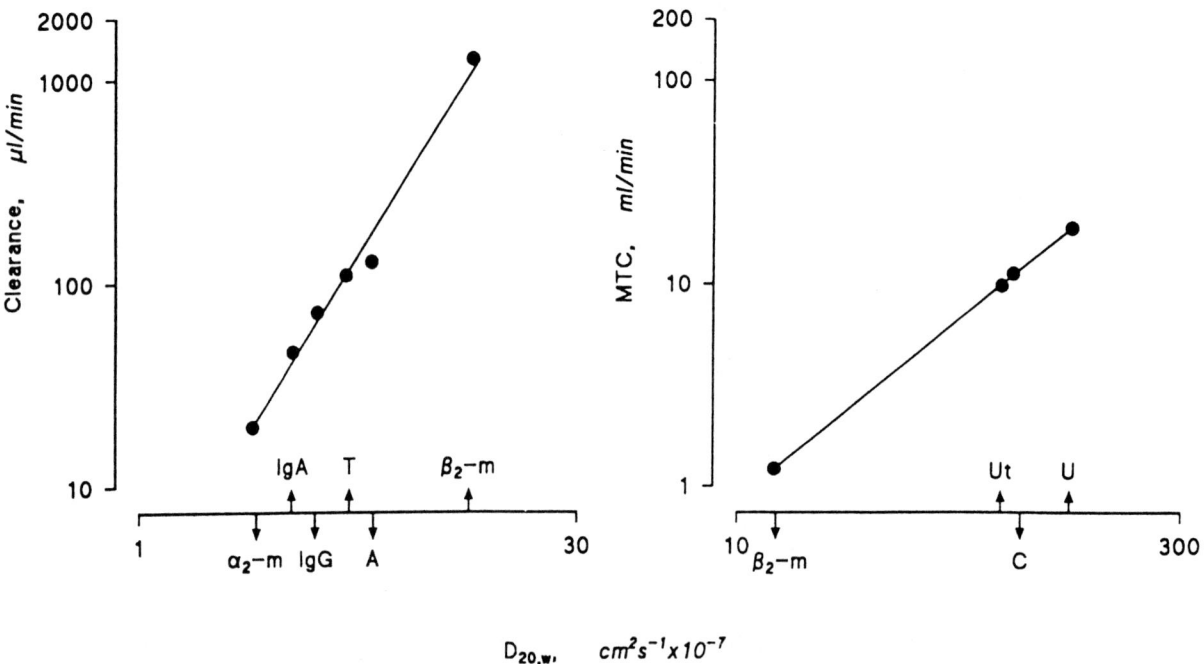

Figure 8. The power relationship between the mass transfer area coefficients of urea (U), creatinine (C), urate (Ut), and β_2-microglobulin (β_2-M) and their free diffusion coefficient in water (D20,w) (right pannel), and the power relationship between the protein clearances of β_2-microglobin (β_2-M), albumin (A), transferrin (T), IgG, IgA and α_2-macroglobulin (α_2-M), and their free diffusion coefficient in water (left pannel). The data are plotted on a double logarithmic scale. The slope of the regression line represents the restriction coefficient (see text): for the low-molecular weight solutes a mean slope of 1.24 and for the proteins a mean slope of 2.37 was found. Published with permission of reference 107 and of Blackwell Scientific Publications, Inc.

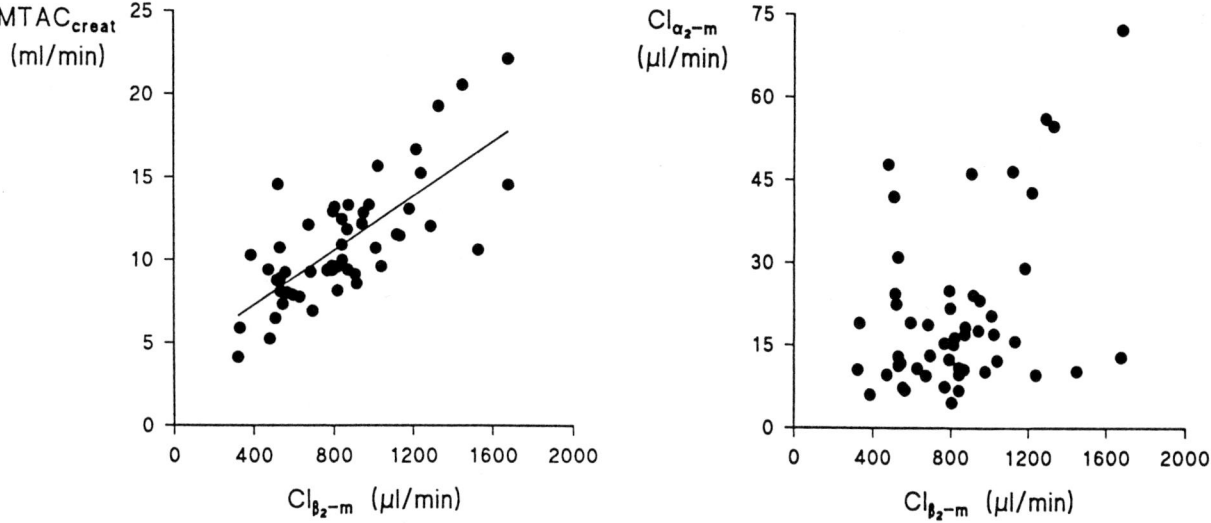

Figure 9. The correlation between the clearance of β_2-microglobulin and the mass transfer area coefficient of creatinine (left panel) and the absence of a correlation between the clearance of β_2-microglobulin and that of α_2-macroglobulin (right panel). Data are taken from references [94] and [117].

times leading to equilibrium between dialysate and blood concentrations, by the clearance of β_2-microglobulin. The latter is correlated with the MTAC of creatinine (Fig. 9), but not with the clearance of larger proteins [142]. The intrinsic permeability can be characterized by the calculation of the restriction coefficient. In this way both membrane characteristics can be established in individual patients and used during follow-up.

6. Solute transport from the peritoneal cavity

6.1. Low molecular weight solutes

The disappearance rate of intraperitoneally administered low molecular weight solutes from the dialysate is dependent on their molecular weights, as shown in Table 2 [116, 145]. This suggests a

Table 2. Mass transfer area coefficients (MTAC, ml/min) of intraperitoneally administered non-protein bound low molecular weight solutes. Data are from references [116] and [145].

Solute	Molecular weight	MTAC after ip administration
Lactate	90	20.5
5-flucytosine	129	19.2
Glucose	180	13.6
Kanamycin	484	12.0
Inulin	5500	4.4

mainly diffusive process. As a consequence the absorption of lactate during a 4 hr dialysis dwell was found to average 82 percent of the instilled quantity [data from ref 116]. For glucose a mean value of 66% has been reported, irrespective of the glucose concentration used in the dialysate [145]. It could range between 51 and 80% in individual patients. When the disappearance of glucose is expressed as the ratio between the dialysate concentration after a 4 hrs dwell and the initial dialysate concentration (D/D_0), as is usually done during PET tests, values ranging from 0.12 to 0.60 can be found [101]. Other low molecular weight solutes that can be used as osmotic agents during peritoneal dialysis, such as glycerol and amino acids, are also absorbed according to their molecular weights. The absorption of glycerol (MW 92) averages 84% after a 6 hrs dwell [147], and that of amino acids (mean MW 145) 73 to 90% [148, 149]. The absorption of these solutes by diffusion occurs mainly in the portal circulation [150].

Babb *et al.* were the first who studied bidirectional solute transport [151]. This was done by comparing mass transfer area coefficients of radiolabelled sucrose and vitamin B12 in the same patients after intravenous and intraperitoneal administration. Higher MTAC values were found after intraperitoneal administration. Similar results have been reported for the clearances of the non-protein bound antibiotics fosfomycine [152] and cefamandole [153], as well as for inulin [118, 154]. A difference between MTAC values after intravenous and intraperitoneal administration of the same order of magnitude is present when transport rates of endogenous creatinine and albumin are compared to those of intraperitoneally administered solutes with an almost identical molecular weight [145, 155]. These data are summarized in Table 3. When we assume that the peritoneal restriction barrier is symmetric in its hindrance to diffusion, i.e., there is bidirectional equivalency to diffusive mass transfer, then a molecular-weight independent, convective transport out of he peritoneal cavity of 1 to 2 ml/min should be present for solutes that are administered intraperitoneally. Although such a bidirectional equivalency to diffusion has not been proven definitely, it is supported by the fact that the absolute difference between i.v. and i.p. administration is always of the same order of magnitude, irrespective of the size of the solutes. However, the relative difference (compared to the MTAC after i.v. administration) ranges from 16% for low molecular weight solutes like creatinine, to more than 1000% for albumin. When diffusion would not occur equally in both directions, but would always be systematically higher for i.p. administered solutes, a constant relative difference would have been expected. Furthermore, Leypoldt et al. compared the bidirectional transport of creatinine in rabbits using a kinetic model that included convective solute transport by lymphatic absorption out of the peritoneal cavity, and found identical MTAC values [156]. This confirms the presence of a size independent transport out of the peritoneal cavity from 1 to 2 ml/min.

The higher solute transport rates after intraperitoneal administration due to convection, imply that MTAC calculations do not represent diffusion only, when they are calculated with simplified models that do not take into account convective transport out of the peritoneal cavity. Whether this convective leak is solely caused by the lymphatic drainage from the peritoneal cavity, or merely by transmesothelial transport to the peritoneal interstitial tissue induced by abdominal pressure, is a matter that is still under debate (see Chapter 5). The contribution of convection to diffusive transport is relatively small for low molecular weight solutes, but becomes increasingly more important the higher the molecular weight of a solute. The convection/diffusion ratio is about 0.1 for glucose, 1.0 for inulin [118], but 10 for intraperitoneally administered autologous haemoglobin [155], making the disappearance rate of macromolecules relatively independent of molecular size (see below).

It can be concluded that the absorption of intraperitoneally administered molecules is partly size selective (diffusion) and partly non-size selective (convection). The relative contribution of convection increases the higher the molecular weight of the solute. Size-selectivity is therefore most pronounced for solutes with a molecular weight of less than 500.

6.2. Macromolecules

Particles, such as blood cells and bacteria, that are introduced into the peritoneal cavity, are absorbed in the diaphragmatic lymphatics [reviewed in 157]. It is therefore not surprising that a proportion of intraperitoneally administered macromolecules during peritoneal dialysis, also disappears from the peritoneal cavity. Gjessing using dextran 70, 60 g/l as a dialysis solution in peritoneal dialysis patients treated with 30 minute dwells. The recovery of dextran 70 in the dialysate averaged 92% after the

Table 3. Comparison of bidirectional transport of solutes with similar molecular weights. Transport rates are expressed as mass transfer area coefficients (MTAC) or clearances (Cl), both in ml/min. Only paired data are used. Note that clearances are always lower than MTAC values for a given molecular weight.

Solute (IV/IP)	Molecular weight	IV administration	IP administration	Difference
MTAC creatinine/5-flucytosine[a]	113/129	16.10	19.20	3.10
Cl fosfomycine[b]	182	4.40	6.79	2.39
MTAC sucrose[c]	360	5.48	7.56	2.08
Cl cefamandole[d]	485	1.48	2.50	1.02
MTAC vitamin B12[c]	1355	3.30	4.85	1.55
MTAC inulin[e]	5500	1.83	3.17	1.35
Cl inulin[f]	5500	1.79	3.13	1.34
Cl albumin/haemoglobin[g]	69000/68000	0.12	1.53	1.43

Data taken from references [a][145], [b][152], [c][151], [d][153], [e][118], [f][154], [g][155].

dwell, while the plasma concentration increased to 1 g/l after 8 hrs dialysis and even to 4 g/l after 24 hrs [158].

Recoveries of intraperitoneally administered macromolecules of 70–90% after 4 to 7 hr dwells in patients have been reported for radio-iodine tagged serum albumin [51, 52, 105, 159–161], for unlabelled human albumin [162], for dextran 70 10 g/l [54] and 1 gl [55] and for autologous haemoglobin [154, 160]. In only one study a recovery of autologous haemoglobin in excess of 95% has been reported [163]. A high recovery of one batch of unlabelled human albumin was found in another study [164]. This was shown to be caused by a high transport of endogenous albumin, because this particular batch contained a high concentration of prekallikrein activator that caused an inflammatory reaction.

The disappearance rate of intraperitoneally administered macromolecules is independent of molecular size, both in animals [45, 165, 166] and in CAPD patients [50]. Furthermore, it is linear in time [55, 167]. In one study, it was influenced by the osmolarity of the dialysis solution [160], but other studies could not confirm this [107, 167]. The disappearance rate is increased after the instillation of large dialysate volumes [116], during peritonitis [163, 168] and after the application of external pressure [169, 170]. It is likely that a proportion of the intraperitoneally administered macromolecules is taken up directly into the subdiaphragmatic lymphatic vessels, as has been shown in experiments using india ink [171]. Transmesothelial uptake, especially in the anterior abdominal wall has been shown in rats using radio-labelled fibrinogen [56] and – albumin [46]. Uptake of radio-labelled albumin in peritoneal tissues is also likely to be present in peritoneal dialysis patients [51–52]. The macromolecules transported to the interstitial tissue are probably taken up slowly in the lymphatic system, as continuous intraperitoneal administration of dextran 70 in CAPD patients had no effect on the magnitude of its disappearance rate from the peritoneal cavity [55].

In summary, the above data from the literature point to the presence of a non-size-selective mechanism for the disappearance of macromolecules from the peritoneal cavity. They are partly taken up directly by the subdiaphragmatic lymphatic vessels and partly in the peritoneal interstitium. Subsequent uptake into the lymphatics that drain the interstitial tissues is likely to occur.

7. The regulation of surface area and permeability

The effective peritoneal surface area is determined by the area of the membrane that is in direct contact with the dialysate and by the number of perfused peritoneal capillaries. Ultrasound studies have shown that dialysate is evenly distributed throughout the peritoneal cavity in the supine position, but it accumulates mainly in the subumbilical region in sitting – or upright position [63]. This may be the explanation that lower solute clearances have been found while sitting or upright, than during recumbency [172, 173].

The number of perfused peritoneal capillaries is dependent on splanchnic blood flow and volume and on its distribution over the various intestinal organs. Splanchnic blood flow averages 1200 ml/min in normal adults [174]. About 10% of it probably passes through the peritoneum. This is supported by experiments in various animals. Using hydrogen gas clearances a mean peritoneal blood flow of 4.2 ml/min/kg body weight was found in rabbits [175]. In cats a mean value of 1.7ml/min/kg has been reported with microspheres. This value increased markedly to 4.0 ml/min/kg after the instillation of commercially available dialysate [134]. Carbon dioxide experiments in rats yielded values of 4.9 ml/min/kg after the instillation of an isotonic solution and 8.1 ml/min/kg with a hyperosmotic dialysis fluid [176]. Mean values of 75 ml/min [177], or even exceeding 100 ml/min [178] have been reported in peritoneal dialysis patients, using mass transfer area coefficients of carbondioxide. In one study a much lower value of 25 ml/min has been suggested, based on the relationship between the hydrostatic pressure and the plasma protein concentration obtained with a hollow-fiber haemofilter [179, 180] and extrapolated to the situation in peritoneal dialysis. It can be concluded that peritoneal blood flow probably is 70–100 ml/min during peritoneal dialysis in man, and is influenced by the osmolarity and the pH of the dialysis fluid [134, 181].

The regulation of splanchnic blood flow is subject to intrinsic and extrinsic control mechanisms [182]. The intrinsic mechanisms include a pressure-flow autoregulation, an effect of the venous pressure, and the well-known increase of splanchnic blood flow after a meal [183]. The intrinsic regulation is mediated by myogenic factors, metabolic factors and locally produced substances such as vasoactive peptides and autocoids, like prostaglandins [182]. Extrinsic control mechanisms are predominantly by the sympathetic noradrenergic nerves and by circulating vasoactive substances, such as catecholamines, vasopressin and angiotensin II [182]. Alpha-adrenergic stimulation causes intestinal vasoconstriction, stimulation of β_2-receptors leads to dilatation. Intra-arterial infusion of nor-epinephrine causes intestinal vasoconstriction and a decrease in capillary density [182]. A similar effect is present for epinephrine in high doses, but β_2-receptor mediated vasodilation prevails after the administration of a low dose. Vasopressin and angiotensin II cause generalized vasoconstriction with disproportionate reduction in mesenteric blood flow [184]. Vasopressin also causes a decrease in the density of perfused capillaries [182]. Angiotensin II is probably mainly involved in the control of mesenteric blood flow after volume depletion [185]. The administration of glucagon leads to splanchnic dilation [186], but its role in the regulation of splanchnic blood flow is not established [182]. The extrinsic control mechanisms of splanchnic blood flow regulation are mainly involved in the decrease that is present during shock and exercise [187].

The possible effects of variations in splanchnic blood flow and volume on the effective peritoneal surface area have been analyzed in (1) studies during conditions known to be associated with altered splanchnic blood flow, (2) studies on relationships between permeability characteristics and solutes known to be involved in splanchnic blood flow, and (3) experiments during the administration of these solutes. A close relationship has been found in dogs with hemorrhagic shock between the decrease in blood pressure and the decrease in peritoneal urea clearance [188]. However, a decrease in mean arterial pressure to 38% of the initial value produced only a fall in urea clearance to 74%. When blood pressure was restored to 68% of control, urea clearance exceeded the control value by 28%. Physical exercise by CAPD patients has been reported to have no effect on dialysate/plasma ratios of low molecular weight solutes in one study [173], but a decrease in the clearances of albumin and IgG was found in another one [95]. The ingestion of a meal only produced a marginal increase in the clearances of these proteins.

Plasma levels of catecholamines, vasopressin, aldosterone and plasma renin activity are elevated in CAPD patients [189–191]. This does not necessarily imply increased sympathetic activity, but could also be the result of a decrease clearance [190]. Dialysate levels of catecholamines have been measured in one study [189]. The dialysate/plasma ratio was 0.69 for epinephrine and 1.17 for norepinephrine, suggesting local production in the peritoneal cavity. A correlation was found between the dialysate levels of norepinephrine and the effective peritoneal surface area, represented by the mass transfer area coefficient of creatinine. Because this finding is the opposite of the effects of intraperitoneally administered norepinephrine, as will be discussed below, it may be that the large effective surface area causes the release of norepinephrine.

Prostaglandins and cytokines are likely to be produced locally in the peritoneal cavity during peritoneal dialysis. This has been shown for the postaglandins 6-keto-PGF1α, PGE2, PGF2α, TXB2 and 13,14-dihydro-15-keto-PGF2α [192–194]. The concentrations of the vasodilating prostaglandins exceeded that of the vasoconstricting ones. Drained peritoneal effluent also contains the cytokines TNFα [195, 196], interleukin-1 (IL-1) [197, 198], IL-6 [199–201] and IL-8 [201]. The presence of TNFα in the dialysate of uninfected CAPD patients is probably caused by diffusion from the circulation [195, 196], while the other cytokines mentioned above are produced locally within the peritoneal cavity. A relationship has been reported between very high dialysate IL-6 levels in stable CAPD patients and a low peritoneal restriction coefficient, representing a high intrinsic permeability to macromolecules [200]. In that study no relationship was found with the effective peritoneal surface area, as judged from the clearance of β_2-microglobulin. Marked elevations of prostaglandins and cytokines in dialysate are present during peritonitis [192–194, 199, 201, 202]. In addition, also local production of TNFα has been reported during the acute phase of the inflammation [202]. It appeared that the increase in effective peritoneal surface area during peritonitis was related to increases in dialysate TNFα and IL-6, while the increased intrinsic permeability to macromolecules was correlated with dialysate IL-6 and PGE2 concentrations [202]. Intraperitoneal administration of indomethacin during peritonitis inhibited the increase of prostaglandins and also the protein loss in the dialysate [194].

Possible effects of solutes, generally considered to be involved in the regulation of the permeability characteristics of the peritoneum, have been analyzed by studying transport kinetics during peritoneal dialysis after their intraperitoneal or intravenous administration. These include (1) the dialysate itself, (2) hormones, such as catecholamines, gastrointestinal hormones and vasopressin, and (3) histamine and prostaglandins.

The administration of hypertonic and acid dialysate in the rat causes arteriolar vasodilation in the cremaster muscle preceded by an initial vasoconstriction [203–205], and also vasodilation of cecum arterioles [206]. This effect was more pronounced for acetate buffered than for lactate buffered dialysate, and also more pronounced for glucose 1.5% than for glucose 0.5% containing dialysate. The instillation of commercial dialysate in cats leads to a redistribution of splanchnic blood flow, especially to an increased flow in the mesentery, omentum, intestinal serosa and parietal peritoneum [134]. The application of an iso-osmotic bicarbonate buffered solution, that was not vasoactive in the rat cremaster muscle model, to patients treated with peritoneal dialysis had no effect on the effective peritoneal surface area when compared with commercial dialysate [207]. However, it led to an increase in the total protein concentration of the dialysate. In further studies it appeared that this effect could not be explained solely by the osmolarity or pH of the dialysis fluid [208]. The vasoactive effects of commercial glucose based dialysis fluids are likely to be most pronounced during the beginning of a CAPD dwell, as the osmolality is maximal and the pH is minimal. This may be the explanation that MTAC values of low molecular weight solutes and peritoneal protein clearances are higher during the first hour of a dwell than during subsequent hours [107, 110], as has been discussed previously in this chapter.

Increasing the glucose concentration of the dialysate from 1.36% to 3.86% has no effect on the indices of the effective peritoneal surface area [107]. A decrease in them has been reported using glycerol based dialysate [147]. The effects of amino acid containing dialysate are not equivocal. In some studies no effect was found on peritoneal solute transport [119, 149, 209], but others reported increased dialysate protein losses [210, 211]. It may therefore be that amino acids have a more pronounced effect on the intrinsic peritoneal permeability to macromolecules than on the effective surface area. Glucose polymers containing dialysate increases the clearance of β_2-microglobulin, probably by increased convective transport, but it has no effect on other permeability characteristics. [212, 213].

Intravenous administration of norepinephrine in rabbits leads to a decrease in effective surface area as judged from the clearances of urea and creatinine [214]. In contrast, intravenous glucagon increases the clearances of urea and creatinine [215, 216]. As glucagon, a peptide with a molecular weight of 3484 D, was not effective after intraperitoneal administration, these findings support a direct effect on the peritoneal microvasculature. The effects of glucagon have also been confirmed in dogs [217]. Vasopressin administered either intraperitoneally [218] or intravenously [219] leads to a fall in solute kinetics consistent with a decreased effective peritoneal surface area. Topical application of histamine causes arteriolar vasodilation with leakage of proteins both in skeletal muscles and in the mesenterial vasculature [220, 221]. This would suggest an action both on the effective peritoneal surface area and on the intrinsic permeability to macromolecules. Intraperitoneal administration of histamine in rats caused a 10 to 20 percent increase in the clearance of urea [222]. This effect was not confirmed in rabbits in another study, but a marked increase was reported for the protein loss in the dialysate [223]. The histamine-induced protein loss could be blocked by H1 and H2 receptor antagonists. These antagonists were not effective when given alone or during desoxycholate induced chemical peritonitis.

The possible role of prostaglandins on the effective peritoneal surface area has been studied by intravenous and intraperitoneal administration of vasodilating and vasoconstricting ones in rabbits [224–226]. In general the effects were most pronounced after intraperitoneal administration. Arachidonic acid and the vasodilating prostaglandins lead to an increase in the effective peritoneal surface area, while the vasoconstricting PGF2α decreases the clearances of urea and creatinine. The oral administration of the cyclooxygenase inhibitor indomethacin had no effect in these animals. Intraperitoneally administered mefanamic acid reduced the clearance of creatinine marginally, but not that of urea. The intraperitoneal administration of indomethacin in CAPD patients during peritonitis leads to a reduction in peritoneal protein loss [193, 194]. This suggests that prostaglandins may be more involved in the regulation of the intrinsic peritoneal permeability than in that of the effective surface area.

It can be concluded that many factors, that are possibly involved in the regulation of effective peritoneal surface area and intrinsic permeability have been identified, but their relative importance and interactions in the day to day variability of these parameters during peritoneal dialysis still remain unclarified.

8. Peritoneal permeability in systemic diseases

8.1. Uremia

The uremic state is probably associated with more permeable serosal membranes, than the non-uremic situation. This is illustrated by the easy development of pleural and pericardial effusions. Increased capillary permeability has also been reported in the lungs during chronic uremia [227]. A similar increase has been found for the permeability characteristics of the peritoneal membrane during three hour dialysis exchanges, when three patients with chronic renal failure were compared to four patients with normal renal function who were dialyzed because of psoriasis [228]. The uremic patients had higher transport rates for uric acid, phosphate and protein than those with psoriasis, indicating a larger effective peritoneal surface area in the uremics. The intrinsic permeability to macromolecules was not investigated in this study. On the other hand decreased clearances of urea and creatinine have been reported during intermittent peritoneal dialysis in patients with severe hyperparathyroidism [229]. Also in acute renal failure due to rhabdomyolysis caused by heat stress and exercise, decreased peritoneal clearances have been reported for creatinine and uric acid, but not for urea [230].

8.2. Diabetes mellitus

Patients with diabetes mellitus have an abnormal microcirculation. Especially capillary basement membrane alterations with thickening and loose areas of the fibrillar meshwork are common [231]. Also increased microvascular leakage to proteins is present [232]. Peritoneal clearances of exogenous administered radiolabelled albumin in rats undergoing peritoneal dialysis have been found higher in animals with alloxan-induced diabetes mellitus, than in those with gentamicin induced renal failure [233]. This was especially the case in the rats with the most severe diabetes.

Low peritoneal clearances of creatinine and urate have been reported in one patient with severe diabetes mellitus treated with intermittent peritoneal dialysis [234]. In contrast, the MTAC values of urea, creatinine and glucose in a larger group of diabetic CAPD patients were similar to those of patients with renal failure due to a primary renal disease [235–237] (Table 4). Peritoneal protein losses in diabetic CAPD patients are not different from those of other patients [237–239]. As serum albumin concentrations are often low in some of them [240], this can mask increased permeability to macromolecules. In accordance with the findings in alloxan-induced diabetes in rats [233], clearances of albumin, transferrin and IgG have been reported 30% higher in diabetic than in non-diabetic CAPD patients [123]. However, when larger numbers of patients were studied, the difference was no longer significant (Table 4). The explanation for this is probably the large variability in the effective peritoneal surface area and intrinsic permeability in the patients with a primary renal disease.

8.3. Systemic lupus erythematosus

Low clearances for urea, creatinine and urate have been reported in one patient with fulminant systemic lupus erythematosus (SLE) and severe hypertension, treated with intermittent peritoneal dialysis [234]. More recent data show that the prognosis of SLE patients on renal replacement therapy is similar to those with a primary renal disease [241]. In the literature more detailed data on CAPD in SLE have only been reported in 16 patients [242–244]. Solute transport rates were published in four CAPD patients, indicating a normal effective surface area and a decreased intrinsic permeability to macromolecules [235, 245]. This could not be confirmed when larger number of patients were studied (Table 4).

8.4. Systemic sclerosis

Patients with systemic sclerosis can be treated with peritoneal dialysis, despite their low life expectancy [241]. Low peritoneal clearances of low molecular weight solutes have been reported in one patient on intermittent peritoneal dialysis [246], but essentially normal values were found in another one [247]. CAPD treatment has also been described to give good metabolic control [248] and acceptable clearances of low molecular weight solutes [249]. Data on solute transport in two patients are given in Table 4.

8.5. Amyloidosis and paraproteinemia

Peritoneal dialysis as renal replacement therapy in patients with amyloidosis and/or paraproteinemia has given satisfactory clinical results [244, 250]. Evidence for a large effective peritoneal surface area has been reported in four patients with amyloidosis [235, 245]. This may be of importance because peritoneal dialysis can be used to remove immunoglobulins and light chains from the body, thereby preventing further amyloid formation, hyperviscosity syndromes and, perhaps in some cases, reverse renal insufficiency in patients with nephrotoxic light chain induced renal failure [251, 252]. Solute transport data in six patients with amyloidosis are given in Table 4.

It can be concluded that the presence of a systemic disease has no uniform effect on the permeability characteristics of the peritoneal membrane during CAPD, although some patients may present with abnormal high or low MTAC values. However, such abnormal values can also be found in patients with a primary renal disease. It implies that peritoneal dialysis should not be abandoned in patients with systemic diseases, because of the expectation of an abnormal peritoneal permeability.

9. Solute transport during peritonitis

9.1. Low molecular weight solutes

Studies on peritoneal solute transport during intermittent peritoneal dialysis are scarce. "Membrane failure", as judged from deteriorating biochemical control has been reported in four out of 35 IPD patients with peritonitis [253]. In contrast an increase in the clearance of urea with 26% and in that of creatinine with 56% has been found in four IPD patients who were studied in the absence and in the presence of peritonitis [254]. As the effluent volume was similar in these patients, increased permeability caused by the inflammation was the most likely explanation. Decreased drainage volumes, leading to weight gain and other signs of fluid overload have been reported already in the first series on peritonitis in CAPD patients [255]. This reduced net ultrafiltration is associated with increased transport of low molecular weight solutes and increased absorption of glucose [78, 115, 254, 256–259]. These phenomena, pointing to an increased effective peritoneal surface area, lead to a rapid disappearance of the osmotic gradient and thus a reduced net ultrafiltration. Using autologous hemoglobin as a volume marker, it was shown that the maximum intraperitoneal volume during peritonitis was reached at about one hour and after recovery at 2.5 hours [115]. This may explain why a decrease in net ultrafiltration has not been observed during peritonitis in IPD patients. In addition, a high lymphatic absorption rate from the peritoneal cavity may also contribute to the decreased net ultrafiltration during peritoneal inflammation [168]. The changes in solute transport are reversible after resolution of peritonitis [115, 259].

9.2. Macromolecules

Protein loss in the dialysis effluent is markedly increased during peritonitis, both in IPD and in CAPD patients [115, 121, 123, 254, 257, 260]. In IPD patients these losses can be as high as 48 grams per dialysis and often remain elevated for several weeks [121]. Protein loss in the effluent of CAPD patients with peritonitis averages about 15 grams per day and generally returns to baseline values within a few days of antibiotic treatment [121]. The proteins could be produced locally [261] or originate from the circulation. The marked elevation of serum proteins in the dialysate favours the last mechanism. The more than 100% increase in the

Table 4. Comparison of peritoneal permeability characteristics between 46 CAPD patients with a primary renal disease and 38 CAPD patients with systemic diseases. Permeability to low molecular weight solutes is expressed as mass transfer area coefficient (MTAC), that of proteins as clearance (Cl). Mean values ± SEM are given.

	Primary renal disease ($n = 46$)	Systemic lupus erythematosus ($n = 7$)	Systemic Sclerosis ($n = 2$)	Diabetes mellitus ($n = 23$)	Amyloidosis ($n = 6$)
MTAC creatinine (ml/min)	9 ± 0.4	10 ± 1	12 ± 1	10 ± 1	14 ± 2*
MTAC glucose (ml/min)	9 ± 0.4	11 ± 1	10 ± 1	11 ± 1	13 ± 2
Cl albumin (μl/min)	92 ± 6	92 ± 19	118 ± 11	97 ± 7	110 ± 21
Cl IgG (μl/min)	50 ± 3	47 ± 12	61 ± 2	53 ± 5	59 ± 13

* $p < 0.05$ versus primary renal disease.

peritoneal clearances of serum proteins [115, 123] during peritonitis, suggest not only the presence of an increased effective surface area, but also increased intrinsic permeability. Further evidence for increased permeability was obtained by studies on the selectivity index or restriction coefficient of the peritoneum [123, 202]. Possible causes of the increase in surface area and permeability include endotoxin and complement activation [262], as well as prostaglandins [192–194], IL-6 [199, 202] and TNFα [202].

9.3. Sclerosing encapsulating peritonitis

Loss of net ultrafiltration is the most prominent sign of changed peritoneal transport in patients with sclerosing peritonitis [263–270]. A reduced clearance of urea and creatinine has been described in two IPD patients who developed this condition [271]. One CAPD patient has been described who initially had loss of net ultrafiltration associated with increased glucose absorption, that was followed by a normal glucose absorption at a stage where sclerosing peritonitis was present [265]. In another study serial measurements of peritoneal transport kinetics were reported in four CAPD patients, who developed sclerosing peritonitis [269]. Loss of net ultrafiltration was associated with an increase in glucose absorption and an increase in transperitoneal solute transport in three of them. In the other patient a decrease in all these parameters was found. The data suggest that sclerosing peritonitis can either be associated with a small – or with a large effective peritoneal surface area. Local production of interleukin-1 has been hypothesized as a pathogenetic mechanism [197, 272]. The secretion of this cytokine in the peritoneal cavity could lead to an increased production of collagen by peritoneal fibroblasts, but also to release of prostacyclin by the vascular endothelium. It is conceivable that the vasodilating properties of this eicosanoid augment the peritoneal permeability characteristics by increasing the number of perfused capillaries. In addition, the formation of connective tissue could lead to an increase in the number of blood vessels in the poorly vascularized parts of the peritoneum. It is possible that the differences in solute transport in patients with sclerosing peritonitis can be explained by interindividual variations in the susceptibility to either formation of collagen, or the effect of prostacyclin and neovascularization. The former would lead to low, and the latter to high transport rates.

10. Solute transport during long-duration peritoneal dialysis

The efficiency of intermittent peritoneal dialysis has been studied by Finkelstein et al. in eight patients during a follow-up of 10 months [273]. A decrease was found for the clearances of urea, creatinine and glucose in all patients. It is unclear whether this was due to decreased drainage volumes or to decreased dialysate/plasma ratios. All other studies on solute transport during long-duration peritoneal dialysis have been done in CAPD patients. The first study in 12 CAPD patients showed no significant differences for one hour clearances of low molecular weight solutes, except for an increased inulin clearance during the first 6 months on CAPD [274].

The last decade at least 9 cross sectional studies [114, 117, 275–281] on the effect of the duration of CAPD on peritoneal solute transport parameters (Table 5) and 16 longitudinal studies [114, 159, 275, 279, 282–293] (Table 6) have been published. The studies that report clearances of low molecular weight solutes are difficult to interpret, since the drained volume can contribute significantly to the result. This may be the explanation of the contrasting finding of a reduced creatinine clearance in combination with an increased glucose absorption in the study of Nikolakakis et al. [276]. In three of the studies only patients were included who were at least treated with CAPD for 3 years [291], 4 years [286], and 5 years [293]. They therefore represents an interesting, but selected population. Most studies only give results on the transport of low molecular weight solutes. Data on middle-molecules are reported in 6 studies [275, 280, 283–285, 293]. The transport of macromolecules was investigated in 7 studies [114, 117, 278, 280, 282, 287, 293], in 4 of them this was limited to the dialysate loss or clearance of total protein [278, 280, 282, 287].

It is evident from Table 5 and Table 6 that reduced MTAC values or D/P ratios are not a normal finding during long-duration CAPD. This implies that the capability of the peritoneum in the removal of uremic toxins remains intact. In 14 studies no effect of time was found [114, 159, 275, 277–280, 281, 283, 284, 286, 288, 290, 293], in the other 11 an increase in the transport of low molecular weight solutes and middle molecules was reported, indicating a large effective peritoneal surfaces area [114, 117, 275, 276, 279, 282, 285, 287, 289, 291, 292]. The discrepancy may be explained by the fact that solute transport parameters, when measured shortly after the initiation of

Table 5. Summary of the published cross sectional studies on the effect of the duration of CAPD on peritoneal solute transport parameters.

Year	Number of patients	Duration of treatment (years)	Solute studied	Methods	Effect of time	References
1984	45	0–2.5	U, C, UA, PTH, I	MTAC	no	[275]
1985	56	0–4.7	C, G	Cl, GA	C↓, GA↑	[276]
1986	38	0–4	U, C, G, A, IgG	MTAC, GA	MTAC =, GA↑	[114]
1989	43	0–5.8	U, C, G	MTAC, GA	no	[277]
1989	35	0–6.4	U, C, G, TP	Cl, GA	no	[278]
1991	87	0– >3	U, C, G	D/P, Dt/Do	U↑, C↑, G↓[a]	[279]
1991[b]	12	0–4	U, C, TP	Cl	no	[280]
1991[c]	40	0–6.3	C, G, I, β_2-M, A, IgG, α_2-M	MTAC	C↑, G↑, I↑ β_2-M=, A=, iGG=, α_2-M↓	[117]
1992[c]	30	0–7.2	C, G	D/P, Dt/Do	no	[281]

U: urea; C: creatinine; UA: uric acid; I: inulin; G: glucose; β_2-M: β_2-microglobulin; A: albumin; TP: total protein; α_2-M: α_2-macroglobulin; MTAC: mass transfer area coefficient; Cl: clearance; GA: glucose absorption; D: dialysate concentration; P: plasma concentration.
[a] a reduced Dt/Do of glucose is equivalent to an increased GA
[b] only patients with diabetes mellitus
[c] case-control studies comparing long-term patients with recently started controls.

Table 6. Summary of the published longitudinal studies on the effect of the duration of CAPD on peritoneal solute transport parameters.

Year	Number of patients	Duration of follow-up (years)	Number of patients at last follow-up	Solute studied	Methods	Effect of time	References
1979	12	1	6	U, C, I, TP	Cl	C↑, I↑	[282]
1980	10	1	6	U, C, B12	MTAC	no	[283]
1981	15	1.5	4	U, C, B12	MTAC	no	[284]
1984	25	1.5	9	U, C, UA, PTH, I	MTAC	UA↑	[275]
1986	18	1	5	U, C	MTAC	no	[159]
1986	15	3	5	U, C, G, A, IgG	MTAC, GA	no	[114]
1986	18	3–4	10	U, C, UA, PTH, I	MTAC	C↑, UA↑, PTH↑	[285]
1989[a]	16	5	14	U, C	MTAC	no	[286]
1989	134	8	?	C, TP	Cl	C↑	[287]
1989	49	2.5	8	U, C, G	D/P, Cl	no	[288]
1990	35	2.5	?	U, C, G	MTAC	C↑	[289]
1990	31	4	5	U, C, G	U, GA	no	[290]
1990[a]	32	3–6	32	U, C, PO4	Cl	U↑	[291]
1991	17	2	7	U, C, G	D/P, Dt/Do	no	[279]
1992	61	2	19	U, C, G, I, β_2-M A, IgG, α_2-M	MTAC	U=, α_2-M= all other↑[b]	[292]
1992[a]	16	5	16	U	Cl	no	[293]

U: urea; C: creatinine; UA: uric acid; I: inulin; G: glucose; β_2-M: β_2-microglobulin; A: albumin; α_2-M: α_2-macroglobulin; B12: vitamin B12; TP: total protein, PO4: phosphate; Cl: clearance; MTAC: mass transfer area coefficient; GA: glucose absorption; D: dialysate concentration; P: plasma concentration.
[a] In these studies only patients were included who were at least treated with CAPD for 4 years [286], 3 years [291] and 5 years [293]. They therefore represent a selected population.
[b] All values measured between 0 and 3 months (median 43 days) were significantly higher than 4 months later (median 161 days), suggesting that baseline values are not reached before 3 months.

CAPD are higher than after 4 months [292], suggesting that real baseline values are not reached before three months on CAPD.

The clearances of serum proteins were in general not increased, despite the development of a large effective peritoneal surface area. It would suggest a decrease in the intrinsic permeability of the peritoneum. This was supported by the finding of a higher restriction coefficient in patients treated with CAPD for more than 4 years, when compared with matched controls who were studied within the first three months of CAPD [117]. It may, however, be a late effect, because the restriction coefficient showed no changes during the first 2 years [292]. Another interpretation of these findings can be made assuming that the peritoneal interstitial diffusion resistances play a significant part in the transperitoneal exchange of small solutes. If, for example, intestitial diffusion resistances would drop during long-term CAPD, then small solute clearances would increase also.

It can be concluded that long-duration CAPD does not lead to a functional deterioration of the peritoneal membrane, as far as solute transport is concerned. The modest alterations found in some studies suggest an increase in the effective peritoneal surface area. This does not lead to increased protein loss in the effluent, because the intrinsic permeability of the membrane to macromolecules tends to decrease.

Acknowledgements

This work was supported by grant no 08285 from the Swedish Medical Research Council and from the Medical Faculty, University of Lund.

References

1. Esperanca MJ. Collins CL. Peritoneal dialysis efficiency in relation to body weight. J Paediatric Surg 1966; 1: 162–9.
2. Wegener G. Chirurgische Bemerkungen über die peritoneal Hole, mit besondere Berücksichtigung des Overiotomie. Arch Klin Chir 1877; 20: 51–9.
3. Putiloff PV. Materials for the study of the laws of growth of the human body in relation to the surface area: the trial in Russian subjects of planigraphic anatomy as a mean of exact anthropometry. Presented at the Siberian branch of the Russian Geographic Society, Omsk, 1886.
4. Rubin JL. Clawson M, Planch A, Jones Q. Measurements of peritoneal surface area in man and rat. Am J Med Sci 1988; 295: 435–8.
5. Albert A, Takamatsu H, Fonkalsrud EW. Absorption of glucose solutions from the peritoneal cavity in rabbits. Arch Surg 1984; 119: 1247–51.
6. Rubin J, Jones Q, Planch A, Stanek K. Systems of membranes involved in peritoneal dialysis. J Lab Clin Med 1987; 110: 448–53.
7. Bell JL, Leypoldt JK, Frigon RP, Henderson LW. Hydraulically-induced convective solute transport across the rabbit peritoneum. Kidney Int 1990; 38: 19–27.
8. Leypoldt JK, Parker HR, Frigon RP, Henderson LW. Molecular size dependence of peritoneal transport. J Lab Clin Med 1987; 110: 207–16.
9. Fox SD, Leypoldt JK, Henderson LW. Visceral peritoneum is not essential for solute transport during peritoneal dialysis. Kidney Int 1991; 40: 612–20.
10. Alon U, Bar-Maor JA, Bar-Joseph G. Effective peritoneal dialysis in an infant with extensive resection of the small intestine. Am J Nephrol 1988; 8: 65–7.
11. Rippe B, Stelin G, Haraldsson B. Understanding the kinetics of peritoneal transport. Nephrology (Proceedings of the XIth International Society of Nephrology meeting. Tokyo, 1990). Springer International Inc. Tokyo. M Hatano (ed) 1991; pp 1563–72.
12. Rippe B, Stelin G, Haraldsson B. Computer simulations of peritoneal fluid transport in CAPD. Kidney Int 1991; 40: 315–25.
13. Clough G, Michel CC. Quantitative comparisons of hydraulic permeability and endothelial intercellular cleft dimensions in single frog capillaries. J Physiol 1988; 405: 563–76.
14. Landis EM, Pappenheimer JR. Exchange of substances through the capillary walls. In: Hamilton WF, Dow P (eds), Handbook of Physiology, Circulation. Washington DC: Am Physiol Soc, 1963; 2: 961–1034.
15. Myrhage R, Hudlicka O. The microvascular bed and capillary surface area in rat extensor hallucis proprius muscle (EHP). Microvasc Res 1976; 11: 315–23.
16. Flessner MF. Peritoneal transport physiology: Insights from basic research. J Am Soc Nephrol 1991; 2: 122–35.
17. Bundgaard M, Frøkjær-Jensen J, Crone C. Endothelial plasmalemmal vesicles as elements in a system of branching invaginations from the cell surface. Pro Natl Acad Sci 1979; 76: 4639–42.
18. Frøkjær-Jensen J. The plasmalemmal vesicular system in capillary endothelium. Conventional electron microscopic (EM) thin sections compared with the picture arising from ultrathin (~140Å) serial sectioning. Prog Appl Microcirc 1983; 1: 17–34.
19. Frøkjær-Jensen J. The vesicle controversy. Prog Appl Microcirc 1985; 9: 21–42.
20. Alvarez OA, Yudilevich DL. Heart capillary permeability to lipid-insoluble molecules. J Physiol 1969; 202: 45–58.
21. Curry FE, Mason JCm Michel CC. Osmotic reflection coefficients of capillary walls to low

molecular weight hydrophilic solutes measured in single perfused capillaries of the frog mesentery. J Physiol (London) 1976; 261: 319–36.
22. Crone C, Levitt DG. Capillary permeability to small solutes. In: Renkin EM, Michel CC (eds), Handbook of Physiology, The cardiovascular system. Microcirculation. Methesda MD: Am Physiol Soc 1984; 4: 411–66.
23. Dempster JA, Van Hoek AN, Van Os CH. The quest for water channels. News Physiol Sci 1992; 7: 172–6.
24. Curry FE. Mechanics and thermodynamics of transcapillary exchange. In: Renkin EM, Michel CC (eds), Handbook of Physiology, The cardiovascular system. Microcirculation. Bethesda MD: Am Physiol Soc 1984; 4: 309–74.
25. Bundgaard M. The three-dimentional organization of tight junctions in a capillary endothelium revealed by serial-section electron microscopy. J. Ultrastruct Res 1984; 88: 1–17.
26. Rippe B, Haraldsson B. How are macromolecules transported across the capillary wall? NIPS 1987; 2: 135–8.
27. Palade GE. Fine structure of blood capillaries. J Appl Physiol 1953; 24: 1424.
28. Simionescu N. Cellular aspects of transcapillary exchange. Physiol Reviews 1983; 63: 1536–79.
29. Simionescu N, Simionescu M, Palade G. Permeability of muscle capillaries to small heme peptides. Evidence for the existence of patent transendothelial channels. J Cell Bio 1975; 64: 568–607.
30. Rippe B, Kamiya A, Folkow B. Transcapillary passage of albumin, effects of tissue cooling and of increases in filtration and plasma colloid osmotic pressure. Acta Physiol Scand 1979; 105: 171–87.
31. Rippe B, Haraldsson B. Fluid and protein fluxes across small and large pores in the microvasculature. Application of two-pore equations. Acta Physiol Scand 1987; 131: 411–28.
32. Rippe B, Haraldsson B. Transport of macromolecules across microvascular walls. The two-pore theory. Physiol Rev 1994; 74: 163–219.
33. Grotte G. Passage of dextran molecules across the blood-lymph barrier. Acta Chir Scand Suppl 1956; 211: 1–84.
34. Taylor AE, Granger DN. Exchange of macromolecules across the microcirculation. In: Renkin EM, Michel CC, editors. Handbook of Physiology. The cardiovascular system. Microcirculation. Methesda MD: Am Physiol Soc 1984; 4: 467–520.
35. Renkin EM. Capillary transport of macromolecules: pores and other endothelial pathways. J Appl Physiol 1985; 58: 315–25.
36. Leypoldt JK, Blindauer KM. Convection does not govern plasma to dialysate transport of protein. Kidney Int 1992; 42: 1412–8.
37. Gerch I, Catchpole HR. The nature of ground substances of connective tissue. Perspect Biol Med 1960; 3: 282–319.
38. Wiederhielm CA. The interstitial space. In: Fung YC, Perrone N, Andeker M, editors. Biomechanis:
Its Foundations and Objectives. Englewood Cliffs, NJ: Prentice-Hall, 1972, pp 273–86.
39. Aukland K, Reed RK. Interstitial-lymphatic mechanisms in the control of extracellular fluid volume. Physiol Rev 1993; 73: 1–78.
40. Barber BJ, Nearing BD. Spatial distribution of protein in interstitial matrix of rat mesenteric tissue. Am J Physiol 258 (Heart Circ. Physiol 27) 1990; H556–64.
41. Watson PD, Grodins FS. An analysis of the effects of the interstitial matrix on plasma-lymph transport. Microvasc Res 1978; 16: 19–41.
42. Schultz JS, Armstrong W. Permeability of interstitial space of muscle (rat diaphragm) to solutes of different molecular weights. J Pharm Sci 1978; 67: 696–700.
43. Flessner MF, Dedrick RL, Schultz JD. A distributed model of peritoneal plasma transport: analysis of experimental data in the rat. Am J Physiol 1985; 248: F413–F24.
44. Flessner MF, Fenstermacher JK, Dedrick RL, Blasberg RG. A distributed model of peritoneal-plasma transport: Tissue concentration gradients. Am J Physiol 1985; 248: F425–35.
45. Flessner MF, Dedrick RL, Schultz JS. Exchange of macromolecules between peritoneal cavity and plasma. Am J Physiol 1985; 248: H15–25.
46. Flessner MF, Fenstermacher JD, Blasberg RG, Dedrick RL. Peritoneal absorption of macromolecules studied by quantitative autoradiography. Am J Physiol 1985; 248: H26–32.
47. Strømme SB, Maggert JE, Scholander PF. Interstitial fluid pressure in terrestrial and semiterrestrial animals. J Appl Physiol 27(1)1961; 123–26.
48. French JE, Florey HW, Morris B. The absorption of particles by the lymphatics of the diaphragm. Q J Exp Physiol 1960; 45: 88–103.
49. Bettendorf U. Lymph flow mechanism of the subperitoneal diaphragmatic lymphatics. Lymphology 1978; 11: 111–6.
50. Krediet RT, Struijk DG, Koomen GCM, Hoek FJ, Arisz L. The disappearance of macromolecules from the peritoneal cavity during continuous ambulatory peritoneal dialysis (CAPD) is not dependent on molecular size. Perit Dial Int 1990; 10: 147–52.
51. Daugirdas JT, Ing TS, Gandhi VC, Hano JE, Chen WT, Yuan L. Kinetics of peritoneal fluid absorption in patients with chronic renal failure. J Lab Clin Med 1980; 95: 351–61.
52. Rippe B, Stelin G, Ahlmen J. Lymph flow from the peritoneal cavity in CAPD patients. In: Maher JF, Winchester JF (eds), Frontiers in peritoneal dialysis. Field, Rich, New York 1986; pp 24–30.
53. Mactier RA, Khanna R, Twardowski ZJ, Moore H, Nolph KD. Contribution of lymphatic absorption to loss of ultrafiltration and solute clearances in continuous ambulatory peritoneal dialysis. J Clin Invest 1987; 80: 1311–6.
54. Krediet RT, Struijk DG, Koomen GCM, Arisz L. Peritoneal fluid kinetics during CAPD measured with intraperitoneal dextran 70. ASAIO Trans 1991; 37: 662–7.

55. Struijk DG, Koomen GCM, Krediet RT, Arisz L. Indirect measurement of lymphatic absorption in CAPD patients is not influenced by trapping. Kidney Int 1992; 41: 1668–75.
56. Flessner MF, Parker RJ, Sieber SM. Peritoneal lymphatic uptake of fibrinogen and erthrocytes in the rat. Am J Physiol 1983; 244: H89–96.
57. Flessner MF, Dedrick RL, Reynolds JC. Bidirectional peritoneal transport of immunoglobulin in rats: compartmental kinetics. Am J Physiol 1992; 262: F275–87.
58. Dobbie JW. Morphology of the peritoneum in CAPD. Blood Purif 1989; 7: 74–85.
59. Nagel W, Kuschinsky W. Study of the permeability of the isolated dog mesentery. Eur J Clin Invest 1970; 1: 149–54.
60. Rasio EA. Metabolic control of permeability in isolated mesentery. Am J Physiol 1974; 226(4): 962–8.
61. Michel CC. Filtration coefficients and osmotic reflection coefficients of the walls of single frog mesenteric capillaries. J Physiol 1980; 309: 341–55.
62. Seames EL, Moncrief JW, Popovich RP. A distributed model of fluid and mass transfer in peritoneal dialysis. Am J Physiol 1990; 258: 958–72.
63. Rippe B, Stelin G. Simulations of peritoneal solute transport during CAPD. Application of two-pore formalism. Kidney Int 1989; 35: 1234–44.
64. Bassingthwaighte JB, Chinard FP, Crone C, Goresky CA, Lassen NA, Reneman RS, Zierler KL. Terminology for mass transport and exchange. Am J Physiol 250 (Heart Circ Physiol 19) 1986; 250: H539–45.
65. Kedem O, Katchalsky A. Thermodynamic analysis of the permeability of biological membranes to nonelectrolytes. Biochem Biophys Acta 1958; 27: 229–46.
66. Patlak CS, Goldstein DA, Hoffman JF. The flow of solute and solvent across a two-membrane system. J Theor Biol 1963; 5: 425–42.
67. Henderson LW, Nolph KD. Altered permeability of the peritoneal membrane after using hypertonic peritoneal dialysis fluid. J Clin Invest 1969; 48: 992–1001.
68. Garred LJ, Canaud B, Farrell P. A simple kinetic model for assessing peritoneal mass transfer in chronic ambulatory peritoneal dialysis. ASAIO J 1983; 6: 131–7.
69. Pyle WK. Mass transfer in peritoneal dialysis [dissertation]. Texas: Univ. of Texas, Austin, 1981.
70. Popovich RP, Pyle WK, Moncrief JW. Kinetics of peritoneal transport. In: Nolph KD (eds), Peritoneal dialysis. Nijhoff, Boston 1981; pp 115–8.
71. Pyle WK, Moncrief JW, Popovich RP. Peritoneal transport evaluation in CAPD. CAPD update, Continuous Ambulatory Peritoneal Dialysis. Masson Publishing, USA, Inc, New York 1981; 35–52.
72. Lysaght MJ, Farrell PC. Membrane phenomena and mass transfer kinetics in peritoneal dialysis. J Membr Sci 1989; 44: 5–23.
73. Waniewski J, Werynski A, Heimbürger O, Lindholm B. Simple models for description of small-solute transport in peritoneal dialysis. Blood Purif 1991; 9: 129–41.
74. Waniewski J, Werynski A, Heimbürger O, Lindholm B. A comparative analysis of mass transfer models in peritoneal dialysis. ASAIO Trans 1991; 37: 65–75.
75. Stelin G, Rippe B. A phenomenological interpretation of the variation in dialysate volume with dwell time in CAPD. Kidney Int 1990; 38: 465–72.
76. Rippe B, Perry MA, Granger DN. Permselectivity of the peritoneal membrane. Microvasc Res 1985; 29: 89–102.
77. Zakaria E, Rippe B. Osmotic barrier characteristics of the rat peritoneal membrane. Acta Physiol Scand 1993; 149: 355–64.
78. Smeby LC, Wideröe T-E, Jörstad S. Individual differences in water transport during peritonitis. ASAIO J 1981; 4: 17–27.
79. Wideröe T-E, Smeby LC, Dahl K, Jörstad S. Definitions of differences and changes in peritoneal membrane transport properties. Kidney Int 1988; 33: S107–13.
80. Krediet RT, Imholz ALT, Struijk DG, Koomen GCM, Arisz L. Ultrafiltration failure in CAPD. Perit Dial Int 1993; 13 (suppl 2): S59–66.
81. Vonesh EF, Lysaght MJ, Moran J, Farrell P. Kinetic modelling as a prescription aid in peritoneal dialysis. Blood Purif 1991; 9: 246–70.
82. Vonesh EF, Rippe B. Net fluid absorption under membrane transport models of peritoneal dialysis. Blood Purif 1992; 10: 209–26.
83. Rippe B. A three-pore model of peritoneal transport. Perit Dial Int 1993; 13 (Suppl 2): S35–8.
84. Mason EA, Wendt RP, Bressler EH. Similarity relations (dimensional analysis) for membrane transport. J Mebr Sci 1980; 6: 283–98.
85. Areekul S. Reflection coefficients of neutral and sulphate-substituted dextran molecules in the isolated perfused rabbit ear. Acta Soc Med Upsal 1969; 74: 139–42.
86. Haraldsson B, Moxham BJ, Rippe B. Capillary permeability to sulphate-substituted and neutral dextran fractions in the rat hindquarter vascular bed. Acta Physiol Scand 1982; 115: 397–404.
87. Haraldsson B, Ekholm C, Rippe B. Importance of molecular charge for the passage of endogenous macromolecules across continuous capillary walls, studied by serum clearance of lactate dehydrogenase (LDH) isoenzymes. Acta Physiol Scand 1983; 117: 123–30.
88. Adamson RH, Huxley VH, Curry FE. Single capillary permeability to proteins having similar size but different charge. Am J Physiol. 254, 1988; H304–12.
89. Haraldsson B, Rippe B. Orosmucoid as one of the serum components contributing to normal capillary permselectivity in rat skeletal muscle. Acta Physiol Scand 1986; 129: 127–35.
90. Haraldsson B, Johnsson E, Rippe B. Glomerular permselectivity is dependent on adequate serum concentrations of orosmucoid. Kidney Int 1992; 41: 310–6.

91. Parker JC, Gilchrist S, Cartledge JT. Plasma – lymph exchange and interstitial distribution volumes of charged macromolecules in the lung. J Appl Physiol 1985; 59: 1128–36.
92. Gilchrist SA, Parker JC. Exclusion of charged macromolecules in the pulmonary interstitium. Microvasc Res 1985; 30: 88–98.
93. Leypoldt JK, Henderson LW. Molecular charge influences transperitoneal macromolecule transport. Kidney Int 1993; 43: 837–44.
94. Krediet RT, Koomen GCM, Koopman MG, Hoek FJ, Struijk DG, Boeschoten EW, Arisz L. The peritoneal transport of serum proteins and neutral dextran in CAPD patients. Kidney Int 1989; 35: 1064–72.
95. Krediet RT, Struijk DG, Koomen GCM, Zemel D, Boeschoten EW, Hoek FJ, Arisz L. Peritoneal transport of macromolecules in patients on CAPD. Contr Nephrol 1991; 89: 161–74.
96. Alavi N, Lianos E, Andres G, Bentzel CJ. Effect of protamine on the permeability and structure of rat peritoneal. Kidney Int 1982; 21: 44–53.
97. Galdi P, Shostak A, Jaichenko J, Fudin R, Gotloib L. Protamine sulfate induces enhanced peritoneal permeability to proteins. Nephron 1991; 57: 45–51.
98. Rippe B, Kamiya A. Folkow B. Simultaneous measurements of capillary diffusion and filtration exchange during shifts in filtration (absorption and at graded alterations in the capillary permeability surface area product (PS). Acta Physiol Scand 1978; 105: 171–87.
99. Gotloib L, Shustak A, Jaichenko J. Loss of mesothelial electronegative fixed charges during murine septic peritonitis. Nephron 1989; 51: 77–83.
100. Munck WD, Zestar LP, Anderson JL. Rejection of polyelectrolytes from microporous membranes. J Membr Sci 1979; 5: 77–102.
101. Twardowski ZJ, Nolph KD, Khanna R, Prowant BF, Ryan LP, Moore HL, Nielsen MP. Peritoneal equilibration test. Perit Dial Bull 1987; 7: 138–47.
102. Krediet RT, Boeschoten EW, Zuyderhoudt FMJ, Strackee J, Arisz L. Simple assessment of the efficiency of peritoneal transport in continuous ambulatory peritoneal dialysis patients. Blood Purif 1986; 4: 194–203.
103. Struijk DG, Krediet RT, Koomen GCM, Boeschoten EW, Arisz L. Measurement of peritoneal transport for low molecular weight solutes; which test should be used? Nephrol Dial Transplant 1990; 5: 721.
104. Heimbürger O, Waniewski J, Weryshi A, Parh MS, Lindholm B. Dialysate to plasma solute concentration (DIP) versus peritoneal transport parameters in CAPD. Nephrol Dial Transplant 1994; 9: 47–59.
105. Heimbürger O, Waniewski J, Werynski A, Traneus A, Lindholm B. Peritoneal transport in CAPD patients with permanent loss of ultrafiltration capacity. Kidney Int 1990; 38: 495–506.
106. Waniewski J, Heimbürger O, Werynski A, Lindholm B. Aqueous solute concentration and evaluation of mass transport coefficients in peritoneal dialysis. Nephrol Dial Transpl 1992; 7: 50–6.
107. Imholz ALT, Koomen GCM, Struijk DG, Arisz L, Krediet RT. The effect of dialysate osmolarity on the transport of low molecular weight solutes and proteins during CAPD. Kidney Int 1993; 43: 1339–46.
108. Lindholm B, Werynski A, Bergsgtröm J. Kinetics of peritoneal dialysis with glycerol and glucose as osmotic agents. ASAIO Trans 1987; 10: 19–27.
109. Rubin J, Nolph K, Arfania D, Brown P, Prowant B. Follow-up of peritoneal clearances in patients undergoing continuous ambulatory peritoneal dialysis. Kidney Int 1979; 16: 619–23.
110. Kagan A, Bar-Khayim Y, Schafer Z, Fainaru M. Kinetics of peritoneal protein loss during CAPD: 1. Different characteristics for low and high molecular weight proteins. Kidney Int 1990; 37: 971–9.
111. Imholz ALT, Koomen GCM, Struijk DG, Arisz L, Krediet RT. Residual volume measurements in CAPD patients with exogenous and endogenous solutes. Adv Perit Dial 1992; 8: 33–8.
112. Crone C. Does 'restricted diffusion' occur in muscle capillaries. Proc Soc Exp Biol Med 1963; 112: 453–5.
113. Rippe B, Stelin G, Ahlmén J. Basal permeability of the peritoneal membrane during continuous ambulatory peritoneal dialysis (CAPD). In: Gahl GM, Kessel M, Nolph KD (eds), Advances in peritoneal dialysis. Proceedings of the 2nd International Symposium on Peritoneal Dialysis. Excerpta Medica, Amsterdam 1981; pp 5–9.
114. Krediet RT, Boeschoten EW, Zuyderhoudt FMJ, Arisz L. Peritoneal transport characteristics of water, low-molecular weight solutes and proteins during long-term continuous ambulatory peritoneal dialysis. Perit Dial Bull 1986; 6: 61–5.
115. Krediet RT, Zuyderhoudt FMJ, Boeschoten EW, Arisz L. Alterations in the peritoneal transport of water and solutes during peritonitis in continuous ambulatory peritoneal dialysis patients. Eur J Clin Invest 1987; 17: 43–52.
116. Krediet RT, Boeschoten EW, Struijk DG, Arisz L. differences in the peritoneal transport of water, solutes and proteins between dialysis with two- and with three-litre exchanges. Nephrol Dial Transplant 1988; 2: 198–204.
117. Struijk DG, Krediet RT, Koomen GCM, Hoek FJ, Boeschoten EW, van der Reijden HJ, Arisz L. Functional characteristics of the peritoneal membrane in long-term continuous ambulatory peritoneal dialysis. Nephron 1991; 59: 213–20.
118. Struijk DG, Krediet RT, Koomen GCM, Boeschoten EW, Reijden JH van der, Arisz L. Indirect measurement of lymphatic absorption with inulin in continuous ambulatory peritoneal dialysis (CAPD) patients. Perit Dial Int 1990; 10: 141–5.
119. Lindholm B, Werynski A, Bergström J. Peritoneal dialysis with amino acid solutions: fluid and solute transport kinetics. Artif Org 1988; 12: 2–10.
120. Heimbürger O, Waniewski J, Werynski A, Lindholm B. A quantitative description of solute

and fluid transport during peritoneal dialysis. Kidney Int 1992; 41: 1320–32.
121. Blumenkrantz MJ, Gahl GM, Kopple JD, Kamdar AV, Jones MR, Kessel M, Coburn JW. Protein losses during peritoneal dialysis. Kidney Int 1981; 19: 593–602.
122. Young GA, Brownjohn AM, Parsons FM. Protein losses in patients receiving continuous ambulatory peritoneal dialysis. Nephron 1986; 45: 196–201.
123. Krediet RT, Zuyderhoudt FMJ, Boeschoten EW, Arisz L. Peritoneal permeability to proteins in diabetic and non-diabetic continuous ambulatory peritoneal dialysis patients. Nephron 1986; 42: 133–40.
124. Davies SJ, Brown B, Bryan J, Russell M. Clinical evaluation of the peritoneal equilibration test: a population based study. Nephrol Dial Transplant 1993; 8: 64–70.
125. Nolph KD, Miller FN, Pyle WK, Popovich RP, Sorkin MI. An hypothesis to explain the ultrafiltration characteristics of peritoneal dialysis. Kidney Int 1981; 20: 543–8.
126. Comper WD, Laurent TC. Physiological function of connective tissue polysaccharides. Physiol Rev 1978; 58: 255–315.
127. Knochel JP. Formation of peritoneal fluid hypertonicity during dialysis with isotonic glucose solutions. J Appl Physiol 1969; 27: 233–6.
128. Fox JR, Wayland H. Interstitial diffusion of macromolecules in the rat mesentery. Microvasc Res 1979; 18: 277–9.
129. Verger C, Luger A, Moore HL, Nolph KD. Acute changes in peritoneal morphology and transport properties with infectious peritonitis and mechanical injury. Kidney Int 1983; 23: 823–31.
130. Brown ST, Ahearn DJ, Nolph KD. Reduced peritoneal clearances in scleroderma increased by intraperitoneal isoproterenol. Ann Intern Med 1973: 78: 891–4.
131. Nolph KD, Ghods, AJ, Van Stone J, Brown PA. The effects of intraperitoneal vasodilators on peritoneal clearances. Trans Am Soc Artif Intern Organs 1976; 22: 586–94.
132. Nolph KD, Ghods A, Brown P, Miller F, Harris P, Pyle K, Popovich R. Effects of nitroprusside on peritoneal mass transfer coefficients and microvascular physiology. Trans Am Soc Artif Inter Organs 1977; 23: 210–8.
133. Miller FN, Joshua IG, Anderson GL. Quantation of vasodilator-induced macromolecular leakage by in vivo fluorescent microscopy. Microvasc Res 1982; 24: 56–67.
134. Granger DN, Ulrich M, Perry MA, Kvietys PR. Peritoneal dialysis solutions and feline splanchnic blood flow. Clin Exp Pharmacol Physiol 1984; 11: 473–82.
135. Pietrzak I. Hirszel P, Shostak A, Welch PG, Lee RE, Maher JF. Splanchnic volume, not to flow rate determines peritoneal permeability. Trans Am Soc Artif Intern Organs 1989; 35: 583–7.
136. Popovich RP, Pyle WK, Moncrief JW, Bomar JB. Peritoneal Dialysis. Chronic Replacement of Kidney Function. Am ChE Symp Series 1987; 75(187): 31–45.
137. Bonomini V, Zucchelli P, Mioli V. Selective and unselective protein loss in peritoneal dialysis. Proc Eur Dial Transplant Ass 1967; 4: 146–9.
138. Leypoldt JK, Parker HR, Frigon RP, Henderson LW. Molecular size dependence of peritoneal transport. J Lab Clin Med 1987; 110: 207–16.
139. Leypoldt JK, Frigon RP, De Vore KW, Henderson LW. A rapid renal clearance methodology for dextran. Kidney Int 1987; 31: 855–60.
140. Granath KA, Kvist BE. Molecular weight distribution analysis by gel chromatography on sephadex. J Chromatogr 1967; 28: 69–81.
141. Krediet RT, Struijk DG, Zemel D, Koomen GCM, Arisz L. The transport of macromolecules across the human peritoneum during CAPD. In: La Graeca G, Ronco C, Feriani M, Chiaramonte S, Conz P (eds), Peritoneal Dialysis. Wichtig, Milano 1991; pp 61–9.
142. Zemel D, Krediet RT, Koomen GCM, Struijk DG, Arisz L. Day-to-day variability of protein transport used as a method for analyzing peritoneal permeability in CAPD. Perit Dial Int 1991; 11: 217–23.
143. Krediet RT, Zemel D, Struijk DG, Koomen GCM, Arisz L. Individual characterization of the peritoneal restriction barrier to macromolecules. Adv Perit Dial 1991; 7: 15–20.
144. Krediet RT, Zemel D, Struijk DG, Koomen GCM, Arisz L. Individual characterization of the peritoneal restriction barrier to the transport of serum proteins. In: Ota K et al. (eds), Current concepts in peritoneal dialysis. Elsevier 1992; pp 49–55.
145. Krediet RT, Boeschoten EW, Struijk DG, Arisz L. Pharmacokinetics of intraperitoneally administered 5-fluorocytosine in continuous ambulatory peritoneal dialysis. Nephrol Dial Transplant 1987; 2: 453.
146. Krediet RT, Boeschoten EW, Zuyderhoudt FMJ, Arisz L. The relationship between peritoneal glucose absorption and body fluid loss by ultrafiltration during continuous ambulatory peritoneal dialysis. Clin Nephrol 1987; 27: 51–5.
147. Heaton A, Ward MK, Johnston DG, Nicholson DV, Alberti KGMM, Kerr DNS. Short-term studies on the use of glycerol as an osmotic agent in continuous ambulatory peritoneal dialysis (CAPD). Clin Sci 1984; 67: 121–30.
148. Williams PF, Marliss EB, Andersson GH, Oren A, Stein AN, Khanna R, Petitt J, Brandes L, Rodella H, Mupas L, Dombros N, Oreopoulos DG. Amino acid absorption following intraperitoneal administration in CAPD patients. Perit Dial Bull 1982; 2: 124–30.
149. Goodship THJ, Lloyd S, McKenzie PW, Earnshaw M, Smeaton I, Bartlett K, Ward MK, Wilkinson R. Short-term studies on the use of amino acids as an osmotic agent in continuous ambulatory peritoneal dialysis. Clin Sci 1987; 73: 471–8.
150. Lukas G, Brindle SD, Greengard P. The route of absorption of intraperitoneally administered compounds. J Pharm Exp Ther 1971; 178: 562–6.

151. Babb AL, Johansen PJ, Strand MJ, Tenckhoff H, Scribner BH. Bi-directional permeability of the human peritoneum to middle molecules. Proc Eur Dial Transplant Ass 1973; 10: 247–61.
152. Bouchet JL, Albin H, Quentin C, De Barbeyrac B, Vinçon G, Martin-Dupont Ph, Potaux L, Aparicio M. Pharmacokinetics of intravenous and intraperitoneal fosfomycin in continuous ambulatory peritoneal dialysis. Clin Nephrol 1988; 29: 35–40.
153. Janicke DM, Morse GD, Apicella MA, Jusko WJ, Walshe JJ. Pharmacokinetic modelling of bidirectional transfer during peritoneal dialysis. Clin Pharmacol Ther 1986; 40: 209–18.
154. Struijk DG, Imholz ALT, Krediet RT, Koomen GCM, Arisz L. The use of the disappearance rate for the measurement of lymphatic absorption during CAPD. Blood Purif 1992; 10: 182–8.
155. Krediet RT, Struijk DG, Boeschoten EW, Hoek FJ, Arisz L. Measurement of intraperitoneal fluid kinetics in CAPD patients by means of autologous hemoglobin. Neth J Med 1988; 33: 281–90.
156. Leypoldt JK, Pust AH, Frigon RP, Henderson LW. Dialysate volume measurements required for determining peritoneal solute transport. Kidney Int 1988; 34: 254–61.
157. Khanna R, Mactier R, Twardowski ZJ, Nolph KD. Peritoneal cavity lymphatics. Perit Dial Bull 1986; 6: 113–21.
158. Gjessing J. The use of dextran as a dialyzing fluid in peritoneal dialysis. Acta Med Scan 1969; 185: 237–9.
159. Spencer PC, Farrell PC. Solute and water transfer kinetics in CAPD. In: Gokal R (ed), Continuous ambulatory peritoneal dialysis. Edinburgh: Churchill Livingstone, 1986; 38–55.
160. De Paepe M, Belpaire F, Schelstraete K, Lameire N. Comparison of different volume markers in peritoneal dialysis. J Lab Clin Med 1988; 111: 421–9.
161. Lindholm B, Heimbürger O, Waniewski J, Werynski A, Bergström J. Peritoneal ultrafiltration and fluid reabsorption during peritoneal dialysis. Nephrol Dial Transplant 1989; 4: 805–13.
162. Mactier RA, Khanna R, Twardowski ZJ, Moore H, Nolph KD. Contribution of lymphatic absorption to loss of ultrafiltration and solute clearances in continuous ambulatory peritoneal dialysis. J Clin Invest 1987; 80: 1311–6.
163. Brouard R, Tozer TN, Baumelou A, Gambertoglio JG. Transfer of autologous haemoglobin from the peritoneal cavity during peritoneal dialysis. Nephrol Dial Transplant 1992; 7: 57–62.
164. Struijk DG, Bakker JC, Krediet RT, Koomen GCM, Stekkinger P, Arisz L. Effect of intraperitoneal administration of two different batches of albumin solutions on peritoneal solute transport in CAPD patients. Nephrol Dial Transplant 1991; 6: 198–202.
165. Hirszel P, Shea-Donohue T, Chakrabarti E, Montcalm E, Maher JF. The role of the capillary wall in restricting diffusion of macromolecules. Nephron 1988; 44: 58–61.
166. Cheek TR, Twardowski ZJ, Moore HL, Nolph KD. Absorption of inulin and high-molecular weight gelatin isocyanate solutions from peritoneal cavity of rats. In: Avram MM, Giordano C (eds), Ambulatory peritoneal dialysis. Plenum, New York 1990; pp 149–52.
167. Nolph KD, Mactier R, Khanna R, Twardowski ZJ, Moore H, McGary T. The kinetics of ultrafiltration during peritoneal dialysis: the role of lymphatics. Kidney Int 1987; 32: 219–26.
168. Krediet RT, Arisz L. Fluid and solute transport across the peritoneum during continuous ambulatory peritoneal dialysis (CAPD). Perit Dial Int 1989; 9: 15–25.
169. Imholz ALT, Koomen GCM, Struijk DG, Arisz L, Krediet RT. The effect of increased intraperitoneal pressure on fluid and protein transport during CAPD. Kidney Int 1993; 44: 1078–83.
170. Rippe B, Zakaria E. Peritoneal fluid and albumin kinetics in the rat; effects of increases in intraperitoneal hydrostatic pressure. Perit Dial Int 1993; 13; suppl 1: S74.
171. Mactier RA, Khanna R, Twardowski ZJ, Moore H, Nolph KD. Influence of phosphatidylcholine on lymphatic absorption during peritoneal dialysis in the rat. Perit Dial Int 1988; 8: 179–86.
172. Curatola G, Zoccali C, Crucitti S, Pastorino D, Siclari F, Cuzzucri A, Maggiore Z. Effect of posture on peritoneal clearance in CAPD patients. Perit Dial Int 1988; 8: 58–9.
173. Zanozi S, Winchester JF, Kloberdanz N, Preuss H, Fox S, Cocker C, Sanders K, Barnard W, Fox L. Upright position and exercise lower peritoneal transport rates. Kidney Int 1983; 23: 165.
174. Bradley SE. Variations in hepatic blood flow in man during health and disease. New Engl J Med 1949; 240: 456–61.
175. Aune S. Transperitoneal exchange. Peritoneal blood flow estimated by hydrogen gas clearance. Scand J Gastroent 1970; 5: 99–104.
176. Grzegorzewska AE, Moore HL, Nolph KD, Chen TW. Ultrafiltration and effective peritoneal blood flow during peritoneal dialysis in the rat. Kidney Int 1991; 39: 608–17.
177. Nolph KD, Popovich RP, Ghods AJ, Twardowski ZJ. Determinants of low clearances of small solutes during peritoneal dialysis. Kidney Int 1978; 13: 117–23.
178. Grzegozewska AE, Antoniewicz K. An indirect estimation of effective peritoneal capillary blood flow (EPBF) in peritoneally dialyzed uremic patients. Perit Dial Int 1992; 12;suppl 2: S3.
179. Ronco C, Brendolan A, Bragantini L, Chiaramonte S, Feriani M, Fabris A, La Greca G. Studies on ultrafiltration in peritoneal dialysis: influence of plasma proteins and capillary blood flow. Perit Dial Bull 1986; 6: 93–7.
180. Ronco C, Feriani M, Chiaramonte S, Brendolan A, Bragantini L, Conz P, Dell'Aquila R, Milan M, La Greca G. Pathophysiology of ultrafiltration in peritoneal dialysis. Perit Dial Int 1990; 10: 119–26.
181. Grzegorzewska AE, Moore HL, Chen TW, Nolph KD. Peritoneal clearances of carbon dioxide in the rat. Adv Perit Dial 1992; 8: 26–9.

182. Crissinger KD, Granger DN. Gastrointestinal blood flow. In: Yamada T (ed), Textbook of gastroenterology. Lippincott, Philadelphia 1991: pp 447–74.
183. Brandt JL, Castleman L, Ruskin HD, Greenwald J, Kelly JJ jr, Jones A. The effect of oral protein and glucose feeding on splanchnic blood flow and oxygen utilization in normal and cirrhotic subjects. J Clin Invest 1955; 34: 1017–25.
184. Rocha E, Silva M, Rosenberg M. The release of vasopressin in response to haemorrhage and its role in the mechanism of blood pressure regulation. J Physiol (London) 1969; 202: 535–57.
185. Suvannapura A, Levens NR. Local control of mesenteric blood flow by the renin-angiotensin system. am J Physiol 1988; 255: G267–74.
186. Rayford PL, Miller TA, Thompson J. Secretin, cholecystokinin and newer gastrointestinal hormones. N Engl J Med 1976; 294: 1093–100.
187. Wade OL, Combes B, Childs AW, Wheeler HO, Cournand A, Bradley SE. The effect of exercise on the splanchinic blood flow and splanchnic blood volume in normal man. Clin Sci 1956; 15: 457–63.
188. Erbe RW, Greene JA jr, Weller JM. Peritoneal dialysis during hemorrhagic shock. J Appl Physiol 1967; 22: 131–5.
189. Selgas R, Munoz IM, Conesa J, Madero R, Gancedo PG, Carmona AR, Martinez ME, Huarte E, Fontan MP, Sicilia L. Endogenous sympathetic activity in CAPD patients: its relationship to peritoneal diffusion capacity. Perit Dial Bull 1986; 6: 205–8.
190. Ratge D, Augustin R, Wisser H. Plasma catecholamines and α- and β-adrenoceptors in circulating blood cells in patients on continuous ambulatory peritoneal dialysis. Clin Nephrol 1987; 28: 15–21.
191. Zabetakis PM, Kumar DN, Gleim GW, Gardenswartz MH, Agrawal M, Robinson AG, Michelis MF. Increased levels of plasma renin, aldosterone, catecholamines and vasopressin in chronic ambulatory peritoneal dialysis (CAPD) patients. Clin Nephrol 1987; 28: 147–51.
192. Steinhauer HB, Grünter B, Schollmeyer P. Stimulation of peritoneal synthesis of vasoactive prostaglandins during peritonitis in patients on continuous ambulatory peritoneal dialysis. Eur J Clin Invest 1985; 15: 1–15.
193. Steinhauer HB, Günter B, Schollmeyer P. Enhanced peritoneal generation of vasoactive prostaglandins during peritonitis in patients undergoing CAPD. In: Maher JF, Winchester JF (eds), Frontiers in peritoneal dialysis. Field, Rich, New York 1986; pp 604–9.
194. Steinhauer HB, Schollmeyer P. Prostaglandin-mediated loss of proteins during peritonitis in continuous ambulatory peritoneal dialysis. Kidney Int 1986; 29: 584–90.
195. Hain H, Jorres A, Gahl M, Pustelnik A, Müller C, Köttgen E. Peritoneal permeability for proteins in uninfected CAPD patients: a kinetic study. In: Ota K et al. (eds), Current concepts in peritoneal dialysis. Excerpta Medica, Amsterdam 1992; pp 59–66.
196. Zemel D, Imholz ALT, Koomen GCM, Struijk DG, Krediet RT. TNFα in stable patients treated with CAPD. Perit Dial Int 1993; suppl 1: S61.
197. Shaldon S, Koch KM, Queelhorst E, Dinarello CA. Hazards of CAPD: interleukin-1 production: In: Maher JF, Winchester JF (eds), Frontiers in peritoneal dialysis. Field, Rich, New York 1986; pp 630–6.
198. Shaldon S, Dinarello CA, Wyler DJ. Induction of interleukin-1 during CAPD. Contr Nephrol 1987; 57: 207–12.
199. Goldman M, Vandelabeele P, Moulart J, Amraoui Z, Abramowicz D, Nortier J, Vanherweghem JL, Fiers W. Intraperitoneal secretion of interleukin-6 during continuous ambulatory peritoneal dialysis. Nephron 1990; 56: 277–80.
200. Zemel D, ten Berge RJM, Struijk DG, Bloemena E, Koomen GCM, Krediet RT. Interleukin-6 in CAPD patients without peritonitis: relationship to the intrinsic permeability of the peritoneal membrane. Clin Nephrol 1992; 37: 97–103.
201. Lin CY, Lin CC, Huang TP. Several changes of interleukin-6 and interleukin-8 levels in drain dialysate of uremic patients with continuous ambulatory peritoneal dialysis during peritonitis. Nephron 1993; 63: 404–8.
202. Zemel D, Koomen GCM, ten Berge RJM, Hart AAM, Struijk DG, van Acker BAC, Krediet RT. Relationship of THF$_\alpha$, interleukin-6 and prostaglandins to peritoneal permeability for macromolecules during longitudinal follow-up of peritonitis in continuous ambulatory peritoneal dialysis. J Lab Clin Med 1993; 122: 686–96.
203. Miller FN. Effects of peritoneal dialysis on rat microcirculation and peritoneal clearances in man. Dial Transplant 1978; 7: 818–38.
204. Miller FN. The peritoneal microcirculation. In: Nolph KD (ed), Peritoneal Dialysis, 2nd ed. Nihoff, Boston 1985: pp 51–93.
205. Miller FN, Nolph KD, Joshua IG, Wiegman DL, Harris PD, Andersen DB. Hyperosmolality, acetate, and lactate: dilatory factors during peritoneal dialysis. Kidney Int 1981; 20: 397–402.
206. Miller FN, Nolph KD, Joshua IG. The osmolality component of peritoneal dialysis solutions. In: Legrain M (ed), Continuous ambulatory peritoneal dialysis. Excerpta Medica Amsterdam 1980: pp 12–7.
207. Rubin J, Nolph KD, Arfania D, Joshua IG, Miller FN, Wiegman DL, Harris PD. Clinical studies with a nonvasoactive peritoneal dialysis solution. J Lab Clin Med 1979; 93: 910–5.
208. Miller FN, Nolph KD, Sorkin ML, Gloor HJ. The influence of solute composition on protein loss during peritoneal dialysis. Kidney Int 1983; 23: 35–9.
209. Bruno M, Bagnis C, Marangella M, Rovera L, Cantaluppi A, Linari F. CAPD with an amino acid dialysis solution: a long term cross-over study. Kidney Int 1989; 35: 1189–94.
210. Young GA, Dibble JB, Taylor AE, Kendall S, Brownjohn AM. A longitudinal study of the effects of amino acid-based CAPD fluid on amino acid

solution and protein losses. Nephrol Dial Transplant 1989; 4: 900–5.
211. Steinhauer HB, Lubrick-Birkner I, Kluthe R, Baumann G, Schollmeyer P. Effect of amino-acid based dialysis solution on peritoneal permeability and prostanoid generation in patients undergoing continuous ambulatory peritoneal dialysis. Am J Nephrol 1991; 12: 61–7.
212. Mistry CD, O'Donoghue DJ, Nelson S, Gokal R, Ballardi FW. Kinetic and clinical studies of β_2-microglobulin in continuous ambulatory peritoneal dialysis: influence of renal and enhanced peritoneal clearances using glucose polymer. Nephrol Dial Transplant 1990; 5: 513–9.
213. Imholz ALT, Brown CB, Koomen GCM, Arisz L, Krediet RT. The effects of glucose polymers on water removal and protein clearances during CAPD. Adv Perit Dial 1993; 9: 25–30.
214. Hirszel P, Lasrich M, Maher JF. Augmentation of peritoneal mass transport by dopamine. J Lab Clin Invest 1979; 94: 747–4.
215. Hirszel P, Maher JF, Le Grow W. Increased peritoneal mass transport with glucagon acting at the vascular surface. Trans Am Soc Artif Intern Organs 1978; 24: 136–8.
216. Maher JF, Hirszel P, Lasrich M. Effects of gastrointestinal hormones on transport by peritoneal dialysis. Kidney Int 1979; 16: 130–6.
217. Felt J, Richard C, McCaffrey C, Levy M. Peritoneal clearance of creatinine and inulin during dialysis in dogs: effect of splanchnic vasodilators. Kidney Int 1979; 16: 459–69.
218. Hare HG, Valtin H, Grosselin RE. Effects of drugs on peritoneal dialysis in the dog. J Pharmacol Exp Ther 1964; 145: 122–9.
219. Henderson LW, Kintzel JE. Influence of antidiuretic hormone on peritoneal membrane area and permeability. J Clin Invest 1971; 40: 2437–43.
220. Fox J, Galey F, Wayland H. Action of histamine on the mesenteric microvasculature. Microvasc Res 1980; 19: 108–26.
221. Miller FN, Joshua IG, Anderson GL. Quantitation of vasodilator-induced macromolecular leakage by in vivo fluorescent microscopy. Microvasc Res 1982; 24: 56–67.
222. Brown EA, Kliger AS, Goffinet J, Finkelstein FO. Effect of hypertonic dialysate and vasodilators on peritoneal dialysis clearances in the rat. Kidney Int 1978; 13: 271–7.
223. Shostak A, Chakrabarti E, Hirszel P, Maher JF. Effects of histamine and its receptor antagonists on peritoneal permeability. Kidney Int 1988; 34: 786–90.
224. Maher JF, Hirszel P, Lasrich M. Modulation of peritoneal transport rates by prostaglandins. Adv Prostaglandin Thromboxane Res 1980; 7: 695–700.
225. Hirszel P, Lasrich M, Maher JF. Arachidonic acid increases peritoneal clearances. Trans Am Soc Artif Intern Organs 1981; 27: 61–3.
226. Maher JF, Hirszel P, Lasrich M. Prostaglandin effects on peritoneal transport. In: Gahl GM, Kessel M, Nolph KD (eds), Adv Perit Dial. Excerpta Medica, Amsterdam 1981; pp 64–9.
227. Crosbie WA, Snowden S, Parsons V. Changes in lung capillary permeability in chronic uremia. Br Med J 1972; 4: 388–90.
228. Rubin J, Rust P, Brown P, Popovich RP, Nolph KD. A comparison of peritoneal transport in patients with psoriasis and uremia. Nephron 1981; 29: 185–9.
229. Diaz-Buxo JA, Farmer CD, Walker PJ, Chandler JT, Holt KL. Effect of hyperparathyroidism on peritoneal clearances. Trans Am Soc Artif Intern Organs 1982; 28: 276–9.
230. Nolph KD, Whitcomb ME, Schrier RW. Mechanisms for inefficient peritoneal dialysis in acute renal failure associated with heat stress and exercise. Ann In Med 1969; 71: 317–26.
231. Østerby R. Basement membrane morphology in diabetes mellitus. In: Ellenberg M, Rifkin H (eds), Diabetes mellitus, theory and practice, 3rd ed. Medical examination publishing Co, New York 1983; pp 323–42.
232. Parving H. Increased microvascular permeability to plasma proteins in short- and longterm juvenile diabetes. Diabetes 1976; 25 (suppl 2): 884–9.
233. Zimmerman AL, Sablay LB, Aynedjian HS, Bank N. Increased peritoneal permeability in rats with alloxan-induced diabetes mellitus. J Lab Clin Med 1984; 103: 720–30.
234. Nolph KD, Stolz ML, Maher JF. Altered peritoneal permeability in patients with systemic vasculitis. Ann Intern Med 1971; 75: 753–5.
235. Krediet RT. Peritoneal permeability in continuous ambulatory peritoneal dialysis [dissertation]. Amsterdam: Univ. of Amsterdam 1986.
236. Selgas R, Madero R, Munoz J, Huarte E, Rinon C, Miquel JL, Sanchez-Sécilia L. Functional peculiarities of the peritoneum in diabetes mellitus. Dial Transplant 1988; 17: 419–36.
237. Rubin J, Nolph KD, Arfania D, Brown P, Moore H, Rust P. Influence of patient characteristics on peritoneal clearances. Nephron 1981; 27: 118–21.
238. Rottembourg J, El Shahat Y, Agrafiotis A, Thuillier Y, de Groq F, Jacobs C, Legrain M. Continuous ambulatory peritoneal dialysis in insulin-dependent diabetic patients: a 40-month experience. Kidney Int. 1983; 23: 40–5.
239. Rubin J, Walsh D, Bower JD, Diabetes, dialysate losses, and serum lipids during continuous ambulatory peritoneal dialysis. Am J Kidney Dis 1987; 10: 104–8.
240. Kaysen G, Schoenfeld PY. Albumin homeostasis in patients undergoing continuous ambulatory peritoneal dialysis. Kidney Int 1984; 25: 107–14.
241. Fassbinder W, Brunner FP, Brynger H, Ehrich JHH, Geerlings W, Raine AEG, Rizzoni G, Selwood NH, Tufveson G, Wing AJ. Combined report on regular dialysis and transplantation in Europe 20, 1989. Nephrol Dial Transplant 1991; 6: 5–35.
242. Correia P, Cameron JS, Ogg CS, Williams DG, Bewick M, Hicks JA. Endstage renal failure in SLE with nephritis. Clin Nephrol 1984; 22: 293–302.
243. Wu GG, Gelbast DR, Hasbargen JA, Inman R, McNamee P, Oreopoulos DG. Reactivation of

systemic lupus in three patients undergoing CAPD. Perit Dial Bull 1986; 6: 6–9.
244. Cantaluppi A. CAPD and systemic diseases. Clin Nephrol 1988; 30;(suppl 1): S8–S12.
245. Krediet RT, Boeschoten EW, Zuyderhoudt FMJ, Arisz L. Permeability of the peritoneum to proteins in CAPD patients with systemic disease. Proc Eur Dial Transplant Ass 1985; 22: 405–9.
246. Brown ST, Ahearn DJ, Nolph KD. Reduced peritoneal clearances in scleroderma increased by intraperitoneal isoproterenol. Ann Intern Med 1973; 78: 891–4.
247. Robson M, Oreopoulos DG. Dialysis in scleroderma. Ann Intern Med 1978; 88: 843.
248. Winfield J, Khanna R, Reynolds WJ, Gordon DA, Finkelstein S, Oreopoulos DG. Management of end-stage scleroderma renal disease with continuous ambulatory peritoneal dialysis. Report of two cases. Perit Dial Bull 1982; 2: 174–7.
249. Copley JB, Smith BJ. Continuous ambulatory peritoneal dialysis and scleroderma. Nephron 1985; 40: 353–6.
250. Browning MJ, Banks RA, Harrison P, Tribe CR, Fraley CT, Zuchary G, Mackenzie C. Continuous ambulatory peritoneal dialysis in systemic amyloidosis and end-stage renal disease. J Royal Soc Med 1984; 77: 189–92.
251. Rosansky SJ, Waddell PH. CAPD in the treatment of primary amyloidosis. Perit Dial Bull 1983; 3: 217–8.
252. Rosansky SJ, Richards FW. Use of peritoneal dialysis in the treatment of patients with renal failure and paraproteinemia. Am J Nephrol 1985; 5: 361–5.
253. Heale WF, Letch KA, Dawborn JK, Evans SM. Long term complications of peritonitis. In: Atkins RC, Thomson NM, Farrell PC (eds), Peritoneal Dialysis. Churchill Livingstone, Edinburgh 1981; pp 284–90.
254. Rubin J. McFarland S, Hellems EW, Bower JD. Peritoneal dialysis during peritonitis. Kidney Int 1981; 19: 460–4.
255. Prowant BF, Nolph KD. Clinical criteria for diagnosis of peritonitis. In: Atkins RC, Thomson NM, Farrell PC (eds), Peritoneal Dialysis. Churchill Livingstone, Edinburgh 1981; pp 257–63.
256. Raja RM, Kramer MS, Rosenbaum JL, Bolisay C, Krug M. Contrasting changes in solute transport and ultrafiltration with peritonitis in CAPD patients. Trans Am Soc Artif Intern Organs 1981; 27: 68–70.
257. Rubin J, Ray R, Barnes T, Bower J. Peritoneal abnormalities during infectious episodes of continuous ambulatory peritoneal dialysis. Nephron 1981; 29: 124–7.
258. Smeby LC, Wideröe T-E, Svartås TM, Jörstad S. Changes in water removal due to peritonitis during continuous ambulatory peritoneal dialysis. In: Gahl GM, Kessel M, Nolph KD (eds), Advances in Peritoneal Dialysis. Excerpta Medica, Amsterdam 1981; pp 287–92.
259. Raja RM, Kramer MS, Barber K. Solute transport and ultrafiltration during peritonitis in CAPD patients. ASAIO J 1984; 7: 8–11.
260. Katirtzoglou A, Oreopoulos DG, Husdan H, Leung M, Ogilvie R, Dombros N. Reappraisal of protein losses in patients undergoing continuous ambulatory peritoneal dialysis. Nephron 1980; 26: 230–3.
261. Dulaney JT, Hatch jr FE. Peritoneal dialysis and loss of proteins: a review. Kidney Int 1984; 26: 253–62.
262. Miller FN, Hammerschmidt DE, Anderson GL, Moore JN. Protein loss induced by complement activation during peritoneal dialysis. Kidney Int 1984; 25: 480–5.
263. Slingeneyer A, Mion C, Mourad G, Canaud B, Faller B, Bérund JJ. Progressive sclerosing peritonitis: a late and severe complication of maintenance peritoneal dialysis. Trans Am Soc Artif Intern Organs 1983; 29: 633–40.
264. Rottembourg J, Gahl GM, Poignet JL, Mertani E, Strippoli P, Langlois P, Tranbaloc P, Legrain M. Severe abdominal complications in patients undergoing continuous ambulatory peritoneal dialysis. Proc Eur Dial Transplant Ass 1983; 20: 236–42.
265. Verger C, Celicout B. Peritoneal permeability and encapsulating peritonitis. Lancet 1985; 1: 986–7.
266. Manos J, Postethwaite RJ, Mallick NP, Gokal R. Sclerosing encapsulating peritonitis and other complications of CAPD peritonitis. In: Maher JF, Winchester JF (eds), Frontiers in peritoneal dialysis. Field, Rich, New York 1986; pp 634–7.
267. McWhinnie DL, Bradley JA, Bramwell SP, Hamilton DNH, Macpherson SG, Cram LP, More IAR, Forwell MA, Smith WGJ, Briggs JD, Junor BJR. Sclerosing peritonitis – a further complication of CAPD. In: Maher JF, Winchester JF (eds), Frontiers in peritoneal dialysis. Field, Rich, New York 1986; pp 638–42.
268. Rottembourg J, Issad B, Langlois P, de Groc F, Legrain M. Sclerosing encapsulating peritonitis during CAPD. Evaluation of the potential risk factors. In: Maher JF, Winchester JF, editors. Frontiers in peritoneal dialysis. New York, Field, Rich 1986; 643–9.
269. Krediet RT, Struijk DG, Boeschoten EW, Koomen GCM, Stouthard JML, Hoek FJ, Arisz L. The time course of peritoneal transport kinetics in continuous ambulatory peritoneal dialysis patients who develop sclerosing peritonitis. Am J Kidney Dis 1989; 13: 299–307.
270. Tanaka Y, Shirai D. Clinical aspects of sclerosing peritonitis. In: Ota K et al. (eds), Current concepts in peritoneal dialysis. Excerpta Medica, Amsterdam 1992; pp 112–5.
271. Gandhi VC, Ing TS, Daugirdus JT, Hagen C, Blumenkrantz MJ, Jablokow VR. Failure of peritoneal dialysis due to peritoneal sclerosis. Int J Artif Organs 1983; 6: 97.
272. Shaldon S, Koch KM, Quellhorst E, Dinarello CA. Pathogenesis of sclerosing peritonitis in CAPD. Trans Am Soc Artif Intern Organs 1984; 30: 193–4.
273. Finkelstein FO, Kliger AS, Bastl C, Yap P. Sequential clearance and dialysance measurements

in chronic peritoneal dialysis patients. Nephron 1977; 18: 342–7.
274. Rubin J, Arfania D, Nolph KD, Prowant B, Fruto L, Brown P, Moore H. Peritoneal clearances after 6–12 months on continuous ambulatory peritoneal dialysis. Trans Am Soc Artif Intern Organs 1979; 25: 104–9.
275. Selgas R, Rodrigues-Carmona A, Martinez ME, Perez-Fontan M, Salinas M, Escuin F, Rinon C, Martinez-Ara J, Sanchez-Sicilia L. Peritoneal mass transfer in patients on long-term CAPD. Perit Dial Bull 1984; 4: 153–6.
276. Nikolakakis N, Rodger RSC, Goodship THJ, Flectcher K, Ashcroft R, Wilkinson R, Ward MK. The assessment of peritoneal function using a single hypertonic exchange. Perit Dial Bull 1985; 5: 186–8.
277. Hallet MD, Kush RD, Lysaght MJ, Farrel PC. The stability and kinetics of peritoneal mass transfer. In: Nolph KD (ed), Peritoneal Dialysis. Kluwer, Dorerecht 1989; pp 380–8.
278. Park MS, Lee J, Lee MS, Baick SH, Hwang SD, Lee HB. Peritoneal solute clearances after four years of continuous ambulatory peritoneal dialysis (CAPD). Perit Dial Int 1989; 9: 75–8.
279. Passlick-Deetjen J, Chlebowski H, Koch M, Ziergelmayer C, Grabensee B. Evaluation of long-term changes in peritoneal membrane function. In: La Graeca G, Ronco C, Feriani M, Chiaramonte S, Cour P (eds), Peritoneal Dialysis. Wichtig, Milano 1991; pp 109–15.
280. Coronel F, Tornero F, Mucia M, Sánchez A, De Oleo P, Naranjo P, Barrientos A. Peritoneal clearances, protein losses and ultrafiltration in diabetic patients after four years on CAPD. Adv Perit Dial 1991; 7: 35–8.
281. Lee HB, Park MS, Chung SH, So IN, Han DC, Lee SK. Hwang SD, Moon C. Peritoneal membrane performance after 5 years on CAPD. In: Ota K et al. (eds), Current Concepts in Peritoneal Dialysis. Excerpta Medica, Amsterdam 1992; pp 84–8.
282. Rubin J, Nolph KD, Arfania D, Brown P, Prowant B. Follow-up of peritoneal clearances in patients undergoing continuous ambulatory peritoneal dialysis. Kidney Int 1979; 16: 619–23.
283. Farrell PC, Randerson JH. Membrane permeability changes in long-term CAPD. Trans Am Soc Artif Intern Organs 1980; 26: 197–200.
284. Randerson DH, Farrell PC. Long-term peritoneal clearance in CAPD. In: Atkins RC, Thomson NM, Farrell PC (eds), Peritoneal Dialysis. Churchill Livingstone, Edinburgh 1981; pp 21–29.
285. Selgas R, Rodrigues-Carmona A, Martinez ME, Conesa J, Perez-Fontan M, Huarte E, Ortega O, Sanchez-Sicilia L. Follow-up of peritoneal mass transfer properties in long-term CAPD patients. In: Maher JF, Winchester JF (eds), Frontiers in Peritoneal Dialysis. Field, Rich, New York 1986; pp 53–5.
286. Selgas R, Muños J, Cigarran S, Ramos P, L-Revuelta K, Escuin F, Miguel JL. Peritoneal functional parameters after five years on continuous ambulatory peritoneal dialysis (CAPD): The effect of late peritonitis. Perit Dial Int 1989; 9: 329–32.
287. Pollock CA, Ibels LS, Caterson RJ, Mahoney JF, Waugh DA, Cocksedge B. Continuous ambulatory peritoneal dialysis. Eight years of experience at a single center. Medicine 1989; 68: 293–308.
288. Blake PG, Abraham G, Sombolos K, Izatt S, Weissgarten J, Ayiomamitis A, Oreopoulos DG. Changes in peritoneal membrane transport rates in patients on long term CAPD. Adv Perit Dial 1989; 5: 3–7.
289. Kush RD, Hallett MD, Ota K, Yamushita A, Kumano K, Watenabe N, Sakai T, Hidai H, Farrell PC. Long-term ambulatory peritoneal dialysis; mass transfer and nutritional and metabolic stability. Blood Purif 1990; 8: 1–13.
290. Bordoni E, Lombardo V, Bibiano L, Carletti P, Francialli E, Gaffi G, Perilli A, Mioli V. Peritoneal clearances, ultrafiltration and diuresis in long-term continuous ambulatory peritoneal dialysis. In: Avram MM, Giordano C (eds), Ambulatory peritoneal dialysis. Plenum, New York 1990; 87–90.
291. Chan PCK, Chan CY, Wu PG, Cheng IKP, Chan MK. Long-term peritoneal clearances in patients on continuous ambulatory peritoneal dialysis. Int J Artif Organs 1990; 13: 707–8.
292. Struijk DG, Krediet RJ, Koomen GCM, Boeschoten EW, Hoeh FJ, Arisz L. A prospective study of peritoneal transport in CAPD patients. Kidney Int 1994, in press.
293. Lameire NH, Vanholder R, Veyt D, Lambert M-C, Ringoir S. A longitudinal, five year survey of urea kinetic parameters in CAPD patients. Kidney Int 1992; 42: 426–32.

5 Peritoneal lymphatics

ROBERT A. MACTIER AND RAMESH KHANNA

1. Introduction 115
2. Translymphatic absorption 115
   2.1. Lymphatic pathways from the peritoneal cavity 115
   2.2 The subdiaphragmatic stomata 116
   2.3. Mechanisms of lymphatic absorption 117
   2.4. Function of the peritoneal cavity lymphatics 118
   2.5. Absorptive capacity of the peritoneal lymphatics 119
   2.6. Factors influencing peritoneal lymphatic absorption 119
3. Transcapillary absorption 119
4. Role of lymphatic absorption in ascites 120
5. Role of lymphatic absorption in peritoneal dialysis kinetics 121
6. Indirect and direct methods of estimating lymphatic absorption in peritoneal dialysis 122
   6.1. Mass transfer rates of intraperitoneal colloids to the blood 123
   6.2. Mass transfer rates of colloids from the peritoneal cavity 123
   6.3. Computer simulations of transperitoneal fluid transport 125
   6.4. Cannulation of the major lymphatics vessels 125
   6.5. Comparison of methods of estimating lymphatic absorption 125
7. Factors controlling backfiltration in peritoneal dialysis 126
8. Consequences of backfiltration in peritoneal dialysis 126
   8.1. Loss of ultrafiltration 126
   8.2. Reduction in solute mass transfer 127
   8.3. Absorption of intraperitoneal bacteria 128
   8.4. Absorption of intraperitoneal polymers and particles 128
9. Conclusion 129
References 129

1. Introduction

The peritoneal lymphatics serve as a route for continuous absorption of fluids and solutes from the peritoneal cavity by convective flow [1, 2]. The important role of lymphatic drainage from the peritoneal cavity in the pathogenesis of ascites due to liver disease or malignancy is well established [3–16] and the considerable absorptive capacity of the peritoneal lymphatics has been utilized to perform intraperitoneal blood transfusions in the fetus and in children [19–21]. However, until recently, kinetic studies of peritoneal dialysis iatrogenic "ascites" have tended to focus only on fluid and solute exchange between the peritoneal microcirculation and the instilled dialysis solution and have neglected the role of the peritoneal lymphatics [22–39]. The efficiency of peritoneal dialysis is assessed by measuring solute clearances and *net* ultrafiltration volumes. These indices of dialysis efficacy represent the cumulative balance of transperitoneal transport into and out of the peritoneal cavity and therefore incorporate the role of backfiltration from the peritoneal cavity. Absorption from the peritoneal cavity can occur by two mechanisms; uptake via the peritoneal cavity lymphatics (translymphatic absorption) or uptake by the peritoneal capillaries (transcapillary absorption).

2. Translymphatic absorption

2.1. Lymphatic pathways of the peritoneal cavity

Lymphatic drainage from the peritoneal cavity is primarily via specialized end lymphatic openings (stomata) located in the subdiaphragmatic peritoneum [40–43]. Moreover, absorption of intraperitoneal fluid is greatest from the right side overlying the liver [42]. In contrast, absorption by the lymphatic capillaries within the interstitium of the mesentery, omentum and parietal peritoneum make a relatively minor contribution to total peritoneal lymphatic drainage [2, 43, 44].

The lymphatic capillaries leading from the subdiaphragmatic stomata coalesce to form a plexus of collecting lymphatics within the muscular portion of the diaphragm. This subperitoneal plexus also communicates with the lymphatics from the pleural surface. From the diaphragm and the diaphragmatic lymph nodes, most of the lymphatic trunks accompany the internal mammary vessels to the anterior mediastinal lymph nodes around the thymus (Fig. 1) and thereafter return almost 80% of the peritoneal lymphatic drainage to the venous circulation via the right lymph duct [2, 45]. Some of the efferent lymphatics from the anterior mediastinal nodes may, however, occasionally drain to the central veins on the left side either in association with or separate from the thoracic duct. The lymphatic drainage from the remainder of the peritoneum, including part of the subdiaphragmatic peritoneum, returns to the systemic circulation through the thoracic duct [2]. Consequently cannulation of the thoracic duct during peritoneal dialysis in the rat collected less than 30% of total estimated lymphatic absorption [46]. The major substernal and other minor lymphatic pathways from the peritoneal cavity are summarized schematically in Fig. 2.

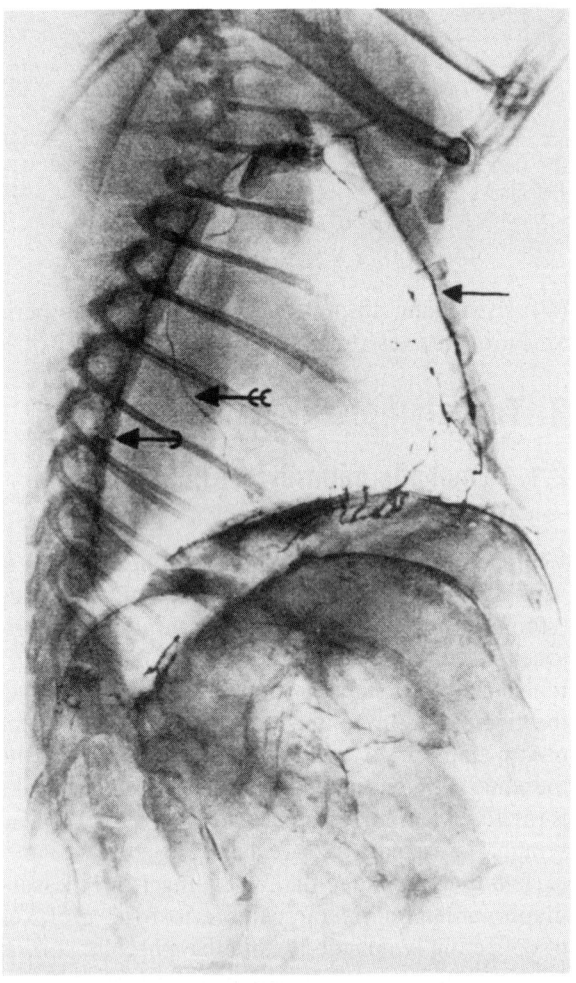

Figure 1. Lateral x-ray following intraperitoneal Thorotrast. The diaphragmatic lymphatics drain predominantly into the parasternal lymphatics (←). The paravertebral lymphatics (↔) and a small tortuous mediastinal lymphatic (←) are also opacified (reproduced with permission from reference [40]).

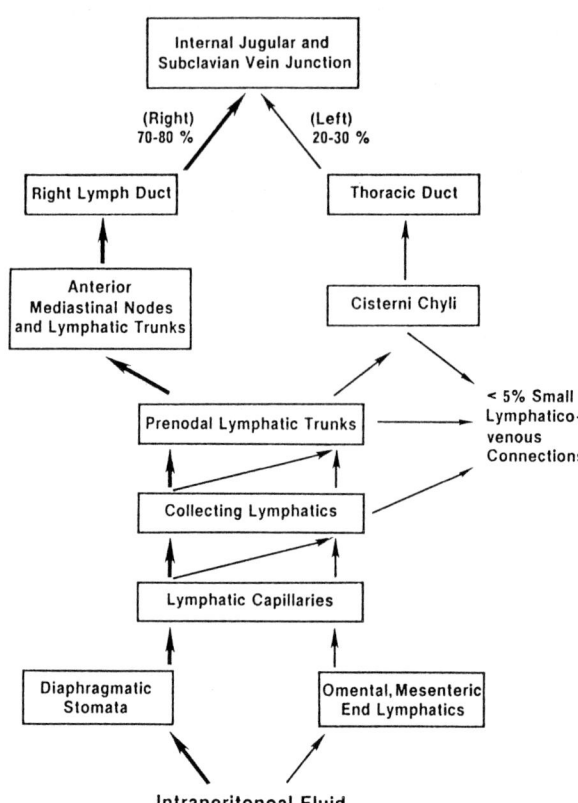

Figure 2. Anatomical pathways of lymphatic absorption of intraperitoneal fluid. (Reproduced with permission from reference [108]).

2.2. The subdiaphragmatic stomata

Von Recklinghausen in 1863 was the first to suggest that carbon particles, red blood cells, proteins and fluid were transported directly from the peritoneal cavity into the lymphatics of the diaphragm via openings in the subdiaphragmatic peritoneum, which he called stomata [47]. Other investigators subsequently claimed that the stomata were artifacts [48–50] but the presence of these specialized terminal lymphatics in animals and man has since been confirmed by light and electron microscopy [51–56].

The lacunae of the terminal lymphatics of the subdiaphragmatic peritoneum are only separated from the peritoneal cavity by a thin triple-layer, consisting of small, rounded, and interdigitating mesothelium, a loose network of connective tissue and lymphatic endothelium [52, 54]. Scanning and transmission electron microscopy have shown that the stomata permit absorption of intraperitoneal particles, cells, colloids and fluid into the underlying lymphatic lacunae via extracellular pathways [52,

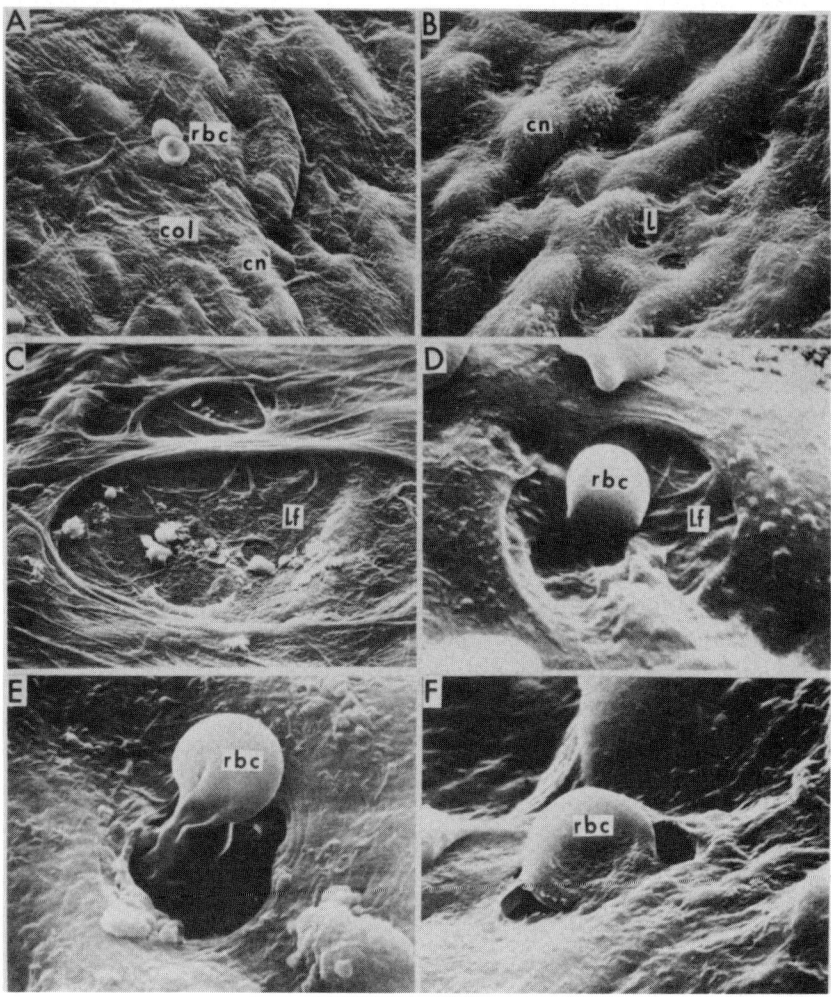

Figure 3. Scanning electron microscopy of red blood cells passing through the subdiphragmatic stomata.
A Non-absorbing surface in the rat diaphragm; rbc, red blood cell; col, collagen fibers; cn, mesothelial cell nucleus. × 780.
B Absorbing surface overlying lymphatic lacunae (L) in the rat diaphragm. × 1200.
C Rabbit diaphragm showing the roof of a lacuna (Lf).
D Red blood cell passing through a slit in the roof of lacuna in the rabbit diaphragm. × 3120.
E Red blood cell passing between mesothelial cells in the rat diaphragm. × 4200.
F As for E. × 3780.
(Reproduced with permission from reference [57]).

57] (Fig. 3). The mesothelial cells which overlie the lymphatic lacunae are smaller and separate from each other more readily than the cells in the surrounding mesothelium [52, 58]. Internally the lacunar mesothelial cells have bands of actin filaments arranged along their base [54]. The stomata are formed by the separation of adjacent mesothelial cells and, in the rat, can accommodate spherical particles up to 22.5μ in diameter [59]. At the stomata the submesothelial basement membrane and the underlying lattice of connective tissue become fenestrated [60] and so allow the mesothelial cells to adjoin the lymphatic endothelial cells to form a channel from the peritoneal cavity to the lumen of the underlying lacuna [61, 62].

2.3. Mechanism of lymphatic absorption

The rate at which intraperitoneal fluid is absorbed by the peritoneal cavity lymphatics depends on the excursions of the diaphragm during respiration [63–65]. As the diaphragm relaxes during expiration, the adjacent mesothelial and endothelial cells in the roofs of the lymphatic lacunae separate from each other and intraperitoneal fluid is absorbed as suction is created by the distension of the lacunae. In inspiration the contraction of the diaphragm closes the gaps between the overlying mesothelial and endothelial cells and the contents of the lacunae are emptied into the efferent lymphatics. The presence of the abundant actin filaments in the cytoplasm of both the mesothelial and endothelial cells, however, suggests that there may be an active as well as a passive mechanism for maintaining the patency of the stomata [63, 64]. Backflow of the absorbed fluid into the peritoneal cavity is prevented during inspiration by the overlapping endothelial cells in the roofs of the lacunae [53, 54] (Fig. 4). Forward flow, induced by lymphatic contractility and changes in intrathoracic pressure, is maintained by the presence of valves in the efferent lymphatics [53, 54, 65]. The higher lymphatic absorption rate from the right hemidiaphragm is probably due to compression of the liver against the subdiaphragmatic stomata during respiration [58]. The ultrastructure and the mechanism of absorption of the peritoneal cavity lymphatics may be reviewed in greater detail elsewhere [66].

2.4. Function of peritoneal cavity lymphatics

The lymphatics draining the peritoneal cavity act as a one-way system returning excess intraperitoneal fluid and protein to the systemic circulation. The sum of the hydrostatic and osmotic pressure gradients across the peritoneum normally favors a minor net inflow of fluid into the peritoneal cavity [31]. Bidirectional transperitoneal transfer of small solutes occurs by diffusion and by solvent drag. However, macromolecules (molecular weight greater than 20,000) exhibit minimal direct reabsorption into the peritoneal capillaries [67] and consequently, after unidirectional transport from the peritoneal microcirculation into the peritoneal cavity, are returned to the venous circulation by convective flow into the lymphatics. Normally peritoneal lymphatic drainage of serous fluid equals its rate of formation and only a small volume of isosmotic fluid is maintained within the peritoneal cavity.

The second major function of the lymphatics is their contribution to the host defenses of the peritoneal cavity. Absorption by the peritoneal cavity lymphatics and phagocytosis by the resident intraperitoneal and omental macrophages are the first

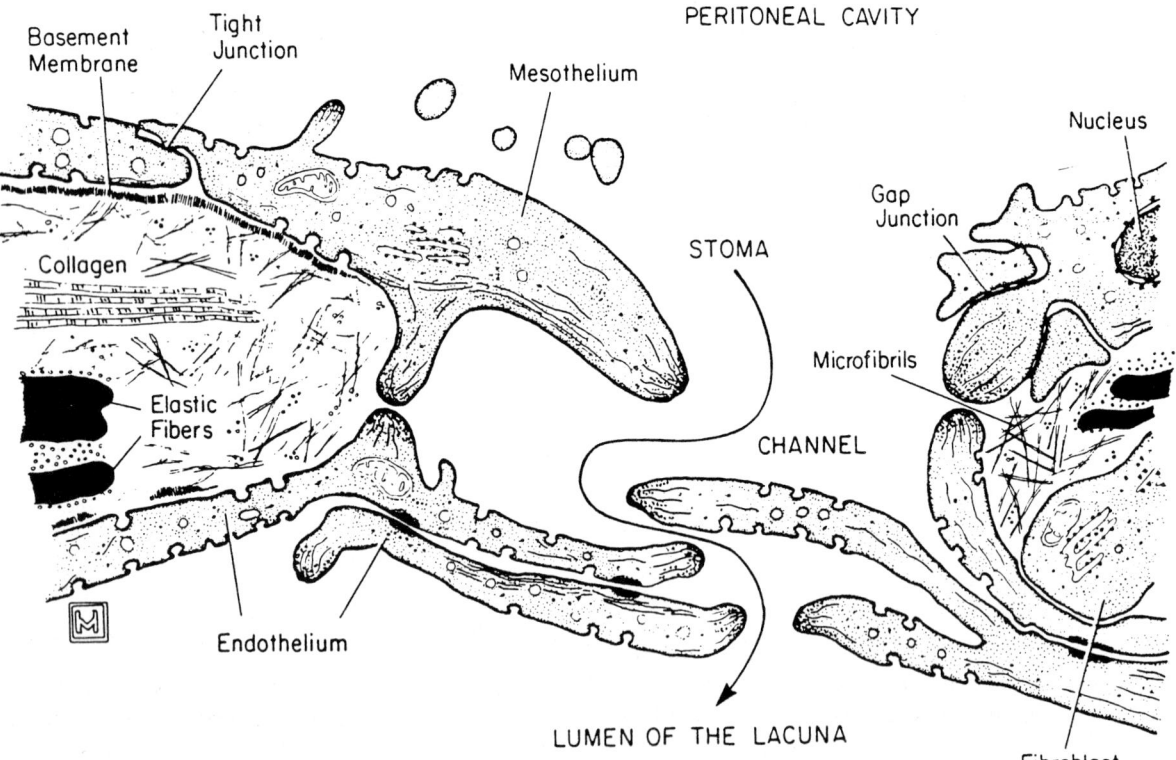

Figure 4. Diagram of a typical stoma and underlying channel linking the peritoneal cavity with the lumen of a lymphatic lacuna. (Reproduced with permission of reference [54]).

lines of defense after the inoculum of bacteria gains entry to the peritoneal cavity [68, 69]. The macrophages in the omentum provide an effective defense against bacteria but the omental lymphatics play only a minor role in the absorption of fluid from the peritoneal cavity [44]. Likewise, it is important to emphasize that although the lymphatics carrying fluid and solutes from the intestinal mucosa traverse the mesentery before draining into the cisterna chyli and the thoracic duct, they are not significantly involved in absorption of isosmotic fluid from the peritoneal cavity per se [2, 43].

2.5. Absorptive capacity of the peritoneal lymphatics

The lymphatics draining the peritoneal cavity, therefore, are virtually the only pathway for absorption of intraperitoneal isosmotic fluid, biologically inert particles, colloids and cells [2, 58, 65, 70]. Consequently the absorptive capacity of the peritoneal cavity lymphatics has been evaluated in normal animals from the rate of uptake of isosmotic fluid (plasma, whole blood, crystalloid solutions) infused into the peritoneal cavity [41–43, 71–80]. Representative values from these studies indicate that lymphatic absorption rates from the peritoneal cavity in animals are considerable (Table 1). Furthermore, obliteration of the subdiaphragmatic peritoneum [43, 73] or ligation of the parasternal lymphatic trunks [74] greatly reduces the rate of intraperitoneal fluid absorption.

2.6. Factors controlling peritoneal lymphatic absorption

From studies performed mainly in animals, several physiological factors have been shown to alter the rate of lymphatic absorption from the peritoneal cavity. Hyperventilation, which was induced by breathing carbon dioxide, increased whereas anesthesia and acute phrenic neurectomy reduced lymphatic absorption [79–82]. Lymphatic and peritoneal transcapillary absorption were both enhanced by increasing intraperitoneal hydrostatic pressure [78] and decreased after paracentesis [83]. Upright posture with small intraperitoneal volumes reduced the rate of lymphatic flow, although absorption still occurred due to propulsion of the intraperitoneal fluid towards the diaphragm by intestinal peristalsis [74]. Indeed, the circulation of intraperitoneal fluid towards the diaphragm is the most likely explanation for the relative frequency of abscess formation in the right subphrenic space following entry of bacteria into the peritoneal cavity [84]. Fowler successfully localized infection in the pelvis of patients with diffuse peritonitis by elevating the head of their beds by twelve to fifteen inches [85]. Even though obstruction of the peritoneal cavity lymphatics by fibrin or fibrosis may decrease lymphatic absorption after infectious peritonitis, chemical peritonitis induced by sodium hypochlorite was observed to increase the rate of lymphatic absorption in the recovery period [86]. This rise in lymphatic flow may be related to rapid regeneration of end lymphatics after injury. Lymphatic flow is reduced if outflow pressure is increased by catheter insertion or raised central venous pressure [87]. The factors known to influence peritoneal lymphatic drainage are summarized in Table 2.

3. Transcapillary absorption

Prior to absorption into the peritoneal capillaries located mainly within the deeper layers of the interstitium intraperitoneal fluid and solutes must traverse at least six identified anatomical resistance sites: fluid films within the peritoneal cavity, mesothelium and its basal lamina, interstitial matrix, endothelial basement membrane, endothelial layer and fluid films within the capillary lumen [22]. Fluid movement between the peritoneal cavity and peritoneal capillaries is determined by the balance of hydrostatic and osmotic pressure gradients across these resistance sites. Transperitoneal absorption is only strictly analogous to transcapillary uptake within other tissue if solutes and water permeate

Table 1. Rates of isosmotic fluid absorption from the peritoneal cavity in different species.

Species	Infusion volumes	Infused solution	Absorption rate	References
Rat	20 ml (per kg)	Homologous plasma	6 ml per kg per hr	[74]
Rabbit	20 ml (per kg)	Homologous plasma	3.5 ml per kg per hr	[74]
Cat	50 ml (2.4–2.7 kg)	Homologous serum	4.2–6.0 ml per hr	[43]

equally in either direction across the peritoneal barrier.

The peritoneum acts as a composite membrane (capillary endothelium, interstitium and mesothelium) which exhibits functional as well as anatomical asymmetry. Phylogenetic evidence indicates that the peritoneum evolved as an excretory organ and therefore may not permit ready absorption of intraperitoneal fluid or solutes [88, 89]. The presence of phospholipids (surfactant) within peritoneal fluid which is synthesized and secreted by the mesothelium suggests that the mesothelial surface has fluid repellant properties [90–92]. Small solutes are absorbed by diffusive transport which is dependent on solute size, charge and configuration whereas large solutes of molecular weight greater than 20,000 demonstrate minimal absorption into the peritoneal capillaries [67]. Macromolecules would accumulate within the peritoneal cavity if there was no alternative absorptive pathway.

4. Role of lymphatic absorption in ascites

Ascites develops when the net transperitoneal inflow of fluid into peritoneal cavity exceeds the rate of fluid efflux via the peritoneal cavity lymphatics [3–8]. The fluid flux rate across the peritoneum (Jw) is determined by the product of peritoneal hydraulic permeability (Lp), the effective membrane area (A) and the sum of osmotic ($\Delta\pi$) and hydrostatic (ΔP) transmembrane pressure gradients. That is:

$$Jw = Lp \cdot A(\Delta\pi + \Delta P).$$

Accordingly, net inflow of fluid into the peritoneal cavity is observed in conditions where there is a rise in hepatic sinusoidal and portal venous hydrostatic pressure, a reduction in serum albumin concentration and/or an increase in peritoneal permeability. The accumulation of intraperitoneal fluid is countered by its continuous reabsorption by the peritoneal cavity lymphatics at a rate influenced by the volume of ascites, the intraperitoneal hydrostatic pressure, the patency of the lymphatic pathways and central venous pressure (Table 2). The continuous bidirectional transport of fluid in ascites, however, precludes direct estimation of lymphatic drainage from the rate of absorption of isosmotic fluid as in normal animals (Table 1).

The peritoneal lymphatic absorption rate in ascites has been estimated indirectly from the rate of mass transfer of labelled colloids from the peritoneal cavity to the systemic circulation. This formulation is dependent on prior observations that intraperitoneal macromolecules (molecular weight grater than 20,000) are returned to the venous circulation almost exclusively by the peritoneal lymphatics [2, 67, 93, 94] and that isosmotic intraperitoneal fluid is drained by the peritoneal lymphatics without change in the concentration of index macromolecules [77, 78, 95–97]. This methodology underestimates lymphatic absorption from the peritoneal cavity for several reasons. A significant proportion of the tracer colloid, absorbed by the peritoneal lymphatics, does not reach the systemic circulation during the study time due to delayed transit or permanent entrapment in the diaphragmatic and mediastinal lymph nodes. Indeed, this physiological function of the draining lymph nodes is utilized in mediastinal lymphoscintigraphy [10–13, 98]. Secondly, the rise in blood concentration of the tracer colloid must be corrected for redistribution of the tracer out of the blood volume during the study interval [46, 67, 97]. Nevertheless, peritoneal to plasma mass transfer rates of radio-iodinated serum albumin [9, 10, 97] and other radio-colloids [10–13] have provided a valid comparison of the relative peritoneal lymphatic flow rates in patients with hepatic [9, 10, 97], malignant [10–13] and dialysis associated ascites [9]. Estimations of peritoneal lymphatic absorption by this method in 10 patients with hepatic ascites ranged from 24 to 223 ml per hour and averaged 80 ml per hour [9, 10, 97]. Presumably the large intraperitoneal fluid volume ensures constant contact of fluid with the undersurface of the diaphragm and the concurrent rise in intraperitoneal pressure enhances convective movement of fluid into the diaphragmatic lymphatics. In contrast, metastatic invasion of the subdiaphragmatic peritoneum is not uncommon in patients with intra-

Table 2. Factors influencing lymphatic absorption from the peritoneal cavity.

1 Intraperitoneal fluid volume.
2 Intraperitoneal hydrostatic pressure.
3 Rate and depth of respiration.
4 Posture.
5 Intestinal peristalsis.
6 Patency of the diaphragmatic and mediastinal lymphatics.
7 Lymphatic vessel outflow pressure.

abdominal malignancy [99, 100] and may at least partially obstruct lymphatic drainage from the peritoneal cavity [14, 15]. Peritoneal lymphatic absorption in 22 patients with malignant ascites ranged from 1 to 63 ml per hour and averaged only 11 ml per hour [10]. Mediastinal lymphoscintigraphy in patients with malignant ascites often failed to demonstrate patent diaphragmatic lymphatics or identify mediastinal lymph nodes [10–13]. Moreover, the calculated lymphatic absorption rate correlated with the concurrently performed lymphoscintigram [10]. Likewise, patients with schistosomal hepatic fibrosis and ascites have significant fibrous thickening of the subdiaphragmatic peritoneum, which most likely limits flow into the diaphragmatic lymphatics [16]. In support of this mechanism, obliteration of the diaphragm with fibrous tissue significantly increased the incidence and severity of ascites in animals with infrahepatic portal hypertension [101]. The role of lymphatic absorption in the pathophysiology of these different forms of ascites is summarized in Table 3.

5. Role of lymphatic absorption in peritoneal dialysis kinetics

The terminology used to describe the kinetics of peritoneal dialysis has been modified to incorporate the role of the peritoneal cavity lymphatics. The measurable net ultrafiltration volume represents the net change in the intraperitoneal fluid volume at the end of the dwell time and, assuming that the residual volume remains constant, equals the dialysate drain volume minus the infusion volume. However, the net ultrafiltration volume, in effect, is the difference between cumulative net transcapillary ultrafiltration into the peritoneal cavity and total lymphatic absorption out of the peritoneal cavity during the dwell time (Fig. 5). These two formulations of net ultrafiltration may be designated directly measured and calculated net ultrafiltration (UF), respectively. That is:

Measured net UF = drain volume – infusion volume

Calculated net UF = cumulative net transcapillary UF – lymphatic absorption

Cumulative net transcapillary ultrafiltration defines the total net influx of fluid from the peritoneal microcirculation into the peritoneal cavity during the dwell time in response to the osmotic pressure of the dialysis solution. This definition allows for bidirectional transcapillary water movement during the dwell time but acknowledges that inflow into the peritoneal cavity dominates and that only the net fluid flux can be measured. The resultant net inflow of fluid would equal measured net ultrafiltration if it was not for cumulative drainage via the lymphatics during the dwell time (Fig. 5).

In patients with ascites lymphatic drainage exceeds 50 ml per hour unless the diaphragmatic or mediastinal lymphatics are obstructed by tumor or fibrosis [10]. Intraperitoneal fluid volumes during peritoneal dialysis are routinely greater than 2 liters and should also ensure continuous contact of fluid with the undersurface of the diaphragm. Furthermore, the patency of the peritoneal cavity lymphatics should be preserved in peritoneal dialysis provided that the subdiaphragmatic parietal peritoneum only undergoes the same minor histological changes as are observed in the parietal peritoneum lining the anterior abdominal wall [102–104]. In peritoneal dialysis as well as chronic hepatic ascites the thoracic duct and other mediastinal lymph vessels may gradually dilate and so promote lymph flow from the peritoneal cavity [6].

Table 3. Transcapillary fluid influx and lymphatic absorption rates in ascites.

Form of ascites	Net transcapillary fluid influx rate	Lymphatic absorption rate
Hepatic	++++	++
Malignant	+	
Nephrogenic	+	–
Peritoneal Dialysis	+++	+?

Abbreviations: + increase; – decreases.

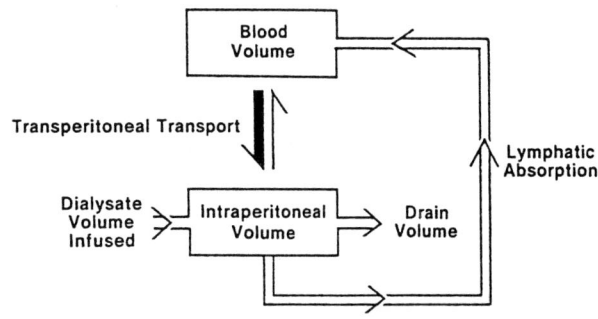

Figure 5. Schematic representation of the role of lymphatic absorption in the kinetics of peritoneal dialysis. (Reproduced with permission from reference [108]).

In hypertonic peritoneal dialysis the intraperitoneal fluid volume begins to decrease before isomolarity of the dialysis solution and plasma is observed [29, 32], indicating that net fluid absorption occurs before net transcapillary ultrafiltration is complete (Fig. 6). In addition, osmolar equilibrium is reached before glucose equilibrium [29]. The dialysis solution becomes isosmolar with the plasma before glucose equilibrium because of solute sieving with transcapillary ultrafiltration [24, 25, 105].

The total transperitoneal osmotic pressure gradient is the sum of products of the concentration gradient and the peritoneal reflection coefficient of each solute. Accordingly, a higher peritoneal reflection coefficient of glucose than other small molecular weight solutes [106] tends to maintain an osmotic pressure gradient into the dialysis solution after isosmolality is reached and thereby allows net transcapillary ultrafiltration to continue at a slow rate until osmotic pressure equilibrium is approached later in the dwell time. This mechanism has also been invoked to explain the net ultrafiltration observed following intraperitoneal infusion of electrolyte-free 5% dextrose solution (252 mOsm/l) [106]. Since the dialysis solution becomes hyposmolar to the plasma towards the end of the dwell time [110], this further suggests that net transcapillary ultrafiltration continues after osmolar equilibrium is first observed. Consequently the reduction in intraperitoneal volume (ΔV) after peak ultrafiltration really represents the lymphatic absorption rate (L) in excess of the concurrent net transcapillary ultrafiltration rate (Jw in equation 1). Thus,

$$V = Lp \cdot A \, (\Delta \pi + \Delta P) - L$$

Direct measurements of drain volumes after sequential dwell times in 29 CAPD patients showed that the rate of decrease in the intraperitoneal volume ranged from 8 to 89 ml per hour and average 39 ml per hour [28, 29]. The net absorption rate was not significantly different, irrespective of whether 2l volumes of 1.5% 2.5% or 4.25% dextrose dialysis solution were instilled [28, 29]. Moreover, net absorption rates during dialysis with 2.5l infusion volumes also averaged 37 ml per hour in 16 CAPD patients [26].

In conclusion, by analogy with ascites and by extrapolation from previous studies of drain volumes after infusion of isotonic and hypertonic solutions, the average daily lymphatic absorption rate during CAPD may be predicted to approach 1 liter per day.

6. Methods of estimating lymphatic absorption in peritoneal dialysis

Indirect methods

Two indirect methods have been described for measuring lymphatic drainage during peritoneal dialysis [46, 67, 107–132]. Both apply the same physiological functions of the peritoneal cavity lymphatics. By assuming that intraperitoneal marker colloids are returned to the systemic circulation exclusively by the lymphatics and that intraperitoneal fluid is drained by the peritoneal lymphatics without increase or decrease in concentration of index colloids [2, 67, 77, 93–97], the lymphatic absorption rate may be estimated either from the mass transfer rate of marker colloids from the peritoneal cavity to the blood [46, 67, 107] or from their rate of disappearance from the peritoneal cavity [108–132].

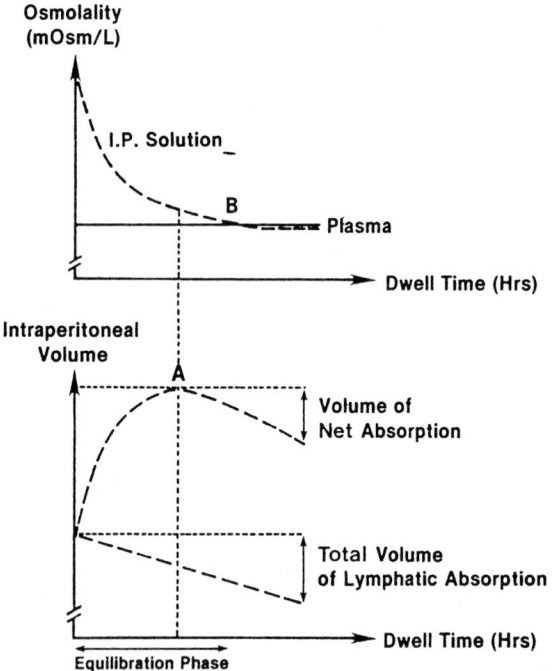

Figure 6. Changes in osmolality and intraperitoneal fluid volume following infusion of a hypertonic dextrose dialysis solution. The peak intraperitoneal volume (point A) precedes osmolar equilibrium (point B). Thereafter net fluid absorption represents lymphatic absorption in excess of net transcapillary ultrafiltration. (Reproduced with permission from reference [108]).

6.1. Mass transfer rates of intraperitoneal colloids to the blood

The first method essentially represents the peritoneal to blood clearance of a radio-labelled colloid. that is:

$$L = \frac{V_D \times \Delta C_D}{\overline{C_P}}$$

where

- L = total lymphatic flow during the time of the study
- V_D = volume of distribution of the tracer colloid (plasma volume)
- ΔC_D = rise in plasma concentration of the tracer colloid
- $\overline{C_p}$ = time averaged mean intraperitoneal concentration of the tracer colloid.

Using this approach, the average lymphatic absorption rate in 10 CAPD patients was only 0.21 ml per min per 1.73m² body surface area [107]. The absolute lymphatic absorption rates during CAPD most likely was underestimated in this study since the plasma volume of the CAPD patients was extrapolated from their body weight and, most importantly, the plasma appearance rate of radio-iodinated serum albumin, as in similar studies in patients with ascites [97, 133, 134] was only 20% of the peritoneal disappearance rate. As well as confirming that there is an initial lag phase before the plasma concentration of the radio-colloid begins to increase linearly [9, 10, 46, 97], Spencer and Farrell have recently shown that the mass transfer of intraperitoneal radio-iodinated albumin to the blood in CAPD patients was significantly greater after 24 hours than after the end of a four hour study exchange [33]. Thus, transfer of radio-colloids continues after the washout exchange at the end of the study time and cannot be accurately timed to the duration of the exchange. These factors may explain why lymphatic flow rates calculated by this method are much lower than direct observations of absorption of intraperitoneal plasma or whole blood in the same animal model [41, 46].

Estimates by this method represent the lower limit of lymphatic absorption rates in peritoneal dialysis.

6.2. Mass transfer rates of colloids from the peritoneal cavity

Alternatively the lymphatic absorption rate (L) may be estimated from the mass transfer rate of intraperitoneal macromolecules from the peritoneal cavity. That is:

$$L = \frac{(V_0 \times C_0) - (V_1 \times C_1)}{\overline{C_P}}$$

where

- V_0 and V_1 = intraperitoneal fluid volumes at time O and t
- C_0 and C_1 = intraperitoneal concentration of marker colloid at time O and t
- $\overline{C_p}$ = time averaged mean intraperitoneal concentration of marker colloid.

This mass balance equation avoids the error in calculating lymphatic flow in the previous method due to delayed transfer of radio-labelled colloids from the diaphragm and interstitial lymphatics to the blood. This method, however, not only depends on the assumption that intraperitoneal macromolecules are absorbed exclusively from the peritoneal cavity by the convective flow via the lymphatics but further assumes that all of the intraperitoneal marker colloid lost form the peritoneal cavity is absorbed by the non-restrictive pathways of the lymphatics. In connective tissue spaces, back diffusion of colloids into capillaries is negligible, the osmolality and the concentration of protein in the tissue fluid and end lymphatic lymph are equal [36, 37] and absorption of tissue protein is fully accounted for by lymphatic flow [135, 138]. Several observations indicate that these findings also pertain to intraperitoneal fluid and colloid kinetics and that intraperitoneal fluid absorption may be estimated from the rate of loss of an intraperitoneal marker colloid.

(a) Cannulation or ligation of both the right lymph duct and thoracic ducts prevents T-1824 labelled protein from reaching the blood [2, 74].
(b) Obliteration of the subdiaphragmatic peritoneum markedly reduces the absorption of intraperitoneal colloid [73, 74].
(c) The concentration of marker colloids remains unchanged during absorption of intraperitoneal isosmotic fluid [41, 46, 47], suggesting that colloids are absorbed with fluid by convective transport presumably through lymphatic pathways.

(d) Fractional peritoneal absorption of albumin and IgG [97] and gelatins and dextrans of different molecular weight [139, 140] are similar, further suggesting that absorption of macromolecules is by convective flow.

(e) The intraperitoneal content of radio-iodinated serum albumin during hypertonic peritoneal dialysis decreases at a linear rate averaging 3% per hour [107] and, late in the dwell time, correlates with net fluid absorption [32, 107, 129].

However, with microquantities of radio-colloid, a significant proportion of the administered dosage may be adsorbed to the peritoneal mesothelium, dialysis bag and administration set or be adsorbed by the adjacent subperitoneal tissues [46, 141]. The addition of a large quantity of unlabelled colloid, such as albumin, instead of microamounts of radio-labelled colloid may obviate this potential error [109–111, 115].

Cumulative net transcapillary ultrafiltration can be estimated concurrently from the dilution of the initial dialysate marker colloid concentration [108] since the intraperitoneal colloid concentration is unchanged by lymphatic absorption of intraperitoneal fluid [93, 94] and thus any decrease in the dialysate colloid lymphatic absorption of intraperitoneal fluid during the dwell time results from net influx of fluid from the peritoneal microcirculation. However allowance must be made for the effect of tracer disappearance on its dilution by the ultrafiltrate [142].

Lymphatic absorption rates estimated from the disappearance rate of intraperitoneal colloids exceed 1 ml per minute in adult CAPD patients (Table 4) [110, 112, 125, 128, 129, 131]. These lymphatic absorption rates are higher than net fluid absorption rates in CAPD patients estimated from sequential drain volumes after exchanges of increasing duration [26, 28]. A transperitoneal glucose and osmolar concentration gradient persists after the peak intraperitoneal volume is attained which may allow transcapillary ultrafiltration to continue at a slow rate provided that the peritoneal reflection coefficient for glucose is sufficient to generate an adequate osmotic pressure gradient. Lymphatic absorption in many of the above studies may be higher than in active CAPD patients since fluid contact with the subdiaphragmatic peritoneum is more extensive with the patient supine than when the patient is ambulatory [74]. Alternatively upright posture may enhance backfiltration by increasing intraperitoneal pressure [143]. In 15 patients who remained in the upright position or sitting throughout the study dwell time, the lymphatic absorption rate calculated from the peritoneal disappearance of dextran 70 averaged 1.03 ± 0.45 ml per minute [131].

The peritoneal disappearance rate may overestimate actual lymph flow if, under non-steady state conditions, tracer enters and accumulates in the adjacent tissues [46, 67, 108]. However, measurements of lymphatic absorption were not reduced after prior administrations of tracer colloid which suggests that there is no significant effect of tracer trapping in the submesothelial tissues [132]. Alternatively lymphatic absorption in CAPD has been evaluated by comparing transperitoneal transport of a lower molecular weight solute following both intravenous (mainly diffusive transport) and intraperitoneal administration (diffusive and lymphatic transport). It was assumed that inulin would be less likely to be trapped in the interstitium and the difference between the mass transfer area coefficients of intraperitoneal and intravenous inulin averaged 1.5ml per minute [123], which corresponds to estimates of lymphatic absorption using the disappearance rate of macromolecules (Table 5). Estimates of lymphatic absorption derived from the

Table 3. Transcapillary fluid influx and lymphatic absorption rates in ascites.

Marker Solute	Molecular Weight	Lymph Flow (ml/min ± SEM)	References
Dextran	30,500	1.56 ± 0.42	[140]
Autologous Haemoglobin	34,500	1.59 ± 0.15	[112]
Dextran	50,500–57000	1.71 ± 0.30	[140]
Unlabelled Human Albumin*	69000	1.47 ± 0.15	[110]
RISA	69000	1.20 ± 0.3	[129]

* Exchange using 2.27% dextrose dialysis solution (all other studies used 1.36% dextrose solution).

mass transfer rates of colloids from the peritoneal cavity represent the upper limit of lymphatic flow in peritoneal dialysis patients.

6.3. Computer simulations of transperitoneal fluid transport

Theoretical lymphatic absorption rates have been derived by a computer model based upon a three-pore model of the peritoneal barrier [144, 145]. Using this model, if fluid reabsorption from the peritoneal cavity to blood is constant at 1.25 ml per min and peritoneal membrane sieving coefficients for small solutes are at least 0.3, theoretical values for lymphatic absorption during peritoneal dialysis in man varied between 0.3 and 0.75 ml per min.

The computer predictions of intraperitoneal volume versus time data make a good fit with clinical measurements in adult patients [145].

6.4. Cannulation of the major lymphatic vessels

Direct measurement of *total* lymph flow from the peritoneal cavity during peritoneal dialysis cannot be performed. Cannulation of the major lymphatics draining the peritoneal cavity has been studied recently during peritoneal dialysis in experimental animals but not in man [146–150]. This approach has provided comparisons of the different methods used for estimating lymphatic absorption and has been used to evaluate the relationship between fluid loss rates and lymphatic absorption rates from the peritoneal cavity. This methodology permits a more direct measurement of lymph flow but has several limitations:

1. It is not possible to cannulate all of the major lymphatic pathway draining the peritoneal cavity. In the sheep model only the thoracic and caudal lymphatic ducts are cannulated and drainage via the right cannulation of two of the major lymphatic vessels, over half of recovered tracer colloid or labelled red blood cells lost from the peritoneal cavity reached the blood compartment via the right lymph duct, other minor lymphatic pathways or direct entry into the bloodstream [146, 147, 150]. Absorption directly into the systemic circulation was unlikely to be significant since the recovery rate in the blood compartment of labelled intraperitoneal red blood cells in the lymphatic cannulation studies was similar to radio-labelled albumin [150].
2. Tracer colloids or cells may be entrapped in the lymph nodes draining the peritoneal cavity [46, 150]. Sieving in the lymphatic stomata and capillaries or lymph nodes is the most likely reason for the lower estimates of lymph drainage when using labelled red blood cells instead of labelled albumin in lymphatic cannulation experiments of peritoneal dialysis [150].
3. Cannulation of lymphatics may alter outflow pressure and lymph flow [151].
4. Anaesthesia reduces lymphatic absorption substantially [81, 82, 146, 147] and therefore the results of studies in conscious animals are more likely to reflect dialysis conditions.

In conscious sheep (n = 6) lymph flow rates measured by cannulation of the thoracic and caudal ducts averaged 1.02 ± 0.21 ml per hour per kg [148]. Much lower estimates of total lymph drainage were observed in anesthetized sheep (n = 6) using 50 ml per kg 1.5% dextrose dialysis solution [147]. Lymph flow values were significantly higher in conscious than in anesthetized animals [148, 149].

6.5. Comparison of methods of estimating lymphatic absorption

None of the above methods directly measures total lymphatic flow from the peritoneal cavity during peritoneal dialysis. Comparative data for each method of measuring peritoneal lymph flow in a sheep model of peritoneal dialysis are summarized in Table 5 [149]. The estimates of lymph flow during peritoneal dialysis in conscious sheep using the same dialysis parameters varied widely but only the estimates from the peritoneal disappearance of

Table 5. Peritoneal lymph flow rates during peritoneal dialysis in conscious sheep.

Method of Estimating Lymph Flow	Lymph Flow (ml per hr per kg)
Plasma appearance rate of tracer	1.42 ± 0.11
Peritoneal disappearance rate of tracer	2.40 ± 0.62
Cannulation of thoracic and caudal ducts (right lymph duct = zero)	1.02 ± 0.19
Cannulation of thoracic and caudal ducts (right lymph duct = caudal)	1.52 ± 0.21

(Data derived from reference [149]).

tracer and the unadjusted cannulation studies differed significantly (Table 5).

The peritoneal disappearance rate of tracer equates with fluid loss via bulk flow (convection) from the peritoneal cavity [152]. Accordingly if the peritoneal disappearance rate of tracer is an accurate estimate of lymph flow, all of the calculated fluid loss from the peritoneal cavity can be ascribed to translymphatic uptake [108, 116, 118–121, 124–128]. If the alternative methods of estimating lymphatic drainage are more precise only a proportion of the fluid losses are considered to leave the peritoneal cavity by true lymphatic flow [46, 107, 145–150].

An unifying interpretation of fluid losses and lymphatic drainage rates from the peritoneal cavity has been proposed [153]. Fluid and macromolecules are transported from the peritoneal cavity by bulk flow (convection) into the peritoneal lymphatics and interstitium due to intraperitoneal hydrostatic pressure but sieving within the interstitium then leads to absorption of much of the fluid into the peritoneal capillaries and the macromolecules are removed by the interstitial lymphatics [153]. However, lymph flow from the caudal lymphatic in sheep increased from 5 ml per hour to almost 30 ml per hour after the intraperitoneal infusion of 50 ml per kg of Ringer's lactate while the draining lymph albumin concentration rapidly equilibrated with and remained similar to the labelled albumin concentration of the intraperitoneal fluid [150].

Fluid losses from the peritoneal cavity during peritoneal dialysis in adult man are acknowledged to approximate 1.0–1.5 ml per min and to be clinically relevant [110–120, 122–129]. The proportion of fluid loss which is attributed to peritoneal lymphatic drainage is dependent upon the method used to measure lymph flow rates. To circumvent this unresolved debate, **convective fluid losses from the peritoneal cavity hitherto are designated as backfiltration.**

7. Factors controlling backfiltration in peritoneal dialysis

The rate of disappearance of tracer macromolecules has been utilized to assess which variables influence fluid absorption rates from the peritoneal cavity in peritoneal dialysis. The elimination rates of radio-colloid during 2 liter exchanges with 1.36%, 2.27% and 3.86% anhydrous dextrose dialysis solutions were not significantly different with values of 1.47 ± 0.15, 1.28 ± 0.16 and 1.30 ± 0.25 ml per min respectively (32). Studies with 2 liter volumes of different osmotic agents (dextrose, amino acids and glycerol) demonstrated similar backfiltration rates [118]. Hence neither the osmolality or osmotic agent of the dialysis solution significantly influence fluid backfiltration rates in peritoneal dialysis.

Backfiltration rates were elevated from 1.87 ± 0.23 to 3.39 ± 0.31 ml per min ($p < 0.01$) when the infusion volume of 1.36% dextrose dialysis solution was increased from 2 to 3 liters [113]. During peritonitis calculated fluid reabsorption rates were 2.11 ± 0.25 ml per min compared with $1.05 \pm$ ml per min in the recovery period 20–40 days later ($p < 0.01$) [114]. During exchanges in adults and children using exchanges with comparable dialysate volumes backfiltration rates in the children were 1.13 ± 0.20 ml per min per m^2 BSA and in the adults 0.75 ± 0.15 ml per min per m^2 BSA [115]. Backfiltration rates in 34 adult CAPD patients were unrelated to patient age, sex, body surface area, duration of peritoneal dialysis or past history of peritonitis [128]. These studies indicate that backfiltration and thus probably lymphatic drainage are increased in peritoneal dialysis using higher dialysate volume [113, 128], during episodes of peritonitis [114], and in childhood [115].

Net ultrafiltration volumes are inversely related to intraperitoneal pressure in CAPD patients [154]. Intraperitoneal pressure has been shown to be inversely related to transcapillary ultrafiltration [154] and to correlate with backfiltration rates [154, 155]. From animal studies raised central venous pressure may be expected to reduce lymphatic flow rates but this has not yet been evaluated in CAPD [87].

8. Consequences of backfiltration during peritoneal dialysis

The physiological roles of the peritoneal cavity lymphatics in the absorption of intraperitoneal isosmotic fluid, macromolecules, particles and bacteria are normally beneficial. However, lymphatic absorption has mainly adverse effects on the clinical application of long-dwell peritoneal dialysis as an effective form of renal replacement therapy.

8.1. Loss of ultrafiltration

Lymphatic drainage of intraperitoneal fluid throughout the dwell time reduces the potential drain volume and, thus net ultrafiltration, in all CAPD patients. Since net transcapillary ultrafiltration occurs mainly during the first hours of each exchange whereas lymphatic absorption is continuous, fluid absorption via the lymphatics has a greater influence on ultrafiltration kinetics in CAPD than in intermittent peritoneal dialysis with rapid exchanges. In short-dwell exchanges cumulative net transcapillary ultrafiltration greatly exceeds lymphatic drainage and consequently the reduction in the dialysate drain volume resulting from lymphatic absorption is relatively minor. Wide inter-individual [35, 36] and intra-individual [37] variations in net ultrafiltration has been observed in CAPD patients even if the dwell time, osmolality and volume of exchanges are standardized. Poor peritoneal ultrafiltration capacity has usually been ascribed to high peritoneal permeability × area, rapid absorption of glucose from the dialysate, early dissipation of the transperitoneal osmolar gradient and thus reduced cumulative net transcapillary ultrafiltration [35–37, 39, 156, 157]. In addition, since transperitoneal osmotic pressure is equivalent to the sum of the products of the osmolar gradient and the peritoneal reflection coefficient of each solute, the lower peritoneal reflection coefficient for glucose in patients with high peritoneal permeability × area will further reduce transcapillary ultrafiltration by generating reduced osmotic pressure at any given glucose concentration gradient. Interpatient differences in peritoneal ultrafiltration capacity after long-dwell exchanges may, however, depend on lymphatic absorption as well as peritoneal permeability × area.

Studies of ultrafiltration kinetics in two groups of CAPD patients with high and average peritoneal transport rates showed that the disappearance rate of intraperitoneal marker macromolecules and backfiltration were similar (83 ± 16 ml per hour in patients with average peritoneal solute transport rates and 89 ± 9 ml per hour in patients with high peritoneal permeability × area) [116]. The former group, as expected had higher net transcapillary ultrafiltration and net ultrafiltration volumes. Therefore, despite equal absolute rates, backfiltration causes a proportionately greater reduction in ultrafiltration capacity in patients with higher than average peritoneal permeability-area (Fig. 7).

Studies in a total of 47 CAPD patients with true loss of peritoneal ultrafiltration capacity have identified 3 patterns of ultrafiltration failure [34, 110, 111, 156–160]. It was not possible to delineate the pattern of ultrafiltration failure in 5 patients [159]. The most common cause of loss of ultrafiltration is a decrease in transcapillary ultrafiltration as a result of rapid absorption of dialysate glucose and early loss of the transperitoneal osmotic gradient (Type 1 membrane failure) whereas failure of ultrafiltration due to a reduction in transcapillary ultrafiltration in patients with low peritoneal permeability × area is uncommon (Type 2; Table 6).

However a significant proportion of patients with loss of ultrafiltration capacity have average transcapillary ultrafiltration but high backfiltration rates from the peritoneal cavity (Type 3; Table 6). Sclerosing peritonitis may be associated with either Type 1 or Type 2 membrane failure. Nevertheless the underlying pathophysiological mechanisms of ultrafiltration failure remain unknown in most patients. The prevalence of ultrafiltration failure in patients using only lactate based dialysis fluids increases with the duration of dialysis; 3% of patients after 1 year of CAPD, 10% after 3 years and 31% after 6 years excluding patients with temporary loss of ultrafiltration capacity due to peritoneal catheter malposition or dialysate leaks [156]. It remains uncertain whether factors such as temporal changes in the mesothelium, the glycation of peritoneal structural proteins or dialysate effluent phospholipid concentrations determine peritoneal ultrafiltration capacity.

8.2. Reduction in solute mass transfer

The continuous absorption of dialysate solutes by convective flow via the peritoneal cavity lymphatics decreases solute mass transfer during CAPD [110, 116, 161]. Peritoneal solute clearances are calculated as the product of daily drain volume and drain dialysate solute concentration divided by the mean serum solute concentration while reverse solute clearances may be estimated from the product of daily backfiltration and mean dialysate solute concentration divided by the mean serum solute concentration. Extrapolated to four exchanges using 2 liters of 2.5% dextrose dialysis solution per day, backfiltration in 18 CAPD patients reduced the potential daily drain volume by $18 \pm 2\%$, potential daily urea clearance by $14 \pm 1.4\%$ and potential daily creatinine clearance by $13.3 \pm 1.5\%$ (Fig. 8) [116]. These findings indicate that estimates of transperitoneal solute transport, which are based on the dialysate drain volume and solute concentration, are erroneously low since no allowance has been made for backfiltration throughout the dwell time. Accordingly the efficiency of the peritoneum as a dialyzing membrane is greater than previously rec-

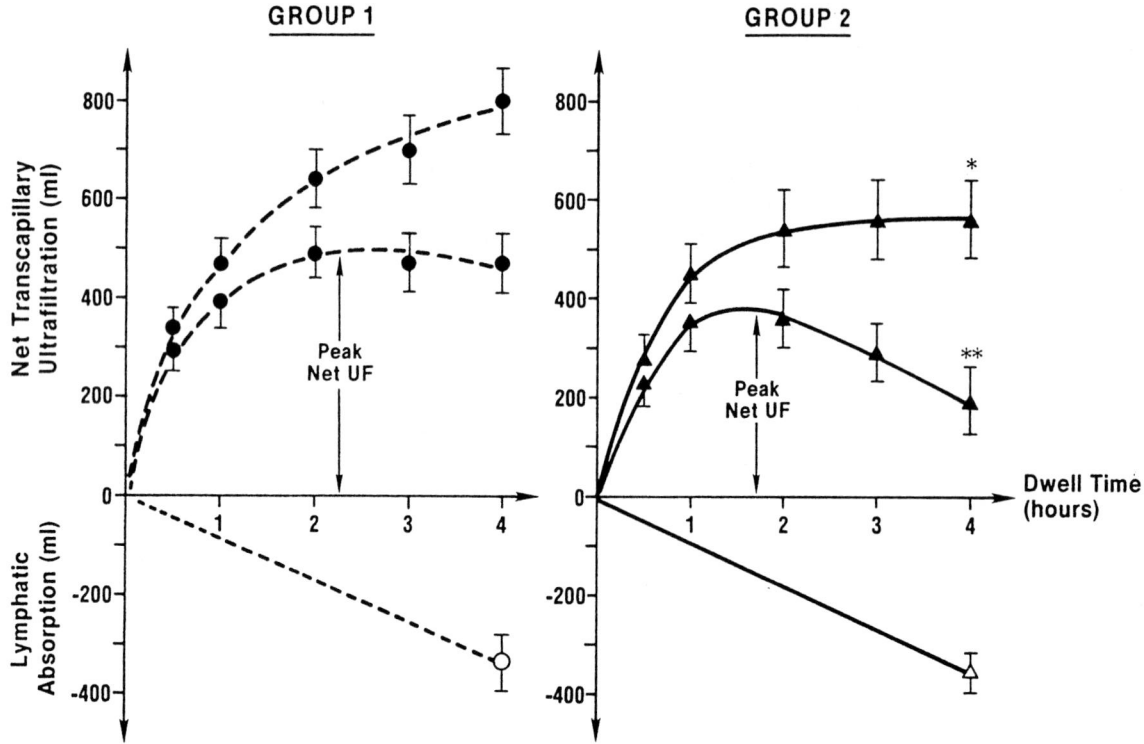

Figure 7. Comparison of cumulative lymphatic absorption, net ultrafiltration and cumulative net transcapillary ultrafiltration (mean SEM) during four hour exchanges using 2 liters of 2.5% dextrose dialysis solution in CAPD patients with average (group 1) and high (group 2) peritoneal permeability × area. (Reproduced with permission from reference [116]). (**$p < 0.01$;*$p < 0.05$).

ognized [27, 33, 34, 162–165]. Practical approaches for decreasing backfiltration from the peritoneal cavity are limited. The clinical results of attempting to use phospholipids or neostigmine to reduce backfiltration and to augment ultrafiltration and solute clearances have been conflicting [120, 124, 130, 166–176].

Table 6. Incidence of different types of ultrafiltration failure in 47 CAPD patients.

	Number of Patients		References
Type 1	Type 2	Type 3	
3	–	2	[34]
4	–	–	[110]
–	–	2	[111]
7	–	2	[156]
3	–	2	[157]
4	1	–	[158]
6	–	5	[159]
5	–	2	[160]
32	1	14	

8.3. Absorption of intraperitoneal bacteria

The uptake of intraperitoneal bacteria by the peritoneal cavity lymphatics is well established [177, 178]. Nevertheless, blood cultures are infrequently positive during CAPD associated peritonitis [179] and secondary pulmonary infections or right sided endocarditis are very rare complications of peritonitis [69, 179]. The bacteria are presumably filtered and effectively trapped by the mediastinal lymph nodes.

8.4. Absorption of intraperitoneal polymers and particles

The uptake of large solutes and particles by convective flow into the peritoneal cavity lymphatics has several implications for peritoneal dialysis. Alternative, less absorbable osmotic agents than glucose have been sought to reduce the undesired metabolic sequelae of dialysate glucose absorption and, most importantly, to induce sustained net transcapillary ultrafiltration [31, 180]. However, lymphatic drainage results in significant systemic absorption of all polymer osmotic agents [180–184],

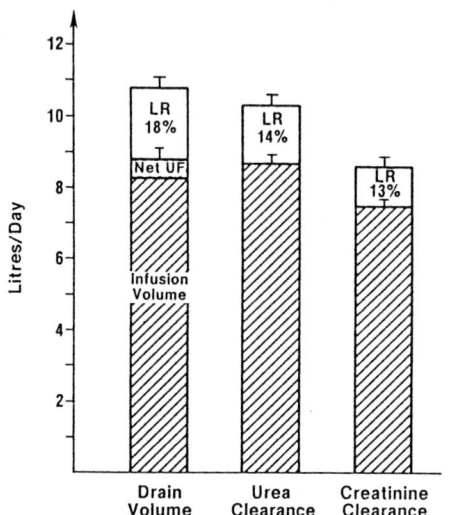

Figure 8. Contribution of backfiltration to loss of potential drain volume, urea clearance and creatinine clearance (mean ±SEM) in adult CAPD patients (n = 18) using 4 exchanges of 2.5% dextrose dialysis solution per day (Reproduced with permission from reference [116]).

regardless of their molecular weight, and has hindered the development of safe and effective alternative osmotic agents to glucose. Human albumin would be an ideal osmotic agent since its systemic absorption would be beneficial rather than potentially harmful.

Particulate material entering the peritoneal cavity in the dialysis solution will also be absorbed by the peritoneal cavity lymphatics. Thus contaminants in commercial dialysis solutions should be avoided to prevent their systemic accumulation and toxicity as well as their potentially adverse effects on the peritoneal membrane [114, 185].

The continuous uptake of tracer macromolecules from the peritoneal cavity requires that estimates of the dialysate volume using the single injection indicator-dilution method must be corrected for the peritoneal disappearance rate of the index colloid [186, 187].

9. Conclusion

Backfiltration rates during peritoneal dialysis are greater than 1.0 ml per min in most patients and have a major influence on the kinetics of ultrafiltration in long-dwell exchanges. The currently available range of glucose containing dialysis solutions has been developed to induce sufficient net transcapillary ultrafiltration to offset backfiltration and so achieve adequate daily peritoneal ultrafiltration in the majority of CAPD patients.

References

1. Allen L. Lymphatics and lymphoid tissues. Ann Rev Physiol 1967; 29: 197.
2. Courtice FC, Steinbeck AW. The lymphatic drainage of plasma from the peritoneal cavity of the cat. Austral J Exp Biol Med Sci 1950; 28: 161.
3. Hyatt RE, Smith JR. The mechanisms of ascites: physiological appraisal. Am J Med 1954; 16: 434.
4. Courtice FC. Ascites: the role of the lymphatics in the accumulation of ascitic fluid. Med J Aust 1959; 26: 945.
5. Witte MH, Witte CL, Dumont AE. Progress in liver disease: physiological factors involved in the causation of cirrhotic ascites. Gastroenterology 1971; 61: 742.
6. Dumont AE, Mulholland JH. Flow rate and composition of thoracic duct lymph in patients with cirrhosis. N Engl J Med 1960; 263: 471.
7. Barrowman JA. Liver lymph. In: Barrowman JA (ed), Physiology of the Gastrointestinal Lymphatic System. Cambridge, Cambridge University Press 1978; p. 229.
8. Witte CL, Witte MH, Dumont AE. Lymph imbalance in the genesis and perpetuation of the ascites syndrome in hepatic cirrhosis. Gastroenterology 1980; 78: 1059.
9. Morgan AG, Terry SI. Impaired peritoneal fluid drainage in nephrogenic ascites. Clin Nephrol 1981; 15: 61.
10. Bronskill MJ, Bush RS, Ege GN. A quantitative measurement of peritoneal drainage in malignant ascites. Cancer 1977; 40: 2375.
11. Coates G, Bush RS, Aspin N. A study of ascites using lymphoscintigraphy with 99m Tc sulfur colloid. Radiology 1973; 107: 577.
12. Atkins HL, Hauser W, Richards P. Visualization of mediastinal lymph nodes after intraperitoneal administrations of 99m Tc sulfur colloid. Nuclearmedizin 1970; 9: 275.
13. Kroon BBR. Overhet ontstaan en de chirurgische behandeling van maligne ascites. M. D. Thesis, University of Amsterdam 1986.
14. Feldman GB, Knapp RD. Lymphatic drainage of the peritoneal cavity and its significance in ovarian cancer. Am J Obstet Gynec 1974; 119: 991.
15. Feldman GB. Lymphatic obstruction in carcinomatous ascites. Cancer Res 1975; 35: 325.
16. Ismail AH, Mohamed FS. Structural changes of the diaphragmatic peritoneum in patients with schistosomal hepatic fibrosis in relation to ascites. Lymphology 1986; 19: 82.
17. Clausen J. Studies on the effect of intraperitoneal blood transfusion. Acta Paediat 1940; 27: 24.
18. Cole WC, Montgomery JC. Intraperitoneal blood transfusion. Report of 237 transfusions in 117

patients in private practice. Am J Dis Child 1929; 37: 497.
19. Siperstein DM, Sansby JM. Intraperitoneal transfusion with citrated blood. Am J Dis Child 1923; 25: 107.
20. Scopes JW. Intraperitoneal transfusion of blood in newborn babies. Lancet 1963; i: 1027.
21. Liley AW. Intrauterine transfusion of the foetus in haemolytic disease. Br Med J 1963; ii: 1107.
22. Nolph KD, Popovich RP, Ghodes AJ, Twardowski ZJ. Determinants of low clearances of small solutes during peritoneal dialysis. Kidney Int 1978; 13: 117.
23. Nolph KD, Miller FN, Rubin J, Popovich R. New directions in peritoneal dialysis concepts and applications. Kidney Int 1980; 18: S111.
24. Nolph KD. Solute and water transport during peritoneal dialysis. Perspect Perit Dial 1983; 1: 4.
25. Nolph KD, Miller FN, Pyle WK, Popovich RP, Sorkin MI. An hypothesis to explain the ultrafiltration characteristics of peritoneal dialysis. Kidney Int 1981; 20: 543.
26. Twardowski ZJ, Janicka L. Three exchanges with a 2.5 liter volume for continuous ambulatory peritoneal dialysis. Kidney Int. 1981; 20: 281.
27. Pyle WK, Popovich RP, Moncrief JW. Mass transfer evaluation in peritoneal dialysis. In: Moncrief JW, Popovich RP (eds), CAPD Update. New York, Masson Publishing USA, Inc 1981; p. 35.
28. Twardowski ZJ, Ksiazek A, Majadan M et al. Kinetics of continuous ambulatory peritoneal dialysis (CAPD) with four exchanges per day. Clin Nephrol 1981; 15: 119.
29. Rubin J, Nolph KD, Popovich RP, Moncrief JW, Prowant B. Drainage volumes during continuous ambulatory peritoneal dialysis. ASAIO J 1979; 2: 54.
30. Krediet RT, Boeschoten EW, Zuyderhoudt RMJ, Arisz L. The relationship between peritoneal glucose absorption and body fluid loss by ultrafiltration during continuous ambulatory peritoneal dialysis. Clin Nephrol 1987; 27: 51.
31. Twardowski ZJ, Khanna R, Nolph KD. Osmotic agents and ultrafiltration in peritoneal dialysis. Nephron 1986; 42: 93.
32. Lindholm B, Werynski A, Bergstrom J. Kinetics of peritoneal dialysis with glycerol and glucose osmotic agents. ASAIO Trans 1987; 33: 19.
33. Spencer PC, Farrell PC. Solute and water kinetics in CAPD. In: Gokal R (ed), Continuous Ambulatory Peritoneal Dialysis. Edinburgh, Churchill Livingstone 1986; p. 38.
34. Krediet RT, Boeschoten EW, Zuyderhoudt FMJ, Arisz L. Peritoneal transport characteristics of water, low-molecular weight solutes and proteins during long-term continuous ambulatory peritoneal dialysis. Perit Dial Bull 1986; 6: 61.
35. Nikolkakis N, Rodger RSC, Goodship THJ et al. The assessment of peritoneal function using a single hypertonic exchange. Perit Dial Bull 1985; 5: 186.
36. Smeby LC, Wideroe TE, Jorstad S. Individual differences in water transport during continuous peritoneal dialysis. ASAIO J 1981; 4: 17.
37. Wideroe TE, Smeby LC, Mjaaland S, Dahl K, Berg KJ, Aas TW. Long-term changes in transperitoneal water transport during continuous ambulatory peritoneal; dialysis. Nephron 1984; 38: 238.
38. Raja RM, Khanna MS, Barber K. Solute transport and ultrafiltration during peritonitis in CAPD patients. ASAIO J 1984; 7: 8.
39. An International Co-operative Study. A survey of ultrafiltration in continuous ambulatory peritoneal dialysis. Perit Dial Bull 1984; 4: 137.
40. Olin T, Saldeen T. The lymphatic pathways from the peritoneal cavity: a lymphangiographic study in the rat. Cancer Res 1964; 24: 1700.
41. Courtice FC, Simmonds WJ. Physiological significance of lymph drainage of the serous cavities and lungs. Physiol Rev 1954; 34: 419.
42. Higgins GM, Graham AS. Lymphatic drainage from the peritoneal cavity in the dog. Arch Surg 1929; 19: 452.
43. Raybuck HE, Allen L, Harms WS. Absorption of serum from the peritoneal cavity. Am J Physiol 1960; 199: 1021.
44. Simer PH. The drainage of particulate matter from the peritoneal cavity by lymphatics. Anat Rec 1944; 88: 175.
45. Courtice FC, Harding J, Steinbeck AW. The removal of free red blood cells from the peritoneal cavity of animals. Aust J Exp Biol Med Sci 1953; 31: 215.
46. Flessner MF, Perker RJ, Sieber SM. Peritoneal lymphatic uptake of fibrinogen and erythrocytes in the rat. Am J Physiol 1983; 244: H89.
47. Von Recklinghausen F. Zur Fettresorption. Archiv fur Pathologische Anatomie und Physiologie und fur Klinische Medicin. 1863; 26: 172.
48. MacCallum WG. On the mechanism of absorption of granular material from the peritoneum. Bull John Hopkins Hosp 1903; 14: 105.
49. Cunningham RS. Studies in absorption from serous cavities IV. On the passage of blood cells and particles of different size through the walls of the lymphatics in the diaphragm. Am J Physiol 1922; 62: 248.
50. Hertzler AE. The morphogenesis of the stigmata and stomata occurring in peritoneal and vascular endothelium. Trans Am Micro Soc 1901; 22: 63.
51. Allen L. The peritoneal stomata. Anat Rec 1937; 67: 89.
52. French JE, Florey HW, Morris B. The absorption of particles by the lymphatics of the diaphragm. Q J Exp Physiol 1960; 45: 88.
53. Casley-Smith JR. Endothelial permeability – the passage of particles into and out of diaphragmatic lymphatics. Q J Exp Physiol 1964; 49: 365.
54. Tsilibary EC, Wissig SL. Light and electron microscope observations of the lymphatic drainage units of the peritoneal cavity of rodents. Am J Anat 1987; 180: 195.
55. Tsilibary EC, Wissig SL. Absorption from the peritoneal cavity: SEM study of mesothelium covering the peritoneal surface of the muscular

55. portion of the diaphragm. Am J Anat 1977; 149: 127.
56. Hedenstedt S. Elliptocyte transfusions as a method in studies on blood destruction, blood volume and peritoneal resorption. Acta Chir Scandinav 1947; 95(Suppl 128): 105.
57. Morris B, Murphy MJ, Bessis M. The passage of red blood cells from the peritoneal cavity. In: Yoffey JM, Courtice FC (eds), Lymphatics, Lymph and Lymphoid Tissue. London, Academic Press 1970; p 303.
58. Florey HW. Reactions of, and absorption by, lymphatics with special reference to those of the diaphragm. Br J Exp Path 1927; 8: 479.
59. Allen L. On the penetrability of the lymphatics of the diaphragm. Anat Rec 1956; 124: 639.
60. Allen L, Weaterwood T. Role of fenestrated basement membrane in lymphatic absorption from the peritoneal cavity. Am J Physiol 1959; 187: 551.
61. Leak LV, Rahil K. Permeability to the diaphragmatic mesothelium: the ultrastructural basis for stomata. Am J Anat 1978; 151: 557.
62. Tsilibary EC, Wissig SL. Structural plasticity in the pathway for lymphatic drainage from the peritoneal cavity. Microvas Res 1979; 17: S144.
63. Bettendorf U. Lymph flow mechanism of the subperitoneal diaphragmatic lymphatics. Lymphology 1978; 11: 111.
64. Tsilibary EC, Wissig SL. Lymphatic absorption from the peritoneal cavity: Regulation of patency of mesothelial stomata. Microvasc Res 1983; 25: 225.
65. Allen L, Vogt E. A mechanism of lymphatic absorption from serous cavities. Am J Physiol 1937; 119: 776.
66. Khanna R, Mactier R, Twardowski ZJ, Nolph KD. Peritoneal cavity lymphatics. Perit Dial Bull 1986; 6: 113.
67. Flessner MF, Dedrick RL, Schultz JS. Exchange of macromolecules between peritoneal cavity and plasma. Am J Physiol 1985; 248: H15.
68. Dunna DL, Barke RA, Knight NB, Humphrey EW, Simmons RL. Role of resident macrophages, peripheral neutrophils and translymphatic absorption in bacterial clearance from the peritoneal cavity. Infect Immun 1985; 49: 257.
69. Keane WF, Peterson PK. Host defence mechanisms of the peritoneal cavity and continuous ambulatory peritoneal dialysis. Perit Dial Bull 1984; 4: 122.
70. Simer PH. The passage of particulate matter from peritoneal cavity into the lymph vessels of the diaphragm. Anat Rec 1948; 101: 333.
71. Clark AJ. Absorption from the peritoneal cavity. J Pharmacol Exp Ther 1920; 16: 415.
72. Courtice FC, Steinbeck AW. The rate of absorption of heparinized plasma and of 0.9% NaCl from the peritoneal cavity of the rabbit and guinea-pig. Austral J Exp Biol Med Sci 1950; 28: 171.
73. Allen L, Raybuck HE. The effects of obliteration of the diaphragmatic lymphatic plexus on serous fluid. Anat Rec 1960; 137: 25.
74. Courtice FC, Steinbeck AW. The effects of lymphatic obstruction and of posture on the absorption of protein from the peritoneal cavity. Austral J Exp Biol Med Sci 1951; 29: 451.
75. Shear L, Castellot J, Barry KG. Peritoneal fluid absorption: effect of dehydration on kinetics. J Lab Clin Med 1965; 66: 232.
76. Shear L, Swartz C, Shinaberger JA, Barry KG. Kinetics of peritoneal fluid absorption in adult man. New Engl J Med 1965; 272: 123.
77. Bolton C. Absorption from the peritoneal cavity. J Path Bact 1921; 24: 429.
78. Zink J, Greenway CV. Control of ascites absorption in anesthetized cats: effects of intraperitoneal pressure, protein and furosemide diuresis. Gastroenterology 1977; 73: 1119.
79. Morris B. The effect of diaphragmatic movement on the absorption of red cells and protein from the peritoneal cavity. Aust J Exp Biol Med Sci 1953; 31: 239.
80. Higgins GM, Beaver MG, Lemon WS. Phrenic neurectomy and peritoneal absorption. Am J Anat 1930; 45: 137.
81. Schad H, Brechtelsbaver H. Thoracic duct lymph flow and composition in conscious dogs and the influence of anesthesia and passive limb movement. Plugers Arch 1977; 371: 25
82. Elk JR, Adair T, Drake RE, Gabel JC. The effect of anesthesia and surgery on diaphragmatic lymph vessel flow after endotoxin in sheep. Lymphology 1990; 23: 145.
83. Shear L, Ching S, Gabuzda GJ. Compartmentalisation of ascites and oedema in patients with hepatic cirrhosis. New Engl J Med 1970; 282: 1391.
84. Hau T, Ahrenholz DH, Simmons RL. Secondary bacterial peritonitis: the biologic basis of treatment. Curr Probl Surg 1979; 16: 1.
85. Fowler GR. Diffuse septic peritonitis, with special reference to a new method of treatment, namely, the elevated head and trunk posture, to facilitate drainage into the pelvis. With a report of nine consecutive cases of recovery. Medical Red 1900; 57: 617.
86. Levine S. Post-inflammatory increase of absorption from peritoneal cavity into lymph nodes: particulate and oily inocula. Exp Mol Path 1985; 43: 124.
87. Drake RE, Gabel JC. Abdominal lymph flow response to intra-peritoneal fluid in awake sheep. Lymphology 1991: 24: 77.
88. Dobbie JW. From philosopher to fish: The comparative anatomy of the peritoneal cavity as an excretory organ and its significance for peritoneal dialysis in man. Perit Dial Int 1988; 8: 3.
89. Di Paolo N. The peritoneal mesothelium: An excretory organ. Perit Dial Int 1989; 9: 151.
90. Dobbie JW, Pavlina T, Lloyd J et al. Phosphatidylcholine synthesis by peritoneal mesothelium: Its implications for peritoneal dialysis. Am J Kidney Dis 1988; 12: 31.
91. Grahame GR, Torchia MC, Dankevich KA et al. Surface active material in peritoneal effluent of CAPD patients. Perit Dial Bull 1985; 5: 109–11.
92. Breborowicz A, Sombolos K, Rodela H et al.

93. Lill SR, Parsons RH, Bohac I. Permeability of the diaphragm and fluid resorption from the peritoneal cavity in the rat. Gastroenterology 1979; 76: 997.
94. Aune S. Transperitoneal exchange IV. The effect of transperitoneal fluid transport on the transfer of solutes. Scand J Gastroenterol 1970; 5: 241.
95. Courtice FC, Steinbeck AW. Absorption of protein from the peritoneal cavity. J Physiol 1951; 114: 336.
96. Nicoll PA, Taylor AE. Lymph formation and flow. Ann Rev Physiol 1977; 39: 73.
97. Henriksen JH, Lassen NA, Parving H, Winkler K. Filtration as the main transport mechanism of protein exchange between plasma and the peritoneal cavity in hepatic cirrhosis. Scand J Clin Invest 1980; 40: 503.
98. Goranson LR, Johsson K, Olin T. Parasternal scintigraphy with technetium – 99m sulfide colloid in human subjects: a comparison between two techniques. Acta Radiol Diagnosis 1974; 15: 639.
99. Bergman F. Carcinoma of the ovary: a clinicopathological study of 86 autopsied cases with special reference to mode of spread. Acta Obstet Gynecol Scand 1966; 45: 211.
100. Baglley CM, Young RC, Schein PS, Chabner BA, DeVita VT. Ovarian carcinoma metastatic to the diaphragm – frequently undiagnosed at laparotomy. Am J Obstet Gynecol 1973; 116: 397.
101. Raybuck HE, Weatherwood T, Allen L. Lymphatics in the rat. Am J Physiol 1960; 198: 1207.
102. Dobbie JW, Zaki M, Wilson L. Ultrastructural studies on the peritoneum with special reference to chronic ambulatory peritoneal dialysis. Scot Med J 1981; 26: 213.
103. Di Paolo N, Sacchi G, De Mia M et al. Morphology of the peritoneal membrane during peritoneal dialysis. Nephron 1986; 44: 204.
104. Verger C, Burnschvigg O, Le Carpentier Y, Laverone A. Structural and ultrastructural peritoneal membrane changes and permeability alterations during CAPD. Proc EDTA 1981; 18: 199.
105. Nolph KD, Hano JE, Teschan PE. Peritoneal sodium transport during hypertonic peritoneal dialysis: Physiologic mechanisms and clinical implications. Ann Intern Med 1969; 70: 931.
106. Knochel JP. Formation of peritoneal fluid hypertonicity during dialysis with isotonic glucose solutions. J Appl Physiol 1969; 27: 233.
107. Rippe B, Stelin G, Ahlmen J. Lymph flow from the peritoneal cavity in CAPD patients. In: Maher JF, Winchester JF (eds), Frontiers in peritoneal dialysis. Field, Rich and Associates Inc., New York 1986; pp 24–30.
108. Mactier RA, Khanna R, Twardowski ZJ, Nolph KD. Role of peritoneal cavity lymphatic absorption in peritoneal dialysis. Kidney Int. 1987; 32: 165.
109. Nolph KD, Mactier RA, Khanna R, Twardowski ZJ, Moore H, McGary T. Kinetics of peritoneal ultrafiltration: The role of lymphatics. Kidney Int 1987; 32: 219.
110. Mactier RA, Khanna R, Twardowski ZJ, Nolph KD. Contribution of lymphatic absorption to loss of ultrafiltration and solute clearances in CAPD. J Clin Invest 1987; 80: 1311.
111. Mactier RA, Khanna R, Twardowski ZJ, Nolph KD. Failure of ultrafiltration in CAPD due to excessive lymphatic absorption. Am J Kidney Dis 1987; 10: 461.
112. Krediet RT, Struijk DG, Boeschoten EW et al. Autologous haemoglobin for the measurement of intraperitoneal volume and lymphatic absorption in CAPD. Perit Dial Int. VIII Annual CAPD Abstracts 1988; 83A.
113. Krediet RT, Boeschoten EW, Struijk DG, Arisz L. Differences in the peritoneal transport of water, solutes and proteins between dialysis with two or with three liter exchanges. Nephrol Dial Transplant 1988; 2: 198–204.
114. Krediet RT, Struijk DG, Boeschoten EW, Arisz L. The effect of peritonitis on lymphatic fluid absorption from the peritoneal cavity. Nephrol Dial Transplant 1988; 3: 556A.
115. Mactier RA, Khanna R, Moore H, Russ J, Nolph KD, Groshong T. Kinetics of peritoneal dialysis in children: Role of lymphatics. Kidney Int 1988; 34: 82.
116. Mactier RA. The role of lymphatic absorption in peritoneal dialysis. MD Thesis, University of Glasgow 1988.
117. Lindholm B, Werynski A, Bergstrom J. Peritoneal dialysis with amino acid solutions: fluid and solute transport kinetics. Artif Organs 1988; 12: 2.
118. De Paepe M, Matthys D, Lameire N. Measurement of peritoneal lymph flow in CAPD using different osmotic agents. Perit Dial Int, IX Annual CAPD abstracts 1989, 44A.
119. Mactier RA, Khanna R. Absorption of fluid and solutes from the peritoneal cavity. Theoretic and therapeutic implications and applications. Trans ASAIO 1989; 35: 122.
120. Struijk DG, Van der Reijden HJ, Krediet RT, Koomen GCM, Arisz L. Effect of phosphatidylcholine on peritoneal transport and lymphatic absorption in a CAPD patient with sclerosing peritonities. Nephron 1989; 51: 577.
121. Breborowicz A, Rodela H, Oreopoulos DG. Effect of various factors on peritoneal lymphatic flow in rabbits. Perit Dial Int 1989; 9: 85.
122. Lindholm B, Heimburger O, Waniewski J, Werynski A, Bergstrom J. Peritoneal ultrafiltration and fluid reabsorption during peritoneal dialysis. Nephrol Dial Transplant 1989; 4: 805.
123. Struijk DG, Krediet RT, Koomen GCM, Boeschoten EW, Reijden JH. Arisz L. Indirect measurement of lymphatic absorption with inulin in CAPD patients. Perit Dial Int 1990; 10: 141.
124. Chan PCK, Tam SCF, Cheng IKP. Oral neostigmine and lymphatic absorption in a myasthenia gravis patient on CAPD. Perit Dial Int 1990; 10: 93.
125. Krediet RT, Struijk DG, Koomen GCM, Arisz L. Peritoneal fluid kinetics during CAPD measured with intraperitoneal dextran 70. ASAIO Transactions 1991; 37: 662.

(Reference 92 continued at top: Mechanism of phosphalidylcholine action during peritoneal dialysis. Perit Dial Bull 1987; 7: 6.)

126. Lysaght MJ, Moran J, Lysaght CG. Plasma water filtration and lymphatic uptake during peritoneal dialysis. ASAIO Trans 1991; 37: M402.
127. Schroder CH, Reddingius RE, Van Dreumel JAM, Theeuwes AGM, Monnens LAH. Transcapillary ultrafiltration and lymphatic absorption during childhood continuous ambulatory peritoneal dialysis. Nephrol Dial Transplant 1991; 6: 571.
128. Chan PCK, Wu PG, Tam SCF, Ip MSM, Fang GX, Cheng IKP. Factors affecting lymphatic absorption in Chinese patients on CAPD. Perit Dial Int 1992; 11: 147.
129. Heimburger O, Waniewski J, Werynski A, Lindholm B. A quantitative description of solute and fluid transport during peritoneal dialysis. Kidney Int 1992; 41: 1320.
130. Hasbargen JA, Hasbargen BJ. Fortenbery EJ. Effect of intraperitoneal neostigmine on peritoneal transport characteristics in CAPD. Kidney Int 1992; 42: 1398.
131. Abensur H, Romad JE, Prado EBA, Kakehashi ET, Sabbaga E, Marcondes M. Use of dextran 70 to estimate peritoneal lymphatic absorption rate in CAPD. Adv Perit Dial 1992; 8: 3.
132. Struijk DG, Koomen GCM, Krediet RT, Arisz L. Indirect measurement of lymphatic absorption in CAPD patients is not influenced by trapping. Kidney Int 1992; 41: 1668.
133. Dykes PW, Jones JH. Albumin exchange between plasma and ascitic fluid. Clin Sci 1968; 34: 185.
134. Daugirdas JR, Ing TS, Gandhi VC, Hano JE, Chen WT, Yuan L. Kinetics of peritoneal fluid absorption (from the peritoneal cavity) in patients with chronic renal failure. J Lab Clin Med 1980; 95: 351.
135. Arfors KE, Rutili G, Svensjo E. Microvascular transport of macromolecules in normal and inflammatory condition. Acta Physiol Scand 1979; 463: S90.
136. Taylor AE, Gibson WH, Granger HJ, Guyton AC. The interaction between intercapillary and tissue forces in the overall regulation of interstitial fluid volume. Lymphology 1973; 6: 192.
137. Rutili G, Arfors KE. Interstitial fluid and lymph protein concentration in the subcutaneous tissue. Bibl Anat 1975; 13: 70.
138. Noer I, Lassen NA. Evidence of active transport (filtration?) of plasma proteins across the capillary walls in muscle and subcuties. Lymphology 1978; 11: 133.
139. Cheek TR, Twardowski ZJ, Moore HL, Nolph KD. Absorption of inulin and high molecular weight gelatin isocyanate solution from peritoneal cavity of rats. In: Avram MM, Girodano C (eds), Ambulatory Peritoneal Dialysis (Proceedings of the Fourth International Congress of Peritoneal Dialysis) New York, Plenum Publishing Corporation, New York 1990; p 149.
140. Krediet RT, Struijk DG, Koomen GCM, Hoek FJ, Arisz L. The disappearance of macromolecules from the peritoneal cavity during CAPD is not dependent on molecular size. Perit Dial Int 1990; 10: 147.
141. Flessner MF, Fentschermacher JD, Blasberg RG, Dedrick RL. Peritoneal absorption of macromolecules studied by quantitative autoradiography. Am J Physiol 1985; 248: H26.
142. Waniewski J, Heimburger O, Park MS, Werynski A, Lindholm B. Impact of tracer disappearance on transcapillary ultrafiltration and net dialysate volume change. Perit Dial Int 1992; 12 (Suppl 2): S14.
143. Twardowski ZJ, Khanna R, Nolph KD et al. Intra-abdominal pressures during natural activities in patients treated with continuous ambulatory peritoneal dialysis. Nephron 1986; 44: 129.
144. Stelin G, Rippe B. A phenomenological interpretation of the variation in dialysate volume with dwell time in CAPD. Kidney Int 1990; 38: 465.
145. Rippe B, Stelin G, Haraldsson B. Computer simmulations of peritoneal fluid transport in CAPD. Kidney Int 1991; 40: 315.
146. Abernethy NJ, Chin W, Hay JB, Rodela H, Oreopoulos D, Johnston MG. Lymphatic drainage of the peritoneal cavity in sheep. Am J Physiol (Renal, Fluid Electrolyte Physiol 29) 1991; 260: 353.
147. Abernethy NJ, Chin W, Hay JB, Rodela H, Oreopoulos D, Johnston MG. Lymphatic removal of dialysate from the peritoneal cavity of anesthetized sheep. Kidney Int 1991; 4D: 174.
148. Tran LP, Rodela H, Abernethy NJ, Yuan ZY, Hay JB, Oreopoulos D, Johnston MF. Lymphatic drainage of hypertonic dialysis solution from the peritoneal cavity of anesthetized and conscious sheep. Am J Physiol 1993; 74: 859.
149. Tran L, Rodel H, Hay JB, Oreopoulos D, Johnston MG. Quantitation of lymphatic drainage of the peritoneal cavity in sheep. Comparison of direct cannulation techniques with indirect methods to estimate lymph flow. Perit Dial Int 1993; 13: 270.
150. Yuan ZY, Rodela H, Hay JB, Oreopoulos D, Johnston MG. Comparison of the use of $51_{Cr-RBCs}$ and ^{125}I-albumin as markers to estimate lymph drainage of the peritoneal cavity in conscious sheep. Am J Physiol (in press).
151. Laine GA, Allen SJ, Katz J, Gabel JC, Drake RE. Outflow pressure reduces lymph flow rate from various tissues. Microvasc Res 1987; 33: 135.
152. Shockley TR, Ofsthun NJ. Pathways for fluid loss from the peritoneal cavity. Perit Dial Int 1992; (S2): S6.
153. Flessner MF. Peritoneal transport physiology: insights from basic research. J Am Soc Nephrol 1991; 2: 122.
154. Imholz ALT, Koomen GCM, Struijk DG, Arisz L, Krediet RT. The effect of increased intraperitoneal pressure on fluid and protein transport during CAPD. Perit Dial Int 1993; 13 (Suppl 1): S62.
155. Abensur H, Romao Jr. JE, Prado EBA, Kakehashi E, Sabbaga E, Marcondes M. Influence of hydrostatic intraperitoneal pressure and cardiac function on the lymphatic absorption rate of the peritoneal cavity in CAPD. Perit Dial Intern 1993; 13 (Suppl 1): 59.

156. Heimburger O, Waniewski J, Werynski A, Tranaeus A, Lindholm B. Peritoneal transport in CAPD patients with permanent loss of ultrafiltration capacity. Kidney Int 1990, 38: 495.
157. Kumano K, Suyama K, Sakai T. Increased lymphatic absorption as a cause of ultrafiltration failure in long-term CAPD patients. Perit Dial Int 1992; 12(S2): S14.
158. Kim D, Maduluko GC, Thome F, Cattran DC, Fenton SSA. The various spectrum of ultrafiltration failure and its pathogenesis among CAPD patients. Kidney Int 1985; 27: 181A.
159. Davies SJ, Brown B, Bryan J, Russell GI. Clinical evaluation of the peritoneal equilibration test: a population-based study. Nephrol Dial Transplant; 1993; 8: 64.
160. Pollock CA, Ibels LS, Hallett MD, Cocksedge B, Caterson RJ, Mahoney JF, Farrell PC. Loss of ultrafiltration in continuous ambulatory peritoneal dialysis. Perit Dial Int 1989; 9: 107.
161. Hallett M, Lysaght M, Farrell P. The role of lymphatic drainage in peritoneal mass transfer. Artif Organs 1989; 13: 28–34.
162. Randerson DH, Farrell PC. Mass transfer properties of the human peritoneum. ASAIO J 1980; 3: 140.
163. Popovich RP, Moncrief JW. Transport kinetics. In: Nolph KD (ed), Peritoneal Dialysis (2nd edition). Boston, Martinus Nijhoff 1985; p 115.
164. Garred LJ, Canaud B, Farrell PC. A simple kinetic model for assessing peritoneal mass transfer in chronic ambulatory peritoneal dialysis. ASAIO J 1983; 6: 131.
165. Selgas R, Rodriguez-Carmona A, Martinez ME et al. Peritoneal mass transfer in patients on long-term CAPD. Perit Dial Bull 1984; 4: 153.
166. Mactier RA, Khanna R, Nolph KD, Twardowski Z, Moore H. Neostigmine increases ultrafiltration and solute clearances in peritoneal dialysis by reducing lymphatic drainage. Perit Dial Bull 1987; 7: S50.
167. Mactier RA, Khanna R, Moore H, Twardowski ZJ, Nolph K. Phosphatidylcholine enhances the efficiency of peritoneal dialysis by reducing lymphatic reabsorption. Kidney Int 1988; 33: 247A.
168. Di Paolo N, Buoncristiani U, Capotondo L, Gaggiotti E, De Mia M, Rossi P, Sansoni E, Bernini M. Phosphatidylcholine and peritoneal transport during peritoneal dialysis. Nephron 1986; 44: 365.
169. Dombros N, Balaskas E, Savidis N, Tourkantonis A, Sombolos K. Phosphatidylcholine increases ultrafiltration in CAPD patients. Perit Dial Bull 1987; 7: S24.
170. Struijk D, Van Der Reijden H, Krediet R, Koomen G, Arisz L. Effect of phosphatidylcholine on peritoneal transport on lymphatic absorption in a patient with sclerosing peritonitis. Nephron 1989; 51: 577.
171. Di Paolo B, Chakrabarti E, Maher JF. Phosphatidylcholine does not affect peritoneal transport of intact rabbits. Perit Dial Int 1989; 9: 211.
172. De Vecchi A, Castelnovo C, Guerra L, Scalamogna A. Phosphatidylcholine administration in CAPD patients with reduced ultrafiltration. Perit Dial Int 1989; 9: 207.
173. Chan H, Abraham G, Oreopoulos DG. Oral lecithin improves ultrafiltration in patients on peritoneal dialysis. Perit Dial Int 1989; 9: 203.
174. Querques M, Procaccini DA, Pappani A, Strippoli P, Passion EA. Influence of phosphatidylcholine on ultrafiltration and solute transfer in CAPD patients. ASAIO Transactions 1990; 36: M581.
175. Chan PC. Effect of phosphatidylcholine on ultrafiltration in patients on CAPD. Nephron 1993; 59: 100.
176. Krack G, Viglino G, Cavalli PL, Gandolfo C, Magliano G, Cantaluppi A, Peluso F. Intraperitoneal administration of phosphatidylcholine improves ultrafiltration in CAPD patients. Perit Dial Int 1992; 12: 359.
177. Steinberg B. Infections of the peritoneum. New York, Paul Hoeber, Inc 1984.
178. Durham HE. The mechanism of reaction to peritoneal infection J Path Bact 1897; 4: 338.
179. Vas SI. Peritonitis. In: Nolph KD (ed), Peritoneal Dialysis (2nd edition). Boston, Marinus Nijhoff Publishers 1985; p. 403.
180. Wu G. Osmotic agents for peritoneal dialysis solutions. Perit Dial Bull 1982; 2: 151.
181. Higgins JT, Gross ML, Somani P. Patient tolerance and dialysis effectiveness of a glucose polymer containing peritoneal dialysis solution. Perit Dial Bull 1984; 4: S131.
182. Mistry CD, Mallick NP, Gokal R. Ultrafiltration with an isosmotic solution during long peritoneal dialysis exchanges. Lancet 1987; ii: 178.
183. Twardowski ZJ, Nolph KD, Khanna R, Hain H, Moore H, McGary TJ. Charged polymers as osmotic agents for peritoneal dialysis. Materials Research Society Symposium Proceedings 1986; 55: 319.
184. Winchester JF, Stegink LD, Ahmad S et al. A comparison of glucose polymer and dextrose as osmotic agents in CAPD. In: Maher JF, Winchester JF (eds), Frontiers in Peritoneal Dialysis. New York, Field, Rich and Associates, Inc 1986; p. 231.
185. Junor BJR, Briggs JD, Forwell MA, Dobbie JW, Henderson IS. Sclerosing peritonitis: role of chlorhexidine in alcohol. Perit Dial Bull 1985; 5: 101.
186. Mactier RA. Measurement of dialysate volumes in peritoneal dialysis. Perit Dial Int 1989; 9: 155.
187. Pust AH, Leypoldt JK, Frigon RP, Henderson LW. Peritoneal dialysate volume determined by indicator dilution measurements. Kidney Int 1988; 33: 64.

6 Ultrafiltration in peritoneal dialysis

JOHN K. LEYPOLDT AND CHANDRA D. MISTRY

1. Introduction 135
2. Fluid movement across the peritoneum 136
   2.1. Membrane characteristics 136
   2.2 The driving force 136
      2.2.1. Kinetics of osmotic pressure 137
      2.2.2. Factors influencing osmotic forces 137
      2.2.3. Osmotic flow between isosmolar solutions 138
      2.2.4. Osmotic flow against the osmolality gradient 138
   2.3. Clinical adaptaton of osmosis in peritoneal dialysis 140
      2.3.1 Crystalloids 140
      2.3.2. Colloids 144
      2.3.3. A combination of crystalloid and colloid osmotic agents 144
      2.3.4. Where are we going? 145
3. Convective solute transport across the peritoneum 145
   3.1. Peritoneal membrane sieving coefficients 146
   3.2. Peritoneal membrane solute reflection coefficients 148
      3.2.1. Theoretical concerns 148
      3.2.2. Experimental summary 152
4. Modeling ultrafiltration during peritoneal dialysis 155
References 157

1. Introduction

There is a clinical requirement to remove excess body water, electrolytes, and other uremic toxins on a regular basis from patients with end-stage renal failure. During extracorporeal artificial kidney treatment, fluid is removed by simply applying a difference in hydrostatic or hydraulic pressure across the synthetic membrane. This approach is impractical during peritoneal dialysis; instead, fluid is removed from the patient by creating a difference in osmotic pressure between dialysis solution and blood. Thus, fluid removal during peritoneal dialysis is primarily by osmosis and is commonly referred to as osmotic ultrafiltration (or simply ultrafiltration) because of the similarities between transmembrane fluid movement by osmosis and ultrafiltration [1]. We will focus in this chapter on describing both the driving forces that move fluid across the peritoneum and the rate of solute transport that accompanies this transperitoneal fluid movement.

The transport pathways for water and solute across the peritoneum are complex and described elsewhere in this book. It is not possible, however, to represent all of these details in a simple model of the peritoneum yet still retain clinical utility. In this chapter we will characterize the peritoneum using more simple models or representations. Figure 1 shows some of the models of the peritoneum that

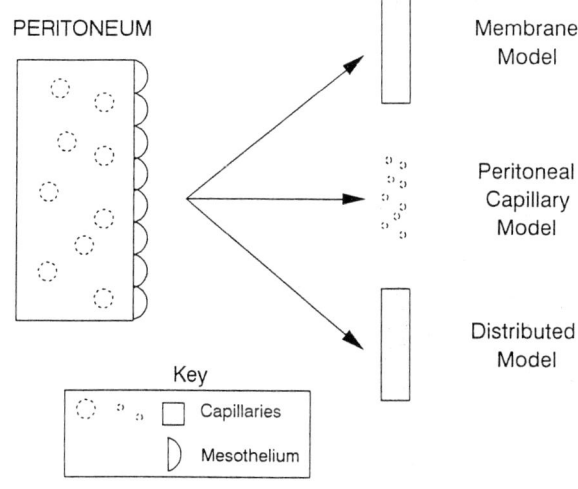

Figure 1. Diagrammatic representation of the peritoneum and the simplified models used in this chapter to describe transperitoneal fluid and solute transport.

have proven useful to describe certain features of transperitoneal fluid and solute transport. For example, we will most commonly define the peritoneum simply as a membrane (or barrier) that represents the resistance to fluid and solute transport separating the bulk phase of plasma water from the bulk phase of well-mixed dialysis solution in the peritoneal cavity. This definition acknowledges our ignorance of the pathways governing transperitoneal transport but has proven useful in describing the kinetics of fluid and solute transport during peritoneal dialysis [2]. The concepts of microcirculatory physiology have been incorporated into more detailed models of the peritoneum, and these models have provided additional insights into the mechanisms governing transperitoneal fluid and solute transport. These more detailed models depict the peritoneum either as peritoneal capillaries suspended in dialysis solution [3–5] or as peritoneal interstitium containing a uniform distribution of peritoneal capillaries [6]. These models will be employed qualitatively below, where necessary, as an aid to explain previous data and certain concepts.

2. Fluid movement across the peritoneum

The transperitoneal ultrafiltration rate in peritoneal dialysis is governed by a complex interplay between the peritoneal membrane and physiological forces across it. This relationship is probably best expressed by the following equations:

$$Q_v = L_p \times A \times (\Delta P - \Delta \pi) \quad (1)$$

Membrane Driving
Characteristic Force

$$Q_v = K_f \times (\Delta P - \Delta \pi) \quad (2)$$

where Q_v represents the transperitoneal ultrafiltration rate (or the volume or water flow [7]), L_p, the peritoneal membrane hydraulic conductivity, A, the peritoneal membrane surface area, ΔP, the hydrostatic pressure difference across the membrane, $\Delta \pi$, the osmotic pressure difference across the membrane and K_f, the peritoneal membrane ultrafiltration coefficient. Since previous work has suggested that transperitoneal ultrafiltration originates from fluid in peritoneal capillaries [8], the quantities ΔP and $\Delta \pi$ refer to differences in hydrostatic and osmotic pressure between blood and dialysis solution in the peritoneal cavity. In like manner, transperitoneal ultrafiltration is predominantly transcapillary ultrafiltration [9]; thus, the peritoneal membrane properties L_p, A, and K_f largely reflect those of peritoneal capillaries.

2.1. Membrane characteristics

Despite the structural uniformity of the human peritoneum, a wide functional variability exists between patients and this is well recognized in clinical practice. Thus, for a given transperitoneal pressure gradient, the difference in transcapillary ultrafiltration occurs primarily as a result of variation in the peritoneal capillary ultrafiltration coefficient, influenced by the hydraulic conductivity and surface area of the membrane.

The hydraulic conductivity is a measure of the intrinsic rate at which water transverses the capillary membrane. It is a function of the intrinsic physicochemical nature of the membrane and is inversely related to its thickness. Both of these parameters are subject to physiological or pathological modification and therefore influence the ultrafiltration rate under different clinical settings. Maher and coworkers [10, 11] have demonstrated that intra-peritoneal administration of certain hormones (i.e. secretin [10]) and drugs (e.g. amphotericin [11]) enhance transperitoneal ultrafiltration by altering the hydraulic conductivity of the peritoneum. Under normal physiological conditions the thickness of the capillary membrane remains fairly constant, but a pathological increase in its thickness occurs in diabetes [12] and sclerosing peritonitis [13] with decline in ultrafiltration capacity.

The surface area of the filtering membrane is an important determinant of ultrafiltration and is likely a function of both the anatomical surface area and that of peritoneal capillaries. In adults, the anatomical surface area of the peritoneum is estimated to vary between 1.72 and 2.08 m^2 [14] but the effective filtering surface area is likely to be smaller due to variation in the distribution of blood supply to the peritoneum. The physiological studies of Henderson [15] have predicted an effective surface area of significantly less than 1 m^2 and this may be reduced further by peritoneal adhesions, cannula malposition and small volume exchanges with a fall in ultrafiltration rate. Alternatively, using larger exchange volumes [16, 17] or intraperitoneal administrations of vasodilators [18] the proportion of effective surface area is increased with greater ultrafiltration.

2.2. The driving force

The driving force across the peritoneum remains the most significant factor influencing water movement in peritoneal dialysis. The two major components of this force are: a) the hydrostatic capillary pressure gradient and b) the osmotic pressure gradient.

The peritoneal capillary hydrostatic pressure probably remains fairly constant during peritoneal dialysis and unlikely to influence the ultrafiltration rate greatly under normal conditions. However, it is susceptible to pharmacological manipulation and this has been demonstrated by intraperitoneal administration of vasoactive drugs, such as dopamine [19], with much improved ultrafiltration.

The osmotic pressure gradient is undoubtedly the major component of the driving force in peritoneal dialysis, and a clear understanding of factors influencing osmotic forces across biological membranes is essential. Osmosis is by no means a modern concept, the principle has been applied empirically since ancient times to dehydrate food by application of salt and sugar. In 1748, Nollet first demonstrated the physiological characteristics of osmosis when he separated chambers containing water and wine with an animal bladder and observed an increased volume in the wine chamber [20]. A century later, Pfeiffer in 1887 examined the process in a more quantitative way by separating water from a sucrose solution by a semipermeable membrane, constructed using a porous wall of an earthware pot on to which was precipitated cupric ferrocyanide. He observed a volume flow from the water side to the sucrose side that could be stopped by applying hydrostatic pressure to the sucrose side and concluded that the magnitude of the water flow was proportional to the sucrose concentration [21]. At about the same time Van't Hoff [22] formulated the relationship between the concentration of impermeable solute on either side of a membrane and hydrostatic pressure required to stop the flow (the osmotic pressure) as:

$$\Delta\pi = -\Delta P = RT\Delta C \qquad (3)$$

where $\Delta\pi$ is the osmotic pressure difference across the membrane, ΔP is the hydrostatic pressure difference across the membrane and ΔC is the difference in solute concentration across the membrane; RT is the product of the universal gas constant and the absolute temperature. The Van't Hoff expression is a good approximation for dilute solutions such as body fluids.

2.2.1. Kinetics of osmotic pressure

In an aqueous solution the concentration of water molecules (chemical potential) is less than in pure water, since the addition of solute to pure water results in a solution which occupies a greater volume than the original pure water. The reduction in chemical potential of water is directly proportional to the concentration of solute. Thus, a chemical potential gradient for water will exist when pure water and aqueous solution, or two aqueous solutions containing different concentrations of same solute, are separated by a membrane permeable to water but impermeable to solute ("ideal" semipermeable membrane). The diffusion of water molecules along the concentration gradient constitutes the osmotic flow [23]. The hydrostatic pressure increment that would have to be imposed on that solution to prevent entry of water through the boundary is, therefore, the osmotic pressure.

2.2.2. Factors influencing osmotic forces

a) *Osmolar concentration*
The reduction in chemical potential of water in solution depends solely on the number of particles (undissociated molecules, ions, colloids, and micelles), and not on the molecular size or weight. A mole of any substance represents the same number (6.023×10^{23}) of molecules, and therefore, the osmolar concentration is conventionally expressed in terms of the unit called an osmole. One osmole is the number of particles (molecules) in one gram molecular weight of undissociated solute. If the solute dissociate into two ions, 1 gram molecular weight of the solute equals 2 osmoles. A solution that has one osmole of solute dissolved in each kilogram of water is said to have an osmolality of 1 osmole/kg and would exert an osmotic pressure of 22.4 atmosphere across an "ideal" semipermeable membrane under ideal conditions. Likewise.

$$1 \text{ mOsm/kg} = 19.3 \text{ mm Hg osmotic pressure.} \qquad (4)$$

When actually measured, osmotic pressures, though linearly related to the concentration of solutes over the range of relatively low values encountered in most physiological situations, are usually less than those calculated on the basis of Van't Hoff equation. This is because the mutual interaction between the molecules of solute leads to their failure to behave as individual units, and the net result is that their effective concentration (number of particles) is reduced. A more precise value of osmotic pressure is therefore given by the equation:

$$\Delta\pi_{actual} = RT\gamma\Delta C \qquad (5)$$

where γ is the activity coefficient for the particular solute.

b) *Membrane permeability*

Even when the effects of mutual interaction between the solute molecules are taken into account, the extent to which a solution achieves the predicted osmotic pressure is greatly influenced by the nature of the separating membrane. The following two membrane types are of interest:

i) An "ideal" semipermeable membrane is one that is permeable to water but not to solutes (irrespective of size and shape). Since all solutes are impermeable through such a membrane, the osmotic flow is directly proportional to the total osmolality gradient across it, i.e. in accordance with the Van't Hoff equation.

ii) A "partially permeable" membrane is one that is permeable to water and some solutes. For osmotic flow through such solute-permeable membranes, as most biological membranes are, a more complex relationship exists. In this situation the flow is a function only of relatively non-permeable solutes, and not necessarily related to the total osmolality (total number of solute particles; diffusable and non-diffusable) of the solution. Furthermore, the ability of solutes to permeate such a membrane is also determined by the physicochemical characteristics of the solute, such as molecular size and shape as well as deformability and ionic charges [24]. To characterize this relationship between solutes and membrane, Staverman [25] introduced the useful concept of the osmotic reflection coefficient whose value ranges from zero for solutes as permeable as water to one for a solute that is completely impermeable. By incorporation of this coefficient into the basic Van't Hoff equation, the flow through a solute-permeable membrane, for solution containing several different solutes (a, b, c, etc.) of differing osmotic reflection coefficients, can be expressed as:

$$Q_v = -RTL_pA[\sigma_a\Delta C_a + \sigma_b\Delta C_b + \sigma_c\Delta C_c + ...] \quad (6)$$

or, more generally,

$$Q_v = L_pA[\Delta P - RT\Sigma^n(\sigma\Delta C)] \quad (7)$$

where $\Sigma^n(\sigma\Delta C)$ is the sum of the products of the osmotic reflection coefficients of the solutes (1 to n) and their differences in molar concentration across the membrane.

It follows, therefore, that the direction of osmotic forces through such a membrane is determined by the differences in the size of the sum of the products of the osmotic reflection coefficients and differences in molar concentration rather than the osmolality gradient [20]. Thus, theoretically it is possible to direct the osmotic flow between isosmolar solutions and even against the conventional osmolality gradient provided an appropriate choice is made of solutes with different osmotic reflection coefficients.

2.2.3. *Osmotic flow between isosmolar solutions*

If the solutions containing identical osmolar concentration (isosmolar solutions) of differing composition are separated by an "ideal" semipermeable membrane, no osmotic flow takes place. However, it may well occur across a solute-permeable membrane provided the sum of the products of solute concentration and osmotic reflection coefficient is higher on one side of the membrane than on the other as shown in Fig. 2a. Thus, isosmolar flow is possible only through a solute-permeable membrane with an appropriate choice of solutes. This is the physiological basis of "colloid" osmotic flow induced by albumin across the capillary wall and proximal tubular transport of isosmolar fluid [26].

2.2.4. *Osmotic flow against the osmolality gradient*

This concept could be extrapolated further when considering the flow from solution of high to low osmolality. Although not readily appreciated, the flow against the conventional osmolality gradient is theoretically possible if a hyposmolar solution contains a greater number of impermeable solutes compared to a hyperosmolar one. In this setting the magnitude of the product of solute concentration and osmotic reflection coefficient would favor the osmotic flow in the direction of a hyposmolar solution, i.e. against the osmolality gradient [26] (Fig. 2b). Meschia and Setniker [27] were first to demonstrate this phenomenon in vitro when they observed water movement from a hyperosmolar solution containing urea (201 mOsm/kg) to a hyposmolar dextran solution (2.3 mOsm/kg) across a collodion membrane, permeable to urea but not to dextran. This phenomenon emphasizes that in the context of a solute-permeable membrane, the direction of osmotic flow cannot always be predicted on the basis of the commonly measured parameter of the total osmolality gradient.

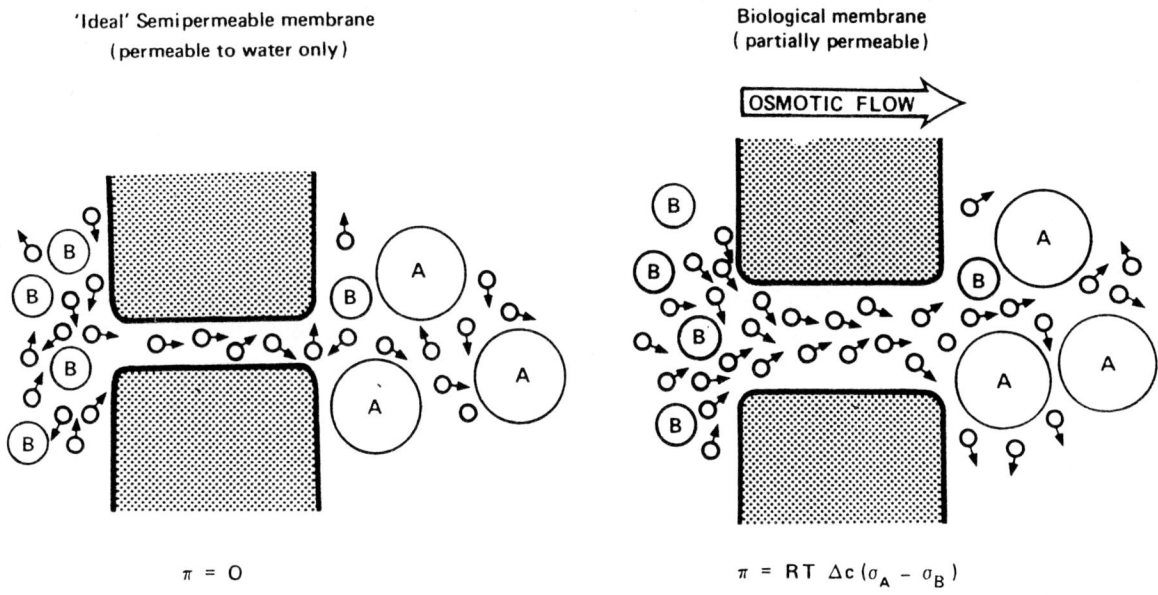

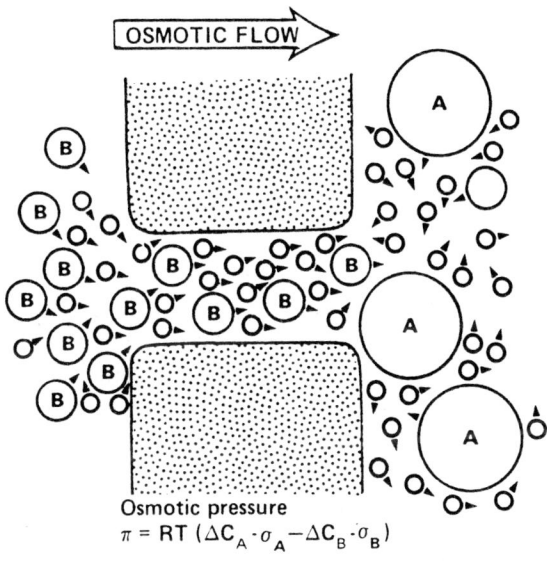

Figure 2. Osmotic flow between isosmolar solutions and from high to low osmolality across a partially permeable membrane. a) Diagrammatic representation of osmotic flow across an "ideal" semipermeable and partially permeable membrane separating isosmotic solutions. No flow occurs across an "ideal" semiphermeable membrane, but the flow proceeds from left to right across the solute-permeable membrane as the reflection coefficient for solute A (s_A) is larger than solute B (σ_B). b) Osmotic flow of water and permeant solute (B) from high to low osmolality as the sum of the products of solute concentration and reflection coefficient ($\sigma_a \Delta C_A$) of the latter solution is greater.

2.3. Clinical adaptation of osmosis in peritoneal dialysis

2.3.1. *Crystalloids*

The early studies in animals and humans demonstrated osmotic flow in the direction of the osmolality gradient across the peritoneal membrane, thus establishing its role as a semipermeable membrane [28–30]. Since the small molecular weight solutes (crystalloids) generated greater osmolality per unit mass, these agents were generally regarded as the most effective osmotic agents. Of the number of small molecular weights agents evaluated in animals, only glucose appeared promising [31]. Glucose-based dialysate became commercially available in 1959 and, in the 1960's, the widespread use of intermittent peritoneal dialysis in the management of patients with both acute and end-stage renal failure confirmed the long term safety of glucose [32]. Over the years glucose-based dialysate has proved to be effective and economical to produce; these unique characteristics have remained unrivaled to this day. The rapid transperitoneal absorption of glucose associated with decline in osmotic gradient was recognized early, but it was of little significance during short dwell (30–60 minutes) intermittent peritoneal dialysis. However, it was not until 1976 when Popovich and Moncrief [33] introduced the fundamental change in the practice of peritoneal dialysis with emphasis on long dwell (4–10 hours) equilibration peritoneal dialysis (i.e. CAPD) that the disadvantage of short duration ultrafiltration profile of glucose was appreciated.

With this new technique the need for regular assessment of volume profile assumed greater importance. The method used for assessing ultrafiltration volume depends to a large degree on the study objective. For routine clinical estimation a simple method of measuring the volume of solution drained from the peritoneal cavity is sufficient. However, its main disadvantages are related to incomplete drainage of the peritoneal cavity with variable residual volumes, inconvenience when sequential estimations are required throughout the dwell period and insensitivity of the direction of fluid movements when more than one competing pathways contribute to the net ultrafiltration. Thus, for physiological studies where more accurate estimation of intraperitoneal dialysate volume profile is required, the majority of investigators have used dilutional principles. The technique involves assessing changes in the dialysate concentration of high molecular weight marker molecules that are minimally absorbed from the peritoneal cavity. The change in volume of the dialysis fluid is calculated based on the change in concentration of the marker molecule. Marker molecules that have been studied include radioiodinated serum albumin (RISA; Mw 68,000; [34]), labelled dextran (Mw 70,000; [35]), "blue" dextran (Mw 2×10^6; [36]) and hemoglobin (Mw 68,000; [37]). Data from these studies indicate that at least 17–20% of the marker is absorbed within 8 hours, predominantly via the lymphatics, irrespective of their size. When corrected for peritoneal absorption, the accuracy of the method is similar for different marker molecules [38]. In human studies the autologous hemoglobin method has the advantage of being cheap, safe and readily available compared to other methods.

Based upon this approach Pyle *et al.* [39, 40] have shown that the dependence of dialysate volume (V) and the transperitoneal ultrafiltration rate on time could be described respectively by the following equations:

$$V(t) = a_1/a_2(\exp[a_2 t] - 1) + a_3 t + V_0 \qquad (8)$$

$$Q_v(t) = a_1 \exp[a_2 t] + a_3 \qquad (9)$$

where a_1, a_2 and a_3 are empirically determined constants and V_0 is the starting volume of dialysis solution.

Using autologous hemoglobin as a volume marker, intraperitoneal volume profiles were determined in 5 CAPD patients receiving 1.36% and 3.86% anhydrous glucose solutions [41]. These are shown graphically in Fig. 3a. With both solutions, the dialysate volumes increase rapidly immediately after the infusions and reach their peak at 120 minutes for 1.36% and 180 minutes for 3.86%. Thereafter, the volumes decrease in response to net intraperitoneal reabsorption. The ultrafiltration profiles, derived using the equations above, are shown in Fig. 3b. This shows that the ultrafiltration rate is maximal at the onset of dialysis and falls exponentially with increasing dwell time, corresponding to changes in dialysate osmolality gradient. On average, 1.36% anhydrous glucose solution induces a maximum ultrafiltration rate of 9.27 ml/min whilst the hypertonic 3.86% anhydrous glucose solution effects a rate of 21.0 ml/min. Since the mean decay constants for ultrafiltration profiles are similar, the higher initial ultrafiltration rate results in net positive ultrafiltration for a longer period. Increasing the dwell time beyond this period

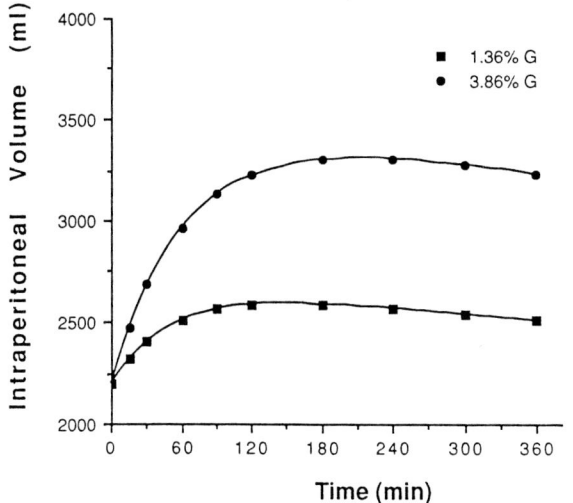

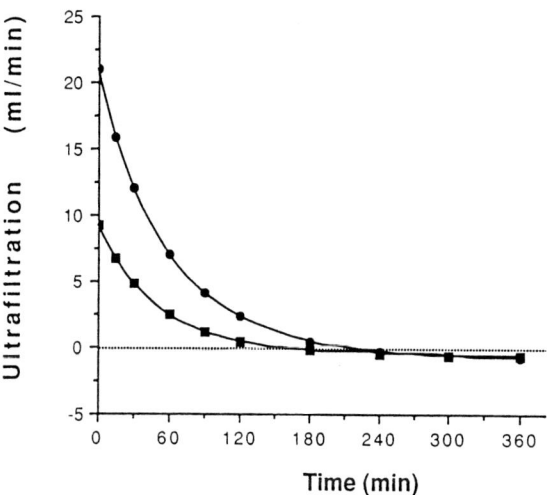

Figure 3. a) Mean intraperitoneal dialysate volume (corrected for the absorption of autologous hemoglobin volume marker) plotted as a function of time for 1.36% and 3.86% anhydrous glucose containing dialysis solutions. Adapted from reference 41. b) The ultrafiltration rate across the peritoneum (derived from the above volume profiles using method described by Pyle *et al.* [39, 40]) plotted as a function of time for 1.36% and 3.86% anhydrous glucose-containing dialysis solutions.

results in net intraperitoneal reabsorption. The mean reabsorption rates for 1.36% and 3.86% glucose solutions are −0.88 and −1.11 ml/mm, respectively [41].

The intraperitoneal reabsorption of dialysate during peritoneal dialysis is likely to be multifactorial and involves at least two different pathways: the lymphatics and transcapillary (venular) fluid absorption in response to Starling forces. The relative contribution of each pathway to overall fluid absorption remains unclear and therefore controversial. But of the two, the lymphatic drainage has received most attention. Using the albumin disappearance rate from the peritoneal cavity to estimate lymphatic absorption, Mactier *et al.* [42, 43] have inferred that lymphatic drainage accounts for nearly all the reabsorption of fluid from the peritoneal cavity. Their assumption is that fluid and albumin losses are coupled and occur through the same pathway. Flessner *et al.* [44] have demonstrated, however, that a significant portion of the apparent protein disappearance from the peritoneal cavity is due to protein equilibration with tissue spaces surrounding the peritoneal cavity and not readily exchangeable with plasma. The rate of this equilibration is of the same order of magnitude as the clearance of fluid from the peritoneal cavity to the blood capillaries, giving the impression of a large unselective bulk absorption of fluid and protein to blood via the lymphatics. However, the peritoneal lymphatic drainage of proteins (and fluid) that reaches the plasma under steady-state conditions represents only a small fraction (20–30%) of these disappearance rates as demonstrated both in CAPD patients [45] and in animal models [44]. As yet, there is no agreement whether the fractional plasma absorption rate or the peritoneal disappearance rate of tracer accurately reflects the true lymphatic flow, but the recent evidence suggests the latter probably represents an overestimation under non-steady state conditions [46].

In contrast, the mechanisms of transcapillary (venular) fluid absorption has received very little attention and its importance largely ignored. The work of Starling established that the movement of fluid across the capillary walls depends on the balance of transcapillary forces [29, 47]: capillary hydrostatic pressure forces fluid out of the capillaries whilst osmotic pressure of the plasma proteins (oncotic pressure) directs the fluid into the capillaries. In normal healthy individuals the balance of forces probably favor exudation of fluid into the peritoneal cavity and this excess fluid is absorbed via the diaphragmatic lymphatics (Fig. 4a). During intraperitoneal infusion of isotonic saline, however, the balance of forces alters in favor of a peritoneal to capillary absorption. This is due to the fact that introduction of an isomolar "crystalloid" solution into the peritoneal cavity causes a dilution of the ascitic protein, thus reducing the interstitial oncotic pressure, as well as increasing the peritoneal hydrostatic pressure. Overall, there is a net transperitoneal pressure gradient (7–14 mm Hg) in favor of capil-

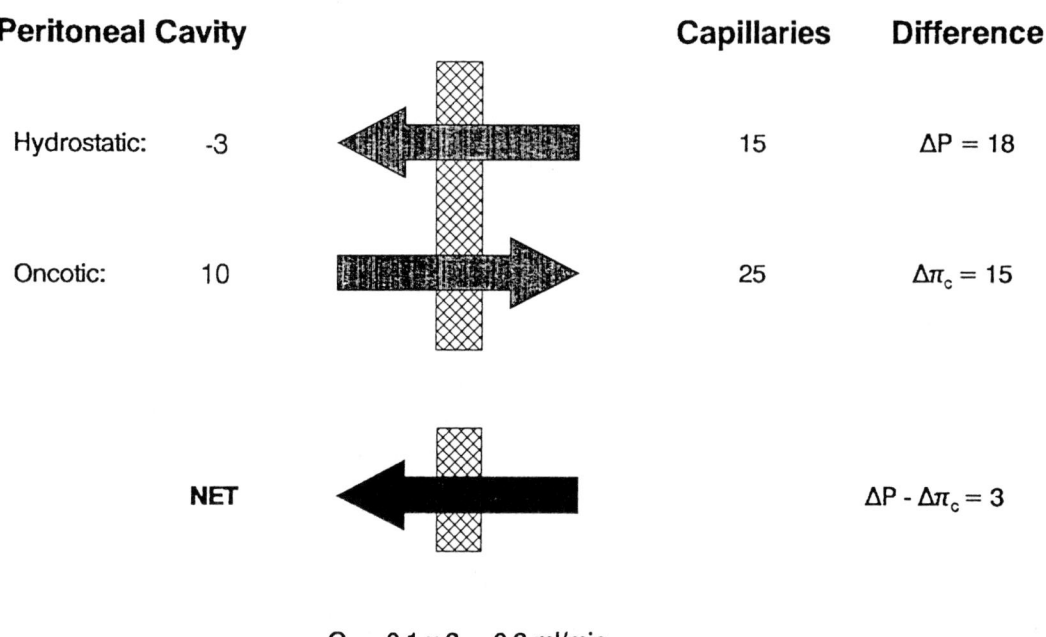

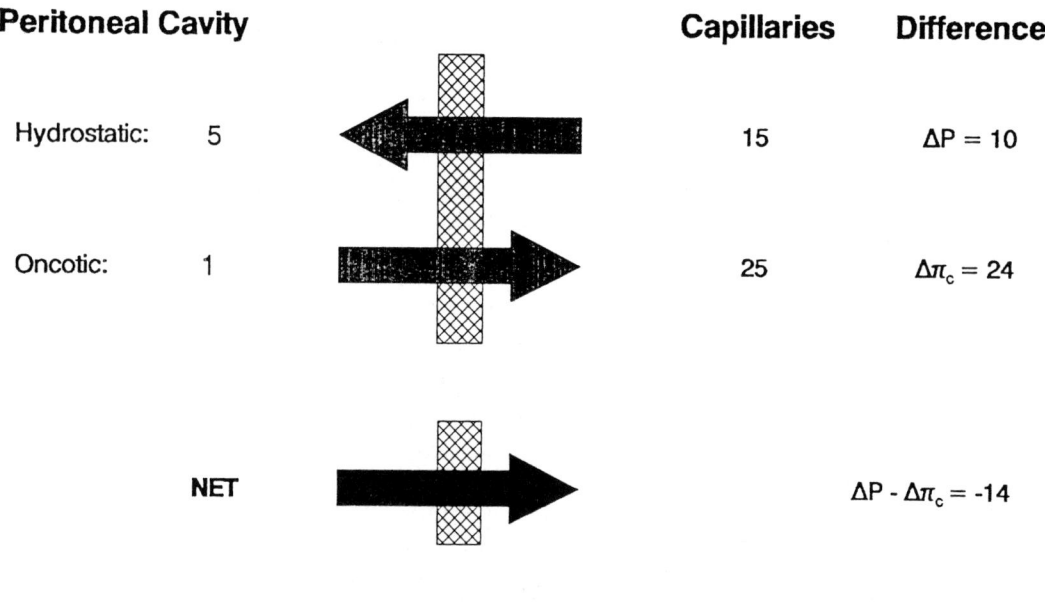

Figure 4. a) Assumed pressure (mmHg) changes across the peritoneal capillary walls. In normal healthy individuals, the net force is probably just in favor of exudation of fluid into the peritoneal cavity. b) Assumed changes in Starling forces after intraperitoneal infusion of approximately 2 liters of isotonic saline. This causes a slight elevation of the intraabdominal pressure and a fall in the intraabdominal oncotic pressure due to protein dilution. Net pressure changes favor transcapillary fluid absorption.

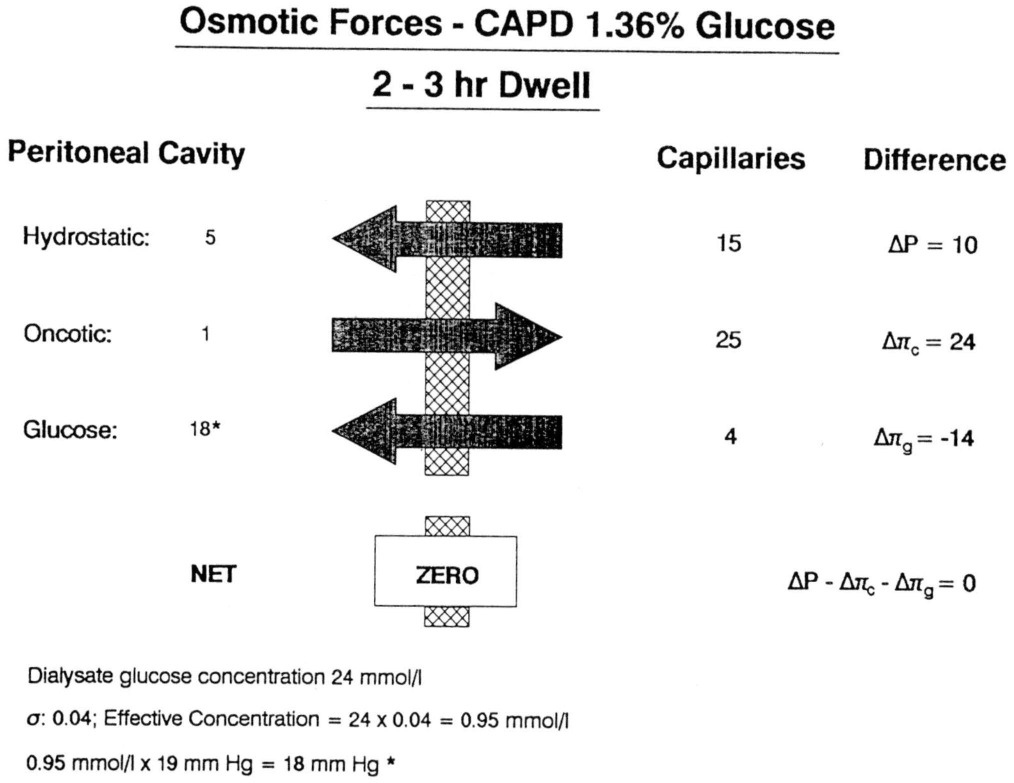

Osmotic Forces - CAPD 1.36% Glucose
2 - 3 hr Dwell

Peritoneal Cavity		Capillaries	Difference
Hydrostatic:	5	15	$\Delta P = 10$
Oncotic:	1	25	$\Delta \pi_c = 24$
Glucose:	18*	4	$\Delta \pi_g = -14$
NET	**ZERO**		$\Delta P - \Delta \pi_c - \Delta \pi_g = 0$

Dialysate glucose concentration 24 mmol/l

σ: 0.04; Effective Concentration = 24 x 0.04 = 0.95 mmol/l

0.95 mmol/l x 19 mm Hg = 18 mm Hg *

Figure 4. c) During peritoneal dialysis with glucose containing solution, the balance of transcapillary forces may occur when the dialysate is relatively hyperosmolar to plasma due to the low osmotic reflection coefficient of glucose.

lary absorption (Fig. 4b). Assuming the hydraulic conductivity of 0.1 ml/min/mmHg, a fluid absorption rate of 0.7–1.4 ml/min can be achieved. Thus, at least 70–90% absorption of isotonic (colloid free) solution from the peritoneal cavity to the blood (1.0–1.5 ml/min) could occur directly across the microvascular wall. In CAPD with conventional glucose solution, the low osmotic reflection coefficient of glucose compared to that of plasma proteins also means that the osmotic balance can occur when the dialysate glucose concentration is substantially higher than in plasma. Hence, transcapillary (venular) oncotic reabsorption may begin when the dialysate is relatively hyperosmolar to plasma (Fig. 4c). Mistry (unpublished observations) has investigated the relationship between the transperitoneal ultrafiltration rate and dialysate osmolality/glucose concentration during a 1.36% anhydrous glucose exchange. He reported that the net transperitoneal absorption occurs when dialysate is hyperosmolar (310 mOsm/kg) with glucose concentration approximately 24–30 mmol/l. Using the values reported by Rippe et al. [3–5, 45] for the capillary hydraulic conductivity (0.1 ml/min/mmHg) and osmotic reflection coefficient of glucose (0.02–0.043) the balance of Starling forces would be in favor of net transcapillary reabsorption as the dialysate glucose concentration falls below 24 mmol/l. It is likely that peritoneal reabsorption involves a number of pathways and to neglect the significance of capillary oncotic pressure on the basis of its low numerical value, would lead to an overestimation of the contribution from other mechanisms, particularly the lymphatic absorption.

In a search for an alternative osmotic agent to glucose, earlier attempts were directed at increasing the osmolality gradient to improve the ultrafiltration profile. Some argued that using agents with molecular weight lower than glucose, such as glycerol [48, 49] and amino acids [50, 51], would generate greater osmolality per unit mass and thereby provide more effective ultrafiltration. However, these agents were more rapidly absorbed, shifting the volume-time profile curve to the left of glucose, with net ultrafiltration of even shorter duration (Fig. 5). Even though the recognition that the peritoneum was not an "ideal" semipermeable membrane but a permeable one and the phenomenon of "colloid" osmosis could be adapted to peritoneal dialysis to generate ultrafiltration, the

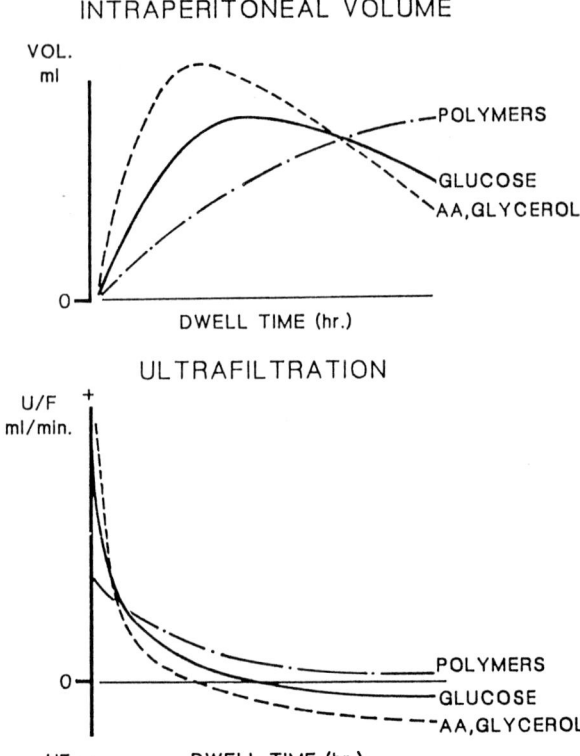

Figure 5. Representative intraperitoneal volume and instantaneous ultrafiltration profiles with osmotic agents of different molecular sizes.

progress in this field has been painstakingly slow due to lack of a suitable macromolecular agent.

2.3.2. Colloids

One of the earliest attempts to explore the potential of large molecular weight substance as an osmotic agent was by Jirka and Kokotvá [52]. They used isosmotic dialysate containing 6% dextran (Mw 70,000) over a 90 minute dwell and demonstrated that while the solution was effective in preventing reabsorption of intraperitoneal fluid in their dog model, it did not produce significant ultrafiltration. Subsequently, Gjessing [53] reported similar findings in 12 IPD patients using an identical solution. Twardowski et al. [54], in an attempt to emulate the physiological characteristics of albumin, sought to optimise ultrafiltration associated with macromolecules by using charged molecules. They demonstrated that both polyanionic and cationic polymers were highly effective in *in vitro* studies but universally toxic to the peritoneum in animal studies [55]. These studies clearly defined the problems associated with the use of non-phys-iological macromolecules, and emphasized the need for a highly soluble, non-allergenic, neutral substance that is readily metabolised.

Using a large molecular weight glucose polymer (Mw 16,000; Mn 5,000), isolated by fractionation of hydrolysed corn starch, with chain length ranging from 4 to >300 units in 5% isosmolar solution, Mistry *et al.* [56] demonstrated sustained ultrafiltration for up to 12 hours in 5 uremic patients. The ultrafiltration kinetics studies show that, in contrast to glucose solution, glucose polymer produced low but sustained ultrafiltration throughout the dwell period resulting in a net intraperitoneal volume significantly greater than 1.36% anhydrous glucose solution [41]. Substantially lower transperitoneal absorption of glucose polymer, indicative of a high osmotic reflection coefficient at the peritoneum, and ultrafiltration rates closely related to the molar concentration of glucose polymer rather than its total osmolality suggest features consistent with "colloid" osmosis. Furthermore, using a larger glucose polymer fraction (Mw 22,000; Mn 7,000), the hypothesis that the osmotic flow could be directed against the conventional osmolality gradient was also tested for the first time in peritoneal dialysis. In 11 uremic patients, hyposmolar dialysis solutions containing 5% (272 ± 1.1 mOsm/kg) and 7.5% (277 ± 2.0 mOsmol/kg) glucose polymer produced net ultrafiltration of 243 ± 53 and 526 ± 59 ml that were significantly greater than −48 ± 96 and 223 ± 84 ml associated with 1.36% and 2.27% anhydrous glucose solutions, respectively, over a 12 hour exchange [57]. This demonstration of osmotic flow with a hyposmolar solution, not only confirms the concept of colloid osmosis, but also provides a potential for addition of a small molecular weight substance (crystalloid) to the solution in a proportion that would raise the osmolality to an isosmolar level whilst maximizing ultrafiltration. In this combination, the small molecular weight agent would initiate the rapid ultrafiltration in the early phase of dialysis with the "colloid" agent maintaining a low but sustained level of ultrafiltration throughout the exchange. The summation of these profiles is likely to generate ultrafiltration greater than either agent alone (Fig. 6).

2.3.3. *A combination of cyrstalloid and colloid osmotic agents*

This hypothesis was investigated in 7 uremic patients by comparing the ultrafiltration performances of hyposmolar 7.5% glucose polymer solution

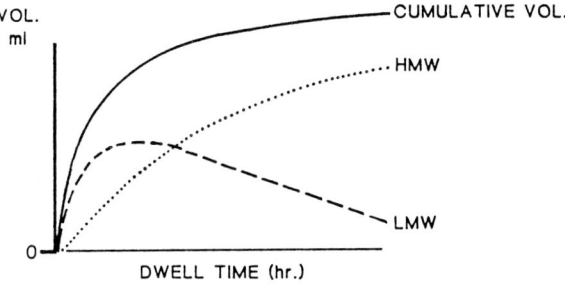

Figure 6. Diagrammatic representation of intraperitoneal volume patterns with an isosmolar combination of high molecular weight (HMW; "colloid") and low molecular weight (LMW; "crystalloid") osmotic agents.

and an isosmolar combination containing 7.5% glucose polymer + 0.35% anhydrous glucose over a 12 hour exchange. The latter solution achieved ultrafiltration 29% greater than the 7.5% solution alone, confirming the superiority of "bimodal" isosmolar formulation [57, 58]. It follows, therefore, that the relative proportion of the two agents could be adjusted with isosmolar limits to achieve a range of ultrafiltration optimised for dwell time, that is, a high small to large molecular weight ratio for short dwell exchanges whilst the converse would be true for long dwell exchanges. In addition, it also provides a further scope for a combination of unrelated but compatible agents (i.e. glucose polymer + amino acids) each with their own metabolic advantages, which would offer a wider spectrum of metabolic correction than a single agent alone.

2.3.4. *Where are we going?*
Over the years we have traditionally relied on crystalloid osmotic forces to provide ultrafiltration in peritoneal dialysis. This requires the use of hypertonic solutions, preparations that have proved to be most effective during short dwell dialysis. However, the introduction of long dwell CAPD has dramatically changed the practice of peritoneal dialysis and the development of osmotic agents has lagged behind. This change in dialysis technique has highlighted some of the disadvantages of continuous use of unphysiological solutions. In an attempt to seek for more physiological solutions adapted for long dwell dialysis, the concept of isosmolar combinations of "crystalloid" and "colloid" osmotic agents looks promising. This has the potential advantage of maintaining the osmolality within the physiological range (isosmolar) while providing a wide range of ultrafiltration (optimised for dwell time) as well as a comprehensive range of metabolic correction.

3. Convective solute transport across the peritoneum

In 1966 Henderson [59] first reported that solute removal during peritoneal dialysis was enhanced when using hypertonic dialysis solutions. Several mechanisms have been proposed to account for these increases in transperitoneal solute transport [59–61]. First, transperitoneal ultrafiltration may directly entrain solute in the solvent stream, transporting the solute by solvent-drag or convection [59]. Second, transperitoneal ultrafiltration may simply dilute the dialysis solution in the peritoneal cavity, resulting in an increased transperitoneal solute concentration gradient and therefore increased diffusive solute transport [59]. Third, hypertonic dialysis fluid may irritate peritoneal tissues and cells, resulting in enhanced diffusive permeability of the peritoneal membrane [60]. Last, hypertonic dialysis solution may increase transperitoneal solute transport since the absorbed glucose can expand extracellular volume and presumably enhance splanchnic blood flow [61]. The present discussion will concentrate primarily on the first mechanism although each may be discussed, where appropriate, below.

In order to define governing transport mechanisms, methods are necessary to differentiate between convective and diffusive transperitoneal solute transport. Simple partitioning of overall solute transport into diffusive and convective components is imprecise and therefore controversial [7]. A more useful approach has been to determine separate properties of the peritoneal membrane that govern diffusive and convective solute transport. The property, or parameter, most commonly employed to characterize peritoneal diffusive solute transport is the permeability-area product (PA). This parameter is also called the mass transfer-area coefficient and defines the rate of transperitoneal solute transport in response to a solute concentration difference between blood and dialysis solution within the peritoneal cavity. This property of the peritoneal membrane is described in detail elsewhere in this book.

Two different parameters have been previously employed to characterize convective solute transport during peritoneal dialysis: the sieving coefficient (S) and the solute (or solvent-drag) reflection coefficient (σ_f). To clarify the difference between these two parameters, consider an in vitro system where ultrafiltration occurs across an ideal homogeneous membrane at a rate Q_v and no unstirred layers exist on either side of the membrane (Fig. 7). The sieving coefficient is defined as the concentration in the ultrafiltrate (C_{uf}) divided by that in the retentate (C_r) and must be between 0 and 1. For example, the sieving coefficient will have a value of 0 when solute is completely rejected by the membrane and will have a value of 1 when the solute is not rejected at all by the membrane. The sieving coefficient is not, however, an intrinsic property of the membrane since it depends on the transmembrane ultrafiltration rate by the relationship first described for a simple homogeneous membrane by Patlak *et al.* [62, 63]

$$S = (1 - \sigma_f) / (1 - \sigma_f \exp[-\beta]) \qquad (10)$$

where β is the membrane Peclet number defined by

$$\beta = Q_v(1 - \sigma_f) / PA. \qquad (11)$$

Thus, the dependence of S on the transmembrane ultrafiltration rate is determined by the values of PA and σ_f for the membrane.

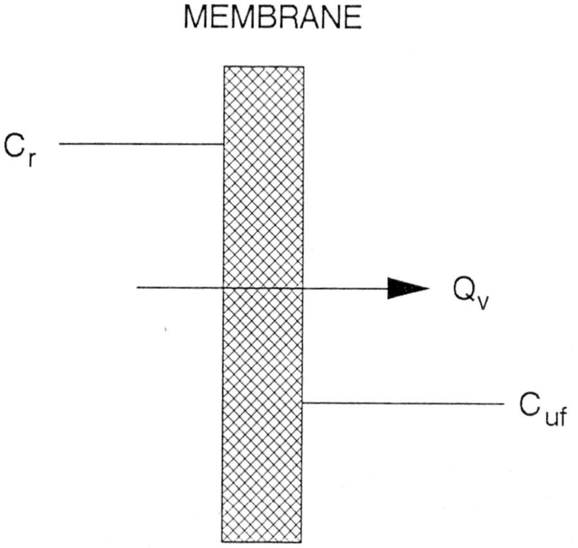

Figure 7. Definition of the sieving coefficient across a membrane. The sieving coefficient is experimentally determined as the ratio of the concentration in the ultrafiltrate (C_{uf}) to that in the retentate (C_r).

An important limiting case of this relationship occurs at high ultrafiltration rates, that is, when the ultrafiltration rate significantly exceeds the diffusive permeability-area product for the membrane. In this case the sieving coefficient can be approximated as

$$S \approx 1 - \sigma_f. \qquad (12)$$

Thus, at high transmembrane ultrafiltration rates the sieving coefficient across a simple homogeneous membrane is approximately equal to one minus the solute reflection coefficient for that membrane. At lower transmembrane ultrafiltration rates, diffusive solute transport is significant and the sieving coefficient is grater than one minus the solute reflection coefficient.

Before proceeding further, it must be emphasized that the above analogy does not apply directly to clinical peritoneal dialysis for at least two reasons. First, the peritoneum is not a simple homogeneous membrane. Second, transperitoneal ultrafiltration and convective solute transport do not occur under the conditions described above. During peritoneal dialysis, the peritoneum is bathing in dialysis solution where the solute concentration is not determined simply by the ultrafiltered solution across the peritoneal membrane. Nonetheless, conditions across the peritoneal membrane can be experimentally manipulated to approximate these conditions and thus permit the determination of the peritoneal membrane sieving coefficient.

3.1. Peritoneal membrane sieving coefficients

Henderson [59] and others [60, 64–66] have determined sieving coefficients for the human peritoneal membrane during hypertonic exchanges using both 7% and 4.25% hydrous glucose-containing dialysis solution. The solutes of interest were added to the infused hypertonic dialysis solution at a concentration equal to those in plasma water to inhibit diffusive solute transport during the exchange. The sieving coefficient was calculated as the ratio of the test solute concentration in the transperitoneal ultrafiltrate to that in plasma water. Previously published values determined for the human peritoneal membrane are shown in Table 1. Sieving coefficients for selected solutes have also been more recently determined in the rat [67, 68]; these values are also shown in Table 1. Measured sieving coefficients generally range between 0.3 and 0.8 and do not depend appreciably on molecular size over the range from urea (Mw of 60) to inulin (approximate Mw of 5000). Note that sieving coefficients for the cations, sodium and potassium, are consistently low.

Based on the above discussion, the sieving coefficient is not expected to be a parameter intrinsic to the peritoneal membrane but is likely a function of the transperitoneal ultrafiltration rate, the peritoneal membrane solute reflection coefficient and the diffusive permeability-area product for the peritoneal membrane. Thus, one cannot completely neglect solute diffusion during these experiments except when the solute reflection coefficient for the peritoneal membrane is identically zero. When the solute reflection coefficient is nonzero, solute is rejected by the peritoneal membrane and a concentration difference will be created by the ultrafiltration process and transperitoneal solute diffusion will occur. An approximate mathematical equation has been derived [69] to illustrate this dependence of the peritoneal membrane sieving coefficient on the transperitoneal ultrafiltration rate and on peritoneal membrane transport properties; however, previously reported sieving coefficients were relatively independent of the transperitoneal ultrafiltration rate [66]. Nonetheless, these measurements of the peritoneal membrane sieving coefficient demonstrate that significant solute rejection occurs during transperitoneal ultrafiltration.

Peritoneal membrane sieving coefficients reported in the above studies were determined when transperitoneal ultrafiltration was induced osmotically using hypertonic dialysis solution. Experiments have also been performed in animals where transperitoneal ultrafiltration was determined predominantly by a hydrostatic pressure driving force (Table 2). Aune [70] determined the sieving coefficient for albumin in the rabbit by collecting naturally-occurring peritoneal ultrafiltrate. He used three different methods for collecting the ultrafiltrate and found similar results using each method. The average transperitoneal ultrafiltration rate was reported as 0.13 ml/min and the albumin sieving coefficient averaged 0.50 in 10 rabbits. Bell et al. [71] determined peritoneal membrane sieving coefficients for creatinine, p-aminohippurate (PAH) and polydispersed neutral dextrans (molecular radii from 13 to 50 Å) in evicerated rabbits by applying a negative hydrostatic pressure within the peritoneal cavity. The transperitoneal ultrafiltration rate in these studies was approximately 0.1 ml/min and selected sieving coefficients are shown in Table 2. Note that sieving coefficients determined during hydraulically-induced transperitoneal ultrafiltration in this model are less than one and do not depend significantly on molecular size. Although it appears conceptually inconsistent for macromolecule sieving coefficients to be both less than one and independent of molecular size, previous studies of transperitoneal protein transport in patients with ascites [72, 73] have demonstrated that ascitic fluid to plasma concentration ratios (i.e. peritoneal membrane sieving coefficients) for albumin (mole-

Table 1. Peritoneal membrane sieving coefficients determined during a hypertonic exchange.

	Species	
Solute	Human [59, 60, 64–66]	Rat [67, 68]
Urea	0.89 ± 0.08 (6) 0.81 ± 0.06 (3) 0.63 ± 0.21 (10)	0.64 ± 0.34 (8)
Creatinine	0.57 ± 0.28 (8)	
Sodium	0.54 ± 0.18 (26) 0.56 ± 0.16 (14)	0.52 ± 0.12 (10) 0.65 ± 0.12 (8)
Potassium	0.36 ± 0.16 (10) 0.40 ± 0.12 (11)	0.45 ± 0.20 (10) 0.27 ± 0.15 (8)
Chloride	0.78 ± 0.21 (26)	
Inulin	0.83 ± 0.13 (7) 0.41 ± 0.18 (6)	

(Mean Values ± SD are shown with the number of observations shown in parentheses).

Table 2. Peritoneal membrane sieving coefficients determined by altering the hydrostatic pressure across the peritoneal membrane.

	Species	
Solute	Rabbit [70, 71]	Rat [76]
Creatinine	0.72 ± 0.11 (13)	
p-aminohippurate (PAH)	0.67 ± 0.18 (13)	
Sodium		0.72 ± 0.10 (6)
Chloride		0.77 ± 0.17 (6)
neutral dextran (15 Å)	0.48 ± 0.10 (13)	
neutral dextran (40 Å)	0.41 ± 0.13 (13)	
albumin	0.50 ± 0.05 (10)	

(Mean Values ± SD are shown with the number of observations shown in parentheses).

cular radius of 36 Å) and immunoglobulin G (molecular radius of 52 Å) were approximately 0.3 and independent of molecular size. Similar observations in the rabbit and in the patient with ascites suggest, therefore, that macromolecule sieving coefficients less than one and independent of molecular size are not artifactual. Further studies to explain these paradoxical observations are necessary [74, 75].

Recently, Chen et al. [76] have determined peritoneal membrane sieving coefficients for sodium and chloride in a rat model using serum as dialysis solution. Transperitoneal ultrafiltration during these experiments was likely driven by differences in hydrostatic pressure since the solution on both sides of the peritoneal membrane were initially identical. Sieving coefficients for sodium and chloride averaged 0.72 and 0.77, respectively, and were significantly less than one (Table 2).

Therefore, peritoneal membrane sieving coefficients determined during hydraulically-induced transperitoneal ultrafiltration are not different from those previously determined during osmotically-induced transperitoneal ultrafiltration. Sieving coefficients are less than one and do not depend significantly on molecular size. Thus, measured sieving coefficients demonstrate that the peritoneal membrane provides a significant resistance to convective solute transport during peritoneal dialysis.

3.2. Peritoneal membrane solute reflection coefficients

3.2.1. Theoretical concerns

To directly evaluate the solute reflection coefficient for the peritoneal membrane, mathematical models must be employed to determine the separate convective and diffusive solute transport properties of the peritoneal membrane. Since this approach is mathematically complex, only a general outline of the procedure will be described. Two different aspects of this procedure are important to evaluate individually: 1) the validity of the mathematical model and 2) the accuracy of the parameter estimation procedure. The former refers to whether the proposed mathematical model of peritoneal fluid and solute transport accurately describes the time dependence of blood and dialysate solute concentrations during the study dwell. The latter refers to whether the solute transport properties of the peritoneal membrane estimated using this procedure are reliable estimates of the true values.

Several different mathematical models have been proposed previously to describe fluid and solute transport during peritoneal dialysis; the differences are most apparent in the equation used to describe solute transport across the peritoneal membrane. Babb et al. [77] and Randerson and Farrell [78] proposed an expression for the solute transport rate across the peritoneal membrane (Q_s) that assumes that overall transport is simply the sum of diffusive and convective components, that is,

$$Q_s = PA(C_b - C_d) + (1 - \sigma_f)Q_v C_i \quad (13)$$

where the subscript i is equal to either b or d depending on the direction of transperitoneal ultrafiltration. When Q_v is in the blood-to-dialysate direction, the subscript is b and when Q_v is in the dialysate-to-blood direction, the subscript is d. Note that the convective solute transport parameter used in the above equation has been previously called either the transmittance coefficient [77] or the sieving coefficient [78]. It should be emphasized, however, that this parameter, when employed in equation (13), is not equal to the peritoneal membrane sieving coefficient as defined above. Because this convective solute transport parameter is an intrinsic property of the peritoneal membrane, it would be more appropriate to define it as one minus the solute reflection coefficient, not the sieving coefficient.

The expression first proposed by Patlak et al. [62] is considered the most rigorous for solute transport across a simple homogeneous membrane and has been employed by Pyle et al. [39, 40] and others [79–81]

$$Q_s = Q_v(1 - \sigma_f)\frac{C_b - C_d \exp[-\beta]}{1 - \exp[-\beta]} \quad (14)$$

where β is defined in equation (11). More recently, Waniewski et al. [81] considered an additional expression, defined as

$$Q_s = PA(C_b - C_d) + (1 - \sigma_f)Q_v[(1 - F)C_b + FC_d] \quad (15)$$

where F is an additional parameter. The relationship between equation (15) and equations (13) and (14) is as follows. Equation (15) is equal to equation (14) if F is assumed as

$$F = 1/\beta - 1/(\exp[-\beta] - 1) \quad (16)$$

Equation (15) is equal to equation (13) if F is equal to either 0 or 1. The above expressions describing solute transport across the peritoneal membrane are then combined with appropriate fluid and solute mass balance relationships to describe the time dependence of the blood and dialysate solute concentrations during the study dwell. Work by Waniewski et al. [81] has demonstrated that all of the above transport equations equally simulate the time dependence of blood and dialysate solute concentrations during peritoneal dialysis using hypertonic dialysis solution. This implies that the expression best describing solute transport across the peritoneal membrane cannot be determined by comparison with the experimental data but must be chosen largely from theoretical considerations.

Use of a mathematical model that accurately simulates the experimental data does not guarantee that the estimated model parameters are reliable however. To further understand these concerns the essential steps involved in the parameter estimation procedure will be briefly reviewed. More details of this estimation procedure can be found in the original literature [39, 40, 79–81]. The proposed mathematical model can predict the time dependence of the blood and dialysate concentrations for any combination of the parameters PA and σ_f. The parameter estimation procedure chooses the optimal parameter combination that "best" fits the experimental blood and dialysate concentrations to predictions of the mathematical model. The criteria for "best" is not unique [82]; however, the most frequent approach is to find the parameter combination that minimizes the squared differences between the time dependence of the dialysate concentration (or the dialysate-to-blood concentration ratio) determined experimentally with that predicted by the mathematical model. This is the same criteria used to compute the "best" straight line through empirical data by linear least squares or linear regression [83]. In the present case, however, the mathematical model depends nonlinearly on the model parameters and the parameter estimation procedure is called nonlinear least squares, nonlinear estimation or nonlinear regression [83].

A major difficulty with using nonlinear regression, unlike linear regression, is that the algorithms employed do not necessarily locate the parameter combination that locates the "best" fit. Several different approaches have been previously formulated [83, 84]; none is ideal. These algorithms start with an initial guess of the parameters and search various parameter combinations until they have found that combination which minimizes the difference between experiment data and that predicted by the mathematical model. These algorithms can be problematic however. Specific algorithms may predict parameter combinations that depend on the search procedure and the initial guess of the parameter values. Waniewski et al. [81] have recently shown how estimation of the solute reflection coefficient for the peritoneal membrane can be performed as a linear regression problem instead of a nonlinear one. This approach is clever and may prove useful because it eliminates a number of concerns when using nonlinear regression. In order to formulate a linear problem, however, these investigators introduced an additional, yet unknown, parameter (F defined in equation (15) above) into the model. Although this approach is simpler than using nonlinear regression, it suffers from the need to choose an optimal value for F.

An essential requirement for using nonlinear regression is that the experimentally measured variables (i.e. dialysate solute concentrations) must be dependent on the parameters to be estimated (i.e. PA and σ). This concern was addressed by Leypoldt [69] in a theoretical study of optimal experimental conditions for estimating both the diffusive and convective solute transport properties of the peritoneal membrane. Leypoldt simulated the time dependence of the dialysate solute concentration (assuming a constant blood concentration) under conditions that have previously been employed to estimate the solute reflection coefficient for the peritoneal membrane. Bidirectional fluid and solute transport was assumed to occur between blood and dialysis solution within the peritoneal cavity across the peritoneum modeled as a membrane using equation (14). Transperitoneal ultrafiltration was assumed to be dependent on time as defined empirically by Pyle [39, 40] (equations (8) and (9)). Figure 8 shows the dialysate concentration normalized by the blood concentration plotted versus dwell time during an exchange using 1.5% hydrous glucose-containing dialysis solution for several values of PA. The dashed lines show the predicted time dependence of the dialysate concentration when the solute reflection coefficient is 0 and the solid lines show the corresponding result when the solute reflection coefficient is 1. During an exchange using 1.5% hydrous glucose-containing dialysis solution, when relatively little transperitoneal ultrafiltration occurs, the time dependence of the dialysate concentration depends almost exclusively on the value of PA and not on the value of the solute reflection coefficient. If the time dependence of the dialysate solute concentration is not significantly altered when the

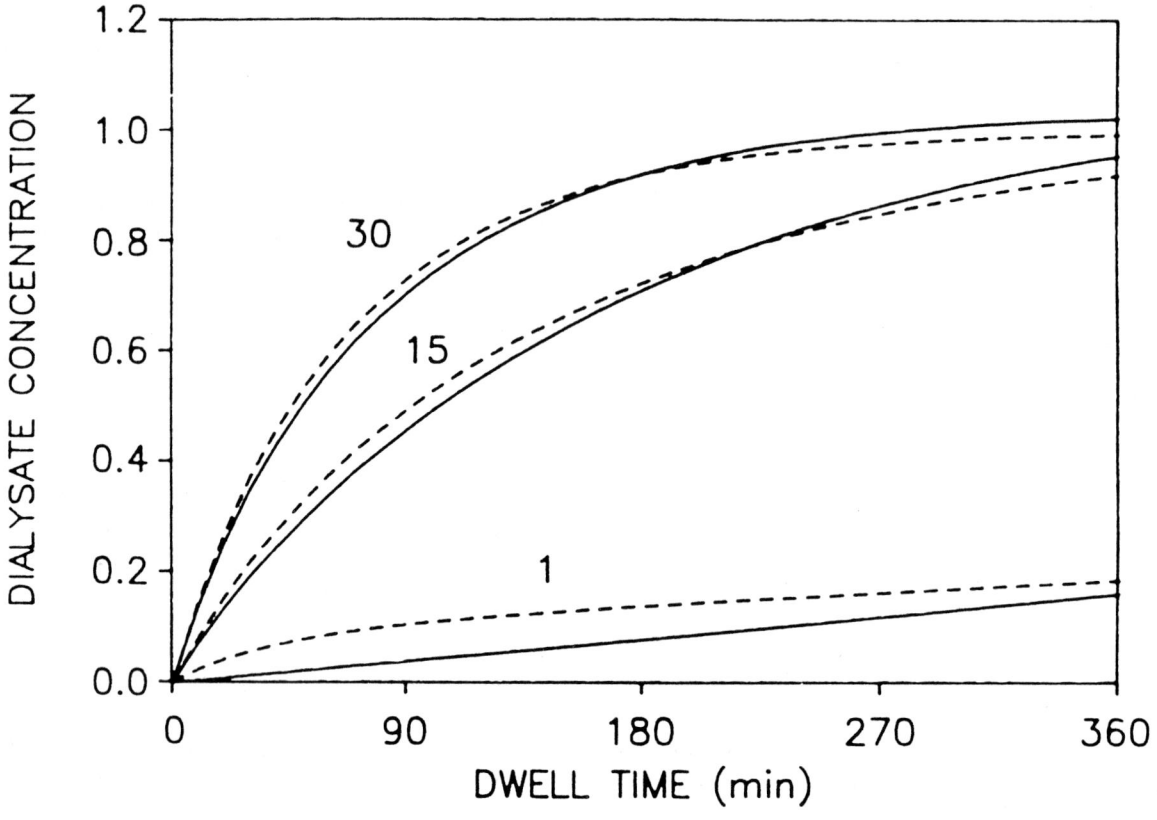

Figure 8. The dependence of the normalized dialysate concentration (i.e. the dialysate-to-plasma concentration ratio) on time when using 1.5% hydrous glucose-containing dialysis solution. Solute transport is in the blood-to-dialysate direction, and the initial dialysate concentration is assumed as zero. Two predictions are shown for each labeled value of PA, that with a solute reflection coefficient of zero (dashed line) and that with a solute reflection coefficient of one (solid line). Reprinted from reference [69] with permission.

solute reflection coefficient is varied between 0 and 1 (i.e. the expected physiologic range), then it is unreasonable to expect that comparing this experimentally determined variable with predictions from the mathematical model can result in meaningful estimates of the convective solute transport properties of the peritoneal membrane. Therefore, solute reflection coefficients determined during exchanges without significant transperitoneal ultrafiltration will not be reliable.

Figure 9 shows results when using 4.25% hydrous glucose-containing dialysis solution under otherwise same conditions as the previous figure. Use of 4.25% hydrous glucose-containing dialysis solution induces significant transperitoneal ultrafiltration, and the time dependence of the dialysate solute concentration depends significantly on the values of both PA and σ. When the solute reflection coefficient is 0, there is significant convective solute transport and the dialysate concentration is higher than when the solute reflection coefficient is 1. These calculated results contrast with those shown in the previous figure and indicate that it is possible to determine the solute reflection coefficient for the peritoneal membrane when there is significant transperitoneal ultrafiltration.

The preceding examples considered only solute transport occurring in the blood-to-dialysate direction. An additional important case is when solute transport is in the dialysate-to-blood direction since these conditions apply to solutes used as osmotic agents during peritoneal dialysis. Figure 10 shows the dialysate solute concentration normalized by its value at time zero plotted as a function of time during an exchange with a 4.25% hydrous glucose-containing dialysis solution for the same conditions as in the previous figure. The differences in the simulated dialysate concentrations when assuming the solute reflection coefficient equal to either 0 and 1 are considered small, and it seems unlikely that such data can be used to determine reliable values of the solute reflection coefficient.

Other studies have also indicated that solute reflection coefficients determined when peritoneal

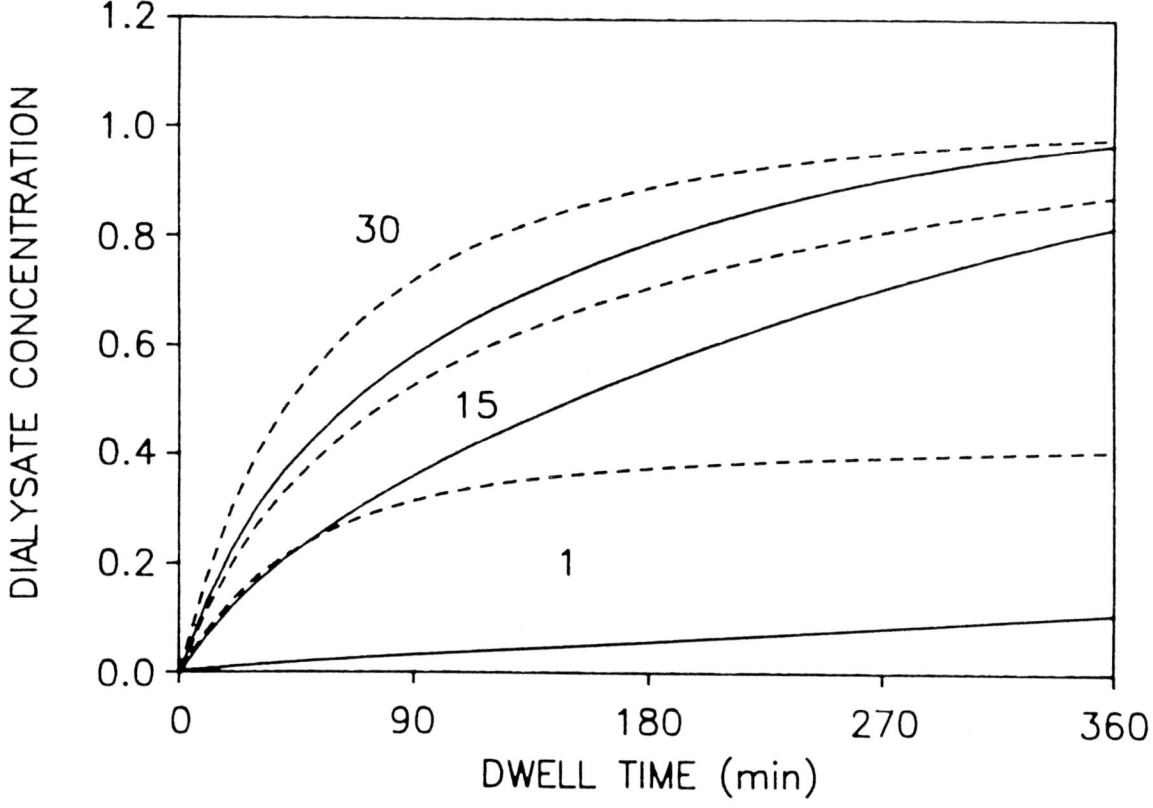

Figure 9. The dependence of the normalized dialysate concentration (i.e. the dialysate-to-plasma concentration ratio) on time when using 4.25% hydrous glucose-containing dialysis solution. Solute transport is in the blood-to-dialysate direction, and the initial dialysate concentration is assumed as zero. Two predictions are shown for each labeled value of PA, that with a solute reflection coefficient of zero (dashed line) and that with a solute reflection coefficient of one (solid line). Reprinted from reference [69] with permission.

solute transport was in the dialysate-to-blood direction may not be very reliable. In 1972, for example, Babb *et al.* [77] estimated mass transfer-area coefficients (or PA values) for the human peritoneum assuming the solute reflection coefficient was equal to either 0 or 1. When solute transport was in the blood-to-dialysate direction, the estimated PA value depended significantly on the assumed value of the solute reflection coefficient; the difference was greater the larger the solute molecular weight. When solute transport was in the dialysate-to-blood direction, however, the estimated PA value was virtually independent of the assumed value of the solute reflection coefficient. This result demonstrates that any value of the solute reflection coefficient between 0 and 1 can equally fit the decrease in the dialysate concentration when solute transport across the peritoneal membrane is in the dialysate-to-blood direction. Furthermore, Nakanishi *et al.* [85] have reported that the solute reflection coefficient for glucose could not be calculated from experiments in peritoneal dialysis patients since the dialysate glucose concentration was much larger than that in plasma. The amount of glucose transferred in the blood-to-dialysate direction by convection was considered too small to measure in the presence of the large amount transferred in the dialysate-to-blood direction by diffusion.

The more recent study by Leypoldt [86] has confirmed and extended the above conclusions by testing the accuracy of solute reflection coefficients estimated from computer experiments. In this study the time dependence of the dialysate concentration was simulated for a 4 hour dwell using a peritoneal membrane model with assumed (or true) vales of PA and σ_f. Values of PA and σ_f were then estimated using nonlinear regression from the simulated data after adding random errors to the dialysate concentrations. When solute transport was in the blood-to-dialysate direction during an isotonic exchange and when solute transport was in the dialysate-to-blood direction during a hypertonic exchange, the estimates of σ_f were shown to be unbiased but highly variable. Such results demonstrate that these con-

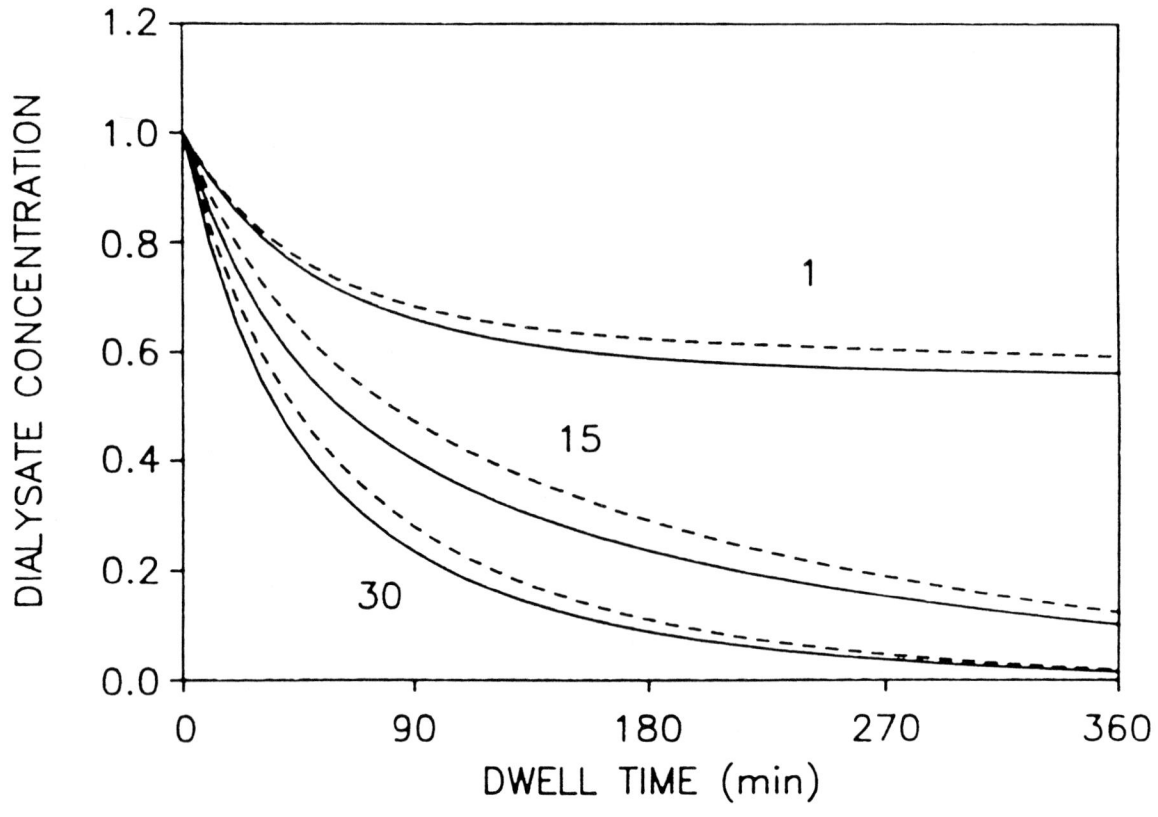

Figure 10. The dependence of the normalized dialysate concentration (i.e. the dialysate concentration divided by its initial value) on time when using 4.25% hydrous glucose-containing dialysis solution. Solute transport is in the dialysate-to-blood direction, and the blood concentration is assumed as zero. Two predictions are shown for each labeled value of PA, that with a solute reflection coefficient of zero (dashed line) and that with a solute reflection coefficient of one (solid line). Reprinted from reference [69] with permission.

ditions are not appropriate for calculating reliable estimates of the solute reflection coefficient for the peritoneal membrane, a conclusion consistent with those from previous studies [69, 77, 85].

When solute transport was simulated in the blood-to-dialysate direction during a hypertonic exchange, however, the estimates of PA and σ_f were shown to be biased for solutes that diffuse rapidly across the peritoneum. Under these conditions the estimates of PA and σ_f were highly correlated such that different parameter combinations could equally simulate the same time dependence of the dialysate concentration. Figure 11 illustrates this difficulty by showing simulated dialysate-to-blood concentration ratios plotted versus dwell time during a hypertonic exchange for 3 different combinations of the parameters PA and σ_f. Experimental discrimination between these 3 parameter combinations would be extremely difficult. It should be noted that an inability to reliably estimate kinetic parameters from experimental data is not unique to models employed in these studies but occurs commonly in biological systems fitted to multiexponential or multicompartmental models [87, 88].

In summary, mathematical models of peritoneal fluid and solute transport can accurately predict the time dependence of the dialysate concentration during exchanges with isotonic and hypertonic dialysis solution. The diffusive permeability-area product and the solute reflection coefficient for the peritoneal membrane can be estimated by comparing predictions of mathematical models for peritoneal transport with the experimental data. These estimates should be interpreted cautiously however. Estimates of the solute reflection coefficient determined during an isotonic exchange and during a hypertonic exchange when solute transport is in the dialysate-to-blood direction are likely unreliable.

3.2.2. *Experimental summary*

Experimentally determined solute reflection coefficients for the peritoneal membrane are summarized in Tables 3 and 4 when solute transport was in the dialysate-to-blood direction and the

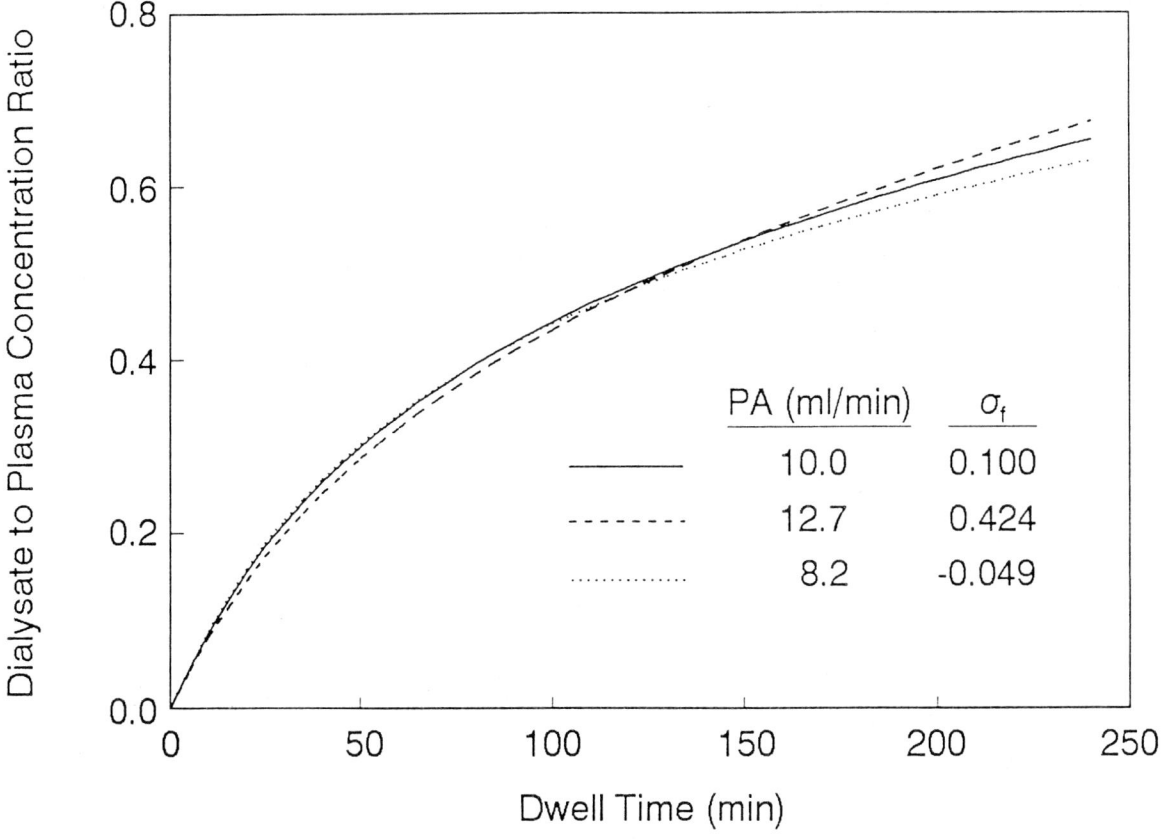

Figure 11. The dependence of the normalized dialysate concentration (i.e. the dialysate-to-plasma concentration ratio) on time when using 4.25% hydrous glucose-containing dialysis solution for the indicated values of PA and σ. Solute transport is in the blood-to dialysate direction. Adapted from reference [86] with the permission of Karger AG.

blood-to-dialysate direction, respectively. Values are expressed as $1 - \sigma_f$ for easy comparison with sieving coefficients listed in Tables 1 and 2 (see equation (12)). Solute reflection coefficients determined when solute transport was in the dialysate-to-blood direction are scattered; some are outside the physiologic range, that is, between 0 and 1. For example, glucose, the most common osmotic agent, has been frequently studied. Values of $1 - \sigma_f$ range between −0.56 and 0.54. Based on the concerns expressed above regarding this approach for estimating peritoneal membrane solute reflection coefficients, such results are not unexpected.

Solute reflection coefficients determined when solute transport was in the blood-to-dialysate direction (Table 4) are comparatively more consistent, but still somewhat variable. For example, $1 - \sigma_f$ values for urea and creatinine have been reported as approximately 0.7–0.8 by certain investigators [39, 40, 89] but as equal to or greater than one by others [80, 81, 90]. Solute reflection coefficients for potassium are also anomalous; values of $1 - \sigma_f$ are greater than one. Peritoneal membrane solute reflection coefficients for sodium and total protein are noteworthy. First, values of $1 - \sigma_f$ for sodium are approximately equal to those reported for peritoneal membrane sieving coefficients. This may not be simply coincidental since the solute reflection coefficient for sodium was determined with initial dialysate sodium concentration approximately equal to those in plasma, conditions identical to those employed when determining the peritoneal membrane sieving coefficient. Second, values of $1 - \sigma_f$ for total protein are approximately zero, indicating little convective protein transport occurs during a hypertonic exchange. This result contrasts sharply with sieving coefficients for proteins and other macromolecules determined by increasing the hydrostatic pressure difference across the peritoneal membrane (Table 2).

The detailed methods used to determine the peritoneal membrane solute reflection coefficient in the above studies were similar overall but differed in several respects. For example, it is necessary to determine the volume of dialysis solution in the peritoneal cavity as a function of dwell time when estimating the solute reflection coefficient during a hypertonic exchange. It has been previously demonstrated [91] that the dilution of a marker macromolecule initially added to peritoneal dialysis solution does not accurately assess the volume of dialysis solution within the peritoneal cavity since the marker macromolecule is lost from the peritoneal cavity via peritoneal lymphatics and directly into the tissues surrounding the peritoneal cavity. Whereas several investigators [80, 92, 93] have assessed the importance of loss of the marker macromolecule on the calculated PA value for the peritoneal membrane, its importance on the calculated solute reflection coefficient has not been studied extensively. Leypoldt et al. [94] have determined the solute reflection coefficient for creatinine in a rabbit model of peritoneal dialysis where the true volume of dialysis solution in the peritoneal cavity and the volume determined by the indicator dilution method without correcting for loss of the marker macromolecule were simultaneously measured. The true value of $1 - \sigma_f$ for creatinine was determined to be 0.54 ± 0.48 (SD) when loss of creatinine and the marker macromolecule from the peritoneal cavity were assessed accurately. If only the true volume of peritoneal dialysate as a function of dwell time was used in the calculations, the value of $1 - \sigma_f$ was 0.42 ± 0.74 (SD) when loss of creatinine from the peritoneal cavity was ignored. If only the indicator dilution volume of peritoneal dialysate as a function of dwell time was used in the calculations, the value of $1 - \sigma_f$ was 0.66 ± 0.26 (SD) when loss of creatinine from the peritoneal cavity was ignored. Such differences are small compared with those observed in Tables 3 and 4.

Waniewski et al. [95] have determined the influence of using plasma water as opposed to plasma concentrations on estimated values of the solute reflection coefficient. In this study values of $1 - \sigma_f$ were computed using measured plasma concentrations and compared with those computed using concentrations corrected for the volume of plasma occupied by protein unavailable to small test solutes. Values of $1 - \sigma_f$ were higher when using plasma water concentrations but the differences were small (33% for urea, 7% for creatinine, 3% for glucose, 5% for potassium, and 2% for sodium). This study demonstrated that any differences in the calculated solute reflection coefficients due to using plasma concentrations are small and corrections to plasma water concentrations do not significantly alter the estimated values.

Table 3. Peritoneal membrane solute reflection coefficients when solute transport was in the dialysate-to-blood direction.

Solute	$1 - \sigma_f$ Species	
	Human [39, 40, 80, 81, 89]	Rat [48]
Glucose	0.54 ± 0.28 (7)	0.63 (3)
	0.51 ± 0.03 (8)	
	-0.38 ± 0.48 (28)	
	-0.56 ± 0.50 (20)	
	-0.40 ± 0.40 (20)	
Glycerol	-1.90 ± 1.50 (4)	0.72 (3)
Inulin	0.42 ± 0.33 (5)	

(Mean Values ± SD are shown with the number of observations shown in parentheses).

Table 4. Peritoneal membrane solute reflection coefficients determined when solute transport was in the blood-to-dialysate direction.

Solute	$1 - \sigma_f$ Species	
	Human [39, 40, 80, 81, 89]	Rabbit [79]
Urea	0.73 ± 0.24 (6)	
	0.86 ± 0.08 (8)	
	1.04 ± 0.33 (28)	
	1.45 ± 0.19 (20)	
Creatinine	0.70 ± 0.26 (9)	0.82 ± 0.52 (7)
	0.72 ± 0.01 (8)	0.54 ± 0.48 (7)
	0.98 ± 0.21 (28)	
	1.05 ± 0.20 (20)	
Uric Acid	0.67 ± 0.15 (9)	
	0.56 ± 0.16 (8)	
Potassium	1.57 ± 0.19 (28)	
	1.67 ± 0.20 (20)	
Sodium	0.58 ± 0.10 (28)	
	0.61 ± 0.11 (20)	
Glucose	0.45 ± 0.38 (9)	
	0.62 ± 0.24 (4)	
p-aminohippurate (PAH)		0.86 ± 0.37 (7)
Total Protein	0.008 ± 0.008 (7)	
	0.05 ± 0.03 (8)	
	0.01 ± 0.01 (28)	
	0.013 ± 0.009 (20)	

(Mean Values ± SD are shown with the number of observations shown in parentheses).

Leypoldt and Blindauer [96] have recently used a new method for determining the solute reflection coefficient of the peritoneal membrane that combines the advantages of those of Henderson [59] and Pyle *et al.* [39, 40] in an attempt to more effectively separate convective and diffusive solute transport during an exchange with hypertonic dialysis solution. Separate isotonic and hypertonic exchanges were performed sequentially and in random order. Test solute was added to the instilled hypertonic dialysis solution to inhibit transperitoneal solute diffusion during the hypertonic exchange as in the method employed by Henderson to measure peritoneal membrane sieving coefficients [59]. The PA value was determined during the isotonic exchange, and the solute reflection coefficient was determined during the hypertonic exchange (assuming a PA value equal to that for the isotonic exchange) by comparing the time dependence of the dialysate concentration with that predicted by a mathematical model as in the method employed by Pyle *et al.* [39, 40]. The advantage of this approach compared to that described above is that only a single parameter (i.e. σ_f) was estimated during the hypertonic exchange. Eight experiments were performed using creatinine as test solute and glucose as osmotic solute, and six experiments were performed with glucose as test solute and mannitol as osmotic solute.

Figure 12 shows the time dependence of the creatinine dialysate-to-plasma concentration ratio for both the isotonic and hypertonic exchanges. The concentration ratios were not highly dependent on the exchange order. When using isotonic dialysis solution, the dialysate-to-plasma concentration ratio increased throughout the 2 hour dwell. When using hypertonic dialysis solution, the initial dialysate creatinine concentration was approximately equal to, but slightly less than, the plasma creatinine concentration at the start of the exchange. The concentration ratio decreased significantly throughout the first 60 minutes. Comparable results were obtained when glucose was the test solute. These observations demonstrated that the transperitoneal ultrafiltrate contains neither creatinine nor glucose at the same concentration as in plasma. The calculated value of $1 - \sigma_f$ for creatinine was 0.62 ± 0.17 (SD) and that for glucose was 0.57 ± 0.12 (SD). These observations support the contention that peritoneal membrane solute reflection coefficients for both creatinine and glucose are within the physiologic range, that is, between 0 and 1.

In summary, experimentally determined solute reflection coefficients for the peritoneal membrane are variable, especially when transport of the test solute is in the dialysate-to-blood direction. The methods previously employed to determine the peritoneal membrane solute reflection coefficient are not optimal; improvements in methodology are desirable. Nevertheless, the majority of reported $1 - \sigma_f$ values are within the physiological range and consistent with previously determined values of the peritoneal membrane sieving coefficient. Therefore, whether determined by either the sieving coefficient or the solute reflection coefficient, all solutes (both small and large) do not appear in transperitoneal ultrafiltrate at their concentration in plasma.

4. Modeling ultrafiltration during peritoneal dialysis

Mathematical models describing transperitoneal fluid and solute transport have been based largely on the assumption that the peritoneum acts as a simple membrane separating blood from dialysis solution in the peritoneal cavity. Such models have proven instrumental in identifying important practical parameters that influence diffusive solute transport across the peritoneum [97]; these early peritoneal membrane models have been reviewed [98]. The work of Pyle *et al.* [39, 40] was noteworthy in demonstrating the importance of ultrafiltration on transperitoneal solute transport; moreover, peritoneal membrane solute reflection coefficients were first determined in these studies. To achieve this goal, Pyle *et al.* determined the dependence of dialysate volume and transperitoneal ultrafiltration on time empirically and fit the empirical results to equations (8) and (9). To further understand the important properties of the peritoneum governing transperitoneal ultrafiltration, mathematical models have also been constructed based on the use of equation (7). Models to date have been largely confined to studies using crystalloids as osmotic agents.

The first model of transperitoneal ultrafiltration that used equation (7) to predict the dependence of dialysate volume on time was described by Smeby *et al.* [99, 100]. This model was complex and required estimates of the peritoneal membrane ultrafiltration coefficient, the osmotic reflection coefficients for all relevant osmotic solutes, and the time dependence of blood and dialysate concentrations for all relevant osmotic solutes. Smeby *et al.* used pore theory for describing membrane transport assuming a mean pore radius of 47–55 Å [100] to

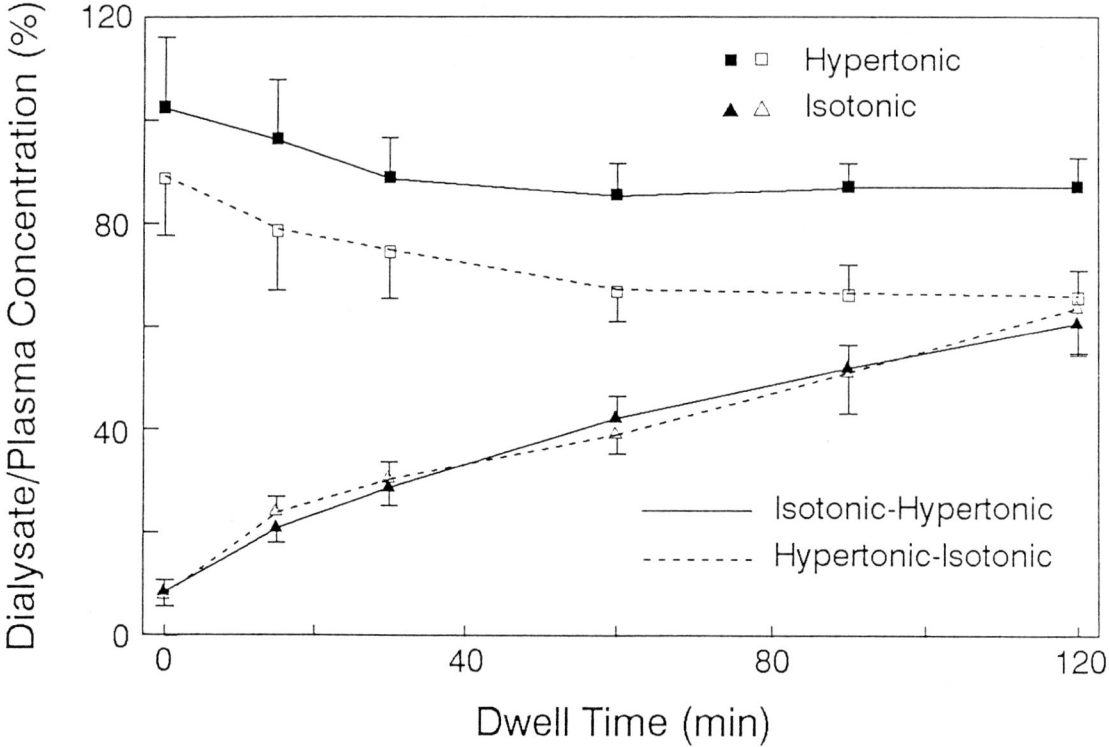

Figure 12. The dependence of the dialysate-to-plasma creatinine concentration ratio during 8 experiments suing glucose as osmotic agent. The isotonic exchange preceded the hypertonic exchange in 4 experiments, and the hypertonic exchange preceded the isotonic exchange in 4 experiments. Results are shown for each exchange sequence separately. Adapted from reference [96] with the permission of Karger AG.

estimate these model parameters. The predictions from this model agreed well with the empirical time dependence of dialysate volume during exchanges with both isotonic and hypertonic dialysis solutions. This work was important in demonstrating the effectiveness of equation (7) to predict transperitoneal ultrafiltration and suggested useful practical guidelines for individualizing CAPD treatment schedules for patients with different peritoneal membrane transport properties.

More recent studies have attempted to simplify this approach. Nakanishi *et al.* [85] used equation (7) to estimate, for the first time, ultrafiltration properties of the peritoneal membrane. These workers compared the time dependence of dialysate volume during 1.5% and 4.25% hydrous dextrose-containing dialysis solutions with equation (7) using nonlinear regression. They assumed that the hydrostatic pressure difference across the peritoneal membrane was zero and limited the number of relevant osmotic solutes to urea, sodium and glucose. Their initial attempt to estimate the osmotic conductance or $K_f\sigma$, that is, the product of the ultrafiltration coefficient times the osmotic reflection coefficient, for urea, sodium and glucose from the time dependence of dialysate volume was unsuccessful. When the contribution from urea was neglected, however, they obtained higher $K_f\sigma$ values for sodium than for glucose during exchanges using both 1.5% and 4.25% hydrous glucose-containing dialysis solution. These observations suggested that the osmotic reflection coefficient for sodium was higher than that for glucose since the peritoneal membrane ultrafiltration coefficient should have a unique, yet unknown, value. Jaffrin *et al.* [101] have described a more simple model of transperitoneal ultrafiltration assuming that glucose is the only osmotic solute determining the dependence of dialysate volume on dwell time. Calculated results from their model predicted accurately the dependence of dialysate volume on time when $K_f\sigma$ was assumed between 3 and 13 µl/min/mm Hg and other peritoneal membrane solute transport properties for glucose were assumed to be similar to those reported in previous studies. This study suggests that the majority of the dependence of dialysate volume on time can be attributed to changes in dialysate glucose concentration.

The above studies did not consider peritoneal lymphatics as an important pathway for fluid loss from the peritoneal cavity. Stelin and Rippe [4] assumed that glucose was the only osmotic solute and mathematically integrated equation (7) including a term for fluid loss from the peritoneal cavity via peritoneal lymphatics. The resulting expression for the time dependence of dialysate volume was identical to equation (8) and permitted a phenomenological interpretation of the parameters in terms of peritoneal membrane transport properties. These investigators also estimated the peritoneal membrane osmotic conductance for glucose two different ways and found a consistent value between 3.5 and 3.8 µl/min/mm Hg. Rippe et al. [5] have extended this model by including glucose, urea, sodium and "sodium anions" (lactate, chloride) as osmotic solutes. The latter model resembles that originally proposed by Smeby et al. [99, 100] and one more recently described by Vonesh et al. [102] except that Rippe et al. have employed peritoneal membrane fluid and solute transport properties calculated using a three-pore model of membrane transport [3]. The models of Vonesh et al. and Rippe et al. have been shown recently to be mathematically equivalent [103].

Further interpretation of the osmotic conductances calculated using these models is problematic. Rippe and Stelin [4] have argued that peritoneal membrane osmotic reflection coefficients can be accurately predicted using a three-pore model of peritoneal transport. Such calculated values are in excellent agreement with measured osmotic reflection coefficients for the cat peritoneal membrane [104] and in continuous capillaries of various organs [105]. The contention that osmotic reflection coefficients for the peritoneal membrane are similar to those for continuous capillaries is consistent with, but cannot be definitely proven, by comparing the dependence of dialysate volume on time with predictions from the mathematical models [103]. Osmotic reflection coefficients for glucose and other small solutes calculated by the three-pore model of peritoneal transport are significantly lower than solute reflection coefficients measured for the peritoneal membrane (Tables 3 and 4). This discrepancy may seem at first to be problematic since it is common to assume that osmotic and solute reflection coefficients are equal [7, 106]. The assumption of equal osmotic and solute reflection coefficients is only applicable to homogeneous membranes [106]; it is therefore unlikely applicable to the peritoneum. Indeed, Rippe and Stelin [3] have demonstrated that the peritoneal membrane can have osmotic reflection coefficients conmensurate with those previously determined for continuous capillaries yet still display transperitoneal solute transport properties consistent with measured solute reflection coefficients.

An alternative explanation for the discrepancy between peritoneal membrane osmotic and solute reflection coefficients may be due to neglecting the importance of peritoneal interstitial tissue in governing transperitoneal diffusive solute transport. When, for example, interstitial tissue is assumed as the dominant diffusive solute transport resistance across the peritoneum, it can be shown using a distributed model of peritoneal transport that the osmotic reflection coefficient for the peritoneal membrane is likely several times less than those for peritoneal capillaries [107]. This occurs because local concentrations within peritoneal tissues are lower than those in the dialysis solution within the peritoneal cavity; thus, the true osmotic concentration difference across peritoneal capillaries is overestimated when using bulk concentrations.

In summary, transperitoneal ultrafiltration can be accurately predicted using mathematical models of peritoneal fluid and solute transport. Osmotic and solute reflection coefficients for the peritoneal membrane are likely different because the peritoneum is not a homogeneous membrane. Further understanding of peritoneal transport physiology will likely result from both improved mathematical models and more detailed expcrimental investigations of the factors that govern peritoneal fluid and solute transport.

References

1. Schultz SG. Basic principles in membrane transport. London, Cambridge University Press, 1980.
2. Henderson LW, Leypoldt JK. Ultrafiltration with peritoneal dialysis. In: Nolph KD (ed), Peritoneal dialysis, 3rd edition. Dordrecht, Kluwer Academic 1989; pp. 117–32.
3. Rippe B, Stelin G. Simulations of peritoneal solute transport during CAPD. Application of two-pore formalism. Kidney Int 1989; 35: 1234–44.
4. Stelin G, Rippe B. A phenomenlogical interpretation of the variation in dialysate volume with dwell time in CAPD. Kidney Int 1990; 38: 465–72.
5. Rippe B, Stelin G, Haraldsson B. Computer simulations of peritoneal fluid transport in CAPD. Kidney Int 1991; 40: 315–25.
6. Dedrick RL, Flessner MF, Collins JM, Schultz JS. Is the peritoneum a membrane? ASAIO J 1982; 5: 1–8.
7. Curry FE. Mechanics and thermodynamics of transcapillary exchange. In: Renkin EM, Michel CC (eds), Handbook of physiology, section 2: the

cardiovascular system, volume IV. Bethesda, American Physiological Society 1984; pp 309–74.
8. Nolph KD, Twardowski ZJ. The peritoneal dialysis system. In: Nolph KD (ed), Peritoneal dialysis, 3rd edition. Dordrecht, Kluwer Academic 1989; pp 13–27.
9. Nolph KD. Peritoneal dialysis. In: Brenner BM, Rector Jr, FC (eds), The kidney, 4th edition. Philadelphia, W. B. Saunders 1991; pp 2299–335.
10. Maher JF, Hirszel P, Lasrich M. Effects of gastrointestinal hormones on transport by peritoneal dialysis. Kidney Int 1979; 16: 130–6.
11. Maher JF, Hirszel P, Bennett RR, Chakrabarti E. Amphotericin selectively increases peritoneal ultrafiltration. Am J Kidney Dis 1984; 4: 285–8.
12. Nolph KD, Stoltz ML. Maher JF. Altered peritoneal permeability in patients with systemic vasculitis. Ann Intern Med 1971; 75: 753–5.
13. Slingeneyer A, Mion C, Mourad G, Canaud B, Faller B, Béraud JJ. Progressive sclerosing peritonitis: a late and severe complication of maintenance peritoneal dialysis. Trans Am Soc Artif Intern Organ 1983; 29: 633–40.
14. Khanna R, Nolph KD. Peritoneal morphology and microcirculation. In: Gokal R (ed), Continuous ambulatory peritoneal dialysis. Edinburgh, Churchill Livingstone 1986; pp 14–37.
15. Henderson LW. The problem of peritoneal membrane area and permeability. Kidney Int 1973; 3: 409–10.
16. Twardowski Z, Janicka L. Three exchanges with a 2.5-liter volume for continuous ambulatory peritoneal dialysis. Kidney Int 1981; 20: 281–4.
17. Kim D, Khanna R, Wu G, Clayton S, Oreopoulos DG. Continuous ambulatory peritoneal dialysis with three-liter exchanges: a prospective study. Perit Dial Bull 1984; 4: 82–5.
18. Miller FN, Nolph KD, Harris PD, Rubin J, Wiegman DL, Joshua IG, Twardowski ZJ, Ghods AJ. Microvascular and clinical effects of altered peritoneal dialysis solutions. Kidney Int 1979; 15: 630–9.
19. Hirszel P, Lasrich M, Maher JF. Augmentation of peritoneal mass transport by dopamine. Comparison with norepinephrine and evaluation of pharmacologic mechanisms. J Lab Clin Med 1979; 94: 747–54.
20. Hebert SC, Schafer JA, Andreoli TE. Principles of membrane transport. In: Brenner BM, Rector Jr FC (eds), The kidney, 2nd edition. Philadelphia, W. B. Saunders 1981; pp 116–43.
21. Dampier WC. A history of science. London, Cambridge University Press 1948; pp 249–51.
22. Van't Hoff JH. Une propriété général de la matière diluée. Svenska Vet Akad Handl 1886; 21: 17–43.
23. Keele CA, Neil E. The regulation of the constancy of the internal environment: body water and fluid. In: Keele CA, Neil E (eds), Samson Wright's applied physiology, 12th edition. London, Oxford University Press 1992; pp 13–7.
24. Ryan GB. Mechanisms of proteinuria. In: Jones NF, Peters KD (eds), Recent advances in renal medicine 2. Edinburgh, Churchill Livingstone 1982; pp 31–53.
25. Staverman AJ. The theory of measurement of osmotic pressure. Rec Trav Chim Pays-Bas 1951; 70: 344–52.
26. Kiil F. Mechanism of osmosis. Kidney Int 1982; 21: 303–8.
27. Meschia G, Setniker I. Experimental study of osmosis through a collodion membrane. J Gen Physiol 1958; 42: 429–44.
28. Wegner G. Chirugische Bemerkungen über die Peritonealhöhle, mit besonderer Berücksichtigung der Ovariotomie. Arch Fur Klin Chir 1877; 20: 51–145.
29. Starling EH, Tubby AH. On absorption from the secretion into the serous cavity. J Physiol 1894; 16: 140–55.
30. Putnam TJ. The living peritoneum as a dialyzing membrane. Am J Physiol 1923; 63: 548–65.
31. Cunningham RS. Studies on absorption from serous cavities. III. The effect of dextrose upon the peritoneal mesothelium. Am J Physiol 1920; 53: 488–94.
32. Palmer RA, Quinton WE, Gray JE. Prolonged peritoneal dialysis for chronic renal failure. Lancet 1964; i: 700–2.
33. Popovich RP, Moncrief JW, Decherd JF, Bomar JB, Pyle WK. The definition of a novel portable/wearable equilibrium peritoneal dialysis technique. [Abstract]. Abs Am Soc Artif Intern Organs 1976; 5: 64.
34. Daugirdas JT, Ing TS, Gandhi VC, Hano JE, Chen W-T, Yuan L. Kinetics of peritoneal fluid absorption in patients with chronic renal failure. J Lab Clin Med 1980; 95: 351–61.
35. Popovich RP, Moncrief JW, Okutan M, Decherd JF. A model of the peritoneal dialysis system. Proc 25th Ann Conf Engr Med Biol 1966; 14: 172.
36. Spencer PC, Farrell PC. Solute and water transfer kinetics in CAPD. In: Gokal R (ed), Continuous ambulatory peritoneal dialysis. Edinburgh, Churchill Livingstone 1986; pp 38–55.
37. Canaud B, Liendo-Liendo C, Claret G, Mion H, Mion C. Etude 'in situ' de la cinétique de l'ultrafiltration, en cours de dialyse péritonéale avec périodes de diffusion prolongée. Nephrologie 1980; 1: 126–32.
38. De Paepe M, Kips J, Belpaire F, Lameire N. Comparison of different volume markers in peritoneal dialysis. In: Maher JF, Winchester JF (eds), Frontiers in peritoneal dialysis. New York, Field, Rich and Associates 1986; pp 279–82.
39. Pyle WK. Mass transfer in peritoneal dialysis. Ph.D. Dissertation. University of Texas at Austin 1981.
40. Pyle WK, Moncrief JW, Popovich RP. Peritoneal transport evaluation in CAPD. In: Moncrief JW, Popovich RP (eds), CAPD update. New York, Masson 1981; pp 35–52.
41. Mistry CD. Glucose polymer as an osmotic agent in continuous peritoneal dialysis. MD Thesis. London, University of London 1989; pp 1–300.
42. Mactier RA, Khanna R, Twardowski Z, Moore H,

Nolph KD. Contribution of lymphatic absorption to loss of ultrafiltration and solute clearances in continuous ambulatory peritoneal dialysis. J Clin Invest 1987; 80: 1311–6.
43. Mactier RA, Khanna R, Twardowski ZJ, Nolph KD. Role of peritoneal cavity lymphatic absorption in peritoneal dialysis. Kidney Int 1987; 32: 165–72.
44. Flessner MF, Parker RJ, Sieber SM. Peritoneal lymphatic uptake of fibrinogen and erythrocytes in the rat. Am J Physiol 1983; 244: H89–96.
45. Rippe B, Stelin G, Ahlmén J. Lymph flow from the peritoneal cavity in CAPD patients. In: Maher JF, Winchester JF (eds), Frontiers in peritoneal dialysis. New York, Field, Rich and Associates 1986; pp 24–30.
46. Flessner MF, Dedrick Rl, Rippe B. Letter to the editor. ASAIO Trans 1989; 35: 178–80.
47. Starling EH. On the absorption of fluids from the connective tissue spaces. J Physiol 1895; 19: 312–26.
48. Daniels FH, Leonard EF, Cortell S. Glucose and glycerol compared as osmotic agents for peritoneal dialysis. Kidney Int 1984; 25: 20–25.
49. Heaton A, Ward MK, Johnston DG, Nicholson DV, Alberti KGMM, Kerr DNS. Short-term studies on the use of glycerol as an osmotic agent in continuous ambulatory peritoneal dialysis (CAPD). Clin Sci 1984; 67: 121–30.
50. Oreopoulos DG, Crassweller P, Katirtzoglou A, Ogilve R, Zellerman G, Rodella H, Vas SL. Amino acids as an osmotic agent (instead of glucose) in continuous ambulatory peritoneal dialysis. In: Legrain M (ed), Continuous ambulatory peritoneal dialysis. Amsterdam, Excerpta Medica 1980; pp 335–40.
51. Williams PF, Marliss EB, Anderson GH, Oren A, Stein AN, Khanna R, Petitt J, Brandes L, Rodella H, Mupas L, Dombros N, Oreopoulos DG. Amino acid absorption following intraperitoneal administration in CAPD patients. Perit Dial Bull 1982; 2: 124–30.
52. Jirka J, Kotková E. Peritoneal dialysis by isooncotic dextran solution in anaesthestised dogs. Intra-peritoneal fluid volume and protein concentration in the irrigation fluid. Proc EDTA 1967; 4: 141–5.
53. Gjessing J. The use of dextran as a dialysing fluid in peritoneal dialysis. Acta Med Scand 1969; 185: 237–9.
54. Twardowski ZJ, Moore HL, McGary TJ, Poskuta M, Stathakis C, Hirszel P. Polymers as osmotic agents for peritoneal dialysis. Perit Dial Bull 1984; 4(Suppl 3): S125–31.
55. Twardowski ZJ, Khanna R, Nolph KD. Osmotic agents and ultrafiltration in peritoneal dialysis. Nephron 1986; 42: 93–101.
56. Mistry CD, Mallick NP, Gokal R. Ultrafiltration with an isosmotic solution during long peritoneal dialysis exchanges. Lancet 1987; ii: 178–82.
57. Mistry CD, Gokal R. Can ultrafiltration occur with a hyosmolar solution in peritoneal dialysis? The role for "colloid" osmosis. Clin Sci 1993; 85: 495–500.
58. Mistry CD, Gokal R. New osmotic agents for peritoneal dialysis: where we are and where we're going. Sem Dial 1991; 4: 9–12.
59. Henderson LW. Peritoneal ultrafiltration dialysis: enhanced urea transfer using hypertonic peritoneal dialysis fluid. J Clin Invest 1966; 45: 950–5.
60. Henderson LW, Nolph KD. Altered permeability of the peritoneal membrane after using hypertonic peritoneal dialysis fluid. J Clin Invest 1969; 48: 992–1001.
61. Maher JF, Bennett RR, Hirzsel P, Chakrabarti E. The mechanism of dextrose-enhanced peritoneal mass transport rates. Kidney Int 1985; 28: 16–20.
62. Patlak CS, Goldstein DA, Hoffman JF. The flow of solute and solvent across a two-membrane system. J Theoret Biol 1963; 5: 426–42.
63. Bresler EH, Groome LJ. On equations for combined convective and diffusive transport of neutral solute across porous membranes. Am J Physiol 1981; 241: F469–76.
64. Nolph KD, Hano JE, Teschan PE. Peritoneal sodium transport during hypertonic peritoneal dialysis. Ann Intern Med 1969; 70: 931–41.
65. Brown ST, Ahearn DJ, Nolph KD. Potassium removal with peritoneal dialysis. Kidney Int 1973; 4: 647–9.
66. Rubin J, Klein E, Bower JD. Investigation of the net sieving coefficient of the peritoneal membrane during peritoneal dialysis. ASAIO J 1982; 5: 9–15.
67. Rubin J, Jones Q, Andrew M. An analysis of ultrafiltration during acute peritoneal dialysis in rats. Am J Med Sci 1989; 298: 383–9.
68. Park MS, Heimbürger O, Waniewski J, Werynski A, Lindholm B, Berström J. Observed net sieving coefficient in experimental peritoneal dialysis in rat. [Abstract]. Perit Dial Int 1993; 13 (Suppl 1): S14.
69. Leypoldt JK. Determining ulatfiltration properties of the peritoneum. ASAIO Trans 1990; 36: 60–6.
70. Aune S. Transperitoneal exchange. III. The influence of transperitoneal fluid flux on the peritoneal plasma clearance of serum albumin in rabbits. Scand J Gastroent 1970; 5: 161–8.
71. Bell JL, Leypoldt JK, Frigon RP, Henderson LW. Hydraulically-induced convective solute transport across the rabbit peritoneum. Kidney Int 1990; 38: 19–27.
72. Henriksen JH, Lassen NA, Parving H-H, Winkler K. Filtration as the main transport mechanism of protein exchange between plasma and the peritoneal cavity in hepatic cirrhosis. Scan J Clin Lab Invest 1980; 40: 503–13.
73. Hoefs JC. Serum protein c and portal pressure determine the ascitic fluid protein concentration in patients with chronic liver disease. J Lab Clin Med 1983; 102: 260–73.
74. Taylor AE, Granger DN. Exchange of macromolecules across the microcirculation. In: Renkin EM, Michel CC (eds), Handbook of physiology, section 2: the cardiovascular system, volume IV, Bethesda, American Physiological Society 1984; pp 467–520.
75. Goresky CA, Groom AC. Microcirculatory events in the liver and the spleen. In: Renkin EM, Michel

CC (eds), Handbook of physiology, section 2: the cardiovascular system, volume IV, Bethesda, American Physiological Society 1984; pp 689–780.
76. Chen TW, Khanna R, Moore H, Twardowski ZJ, Nolph KD. Sieving and reflection coefficients for sodium salts and glucose during peritoneal dialysis in rats. J Am Soc Nephrol 1991; 2: 1091–100.
77. Babb AL, Johansen PJ, Strand MJ, Tenkhoff H, Scribner BH. Bidirectional permeability of the human peritoneum to middle molecules. Proc EDTA 1973; 10: 247–61.
78. Randerson DH, Farrell PC. Mass transfer properties of the human peritoneum. ASAIO J 1980; 3: 140–6.
79. Leypoldt JK, Parker HR, Frigon RP, Henderson LW. Molecular size dependence of peritoneal transport. J Lab Clin Med 1987; 110: 207–16.
80. Waniewski J, Werynski A, Heimbürger O, Lindholm B. A comparative analysis of mass transport models in peritoneal dialysis. ASAIO Trans 1991; 37: 65–75.
81. Waniewski J, Werynski A, Heimbürger O, Lindholm B. Simple membrane models for peritoneal dialysis. Evaluation of diffusive and convective solute transport ASAIO J 1992; 38: 788–96.
82. Sorenson HW. Parameter estimation. New York, Marcel Dekker 1980.
83. Draper NR, Smith H. Applied regression analysis, 2nd edition. New York, John Wiley & Sons 1981.
84. Garfinkel D, Fegley KA. Fitting physiological models to data. Am J Physiol 1984; 246: R641–50.
85. Nakanishi T, Tanaka Y, Fujii M, Fukuhara Y, Orita Y. Nonequilibrium thermodynamics of glucose transport in continuous ambulatory peritoneal dialysis. In: Maekawa M, Kishimoto T, Nolph KD, Moncrief JW (eds), Machine free dialysis for patient convenience: the fourth ISAO official satellite symposium on CAPD, Cleveland, ISAO Press 1984; pp 39–44.
86. Leypoldt JK. Accuracy of peritoneal membrane solute reflection coefficients. Blood Purif 1992; 10: 254–61.
87. DiStefano III JJ, Landaw EM. Multiexponential, multicompartmental, and noncompartmental modeling. I. Methodological limitations and physiological interpretations. Am J Physiol 1984; 246: R651–64.
88. Landaw EM, DiStefano III JJ. Multiexponential, multicompartmental, and noncompartmental modeling. II. Data analysis and statistical considerations. Am J Physiol 1984; 246: R665–77.
89. Morgenstern BZ, Pyle WK, Gruskin AB, Kaiser BA, Perlman SA, Polinsky MS, Baluarte HJ. Convective characteristics of pediatric peritoneal dialysis. Perit Dial Bull 1984; 4 (Suppl 3): S155–8.
90. Waniewski J, Werynski A, Heimbürger O, Berström J, Lindholm B. Diffusive and convective characteristics of bidirectional glucose transport in peritoneal dialysis. [Abstract]. Artif Organs 1991; 15: 332.
91. Pust AH, Leypoldt JK, Frigon RP, Henderson LW. Peritoneal dialysate volume determined by indicator dilution measurements. Kidney Int 1988; 33: 64–70.
92. Hallett MD, Lysaght MJ, Farrell PC. The role of lymphatic drainage in peritoneal mass transfer. Artif Organs 1989; 13: 28–34.
93. Heimbürger O, Waniewski J, Werynski A, TranH1Aus A, Lindholm B. Peritoneal transport in CAPD patients with permanent loss of ultrafiltration capacity. Kidney Int 1990; 38: 495–506.
94. Leypoldt JK, Pust AH, Frigon RP, Henderson LW. Dialysate volume measurements required for determining peritoneal solute transport. Kidney Int 1988; 34: 254–61.
95. Waniewski J, Heimbürger O, Werynski A, Lindholm B. Aqueous solute concentrations and evaluation of mass transport coefficients in peritoneal dialysis. Nephrol Dial Transplant 1992; 7: 50–6.
96. Leypoldt JK, Blindauer KM. Peritoneal solvent drag reflection coefficients are within the physiological range. Blood Purif (in press).
97. Popovich RP, Moncrief JW, Pyle WK. Transport kinetics. In: Nolph KD (ed), Peritoneal dialysis, 3rd edition. Dordrecht, Kluwer Academic 1989; pp 96–116.
98. Popovich RP, Pyle WK, Bomar JB, Moncrief JW. Peritoneal dialysis. In: Villarroel F, Dedrick RL (eds), Chronic replacement of kidney function, New York, American Institute of Chemical Engineers 1979; pp 31–45.
99. Smeby LC, Wideröe T-E, Jörstad S. Individual differences in water transport during continuous peritoneal dialysis. ASAIO J 1981; 4: 17–27.
100. Smeby LC, Wideröe T-E, Mjaaland S, Dahl K. Changes in ultrafiltration and solute transport during CAPD. In: Maher JF, Winchester JF (eds), Frontiers in peritoneal dialysis. New York, Field, Rich and Associates 1986; pp 68–74.
101. Jaffrin MY. Odell RA, Farrell PC. A model of ultrafiltration and glucose mass transfer kinetics in peritoneal dialysis. Artif Organs 1987; 11: 198–207.
102. Vonesh EF, Lysaght MJ, Moran J, Farrell P. Kinetic modeling as a prescription aid in peritoneal dialysis. Blood Purif 1991; 9: 246–70.
103. Vonesh EF, Rippe B. Net fluid absorption under membrane transport models of peritoneal dialysis. Blood Purif 1992; 10: 209–26.
104. Rippe B, Perry MA, Granger DN. Permselectivity of the peritoneal membrane. Microvasc Res 1985; 29: 89–102.
105. Crone C, Levitt DG. Capillary permeability to small solutes. In: Renkin EM, Michel CC (Eds), Handbook of physiology, section 2: the cardiovascular system, volume IV, Bethesda, American Physiological Society 1984; pp 411–66.
106. Katchalsky A, Curran PF. Nonequilibrium thermodynamics in biophysics. Cambridge, Harvard University Press 1965; pp 113–32.
107. Leypoldt JK. Interpreting peritoneal membrane osmotic reflection coefficients using a distributed model of peritoneal transport. Adv Perit Dial 1993; 9: 3–7.

7. Pharmacologic alterations of peritoneal transport rates and pharmacokinetics of the peritoneum

PRZEMYSLAW HIRSZEL, NORBERT LAMEIRE AND MARC BOGAERT

1.	1.1.	Rationale for augmenting rates	161
	1.2.	Mechanisms of transport	162
	1.3.	Diffusion	162
	1.4.	Dialysate flow rate	163
	1.5.	Mesenteric blood flow	163
	1.6.	Convective transport	164
	1.7.	Transport of lipids	165
	1.8.	Lymphatic absorption	166
	1.9.	Mechanisms of accelerating peritoneal transport	166
	1.10.	Restoration of decreased transport rates toward normal	168
	1.11.	Increasing peritoneal transport above normal values	168
	1.12.	Isoproterenol enhancement of peritoneal mass transport	169
	1.13.	Nitroprusside augmentation of peritoneal mass transfer	169
	1.14.	Dipyridamole effects on peritoneal dialysis efficiency	169
	1.15.	Influence of catecholamines on peritoneal transport kinetics	170
	1.16.	Other vasodilators that affect peritoneal transport	170
	1.17.	Prostaglandin modulation of peritoneal transport	171
	1.18.	Vasodilator gastrointestinal hormones	172
	1.19.	Other hormones and drugs affecting peritoneal blood flow and diffusion	173
	1.20.	Membrane surface-active agents	173
	1.21.	Increasing ultrafiltration rates	174
	1.22.	Transport acceleration of specific solutes	175
	1.23.	Peritoneal protein loss attenuation	176
	1.24.	Conclusion	176
2.		Pharmacokinetic aspects of peritoneal transport of drugs	177
	2.1.	Basic pharmacokinetics	177
	2.1.1.	Compartmental models	177
	2.1.2.	Plasma concentration – time course	178
	2.2.	Pharmacokinetic alterations in patients with decreased renal function	180
	2.3.	Pharmacokinetic alterations in patients on peritoneal dialysis	181
	2.3.1.	Pharmacokinetics of drugs after systemic administration	181
	2.3.2.	Factors influencing the peritoneal drug clearance	181
	2.3.3.	Need for dose adaptation	182
	2.3.4.	Bidirectional transfer	183
	2.3.5.	Pharmacokinetics of drugs after intraperitoneal administration	183
	2.3.6.	Factors affecting transperitoneal drug absorption after intraperitoneal administration	183
	2.4.	Effect of peritoneal dialysis on drug protein binding	185
	2.5.	Peritoneal pharmacokinetics of common drugs and dose recommendations	186
	2.5.1.	Description of the tables	186
	2.5.2.	Pharmacokinetic data in intermittent peritoneal dialysis (IPD)	186
	2.5.3.	Pharmacokinetic data in CAPD	191
	2.5.4.	Antiviral drugs	205
	2.5.5.	Antifungal drugs	205
	2.6.	Insulin	208
	2.7.	Heparin	211
	2.8.	Desferrioxamine	211
	2.9.	Vitamins D3 and its metabolites	212
	2.10.	Other vitamins	212
	2.11.	Miscellaneous	212
Dedication			214
Acknowledgements			214
References			214

Peritoneal dialysis has become an increasingly popular alternative to hemodialysis for therapy of chronic renal failure [1–3]. In the first part of this chapter, the effects of pharmacological and physiological manipulations on peritoneal transport, seeking enhanced understanding of transport mechanisms and clinically useful methods to augment transport will be discussed. In the second part, the pharmacokinetic mechanisms of transperitoneal drug transport and their implications for rational and safe use of drugs in patients on peritoneal dialysis will be reviewed.

1.1. Rationale for augmenting rates

Mass transport rates of small solutes by peritoneal dialysis are slower than those by hemodialysis. Hence, peritoneal dialysis consumes more time to achieve a given control of the plasma concentration of a solute such as urea. Insufficient transport can contribute to the risk of peritonitis because more exchanges of dialysis solution are required. Once peritonitis occurs solute transport may increase, but the ultrafiltration rate decreases because of more rapid dissipation of the osmotic gradient. Thereafter, transport should return to baseline rates unless inadequate treatment allows loss of peritoneal surface area or decreased permeability. Marginal transport rates after peritonitis may lower the ultrafiltration capacity to an unacceptable level [4]. Moreover, for hypercatabolic or hyperkalemic patients the transport inefficiency for small solutes may be quite significant, even when the peritoneal surface area and permeability have not been reduced. The efficiency of peritoneal mass transport may be particularly impaired by systemic vascular disease [5].

Continuous ambulatory peritoneal dialysis (CAPD) does not have the disadvantage of being overly time consuming because treatment time does not inhibit rehabilitation [6]. But CAPD also requires adequate efficiency to be clinically satisfactory. With coexistent vascular disease or after many episodes of peritonitis, peritoneal mass transport may be so borderline as to render the procedure inadequate unless more frequent exchanges are used, with the attendant hazards of multiple tubing disconnections. Moreover, some patients undergoing CAPD have low rates of ultrafiltration or acquire this abnormality, which is an important limiting factor for effective dialysis therapy. Under other circumstances increased catabolism may increase the nitrogen load. Despite continuous peritoneal dialysis, augmented transport may be required whenever there is decreased transport efficiency or increased catabolism.

When peritoneal dialysis is used to remove exogenous toxins, it is usually mandatory that removal rates be maximal. Conversely, when protein loss is excessive, it may be judicious to decrease the transport rates, at least of larger solutes. Hence, further understanding of the mechanisms of mass transport and the influence of pharmacologic and physiologic manipulations on them is important for accelerating or decreasing transport rates as clinically indicated. It has been postulated that the major sites of ultrafiltration and of diffusion across the peritoneum differ [7] and these transport sites can be modulated selectively [8, 9]. Recent evidence suggests that lymphatic flow is an important determinant of the net peritoneal ultrafiltration [10]. Frequently, patients undergoing peritoneal dialysis also require a variety of drugs that have specific vasoactive or membrane effects. Knowledge of the effects of such agents on transport parameters can influence the appropriate choice of a drug.

1.2. Mechanisms of transport

A dialysis solution in the peritoneal cavity approaches concentration equilibrium with plasma by diffusion. Additionally, net osmotic and hydrostatic forces promote the movement of water, usually from plasma to dialysate. Such ultrafiltration also convectively removes solutes. Solutes also can enter dialysate from adjacent tissue rather than from plasma [11]. Finally, solutes absorbed from peritoneal dialysate into the portal vasculature may undergo hepatic metabolism before reaching the systemic circulation decreasing the absorbed concentration [12]. The bulk of absorption which reduces the net solute and water transfer presumably occurs through lymphatics.

1.3. Diffusion

Diffusion occurs by random kinetic movement of molecules and tends to spread any substance evenly through the space available to it. this process is not affected by drugs directly, but the barriers to diffusion can be influenced pharmacologically. Diffusion rates correlate directly with temperature, however.

The rate of linear diffusion of a solute in any direction throughout a cross-sectional area, expressed as mass transport or quantity per unit time, is proportional to the concentration gradient. Interposing a membrane with pores that are large in relation to the diffusing molecules merely restricts the total area available for free diffusion. Dividing the mass transport rate by the gradient, or more simply by the plasma concentration, yields a clearance value. Prolonged intraperitoneal dwell dissipates the concentration gradient, decreasing the mass transport rate. Hence, unless clearances are calculated on short-time exchanges, e.g., hourly, they are misleadingly low and the dialysance [13] or mass transfer coefficient must be determined. [14].

Free diffusion across capillary walls becomes progressively restricted as the square root of the molecular mass of the solute increases [15]. Accordingly, peritoneal permeability area coefficients decrease as the square root of the molecular mass increases, while clearances bear a slightly different relationship as concentration equilibrium is approached [16]. Many other factors affect the multiple diffusion coefficients that characterize multicomponent mass transfer across macroscopic biologic membranes.

Water soluble solutes traverse intercellular channels, whereas lipid soluble dissolve in plasma membranes readily permeating cells. The diffusion of small water soluble solutes is so rapid that the observed peritoneal transport rates can be accounted for by intercellular pores that total only 0.2% of the estimated surface area [17]. At the exchange rate of dialysis solution of 2 liters hourly and with a peritoneal blood flow rate of 60–100 ml/min [18], the clearances of small solutes such as urea and creatinine are much lower than by hemodialysis, but large solutes like inulin are removed relatively faster, which suggests that the total pore area of the peritoneum is less than that of cellulosic membranes but that the pores are larger [19]. Studies of the transport of neutral dextrans are consistent with heteroporosity of the peritoneum with some pores larger that 40Å [20]. Larger solutes such as polypeptides and small proteins appear to traverse the capillary wall in vesicles adjoining or contiguous with intercellular clefts [21–23]. The effective size of the pores in capillaries can be influenced by the protein concentration of the perfusate, by the capillary blood pressure and volume, and by drugs.

The thickest layer of transport resistance is the dense interstitial connective tissue between the capillary endothelim and the mesothelium. This unstirred layer of gelatinous fluid impedes transport of solutes that permeate the capillary wall. Dehydration increases this resistance because of the resultant distortion of the porous channels of this layer [24].

Studies of transport across isolated mesentery suggest that the mesothelial cells also contribute to transport resistance [25]. It has been demonstrated that permeation of solutes into the isolated hemidiaphragm is lower in areas covered by the mesothelium compared to bare areas. This impedance is offset by the addition of a redox dye to the system and is restored by adding malate or succinate, but lost again when malonate is added [26]. These results suggest that oxidative metabolism and ATP formation are intimately linked in regulating diffusion through this cell layer; it should respond to pharmacologic manipulation. Furthermore, mesothelial cells are capable of synthetizing phosphatidylcholine in a similar manner to type II pneumocytes, thereby they may play a role in the regulation of peritoneal permeability and the rate of ultrafiltration [27].

1.4. Dialysate flow rate

The diffusive transport rate of any given solute depends mostly on the electrochemical concentration gradient. This gradient dissipates as solute leaves the plasma and accumulates in dialysate. Obviously impractical, infinitely high blood and dialysate flow rates would maintain maximal concentration gradients. Large, poorly diffusible solutes accumulate in dialysate so slowly that increasing the rate of dialysis solution exchange above 2 liters per hour adds little to the gradient and the clearance. With intermittent peritoneal dialysis the usual drainage rate of dialysate is about 2,100 ml/h or 35 ml/min. Under this circumstance the clearance of a small, highly diffusible solute such as urea is about 20 ml/min, indicating incomplete equilibration, i.e., a dialysate/plasma concentration ratio of 20/35 or about 0.6. Increasing the dialysate exchange rate can only increase the clearance by about 30% [28]. When dialysate volume is insufficient to contact the entire peritoneal surface, however, clearances are suboptimal until the exchange volume is increased [29]. Accordingly, clearance decreases as fluid is being exchanged and can be augmented by leaving a residual volume in the peritoneum as the excess volume is exchanged in a technique named tidal peritoneal dialysis [30]. But, greatly improved mass transport must depend on augmentation of blood flow or peritoneal permeability or area, just as hemodialyzer efficiency has increased with larger surface area dialyzers, more permeable membranes and higher blood flow rates. Recognition of the limited value of high dialysate flow rates prompted Popovich and colleagues [6] to develop CAPD which prolongs diffusion time rather than increasing the volume or exchange rate of dialysis solution. The procedural variant, continuous cyclic peritoneal dialysis (CCPD), is also based on this concept. [31, 32].

1.5. Mesenteric blood flow

Blood flow to the visceral peritoneum derives predominantly from the mesenteric circulation. About 60% of peritoneal surface can be ascribed to the mesentery of the esophago-rectal viscera, with nearly 15% covering the liver and approximately 15% being parietal [33]. The parietal peritoneum is perfused by vasculature of the abdominal wall. Mesenteric blood flow rates average about 10% of the cardiac output or 40 ml/min/100 g [34, 35], while the effective blood flow rate to the human peritoneum averages 60 to 100 ml/min [18]. When mesenteric blood flow is doubled, the clearances of small solutes such as urea increase by 30% to 50% [36], consistent with a resting blood flow that exceeds the maximal rate at which the capillary diffusion capacity can completely clear the perfusing blood [37]. It is noteworthy that peritoneal transfer of water and small solutes is not affected by the increase in hematocrit and platelet aggregation following erthropoietin therapy [38, 39].

The splanchnic vascular bed can sequester blood, excluding it from or releasing it into the circulation as systemic volume changes. Thus, hemodynamic effects of drugs can influence splanchnic blood volume and flow rate considerably. Because drugs usually affect the splanchnic blood flow and volume *pari passu*, changes in peritoneal transport that result from the altered volume can be misinterpreted as flow rate mediated. The mesenteric vasculature is accompanied by autonomic neuroelements from the celiac plexus with primary neurocontrol by sympathetic innervation. Both alpha- and beta-adrenergic receptors are located in mesenteric vessels [40]. These vessels also contain dopaminergic receptors. Vasoactive responses of the mesenteric vascular bed to pharmacologic manipulations are well established. The vasocontrictor response that normally occurs with appropriate stimuli can be prevented by blocking alpha receptors of the mesenteric vascular bed with phenoxybenzamine. Moreover, prostaglandins are intimately involved in the fine control of vascular dynamics by modifying vasoconstrictor responses [41]. Indeed, during peritonitis peritoneal generation of prostaglandins (especially vasodilators) increases contributing importantly to the protein loss and other flux abnormalities [42]. There is also evidence to suggest that the splanchnic blood volume rather than the flow rate determines the degree of peritoneal mass transfer [43]. The opportunities for increasing peritoneal mass transport by pharmacologic modulation of blood flow to the peritoneum are numerous [44].

1.6. Convective transport

Solute is also convected into the peritoneum by ultrafiltration. The pores through capillary walls restrict the passage of protein but little compositional change occurs with smaller solutes such as urea. Solutes as large as inulin are sieved appreciably during peritoneal ultrafiltration. The hydrostatic pressure of the blood, which decreases from 32 to 15 mm Hg from the arterial to the venous end of the capillary, is opposed by the plasma oncotic pressure, normally 25 mm Hg, and by the interstitial hydrostatic pressure minus the interstitial osmotic pressure. Hence, the ultrafiltration rate through mesenteric capillaries at normal pressure is only about 3.0 ml/min/M^2 of surface area. This ultrafiltrate returns promptly to venules and lymphatics. Normally, peritoneal fluid resembles lymph from the leg rather than from the hepatic or thoracic duct [45] and is derived from mesenteric capillaries. With increased hepatic venous pressure the surface of the liver contributes predominately to ascites formation.

When 2 liters of isotonic fluid is infused intraperitoneally, it raises extravascular hydrostatic pressure promoting the absorption of fluid at a rate of about 10% of residual volume per hour [46]. Added dextrose raises the dialysate osmotic pressure sufficiently to induce net ultrafiltration in proportion to the dextrose concentration of the instilled fluid. Because of the restricted diffusion coefficient of dextrose relative to the solvent, 1.5% dextrose dialysis fluid yields about 3.0 ml/min/M^2 of ultrafiltrate. Inward diffusion of dextrose dissipates the osmotic pressure gradient rapidly, despite metabolism of the absorbed glucose, and lymphatic absorption further decreases the rate of the net ultrafiltration. Hence, the ultrafiltration rate decreases with time. The ultrafiltration rate can be increased by using a higher concentration of dextrose, a less permeant solute of comparable osmotic activity, or by drugs that increase the capillary filtration coefficient [47] or raise the capillary hydrostatic pressure by venular constriction, which may be the case with dopamine [48].

In uremic patients hypertonic dextrose dialysis solution increases rates of solute loss, which has been attributed to enhanced permeability [49]. Most of the increased solute removal with hypertonic dextrose dialysis fluid can be accounted for by increased convective transport, however. Moreover, plasma volume expansion due to retention of absorbed dextrose contributes importantly to the higher mass transport rates [50]. Indeed, in the intact rabbit convective transport increases but diffusion does not as the volume expansion by hypertonic dialysis fluid is promptly excreted. Unlike diffusion which separates solutes according to molecular size, convection does not discriminate by size until sieving occurs as the dimensions of the effective pores are approached. Since convection adds more to the transport rate of slowly diffusible solutes, it mimics an increase in permeability of the diffusion barrier.

Biologic membranes have interstices and discontinuities between their lipid and protein complexes so that pores of a sort exist for diffusion and ultrafiltration. The Pappenheimer theory of restricted diffusion across capillaries takes into account (1) the stearic hindrance at the entrance of a pore, (2) friction between molecules moving within a pore and, (3) molecular friction with the stationary walls of a pore as factors impeding the passage of molecules through pores of molecular dimensions. Such pores are lined by the fixed ionic charge groups of protein (amino-, imino- and carboxyl) and of lipid (phosphate and choline) [51].

Anionic sites predominantly composed of heparan sulfate and chondroitin sulfate are a constant feature of basement membranes of the microvasculature [52]. They are particularly abundant in fenestrated capillaries, some of which have been identified in human parietal and diaphragmatic peritoneum [53]. Anionic sites are also found on the luminal surface of fenestrated endothelia, in the amorphous interstitial connective substance and at the peritoneal surface of the mesothelial plasmalemma, all of which contribute to the structure of peritoneal membrane [53]. Lastly, the lymphatic endothelium and intercellular clefts of lymphatic endothelial cells contain abundant anionic sites [54].

These anionic charges restrict the diffusive and connective passage of charged solutes through the membrane. For example, the rate of absorption of acids and bases from peritoneal fluid decreases to the extent of the ionization at physiological pH [46]. Diffusive rates of potassium, lithium and phosphate into the peritoneum are slower than the rates of uncharged solutes of similar size, unlike the transport across synthetic hemodialysis membranes [16]. Moreover, in the absence of a diffusion gradient, the sodium concentration of osmotically induced peritoneal ultrafiltrate is much lower than that of plasma, i.e., about 75 mEq/L [55]. The addition of furosemide to the dialysis solution raises the peritoneal ultrafiltrate sodium concentration [56], consistent with a drug effect on the membrane. A significant decrease in dialysate sodium during dextrose-induced ultrafiltration reflects an appropriate transcapillary water movement and can be used in the differential diagnosis of ultrafiltration loss in CAPD patients [57].

There is a paucity of data concerning the influence of the peritoneal membrane anionic sites on transport of charged macromolecules across the peritoneum. Peritoneal transfer of heparin is negligible, which may relate to its negative charge [58]. With higher amounts of intraperitoneal heparin, absorption may reach 15% to 20% of the administered dose [59].

The charge issue is further complicated by the presence of a surface-active material lining the peritoneal membrane which is mostly composed of phosphatidylcholine (lecithin) [60]. A decrease in dialysate phospholipids was reported in patients with a low ultrafiltration capacity and in those with peritonitis [61]. Intraperitoneal phosphatidylcholine promptly raised the ultrafiltration rate while the oral route required about 30 days to achieve this effect. The authors suggest that lecithin administration restored the normal peritoneal surfactant lining [61]. To explain augmentation of ultrafiltration after phosphatidylcholine, another group proposed that these phospholipid molecules bind to the anionic sites on the luminal side of the mesothelium, creating a water repellent surface which diminishes the thickness of the unstirred dialysate. This would augment diffusion of solutes from blood to the peritoneum while the hydorphobic lecithin molecules would impede water absorption, favoring ultrafiltration [62]. A recent review by Maher presents an in-depth discussion of the lubricant and surfactant properties of phosphatidlycholine in peritoneal fluid [63].

1.7. Transport of lipids

Transport of fatty acids into peritoneal fluid does not proceed by simple diffusion and convection from plasma. These lipids rapidly diffuse through cell membranes reaching concentration equilibrium across biological membranes within a few minutes. The concentration ratio dialysate/plasma water, however, is far above unity for several fatty acids. Diffusion equilibrium does not occur from plasma to dialysate or from gastrointestinal luminal contents to dialysate and is uninfluenced by circulating concentrations of lipases [11]. Rather, non-esterified fatty acids flux from adjacent adipose tissues to peritoneal fluid and thereafter into portal venous blood [64]. Moreover, peritoneal absorption of barbiturates of comparable size depends on their lipid partition coefficient [46]. Whether lipid soluble drugs can be removed from fat stores in the mesentery by this process remains to be established and methods to exploit this transport mechanism should be studied.

With regard to the triglyceride transport from the peritoneal cavity, animal studies indicate that the major triglyceride absorption occurs across the visceral peritoneum through lymphatic vessels, with little participation of the portal vein system [65].

1.8. Lymphatic absorption

Lymphatics are the primary route for absorption from the peritoneum of isotonic dialysate including macromolecules, particles and formed blood elements [66]. Most absorption occurs via the subdiaphragmatic lymphatics with lesser amounts via the mesenteric lymphatic vessels [67]. Yet, before reaching lymphatic channels macromolecules are probably distributed in the large peritoneal tissue compartment [68]. Absorption from the peritoneum of macromolecules such as albumin, hemoglobin fibrinogen and polydisperse dextran 70 has been reported [69–74] and used as a measure of peritoneal lymphatic flow rates [71, 72, 75–77]. The lymphatic flow rate in CAPD patients is about 11 ml/hr based on radioiodinated serum albumin studies [71], or is about 1 to 2.5 ml/min based on the disappearance rate of intraperitoneal macromolecules [76, 77]. Peritoneal lymph flow is significantly increased during peritonitis [72].

The peritoneal absorption of polydispersed neutral dextrans does not show size discrimination, adding evidence that the major route is by lymphatic transport [74, 78]. The rate of lymphatic flow from the peritoneum correlates positively with ventilation (diaphragmatic movement) and negatively with end expiratory pressure; it decreases with erect posture and with dehydration [79]. Lymphatic absorption subtracts from the gross peritoneal ultrafiltration volume and may be an especially important negative quantity in patients with clinically significant loss of net ultrafiltration. In the rat peritoneal dialysis model, neostigmine increased net ultrafiltration and solute transport by reducing the cumulative lymphatic absorption and without an increase in total transcapillary ultrafiltration [80]. Lower doses of intraperitoneal neostigmine failed to influence lymphatic absorption in CAPD patients [81], but the animal data were confirmed by a case report of a CAPD patient who required high oral dosage of this drug for therapy of myasthenia gravis [82]. In another animal study, phosphatidylcholine augmented net ultrafiltration and solute clearances without increasing flux of water and solutes into the peritoneal cavity, thus acting by reducing lymphatic reabsorption [83].

Similar results were reported in a recent clinical study [84] and preliminary data suggest that phosphatidylcholine affects peritoneal fluid kinetics through its cholinergic action [85]. These studies suggest that limiting lymphatic absorption is a potential mechanism for augmenting peritoneal clearances that should be explored further.

1.9. Mechanisms of accelerating peritoneal transport

An adequate rate of transport by peritoneal dialysis requires enough blood flow to the dialyzing surface, sufficient area and permeability of the membrane for rapid permeation of solutes and ultrafiltration of fluid, as well as rapid diffusion throughout the dialysate which is periodically replaced, thereby maintaining electrochemical gradients.

Mechanisms whereby peritoneal transport might be augmented are outlined below and conceptually presented in Fig. 1. Increasing blood flow to the peritoneum accelerates the rate of solute delivery to the membrane augmenting transport of small highly diffusible solutes, but only modestly.

Increased splanchnic perfusion, however, augments peritoneal clearances of larger solutes at least as much as the transport of smaller solutes. This suggests an increase in peritoneal surface area or permeability resulting from vasodilation, attributed to dilation of the functional peritoneal capillaries combined with perfusion of more capillaries. Spreading the same wall mass over a larger circumference decreases the wall thickness and stretches pores. Intercellular junctions widen, accelerating mass transport [24]. Raising blood flow by local application of vasodilators also opens previously closed capillaries, increasing the surface area available for transport [86, 87]. In the resting state, blood may circulate predominantly through metarterioles. Enhanced perfusion opens more capillaries exposing blood to a more permeable surface. Furthermore, vasodilators with a predominant venular site of action may cause greater increases in diffusion rates but arteriolar dilators may increase the ultrafiltration rate. By increasing blood flow, diffusion and ultrafiltration may occur throughout a greater length of the capillaries than occurs under resting conditions.

Depending on the nature of the vasodilating agent there may be an increase (arteriolar relaxation), decrease (lowered venular tone), or no change (balanced effects) in capillary hydrostatic pressure. This hydrostatic pressure may affect cap-

MECHANISMS OF ACCELERATED PERITONEAL SOLUTE TRANSPORT

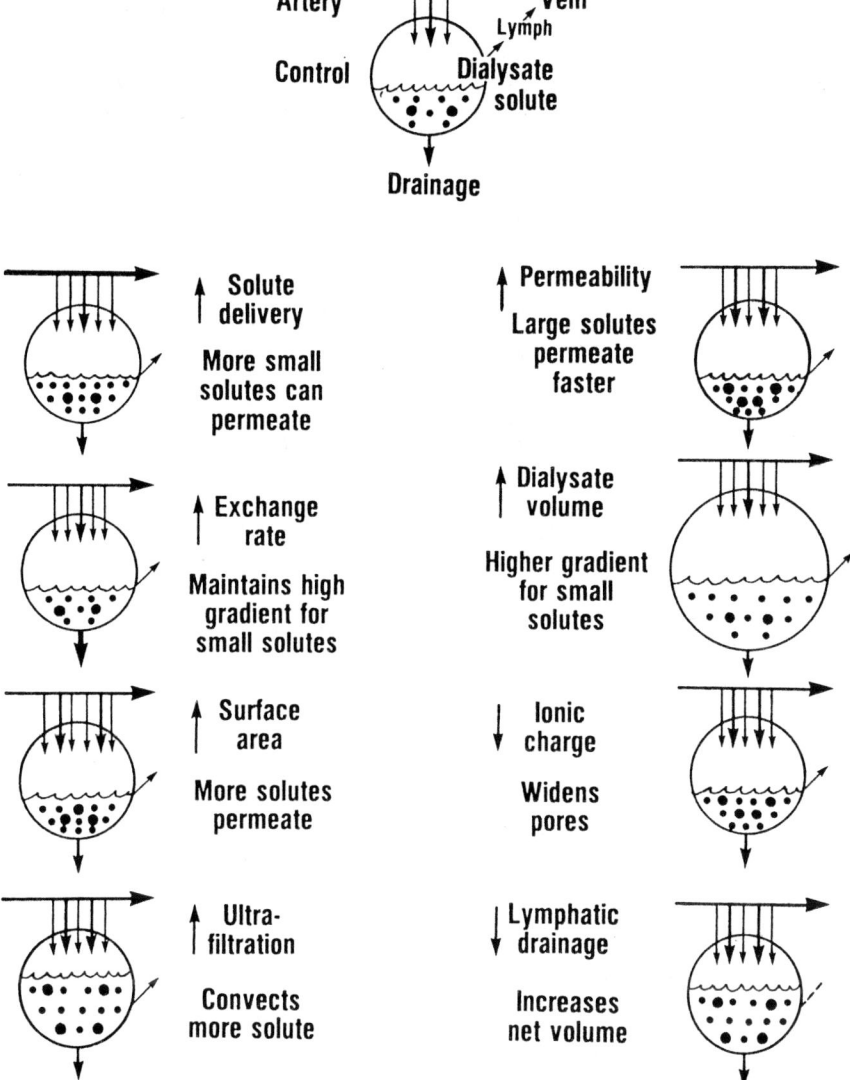

Figure 1. A schematic representation of solute removal by peritoneal dialysis. The circles represent the peritoneum containing small solutes (dots) and larger compounds. The long horizontal arrow above the circle represents peritoneal blood flow. Vertical arrows above the circle display transfer of small (thin lines) and large (thick lines) solutes. The lower arrow indicates drainage, and the side arrow indicates lymphatic absorption.

illary diameter, volume and permeability and is a major determinant of the filtration rate through the capillary. Certain drugs can affect specifically the capillary filtration coefficient, i.e., the volume filtered per unit of pressure per unit of time (ml/mm Hg/min). The rate of ultrafiltration is largely determined, however, by the osmotic gradient across the peritoneum customarily induced by dextrose. As dextrose diffuses, the gradient dissipates rapidly. Increased solute permeability of the peritoneum increases the rate of glucose absorption so a constant fluid flux may represent increased fluid flux/gradient.

The gross ultrafiltration rate and solute mass transfer are offset by dialysate absorption; hence, lowering lymphatic flow rates raises net ultrafiltration and peritoneal clearance of solutes.

Specific drugs may affect directly the permeability of the capillary or the mesothelium [88]. Drugs that influence membrane charge, cell volume, cell metabolism or intercellular junction may directly influence peritoneal permeability without affecting flow rates.

The flow rate of dialysate determines the transport rate, at least of very diffusible solutes by maintaining the chemical gradient. Transport requires dialysate contact with the membrane, which is adequate when fluid volume reaches 1.5 L/M^2 [29]. Rapid exchange of small volumes enhances mixing and increases transport by decreasing the impedance due to unstirred layers. Tidal exchange techniques that leave a residual volume of dialysate in the peritoneum maintain peritoneal surface contact throughout the fluid exchange, also increasing efficiency [30]. Although clinically impractical, vibration used to disrupt stagnant fluid films raised peritoneal transport of urea and glucose in rats [89].

Finally, the transport rate of specific solutes may be accelerated, e.g., by chelating agents or adsorbents, by changing pH thereby influencing nonionic diffusion, by adding protein to dialysate to bind toxins, or by intraperitoneal charged macromolecules [90]. It is likely that maximal transport rates will only be achieved by combinations of maneuvers affecting different resistances to transport as exemplified by the additive transport acceleration effects of intraperitoneal nitroprusside, increased dialysis fluid flow rate, temperature and dextrose concentration [91].

1.10. Restoration of decreased transport rates toward normal

When peritoneal blood flow and clearances have been reduced by disease, transport rates may be restored toward normal by treating the specific abnormality. For example, the mesenteric blood flow rate varies directly with cardiac output. Treatment of heart failure should improve peritoneal clearances, although digoxin is a mesenteric vasoconstrictor. Treatment of heart failure in our patients increased mean clearances of creatinine and urea by 37% and 47% respectively. Chronic congestive heart failure with hepatic congestion may raise portal venous pressure, however, increasing splanchnic volume, capillary diameter and peritoneal permeability.

Loss of blood volume by hemorrhage reduces peritoneal transport of urea and potassium in the dog [92]. When blood pressure and volume are restored toward normal by infusing blood or saline, clearances return to normal. After hemorrhagic hypotension, clearances are not increased by raising blood pressure with norepinephrine nor is transport affected adversely by lowering the blood pressure further with phenoxybenzamine [93]. These studies suggest that blood pressure per se does not influence importantly the efficiency of peritoneal dialysis which does depend, however, on adequate splanchnic volume and perfusion.

Several vascular diseases can impair the mesenteric arterial circulation, so reducing peritoneal transport rates [5]. Vascular damage secondary to diabetes mellitus is not considered reversible and the vasculitis of systemic lupus erythematosus does not readily respond to therapy. Some diseases that cause renal failure, such as malignant hypertension and hemolytic uremic syndrome, cause widespread vascular endothelial injury, inducing platelet thrombi [94]. Reduced peritoneal transport rates complicating these disease are improved by dipyridamole [95]. The augmentation of peritoneal transport rates persists after dipyridamole vasodilation abates and is attributed to its antiplatelet aggregating effect. Peritoneal clearances of patient with normal vasculature improve only minimally and transiently with dipyridamole administered orally or intraperitoneally, and only a modest increment in peritoneal solute transport occurs in animals given dipyridamole intraperitoneally or intravenously [96].

The impaired peritoneal transport that complicates irreversible systemic vascular lesions can also improve toward normal with the local application of vasodilators such as isoproterenol [97, 98]. There is no evidence that increased clearances result from improvement in the vascular disease but rather may be attributed to vasodilation of diseased vessels.

1.11. Increasing peritoneal transport above normal values

Drugs may increase peritoneal transport rates to values exceeding normal, both in patients without vascular disease [99] and in animal models [100–102]. Evidence against a nonspecific effect due to an intraperitoneal inflammatory reaction includes the following. Effects on mass transport can be separated from those on fluid flux and solvent drag [8, 9, 56, 103]. Transport rates increase without the vasodilator inducing an intraperitoneal inflammatory exudate [99]. Certain drugs accelerate transport when given either intravenously or intraperitoneally [96, 104]. Peritoneal transport rates respond in accord with the known vasoactive properties, increasing with vasodilators and decreasing with vasoconstrictor agents [104, 105]. Solute response may be selective, based for example on ionic charge. Finally, inactive metabolites and drug vehicles do not affect peritoneal transport rates [8, 105].

Many studies suggest that peritoneal clearances will increase only if a vasodilator selectively affects the splanchnic vasculature or is applied locally, e.g., by intraperitoneal instillation. Intravenously such drugs may cause widespread vasodilation, decreasing blood pressure, splanchnic perfusion and splanchnic volume, thereby lowering peritoneal transport rates. To date, membrane-active agents have only augmented transport when applied locally, i.e. instilled intraperitoneally.

1.12. Isproterenol enhancement of peritoneal mass transport

In patients with reduced peritoneal clearance, Nolph et al. improved transport rates by adding isoproterenol (0.06 mg/L) to the dialysis solution [97, 98]. Mean clearances increased to the lower range of normal but only transiently and not all patients improved significantly [106]. No systemic effects of intraperitoneal isoproterenol were detected even with cardiac monitoring. Such use of isoproterenol has been explored in greater detail in animals. In acute studies in anesthetized dogs, intraperitoneal isoproterenol increased urea and creatinine clearance by 45% and 30%, respectively, but subpressor intravenous doses of isoproterenol did not augment transport [101]. In normal, unanesthetized rabbits, 0.04 μmol/kg of intraperitoneal isoproterenol raised urea and creatinine clearance by 50%, but osmotically induced water flux was unaffected [107]. No systemic effects were observed. On exposure to light and air, isoproterenol rapidly became ineffective.

Despite raising mesenteric blood flow to 188% of control by intravenous isoproterenol, Felt et al. [36] showed that clearances did not increase. With intraperitoneal isoproterenol, a comparable flow increase raised peritoneal inulin and creatinine clearances by 27% and 18%, respectively. The disparity in blood flow and clearance changes suggests that capillary blood volume may be as important as blood flow in mediating changes in permeability.

Isoproterenol, a beta adrenergic agonist, relaxes the mesenteric vascular bed. When used clinically to accelerate peritoneal transport, no systemic toxicity was shown, despite continuous use of isoproterenol for 20 exchanges [108]. Yet, a better transport accelerator continues to be sought because of the potential cardiotoxicity and the need to apply the drug topically.

1.13. Nitroprusside augmentation of peritoneal mass transfer

The observations by Nolph et al. [106] that intraperitoneal nitroprusside increases peritoneal mass transport have been confirmed in multiple laboratories in several species [109–112]. Urea and creatinine clearances increase as much as 50% above control with greater increments in inulin clearances and protein loss, consistent with enhanced peritoneal permeability or area or both rather than simply increased solute delivery. Osmotic ultrafiltration increases slightly [110] or not at all as rapid glucose absorption dissipates the osmotic gradient. Nitroprusside-induced increases in mass transport are dose dependent and can be seen with as little as 1.0 mg/L [113]. It has also been suggested that increments in peritoneal mass transfer coefficients with topical nitroprusside can indicate peritoneal vascular reserve [114]. Systemic effects of nitroprusside have not been detected in most studies and intravenously the drug does not accelerate peritoneal mass transport. The transport increment is sustained for several exchanges, and on discontinuation may persist somewhat for up to 2 hours [115]. Augmented transport represents an increase in permeance of the peritoneum (mass transfer coefficient x area) due to capillary, especially venular, dilation and from opening of previously nonperfused capillaries [86, 113]. Although it is metabolized to thiocyanate, this toxic metabolite is rapidly dialyzed and no evidence of accumulation has been observed with repeated nitroprusside instillation.

1.14. Dipyridamole effects on peritoneal dialysis efficiency

Dipyridamole is an orally effective general smooth muscle relaxant with pharmacologic properties similar to those of papaverine. It rapidly but transiently vasodilates [116] and has a sustained antiplatelet aggregating effect, which may explain the restoration of clearances toward normal in patient with intravascular platelet aggregations [96]. Peritoneal transport of urea and creatinine increase by 43% and 70%, respectively, in patients with normal vasculature given 300 mg/day of dipyridamole orally [117, 118]. The clearance of radiolabeled EDTA and DPTA increase by 75% and 41%, respectively [118]. Modest increments in the clearances of uric acid and inulin also occur but are delayed for a few days [119]. In normal rabbits, dipyridamole given intravenously (0.5 mg/kg) or intraperitoneally (2.5 mg/kg) increased urea and creatinine clearances by 39% and 16%, respectively [96, 120]. The limited effectiveness and the transient vasodilator response of dipyridamole are reflected by two randomized control studies which did not demonstrate significant increases in peritoneal transport [121, 122]. Nevertheless, dipyridamole may be useful for selected patients when systemic disease with platelet thrombi affects mesenteric vessels and an oral agent is preferred.

1.15. Influence of cathecholamines on peritoneal transport kinetics

To explore further vasoactive effects on peritoneal transport, catecholamines have been studied in animals undergoing peritoneal dialysis. Gutman *et al.* [101] noted lower increments in dialysate urea with large intraperitoneal doses of dopamine in dogs, but did not measure dialysate volume. Because blood pressure increased, the lower urea accumulation in the dialysate was attributed to splanchnic vasoconstriction. To offset vasoconstriction, Parker *et al.* [123] added alpha adrenergic blocker to the dialysis fluid. With intraperitoneal phentolamine and intravenous dopamine, peritoneal clearances increased in dogs. In patients, however, Chan *et al.* [124] observed no effect of low (4 mg/L) or high doses (20–160 mg/L) of intraperitoneal dopamine on dialysate urea, creatinine or phosphate. They did not measure dialysate volume, so the effect on ultrafiltration rate could not be discerned. In rabbits, intraperitoneal dopamine caused dose-related (0.6 to 1.8 mg/kg) increases in peritoneal urea clearance [104]. The increments occurred with lower doses than those used by Gutman *et al.* [101] and drug concentrations (10 to 30 mg/L) within the range studied by Chan *et al.* [124]. Species differences may account for the discrepant results.

Intravenous 1-norepinephrine significantly decreased peritoneal clearances of urea and creatinine in unanesthetized rabbits [104, 124]. Dose dependent decrements correlated with the pressor response [125]. Comparable pressor doses of intravenous dopamine increased clearances of urea and creatinine to 145% of control values, whereas low doses had minimal and inconsistent effects [125].

Osmotic water flux increased only slightly (from 0.18 to 0.24 ml/kg/min) but significantly ($p < 0.02$). Because dopamine vasoconstricts venules relatively more than arterioles as compared to norepinephrine [48], augmented water flux could be mediated by increased hydrostatic pressure rather than a change in hydraulic permeability. Dopamine-augmented solute transport was unaffected by concurrent beta blockade with propranolol, was decreased by simultaneous alpha adrenergic receptor blockade by phentolamine, and was abolished by haloperidol blockade of dopaminergic receptors [125]. Accordingly, the augmented transport is attributed to dopamine receptor mediated mesenteric vasodilation and in part, alpha adrenergic somatic vasoconstriction increasing blood pressure while mesenteric blood flow is maintained. Although dopamine may not be suitable for augmenting efficiency of routine peritoneal dialysis, these data argue strongly that it should be preferable to 1-norephinephrine when vasopressor therapy is required during peritoneal dialysis. Seeking an effective oral agent we studied the influence of ibopamine, an analogue. Only minimal increments in fluid and solute flux occurred with ibopamine, whether given by mouth, intravenously or intraperitoneally to normal rabbits [126].

1.16. Other vasodilators that affect peritoneal transport

No consistent change in peritoneal clearance of urea or creatinine was observed in patients given 20 to 40 mg of hydralazine intraperitoneally, which decreased blood pressure slightly [106]. Hydralazine (168 daltons) should be rapidly absorbed from the peritoneal fluid, but its pharmacologic action may depend on biotransformation to an active compound. Hence, widespread vasodilation may occur despite local application with no preferential effect on splanchnic blood flow or volume.

Theophylline acts as a nonselective antagonist of two types of adenosine receptors which mediate opposite effects on vascular tone [127]. In rabbits, changes in solute and water fluxes were inconsistent after intraperitoneal or intravenous aminophylline in doses exceeding the therapeutic range [128]. Presumably widespread vasodilation blunted any potential gain in peritoneal blood flow.

Diazoxide caused a modest increase in peritoneal clearances of urea and creatinine and a significant decrement in blood pressure when administered intraperitoneally to patients at a dose of 100 to 300 mg [106]. An increase in ultrafiltration rate approaching 50% of control values was found inconsistently. In another study, 150 mg of diazoxide increased peritoneal clearances of urea, creatinine and phosphate by 58%, 48% and 39%, respectively [118].

The intraperitoneal administration of 5 mg of phentolamine did not influence peritoneal solute transport rates in five patients so investigated, nor did it affect osmotic water flux [106].

In anesthetized rats, histamine (4 to 8 μg) raised only modestly (9% to 16%) the clearances of urea and inulin, whereas 3 μg of bradykinin augmented these clearances by 13% and 25%, respectively [109]. Histamine causes overt capillary dilation and increased permeability with protein exudation, which can be blocked in rabbits by both H_1 and H_2 receptor antagonists [129]. Minimal effects of histamine on small solute transport may reflect decreased plasma volume due to protein loss. In isolated rat mesentery, viewed by television microscopy after fluorescein labeling, protein exudation is also demonstrable [24]. Dilation is most prominent in the venous end of the capillary and similar changes are noted with nitroprusside.

The effects of calcium channel blockers on peritoneal mass transport have been evaluated by several investigators. In the anesthetized rat model, verapamil and diltiazem given locally, modestly but significantly increased peritoneal clearances of urea without enhancing protein losses [130]. Significantly augmentation of small solutes clearances and ultrafiltration associated with diminished glucose reabsorption were reported with intraperitoneal verapamil in CAPD patients [131]. Similarly, in another clinical study, intraperitoneal administration of nifedipine resulted in increased urea and creatinine clearances and higher ultrafiltration rates due to the decreased peritoneal glucose transfer [132]. In hypertensive CAPD patients, oral nifedipine administered in blood pressure controlling dosage brought about significant augmentation of peritoneal clearance of creatinine, and β_2-microglobulin associated with higher glucose reabsorption, while the rate of ultrafiltration remained unaffected [133]. These studies suggest calcium channel blockers action on the arteriolar end of peritoneal capillaries without a consistent effect on the venular permeability. It is noteworthy that Lamperi et al. [134] proposed an immunologic mechanism to account for verapamil action in CAPD patients. They demonstrated that in patients with low peritoneal permeability, improvement in ultrafiltration rates after intraperitoneal verapamil is associated with normalization of elevated lymphomonokines production by peritoneal lymphocytes and macrophages.

Modest increases in urea clearance and glucose absorption and a marked exaggeration of protein loss followed intraperitoneal instillation of very large doses of captopril, an angiotension converting enzyme inhibitor in rats [135]. These increments, despite drug induced systemic hypotension, may reflect increased blood flow, surface area, or permeability. Similarly, glucose, creatinine and β_2-microglobulin transport rates were meaningfully increased after oral administration of hypotensive doses of enalapril in a study performed in CAPD patients [133]. Yet, smaller doses of oral captopril significantly reduced peritoneal protein loss in diabetic CAPD patients, with only a small decrease in their mean blood pressure [136]. It is uncertain whether this change in peritoneal permeability reflects the blockade of a baseline level of angiotension II activity or the action of the drug on kinins.

It is thus apparent that many vasoactive drugs can affect peritoneal transport rates. Some have been studied in a limited number of species, only in a few animals, or at only one dose. Isoproterenol and nitroprusside consistently augmented clearances in several studies from multiple laboratories. Dipyridamole advantageously can be given by mouth and is particularly effective when platelet aggregation limits capillary filling.

Norepinephrine as anticipated consistently decreased clearances, whereas dopamine did and at certain doses appreciably increased transport rates. Interestingly, dihydroergotamine, an agent that accelerates blood flow by causing somatic venoconstriction, reduces peritoneal ultrafiltration rates and urea clearance, presumably due to the decreased plasma volume [126, 137]. No consistent change in small solutes transport was seen after modest doses of intraperitoneal papaverine [138].

Because numerous other drugs are administered for various indications to patients undergoing peritoneal dialysis, the influences of a variety of other agents on peritoneal mass transport have been explored.

1.17. Prostaglandin modulation of peritoneal transport

Prostaglandins control regional blood flow by virtue of their capability of modulating vasoconstrictor responses [41]. The prostaglandins are unsaturated

20 carbon lipids biosynthesized from arachidonic acid and other precursors by prostaglandin synthetase, an enzyme present in tissues [139]. Depending on the local concentration of the specific terminal enzymes, e.g. endoperoxide reductase leading to PGF_{2a} or endoperoxide isomerase leading to PGE_2, a given product predominates in a given tissue. Regional blood flow is one determinant of enzyme activity. In circulation the prostaglandins are degraded during a single passage through the lung, thereby acting only locally with the exception of prostacyclin and thromboxanes which have half-lives of a few minutes. Biosynthesis of these compounds can be inhibited by various drugs at varied sites in the synthetic pathway. Prostaglandins of the PGA, PGE or PGI series vasodilate, whereas PGF_{2a} and thromboxanes are potent vasoconstrictors [140, 141]. These prostaglandins act locally in arterial walls to influence vascular tone and modulate the response of vascular smooth muscle to other vasoactive agents [142].

Intraperitoneal instillation of PGA_1 or PGE_1 increased peritoneal clearances of urea and creatinine modestly in alert normal rabbits, whereas 125 μg/kg of PGE_2 significantly raised creatinine clearance to 132% and urea clearance to 180% of control values [100, 105, 143]. In contrast, intraperitoneally the vasoconstrictor PGF_{2a} (125 μg/kg) decreased peritoneal clearances to 80% (urea) and 82% (creatinine) of control [105]. These prostaglandins did not affect fluid flux and were totally ineffective when given intravenously. Neither intravenous nor intraperitoneal administration of prostacyclin affected peritoneal solute or water transport significantly over a dose range from 25 to 125 μg/kg [105]. It is interpreted that prostacyclin caused widespread vasodilation so that mesenteric blood flow and volume were not selectively increased. Hence, transport remained unaffected.

Prostaglandin synthetase stimulators and inhibitors have not had pronounced effects on peritoneal transport under baseline conditions. Oral pretreatment with 10 to 21 mg/kg of sulfinpyrazone, a potent stimulator of prostaglandin synthetase, did not alter peritoneal clearances significantly [143]. When mefenamic acid, a prostaglandin synthetase inhibitor, is administered intravenously or intraperitoneally to alert intact rabbits in doses sufficient to inhibit platelet function, neither the peritoneal clearances of creatinine or urea nor water flux changed [143]. Oral pretreatment of rabbits with indomethacin blocked platelet aggregation but did not change clearance or ultrafiltration rates significantly [143]. Intraperitoneal indomethacin increases the size of pinocytotic vesicles and narrows intercellular spaces in the rabbit, however [144]. Alteration of prostaglandin synthetase affects both vasoconstrictor and vasodilator prostaglandins. Hence, regional blood flow may not change. Yet, when vasodilator prostaglandin activity predominates to compensate for increased renin-angiotensin activity or ischemic vascular disease, aspirin or indomethacin decreases regional blood flow [145]. However, the reduction of clearances induced by intravenous 1-norepinephrine, which should be accompanied by vasodilator prostaglandin stimulation, is exaggerated by pretreatment with indomethacin in only half of the animals so studied. These results suggest that endogenous prostaglandins do not play a major role in regulating peritoneal blood flow under ordinary circumstances. But in patients that depend on vasodilator prostaglandins to maintain organ perfusion, blockade of prostaglandin synthetase could impair transport and a history of exposure to such drugs should be sought if clearances are low. Intraperitoneally, the prostaglandin precursor arachidonic acid (1.5 to 5.6 mg/kg) increased creatinine clearance by 36% and urea clearance by 24%, however, suggesting an effect of endogenous prostaglandins, but systemic use of indomethacin did not block this increase [143, 146]. With peritonitis the increased solute transport rates are accompanied by augmented prostaglandin release, abnormalities that can be blocked by indomethacin [42].

1.18. Vasodilator gastrointestinal hormones

Glucagon and secretin are structurally similar polypeptide gastrointestinal hormones that increase mesenteric blood flow by as much as 100% above baseline when pharmacologic doses are given, but augment different gastrointestinal functions [147]. Secretin, like cholecystokinin, increases predominantly hepatic blood flow, but glucagon has the more potent effect on the mesenteric circulation. Gastrin, structurally similar to cholecystokinin, also increases mesenteric blood flow [147]. The augmented mesenteric circulation can be induced by intraduodenal instillation of corn oil, 1-phenylalanine or acid, after a short latency consistent with the physiologic release of secretin or cholecystokinin [148]. Similar changes can be induced by low intravenous doses of these hormone. The effects of secretin and cholecystokinin on mesenteric blood flow are additive and potentiated by theophylline [149]. This hormonal mesenteric vasodilation is attributed to direct relaxation of vascular tone presumably mediated by cyclic AMP.

When administered intravenously immediately predialysis, 30 µg/kg of glucagon significantly increased peritoneal clearances of urea and creatinine in alert rabbits [103, 150]. The same dose of glucagon intraperitoneally did not augment clearances significantly. Since this large peptide should traverse the peritoneum slowly, hormonal activity presumably occurs at the endothelial rather than the mesothelial surface. Nevertheless, much higher doses given intraperitoneally do increase clearance somewhat.

Bolus administration of these hormones is more effective than continuous infusion despite their short half-lives [151]. Nevertheless, intravenous infusion of about 30 µg/kg/hr increased mesenteric arterial blood flow and peritoneal inulin clearance (but no creatinine) in dogs, unlike intraperitoneal instillation [36]. Slight increments in urea and creatinine clearances occurred with intravenous secretin or cholecystokinin [103]. Intravenously, but not intraperitoneally, secretin (10 U/kg) increased osmotic water flux in rabbits from 0.19 to 0.29 ml/kg/min [103]. The endogenous release of cholecystokinin or secretin or their intra-arterial infusion relaxes precapillary sphincters and increases the capillary filtration coefficient from 0.05 to 0.10 ml/min/mm Hg/100 g [152]. Secretin also increases the capillary filtration coefficient in the mesenteric vasculature of the cat [47]. Neither glucagon nor cholecystokinin affected peritoneal water flux during dialysis in rabbits, however [103]. The separation of the effects of gastrointestinal hormones on diffusive and on convective transport suggests the possible use of separate pharmacologic agents acting additively.

1.19. Other hormones and drugs affecting peritoneal blood flow and diffusion

Parenteral administration of vasopressin to anesthetized dogs decreased peritoneal clearances of small solutes, consistent with a hormonally mediated reduction in mesenteric blood flow [153, 154]. Since inulin clearance increased slightly under such circumstances, a concurrent increase in membrane permeability has been postulated [122], in accord with the accelerated transport that occurs in isolated membrane preparations [155].

In preliminary studies in rabbits and patients, large doses of methyl prednisolone increased peritoneal clearances by as much as 69%, but such augmented transport was observed inconsistently [156].

The peritoneal transport rates of potassium and ^{131}iodide increased when streptokinase or serotonin were administered systemically to anesthetized dogs [153]. Whether these agents affect peritoneal permeability directly or augment blood flow remains to be determined.

In sedated rabbits dialyzed with a hypertonic dialysis solution containing 0.25% procaine hydrochloride, peritoneal urea and inulin clearances increased by more than 60% [157]. The effect persisted for at least an hour after procaine was discontinued. Procaine vasodilates, which may augment transport. However, the addition of procaine to either side of the isolated mesothelium increased transport after a transient decrease. This effect may be due to disruption of the microfilaments of tight junctions between cells.

Variations in electrolyte concentrations also influence peritoneal blood flow and permeability. For example, topically applied low potassium solutions vasoconstrict several vascular beds including the mesentric, interfering with normal Na-K-ATPase activity and should thereby decrease peritoneal transport efficiency. Modest increments in potassium concentration vasodilate, an effect that is inhibited by oubain [158].

The dialysis solution itself affects the peritoneal vasculature. Miller and colleagues [86, 159] have shown that the mesenteric vasculature transiently vasoconstricts and then vasodilates when exposed to peritoneal dialysis solution. The prolonged vasodilation depends on the presence of hyperosmolar dialysis fluid containing either acetate or lactate. Bicarbonate buffered isotonic Krebs solution did not induce vasodilation.

1.20. Membrane surface-active agents

Penzotti and Mattocks [102, 160, 161] accelerated peritoneal transport of labeled urea and creatinine in sedated rabbits by adding a variety of surface-acting agents including dioctyl sodium sulfosuccinate, cetyl trimethyl ammonium chloride, and N-myristyl-β-amino-proprionate. These compounds have not been employed clinically but may help identify agents for clinical use. More recently, Dunham et al. [162] verified a dose-dependent rise in creatinine and urea clearances when docusate sodium was given intraperitoneally to tranquilized rabbits. The effect persisted for 5 hr.

The solvent dimethyl sulfoxide did not augment clearance of potassium or urea in rabbits, however, except to the extent that large doses intraperitoneally created an osmotic gradient and increased convective transport [163].

Cytochalasins disrupt microfilaments of cellular junctions. Cytochalasin D given intraperitoneally raises the clearances of creatinine and urea in the rabbit, consistent with augmented diffusion through intercellular gaps [8]. Concurrently the ultrafiltration rate decreases, attributed to accelerated glucose transport, diminishing the osmotic gradient more rapidly, as occurs in acute peritonitis [164]. Similarly, cytochalasin B, D and E increase permeability of the peritoneum to urea, inulin and albumin in rats [165]. Only cytochalasin B actions were significantly reversible, which may relate to the unique ability to affect carrier proteins of the cell membrane.

The addition of 1 mg/kg of furosemide to hypertonic peritoneal dialysis solution augmented sodium movement, accompanying osmotically induced water flux in rabbits [56]. Normally, electrolytes do not accompany water in the same concentration as exists in plasma water, suggesting that membrane charge impedes transport, a phenomenon that is interrupted by furosemide. Intraperitoneal furosemide also caused a 27% increase in peritoneal urea clearance, but no demonstrable changes in transport rates occur in patients undergoing intermittent peritoneal dialysis when treated systemically with this diuretic. Moreover, oral use of furosemide did not affect sodium, potassium or water transport in patients undergoing continuous ambulatory peritoneal dialysis [166]. But, furosemide does increase the peritoneal transport of uric acid and of barbiturates [167]. Intraperitoneally, 1.25 mg/kg of ethacrynic acid did not affect sodium flux with the bulk flow of water across the peritoneum but augmented urea clearance to about 165% of baseline [56]. Patients treated by CAPD may experience a restoration of lost ultrafiltration capacity after treatment by furosemide or by hemofiltration [168]. A specific effect of furosemide has been postulated, but correction of an overexpanded splanchnic volume by decreasing glucose absorption could restore ultrafiltration capacity.

Charged macromolecules may also interact with peritoneal anionic sites, altering membrane ultrastructure and permeability. In rats, local administration of protamine, a polycation, markedly increases peritoneal permeability to inulin and to a lesser extent urea, associated with a partial disruption of the mesothelial junctions [169]. In rabbits, protamine-induced rise in peritoneal permeability to proteins can be reversed by heparin, which provides additional evidence for the physiological importance of negative electric charges on the membrane [170]. Similarly in rats, cationic poly-1-lysine augments peritoneal permeability for urea, inulin and albumin, while with the anionic poly-1-glutamic acid there was an opposite trend [171]. These results were confirmed in a rabbit model by Pietrzak et al. [172] who showed that intraperitoneal administration of poly-1-lysine is associated with a significant increase in ultrafiltration rate and higher peritoneal permeability to protein and dextran. The ultrafiltrate sodium concentration was also increased, implying that elimination of the hindrance of anionic charges on the peritoneal transport barrier allowed sodium to follow water flux more proportionately. These findings contrast with those of Breborowicz et al. [173] who found decreased hydraulic permeability of the mesothelium in vitro when exposed to cationic ferritin or alcian blue. In vitro studies of isolated mesothelium, however, may not relate closely to in vivo conditions, where the capillary wall and interstitium are the more important transfer barriers. Further evaluation of polycations as transport accelerators, particularly for patients with impaired peritoneal transfer capacity is undoubtedly warranted.

1.21. Increasing ultrafiltration rates

Because the peritoneal ultrafiltration rate is normally low compared to the clearance of low molecular weight solute (10% to 20%), even doubling this rate has only a modest effect on removal of such substances as urea and drugs [174]. Ultrafiltration contributes importantly, however, to the removal of large, poorly diffusible solutes as occurs with hemodialysis [175]. Mechanisms of pharmacological alteration of ultrafiltration rates have been recently reviewed by Khanna et al. [176].

The ultrafiltration rate can be increased by raising the capillary hydrostatic pressure, by venular constriction, or by arteriolar relaxation. Few drugs appear to increase capillary hydrostatic pressure, but this mechanism can account for increased ultrafiltration by dopamine [125]. Surface-active agents can increase ultrafiltration by narrowing the stagnant dialysate layer and creating a water-repellent lining on the surface of the peritoneum

[62]. Factors that diminish peritoneal lymph flow raise net ultrafiltration rate by minimizing the loss of fluid by absorption [80].

Secretin increases the hydraulic permeability of the peritoneal membrane [99]. This selective action on the splanchnic bed occurs from the vascular side only. The aminonucleoside, puromycin, which causes glomerular lesions with increased macromolecular permeability, also induces this effect on peritoneal capillaries [177]. After a few days, puromycin causes a proteinaceous ascites in rats with faster permeation of labeled test solutes than in control rats. The prolonged effect of such a permeability augmenting drug could be commendable, but other nonglomerular capillary beds are probably also affected, which would make it hazardous even in anephric patients.

Amphotericin B increases the rate of ultrafiltration per osmotic gradient, i.e. the ultrafiltration coefficient [9]. Above 0.5 mg/kg there is no dose effect, and it is effective only from the serosal side [9, 178]. Amphotericin B creates channels in biological membranes for solute and water penetration. Increments in peritoneal solute clearances with amphotericin B are only modest and can be accounted for by enhanced convection [9]. However, peritoneal mass transport of sodium also increases. Because osmotic ultrafiltrate during peritoneal dialysis is hyponatric, the sodium gradient so established is an impediment to water transport that amphotericin B cancels [178]. Amphotericin B or safer analogues could help treat the reduced ultrafiltration capacity that occasionally complicates long-term peritoneal dialysis.

Phosphatidylcholine increases ultrafiltration rates in patients with peritonitis and those who acquire low filtration capacity, presumably by restoring mesothelial surfactant [61]. In rabbits, phosphatidylcholine increases net ultrafiltrate volume [62], an effect that only becomes significant after hours of peritoneal dialysis in accord with our studies, showing ineffectiveness during hourly exchanges. Rather than the surfactant effect, phosphatidylcholine may impede lymphatic absorption [83].

Chlorpromazine (2 mg/L) intraperitoneally also increases the ultrafiltration rate and solute clearance, largely by increased convection and presumably by its surfactant effect [179]. This drug decreased surface tension of the dialysate.

Neostigmine decreases the rate of lymphatic flow and thereby increases net ultrafiltration in rats [80]. Anticholinesterase agents also have complex hemodynamic effects which could influence peritoneal transport and increase gastrointestinal motility which would enhance dialysate mixing.

The osmotic gradient across the peritoneum is the major determinant of the rate of ultrafiltration per surface area. This gradient depends mainly on the dialysate dextrose concentration but is also influenced by sodium and urea gradients, plasma oncotic pressure and the rate of dextrose absorption. Higher ultrafiltration rates due to diminished glucose reabsorption were reported with intraperitoneal calcium channel blockers in CAPD patients [131, 132]. Ronco et al. [180] suggested that maximal rates of ultrafiltration are inhibited by the steep curvilinear rise in plasma protein oncotic pressure in the peritoneal capillaries, reflecting the limited blood flow rate. Nitroprusside vasodilation did not raise the ultrafiltration ceiling, however [181]. We demonstrated that the ultrafiltration coefficient decrease in rabbits as intraperitoneal dwell is prolonged, suggesting some concentration polarization, which could be corrected by increasing turbulence at the membrane interfaces [182]. Increased absorption of dextrose will accompany most manipulations that enhance solute permeability and hence dissipate the glucose osmotic gradient faster, reducing ultrafiltration. Insulin is required to maintain low plasma glucose levels and achieve the maximal gradient. Exogenous insulin added intraperitoneally does not increase the glucose mass transfer coefficient [183]. Because excessive glucose absorption can be hazardous, alternative osmotic agents have been evaluated. Amino acids added to the dialysate offer a nutritional advantage but may be costly. Dextrans, glucose polymers and cross-linked gelatins are large enough to permeate the peritoneum poorly, thereby maintaining the osmotic gradient throughout long dwell exchange [184], but are eliminated slowly after absorption. An ideal agent for achieving maximal ultrafiltration has not been identified.

1.22. Transport acceleration of specific solutes

Removal of barbiturates may be accelerated by increasing dialysate pH with tris buffer, thereby influencing the rate of non-inionic diffusion [184]. Alkalinization of peritoneal dialysate by THAM also raised uric acid transport [185]. Drugs that counteract the membrane anionic charge should enhance removal of charged solutes. For example, hexadimethrine bromide increases peritoneal phosphate clearances but does not affect urea or glucose transport [126] and a polycation especially augments phosphate transfer [90]. Adding albumin to peritoneal dialysis solution enhances removal of barbiturates [187], etchlorvynol [188] and salicylate [189], and predictably should augment the clearance of numerous other drugs that circulate bound to plasma proteins, such as some aminoglycoside antibiotics, quinine and phenytoin. Increases in peritoneal clearance of barbiturates, phenytoin and salicylates have been achieved by agents that displace protein binding [190]. Albumin enriched peritoneal dialysis fluid also augments removal of trace metals such as copper [191]. Enhanced removal of trace elements can also be accomplished by chelation [192–194]. For lipophilic drugs such as glutethimide and short-acting barbiturates, transport can be enhanced by adding lipid to the dialysate [195]. In general, the removal of drugs is too slow by peritoneal dialysis for treating severe overdosage. These specific effects such as chelation, however, may influence therapeutic drug concentrations and certain uremic metabolites.

1.23. Peritoneal protein loss attenuation

Protein loss is a cumbersome complication of CAPD [196] particularly in patients with efficient peritoneal mass transport. Since long dwell times have more effect on the removal of macromolecules than on the small solute clearances, CCPD with the use of increased number of short dialysis cycles may be helpful in patients with an excessive peritoneal protein leakage [197].

Augmented protein loss is associated with peritonitis and it can be reduced by inhibition of prostaglandin synthetase [42], suggesting that prostaglandins play a role in the control of peritoneal capillary permeability. In a preliminary study captopril significantly reduced protein loss into the peritoneum in diabetic CAPD patients, presumably by modulating vasoconstrictive responses of peritoneal capillaries [136]. In rabbits a marked increase in protein elimination into the peritoneum occurred after addition of histamine, an effect blocked by its antagonist [129]. Because histamine may be involved in the pathogenesis of hypersensitivity reactions to drugs, leachables or contaminants of the dialysis solution, anti-histamine agents could be therapeutic in such circumstances.

Several lines of evidence support the important role of intact anionic sites on the peritoneal transport barrier in the restriction of the passage of charged macromolecules to the peritoneal cavity. Partial neutralization of anionic sites may account for the findings from the animal study in which the dialysate pH adjustment from 5.6 up to 7.4 significantly increased peritoneal protein loss in the presence of nitroprusside [86]. Another group demonstrated that transperitoneal protein loss was substantially enhanced by protamine in rabbits. Neutralization of protamine with heparin prevented this effect [170]. Blood to peritoneum transport rates of cationic DEAE dextran were less that those for both neutral dextran and dextran sulfate in a recent animal study [198].

Augmentation of the anionic charges could be expected to have a beneficial effect on the peritoneal protein loss. Indeed, local administration of polyanionic chondroitin sulfate diminished bidirectional transport of protein during peritoneal dialysis in rats [199]. The authors postulate that this action could be due to the trapping of the molecules of the polymer in the peritoneal interstitium.

These early studies suggest that attenuation of peritoneal protein loss by pharmacologic agents is likely to become clinically useful in the future.

1.24. Conclusions

It is easy for clinicians as well as bioengineers to forget that the peritoneum, unlike synthetic hemodialysis membranes, is alive. The mesenteric circulation is remarkable for its size and complexity, and until recently for the paucity of knowledge about its physiology. The numerous drugs and hormones that affect mesenteric blood flow and membrane physiology should have predictable effects on peritoneal transport parameters (44,200). Patients undergoing chronic dialysis characteristically receive several drugs regularly, many of which have hemodynamic and membrane transport effects. The influences of these agents on the peritoneum must be ascertained. Those treated for acute problems, for example in an intensive care unit, are exposed to even a greater abundance of drugs potentially altering transport. Rational use of drugs and other physiological manipulations in patients maintained by peritoneal dialysis requires an understanding of their effects on peritoneal blood flow and permeability. It is naive to consider the peritoneum as an inert membrane with constant blood flow and transport characteristics. Further investigation of the interactions of drugs and the peritoneum may identify optimal methods for augmenting transport efficiency safely.

2. Pharmacokinetic aspects of peritoneal transport of drugs

The second part of this chapter has been divided in two major sections: the first section covers some basic pharmacokinetic concepts in the presence of normal and abnormal renal function. More detailed information on this subject is available in standard textbooks and reviews on pharmacokinetics [201–204].

In addition, a general discussion on the major factors determining the transperitoneal transport after systemic and intraperitoneal administration of drugs will be provided.

In the second section, the pharmacokinetic data obtained with drugs, commonly used in either intermittent or continuous ambulatory peritoneal dialysis patients, have been collected in tables. Following each table, recommendations for eventual dose adaptations in peritoneal dialysis patients are provided.

2.1. Basic pharmacokinetics

Drugs produce their therapeutic or toxic effects in biological systems by reacting with receptor sites or other sites of action located in target tissues. The intensity of these effects is, in most cases, determined by the concentration of the drug in the direct environment of the site of action (the "biophase"). It is not possible to determine drug concentrations in the biophase. However, all tissues are supplied by blood (or plasma) and often a complex relationship exists between the drug concentration in the biophase and that in plasma water; the latter can be measured to approach the former. Drug responses to a particular dose are therefore commonly related to the concentration of the drug (or in some cases of its metabolites), in plasma water. With the usual methods, however, total plasma drug concentrations are measured, i.e. drug bound to plasma proteins, as well as free drug, dissolved in plasma water. If the protein binding of the drug is constant, total drug concentration in plasma water will reflect free drug concentration. If however, the protein binding of the drug has changed, this relationship will change and the intensity of effect will be smaller or larger than expected for a particular total plasma drug concentration. After administration of a drug, absorption from the site of administration to the plasma (in case of extravascular administration), distribution from the plasma to organs and tissues, elimination by biotransformation (predominantly in the liver) or by excretion (predominantly via the kidneys), take place. As a consequence of these events, drug concentrations in plasma water and in the biophase, change with time as does the pharmacological effect.

2.1.1. Compartmental models

Pharmacokinetics involves the mathematical description of the time course of the concentration of the drug (and, in some cases, its metabolites), in biologic fluids after drug administration. In most models, compartments are used; it is important to realize that a pharmacokinetic compartment does not necessarily correspond to a given anatomical body fluid compartment. The time course of the plasma drug concentrations can usually be adequately described by a one-compartment model; the body is viewed as one space, in which the drug is distributed rapidly and homogenously.

Although this is an oversimplification, such a one-compartment model is often satisfactory for the study of the pharmacokinetics of a drug, e.g., in order to determine its optimal dosage.

A two-compartment model (Fig. 2) consists of a central and a peripheral compartment. The central compartment includes the plasma, but also the extracellular fluid of highly perfused organs such as heart, lung, liver and kidney. The peripheral compartment involves the compartment in which

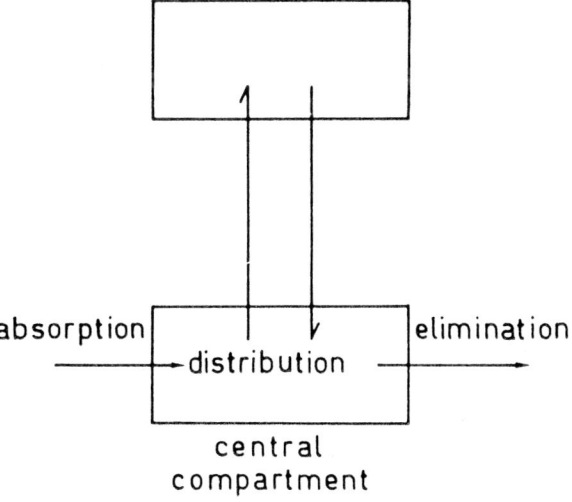

Figure 2. Schematic representation of a two-compartment open model.

the drug is distributed at a slower rate. What parts of the organism belong to the central or to the peripheral compartment will depend upon the physico-chemical characteristics of the drug. Although three- and even more-compartmental models describe the situation more correctly, they are difficult to handle and their use is usually not needed.

2.1.2. *Plasma concentration – time course*

In Fig. 3 the time course of the plasma concentrations of a drug after intravenous injection of a single dose is shown for both a one-compartmental and a two-compartmental models. Factors such as absorption, distribution, elimination and excretion usually follow first-order kinetics. When first-order kinetics indeed apply, the concentration changes which occur are proportional to the drug concentration at that particular moment. After absorption and distribution, the fall of plasma concentration is only determined by elimination. If elimination follows first-order kinetics, the log concentration-versus-time curve is a straight line. From the plasma concentration-time curve, a number of pharmacokinetic parameters can be calculated. These are useful in the search for dose adaptation in different situations.

The elimination half-life of the drug ($t^{1}/_{2}$), is the time needed for the organism to decrease the amount of the drug in the organism by fifty percent. This corresponds with the time required for any given drug concentration in the plasma to decrease by half. A closely related parameter is the elimination constant (Ke), where

$$Ke = 0.693 / t^{1}/_{2}. \tag{1}$$

The apparent volume of distribution (Vd) of a drug relates the total amount of drug in the body to the concentration of drug in plasma.

The volume of distribution (Vd) can be calculated from

$$Vd = D/C_0 \tag{2}$$

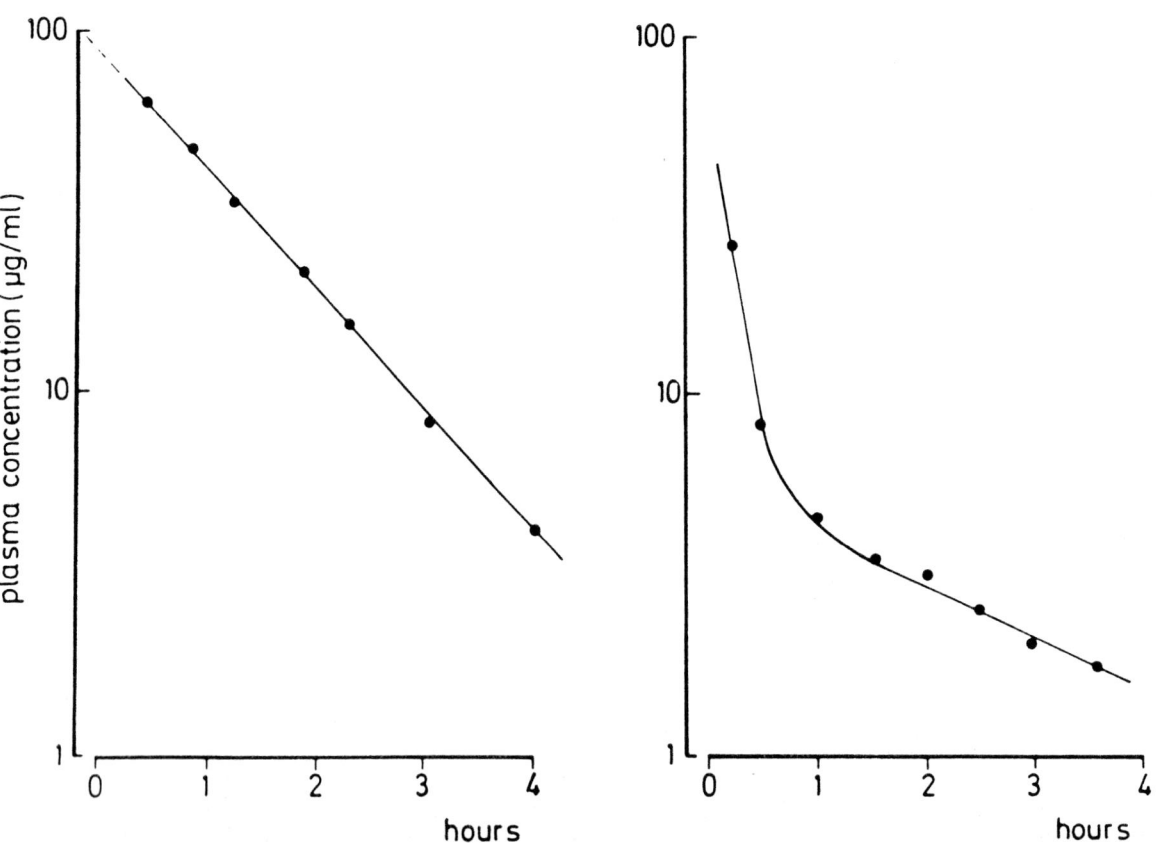

Figure 3. Plasma concentrations as a function of time; in the left panel the logarithm of the plasma concentration is plotted for a drug for which a one-compartmental analysis is appropriate. In the right panel, log plasma concentrations are shown for a two-compartmental analysis. After the distribution phase, there is a linear decay of the concentration, corresponding to the elimination phase.

where D equals the dose given and C_0 equals the plasma concentration at the time 0, the time of administration. The volume of distribution can only be calculated when the dose of the drug entering the body is known, that means when the drug is either given intravenously or if the exact amount absorbed is known.

The distribution volume provides an estimate of the extent of distribution of the drug throughout the body. If there is important uptake of the drug by the tissues, a distribution volume several times larger than the total body fluid volume (approximately 42 L for a man of 70 kg) can be found.

One of the important factors determining the size of the apparent distribution volume is the degree of plasma protein binding. The relationship between the apparent volume of distribution of a drug and its protein binding is as follows:

$$VD = V_B + V_T (F_B/F_T) \qquad (3)$$

V_B and V_T are the volumes of water in blood and in tissues, respectively, and F_B and F_T are the fractions of free drug in blood and tissues, respectively. An increase in F_B without a proportional increase in F_T would produce an increase in the apparent volume of distribution. The apparent distribution volume can also be calculated from the area under the plasma concentration versus time-curve (AUC), and Ke.

$$Vd = D/\text{AUC} \times Ke \quad \text{or} \\ D/\text{AUC} \cdot 0.693/t^{1}\!/_{2}. \qquad (4)$$

Total body clearance or total plasma clearance is the volume of plasma which is cleared completely of the drug per unit time: it gives an estimate of the efficiency of the elimination of the drug by organs such as liver or kidney. Total body or plasma clearance is the sum of the clearances by the individual elimination routes, mainly biotransformation in the liver and renal excretion. For some substances, elimination takes place only via the kidney, and total body clearance equals renal clearance. Total body clearance (Cl_{tot}) can be calculated by means of the equations:

$$Cl_{\text{tot}} = 0.693 \; Vd/t^{1}\!/_{2} \qquad (5)$$

or

$$Cl_{\text{tot}} = D/\text{AUC}. \qquad (6)$$

Although clearance can be calculated from Vd and $t^{1}\!/_{2}$, it does not depend on these parameters. On the other hand, half-life of elimination is dependent not only upon the clearance, but also upon the volume of distribution. Although gentamicin and digoxin are both cleared by the kidneys to approximately the same extent as creatinine, this means at a rate of 120 ml/min in a normal situation, the half-life of elimination for digoxin is 36 hours, while that of gentamicin is only 2 hours: this is due to the fact that the distribution volume of digoxin is more than 500 liters, while gentamicin is only about 15 liters. When elimination in different situations is compared (for example patients with renal failure compared to normals, or predialysis patients compared to those on dialysis), clearances should be calculated wherever possible.

Elimination half-life should not be confused with duration of action. The latter is determined by the time during which drug concentrations are above the minimal effective concentration (MEC). In case of antibiotics, for example, the MEC may be the minimal inhibitory drug concentration where 90% of the microorganisms are killed (MIC_{90}). The duration of drug action is not only dependent on the elimination half-life of the drug but also of the dose given, and of the drug distribution. A drug with a longer elimination half-life can exhibit a shorter duration of action than a drug with a shorter half-life depending on the distribution kinetics of the two drugs.

Total body clearance can only be measured exactly after intravenous drug administration or when the bioavailability, f, is known to be complete. Drugs are, however, often administered orally without knowing exactly their bioavailability. "Oral plasma clearance" can be used to estimate total body clearance, irrespective of bioavailability. Oral plasma clearance is usually indicated by "Cl/f".

While pharmacokinetics of a drug are usually studied after single dose administration, it is of utmost importance to know what happens after chronic administration of a drug. For some drugs at the moment of the second administration, the amount still present in the body is negligible, so that after the second administration, concentrations in the plasma will be similar to those after the first administration. This is the case when gentamicin, with an elimination half-life of two hours in patients with normal renal function, is administered three times a day. When however a drug with a longer half-life is administered or if the dosing interval is short (i.e., less than 4 half-lives), an important fraction of what was introduced with the first administration, is still present at the time of the second dosage.

Consequently, the concentration after the second dose will be higher than that after the first dose, and accumulation of the drug occurs. In that case, steady-state concentrations are only obtained after a number of administrations. The time to reach steady-state plasma concentrations depends only on the half-life, and is approximately four to five times the half-life of the drug. For example, for digoxin with its half-life of 1.5 days, this works out at approximately one week. If the steady-state levels are to be achieved earlier, a loading dose of the drug must be given. The extent of accumulation (i.e., how much higher steady-state levels will be than those after the first administration) depends on the half-life and the dosing interval.

2.2. Pharmacokinetic alterations in patients with decreased renal function

In patients with renal failure, the fate of a drug can be altered profoundly. Most important of course is the decrease in renal excretion of the drug; other processes can, however, also be affected. Gastro-intestinal absorption after oral administration of a drug may be impaired in uremic patients because gastro-intestinal pH or motility are altered, or by binding of the drug to co-administered chelators. Biotransformation of drugs can be decreased or increased in uremic patients. There is much interest for alterations in plasma protein binding of drugs in these patients. For a number of acidic drugs, which are mainly bound to plasma albumin, binding is often markedly decreased, due to either a decrease in albumin concentration in the plasma or to a decrease in the affinity at the binding sites; the decrease in affinity can be due to structural changes of the albumin molecules or to the presence of endogenous inhibitors. These changes in protein binding can markedly affect the calculated pharmacokinetic parameters, and they can in some circumstances lead to changes in free drug concentration in plasma, and to side effects. Some basic drugs bind mainly to alpha-1-acid glycoprotein (alpha-1-AGP). In renal failure, the binding of these drugs may be increased due to the elevated alpha-1-AGP concentrations in the plasma.

The renal clearance of a drug is usually decreased proportionally to the decrease in creatinine clearance. If renal excretion is the only elimination route of the drug, total body or plasma clearance will be reduced to the same extent. For substances which are only partly eliminated by the kidneys, the alteration in total body clearance will depend upon the relative importance of the renal versus the non-renal elimination. It should, however, not be assumed that for a drug which is not eliminated via the kidney, total body clearance is not altered in patients with renal failure: indeed, hepatic clearance can also be affected.

In patients with renal failure, the half-life of drugs, which are excreted wholly or in part by renal excretion is prolonged and is inversely related to the decrease in total body clearance. However, the volume of distribution of drugs in these patients is often also different due to the changes in binding in plasma or in tissues. The plasma half-life, which depends on both Vd and Cl, is therefore not always a good parameter of the drug clearance in these patients. Digoxin is not bound to a significant extent to plasma proteins, but it is bound extensively to tissues of the kidneys, liver and myocardium. This binding is decreased in patients with renal failure. As apparent from formula [3], a decrease in drug tissue binding without a corresponding decrease in drug plasma binding results in a decrease in the apparent volume of distribution. In several studies it has indeed been observed that the volume of distribution of digoxin is significantly smaller in patients with chronic renal failure (230 to 280 L vs 500 L in normals).

The pharmacokinetic changes in chronic renal failure can, mainly after chronic administration of a drug, lead to important changes in plasma concentrations, if the dose is not adjusted. Drug concentrations in the body can be much higher and the time to reach steady-state can be increased, if the half-life is prolonged. This explains why in patients with renal failure a loading dose is often needed. Thus, for many drugs dose adjustments will be necessary in chronic renal failure. The mean steady-state levels (Css) which will be achieved in a given situation, can be calculated with the following equation:

$$Css = \frac{F \times D}{Cl_{tot} \times T} \quad (7)$$

where F = fraction absorbed, and T = the dosing interval and D the maintenance dose.

This can also be expressed as:

$$Css = \frac{1.44 F \times D \times T^{1/2}}{Vd \times T}. \quad (8)$$

From these equations, the maintenance dose needed for a given Css can be calculated.

The many nomograms available for calculation of maintenance doses are based on these principles.

The loading dose (D^*), i.e., the dose needed to obtain a given Css at once, can be calculated by the equation

$$D^* = Vd \times Css. \qquad (9)$$

2.3. Pharmacokinetic alterations in patients on peritoneal dialysis

Peritoneal dialysis can alter the pharmacokinetics of a drug, depending upon the route of administration of the drug and rate of removal via the dialysate for some agents. This can necessitate dose adaptations.

2.3.1. Pharmacokinetics of drugs after systemic administration

Assessment Plasma and dialysate concentrations can be measured as a function of time. To evaluate whether systemic kinetics are affected by dialysis, serum half-life, volume of distribution and total body clearance (and in some cases residual renal clearance) can be calculated and compared to the values obtained in terminal chronic renal failure without dialysis.

The amount recovered from the peritoneal dialysate over the period of time (A_{per}), can be used to assess the need for dose adaptation. This amount should be viewed in relation to that lost in the body over the same period of time by other routes, such as hepatic biotransformation or residual renal excretion.

The peritoneal dialysis clearance (Cl_{per}) can be calculated from the equation:

$$Cl_{per} = \frac{A_{per}\ t_1 - t_2}{AUC\ t_1 - t_2} \qquad (10)$$

where $A_{per}\ t_1 - t_2$ is the amount recovered in the dialysate over a given time period and AUC $t_1 - t_2$ is the area under the plasma concentration curve over the same time period. The peritoneal clearance should be compared to the total body clearance (Cl_{tot}). Indeed, the increased plasma clearance which can be found with dialysis is dependent of the peritoneal clearance of the drug, the renal clearance and the non-renal clearance.

2.3.2. Factors influencing the peritoneal drug clearance

The dialysis clearance of a systemically administered drug in the peritoneal dialysis setting will depend upon a number of factors that are summarized in Table 1. The peritoneal membrane characteristics have been described in the first part of this chapter. Only some of the other factors will be discussed below.

The most important factor in determining the magnitude of the peritoneal clearance of a drug, is the dialysate flow rate which is around 6–7 ml/min in CAPD. Small solute peritoneal clearances are largely dialysate flow dependent. This explains why rapid exchange peritoneal dialysis, as in intermittent peritoneal dialysis, increases low clearances of solutes with low molecular weight. In CAPD on the other hand, the transport of small solutes per unit of time is small, because diffusion equilibrium is either obtained or approached before the dialysate is changed.

An important factor determining the rate of diffusion across the peritoneal membrane is the molecular weight of the drug. The molecular weights of most drugs lie within the narrow range of 100 to 700 daltons, with some notable exceptions as vancomycin (MW of 1450), insulin (MW 6000) and erythropoietin (MW 30,400). The diffusion of a solute from blood to dialysate is inversely pro-

Table 1. Factors affecting peritoneal drug clearance after systemic administration.

Dialysate properties
    Flow rate
    Temperature
    pH
    Osmotic content

Drug properties
    Molecular weight
    Ionic charge
    Volume of distribution
    Protein binding
    Extrarenal clearance
    Lipid or water solubility

Characteristics of the peritoneal membrane
    Surface and charge
    Permeability
        Peritonitis
        Sclerosis
    Peritoneal blood flow
    Stagnant layers
    Ultrafiltration

portional to the square root of the solute mass, both in hemo- and peritoneal dialysis [16, 205].

Another factor is the extent of drug-protein binding, since only unbound, free drug is available for diffusion. A drug with a high plasma protein binding usually shows a low peritoneal clearance. Recently, the effect of plasma protein binding on the peritoneal transport of intravenously administered beta-lactam antibiotics was investigated in rats [206]. The antibiotic concentration-time profiles obtained in the dialysate were compatible with the model in which only the unbound antibiotic is available for peritoneal transport. Although Flessner et al. [207] reported that bovine serum albumin transferred through the peritoneal tissues from plasma to the peritoneal cavity in rats, the capillary membrane permeability of cephalosporins was 5 to 17-fold higher than that of albumin. Therefore, even if drugs bound to albumin can be transported through the peritoneal membrane, the contribution of this fraction is probably minor. For practical purposes, this implies that the peritoneal membrane plays no important role in the transport of endogenous substances highly bound to proteins [208]. Dialysate concentrations of proteins are lower than serum concentrations and the protein binding of drug molecules in the peritoneal compartment is believed to be of minor clinical significance [209]. Based upon these considerations, a reasonably accurate formula for the prediction of the peritoneal clearance in CAPD after systemic administration of drugs has been proposed [210].

$$Cl_{per} \text{ (ml/min)} = 75 \sqrt{fU}/\sqrt{MW}$$

where fU represents the free fraction in the serum and MW the molecular weight of the drug. This formula is valid for a 2 L-dialysate and a 6 h dwell, in the absence of peritonitis. Erythromycin e.g., has a molecular weight of 730 and a free fraction of 0.30; therefore, the peritoneal clearance is estimated to be 1.52 ml/min. The validity of the formula was tested by comparing the predicted values with the observed clearances in 19 clinical studies. A linear regression analysis yielded a correlation coefficient of 0.958.

A drug with a low molecular weight (< 500 kilodalton) and with a low plasma protein binding may have a clinically relevant peritoneal dialysis clearance.

2.3.3. *Need for dose adaptation*

One accepts that the dialysability of a drug in any dialysis strategy is only clinically relevant when at least two conditions are fulfilled. First, the dialysis clearance should be at least 30% higher than the endogenous total plasma clearance; otherwise the additive effect of dialysis clearance on overall drug elimination is negligible [211]. Second, the distribution volume of the drug should be less than 1 L/kg bodyweight. If Vd is larger, only a small fraction of the drug is available in the plasma for elimination via dialysis, and the amount of drug removed is small, even for a high clearance. Since in terminal chronic renal failure, the total endogenous drug plasma clearance is usually higher than 20–30 ml/min, and for most drugs the distribution volume is more than 1 L/kg body weight, the peritoneal drug clearance hardly ever contributes significantly to drug removal in the CAPD setting. Therefore, additional dose adaptations for CAPD beyond the recommendations for terminal chronic renal failure are almost never necessary. Notable exceptions are drugs with a small distribution volume, low protein binding and a small total plasma clearance in uremia, such as the aminoglycosides, vancomycin, fosfomycin, amantadine, flucytosine, atenolol, sotalol and lithium. The presence of peritonitis does not significantly influence the magnitude or rapidity of drug transport into the peritoneal cavity after systemic administration. Vancomycin is, however, an exception. After intravenous administration, therapeutic vancomycin concentrations in the dialysate are reached after 30 minutes of dwell in peritonitis, versus 2 to 4 hours in a non-inflamed peritoneum, with an increase in the peritoneal vancomycin clearance from 3 to 4 ml/min during a 5 hour dwell [212]. On the other hand, the peritoneal clearances of netilmicin and of ciprofloxacin in patients, with or without peritonitis were not different [213, 214].

Studies after systemic administration are of interest not only to evaluate the need for dose adaptations to maintain adequate systemic concentrations of a drug, but also for knowing the dialysate concentrations of the drug. The low peritoneal drug clearance does not exclude that therapeutically effective concentrations in the dialysate, e.g., for an antibiotic, can be achieved after systemic administration, due to the low volume (2–3 liters), in which the drug diffuses. The concentrations of antibiotic drugs that are achieved in the dialysate after systemic (and intraperitoneal) administration must be viewed against their activities against the strains that are isolated from patients with peritonitis. As recently pointed out by several workers, used peritoneal dialysis fluid is a better medium to test these activities than the classically used broth [215–218]. Furthermore, recent work has shown that culture conditions, dialysate manipulations, and adherence capacity of germs are critical factors affecting the antibiotic activity [219].

2.3.4. Bidirectional transfer

After a dwell time of 5 to 6 hours, equilibrium between plasma and dialysate is approached and the calculated clearances give the difference between transfer to and from the body and the dialysate bag. According to the pharmacokinetic model of Janicke et al. [220] it is possible to evaluate the bidirectional transport. Based on simple mass balance, one can calculate the time-independent, one-way instantaneous clearances between the peritoneal cavity and the circulation. These unidirectional clearances are called distributional clearances, where ClD_1 describes the transport from body to dialysate and ClD_2 the transport from dialysate to body. For example, for Cefamandole, both distributional clearances were approximately 16 ml/min, although the net clearance was only 2 ml/min. In children treated with intermittent peritoneal dialysis, ClD_1 values for gentamicin 2 to 3-fold greater than ClD_2 values have been reported [221]. In a recent study with cefotiam and cefsulodine, distributional clearances were 15 and 17 ml/min respectively with net peritoneal clearances ranging between 3.3 and 4.3 ml/min [222]. This method of calculation is simple, does not require computer-fitting of the model equations, and is independent of the number of compartments of the model used. The data can be derived from analysis during one dwell period only.

2.3.5. Pharmacokinetics of drugs after intraperitoneal administration

Peritoneal transport is also of interest with regard to intraperitoneal administration of drugs. For example, the intraperitoneal doses of insulin or erythropoietin required to achieve adequate systemic concentrations, or of antibiotics for local treatment of peritonitis, need to be carefully worked out. There are two sources of blood supply to the organs of the peritoneal cavity, one to the parietal and the other to the visceral peritoneum; both layers are rich in lymphatic circulation. The venous blood of visceral peritoneum returns to the portal circulation, while the venous return from the parietal peritoneum drains into the systemic rather than the portal circulation. Earlier pharmacokinetic studies have indicated that drugs such as atropine, caffeine, glucose, glycine and progesterone are absorbed predominantly via the visceral peritoneum after intraperitoneal injection [223]. Therefore these drugs, when introduced intraperitoneally, are subject to immediate handling by the liver. Some of these drugs might undergo a first pass metabolism.

After intraperitoneal administration of drugs, concentrations can be measured as a function of time in both dialysate and plasma. In view of the low peritoneal clearance of drugs after systemic administration, the rapid drug disappearance out of the peritoneum when the drug is given via the intraperitoneal route is at first sight surprising. This has been explained by assuming a mainly unidirectional transperitoneal drug movement from the peritoneal cavity towards the blood [224]. It is, however, merely the consequence of pharmacokinetic factors, i.e., volume of distribution and protein binding. The contrast between the small dialysate volume and the very large distribution volume of the drug in the body, leads to a high concentration gradient. This is well illustrated by the much greater systemic availability of drugs like insulin or erythropoietin when they are given into an empty abdominal cavity or in a small (50 ml) volume of saline, than when these drugs are added to the two liters of dialysate [225, 226]. Furthermore, the high protein binding of some drugs in the plasma, versus a negligible protein binding in the dialysate, further promotes this apparent one-way diffusion from dialysate to blood.

2.3.6. Factors affecting transperitoneal drug absorption after intraperitoneal administration

These factors are summarized in Table 2. Only a few of them will be discussed here; some of these factors have been described in the first part of this chapter.

Electric charge Among the factors influencing intraperitoneally administered drug transport, to which attention has been paid only recently are the electric charges of a drug. Studies using electron dense tracers have shown the existence of anionic charges on the peritoneal basement membrane and capillaries subjacent to it [53, 227]. These charges are known to reside on the heparan or chondroitin sulfate components of cellular membranes.

They are greatly reduced under conditions of

local or generalized inflammation (i.e., during peritonitis and sepsis) [228]. Intraperitoneal protamine, a highly cationic molecule, neutralizes these anionic fixed charges and enhances the peritoneal permeability to anionic plasma proteins [170]. The presence or absence of these peritoneal anionic charges can influence transperitoneal absorption of cationic drug molecules such as aminoglycosides. We and others have, however, shown a much enhanced transperitoneal absorption of gentamicin, netilmicin and tobramycin during peritonitis [213, 229, 230] (see below). These observations are difficult to explain if electric charges are important in their transport. Similarly, conflicting effects on the transport of gentamicin with intraperitoneal heparin, a negatively charged drug, have been reported. One earlier study reported lower blood gentamicin concentrations with intraperitoneal heparin [231], while a more recent study revealed that heparin caused an improvement in transport of uncharged molecules such as urea and creatinine and of the positively charged gentamicin [232].

Peritoneal lymphatic drug absorption Studies in rats have shown that a significant proportion of the peritoneal cavity to plasma transport of macromolecules e.g., insulin, is via convective transport [233]. Recombinant human growth hormone (GH), (MW 21,000) was intraperitoneally instilled and showed an immediate absorption with peak serum GH levels obtained between 4 and 8 h following administration [234]. It is highly probable that this drug is, at least partly, transported via the lymphatics. The pharmacokinetics of erythropoietin an heparin will be described later.

Drug degradation and interaction As reviewed by a number of authors [208, 235–237] intraperitoneal antibiotics show a systemic absorption varying from 50 to 80% within a dwell period of 6 hours in CAPD. The amount absorbed can easily be obtained by subtracting from the amount of drug initially instilled, the total amount of drug that is present in the first peritoneal outflow. This, however, assumes that there is no degradation of the drug over the time interval in the dialysate. Most commonly used antibiotics are stable in peritoneal dialysate either alone or in combination, or in the presence of additives such as insulin or heparin [238–242]. Some cephalosporins, however, showed a degradation of 12 to 16%, and rifampicin a degradation of 6% in CAPD solutions or in effluent over 6 hr [240]. This may lead to an overestimation of the amount of drug absorbed after intraperitoneal administration.

Peritonitis Studies by us and others have demonstrated a faster and more important absorption of antibiotics such as aminoglycosides, vancomycin, piperacillin and various beta-lactam antibiotics during peritonitis compared to non-peritonitis [213, 229, 230, 243–245]. This has not been observed with other antibiotics, such as cefsulodin [14]. Fig. 4, taken from the paper by De Paepe et al. [229], illustrates the difference between peritonitis and non-peritonitis. It is also apparent that after intraperitoneal administration of gentamicin, the fall in dialysate concentration is much more pronounced than the rise in plasma concentrations. This not surprising as the volume of distribution of the body is much larger than the volume of the peritoneal dialysis fluid. Equal concentrations of gentamicin in serum and dialysate were achieved at approximately 24 hours. The clinical relevance of the higher systemic availability during peritonitis is questionable for drugs with a wide therapeutic toxic margin. However, if a drug with a narrow therapeutic index is only negligibly cleared after transport to the systemic circulation, systemic accumulation after repetitive intraperitoneal administration of the drug could occur. After chronic administration of gentamicin into the peritoneal dialysis fluid for 2 to 3 weeks, plasma concentrations approach end of dwell-time dialysate concen-

Table 2. Factors affecting transperitoneal drug absorption after intraperitoneal administration.

Dialysate properties
 Flow rate
 Temperature
 Volume
 Chemical composition

Drug properties
 Molecular weight
 Ionic charge
 Volume of distribution
 Binding to membrane
 Lipid or water solubility

Characteristics of the peritoneal membrane
 Surface and charge
 Permeability
  Peritonitis
  Sclerosis
 Peritoneal blood flow
 Lymphatic absorption
 Stagnant layers

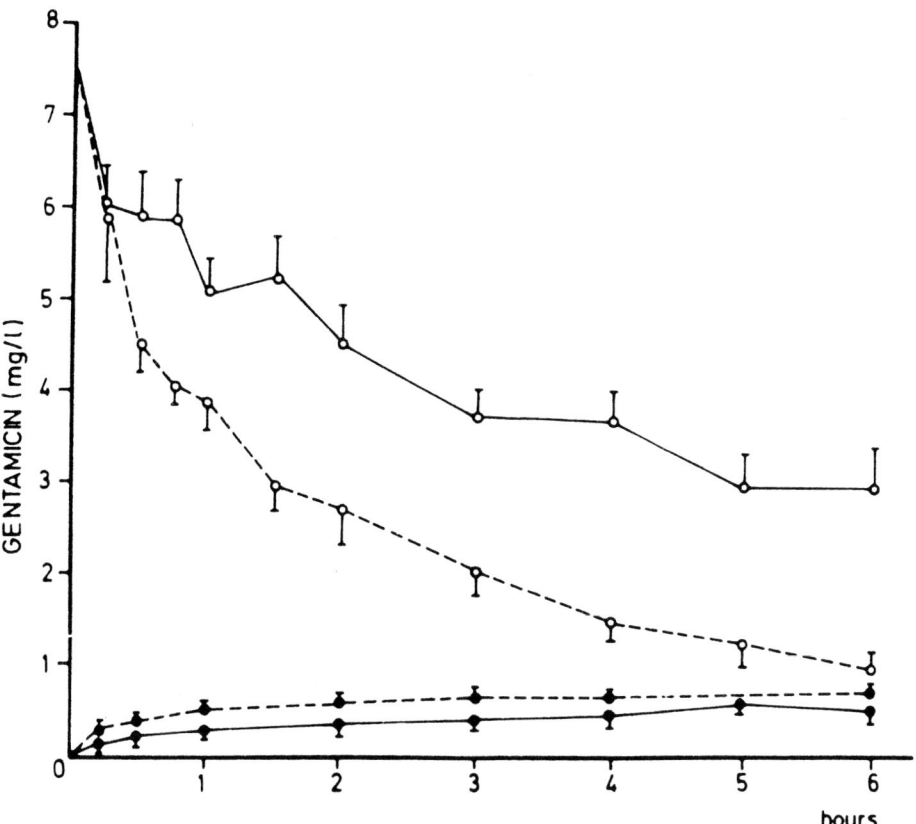

Figure 4. Concentrations (mean ± SEM) of gentamicin in serum (○) and dialysate (●) in 5 patients without peritonitis (—) and 5 patients with peritonitis (---). Gentamicin was added in a concentration of 7.5 mg/L to the dialysate at time 0.

trations [229]. This can lead to potentially toxic concentrations and necessitates dose reduction.

Adverse effects Rapid transperitoneal drug absorption may also cause adverse systemic effects. The "red man syndrome" has been described after rapid intraperitoneal administration of 1 g of vancomycin diluted in 2 L of dialysate [246].

Drugs, when given intraperitoneally in therapeutic doses may also cause peritoneal irritation. This has been described with a fixed combination of cilastatin/imipenem [208], amphotericin B [247–250], certain brands of vancomycin [251], methylene blue [252] and antiotension I [253].

2.4. Effect of peritoneal dialysis on drug protein binding

There exist only few studies where the influence of peritoneal dialysis, notably CAPD, on drug binding has been assessed. Drug protein binding of acid drugs in peritoneal dialysis patients is expected to be lower than in undialysed or hemodialysis patients. This may be secondary to the often poor nutritional status of these patients, as reflected by serum albumin concentrations in the lower normal range, the continuous peritoneal losses of proteins during the dialysis process, and accumulating endogenous compounds competing for occupation of binding sites. Changes in protein binding and total and free concentrations of digitoxin have been reported for CAPD and hemodialysis patients. The binding of digitoxin was 94.7% ± 1.5% in CAPD, significantly less than that observed in hemodialysis patients (96.2 ± 1.3%). Following a 0.1 mg oral dose of digitoxin, the mean free serum concentrations in CAPD and hemodialysis were 0.8 and 0.9 ng/ml respectively, which is not significantly different [254].

Relevant to this problem is the case of severe toxic myopathy and associated hyperkalemia that we observed in a CAPD patient treated with a dose of clofibrate that was not adapted to the decrease in protein binding of that drug [255]. We may expect that in some malnourished peritoneal dialysis patients, the binding to serum albumin of several acid drugs may be lowered, possibly leading to elevated free drug concentrations. Protein binding of the antifungal drug ketoconazole was also lower in CAPD patients (98.5%) than in control subjects (99%) [256].

The influence of CAPD on the concentrations of alpha-1-AGP in serum and dialysate and on the serum binding of two basic drugs (oxprenolol and propranolol) and of one acidic drug (phenytoin) has been reported [257]. Before starting CAPD treatment, the protein binding of oxprenolol and propranolol was higher, related to the elevated serum levels of alpha-1-AGP concentrations in uremia [258], while the binding of phenytoin was lower than in healthy volunteers. During the first week after starting CAPD, the serum alpha-1-AGP concentrations rose with a concomitant increase in the binding of oxprenolol and propranolol. Subsequently however, the alpha-1-AGP levels and the binding of oxprenolol and propranolol decreased to the values found before starting CAPD. The binding of phenytoin, which was lower than in normal healthy volunteers did not show any change during CAPD.

2.5. Peritoneal pharmacokinetics of common drugs and dose recommendations

2.5.1. *Description of the tables*

In the following tables, the pharmacokinetics are described per class of drugs studied during intermittent peritoneal dialysis (IPD) or during CAPD or continuous cycling peritoneal dialysis (CCPD). The tables also provide data on protein binding, elimination half-life, distribution volume and total plasma clearance for each drug in the presence of normal renal function, and on elimination half life and total plasma clearance in end-stage chronic renal disease (ESRD). For this information we have used, with kind permission, the data recently collected by St. John Hammond *et al.* [259]. Many of these data have also been published in standard textbooks [203, 204, 260, 261].

The pharmacokinetic data for IPD, CAPD and CCPD have been collected from reports published up to the end of 1992. Many papers contain results obtained in cross-over studies after either intravenous, oral or intraperitoneal administration. therefore, the data published per individual paper have been included in the tables. The dose/route column indicates the dose and the route of drug administration in each respective study. When available, the loading dose or maintenance dose are given. Data on serum half-life ($T^1/_2$), maximal – or, occasionally, steady state (SS) – serum concentrations achieved, total plasma clearance and peritoneal clearance are given. A comparison of these values with data obtained in normal renal function and in terminal renal failure shows the effect of peritoneal dialysis on these parameters. Finally, the percentage of dose either removed from the body by PD (in case of systemic administration) or absorbed across the peritoneal membrane (after IP administration) is provided, whenever it has been calculated.

Data are expressed as means ± either standard errors of means or standard deviations.

Each table is accompanied by a brief discussion of the need for dose adjustment in peritoneal dialysis, for the drugs that are frequently used in these patients.

Table 3 provides a glossary of the abbreviations used in the tables.

2.5.2. *Pharmacokinetic data in intermittent peritoneal dialysis (IPD)*

Table 4 summarizes the data after systemic or intraperitoneal drug administration in intermittent peritoneal dialysis. Several generalisations can be made: All beta-lactams penetrate well [316–319], whilst the aminoglycosides have relatively high recovery in the dialysate.

Amongst the cephalosporins, cephaloxin, cefuroxime and ceftazidime require dosage modifications beyond those required in end-stage renal disease. The results obtained with vancomycin are conflicting [283, 285, 286]. For all other drugs examined during IPD, the peritoneal clearance contributes little to the total plasma clearance.

Table 3. Abbreviations used in the Tables 4–11.

All data are given as mean ± standard error or standard error of mean

- SD : single dose
- MTC : mass transfer coefficient
- LD : loading dose
- MD : maintenance dose
- perit +: in presence of peritonitis
- IV : intravenous administration
- IP : intraperitoneal administration
- 0 : oral administration

Table 4. Pharmacokinetic studies in intermittent peritoneal dialysis.

	Normal renal function				ESRD		Dos/route	IPD					References
	PB %	$T^{1/2}$ h	V_d L/kg	Cl_{tot} ml/min	$T^{1/2}$ h	Cl_{tot} ml/min		$T^{1/2}$ h	C_{max} μg/ml	Cl_{tot} ml/min	Cl_{per} ml/min	% dos removed or absorbed	
I. Penicillins													
Amoxycillin	15–25	1	0.2	160	9	25	O 750 mg	15 (8.6–22)	16.95 /2–8 h	–	–	–	[262]
Ampicillin	16–20	1.2	0.48	325	14	30	O 750 mg IP 25 mg/L	13.5 (10.9–14.6) 7.5±1.2 /12h	–	–	–	7/12 h 75	[263]
Azlocillin	28	1	0.22	175	6	40	IV 3 g	2.46 ±0.25	–	–	–	5.4/7.5h	[264]
Carbenicillin	50	1	0.19	155	15	10	IV 1 g (n=2)	4.2–7.4	–	–	6.8	–	[265]
Mezlocillin Oxacillin	16–42 93	1 0.5	0.2 0.21	250 335	3.6 1	50 170	IV 60 mg/kg O 500 mg	2.1±0.6 1.4 (1.2–1.5)	–	96±51	7.4±3.9 –	<3/8 h 5/12 h	[266] [263]
Ticarcillin	45	1.2	0.21	140	11	15	IV 50 mg/kg	10.6±0.8	–	–	7.2±1.8	–	[267]
II. Cephalosporins													
Cefamandole	67–80	0.7	0.16	109	15	9	IM 1 g (n=4) IM 1 g (n=2)	7±1.4 (6–9) 10±13 (10–13)	–	–	10±1 (8–12)	14/12 h	[268]
Cefazolin	70–85	1.8	0.14	60	27	5	IV 1 g (n=3) IV 500 mg (n=2) IP 50 mg/L IP 150 mg/L	32±4 (27–38) 20–46 (20–46) – –	– – 30.3±12.8 /24h 71.9±43 /24h	–	–	19.6/30 hr – – –	[269] [270] [271] [272]
Cefotaxime	36	1	0.28	322	2.5	135	IV IV 1 g IV 1 g	3.8±1.4 2.9±1 –	–	39±16	5.5±3	6/8 h – 10.2/8 h	[273] [274] [275]
Cefoxitin	50–60	0.9	0.3	290	22	12	IP 50 mg/L	7–10/8–12 h	–	–	–	–	

Table 4. *(Continued)*

	Normal renal function				ESRD			IPD					
	PB %	$T^{1/2}$ h	V_d L/kg	Cl_{tot} ml/min	$T^{1/2}$ h	Cl_{tot} ml/min	Dos/route	$T^{1/2}$ h	C_{max} µg/ml	Cl_{tot} ml/min	Cl_{per} ml/min	% dos removed or absorbed	References
Cefuroxime	33	1.3	0.2	140	20	15	IV 500 mg	11.8±2.2	—	15.8±2 (14–18)	4.6±1.84	20.8/24 h	[277]
							IP 50 mg/L		14±8.1 /24 h	—	—	44±20	[278]
							IM 1 g	13.6±4.4	61.9 /2–3 h	—	—	—	[279]
							IV 1 g	3–4	—	—	—	—	[280]
							IP 250 mg/L	—	60.9/6 h	—	—	—	
							IV 15 mg/Kg cont. lavage	—	—	—	—	0.15–0.75%	
Cephalexin	10–50	0.8	0.26	263	20	10	IV	6.4	—	—	—	30/7 h	[281]
Cephaloridine		1–1.5	0.18–0.26			10–23		IV	8.3	—	16.3	7.5	
Cephalotin	60–65	0.6	0.26	350	10	21	IV	5.1	—	—	—	—	
Ceftazidime	10–17	2	0.24	130	25	7	IV 1 g	8.7±3.1	25.3±3.1 /12 h	—	8.5±2.7	16.6/12 h	[276]
							IP 100 mg/L	—	44.7±10.5	—	—	—	
Moxalactam							IP 1 g (empty abdomen)	— /2.75 h	2/5±0.9 /1 h	—	—	—	[282]
							IP 100 mg/L LD	—	10.3±4.8 /24 h	—	—	—	
							IP 30 mg/L MD	—		—	—	—	
III. Glycopeptides													
Vancomycin	10	7	0.47	55	240	2	IV 1 g	18	—	—	6.1 (4.2–9.8)	39.7/15 h	[283]
							IV 1 g	7.7–10.9 days	—	2.3	9.8±7.3	—	[284]
							IV 1 or 2 g (+ perit)	205.2±64.24	—	4.25±0.6	2.4	—	[285]
							IV 1 g LD MD 1 g/week	30.1	—	14.2±5.7	—	—	[286]
IV. Aminoglycosides													
Amikacin	40	2.5	0.25	90	70	3	IV 300 mg	29	—	—	—	20/12 h	[287]
							IV 125 mg	18.0±3.2	—	6.4±2	3.9±2.1	—	[288]
							IV 300 mg	25.8±12.9	—	9.7 (5.4±1.9)	6.7±6	23.1/8 h	[289]

Table 4. (Continued)

	Normal renal function					ESRD		Dos/route	IPD					
	PB %	T½ h	V$_d$ L/kg	Cl$_{tot}$ ml/min		T½ h	Cl$_{tot}$ ml/min		T½ h	C$_{max}$ μg/ml	Cl$_{tot}$ ml/min	Cl$_{per}$ ml/min	% dos removed or absorbed	References
Gentamicin	<10	2	0.24	95		60	2	IM 2 × 80 mg/d	—	—	—	13.5 (8–19)	4/22	[290]
								IM 80 mg/12 h	14.7	—	—	9 (5–12)	—	[291]
								IP 5 mg/L	—	1.7–5 /12–24 h	—	—	—	[292]
								IV 1 mg/Kg	6.5–7	—	21.2 (19.8–22.6)	—	—	[221]
								IP 15 mg/L	21 ≠ 12	—	5.5 ± 2.6	4 ± 2.6	—	
									74 ± 44.4	3.76–10.2 /10 h	—	—	—	
Tobramycin	<10	2.5	0.23	80		60	3	IV	14.08 ± 3.57	—	12.85 ± 3.96	9.75 ± 3.78	—	[293]
								IV 64–80 mg	25.4 (18–37)	—	—	—	30–69/36 h	[294]
								IM 1.5 mg/Kg						[295]
								IV 1 mg/Kg	16 ± 4	—	—	15 ± 4	34/12 h	[296]
								IV 1.5 mg/Kg LD	18–50	—	—	—	23–38/48 h	[297]
								IP 10 mg/L	—	6.8–8.4 SS	—	—	—	
Kanamycin	<10	2	0.23	85		80	2	IM 0.5 g	48	—	—	5 ± 2	4.4/1 h	[298]
								IM 7 mg/Kg	12.1 (8–17)	18.5/2 h	—	8.3 (6–11)	31.6 (23.9–41.1) /22 h	[299]
								IP 15 mg/L	—	6.7/16 h	—	—	32/22 h	
								IP 7 mg/Kg	—	S/D = 40% /4 h	—	—	—	
V. Other antimicrobial agents														
Chloramphenicol	25–60	3	0.9	245		5	147	IV 0.5–1 g	3.8 ± 1	—	—	—	—	[298]
Clindamycin	94	2.3	0.7	250		4	150	IV 600 mg	4.6 ± 1.2	—	—	4	—	[296]
Colistin sulfomethate	—	3–8	0.54	—		10–20	—	IV 5 mg/Kg	14 ± 6.8 (6.4–20)	—	31	11 ± 6.8	16/48 h	[298]
								IM 75 mg	—	—	—	5.8 ± 1.9	0.91 mg/1 h	[300]
								IV 2–3 mg/Kg	—	—	—	9.8 (3–16)	—	[301]
Lincomycin	72	5	0.44	72		10	35	IM 600 mg	13.2 (103–15.4)	—	—	—	—	[302]
Metronidazole	20	7	0.7	82		7	82	IV 500 mg	5.6 ± 1	—	80.1 ± 17.1	15.8 ± 1.6	10.2/7.5 h	[303]

Table 4. *(Continued)*

	Normal renal function				ESRD				IPD					
	PB %	$T^{1/2}$ h	V_d L/kg	Cl_{tot} ml/min	$T^{1/2}$ h	Cl_{tot} ml/min	Dos/route	$T^{1/2}$ h	C_{max} µg/ml	Cl_{tot} ml/min	Cl_{per} ml/min	% dos removed or absorbed	References
Sulfamethoxazole	60–68	10	0.36	30	35	10	0.20 mg/Kg	18±3.5	28±4.1 /6 h	26±5.7	1.2±0.2	2/12 h	[304]
							IP 80 mg/L						
							– perit	–	12/24 h	–	–	39/12 h	
							+ perit	–	26/24 h	–	–	55/12 h	
Trimethoprim	40–70	13	2	125	25	65	0.4 mg/Kg	23.7±4	1.98±0.32 /4 h	66.2±11.5	5.1±0.5	3/12 h	
							IP 16 mg/L						
							– perit	–	0.6/12 h	–	–	89/12 h	
							+ perit	–	1.2/12 h	–	–	93/12 h	
Tetracycline	25–65	9	1.5	131	80	14	0.500 mg	60 (45–72)	–	–	–	7/12 h	[263]
							IV 0.5–1 g (n = 3)	67±5.7 (30–128)	–	–	5.6±3.9	–	[298]
							0.500 mg	68	–	–	–	–	[305]
Miscellaneous													
Valproic acid	90–95	12	0.15–0.4	10	–	–	0.500 mg	27.2	–	2.48 ml/kg	0.04 ml/kg	4.3/1 h	[313]
Aminocaproic acid	–	1–2	0.9	–	–	–	IV 36–24 g/d 0.6–24 g/d	31	–	24–29	13.8	–	[306]
Cimetidine	13–25	2	0.81	330	5	132	IV 300 mg (n = 1) 0.4 × 300 mg/d (n = 1)	–	–	–	3.1–9.98	–	[308]
Theophylline	60	8.7	0.45	46	7.3	67	IV 300 mg	3.4–5	–	129±32	5.3	–	[309]
Digoxin	20–30	36	7.1	160	100	35	Cont. Infusion	–	–	–	11.7±2.4	384 mg/48 h	[312]
							0	88 (52–118)	–	–	8 (3–14)	3/32 h	[310]
Quinidine	80–85	6	2	270	6	270	0.200 mg/6 h	–	–	277	1.2	4.5/6 h	[311]
Atenolol	<5	5.5	0.7	176	73	13	0.100 mg	23	–	–	–	26% in steady state	[307]
Verapamil	90	3.5	5	1000	3.8	1000	0.120–480 mg several days	–	–	–	4.0 (0.3–8.1)	–	[314]

2.5.3. Pharmacokinetic data in CAPD

Tables 5 to 11 summarize the pharmacokinetic data on systemic and intraperitoneal drug administration in CAPD. Only a few studies have been performed in continuous cycling peritoneal dialysis (CCPD).

Table 5 summarizes the pharmacokinetic data obtained for cardiovascular drugs and Table 6 summarizes the pharmacokinetic data obtained with the beta-lactam antibiotics and glycopeptides.

In general, the amount of penicillin lost in the peritoneal cavity after systemic administration is negligible; on the other hand, their transperitoneal absorption can be as high as 90%, in the presence of peritonitis. Many semisynthetic penicillins have good anti-pseudomonas activity (i.e., piperacillin) and are used as initial treatment in combination with at least one other anti-pseudomonas drug, such as ceftazidime or an aminoglycoside [410].

First, second and third generation cephalosporins have also been studied. Based on the satisfactory dialysate levels that are achieved even after oral administration (cephadrine or cephalexin) some have used this group of antibiotics as first choice for initial treatment of peritonitis either singly or in combination [411, 412, 414, 418, 419, 420]. Ceftazidime (125 mg/L) in combination with tobramycin (8 mg/L) remains stable for up to 16 hours at room temperature and for an additional 8 hours at 37°C [416]. The intraperitoneal combination of ceftazidime and vancomycin as initial treatment for peritonitis was proven to be effective and safe in 2 British institutions [418, 419] and recommended by the Ad Hoc Advisory Committee [419].

Moxolactam is a semisynthetic beta-lactam antibiotic with activity against a broad range of gram-positive and gram-negative aerobic and anaerobic bacteriae. This antibiotic exists as a pair of stereoisomers which have different antimicrobial activities and kinetics. Several pharmacokinetic studies in CAPD patients have shown that after IV administration, dosage adjustment to account for loss of moxalactam via the peritoneal cavity appears unnecessary. It appears further that there are no significant differences in the kinetics of R-Mox and S-Mox in CAPD patients [393].

The two major substances in the class of glycopeptide antibiotics are vancomycin and teicoplanin.

Vancomycin is a widely used antibiotic in the treatment of Gram-positive infections and is popular as therapy of peritonitis in peritoneal dialysis. Staphylococcus aureus and staphylococcus epidermidis are almost always susceptible to vancomycin. Concentrations of 5 ug/ml or less are inhibitory although a small proportion of strains require 10–20 ug/ml for inhibition. Vancomycin is a large molecule (around 1500 daltons) and has a low serum binding. It has a very prolonged half life in end-stage renal disease [200–250 hr]. Pharmacokinetic studies after IV administration in CAPD patients, show a low peritoneal clearance, which increases during peritonitis. Although it has been asserted that CAPD does not require dosage adjustment, serum drug levels should be followed. Intravenous vancomycin as the sole therapy for peritonitis has been shown to be both safe and effective [212, 421, 422] as has intraperitoneal therapy alone or in combination with cephalosporins, aztreonam and aminoglycosides (Chapter 16).

The existence of chemical peritonitis resulting from intraperitoneal administration of vancomycin remains controversial [251, 423]; it rarely occurs with vancomycin commercialized by the Lilly company [424].

Teicoplanin is a relatively new glycopeptide antimicrobial agent that has a prolonged terminal half life and is mainly excreted via the renal route. The pharmacokinetic data in normal and severely impaired renal function in Table 5 are derived from a review by Rowland [411].

The pharmacokinetic data obtained with fluoroquinolones, aztreonam, aminoglycosides, trimethoprim-sulfamethoxazole and fosfomycin in CAPD are summarized in Table 7.

Fluoroquinolones Fluoroquinolones have a wide antibacterial spectrum, including Gram-negative bacteriae and staphylococci. Most fluoroquinolones are well absorbed after oral administration and have a favourable pharmacokinetic profile. Several of the newer fluoroquinolones have been administered to CAPD patients either for pharmacokinetic studies or as treatment for CAPD-related infections. Janknegt [454] has recently summarized the pharmacokinetic and clinical studies with ciprofloxacin, ofloxacin, pefloxacin and fleroxacin in CAPD patients.

In a CAPD patient therapy with quinolones requires dose adjustment as for patients with end-stage renal failure. However, high drug intraperitoneal concentrations can be achieved after IV or oral administration, making these substances, at least theoretically, attractive alternatives to conventional treatment of CAPD peritonitis (for

Table 5. Pharmacokinetic studies with cardiovascular drugs in CAPD.

	Normal renal function				ESRD		IPD						
	PB %	T½ h	V_d L/kg	Cl_tot ml/min	T½ h	Cl_tot ml/min	Dos/route	T½ h	C_max μg/ml	Cl_tot ml/min	Cl_per ml/min	% dose removed or absorbed	References
Digoxin	20–30	36	7.1 ESRD 4.2!	160	100	35	0 0.125 mg daily 5 days SS (n=1)	97.9	3.2 ng/ml at 2 h	12.6	2.0	<4/24 h	[320]
							0 0.50 mg	–	3.8±2.3 ng/ml at 0.56 h	–	3.0±1	1/24 h	[321]
							0 0.1 mg/d SS	–	–	–	3.9±1.3	<2/24 h	[322]
							0 0.125 mg every 2–3 d	54–141	–	11–52	2.3–3.1	<10/4 d	[323]
							0 0.125 mg per day	–	–	–	3.6±0.4	7.6±0.9/24 h	[324]
Digitoxin	90 86–89 ESRD	145	0.5	3	200	2	0.1 mg/d SS	7.5 days	–	3.5	0.7±0.3	<2/24 h	[322]
Quinidine	80–85	6	2	270	6	270	0 350 mg 4x/day	5.4	–	154.2	0.79	0.6/24h	[325]
Denopamine							0 10 mg SD	4.6±2.5	0.0123±0.0067	–	0.10±0.05	<0.1/6 h	[326]
Labetalol	50	7	5.6	1700	13	1198	IV 0.7–1 mg/kg	13.05±6.32	–	1397.2±372.3	1.94±0.65	0.14/72 h	[327]
Propranolol	93	3.5	3	695	3.5	695	0 320 mg/d	–	–	–	–	3.3/24 h	[328]
							0 20 mg/d	–	–	–	–	5.2/24 h	
Atenolol	<5	5.5	0.7	176	73	13	IV 20 mg	27.6±2.18	–	21±1.4	2.53±0.3	6/24 h	[329]
Esmolol	–	0.2	3.2	19950	–	–	IV 150 μg/kg/min for 4 h	0.1±0.06	0.8 (0.5) C_ss	20504±11448 (80 kg)	0	0	[330]
ASL8123	4.1±1.2							42±20					
Betaxolol	55	14–22	6	327	30	200	–	27	87.1±20.4	–	2.7	<1/24 h	[331] [332]
Nifedipine	90–95	2	1.4	1100	2.6	1100	0 2×20 mg/d	–	–	–	–		[333]
Isosorbide-5-nitrate	16–28	0.2–0.5	1.8	–	0.2–0.5	–	0 3×20 mg/d	4.2±1.1	448±118	–	4.3±2.7	1–6/24 h	
Diltiazem	80–85	4.0	5.3	1400	3.4	1400	0 60 mg	3.09±1.15	95.8±63.8 (3 h)	2653 1316 (70 kg)	1.5±1.0	<0.1/24 h	[334]

Table 5. (Continued)

	Normal renal function				ESRD		Dose/route	IPD					References
	PB %	T½ h	Vd L/kg	Cl_tot ml/min	T½ h	Cl_tot ml/min		T½ h	C_{max} μg/ml	Cl_tot ml/min	Cl_per ml/min	% dose removed or absorbed	
Captopril Free Captopril	25–30	1.9	3	1277	35	69	0 50 mg SD	1 ± 0.3	0.387 ±0.075 2.77±0.43			<1%/6 h	[335]
Total Quinapril*	–	1*	–	–	0.9*	–	0 20 mg SD	1.0 ± 0.3	0.107 ±0.067	2207 ±1621	–	0	[337]
Quinaprilat	97*	–	–	–	12.5*	–		20.1 ± 10.1	0.689 ±0.124	19 ± 8.3		2.6 ± 1.2/24 h	
Osinoprilate	95	15	0.15	–	19–28	–	0 10 mg fosinopril	19.5 ± 7.5	0.202 ±0.071	70.6 ±38.5	0.09 ±0.07	2 ± 1.4/48 h	[338]
Guanfacine	30	17	4	–	14	–	?	–	–	–	1.5	–	[339]
Tocainide	10–15	11–14	3.2	182	17–43	100	0 400 mg SD	15 ± 5	3.2 ± 1	83 ± 36	<5 ml/min	2.2 ± 2/24 h	[340]
Flecainide	40	14–26	8.7	567	19–26	357	0 100 mg/d	40	–	30	2.2	1/24 h	[341]
							0 200 mg (n=1)	–	–	50	–	–	
Procainamide	15	2	2	810	8	200	0 625 mg SD	26	1.9–4.8	143	0.28–5.55	<5/d	[342]
N-acetylprocainamide	10	6	1.5	200	4.2	29		42.8	–	29.8	1.74–7.20	<5	
Furosemide	95	0.5	0.12	162	1.4	105	0 500 mg SD – perit + perit	10.5 ± 1.2 11.6 ± 3.3	12.8 ± 2.1 6.6 ± 0.4	– –	0.5 ± 0.1 0.5 ± 0.1	0.9 ± 0.2/24 h 0.6 ± 0.1/24 h	[343]
							0 500 mg SD – perit 0 80 mg	12.5 ± 3.4	7.7 ± 06	–	0.4 ± 0.1	0.6 ± 0.1/24 h	[344]
							SD – perit IV 80 mg	3.87 ± 1.26	3.2 ± 1.4	–	–	–	[345]
Theophylline	60	8.7	0.45	46	7.3	67	SD – perit	2.7 ± 0.83	–	60 ± 18	–	<1/24 h	[346]
Mexiletine	64	5–9	5–6	846	22	200	IV 250 mg	4.7 10.5	– –	– 25.6/kg	1.5 9.22/kg	– <1%	[347]

* Data from ref. 336.

Table 6. Pharmacokinetic studies with beta-lactams and glycopeptide antibiotics in CAPD.

	Normal renal function			ESRD			IPD						
	PB %	$T^{1/2}$ h	V_d L/kg	Cl_{tot} ml/min	$T^{1/2}$ h	Cl_{tot} ml/min	Dose/route	$T^{1/2}$ h	C_{max} µg/ml	Cl_{tot} ml/min	Cl_{per} ml/min	% dose removed or absorbed	References
I. Beta-lactams													
Ampicillin	16–20	1.2	0.48	325	14	30	IV 2 g	9.5 ±2.2	170.3 ±56.6	25 ±7.7	2.7 ±0.5	11.3 ±2.2 /48 h	[348]
							IP 1 g/L	9.6 ±2.6	48 ±7.6	25 ±7.7	–	60 ±13 /48 h	
Sulbactam	–	0.25	0.2	250	21	–	IV 1 g	9.7 ±2.2	87.5 ±29.9 /5–6 h	22.6 ±3.2	3.4 ±0.4	152 ±1.9 /48 h	[349]
							IP 1 g	9.4 ±3.2	27.8 ±4.1 /5–6 h	22.6 ±3.2	–	68 ±13 /48 h	
Imipenem	13–21	1	–	205	1	205	IV 500 mg SD	3.28 ±0.59	29.3 ±10.5	66.8 ±18.1	–	3.2 ±0.5	[350]
							IP 500 mg/L			–	–	79 ±8	
Cilastatin	13–21	1	0.31	238	3.7–4.8	54	IV 500 mg SD	8.84 ±3.8	34.8 ±6.5	24 ±14.9	–	5.2 ±0.5	
Imipenem							IV 500 mg SD	6.2 ±1.4	29.5 ±12.2	76.3 ±23.5	4.8 ±0.6	–	
							IV 1000 mg SD	6.9 ±1.1	69.5 ±9.5	50.6 ±15.6	5.4 ±0	–	
Cilastatin							IV 500 mg	22.6 ±6.4	51.9 ±13.4	8.1 ±1.8	5.4 ±0.6	–	[245]
							IV 1000 mg	15.4 ±5.0	110.8 ±20.3	10.7 ±1.4	5.4 ±1.2	–	
Piperacillin	21	1	0.21	188	3.3	57	IV 2 g SD	2.43 ±0.84	104.4 ±26.1	104 ±37.7	3.17 ±0.67	2.5 ±0.7/6 h	
							IP 500 mg/L – perit	–	6.8 ±2.9 /2.6 h	–	–	67.8 ±8.5 /6 h	
							+ perit IV 1 g SD	2.41 ±0.49	8.9 ±2	100.2 ±13.8	2.7 ±0.8	83.4 ±4.6/6 h	[351]
							IP 1 g/L + perit	–	–	–	–	96.3/6 h	
Tazobactam	–	0.89 ±4.5	15.91 ±1.9	219 ±25	3.58 ±46.5	49.5 ±8.9	IV 3 g SD	2.12 ±26.3 ±876.1	270 ±31	65 ±12.9	3.6	5.5/28 h	[352]
							IV 0.375 g	6.36	28.6	36.9 ±11.8	3.8	10.7/28 h	
Temocillin	63–88	5–6	0.29	44	16–28		IV 15 mg/kg SD	13.4 ±3.9	±5.7	9.3 ±1.8	–	8 ±2.6 /24 h	[353]

Table 6. *(Continued)*

	Normal renal function				ESRD			IPD				% dose removed or absorbed	References
	PB %	T½ h	V_d L/kg	Cl_tot ml/min	T½ h	Cl_tot ml/min	Dose/route	T½ h	C_max µg/ml	Cl_tot ml/min	Cl_per ml/min		
Cefamandole	67–80	0.7	0.16	109	15	9	IP 500 mg/L SD	10.4±7.3	31.3±4.7 /6 h	20±6.2	3.2±1.6	71.7±12.8 /6 h	[354]
							IV 1 g SD	9.02±1.0 /1 h	65±10	24.4±6.4	1.48 ±0.41	5±2/24 h	[220]
							IP 500 mg	8.1±1.2	33±3/6 h	25.4±6.6	2.5±0.7	71±10/6 h	[355]
							IV 1 g	6.1±1.7	—	21.9±9.7	0.92 ±0.25	5±2.4/54 h	
Cefazolin	70–85	1.8	0.14	60	27	5	IV 10 mg/kg	33.1±1.0	—	5.7±0.6	1.0±0.4	—	[356]
							IP 10 mg/kg	—	30	5.85±0.7	0.81±0.14	73.7/4 h	[357]
							IP 500 mg/L LD	—	54.8±6.7	7.8	—	88/6 h	
							250 mg/L MD perit +	—	110.9±6.7 ±6.7	—	—	65/24 h	[358]
							125 mg/L perit +	29.2 ±16.2	141.3 ±51.9	—	—	—	
Cefepime							IV 1 g SD	17.6 ±2.9	62.9 +15.8	15.4 ±4.9	3.86 ±0.59	25/72 h	[359]
							IV 2 g SD	18.8 ±1.6	124 ±14	14 ±1.3	4.35 ±0.69	—	
Cefodizime	88						IV 1 g SD	4.1–6.8	—	16.1–31.7	0.3–0.9	1.2–6.4/24 h	[360]
							IP 500 mg/L SD	4–9.8	—	19.7–39.2	—	41–100/24 h	
Cefoperazone	65–90	1.8	0.22	100	2.9	78	IV 1 g	—	104.2 ±29.1	80±20	—	—	[361]
							IP 1 g/L		33.2 ±5.3/6 h	—	—	95±12/10 h	
							IV 1 g day 1–3	2.65 ±0.39	—	70.1 ±19.2	6.9 ±1.0	—	[362]
							IP 2 × 1 g/2L 2 days	—	—	—	—	63.8±4.8	
Cefoperazone Sulbactam													
Cefoperazone							IV 2 g ±0.82	2.08 ±21.2	280.9 ±33.4	71.9	0.55 ±0.08	1.0/48 h	[363]
							IV 1 g/L	2.33 ±0.96	38.9 ±12.4/2–4 h	71.9 ±33.4	—	61±14/6 h	

Table 6. *(Continued)*

	Normal renal function				ESRD			IPD					References
	PB %	$T\frac{1}{2}$ h	V_d L/kg	Cl_{tot} ml/min	$T\frac{1}{2}$ h	Cl_{tot} ml/min	Dose/route	$T\frac{1}{2}$ h	C_{max} µg/ml	Cl_{tot} ml/min	Cl_{per} ml/min	% dose removed or absorbed	
Sulbactam							IV 1 g	6.86 ±1.67	82.2 ±16.2	33.4 ±5.3	3.6 ±0.2	11.1±1.4 /48 h	
							IP 0.5 g/L	6.26 ±1.45	82.2 ±2.0	33.4 ±5.3	—	70±10/6 h	
Cefoperazone							IP 62.5 mg/L for 10 days + perit	—	10 at 24 h	—	—	—	[364]
Cefotaxime	36	1	0.28	322	2.5	135	IV 30 mg/kg	1.8±1.2	—	65±25	3.2	—	[273]
							IV 2 g	2.6±0.3	—	88±39	2.4±0.8	—	[365]
							IP 1 g/L	3.1±1.3	—	87.2 ±34.3	1.93±1.0	2.18/6 h	[366]
Cefotaxime (CFT)							IV 1 g						
							IP 0.5 g/L	—	10–12 /2–3 h	—	—	90/9 h	
						CFT	IV 1 g	2.31±0.20	—	118.7 ±12.3	6.7±1.3	4.9±0.7/24 h	[367]
						DAC*	IP 0.5 g/L	11.4±1.9	—	—	3.6±0.9	2.6±0.6/24 h	
						CFT		2.3±0.3	15±1.5/2 h	—	—	58.7±6.4/4 h	
						DAC		13.2±4.3	9.7±1.4/6 h	—	—	—	
						CFT	IV 2 g	2.24±1.04	322.9 ±105.2	81±31	1.82 ±0.43	—	[368]
						DAC	IP 1 g/L	18.9±21.7	37.8±19.4	—	2.84±0.7	—	
						CFT		2.57±1.03	29.7±9.2/ 4–8 h	71.2 ±29.3	11.5±6.9	74.6±21.3/6 h	
						DAC		25.3±33.8	19.5±12.6 /7.1 h	—	3.46±1.03	—	
						CFT	IV 1 g	1.59±0.47	156/5 min	—	—	3.5/6 h	[369]
						DAC		—	17.4/2 h	—	—	65/6 h	
						CFT	IP 0.5 g/L	—	9.1/2 h	—	—	—	[370]
						CFT	IP 250 mg/L + perit	—	—	250.8 ±59.5	—	90/24 h	
							– perit	—	—	94.8 ±23.4	—	67/24 h	
						CFT	IV 1 g	2.3–8.2	10–60	11–103	—	1.4–4.2/6 h	[371]
						DAC		—	—	—	—	—	

* Desacetyl Cefotaxime.

Table 6. *(Continued)*

	Normal renal function				ESRD			IPD					
	PB %	T½ h	V_d L/kg	Cl_{tot} ml/min	T½ h	Cl_{tot} ml/min	Dose/route	T½ h	C_{max} μg/ml	Cl_{tot} ml/min	Cl_{per} ml/min	% dose removed or absorbed	References
Cefotaxime						CFT	IP 500 mg/L (2 children)	1.83–2.49	11.9–13.1 /4.08 and 2.22 h	79–62	1.14–2.81	56.6 and 64.8 /5 h	[372]
						DAC		11–8.1	5.16–9.29 /5.73–5.33 h		1.88–4.15		
						CFT	IP 500 mg/L + perit (children)	–	26.9 ± 7.8	–	–	–	[373]
Cefotetan	78–91	3.7	0.15	39	35	4	IV 1 g	15.5 ± 1.9	–	6.5–20	1.1–3.2	5–9/24 h	[374]
Cefotiam							IV 1 g	8.1 ± 2.4	–	20.9 ± 3.8	3.3 ± 0.2	6 ± 1.1/5 h	[222]
							IV 1 g	5.1	103	20.4 ±1.45	1.44 ±0.25	–	[244]
Cefoxitin	50–60	0.9	0.3	290	22	12	IV 2 g	7.8 ± 1.1	197			–	[375]
							IP 4 × 50 mg/L 4 × 100 mg/L /24 h	20.2 ±3.7	15 7	13 ±3.3	4.1 ±2.3	71.2/24 h	[376]
Cefpirome							IV 1 g SD	15.4 ± 1.9	–	15.4 ± 2.4	1.62 ± 1.5	12.4/96 h	[377]
Cefsulodin							IV 1 g	11.6 ± 4.7	–	14.7 ± 5.4	4.3 ± 1.7	8.7 ± 3.6/5 h	[222]
							IP 1 g – perit	11.2 ± 1.9	–	26.5 ± 9	–	81 ± 13/5 h	
							+ perit	9.4 ± 1.3	–	23.9 ± 11.1	–	84 ± 6/5 h	
Ceftazidime	10–17	2	0.24	130	25	7	IP 4 × 125 mg/L – perit	–	9.27–22.24 (6–24 h)	–	1.47–4.13	–	[378]
							+ perit	–	13.1–25.3 (6–24 h)	–	2.43–3.89	65–75/24 h	
Ceftizoxime	31	1.4	0.4	190	35	6	IV 1 g	–	–	–	3–4	4.3–7/4–6 h	[379]
							IV 500 mg	10.2 ± 5.8	–	27.7	2.9	4.8 ± 2.1/6 h	[380]
							IV 1 g	12 ± 4.8	–	22.8	3.4	4.4/6 h	
							IP 250 mg/L	–	12.5/5 h	–	–	78 ± 4	
							IV 3 g	9.7 ± 5.1	411 ± 137 /0.25 h	17.1 ± 7.4	2.8 ± 0.7	–	[381]
Ceftriaxone	85–95	6–9	0.09	15	12–57	8	IV 1 g	12.3 ± 4.4	412 ± 354	14 ± 5.6	0.6 ± 0.4	4.5 ± 2.9/72 h	[382]
							IP 1 g	13.7 ± 10.1 /42 h	38.8 ± 11.6	–	–	44 ± 13/4 h	

Table 6. (Continued)

	Normal renal function				ESRD		IPD					
	PB %	$T^{1/2}$ h	V_d L/kg	Cl_{tot} ml/min	$T^{1/2}$ h	Cl_{tot} ml/min	Dose/route	$T^{1/2}$ h	C_{max} μg/ml	Cl_{tot} ml/min	Cl_{per} ml/min	% dose removed or absorbed	References
Ceftriaxone							IV 2 × 2 g at 24 h interval						
							– perit	9.8 ± 1.9	285 ± 69	13.3 ± 5	0.67 ± 0.5	–	[383]
							+ perit	14.8 ± 12.7	272 ± 54	15 ± 10	2.05 ± 1	–	[384]
							IP 1 g/L	10.5 ± 2.3	58.9	14.8	–	70.6 ± 7.9/4–6 h	[385]
							IP 1 g/L	–	71.1	10.1 ± 3.0 ml/kg/h	0.69 ± 0.2 ml/kg/h	71.4/5 h	
							IV 1 g	12.7 ± 2.9	–	7.4 (4–12.9)	–	–	[386]
								12.2					
Cefuroxime	33	1.3	0.2	140	20	15	IV 15 mg/kg	14.7 ± 1.1	–	–	3.59 ± 0.8	–	[280]
							IV 500 mg – perit	15.1 ± 1.9	24.2 ± 6.4	21.5 ± 1.2	4.2–2.9 ±1.2–1.3	–	[387]
							IP 250 mg/L – perit	14.4 ± 2.1	12.1 ± 2.2	20.3 ± 1.4	2.3–6.5	70	
							IP 1 × 250 mg/l LD + 125 mg/L MD	–	43.2 ± 7.5	–	9.9–12.4		
Cephalexin	10–50	0.8	0.26	263	20	10	0.500 mg SD	8.6 ± 0.9	SS	18.4 ±2.71	2.29 ± 0.63	–	[356]
							0.1–2 g/d for 3 days	–	–	–	55 ± 19.4 in dialysate day 1	16.5/day 1 –25.5/day 2	[388]
Cephalothin	60–65	0.6	0.26	350	10	21	IP 100 mg/L 4 exch/24 h	–	5.6 ± 2.2 24/h	–	–	–	[389]
							IV 1 g + IP 250 mg/l	17.1 ± 6.0 ± 6.0	100.3 ± 39.2	11.1 ± 12.7	–	–	[358]
							IV 1 g	3.0	111.0	–	–	–	[244]
							IP 0.5 g/L 0.500 mg SD	–	18.4/2h	–	–	–	
Cephradine	8–20	1.0	0.31	323	12	20		–	–	–	2.8–3.5	6.9/48 h	[390]
Moxolactam	50	2.5	0.3	97	20	12	IV 1 g	16.7 ± 2.9	123 ± 9	10.6 ± 2.0	2.7 ± 0.5	17.4 ± 3.1/24 h	[391]
							IP 0.5 g/L	13.2 ± 2.9	38.6 ± 12.7 /4 h	11.5 ± 2.4	2.3 ± 0.5	±60/4 h	[392]
							IV 1–2 g SD R MOX	17.3 ± 3.4	–	12.9 ± 6.9 (ml/h/Kg)	1.1 ± 0.6 (ml/h/Kg)	–	[393]
							S MOX	18 ± 3.3	–	13 ± 5.5	1.27 ± 0.62	–	

Table 6. (Continued)

	Normal renal function				ESRD		IPD					
	PB %	$T^{1/2}$ h	V_d L/kg	Cl_{tot} ml/min	$T^{1/2}$ h	Cl_{tot} ml/min	Dose/route	$T^{1/2}$ h	C_{max} µg/ml	Cl_{tot} ml/min	Cl_{per} ml/min	% dose removed or absorbed	References
Moxolactam							IP 0.5–1 g/L SD R MOX	–	–	–	–	71 ± 18	[394]
							S MOX	–	–	–	–	79 ± 18	
							IV 1 g SD	17.9 ± 4.2	171 ± 62 /0.08 h	12.8 ± 7.7	2.1 ± 0.5	20.2 ± 8.3/48 h	
							IP 0.5 g/l SD	15.4 ± 4.1	34.1 ± 8.5 /4.3 h	–	–	57 ± 16/4 h	
II. Glycopeptides													
Vancomycin	10	7	0.47	55	240	2	IP 500 mg/L	–	23.7 ± 6.5	–	2.4 ± 0.08	53/6 h	[395]
							IV 10 mg/kg	81		9.4 ± 1.9	1.48 ± 3.6	–	[396]
							IP 10 mg/kg 2 L	65.8 ± 10.7	6.3	15.1 ± 2.0	2.50 ± 0.33	65/4 h	[397]
							IV 10 mg/kg	90.2 ± 24.2		6.45 ± 1.1	1.35 ± 0.35		
							IP 500 mg/L LD	–	9.1/5 h	–	–	71.3/6 h	[398]
							IP 500 mg/L + perit	62.3	35.3 ± 19.1 /6 h	–	–	–	[399]
							300 mg/kg per 2 L IP – perit	–	–	–	–	50.8/6 h	[243]
							300 mg/kg per 2 L IP ±perit	–	–	–	–	73.9/6 h	
							IV 25 mg/kg + perit	115 ± 6	56.8 ± 4.7	7.2 ± 0.3	1.4 ± 1.05	–	[400]
							IV 15 mg/kg	111 ± 22	S57.1 ± 9.3	5.0 ± 1.4	1.2 ± 0.5		[401]
							IP 30 mg/kg	91.7 ± 28	S30.4 ± 7.2	5.0 ± 1.3	1.7 ± 0.9	46/6 h	[402]
							IP 1 g/2 L LD		15.5 ± 12.3 /4 h	8.52		–	
							IP 15 mg/kg LD		16.2 ± 1.75				
							IP 37.5 mg/L CAPD + perit	–	13.3 ± 4.5	–	–	70 ± 15/3 h	[403]

Table 6. *(Continued)*

	Normal renal function				ESRD		IPD					References
	PB %	$T_{1/2}$ h	V_d L/kg	Cl_{tot} ml/min	$T_{1/2}$ h	Cl_{tot} ml/min	Dose/route	$T_{1/2}$ h	C_{max} µg/ml	Cl_{tot} ml/min	Cl_{per} ml/min	% dose removed or absorbed	
Vancomycin							IP 37.5 mg/L CAPD –perit	–	8.8 ± 2.5	–	–	39 ± 13/3 h	[404]
							IP 15 mg/kg/2 L LD +MD 25 mg/L		17.8 ± 2.2 /1–6 h			63 ± 10.1/4 h	
							IP 25 mg/L no LD		0.27 ± 0.42 /6 h			71.9 ± 17.5/4 h	
							IV 1 g Perit +	103.9 ± 57.2	–	4.09 ± 0.45	3.84* ± 0.75 * max. perit.	–	[212]
Teicoplanin	95	41–62	0.84–1.13	5–10	124	<2	IV 3 mg/kg	162 ± 52	–	5.15 ± 1.34 ml/h.Kg	0.34 ± 0.02 ml/h.Kg	6.8 ± 1.2/6 days	[405]
							IV 6 mg/kg	242 (202–273)	–	5.7 ± 2.0 0.2 — 0.4		–	[406]
							IV 3 mg/kg	135	4.84 ± 1.43 /6 h	–	–	7.1 ± 1.2/6 h	[409]
							IP 6 mg/kg		8.0 ± 0.6			81.5 ± 10.7 3/5 h 9/2 weeks	[407]
							IV 3 mg/kg	377 ± 109	31.6 ± 5.2	2.76 ± 1.08	0.25 ± 0.21		[408]
							IV 6 mg/kg	266.4 ± 51.9	56.5 ± 7.0	0.04/kg	0.007/kg	6.1 ± 0.7/46 h	[407]
							IP 3 mg/kg	338 ± 60	6.6 ± 1.8/4 h	–	0.13 ± 0.07	77 ± 21	[408]

Table 7. Pharmacokinetic studies with quinolones, aztreonam, aminoglycosides, trimethoprm-sulfamethoxazole and fosfomycin.

	Normal renal function				ESRD			IPD					
	PB %	$T\frac{1}{2}$ h	V_d L/kg	Cl_{tot} ml/min	$T\frac{1}{2}$ h	Cl_{tot} ml/min	Dose/route	$T\frac{1}{2}$ h	C_{max} µg/ml	Cl_{tot} ml/min	Cl_{per} ml/min	% dose removed or absorbed	References
Ciprofloxacin	40	3–4	2.8	652	16.8	300	0 750 mg (n=6)	16.8±5.1	3.61±1.56	373.5 ±213.4	—	0.4–1.6/48 h	[426]
							0.4 × 250 mg – perit	8.44±3.23	—	—	—	1/48 h	[214]
							0.4 × 250 mg + perit	7.19±1.75	—	—	—	1.5/48 h	[427]
							every 12 h	11±1	2.3±0.2	256±47	4.16 ±0.33	2/48 h	
Fleroxacin	18	8.6	1.5	168	24.7 ±9.3	63	IV 100 mg SD	28.6±6.7	—	0.58 ±0.13/kg	0.05 ±0.01/kg	7.8±3.6/96 h	[428]
							0 400 mg SD	—	4.9±0.06	—	—	—	
Ofloxacin	25–30	6* ±1.2	1.23* ±0.11	180.5* ±32.1	18.4* ±12.1	68.4* ±35.1	0 300 mg	25.1±2.54	—	3.55 ±0.43	—	4.2/24 h ±0.5	[431]
							0 200 mg	26.8±2.5	—	35.2±8.2	4.0±0.5	5.8/24 h	[432]
							0 250 mg	—	—	—	—	5/24 h	[433]
							0 200 mg SD	35±4.19	—	29.3 ±11.2	4.5±0.8	15/96 h	[434]
							IP 10 mg/L SD – perit	—	—	—	—	81.9±1.5/4 h	[435]
							4 × 20 mg/2 L MD	—	0.57±0.07 /24 h	—	—	—	
							IP 10 mg/L SD – perit	—	—	—	—	84.7±1.5/3 h	
							4 × 20 mg/2 L MD	—	17.8±0.17	—	—	—	
Pefloxacin	25*	8*	1.9*	137*	12.1* ±1.7	117*	0 400 mg SD	19.2±3.3	—	1.0 ±0.2 (ml/min/Kg)	0.06 ±0.01	—	[436]
							IV 400 mg SD	17.4±2.3	6.4±0.4	—	—	—	

*Data from reference 429 & 430

Table 7. *(Continued)*

	Normal renal function				ESRD			IPD					
	PB %	$T^{1/2}$ h	V_d L/kg	Cl_{tot} ml/min	$T^{1/2}$ h	Cl_{tot} ml/min	Dose/route	$T^{1/2}$ h	C_{max} μg/ml	Cl_{tot} ml/min	Cl_{per} ml/min	% dose removed or absorbed	References
Pefloxacin							IP 200 mg/L	—	3.5 ± 0.8 /65 kg	1.3 ± 0.3	0.09 ± 0.02 (ml/min/Kg)	—	[437]
							0 400 mg SD	19 ± 5.8	5.6 ± 1.3	39.1 ± 11.1	2.7	2.3–3.7/24 h	
* Data from reference [430]													
Aztreonam	50–60	1.8	0.2	80	7.2	22	IV 1 g	—	—	23.8 ± 2.5	2.1 ± 0.29	9/48 h	[438]
							IP 500 mg/L		30 ± 3.3/3 h	—	—	72.9 ± 2.4/6 h	[439]
							IP 500 mg/L		42.5 ± 12.4 /6 h	—	10.05 ± 3.7	90.8 ± 3/8 h	
							IP 1.5 g/L single LD + perit	9.3 (6–14)	83 (61–96)/2 h	30.4	—	86–95	[440]
Gentamicin	<10	2	0.24	95	60	2	IV 1 mg/Kg	27.4 ± 11.7	4.5 ± 1.0	—	—	0 in 3/5 pts	[224]
							IP 1 mg/Kg	27.9	3.64 (6 h)	—	—	84/6 h	[441]
							IP 50 mg/L	36 ± 9	3.9 ± 1.5 (6 h)	—	2.94 ± 0.4	20.2 ± 9/24 h	
							IP 7.5 mg/L		0.6 (6 h)	—	5.7 ± 0.4	64/6 h	[229]
							– perit	—		—	mass transfer		
							+ perit	—	0.8 (6 h)	—	16.4 ± 1.9	79.3/6 h	
											mass transfer		
Tobramycin	<10	2.5	0.23	80	60	3	IV 1.1–1.5 mg/kg	34.6 ± 7.4	—	8.0 ± 1.0	3.8 ± 0.4	13–26/24 h	[442]
							IV 1.5 mg/kg	39.5 ± 18	—	7.6 ± 3.1	1.11 ± 0.8	—	[443]
							IP 1.5mg/Kg/2L	35.1 ± 12	1.8	9.8 ± 4.0	1.96 ± 1.6	52/6 h	[444]
							IV 2 mg/Kg	25.7 ± 46.5	9.8 ± 3 /0.3 h	7.3 ± 2 70 kg	3.4 ± 1 70 kg	30/48 h	
							IP 2 mg/Kg/2L CCPD 2L cycles per hour		5.6 ± 2/6 h	—	—	73 ± 10.6 h	
							IP 160 mg/2L – perit	—	5.9 ± 1.4 /40 h	—	12.8 ± 1.2	44 ± 4.4/48 h	[230]
							+ perit	—	6.5 ± 1.3 /40 h	—	17.4 ± 1.1	55 ± 3.6/48 h	
							IP 5 mg/L	—	1.3–2.1 ± 0.12/24 h	6.8	—	48/48 h	[357]

Table 7. *(Continued)*

	Normal renal function				ESRD		Dose/route	IPD					References
	PB %	T½ h	V_d L/kg	Cl_tot ml/min	T½ h	Cl_tot ml/min		T½ h	C_max µg/ml	Cl_tot ml/min	Cl_per ml/min	% dose removed or absorbed	
Tobramycin							IP 50 mg/L LD	—	4.3/6 h	5.6	—	85/6 h	
							IP 7.5 mg/L MD	—	3.7	—	—	50 ss	[445]
							IP 1.93 mg/Kg/2L LD	38.7±10.6	6.6±1.1	6.9±1.2	—	—	
							IP 0.96 mg/Kg/2L MD						
							IP 20 mg/2L −perit	—	—	—	6.5±3.1 mass transfer	—	[446]
							+perit	—	—	—	18.5±8.2 mass transfer	—	
Streptomycin	35	2.5	0.26	85	80	3	IP 100 mg/L LD	—	5.5/5 h	—	7.3	75/6 h	[447]
							IP 30 mg/L MD	—	4.8	—	—	—	
Amikacin	<10	2.5	0.25	90	70	3	IV 7.5 mg/Kg	42.2±14.2	18.6–26.8 /24 h	3.9±1.0 /1.73 m2	2.0±1.0 /1.73 m2	—	[448]
							IP 7.5 mg/Kg/2L	37.2±13.2	19.6±6.1 /5.6 h	4.6±1.2	2.7±0.4	53±14/5 h	
Netilmicin	<10	2.0	0.25	88	40	5	IV 100 mg −perit	18.1±3.7	—	16.8±2.3	3.38 ±0.37	23±2.7/48 h	[213]
							+perit	19.6±2.0	—	18.5±3.2	4.9±1.1	27.9±5.2/48 h	
Kanamycin	<10	2	0.23	95	80	2	IP 50 mg/L −perit	—	3.1±0.3	—	11.4±0.9 mass transfer	67±4/4 h	[449]
							+perit	—	4.3±0.4	—	17.2±2.1 mass transfer	83±2/4 h	

Table 7. *(Continued)*

	Normal renal function				ESRD			IPD					
	PB %	T½ h	V_d L/kg	Cl_{tot} ml/min	T½ h	Cl_{tot} ml/min	Dose/route	T½ h	C_{max} µg/ml	Cl_{tot} ml/min	Cl_{per} ml/min	% dose removed or absorbed	References
Trimethoprim	40–70	13	2	125	25	65	O 80 mg	24	–	–	2.32 ±0.39 (night) 4.65 ±1.25 (day)	–	[450]
Sulfamethoxazole	40–90	10	0.2	30	35	10	O 400 mg 4 × day	15	–	–	1.64 ±0.58 (night) 4.29 ±0.95 (day)	–	
Trimethoprim							O 320 mg	27.7	–	31.1	0.88	2.75/24 h	[451]
							IV 320 mg	28.6 ±10.6	–	29.3 ±11	0.77 ±0.36	2.7/24 h	
							IP 320 mg	27 ±8.8		39.1 ±20	0.77 ±0.35	73	
Sulfamethoxazole							O 1600 mg	12.8 ±1.9		11.9 ±3.2	0.62 ±0.25	5.24/24 h	
							IV 1600 mg	13.0		11.8 ±3.1	0.62 ±0.25	5.17/24 h	
							IP 1600 mg	11.8 ±2.2		15.3 ±5.0	0.53 ±0.08	65	
Fosfomycin	<10%	1.5–2	–	–	4.88 ±17.5	–	IP	–	–	–	14 ±2.5	60/3 h	[452]
							IV 1 g	38.4 ±8.7	32.6 ±2.8 /4 h	7.0 ±1.4	3.2 ±0.2	37.2 ±3.6	[453]
							IP 0.5 g	–	34.7 ±2.3 /5 h	–	–	68.4 ±6.0	

review and dose recommendations see reference [454]).

The pharmacokinetics after IP administration have only been studied for ofloxacin and pefloxacin, and for ciprofloxacin in CCPD [455]. Ciprofloxacin as single agent therapy was evaluated for the empirical treatment of CAPD peritonitis [456]. The treatment was successful in 83% of the 75 episodes. No accumulation occurred.

Aztreonam Aztreonam, a monobactam antibiotic, is effective against Gram-negative bacteriae, with the advantage of greater safety and a more predictable action in dialysate, compared to aminoglycosides. The pharmacokinetics of aztreonam, have been studied after both intravenous and intraperitoneal administration in CAPD patients. Based on these data, several authors have recently described their favourable results in Gram-negative peritonitis, including some pseudomonas infections, with the intraperitoneal administration of aztreonam [440, 457, 458] or in combination with cefuroxime [415] and vancomycin [457–459].

Aminoglycosides After systemic administration, a substantial fraction of the administered dose of the aminoglycoside is removed over 24–48 hours. The peritoneal clearance adds approximately 20–30% to the total removal from the body and clinically relevant concentrations in the dialysate are achieved after intravenous administration. This significant peritoneal clearance is due to the low protein binding and the small volume of distribution of these drugs. It is recommended that plasma levels should be measured regularly, especially in repeated usage.

Important absorption of these drugs after intraperitoneal administration has been noted; for all aminoglycosides tested, there was a significantly higher systemic bioavailability in peritonitis than in non-peritonitis patients. Continuous intraperitoneal administration of aminoglycosides in patients with peritonitis, leads to more or less constant plasma levels and carries the risk for otovestibular toxicity [460]. Others have found its use safe without ototoxicity [461].

Studies on stability of aminoglycoside antibiotics in peritoneal dialysate have also been performed [462]. Netilmicin, sisomicin and gentamicin were moderately stable (51–76% activity at 24 hr), Amikacin was less stable (38–50% activity at 24 hr) and Tobramycin was the least stable antibiotic (15–30% activity at 24 hr).

Table 8 summarizes the data on antiviral drugs and antifungal drugs.

2.5.4. Antiviral drugs

Acyclovir has significant activity against HSV-1, HSV-2 and Varicella-zoster virus (VZV). All the pharmacokinetic studies indicate that for systemic administration in CAPD patients, no dose adaptations beyond those for ESRD are necessary.

Studies in a limited number of patients on Zidovudine (ZDV) suggest that adjustment of a prescribed renal failure dosage regimen is not necessary during CAPD [468, 469] but great inter-patient variability in the pharmacokinetics was noted [468].

2.5.5. Antifungal drugs

Information on the pharmacokinetics of antifungal drugs in peritoneal dialysis patients is disappointingly scarce. Most studies are limited to occasional measurements of serum and/or dialysate levels during treatment for fungal peritonities. Amphotericin B which is a highly protein bound and circulates in the blood in a complex of high molecular weight (200,000–300,000) penetrates very poorly in the peritoneal fluid after systemic administration. The data are however conflicting [484, 485, 486]. Chemical peritonitis causing abdominal pain after intraperitoneal administration of amphotericin B has been observed [247–250, 487]. It has been proposed that for intraperitoneal use the dialysate should be adjusted to a neutral pH to prevent aggregation [487]. Amphotericin B has been used in an intravenous dose of 0.5 to 1 mg/kg body weight, combined with an intraperitoneal dose of 2 to 3 mg/L dialysate [488].

Fluconazole is a recently introduced antifungal agent, effective for both superficial and systemic fungal infections. The pharmacokinetic profile of orally administered fluconazole shows a low plasma protein binding, and a long plasma half-life, allowing once-daily dosing. The bioavailability is excellent. A good penetration of fluconazole into the peritoneal dialysate after a single oral dose of 100 mg in CAPD patients has been found [472]. When given systemically the dose should be the same as in undialysed patients [489].

Systemically administered fluorocytosine penetrates well into the peritoneal fluid [484]. The usual dose in uremic patients is a loading dose of 20–30 mg/kg, followed by maintenance doses of 15 mg/kg. Serum levels of fluorocytosine should be monitored since toxicity is to be expected when serum levels

Table 8. Pharmacokinetic data with antiviral and antifungal drugs in CAPD.

	Normal renal function					ESRD		Dose/route	IPD				% dose removed or absorbed	References
	PB %	$T^{1}/_{2}$ h	V_d L/kg	Cl_{tot} ml/min		$T^{1}/_{2}$ h	Cl_{tot} ml/min		$T^{1}/_{2}$ h	C_{max} µg/ml	Cl_{tot} ml/min	Cl_{per} ml/min		
Acyclovir	15	2–3	0.6	300		19.5	25	IV 200 mg/kg (n = 1)	14.7	–	48.6	3.6	7.3/24 h	[464]
								IV 5 mg/kg (n = 1) SD	17.1	7.7	48.3	4.4	5.7/24 h	[465]
								IV 1 g (n = 2) 0.5 g (n = 2)	13.2 ± 4.7	–	39.7 ± 10	3.4 ± 0.2	–	[466]
								IP 1 g/2 L	10.8 ± 2.9	≠	64.6 ± 7.5	–	61 ± 10	[467]
Zidovudine								O 200 mg SD				0	0	
Zidovudine								O 200 mg (n = 5) SD	1.8 ± 0.5	5.3 ± 2.4	1059 ± 511	5	< 1/24 h	[467]
GZVD*												15	20/24 h	
* GZVD*: glucuronide metabolite														
Zidovudine	30	1.1	1.4	1500		1.4	737	SD 200 mg	7.9	1.36	856	4.2	0.5/14 h	[469]
								SD 200 mg O (n = 1)						
								SD 100 mg O	26	0.2	2079	5.8	0.14/14 h	
								SD 200 mg ZVD	19.9	9.06	–	3.6	8.5/14 h	
GZVD								100 mg ZVD	7.1	6.78	–	3.7	4/14 h	
Antifungal drugs														
Amphotericin B	90–95	24	0.46	15		40	9	50 mg IV/4 h	S: 10* D: 0.1–0.2 *					[470]
								10 mg IV	S: 0.2 (1–12 h) D: 0.2					[471]
Fluconazole	11	33	0.71	–		98	–	O 100 mg	85	S: 1439 ±246 D: 1050 (6–24) 790 (24–48 h)	–	5.53 ±1.03	18/48 h	[472]
								IP 150 mg/2 L	80	S: 2123 ±360	8.75 ±2	4.3 ±0.4		[473]
								IP 50 mg/2 L	72	S: 885 ±136	7.63 ±1.2	4.41 ±0.49		

Table 8. (Continued)

	Normal renal function				ESRD			IPD					
	PB %	T½ h	V_d L/kg	Cl_tot ml/min	T½ h	Cl_tot ml/min	Dose/route	T½ h	C_max μg/ml	Cl_tot ml/min	Cl_per ml/min	% dose removed or absorbed	References
Fluorocytosine	4	5	0.7	113	85	7	LD 30–40 mg/kg 4 days MD 15 mg/kg 0		S ?				[474]
							LD 3.5 g 2 days 2.5 g 2 days MD 1 g day		D ? SS_s: 24–86				[475]
							IP 100 mg/L		SS_s: 25–33				
							– perit	–	1.78	–	16.1 ±2 81 ±2/4 h mas transfer		[476]
							+ perit	–	–	–	19.0 93/4 h mass transfer		
Itraconazole	99.8	21–38	–	–	25		LD 0 2 g + IP 100 mg/2 L	–	S: 25–33 D: 29–43	–	0		[478]
Ketoconazole	99	3	–	–	–	–	0 200 mg SD 0 400 mg/d (n=1)	3.51	S: 0.08 –	–	–		[479]
							0 200 mg/d for 4 days		SCmax 2.0 ±11.3 DCmax: < 0.1				[480]
							0 400 mg/D for 4 days		SCmax 1.6 ±0.5 DCmax: < 0.1				
							0 200 mg SD – perit + perit		DCmax 0.021 (ND-0.073) DCmax 0.015 (0.010–0.019)				[481]
							400 mg SD – perit + perit		Cmax D: 0.029 (0.014–0.056) D: 0.074 (0.032–0.115)				
							0 400 mg SD	2.4 ±0.8	Cmax 2.3 ±1.7		<1		[258]

exceed 100–125 ug/ml. It has mainly been tried with IP administration of 100–200 mg/2 L together with amphotericin B intravenously [249, 477] or in a dose of 150 mg/L in combination with oral ketoconazole 400 mg daily [490]. A single dose pharmacokinetic study of intraconazole has been performed in patients with ESRD, including 5 CAPD patients [478]. the systemic pharmacokinetics of intraconazole were not affected by CAPD and the drug could not be detected in the peritoneal dialysate.

Oral administration of ketoconazole in CAPD patients revealed extremely low peritoneal clearances, but due to its low protein binding in CAPD therapeutic free drug levels can be achieved in the peritoneal cavity, even after oral administration [256].

Table 9 summarizes the data obtained with drugs used in gastroenterology.

H_2-antagonists are frequently described in patients with ESRD and treated with dialysis, including chronic peritoneal dialysis. Studies have been performed with cimetidine, rantidine and famotidine [491–494]. Dosage reduction necessary for undialyzed patients, should be applied for patients on peritoneal dialysis. No pharmacokinetic data on nizatidine and roxatidine in CAPD are available. These drugs have however been studied in chronic renal failure [499]. It can be presumed that these drugs have a negligible peritoneal clearance.

To our knowledge, omeprazole, an inhibitor of the proton pump of the gastric parietal cell, has not been studied in CAPD patients. In patients with severe chronic renal failure, the pharmacokinetics are not significantly different from those in healthy subjects [500] and the drug is not detected in dialysis fluid during hemodialysis [501]. One can therefore expect that omeprazole could be administered in uremic and CAPD patients with the usual dosage regimen of 20 mg/day.

With cisapride, a gastrokinetic drug, in a dose of 5 mg/L dialysate 4 times per day, excellent results were obtained in two diabetic CAPD patients suffering from gastroparesis. The IP dose produced the same plasma levels as the oral or IV doses of 30 mg and 10 mg, respectively [497].

Tables 10a–c summarize the pharmacokinetic data with intravenous, subcutaneous and intraperitoneal administration of erythropoietin.

Recombinant human erythropoietin (Epo) is now established as an effective theraupeutic agent for anemia in patients undergoing longterm dialysis.

A number of interesting pharmacokinetic studies have been performed with Epo in peritoneal dialysis. For sake of clarity, the single study where the pharmacokinetics of Epo have been studied in IPD, has been included in the tables and in this discussion.

After IV administration, the kinetics can be described by a one-compartmental model, and there is a monoexponential concentration decay with a half-life ranging between 6 and 11 hours. Peritoneal dialysis itself has no significant effect on the removal of erythropoietin. When administered subcutaneouslsy (s.c.), Epo is slowly reabsorbed with a T_{max} around 20–24 hours. The s.c. bioavailability compared to intravenous dosing ranges between 10–36%.

There are theoretical benefits and enhanced absorption in animals associated with the intraperitoneal administration of erythropoietin [510, 511]. However in human pharmacokinetic studies on intraperitoneal administration of erythropoietin, a very low bioavailability (ranging from 2.5 to 8.5%) was found when diluted in 2 L of dialysate but this increased to 41.4 ± 7.2%, when administered into a dry abdomen [226, 506].

The problem of low bioavailability of intraperitoneal erythropoietin when diluted in dialysate, can be overcome by using high dosages of Epo or low volumes of dialysate. Frenken et al. [512] utilized 100 U/kg IP diluted in 1 L of dialysate over an 9-hour dwell thrice weekly and observed a slow but significant increase in hematocrit; Nasu et al. [513] reported an excellent hematocrit response when Epo in a high dose of 300 U/kg, diluted in 2 L dialysate, was given. In CAPD patients with a dry night, or CCPD patients with a dry day, daily IP erythropoietin might be a very efficacous therapy.

2.6. Insulin

Earlier studies demonstrated that intraperitoneal insulin is absorbed into the portal venous circulation [514, 515] and that IP insulin leads to a persistent positive portal-systemic difference [516]. A substantial portion (50%) of the portal venous insulin is degraded during first passage through the liver. Such IP treatment appears to improve glucose control and glucose stability without increasing the risk of hypoglycemia [517–521]. Recent studies have shown that the intrapatient variation of the plasma-free-insulin was markedly lower with continuous intraperitoneal than with continuous subcutaneous or intramuscular insulin administration

Table 9. Pharmacokinetic data with H_2-antagonists, metoclopramide and cispramide.

	Normal renal function				ESRD		Dose/route	IPD					References
	PB %	T½ h	V_d L/kg	Cl_{tot} ml/min	T½ h	Cl_{tot} ml/min		T½ h	C_{max} μg/ml	Cl_{tot} ml/min	Cl_{per} ml/min	% dose removed or absorbed	
Cimetidine	13–25	1.5–2	0.8–1.2	313–808	3–5	193	IV 300 mg	6.9±0.18	–	167.1 ±8.06	3.01 ±0.57	1.6±0.23/24 h	[491]
Ranitidine	15	1.5–3	1.1–1.9	568–709	6–9	103–230	IV 300 mg IV 50 mg	4.3 7.06±0.96	– –	191±55 126 ±67.5	4.2±3.1 3.2±0.7	2.2±1.4/24 h 1.3/24 h	[492] [493]
							O 150 mg	10.02±1.71	904±529 /4.2 h		2.6±0.6	0.9/24 h	
Famotidine	15–20	2.5–3.5	1.1–1.4	412	9–18	40–60	IV 20 mg O 30 mg every 6 h	15.5±4.0 –	– 0.031–0.04 (serum)	– –	– –	4.5±1.1/24 h –	[494]
Cisapride	98*	7–10*	2.4*	–	15*	385*	IV 10 mg every 6 h IP 5 mg/L every 6 h	– –	0.007–0.008 (dialysate) 0.028–0.053 (serum)	– –	– –	– –	[497]
Metoclopramide	–	3	3.4	916	14	196	O 15 mg (n=1) IV 15 mg (n=1) IP 15 mg/2 L (n=1)	34.65 30.13 30.13	66.4 329 146.2	– 61.6 –	3.54 1.47 –	– 3/6 h 97/6 h	[498]

* From references 495 & 496

Table 10A. Pharmacokinetics of intravenously administered erythropoietin in peritoneal dialysis.

PD regimen	Dose	C_{max} U/L	T_{max} h	$T^{1}/_{2}$ h	AUC U/1 hr	Vd (L)	Cl_{tot}	% dose lost	References
6 CAPD	300	7688 ± 1103	0.5	11.2 ± 0.4	81004 ± 9523	5.0 ± 1.0/24 h	0.52 ± 0.008 ml/min/Kg	2.63 ± 0.45 /24 h	[502]
9 CAPD	100	1595 ± 104 (11–145)	0.4 ± 0.1	8.7 ± 1.0	16909 ± 1217	4.9 ± 0.6	6.7 ± 0.5 ml/min	–	[503]
10 CAPD	100	2000	–	5.1 ± 0.6	–	–	–	–	[504]
7 CAPD	100	1440 (1088–1994)	–	8.3 (6.6–13)	14623 (10286–19562)	4.5	6.0 (4.7–9.7) ml/min/1.73 m^2	–	[505]
12 IPD	100	1923 ± 197	0.3	5.6 ± 0.3	–	3.7 ± 0.6	8.1 ± 1.4 ml/min	–	[506]
8 CAPD	120	3959 ± 758	0.25	8 ± 2 (6.2–10.2)	45102 ± 11405 (0–)	0.033 ± 0.013 1/Kg	0.047 ± 0.017 ml/min.Kg	2.3/24 h (1.7–3)	[507]
6 CAPD	100	1602	–	6.1	13592	–	–	–	[508]

Table 10B. Pharmacokinetics of subcutaneously administered erythropoietin in peritoneal dialysis.

PD regimen	Dose	C_{max} U/L	T_{max} h	AUC U/1 h	Bioavailability %	References
6 CAPD	300	484 ± 75	24	8230 ± 1312 (0–24 h)	10.2 ± 1.0/24 h	[502]
9 CAPD	100	81 (11–145)	12	–	14/24 h; 31/72 h	[504]
12 IPD	100	32 ± 4	28 ± 5	–	14.9 ± 4.8	[506]
8 CAPD	120	176 ± 75	18	9610 ± 4862 (0–)	21.5 (11.3–36)	[507]
6 CAPD	100	114	–	3316	24.0	[508]
10 CAPD	50	81 ± 13 mU/L	24	1492 ± 165 mU/1 h	–	[509]

Table 10C. Pharmacokinetics of intraperitoneally administered erythropoietin in peritoneal dialysis.

	Dose U/kg	Vol Dialysate	Dwell (h)	C_{max} U/L	T_{max} (h)	AUC U/1 h	Bioavailability %	References
6 CAPD	300	2	4	108 ± 18	8–12	1981 ± 271 (0–24 h)	2.5 ± 0.2	[502]
3 CAPD	300	2	12	170 ± 13	12	2933 ± 413 (0–24 h)	3.6 ± 0.5	
9 CAPD	100		12	52 ± 14	12 ± 0.2	1426 ± 366	8.5 ± 1.9	[503]
3 CAPD	100	2	10	80	12	56% of AUC after SC inj.	–	[504]
7 CAPD	100	2	12	23 (18–55)	14 (6.3–18)	808 (426–1652)	6.8 (2.2–12)	[505]
12 IPD	100	dry cavity	–	213 ± 27	17 ± 2.3	–	41.4 ± 7.2	[506]
8 CAPD	50.000 U	1.5–2	8	375 ± 123	12	6432 ± 2150 (0–24 h)	2.9 (1.2–6.8)	[507]
10 CAPD	50	2	8	36 ± 4	12–24	803 ± 67 mU/1 h	–	[509]
6 CAPD	400	50 ml of (saline undiluted)	8	1500 (estimated)	12	52399 ± 6865 mU/ml/h	> 9-fold increase vs diluted	[226]
6 CAPD	400	2 diluted	8	300 (estimated)	12	5739 ± 1292 mU/ml/h	–	

[522, 523]. this could be attributed to the considerably smaller insulin depot after IP than after subcutaneous administration.

Insulin is one of the most commonly administered intraperitoneal drugs in peritoneal dialysis patients. As already been pointed out in the introductory section of this chapter, IP insulin administration is most effective in patients on peritoneal dialysis if it is given into an empty peritoneal cavity, at least 30 minutes before the dialysate is instilled [225]; this creates a high peritoneum to plasma concentration gradient and avoids the absorption of insulin to the peritoneal fluid bags. When radiolabeled insulin was added to the 2 L dialysate bags, only 35% of the dose entered the peritoneal cavity [524]. In contrast, about 84 percent of 16 U of unlabelled insulin added per bag reached the peritoneal cavity [525]. Intraperitoneal insulin is rapidly absorbed and is detected in the peripheral blood within 15 minutes of administration and peak serum insulin levels are observed 30 to 45 minutes after administration into an empty peritoneal cavity [526]. These peak values are delayed until 90 to 120 minutes when insulin is added to the dialysate [527]. However, due to the partial hepatic inactivation of IP insulin, absorption kinetics and efficacy of IP and systemic insulin are difficult to compare by measurement of peripheral blood insulin levels.

At least in the experimental animal, the magnitude of the serum level is dependent on the intraperitoneal dose [528]. Studies by Rubin et al. [183] have shown that the addition of IP insulin has no effect on solute clearances, ultrafiltration volume or glucose absorption from the dialysis solution in CAPD patients. Several protocols for administration of intraperitoneal insulin during CAPD have been reviewed [529].

2.7. Heparin

Heparin has an average MW of 15,000 daltons and consists of a heterogeneous group of anionic mucopolysaccharides, called glycosaminoglycans. Heparin is the most frequently used drug in peritoneal dialysis, for the apparent purpose of preventing fibrin formation and catheter obstruction.

In the period when mainly IPD was used, doses from 100 U to 2500 U or more per liter dialysate over varying lengths of time from a few days to many months have been recommended [530–534]. Furman et al. [58] performed a pharmacokinetic study of IP heparin. The IP heparin was assayed as the activated-partial-thromboplastin time (APTT) of dialysate added to control plasma. The half life of disappearance from the peritoneal cavity ranged between 8.26 and 12.77 hours in 4 patients. This study was one of the first to show that systemic blood coagulation was unaffected by a single intraperitoneal dose of 10,000 U of heparin. The authors doubted the usefulness of IP heparin as an anticoagulant because of the low dialysate concentrations of the heparin cofactor anti-thrombin III (ATIII). Oreopoulos [2] confirmed this but other investigators [59, 535] showed that heparin did transfer across the rabbit peritoneal membrane and to a slight extent in CAPD patients [536]. In a CAPD patient with deep vein thrombosis, long-term intraperitoneal application of low molecular weight heparin in a dose of 8,000 antifactor Xa units/2 liter, resulted in adequate and therapeutic plasma levels as measured by antifactor Xa units [537]. Recently, it was demonstrated that the IP administration of heparin (1000 U/L to 2500 U/L) without addition of ATIII was sufficient for prevention of intraperitoneal fibrin formation in CAPD patients [536, 538].

2.8. Desferrioxamine

A pharmacokinetic study of desferrioxamine and its iron and aluminum chelates has been performed in CAPD patients [539].

Ten mg/kg desferrioxamine was administered either intramuscularly or intraperitoneally. The AUC calculated from 0–12 h was about 20% lower after the intraperitoneal than after the intramuscular administration. An advantage of the peritoneal administration was, however, the progressive increase in plasma concentrations, without an unduly high peak. The fact that 8–12 hours after administration the concentrations of desferrioxamine in the plasma and the peritoneal fluid were approximately the same, is consistent with the low binding of desferrioxamine to plasma proteins.

Desferrioxamine was given IV and IP in a CAPD patient in order to remove iron. Forty five percent of the total amount instilled was recovered in the outflow dialysate [540]. An intraperitoneal dose of 750 mg/day or 1250 mg on alternate days led to removal of 73 mg and 39.6 mg iron, respectively, as compared with 75 mg removal per week after an IV dose of 1500 mg thrice weekly.

Several authors have used intraperitoneal desferrioxamine successfully to remove aluminum in peritoneal dialysis patients [541–543]. IP doses of

40 mg/kg were used over a 10 hr dwell in one study [543] and 0.5 g into each 2 L dialysate to a total dose of 6 g was applied in another study [544]. In the latter study, the aluminum clearance with desferrioxamine was 3.1 ml/min vs 2.5 ml/min without desferrioxamine. The enhanced removal of aluminum by peritoneal dialysis persists for several days after single administration of the chelator.

2.9. Vitamin D3 and its metabolites

CAPD treatment is associated with peritoneal losses of vitamin D metabolites, contributing to the low serum levels of 25-OH-D_3 and 25-OH-D binding capacity [545, 546]; losses of 1,25$(OH)_2D_3$ and 24,25$(OH)_2D_3$ in the dialysate average 6 to 8% of the plasma pool per day [547].

Intraperitoneal calcitriol raises serum calcium and depresses serum PTH more effectively than increasing dialysis fluid calcium [548].

Salusky *et al.* [549] have studied the pharmacokinetics of calcitriol after IV, oral and IP administration in CAPD and CCPD patients. Doses of 60 ng/kg were given and the serum calcitriol levels were similar after 24 hours for the different routes of administration (55.6 ± 14.6 pg/ml after oral, 56.4 ± 17.6 pg/ml after IV and 53.8 ± 20.1 pg/ml after IP). The bioavailability of calcitriol (AUC 0–24 hr) was 50 to 60% greater after IV than after oral or IP administration. Radioisotope tracer studies indicated that 35% to 40% of the hormone adheres to plastic components of the peritoneal dialysate delivery system. the authors modified the technique of IP calcitriol administration by direct instillation of the drug in the Tenckhoff catheter and by increasing the IP dose to 120 ng/kg. With this method an AUC equal to the AUC obtained after IV injection was observed.

2.10. Other vitamins

Boeschoten *et al.* [550] have summarized earlier studies on vitamin status and vitamin losses in the dialysate in IPD and CAPD patients. They have recently performed a more complete analysis of plasma and 24 hours dialysate losses of vitamin A, B1, B2, B6, B12, C, folic acid, E and beta-carotene in 44 CAPD patients. Vitamins B12, A and E and carotenoids were not detectable in dialysate. In contrast, vit B2, B3, B6, C and folic acid were excreted in the 24 hr dialysate in amounts higher than in 24 hr urine of individuals with normal renal function. The loss of vit B1 in dialysate was low. These authors recommend vitamin supplementations in CAPD patients for vit B1, B6, C and folic acid.

2.11. Miscellaneous

Table 11 summarizes pharmacokinetic data obtained with a variety of drugs. Recently, an interesting observation on the removal of ethosuximide and phenobarbital by peritoneal dialysis in an epileptic child was made [551]. During a peritonitis episode, the daily dialysis time of 8 hours (CCPD) was increased to 24 hours and the patient developed convulsions. Apparently a substantial amount of both anticonvulsant medications was removed via the peritoneal dialysate and supplementary doses of both drugs were needed to stabilize the patient.

The two agents used in anaerobic infections, metronidazole and ornidazole have a low peritoneal clearance and only 10 and 6% of the dose respectively, are removed by the peritoneum [552, 553]. The dosage in CAPD patients is therefore the same as in undialyzed, uremic patients.

Leaky *et al.* [555] described a 3 year old asthmatic boy who developed acute renal failure necessitating acute peritoneal dialysis. His plasma theophylline concentrations remained therapeutic; yet, the child developed the symptoms of theophylline toxicity while undergoing peritoneal dialysis. Excessively high plasma concentrations of the principal theophylline metabolite, 1, 3-dimethyluric acid, were found. The high concentrations decreased only when renal function recovered. Apparently, peritoneal dialysis is not able to remove this theophylline metabolite.

In a pharmacokinetic study of flurbiprofen, CAPD patients were used as representative patients with end-stage renal disease. Neither flurbiprofen nor its metabolites were detected in dialysate [556].

Alprazolam is a triazolobenzodiazepine and has been studied in a pharmacokinetic and pharmacodynamic evaluation in normal subjects and in dialysis patients, including CAPD patients [557]. Dialysate measurements were not performed but the authors noted that CAPD patients, compared to controls and hemodialysis patients, had significantly longer serum half-lives and lower total clearances. There were also significantly higher free fractions of the drug in the dialysis patients, compared to normal subjects. Although no dosage adjustments for hemodialysis patients are needed compared to normal subjects, CAPD patients should be monitored for side effects and the dose should be

Table 11. Pharmacokinetics of miscellaneous drugs in CAPD.

	Normal renal function				ESRD			IPD				% dose removed or absorbed	References
	PB %	$T^{1/2}$ h	V_d L/kg	Cl_{tot} ml/min	$T^{1/2}$ h	Cl_{tot} ml/min	Dose/route	$T^{1/2}$ h	C_{max} µg/ml	Cl_{tot} ml/min	Cl_{per} ml/min		
Ethosuximide	0	60	–	10	–	–	0.3 × 400 mg CCPD (child)	–	–	–	–	50/24 h	
Metronidazole	20	7	0.7	82	7	82	IV 750 mg	10.93 ±2.01	–	50.17 ±18.6 (ml/Kg/h)	4.49 ±0.88	10/48 h	[552]
Ornidazole							IV 500 mg	11.8 ±0.9	–	47.9 ±6.3	3.0 ±0.4	6.2 ±1.1/48 h	[553]
Phenobarbital	66	70	0.75	9	100	6	0.2 × 250 mg day 6 CCPD (child)	–	[21]	–	–	40/24 h	[551]
Phenytoin	87–93	18	0.57	25	9	125	0.3 × 100 mg	–	16.6 µm/L SS	–	1.77	–	[554]
							0.3 × 200 mg	–	22.6 µm/L SS	–	1.70	–	
							0.4 × 100 mg	–	26.1	–	1.60	–	

adjusted accordingly. Data on other benzodiazepines in CAPD are not available.

Dedication

In memory of John F. Maher, our dear friend and teacher, a pioneer in the field of peritoneal dialysis physiology, who brought the rigorous scientific methodology to this exciting arena.

Acknowledgements

The authors greatly appreciate the secretarial skills of Mrs. Barbara Fitzgerald and Mrs. Ingrid Verslycken. We also thank Dr. Ralph E. Cutler and Mosby Year Book, Inc., for permission to use their data (reference [259]) in the pharmacokinetics tables of this chapter. The opinions and assertions contained herein are private ones of the authors and are not to be construed as official or reflecting the views of the Department of Defense or the Uniformed Services University of the Health Sciences.

References

1. Broyer M, Brunner FP, Brynger H, Donckerwolcke RA, Jacobs C, Kramer P, Selwood NH, Wing AJ. Combined report on regular dialysis and transplantation in Europe, XII, 1981. Proc EDTA 1982; 19: 3–59.
2. Oreopoulos DG. Chronic peritoneal dialysis. Clin Nephrol 1978; 9: 165–173.
3. Nolph KD. Continuous ambulatory peritoneal dialysis. Am J Nephrol 1981; 1: 1–10.
4. Verger C, Brunschvicg O, Le Charpentier Y, Lavergne A, Vantelon J. Structural and ultrastructural peritoneal membrane changes and permeability alterations during continuous ambulatory peritoneal dialysis. Proc EDTA 1981; 18: 199–203.
5. Nolph KD, Stoltz ML, Maher JF. Altered peritoneal permeability in patients with systemic vasculitis. Ann Intern Med 1973; 75: 753–5.
6. Popovich RP, Moncrief JW, Nolph KD, Ghods AJ, Twardowski ZJ, Pyle WK. Continuous ambulatory peritoneal dialysis. Ann Intern Med 1978; 88: 449–56.
7. Nolph KD, Miller FN, Pyle WK, Popovich RP, Sorkin MI. An hypothesis to explain the ultrafiltration characteristics of peritoneal dialysis. Kidney Int 1981; 20: 543–8.
8. Hirszel P, Dodge K, Maher JF. Acceleration of peritoneal solute transport by cytochalasin D. Uremia Invest 1985; 8: 85–9.
9. Maher JF, Hirszel P, Bennett RR, Chakrabarti E. Amphotericin B selectively increases peritoneal ultrafiltration. Am J Kidney Dis 1984; 4: 285–8.
10. Mactier RA, Khanna R, Twardowski ZJ, Nolph KD. Role of peritoneal cavity absorption in peritoneal dialysis. Kidney Int 1987; 32: 165–72.
11. Maher JF, Hirszel P, Hohnadel DC, Abraham J, Lasrich M. Fatty acid removal during peritoneal dialysis. Mechanisms, rates and significance. ASAIO J 1978; 1: 8–14.
12. Dedrick RL, Myers CE, Bungay PM. DeVita VT Jr. Pharmacokinetic rationale for peritoneal drug administration in the treatment of ovarian cancer. Cancer Treat Rep 1978; 62: 1–9.
13. Henderson LW, Cheung AK, Chenoweth DE. Choosing a membrane. Am J Kidney Dis 1983; 3: 5–20.
14. Garred LJ, Canaud B, Farrell PC. A simple kinetic model for assessing peritoneal mass transfer in chronic ambulatory peritoneal dialysis. ASAIO J 1983; 6: 131–7.
15. Pappenheimer JR, Renkin EM, Borrero LM. Filtration, diffusion and molecular sieving through peripheral capillaries; a contribution to the pore theory of capillary permeability. Am J Physiol 1961; 167: 13–46.
16. Lasrich M, Maher JM. Hirszel P, Maher JF. Correlation of peritoneal transport rates with molecular weight: a method for predicting clearances. ASAIO J 1979; 2: 107–13.
17. Gosselin RE, Berndt WO. Diffusional transport of solutes through mesentery and peritoneum. J Theor Biol 1962; 3: 487–95.
18. Aune S. Transperitoneal exchange II: Peritoneal blood flow estimated by hydrogen gas clearances. Scan J Gastroenterol 1970; 5: 99–104.
19. Nolph KD. The first hemodialyzer. ASAIO J 1978; 1: 2–7.
20. Hirszel P, Chakrabarti EK, Bennett RR, Maher JF. Permselectivity of peritoneum to neutral dextrans. Trans Am Soc Artif Intern Organs 1984; 30: 625–8.
21. Casley-Smith JR. An electron microscopical study of the passage of ions through the endothelium of lymphatic and blood capillaries and through the mesothelium. QJ Exp Physiol 1967; 52: 105–13.
22. Cotran RS, Karnovsky MJ. Ultrastructural studies of the permeability of the mesothelium to horseradish peroxidase. J Cell Biol 1968; 37: 123–37.
23. Gotloib L, Digenes GE, Rabinovich S, Medline A, Oreopoulos DG. Ultrastructure of normal rabbit mesentery. Nephron 1983; 34: 248–55.
24. Wayland H. Transmural and interstitial molecular transport. In: Legrain M (ed), Proc Int Symposium Continuous Ambulatory Peritoneal Dialysis. Excerpta Medica, Amsterdam 1980; pp 18–27.
25. Breborowicz A, Knapowski J. Studies on the resistance of the peritoneal mesothelium to solute transport. Perit Dial Bull 1984; 4: 37–9.
26. Cascarano J, Rubin AD, Chick WL, Zweifach BW. Metabolically induced permeability changes across mesothelium and endothelium. Am J Physiol 1964; 206: 373–82.
27. Dobbie JW, Lloyd JK. Mesothelium secretes lamellar bodies in a similar manner to type II pneumocyte secretion of surfactant. Perit Dial Int 1989; 9: 215–9.

28. Robson M, Oreopoulos DG, Izatt S, Ogilvie R, Rapaport A, DeVeber GA. Influence of exchange volume and dialysate flow rate on solute clearance in peritoneal dialysis. Kidney Int 1978; 14: 486–90.
29. Twardowski Z, Nolph KD, Prowant BF, Moore HL. Efficiency of high volume low frequency continuous ambulatory peritoneal dialysis (CAPD). Trans Am Soc Artif Intern Organs 1983; 29: 53–7.
30. Twardowski ZJ, Nolph KD, Khanna R, Prowant BF, Frock JT, Dobbie JW, Kenley RS, Serkes KD, Witsoe DA, Garber JW. Tidal peritoneal dialysis. In: Avram MM, Girodano C (eds), Ambulatory Peritoneal Dialysis. Plenum Publ. Corp, New York, 1990; pp 145–9.
31. Diaz-Buxo JA, Walker PJ, Farmer CD, Chandler JT, Holt KL, Cox P. Continuous cyclic peritoneal dialysis. Trans Am Soc Artif Intern Organs 1981; 27: 51–4.
32. Nakagawa D, Price C, Steinbaugh B, Suki W. Continuous cycling peritoneal dialysis: a viable option in the treatment of chronic renal failure. Trans Am Soc Artif Intern Organs 1981; 23: 55–7.
33. Rubin J, Clawson M, Planch A, Jones Q. Measurements of peritoneal surface area in man and rat. Am J Med Sci 1988; 295: 453–8.
34. Grayson J, Mendel D. Physiology of the Splanchnic Circulation. Baltimore: Williams and Wilkins Co, 1965.
35. Lanciault G, Jacobson ED. The gastrointestinal circulation. Gastroenterology 1976; 71: 851–73.
36. Felt J, Richard C, McCaffrey C, Levy M. Peritoneal clearance of creatinine and inulin during dialysis in dogs: effect of splanchnic vasodilators. Kidney Int 1979; 16: 459–69.
37. Renkin EM. Exchange of substances through capillary walls. In: Wolstenholme GEW (ed), Ciba Foundation Symposium. Little, Brown and Co, Boston 1969; pp 50–66.
38. Taylor JE, MacTier RA, Henderson IA, Belch JJF, Stewart WK. Dialysis efficiency in continuous ambulatory peritoneal dialysis patients treated with erythropoietin. Perit Dial Int 1992; 12: 221–6.
39. Hutchinson AJ, Ofsthun NJ, Howarth D, Gokal R. The effect of hemoglobin concentration on peritoneal mass transfer and drain volumes in continuous ambulatory peritoneal dialysis. Perit Dial Int 1992; 12: 230–3.
40. Swan KG, Reynolds DG. Adrenergic mechanisms in the canine mesenteric circulation. Am J Physiol 1971; 220: 1779–85.
41. Messina EJ, Weiner R, Kaley G. Prostaglandins and local circulatory control. Fed Proc 1976; 35: 2367–75.
42. Steinhauer HB, Schollmeyer P. Prostaglandin-mediated loss of proteins during peritonitis in continuous ambulatory peritoneal dialysis. Kidney Int 1986; 29: 584–90.
43. Pietrzak I, Hirszel P, Shostak A, Welch PG, Lee RE, Maher JF. Splanchnic volume, not flow rate, determines peritoneal permeability. Am Soc Artif Int Organs Transactions 1989; 35: 583–7.
44. Maher JF. Blood flow to the peritoneum: physiological and pharmacological influences. In: Moncrief JW, Popovich RP (eds), CAPD update Continuous Ambulatory Peritoneal Dialysis. Masson Publ USA, New York 1981; 53–62.
45. Courtice FC, Roberts DCK. Peritoneal fluid in the rabbit: permeability of the mesotheliumn to proteins, lipoproteins and acid hydrolases. Lymphology 1975; 8: 1–10.
46. Torres IJ, Litterst CL, Guarino AM. Transport of model compounds across the peritoneal membrane in the rat. Pharmacology 1978; 17: 330–40.
47. Richardson PDI. The actions of natural secretin on the small intestinal vasculature of the anesthetized cat. Br J Pharmacol 1976; 58: 127–35.
48. Goldbert LI. Cardiovascular and renal actions of dopamine: potential clinical applications. Pharmacol Rev 1972; 24: 1–29.
49. Henderson LW, Nolph KD. Altered permeability of the peritoneal membrane after using hypertonic peritoneal dialysis. J Clin Inves 1969; 48: 992–1001.
50. Maher JF, Bennett RR, Hirszel P, Chakrabarti E. The mechanism of dextrose-enhanced peritoneal mass transport rates. Kidney Int 1985; 28: 16–20.
51. Harris EJ. Transport and Accumulation in Biological Systems, Third Edition. Butterworths, London 1972.
52. Charonis AS, Wissig SL. Anionic sites in basement membranes. Differences in their electrostatic properties in continuous and fenestrated capillaries. Microvasc Res 1983; 25: 265–85.
53. Gotloib L, Shustack A, Jaichenko J. Ruthenium-red-stained anionic charges of rat and mice mesothelial cells and basal lamina: The peritoneum is a negatively charged dialyzing membrane. Nephron 1988;48: 65–70.
54. Leak LV. Distribution of cell surface charges on mesothelium and lymphatic endothelium. Microvasc Res 1986; 31: 18–30.
55. Ahearn DJ, Nolph KD. Controlled sodium removal with peritoneal dialysis. Trans Am Soc Artif Intern Organs 1972; 18: 423–8.
56. Maher JF, Hohnadel DC, Shea C, DiSanzo F, Cassetta M. Effects of intraperitoneal diuretics on solute transport during hypertonic dialysis. Clin Nephrol 1977; 7: 96–100.
57. Pollock CA, Ibels LS, Hallett MD, Cocksedge B, Caterson RJ, Mahony JF, Farrell PC. Loss of ultrafiltration in continuous ambulatory peritoneal dialysis (CAPD). Perit Dial Int 1989; 9: 107–10.
58. Furman KI, Gomperts ED, Hockley J. Activity of intraperitoneal heparin during peritoneal dialysis. Clin Nephrol 1978; 9: 15–8.
59. Canavese C, Salomone M, Mangiorotti G, Pacitti A, Trucco S, Scaglia C, Assone F, Lunghi F, Vercellone A. Herparin transfer across the rabbit peritoneal membrane. Clin Nephrol 1986; 26: 116–20.
60. Grahame GR, Torchia MG, Dankewich KA, Ferguson IA. Surface-active material in peritoneal effluent of CAPD patients. Perit Dial Bull 1985; 5: 109–11.
61. DiPaolo N, Buoncristiani U, Capotundo L, Saggiotti E, DeMia M, Rossi P, Sansoni E, Bernini

M. Phosphatidylcholine and peritoneal transport during peritoneal dialysis. Nephron 1986; 44: 365–70.
62. Breborowicz A, Sombolos K, RodeIa H, Ogilvie R, Bargman J, Oreopoulos DG. Mechanism of phosphatidylcholine action during peritoneal dialysis. Perit Dial Bull 1987; 7: 6–9.
63. Maher JF. Lubrication of the peritoneum. Perit Dial Int 1992; 12: 346–9.
64. Mermier P, Baker H. Flux of free fatty acids among host tissues, ascitic fluid and Ehrlich ascites carcinoma cells. J Lipid Res 1974; 15: 339–51.
65. Adkins ES, Salman FT, Fonkalsrud EW. Triglyceride absorption in transperitoneal alimentation. Am J Surg 1990; 159: 237–40.
66. Dumont AE, Robbins E, Martelli A, Iliescu H. Platelet blockade of particle absorption from the peritoneal surface of the diaphragm. Proc Soc Exp Biol Med 1981; 167: 137–42.
67. Flessner MF, Dedrick RL, Fenstermacher JD, Blasberg RG, Sieber SM. Peritoneal absorption of macromolecules. In: Maher JF, Winchester JF (eds), Frontiers in Peritoneal Dialysis. Field Rich and Assoc, New York 1986; pp 41–6.
68. Lindholm B, Werynski A, Bergstrom J. Fluid transport in peritoneal dialysis. Int J Artif Organs 1990; 13: 352–8.
69. Daugirdas JT, Ing TS, Gandhi VC, Hano JE, Chen WT, Yuan L. Kinetics of peritoneal fluid absorption in patients with chronic renal failure. J Lab Clin Med 1980; 95: 351–61.
70. Flessner MF, Parker RJ, Sieber SM. Peritoneal lymphatic uptake of fibrinogen and erythrocytes in the rat. Am J Physiol 1983; 224: H89–96.
71. Rippe B, Stelin G, Ahlmen J. Lymph flow from the peritoneal cavity in CAPD patients. In: Maher JF, Winchester JF (eds), Frontiers in peritoneal Dialysis. Field Rich and Assoc, New York 1986; pp 24–30.
72. Brouard R, Tozer TN, Bameolou A, Gambertoglio JF. Transfer of autologous haemoglobin from peritoneal cavity during peritoneal dialysis. Nephrol Dial Transplant 1992; 7: 57–62.
73. De Paepe M, Belpaire F, Schelstraete K, Lameire N. Comparison of different volume markers in peritoneal dialysis. J Lab Clin Med 1988; 111: 421–9.
74. Krediet RT, Struijk DG, Koomen GCM, Hoek FJ, Arisz L: The disappearance of macromolecules from the peritoneal cavity during continuous ambulatory peritoneal dialysis (CAPD) is not dependent on molecular size. Perit Dial Int 1990; 10: 147–52.
75. Mactier RA, Nolph KD, Khanna R, Twardowski ZJ, Moore H, McGary T. Lymphatic absorption in peritoneal dialysis in the rat. Lymphology 1987; 20: 47.
76. De Paepe M, Matthys D, Lameire N. Measurement of peritoneal lymph flow in CAPD using different osmotic agents. In: Khanna R, Nolph KD, Prowant BF, Twardowski ZJ, Oreopoulos G (eds), Advances in CAPD 1989; 5: 2–15.
77. Koomen GCM, Krediet RT, Leegwater ACJ, Struijk DG, Arisz L, Hoek FJ. A fast reliable method for the measurement of intraperitoneal dextran used to calculate lymphatic absorption. In: Khanna R, Nolph KD, Prowant BF, Twardowski ZJ, Oreopoulos G (eds), Advances in CAPD 1991; 7: 10–4.
78. Hirszel P, Shea-Donohue T, Chakrabarti E, Montcalm E, Maher JF. The role of the capillary wall in restricting diffusion of macromolecules. A study of peritoneal clearance of dextrans. Nephron 1988; 49: 58–61.
79. Khanna R, Mactier R, Twardowski ZJ, Nolph KD. Peritoneal cavity lymphatics. Perit Dial Bull 1986; 6: 113–21.
80. Mactier RA, Khanna , Moore H, Twardowski ZJ, Nolph KD. Pharmacological reduction of lymphatic absorption from the peritoneal cavity increases net ultrafiltration and solute clearances in peritoneal dialysis. Nephron 1988; 50: 229–32.
81. Hasbargen JA, Hasbargen BJ, Fortenberg EJ, James MK. Effect of intraperitoneal neostigmine on peritoneal transport characteristics in CAPD. Kidney Int 1992; 42: 1398–400.
82. Chan PCK, Tam SCF, Cheng IKP. Oral neostigmine and lymphatic absorption in a myasthenia gravis patient on continuous ambulatory peritoneal dialysis (CAPD). Perit Dial Int 1990; 10: 93–6.
83. Mactier R, Khanna R, Twardowski Z, Moore H, Nolph K. Influence of phosphatidylcholine on lymphatic absorption during peritoneal dialysis in the rat. Perit Dial Int 1988; 8: 179–86.
84. Krack G, Viglino G, Cavalli PL, Gandolfo C, Magliano G, Cantaluppi A, Peluso F. Intraperitoneal administration of phosphatidylcholine improves ultrafiltration in continuous ambulatory peritoneal dialysis patients. Perit Dial Int 1992; 12: 359–64.
85. Ersoy FF, Khanna R, Moore H. Effect of phosphatidylcholine (PC) on peritoneal fluid kinetics (PFK). Peritoneal Dial Int 1992; 12 (suppl 2): S3.
86. Miller FN, Nolph KD, Harris PD, Rubin J, Wiegman DL, Joshua IG, Twardowski ZJ, Ghods AJ. Microvascular and clinical effects of altered peritoneal dialysis solutions. Kidney Int 1979; 15: 630–9.
87. Nolph KD. Peritoneal anatomy and transport physiology. In: Drukker W, Parsons FM, Maher JF (eds), Replacement of Renal Function by Dialysis. Second Edition. Martinus Nijhoff, The Hague: 1983; pp 440–56.
88. Breborowicz A, Knapowski J. Local anesthetic-bupivicaine increases the transperitoneal transport of solutes. Part II: In vitro study. Perit Dial Bull 1984; 4: 224–8.
89. Rubin J, Jones Q, Planch A, Lockard V, Bower J. Enhancement of peritoneal transport in rats by disrupting stagnant fluid films. Am J Med Sci 1988; 295: 108–13.
90. McGary TJ, Nolph KD, Moore H, Kartinos NJ. Polycation as an alternative osmotic agent and phosphate binder in peritoneal dialysis. Uremia Invest 1984; 8: 79–84.
91. DeSanto NC, Capodicasa C, Capasso G, Giordano

C. Development of means to augment peritoneal urea clearances: The synergistic effects of combining high dialysate temperature and high dialysate flow rates with dextrose and nitroprusside. Artif Organs 1981; 5: 409–14.
92. Erbe RW, Greene JA Jr, Weller JM. Peritoneal dialysis during hemorrhagic shock. J Appl Physiol 1967; 22: 131–5.
93. Greene JA Jr, Lapco, Weller JM. Effect of drug therapy of hemorrhagic hypotension on kinetics of peritoneal dialysis in the dog. Nephron 1970; 7: 178–83.
94. Kincaid-Smith P. Participation of intravascular coagulation in the pathogenesis of glomerular and vascular lesions. Kidney Int 1975; 7: 242–53.
95. Maher JF, Hirszel P. Augmentation of peritoneal clearances by drugs. In: Legrain M (ed), Proc Int Symposium Continuous Ambulatory Peritoneal Dialysis. Excerpta Med, Amsterdam 1980; pp 42–6.
96. Maher JF, Hirszel P, Abraham JE, Galen MA, Chamberlin M, Hohnadel DC. The effect of dipyridamole on peritoneal mass transport. Trans Am Soc Artif Intern Organs 1977; 23: 219–23.
97. Brown ST, Ahearn DJ, Nolph KD. Reduced peritoneal clearance in scleroderma increased by intraperitoneal isoproterenol. Ann Intern Med 1973; 78: 891–4.
98. Nolph KD, Miller L, Husted FC, Hirszel P. Peritoneal clearance in scleroderma and diabetes mellitus: effects of intraperitoneal isoproterenol. Int Urol Nephrol 1976; 8: 161–9.
99. Nolph KD, Ghods AJ, Brown PA, Twardowski ZJ. Effects of intraperitoneal nitroprusside on peritoneal clearance in man with variations of dose, frequency of administration and dwell times. Nephron 1979; 24: 114–20.
100. Maher JF, Hirszel P, Lasrich M. An experimental model for study of pharmacologic and hormonal influences on peritoneal dialysis. Contrib Nephrol 1979; 17: 131–8.
101. Gutman RA, Nixon WP, McRae R, Spencer HW. Effect of intraperitoneal and intravenous vasoactive amines on peritoneal dialysis: study in anephric dogs. Trans Am Soc Artif Intern Organs 1976; 22: 570–3.
102. Penzotti SC, Mattocks AM. Effects of dwell time, volume of dialysis fluid and added accelerators on peritoneal dialysis of urea. J Pharm Sci 1975; 60: 1520–22.
103. Maher JF, Hirszel P, Lasrich M. The effects of gastrointestinal hormones on transport by peritoneal dialysis. Kidney Int 1979; 16: 131–6.
104. Hirszel P, Lasrich M, Maher JF. Divergent effects of catecholamines on peritoneal mass transport. Trans Am Soc Artif Intern Organs 1979; 25: 110–2.
105. Maher JF, Hirszel P, Lasrich M. Modulation of peritoneal transport rates by prostaglandins. Adv Prostaglandin Thromboxane Res 1 1980; 7: 695–700.
106. Nolph KD, Ghods AJ, Van Stone J, Brown PA. The effects of intraperitoneal vasodilators on peritoneal clearances. Trans Am Soc Artif Intern Organs 1976; 22: 586–93.
107. Maher JF, Shea C, Cassetta M, Hohnadel DC. Isoproterenol enhancement of peritoneal permeability. J Dial 1977; 1: 319–31.
108. Vanichayakornkul S, Nimmanit S, Chirawong P, Nilwarangkur S. Accelerated peritoneal dialysis with intraperitoneal isoproterenol. J Med Assoc Thailand 1978; 61 (suppl 1): 127–9.
109. Brown EA, Kliger AS, Goffinet J, Finkelstein FO. Effect of hypertonic dialysate and vasodilators on peritoneal dialysis clearances in the rat. Kidney Int 1978; 13: 271–7.
110. Nolph K, Ghods A, Brown P, Miller F, Harris P, Pyle K, Popovich R. Effects of nitroprusside on peritoneal mass transfer coefficients and microvascular physiology. Trans Am Soc Artif Intern Organs 1977; 23: 210–7.
111. Hirszel P, Maher JF, Chamberlin M. Augmented peritoneal mass transport with intraperitoneal nitroprusside. J Dial 1978; 2: 131–42.
112. Raja RM, Kramer MS, Rosenbaum J. Enhanced clearance with intraperitoneal nitroprusside in high flow recirculation peritoneal dialysis. Trans Am Soc Artif Intern Organs 1978; 24: 133–5.
113. Nolph KD, Ghods AJ, Brown PA, Twardowski PA. Effects of intraperitoneal nitroprusside on peritoneal clearances in man with variations of dose frequency of administration and dwell times. Nephron 1979; 24: 114–20.
114. Selgas R, Carmona AR, Martinez ME, Perez-Fontan M, Salinas M, Conesa J, Martinez Ara J, Sicilia LS. Peritoneal vascular reserve characterization through nitroprusside-induced modification of peritoneal mass transfer coefficients. Int J Artif Organs 1985; 8: 181–6.
115. Riembau E, Lloveras J, Aubia J, Masramon J, Garcia C, Orfila MA, Llorach M. Sequential intraperitoneal administration of nitroprusside in patients maintained on peritoneal dialysis. J Dial 1980; 4: 203–17.
116. Sano N, Satoh S, Hashimoto K. Differences among dipyridamole, carbochromen and lidoflazine in responses of the coronary and the renal arteries. Jpn J Pharmacol 1972; 22: 857–65.
117. Ryckelynck JP, Pierre D, DeMartin A, Rottembourg J. Amélioration des clairances peritonéales par le dipyridamole. Nouv Presse Med 1978; 7: 472.
118. Limido A, Cantu P, Allaria P, Colombo L, Giangrande G. Velocita di flusso ed effetto dei farmaci nella valutazione dell'efficienza della dialisi peritoneale. Minerva Nephrol 1979; 26: 161–4.
119. Rubin J, Adair C, Barnes T, Bower JD. Augmentation of peritoneal clearance by dipyridamole. Kidney Int 1982; 22: 658–61.
120. Maher JF, Hirszel P. Augmenting peritoneal mass transport. Int J Artif Organs 1979; 2: 59–63.
121. Reams GP, Young M, Sorkin M, Twardowski Z, Gloor H, Nolph KD. Effects of dipyridamole on peritoneal clearances. Uremia Invest 1986; 9: 27–33.
122. Rubin J, Adair C, Bower J. A double-blind trial of

dipyridamole in CAPD. Am J Kidney Dis 1985; 5: 262–6.
123. Parker HR, Schroeder JP, Henderson LW. Influence of dopamine and regitine on peritoneal dialysis in unanesthetized dogs. Abstracts Am Soc Artif Intern Organs 1978; 7: 43.
124. Chan MK, Varghese Z, Baillod RA, Moorhead JF. Peritoneal dialysis: effect of intraperitoneal dopamine. Dial Transplant 1980; 9: 380–4.
125. Hirszel P, Lasrich M, Maher JF. Augmentation of peritoneal mass transport by dopamine. Comparison with norepinephrine and evaluation of pharmacologic mechanisms. J Lab Clin Med 1979; 94: 747–54.
126. Maher JF, DiPaolo B, Shostak A, Hirszel P. Pharmacology of peritoneal transport. In: Khanna R, Nolph KD, Prowant B, Twardowski ZJ, Oreopoulos DG (eds), Advances in CAPD 1987. Univ Toronto Press, Toronto 1987; 3–6.
127. Londos C, Cooper DMF, Wolff J. Subclasses of external adenosine receptors. Proc Natl Acad Sci USA 1980; 77: 2551–4.
128. Maher JF, Cassetta M, Shea C, Hohnadel DC. Peritoneal dialysis in rabbits. A study of transperitoneal theophylline flux and peritoneal permeability. Nephron 1978; 20: 18–23.
129. Shostak A, Chakrabarti E, Hirszel P, Maher JF. Effects of histamine and its receptor antagonists on peritoneal permeability. Kidney Int 1988; 34: 786–90.
130. Lal SM. Nolph KD, Moore FL, Khanna R. Effects of calcium channel blockers (Verapamil, Diltiazem) on peritoneal transport. Trans Am Soc Artif Intern Organs 1986; 32: 564–6.
131. Vargemezis V, Pasadakis P, Thodis E. Effect of a calcium antagonist (Verapamil) on the permeability of the peritoneal membrane in patients on continuous ambulatory peritoneal dialysis. Blood Purif 1989; 7: 309–13.
132. Balaskas E, Dombros N, Savidis N, Pidonia I, Lazaridis A, Tourkantonis A. Nifedipine intraperitoneally increases ultrafiltration in CAPD patients. In: Ota K, Maher J, Winchester J, Hirszel P (eds), Current Concepts in Peritoneal Dialysis. Excerpta Medica, Amsterdam 1992; 427–32.
133. Favazza A, Montanaro D, Messa P, Antonucci F, Gropuzzo M, Mioni G. Peritoneal clearances in hypertensive CAPD patients after oral administration of Clonidine, Enalapril and Nifedipine. Perit Dial Int 1992; 12: 287–91.
134. Lamperi S, Carozzi S, Nasini MG, Canepa M, Zanin T. Intreperitoneal Verapamil therapy in CAPD patients with peritoneal hypopermeability. Effects on ultrafiltration. Am Soc Artif Int Organs Trans 1988; 34: 425–8.
135. Lal SM, Moore HL, Nolph KD. Effects of intraperitoneal captopril on peritoneal transport in rats. Perit Dial Bull 1987; 7: 80–5.
136. Coronel F, Hortal L, Naranjo P, Cruceyra A, Barrientos A. Captopril, Proteinuria and peritoneal protein leakage in diabetic patients. Nephron 1989; 51: 443.
137. Shostak A, Hirszel P, Chakrabarti E, Maher JF. Dihydroergotamine lowers peritoneal transfer rates. A hypovolemic transport decrease. Perit Dial Bull 1987; 7: S69.
138. Ilker NY, Ozgur S, Cetin S. Effects of papaverine on solute transport in peritoneal dialysis. Int Urol Nephrol 1989; 21: 11901.
139. Pace Asciak CR. Oxidative biotransformation of arachidonic acid. Prostaglandins 1977; 13: 811–7.
140. Nakano J, McCurdy JR. Hemodynamic effects of prostaglandins E_1, A_1 and F_2 in dogs. Proc Soc Exp Biol Med 1968; 128: 39–42.
141. Messina EJ, Kaley G. Microcircuatory responses to prostacyclin and PGE_2 in the rat cremaster muscle. Adv Prostagandin Thromboxane Res 1980; 7: 719–22.
142. Vane JR, McGiff JC. Possible contributions of endogenous prostaglandins to the control of blood pressure. Circ Res 1975; 36, 37 (suppl 1): 68–75.
143. Maher JF, Hirszel P, Lasrich M. Prostaglandin effects on peritoneal transport. Proc 2nd Int Symposium on Peritoneal Dial 1981; 2: 65–9.
144. Mileti M, Bufano G, Scaravonati P, Pecchnini F, Carnevale G, Lanzarini P. Effect of indomethacin on the peritoneum of rabbits on peritoneal dialysis. Perit Dial Bull 1983; 3: 194–5.
145. Strong CG, Romero JC. Effects of indomethacin in rabbit renovascular hypertension. Clin Sci Mol Med 1976; 51: 249s–51s.
146. Hirszel P, Lasrich M, Maher JF. Arachidonic acid increases peritoneal clearances. Trans Am Soc Artif Intern Organs 1981; 27: 61–3.
147. Thulin L, Samnegard H. Circulatory effects of gastrointestinal hormones and related peptides. Acta Chir Scand (Suppl) 1978; 482: 73–4.
148. Fara JW, Rubenstein EH, Sonneschein RR. Intestinal hormones in mesenteric vasodilation after intraduodenal agents. Am J Physiol 1972; 223: 1058–67.
149. Fara JW. Effects of gastrointestinal hormones on vascular smooth muscle. Am J Dig Dis 1975; 20: 346–53.
150. Hirszel P, Maher JF, LeGrow W. Increased peritoneal mass transport with glucagon acting at the vascular surface. Trans Am Soc Artif Intern Organs 1978; 24: 136–8.
151. Farini R, Del Favero G, Adorati M, Pedrazzoli S, Fabris G, Giordano P, D'Angelo A, Zotti E, Lise M, Chiaramonte M, Savagini M, Naccarato R. Comparison between bolus injection and infusion of Secretin and Pancreozymin in the diagnosis of chronic pancreatic disease (one-hour test). Acta Hepatogastroenterol (Stuttg) 1977; 24: 462–8.
152. Biber B, Fara J, Lundgren O. Vascular reactions in the small intestine during vasodilation. Acta Physiol Scand 1973; 89: 449–56.
153. Hare HG, Valtin H, Gosselin RE. Effect of drugs on peritoneal dialysis in the dog. J. Pharmacol Exp Ther 1964; 145: 122–9.
154. Henderson LW, Kintzel JE. Influence of antidiuretic hormone on peritoneal area and permeability. J Clin Invest 1971; 50: 2437–43.
155. Shear L, Harvey JD, Barry KG. Peritoneal sodium transport: enhancement by pharmacologic and

physical agents. J Lab Clin Med 1966; 67: 181–8.
156. Maher JF, Hirszel P, LeGrow W. Enhanced peritoneal permeability with methyl prednisolone. Clin Res 1978; 26: 64A.
157. Breborowicz A, Knapowski J. Augmentation of peritoneal dialysis clearance with procaine. Kidney Int 1984; 26: 392–6.
158. Haddy F. The mechanism of potassium vasodilation. In: Vanhoutte PM, Leusen I (eds), Mechanisms of Vasodilation. S Karger, Basel 1978; 200–5.
159. Miller FN, Nolph KD, Joshua IG, Wiegman DL, Harris PD, Anderson DB. Hyperosmolality, acetate and actate: Dilatory factors during peritoneal dialysis. Kidney Int 1981; 20: 397–402.
160. Penzotti SC, Mattocks AM. Acceleration of peritoneal dialysis by surface-active agents. J Pharm Sci 1968; 57: 1192–5.
161. El-Bassiouni EA, Mattocks AM. Acceleration of peritoneal dialysis with minimal N-myristyl-β-aminoproprionate. J Pharm Sci 1973; 62: 1314–7.
162. Dunham CB, Hak LJ, Hull JH, Mattocks AM. Enhancement of peritoneal permeability of the rat by intraperitoneal use of docusate sodium. Kidney Int 1981; 20: 563–8.
163. Maher JF, Chakarabarti E. Ultrafiltration by hyperosmotic peritoneal dialysis fluid excludes intracellular solutes. Am J Nephrol 1984; 4: 169–72.
164. Raja RM, Kramer MS, Rosenbaum JL, Bolisay C, Krug M. Contrasting changes in solute transport and ultrafiltration with peritonitis in CAPD patients. Trans Am Soc Artif Intern Organs 1981; 27: 68–70.
165. Alavi N, Lianos E, Van Liew JB, Mookerjee BK, Bentzel CJ. Peritoneal permeability in the rat: Modulation by microfilament-active agents. Kidney Int 1985; 27: 411–9.
166. Scarpioni L, Ballocchi S, Bergonzi G, Fontana F, Poisetti P, Zanazzi MA. High-dose diuretics in CAPD. Perit Dial Bull 1982; 2: 177–8.
167. Grzegorzewska A, Baczyk K. Furosemide-induced increase in urinary and peritoneal excretion of uric acid during peritoneal dialysis in patients with chronic uremia. Artif Organs 1982; 6: 220–4.
168. Bazzato G, Coli U, Landini S, Lucatello S, Fracasso A, Righetto F, Scanfera F, Morachiello P. Restoration of ultrafiltration capacity of peritoneal membrane in patients on CAPD. Int J Artif Organs 1984; 7: 93–6.
169. Alvai H, Lianos E, Andres G, Bentzel CJ. Effect of protamine on the permeability and structure of rat peritoneum. Kidney Int 1982; 21: 44–53.
170. Galdi P, Shostak A, Jaichenko J, Fudin R, Gotloib L. Protamine sulfate induces enhanced peritoneal permeability to proteins. Nephron 1991; 57: 45–51.
171. Capodicasa G, Capasso G, Anastasio P, Lanzetti N, Giordano C. Changes on peritoneal permeability by charged poly-amino acids. Perit Dial Bull 1987; 7: S13.
172. Pietrzak I, Hirszel P, Maher JF. Poly-1-lysine, a cationic macromolecule, increases peritoneal hydraulic and solute permeability. In: Ota K, Maher J, Winchester J, Hirszel P (eds), Current Concepts in Peritoneal Dialysis. Excerpta Medica, Amsterdam 1992; pp 433–8.
173. Breborowicz A, Rodela H, Bargman J, Oreopoulos DG. Effect of cationic molecules on the permeability of the mesothelium in vitro. Perit Dial Bull 1987; 7: S9.
174. Lau AH, Chow Tung E, Assadi FK, Fornell L, John E. Effect of ultrafiltration on peritoneal dialysis drug clearances. Pharmacology 1985; 31: 284.
175. Nolph KD, Nothum RJ, Maher JF. Ultrafiltration: a mechanism for removal of intermediate molecular weight substances in coil dialyzers. Kidney Int 1974; 6: 55–60.
176. Khanna R, Nolph KD, Twardowski ZJ. Pharmacological alteration of ultrafiltration. Contrib Nephrol 1990; 85: 150–8.
177. Avasthi PS. Effects of aminonucleoside on rat blood-peritoneal barrier permeability. J Lab Clin Med 1979; 94: 295–302.
178. Maher JF, Hirszel P, Bennett RR, Chakrabarti E. Augmentation of peritoneal hydraulic permeability by amphotericin B: locus of action. Perit Dial Bull 1984; 4: 229–31.
179. Indrapasit S, Sooksriwongse C. Effect of chlorpromazine on peritoneal clearances. Nephron 1985; 40: 341–3.
180. Ronco C, Brendolan A, Bragantini L, Chiaramonte S, Feriani M, Fabris A, LaGreca G. Studies on ultrafiltration in peritoneal dialysis: influence of plasma proteins and capillary blood flow. Perit Dial Bull 1986; 6: 93–7.
181. Levin TN, Rigden LR, Bielsen LH, Moore KL, Twardowski ZJ, Khanna R, Nolph KD. Maximal ultrafiltration rates during peritoneal dialysis in rats. Kidney Int 1987; 31: 731–5.
182. Maher JF, Hirszel P, Shostak A, DiPaolo B, Chakrabarti E. Prolonged intraperitoneal dwell decreases ultrafiltration coefficient in rabbits. Am J Kidney Dis 1988; 12: 62–5.
183. Rubin J, Reed V, Adair C, Bower J, Klein E. Effect of intraperitoneal insulin on solute kinetics in CAPD: insulin kinetics in CAPD. Am J Med Sci 1986; 291: 81–7.
184. Twardowski ZJ, Khanna R, Nolph KD. Osmotic agents and ultrafiltration in peritoneal dialysis. Nephron 1986; 42: 93–101.
185. Knochel JP, Clayton LE, Smith WL, Barry KG. Intraperitoneal THAM: an effective method to enhance phenobarbital removal during peritoneal dialysis. J Lab Cin Med 1964; 64: 257–68.
186. Knochel JP, Mason AD. Effect of alkalinization on peritoneal diffusion of uric acid. Am J Physiol 1966; 210: 1160–4.
187. Campion DAS, North JDK. Effect of protein binding of barbiturates on their rate of removal during peritoneal dialysis. J Lab Clin Med 1965; 66: 549–63.
188. Schultz JC, Crouder DG, Medart WS. Excretion studies in ethchlorvynol (Placidyl) intoxication. Arch Intern Med 1966; 117: 409–11.
189. Etteldorf JN, Dobbins WT, Summit RL, Rainwater

WT, Fischer RL. Intermittent peritoneal dialysis using 5% albumin in the treatment of salicylate intoxication in children. J Pediatr 1961; 58: 226–36.
190. Kudla RM, El-Bassiouni EA, Mattocks AM. Accelerated peritoneal dialysis of barbiturates, diphenylhydantoin and salicylate. J Pharm Sci 1971; 60: 1065–7.
191. Cole DEC, Lirenman DS. Role of albumin enriched peritoneal dialysate in acute copper poisoning. J Pediatr 1978; 92: 955–7.
192. Mehbod H. Treatment of lead intoxication. combined use of peritoneal dialysis and edetate calcium disodium. JAMA 1967; 201: 972–4.
193. Lowenthal DT, Chardo F, Reidenberg MM. Removal of mercury by peritoneal dialysis. Arch Intern Med 1974; 134: 139–41.
194. Falk RJ, Mattern WD, Lamanna RW, Gitelman JH, Parker NC, Cross RE, Rastall JR. Iron removal during continuous ambulatory peritoneal dialysis using desferrioxamine. Kidney Int 1983; 24: 110–2.
195. Shinaberger JH, Shear L, Clayton LE, Barry KG, Knowlton M, Goldbaum LR. Dialysis for intoxication with lipid soluble drugs: enhancement of glutethimide extraction with lipid dialysate. Trans Am Soc Artif Intern Organs 1965; 11: 173–7.
196. Dulaney JT, Hatch FE. Peritoneal dialysis and loss of proteins: A review. Kidney Int 1984; 26: 253–62.
197. Kagan A, Bar-Khaim Y, Schafer Z, Fainaru M. Kinetics of peritoneal protein loss during CAPD: I. Different characteristics for low and high molecular weight proteins. Kidney Int 1990; 37: 971–9.
198. Leypoldt JK, Henderson LW. Molecular charge influences transperitoneal macromolecule transport. Kidney Int 1993; 43: 837–44.
199. Breborowicz A, Radkowski M, Knapowski J, Oreopoulos DG. Effects of chondroitin sulphate on fluid and solute transport during peritoneal dialysis in rats. Perit Dial Int 1991; 11: 351–4.
200. Maher JF. Characteristics of peritoneal transport: physiological and clinical implications. Mineral Electrolyte Metab 1981; 5: 201–11.
201. Rowland M, Tozer TN. Clinical pharmacokinetics: concepts and applications. Lea & Febiger, Philadelphia 1989.
202. Greenblatt DJ, Koch-Weser J. Clinical pharmacokinetics. New Eng J Med 1975; 293: 702–5 and 964–70.
203. Bennett WM, Aronoff GR, Golper TA, Morrison G, Singer I, Brater DC. Drug prescribing in renal failure dosing guidelines for adults. Am Coll Physicians 1991; 2nd ed, Philadelphia.
204. Bennett LZ, Williams RL. Appendix II: Design and optimization of dosage regiments; pharmacokinetic data. In: Gilman AG, Rall TW, Niess AS (eds), The pharmacological basis of therapeutics. Pergamon Press New York, 1990; pp 1650–735.
205. Maher JF. Peritoneal transport rates: mechanisms, limitations and methods for augmentation. Kidney Int 1980; 18: S117–20.
206. Deguchi Y, Nakashima E, Ishikawa F, Sato H, Tamai I, Matsushita R, Tofuku Y, Ichimura F, Tsuji A. Peritoneal transport of betalactam antibiotics: effects of plasma protein binding and the interspecies relationship. J. Pharmaceut Sciences 1988; 77: 559–64.
207. Flessner MF, Dedrick RL, Schultz JS. Exchange of macromolecules between peritoneal cavity and plasma. Am J Physiol 1985; 248: H21–5.
208. Keller E, Reetze P, Schollmeyer P. Drug therapy in patients undergoing continuous ambulatory peritoneal dialysis. Clinical pharmacokinetic considerations. Clin Pharmacokinet 1990; 18: 104–17.
209. Morse GD, Rowinski CA, Lieveld PE, Walshe JJ. Drug protein binding during continuous ambulatory peritoneal dialysis. Perit Dial Int 1988; 6: 144–7.
210. Janknegt R, Nube MJ. A simple method for predicting drug clearances during CAPD. Perit Dial Bull 1985; 5: 254–5.
211. Lee CC, Marbury TC. Drug therapy in patients undergoing hemodialysis. Clinical pharmacokinetic considerations. Clin Pharmacokinetics 1984; 9: 42–66.
212. Harford AM, Sica DA, Tartaglione T, Polk RE, Dalton HP, Poynor W. Vancomycin pharmacokinetics in continuous ambulatory peritoneal dialysis patients with peritonitis. Nephron 1986; 43: 217–22.
213. Lameire N, Belpaire F. Pharmacokinetics of antibiotics against Gram-negative infections in CAPD patients. Proc. ISPD meeting, Thessaloniki, Perit Dial Int 1993; 13 (suppl 2): S371–6.
214. Fleming LW, Moreland TA, Scott AC, Stewart WK, White LD. Ciprofloxacin in plasma and peritoneal dialysate after oral therapy in patients in CAPD. J Antimicrob Chemother 1987; 19: 494–503.
215. Verbrugh HA, Keane WF, Conroy WE, Peterson PK. Bacterial growth and killing chronic ambulatory peritoneal dialysis fluids. J Clin Microbiol 1984; 20: 199–203.
216. Guay D, Klicker R, Pence T, Peterson P. In vitro antistaphylococcal activity of teicoplanin and ciprofloxacin in peritoneal dialysis effluent. Eur J Clin Microbiol 1986; 5: 551–3.
217. Weissauer-Condon C, Engels I, Daschner FD. In vitro activity of four new quinolone in Mueller-Hinton broth and peritoneal dialysis fluid. Eur J Clin Microbiol 1987; 6: 324–6.
218. Halstead DC, Guzzo J, Giardina JA, Geshan AE. In vitro bactericidal activities and gentamicin cefazolin and imipenem in peritoneal dialysis fluids. Antimicrob Agents Chemother 1989; 33: 1553–6.
219. Wilcox MH, Smith DGE, Evans JA, Denyer SP, Finck RG, Williams P. Influence of carbon dioxide on growth and antibiotic susceptibility of coagulase-negative staphylococci cultures in human peritoneal dialysate. J Clin Microbiol 1990; 28: 2183–6.
220. Janicke DM, Morse GD, Apicella MA, Jusko WJ, Walshe JJ. Pharmacokinetic modeling of bidirectional transfer during peritoneal dialysis. Clin Pharmacol Ther 1986; 40: 209–18.

221. Jusko WJ, Baliah T, Kim KH, Gerbracht LM, Yaffe SJ. Pharmacokinetics of gentamicin during peritoneal dialysis in children. Kidney Int 1976; 9: 430–8.
222. Brouard R, Tozer TN, Merdjan H, Guillemin A, Beaumelou A. Transperitoneal movement and pharmacokinetics of cefotiam and cefsulodin in patients on continuous ambulatory peritoneal dialysis. Clin Nephrol 1988; 30: 197–206.
223. Lukas G, Brindle SD, Greengard P. The route of absorption of intraperitoneally administered compounds. J Pharmacol Exp Ther 1971; 178: 562–6.
224. Somani P, Shapiro RS, Stockard H, Higgins JT. Unidirectional absorption of gentamicin from the peritoneum during continuous ambulatory peritoneal dialysis. Clin Pharmacol Ther 1982; 32: 113–21.
225. Balducci A, Slama G, Rottembourg J, Baumelou A, Delage A. Intraperitoneal insulin in uraemic diabetics undergoing continuous ambulatory peritoneal dialysis. Brit Med J 1981; 283: 1021–3.
226. Bargman J, Jones JE, Petro JM. The pharmacokinetics of intraperitoneal erythropoietin administered undiluted or diluted in dialysate. Perit Dial Int 1992; 12: 296–72.
227. Gotloib L, Bar-Sella P, Jaichenko J, Shostak A. Ruthenium – red-stained polyanionic fixed charges in peritoneal microvessels. Nephron 1987; 47: 22–8.
228. Gotloib L, Shostak A, Jaichenko J. Loss of mesothelial and microvascular fixed anionic charges during murine experimentally induced septic peritonitis. Nephron 1989; 51: 77–83.
229. De Paepe M, Lameire N, Belpaire F, Bogaert M. Peritoneal pharmacokinetics of gentamicin in man. Clin Nephrol 1983; 19: 107–9.
230. Rubin J, Deraps GD, Walsh D, Adair C, Bower J. Protein losses and tobramycin absorption in peritonitis treated by hourly peritoneal dialysis. Am J Kidney Dis 1986; 8: 124–7.
231. Regany C, Schaberg D, Kiroy W. Inhibitory effect of heparin on gentamicin concentrations of blood. Antimicrob Agents Chemother 1972; 4: 329–32.
232. Ponce SP, Barata JD, Santos R. Interference of heparin with peritoneal solute transport. Nephron 1985; 39: 47–9.
233. Mactier RA, Moore H, Khanna R, Shah J. Effect of peritonitis on insulin and glucose absorption during peritoneal dialysis in diabetic rats. Nephron 1990; 54: 240–4.
234. Fine RN, Fine SE, Sherman BM. Absorption of recombinant human growth hormone (rhGH) following intraperitoneal instillation. Perit Dial Int 1989; 9: 91–3.
235. Paton TW, Cornish WR, Manuel MA, Hardy BG. Drug therapy in patients undergoing peritoneal dialysis. Clinical pharmacokinetic considerations. Clin Pharmacokinet 1985; 10: 404–26.
236. Lameire N, Bogaert MA, Belpaire FM. Peritoneal pharmacokinetics and pharmacological manipulation of peritoneal transport. In: Gokal R. (ed), Continuous ambulatory peritoneal dialysis. Churchill Livingstone, Edinburgh 1986; pp 56–93.
237. Maher JF. Influence of continuous ambulatory peritoneal dialysis on elimination of drugs. Perit Dial Bull 1987; 7: 159–67.
238. Sewell DL, Golper TA. Stability of antimicrobial agents in peritoneal dialysate. Antimicrob Agents Chemother 1982; 21: 528–9.
239. Sewell DL, Golper TA, Brown SD, Nelson E, Knower M, Kimbrough RD. Stability of single and combination antimicrobial agents in various peritoneal dialysates in the presence of insulin and heparin. Am J Kidney Dis 1983; 3: 209–12.
240. Janknegt R, Koks CHW, Nube MJ. Stability of antibiotics in CAPD fluid. Perit Dial Bull 1985; 5: 78.
241. Kehoe WA, Weber JN, Fries DS. The stability and compatibility of clindamycin phosphate and gentamicin sulfate alone and in combination with peritoneal dialysis solution. Perit Dial Bull 1988; 8: 153–4.
242. Mason NA, Johnson CE, O'Biren MA. Stability of ceftazidime and tobramycin sulfate in peritoneal dialysis solution. Am J Hosp Pharmacy 1993; 49: 1139–42.
243. Bastani B, Spijker DA, Westervelt FB. Peritoneal absorption of vancomycin during and after resolution of peritonitis in continuous ambulatory peritoneal dialysis (CAPD) patients. Perit Dial Bull 1988; 8: 135–6.
244. Imada A, Itagaki N, Hasegawa H, Horiuchi A. Comparative study of the pharmacokinetics of various beta-lactams after intravenous and intraperitoneal administration in patients undergoing continuous ambulatory peritoneal dialysis. Drugs 1988; 35: 82–7.
245. Ryckelynck JP, Debruyne D, Hurault de Ligny B, Moulin M. Pharmacocinétique de la pipéracilline en dialyse péritonéale continue ambulatoire. Pathologie Biologie 1988; 36: 507–10.
246. Husserl F, Back S. Intraperitoneal vancomycin and the "red man" syndrome. Perit Dial Bull 1987; 7: 262 (letter).
247. Fabris A, Biasoli S, Borin D, Brendolan A, Chiaramonte S. Fungal peritonitis in peritoneal dialysis: our experience and review of treatment. Perit Dial Bull 1984; 4: 75–7.
248. Mandell IN, Ahern MJ, Klier AS, Andriole VI. Candida peritonitis complicating peritoneal dialysis: successful treatment with low dose amphotericin B therapy. Clin Nephrol 1976; 6: 192–6.
249. Struijk DG, Krediet RT, Boeschoten EW, Rietra P, Arisz L. Antifungal treatment of Candida peritonitis in continuous ambulatory peritoneal dialysis. Am J Kidney Dis 1987; 9: 66–70.
250. Benevent D, El Akoum N, Lagarde C. Danger de l'administration intrapéritonéale de l'amphotéricine B au cours de la dialyse péritonéale continue ambulatoire. La Presse Médicale 1984; 13: 1844.
251. Piraino B, Bernardini J, Johnston J, Sorkin M. Chemical peritonitis due to intraperitoneal vancomycin (Vancoled). Perit Dial Bull 1987; 7: 156–9.
252. Steiner RW. Adverse effects of intraperitoneal methylene blue. Perit Dial Bull 1983; 3: 43 (letter).

253. Bonner G, Lukowski K. Angiotension I in peritoneal dialysis fluid improved hypotension. Clin Nephrol 1987; 27: 99–101.
254. Peters U, Risler T, Grabensee B. Pharmacokinetics of digoxin with end-stage renal failure treated with continuous ambulatory peritoneal dialysis. Kidney Int 1981; 20: 159 (abstract).
255. Demedts W, Desaer JP, Belpaire F, Ringoir S, Lameire N. Life-threatening hyperkalemia associated with clofibrate-induced myopathy in a CAPD patient. Perit Dial Bull 1983; 3: 15–6.
256. Johnson RJ, Blair AD, Ahmad S. Ketoconazole kinetics in chronic peritoneal dialysis. Clin Pharmacol Ther 1985; 37: 325–7.
257. Belpaire FM, Van de Velde EJ, Fraeyman NH, Bogaert MG, Lameire N. Influence of continuous ambulatory peritoneal dialysis on serum alpha-1-acid glycoprotein concentration and drug binding. Eur J Clin Pharmacol 1988; 35: 339–43.
258. Haughy DB, Krafat CJ, Matzke GR, Keane WF, Halstenson CE. Protein binding of disopyramide and elevated alpha-1-acid glycoprotein concentrations in serum obtained from dialysis patients and renal transplant recipients. Am J Nephrol 1985; 5: 35–9.
259. St. John Hammond PG, Forland SG, Erlanger H, Cutler RE. Drugs and the Kidney. In: Gonick HC (ed), Current Nephrology. St. Louis, Mosby Year Book 1992; 15: 245–92.
260. Bennet WM, Swan SK. Drug therapy in renal disease. In: Rubenstein E, Federman DD (eds), Scientific American Medicine. Scientific American, New York 1992; 10: A1–37.
261. Schrier RW, Gambertoglio JG (eds). Handbook of drug therapy in liver and kidney disease. Boston, Little, Brown & Company, 1991.
262. Jones RH, Cundy T, Bullock R, Brown CN, Dafton J, Majer R, Parsons V, Bridgman KM. Concentrations of amoxycillin in serum and dialysate of uraemic patients undergoing peritoneal dialysis. J Infection 1979; 1: 235–42.
263. Reudy J. The effects of peritoneal dialysis on the physiological disposition of oxacillin, ampicillin and tetracycline in patients with renal disease. Can Med Assoc J 1966; 94: 257–61.
264. Whelton A, Stout RL, Delgado FA. Azlocillin kinetics during extracorporeal hemodialysis and peritoneal dialysis. J Antimicrob Chemother 1983; 11 (suppl. B): 89–95.
265. Eastwood JB, Curtis JR. Carbenicillin administration in patients with severe renal failure. Brit Med J 1968; I: 486–7.
266. Kampf D, Schurig R, Weihermuller K, Forster D. Effects of impaired renal function, hemodialysis and peritoneal dialysis on the pharmacokinetics of mezlocillin. Antimicrob Agents Chemother 1980; 18: 81–7.
267. Parry MF, Neu HC. Pharmacokinetics of ticarcillin in patients with abnormal renal function. J Infect Dis 1976; 133: 46–9.
268. Ahern MJ, Finkelstein FO, Andriole VT. Pharmacokinetics of cefamandole in patients undergoing hemodialysis and peritoneal dialysis. Antimicrob Agents Chemother 1976; 10: 457–61.
269. Meyers BR, Hirschman SZ. Pharmacokinetics of cefamandole in patients with renal failure. Antimicrob Agents Chemother 1977; 11: 248–50.
270. Madhaven T, Yaremchuk K, Levin N. Effects of renal failure and dialysis on cefazolin pharmacokinetics. Antimicrob Agents Chemother 1975; 8: 63–6.
271. Levison ME, Levison SP, Ries K. Pharmacology of cefazolin in patients with normal and abnormal renal function. J Infect Dis 1973; 128: S354–7.
272. Kaye D, Wenger N, Agarwal B. Pharmacology of intraperitoneal cefazolin in patients undergoing peritoneal dialysis. Antimicrob Agents Chemother 1978; 14: 318–21.
273. Schurig R, Kampf D, Spieber W, Weihermuller K, Becker H. Cefotaxime pharmacokinetics in peritoneal dialysis. In: Gokal GM, Kessel M, Nolph KD (eds), Advances in peritoneal dialysis. Excerpta Medica, Amsterdam, 1981; pp 96–8.
274. Wise R, Wright N, Willis PJ. Pharmacology of cefotaxime and its desacetyl metabolite in renal and hepatic disease. Antimicrob Agents Chemother, 1981; 19: 526–31.
275. Vlasses PH, D'Silver H, Rocci ML, Koplin JR, Bland JA, Siciliano EG, Ferguson RK. Disposition of intravenous and intraperitoneal cefoxitin during chronic intermittent peritoneal dialysis. Am J Kid Dis 1983; 3: 67–70.
276. Tourkantonis A, Nicolaidis P. Pharmacokinetics of ceftazidime in patients undergoing peritoneal dialysis. J Antimicrob Chemother 1983; 12 (suppl A): 263–7.
277. Local FK, Munro AJ, Kerr DNS, Sussman M. Pharmacokinetics of intravenous and intraperitoneal cefuroxime in patients undergoing peritoneal dialysis. Clin Nephrol 1981; 16: 40–3.
278. Kosmidis J, Stathakis C, Anyfantis A, Daikos GK. Cefuroxime in renal insufficiency: therapeutic results in various infections and pharmacokinetics including the effects of dialysis. Proc Roy Soc Med 1977; 10: S139–43.
279. LaGreca G, Biasioli S, Chiaramonte S. Pharmacokinetics of intravenous and intraperitoneal cefuroxime during peritoneal dialysis. Int J Clin Pharmacol Ther Toxicol 1982; 20: 92–4.
280. Chan MK, Browning AK, Poole CMJ, Matheson LA, Li CS, Baillod RA, Moorhead JF. Cefuroxime pharmacokinetics in continuous and intermittent peritoneal dialysis. Nephron 1985; 41: 161–5.
281. Yamasaku F, Tsuchida R, Usuda Y. A study of kinetics of cephalosporins in renal impairment. J Postgrad Med 1970; 46: S57–9.
282. Stephens NM, Kronfol NO, Kline BJ, Polk RE. Peritoneal absorption of moxalactam. Antimicrob Agents Chemother 1983; 24: 39–41.
283. Nielson HE, Sorensen I, Hansen HE. Peritoneal transport of vancomycin during peritoneal dialysis. Nephron 1979; 24: 274–7.
284. Ayus JC, Eneas JF, Tong TG, Benowitz NL, Schoenfeld PY, Hadley KL, Becker CE, Humphreys MH. Peritoneal clearance and total

body elimination of vancomycin during chronic intermittent peritoneal dialysis. Clin Nephrol 1979; 11: 129–32.
285. Magera BE, Arroyo JC, Rosansky SJ, Postic B. Vancomycin pharmacokinetics in patients with peritonitis on peritoneal dialysis. Antimicrob Agents Chemother 1983; 23: 710–4.
286. Glew RH, Pavuk RA, Shuster A, Alfred JH. Vancomycin pharmacokinetics in patients undergoing chronic intermittent peritoneal dialysis. Int J Clin Pharmacol Therapy Toxicol 1982; 20: 559–63.
287. Madhaven T, Yaremchuk K, Levin N. Effect of renal failure and dialysis on the serum concentration of the aminoglycoside amikacin. Antimicrob Agents Chemother 1976; 10: 464–6.
288. Reguer L, Golding H, Jensen H, Kampman JP. Pharmacokinetics of amikacin during hemodialysis and peritoneal dialysis. Antimicrob Agents Chemother 1977; 11: 214–8.
289. Matzke GR, Salem H, Bockbrader H. The effect of peritoneal dialysis on the pharmacokinetics of amikacin. Proc Dial Transplant Forum 1980; 10: 302–4.
290. Gary NE. Peritoneal clearance and removal of gentamicin. J Infect Dis 1971; 124: S96–7.
291. Smithivas T, Hyams PJ, Matalon R, Simberkoff MJ, Rahal JJ. The use of gentamicin in peritoneal dialysis. I. Pharmacologic results. J Infect Dis 1971; 124: S77–83.
292. Hamann SR, Oeltgen PR, Shank WA. Evaluation of gentamicin pharmacokinetics during peritoneal dialysis. Ther Drug Monit 1982; 4: 297–300.
293. Indrapasit S, Arkaravichienw, Pummangura C, Kaojarern S. Gentamicin removal during intermittent peritoneal dialysis. Nephron 1986; 44: 18–21.
294. Kaojareen S, Arkaravichien W, Indrapasit S, Pummangura C. Dosing regimen of gentamicin during intermittent peritoneal dialysis. J Clin Pharmacol 1989; 29: 140–3.
295. Jaffe G, Meyers BR, Hirschman SZ. Pharmacokinetics of tobramycin in patients with stable renal impairment, patients undergoing peritoneal dialysis and patients on chronic hemodialysis. Antimicrob Agents Chemother 1974; 5: 61–6.
296. Malacoff RF, Finkelstein FO, Andriole VT. Effect of peritoneal dialysis on serum levels of tobramycin and clindamycin. Antimicrob Agents Chemother 1975; 8: 574–80.
297. Ramos E, Adir JA, Shen YL, Leslie J, Atkins J, Sadler JH. Pharmacokinetics of tobramycin in patients undergoing peritoneal dialysis. Kidney Int 1979; 16: 896 (abstract).
298. Greenberg PA, Sanford JP. Removal and absorption of antibiotics in patients with renal failure undergoing peritoneal dialysis. Ann Int Med 1967; 66: 465–78.
299. Atkins RC, Mion C, Despaux E, Van-Hai N, Julian C, Mion H. Peritoneal transfer of kanamycin and its use in peritoneal dialysis. Kidney Int 1973; 3: 391–6.
300. Goodwin NJ, Friedman EA. The effect of renal impairment, peritoneal dialysis and hemodialysis on serum colistimethate levels. Ann Int Med 1968; 68: 984–94.
301. Curtis JR, Eastwood JB. Colistin sulphomethate sodium administration in the presence of severe renal failure and during hemodialysis and peritoneal dialysis. Brit Med J 1968; I: 484–5.
302. Reinarz JA, McIntosh D. Lincomycin excretion in patients with normal renal function, severe azotemia, and with hemodialysis and peritoneal dialysis. Antimicrob Agents Chemother 1965; 5: 232–8.
303. Cassey JG, Clark DA, Merrick P, Jobes B. Pharmacokinetics of metronidiazole in patients undergoing peritoneal dialysis. Antimicrob Agents Chemother 1983; 24: 950–1.
304. Singlas E, Colin JN, Rottembourg J, Meessen JP, De Martin A, Legrain M, Simon P. Pharmacokinetics of sulfamethoxazole-trimetoprim combination during chronic peritoneal dialysis: effect of peritonitis. Eur J Clin Pharmacol 1982; 21: 409–15.
305. Rose HP, Roth DA, Koch ML. Serum tetracycline levels during peritoneal dialysis. Am J Med Sci 1965; 250: 66–8.
306. Fish SS, Pancorbo S, Berkseth R. Pharmacokinetics of epsilonaminocaproic acid during peritoneal dialysis. J Neurosurg, 1981; 54: 736–9.
307. Campese VM, Feinstein EI, Gura V, Mason WD, Massry SG. Pharmacokinetics of atenolol in patients treated with chronic hemodialysis or peritoneal dialysis. J Clin Pharmacol 1985; 25: 393–5.
308. Vaziri D, Ness RL, Barton CH. Peritoneal dialysis of cimetidine. Am J Gastroenterol 1979; 71: 572–6.
309. Pizzella KM, Moore MC, Schultz RW, Walshe J, Schentag JJ. Removal of cimetidine by peritoneal dialysis, hemodialysis and charcoal hemoperfusion. Ther Drug Monit 1980; 2: 273–81.
310. Ackerman GL, Doherty JE, Flanigan WJ. Peritoneal dialysis and hemodialysis of tritiated digoxin. Ann Intern Med 1967; 67: 718–23.
311. Hall K, Meatherall B, Krahn J, Penner B, Rabson JL. Clearance of quinidine during peritoneal dialysis. Am Heart J 1982; 104: 646–7.
312. Brown GS, Lohr TO, Mayor HG, Freitag JJ, Sanchez TV, Prasad JM. Peritoneal clearance of theophylline. Am J Kid Dis 1981; 1: 24–6.
313. Orr JM, Farrell K, Abbott FS, Ferguson S, Godolphin WJ. The effects of peritoneal dialysis on the single dose and steady state pharmacokinetics of valproic acid in an uremic epileptic child. Eur J Clin Pharmacol 1983; 24: 387–90.
314. Beyerlein C, Csaszar G, Hollmann M, Schumacher A. Verapamil in antihypertensive treatment of patients on renal replacement therapy – clinical implications and pharmacokinetics. Eur J Clin Pharmacol 1990; 39: S35–7.
315. Andrews JM, Wise R, Donovan IA, Drumm J. The intraperitoneal penetration of amoxycillin/clavulanic acid. Proc. 3rd ICC Vienna, 1983; 97: 31–4.
316. Wise R, Donovan A, Drumm J, Dyas A, Cross C. The intraperitoneal penetration of temocillin. J Antimicrob Chemother 1983; 12: 93–6.
317. Wise R, Donovan IA, Lockley MR, Dumm J,

Andrews JM. The pharmacokinetics and tissue penetration of imipenem. J Antimicrob Chemother 1986; 18 (suppl E): 93–101.
318. Kavi J, Ashby JP, Wise R, Donovan IA. Intraperitoneal penetration of cefpirome. Eur J Clin Microbiol Inf Dis 1989; 8: 556–8.
319. Hextall A, Andrews JM, Donovan IA, Wise R. Intraperitoneal penetration of meropenem. J Antimicrob Chemother 1991; 28: 314–6.
320. Pancorbo S, Comty C. Digoxin pharmacokinetics in continuous ambulatory peritoneal dialysis. Ann Int Med 1980; 93: 639.
321. De Paoli Vitali E, Casol D, Tessarin C, Tisone GF, Cavogna R. Pharmacokinetics of digoxin in CAPD. In: Gahl GM, Kessel M, Nolph KD (eds). Advances in peritoneal dialysis. Excerpta Med., Amsterdam 1981; 85–7.
322. Risler T, Peters U, Passlick J, Grabensee B, Krokou J. Pharmacokinetics of digoxin and digitoxin in patients on chronic ambulatory peritoneal dialysis. In: Gahl GM, Kessel M, Nolph KD (eds). Advances in peritoneal dialysis. Excerpta Med., Amsterdam 1981; pp 88–9.
323. De Paepe M, Belpaire F, Bogaerts Y. Pharmacokinetics of digoxin in CAPD. Clin Exper Dial Apheresis 1982; 6: 65–73.
324. Gloor HJ, Moore H, Nolph KD. The peritoneal handling of digoxin during CAPD. Perit Dial Bull 1982; 2: 13–6.
325. Chin TWF, Pancorbo S, Comty C. Quinidine pharmacokinetics in continuous ambulatory peritoneal dialysis. Clin Exp Dial Apheresis 1981; 5: 391–7.
326. Yamakado M, Umezu M, Nagano M, Tagawa H. Pharmacokinetics of denopamine in patients on continuous ambulatory peritoneal dialysis. In: Current concepts in peritoneal dialysis. Ota K, Maher J, Winchester J, Hirszel P (eds), Excerpta Med., Amsterdam 1992; 441–4.
327. Halstenson CE, Opsahl JA, Pence TV, Luke DR, Sirgo MA, Plachetka JR, Abraham PA, Matzke GR. The disposition and dynamics of labetalol in patients on dialysis. Clin Pharmacol Ther 1986; 40: 462–8.
328. Parrott KA, Alexander SE, Stennett DJ. Loss of propranolol via CAPD in two patients. Perit Dial Bull 1984; 2: 110 (abstract).
329. Salahudeen AK, Wilkinson R, McAinsh J, Batemax DN. Atenolol pharmacokinetics in patients on continuous ambulatory peritoneal dialysis. Br J Clin Pharmacol 1984; 18: 457–60.
330. Flaherty JF, Wong B, La Follette G, Warnock DG, Hulse JD, Gambertoglio JG. Pharmacokinetics of esmolol and ASL-8123 in renal failure. Clin Pharmacol Ther 1989; 45: 321–7.
331. Bianchetti G, Padovani P, Thenot JP, Thiercelin JF, Fries F, Martin-Dupont C, Bouche JL, Morselli L. Betaxolol disposition in chronic renal insufficiency hemodialysis and ambulatory peritoneal dialysis. Eur J Clin Invest 1982; 12S, 3A (abstract).
332. Spital A, Scandling JD. Nifedipine in continuous ambulatory peritoneal dialysis. Arch Int Med 1983; 143: 2025 (letter).
333. Evers J, Bonn R, Boertz A, Cavello W, Luckow V, Fey M, Aboudan F, Dickmans HA. Pharmacokinetics of isosorbide-5-nitrate during haemodialysis and peritoneal dialysis. Eur J Clin Pharmacol 1987; 32: 503–5.
334. Grech-Belanger O, Langlois S, Leboeuf E. Pharmacokinetics of diltiazem in patients undergoing continuous ambulatory peritoneal dialysis. J Clin Pharmacol 1988; 28: 477–80.
335. Fujimora a, Kajiyama H, Ebihara A, Iwashita K, Nomura Y, Kawahara Y. Pharmacokinetics and pharmacodynamics of captopril in patients undergoing continuous ambulatory peritoneal dialysis. Nephron 1986; 44: 324–8.
336. Olson S, Horvath A, Michniewicz B. The clinical pharmacokinetics of quinapril. Angiology 1989; 40: 351–9.
337. Swartz RD, Starmann B, Horbath AM, Olson SC, Posvar EL. Pharmacokinetics of quinapril and its active metabolite quinaprilat during continuous ambulatory peritoneal dialysis. J Clin Pharmacol 1990; 30: 1136–41.
338. Gehr TWB, Sica DA, Grasela DM, Fakhry I, Davis J, Duchin KL. Fosinopril pharmacokinetics and pharmacodynamics in chronic ambulatory peritoneal dialysis. Eur J Clin Pharmacol 1991; 41: 165–9.
339. Rottembourg J, Issad B, Guerret M, Lavene D, Baumelou A, Kiechel JR. Particularités d'utilisation de la guanfacine chez l'insuffisant rénal traité par dialyse péritonéale continue ambulatoire. In: Structures cérébrales et contrôle tensionnel. Sandoz, Paris, 1983; pp 165–72.
340. Raehl CL, Beirne GJ, Moorthy AV, Patel AK. Tocainide pharmacokinetics during continuous ambulatory peritoneal dialysis. Am J Cardiol 1987; 60: 747–50.
341. Bailie GR, Waldek S. Pharmacokinetics of flecainide in a patient undergoing continuous ambulatory peritoneal dialysis. J Clin Pharmacy and Therapeutics 1988; 13: 121–4.
342. Sica DA, Yonce C, Small R, Cefali E, Harford A, Poynor W. Pharmacokinetics of procainamide in continuous ambulatory peritoneal dialysis. Int J Clin Pharmacol Ther Toxicol 1988; 26: 59–64.
343. Bourtron H, Singlas E, Brocard JF, Charpentier B, Fried D. Pharmacocinétique clinique du furosemide au cours de la dialyse péritonéale continue ambulatoire. Thérapie 1985; 40: 155–9.
344. Baumelou A, Singlas E, Merdjan H, Martre JH, Brouard R, Benthcikon A, Rottembourg J. Pharmacocinétique des médicaments administrés par voie générale chez les malades traités par dialyse péritonéale continue ambulatoire. Sém Urol Néphrol 1985; 11: 124–36.
345. Martin V, Winne R, Prescott LF. Frusemide disposition in patients on continuous ambulatory peritoneal dialysis (CAPD). Brit J Clin Pharmacol 1991; 31: 227–8.
346. Lee CSG, Peterson JC, Marbury TC. Comparative pharmacokinetics of theophylline in peritoneal dialysis and hemodialysis. J Clin Pharmacol 1983; 23: 274–80.
347. Jones TE, Reece PA, Fisher GC. Mexiletine

removal by peritoneal dialysis. Eur J Clin Pharmacol 1983; 25: 839–40.
348. Blackwell BG, Leggett JE, Johnson CA, Zimmerman SW, Craig WA. Ampicillin and Sulbactam pharmacokinetics and pharmacodynamics in continuous ambulatory peritoneal dialysis. Perit Dial Int 1990; 10: 221–6.
349. Somani P, Freimer EH, Gross ML, Higgins JT. Pharmacokinetics of Imipenem-Cilastatin in patients with renal insufficiency undergoing continuous ambulatory peritoneal dialysis. Antimicrob Agents Chemother 1988; 36: 530–4.
350. Chan CY, Lai KN, Lam AW, Li PKT, Chung WWM, French GL. Pharmacokinetics of parenteral imipenem/cilastatin in patients on continuous ambulatory peritoneal dialysis. J Antimicrob Chemother 1991; 27: 225–32.
351. Debruyne D, Ryckelynck JP, Hurault de Ligny B, Moulin M. Pharmacokinetics of piperacillin in patients on peritoneal dialysis with and without peritonitis. J Pharmacokinet Sciences 1990; 79: 99–102.
352. Johnson CA, Halstenson CE, Kelloway JS, Shapiro BE, Zimmerman SW, Tonelli A, Faulkner R, Dutta A, Haynes J, Greene DS, Kuye O. Single dose pharmacokinetics of piperacillin and tazobactam in patients with renal disease. Clin Pharmacol Ther 1992; 51: 32–41.
353. Boelaert J, Daneels R, Schurgers M, Mellows G, Swaisland AJ, Lambert AM, Van Landuyt HW. Effect of renal function and dialysis on temocillin pharmacokinetics. Drugs 1985; 29 (suppl 5): 109–13.
354. Pancorbo S, Compty C. Pharmacokinetics of cefamandole in patients undergoing continuous ambulatory peritoneal dialysis. Perit Dial Bull 1983; 3: 135–7.
355. Bliss M, Mayersohn M, Arnold T, Logan J, Michael UF, Jones W. Disposition kinetics of cefamandole during continuous ambulatory peritoneal dialysis Antimicrob Agents Chemother 1986; 29: 649–53.
356. Bunke CM, Aronoff GR, Brier ME, Sloan R, Luft FC. Cefalozin and cephalexin kinetics in continuous ambulatory peritoneal dialysis. Clin Pharmacol Ther 1983; 33: 66–72.
357. Paton TW, Manuel A, Cohen LB, Walker SE. The disposition of cefazolin and tobramycin following intraperitoneal administration in patients on CAPD. Perit Dial Bull, 1983; 3: 73–6.
358. Morrison G, Audet P, Peingold R, Murray T. Cefazolin: the cephalosporin antibiotic of choice in CAPD patients. Kidney Int 1982; 21: 174 (abstract).
359. Barbhaiya RH, Knupp CA, Pfeffer M, Zaccardelli D, Dukes GM, Mattern W, Pittman KA, Hak LJ. Pharmacokinetics of cefepime in patients undergoing continuous ambulatory peritoneal dialysis. Antimicrob Agents Chemother 1992; 36: 1387–91.
360. Mendes P, Lameire N, Rosenkranz B, Malerczyk V, Damm D. Pharmacokinetics of cefodizime during continuous ambulatory peritoneal dialysis.
J Antimicrob Chemother 1990; 26 (suppl C): 89–93.
361. Keller E, Jansen A, Pels K, Hoppe-Seyler G, Scholllmeyer P. Intraperitoneal and intravenous cefaperazone kinetics during continuous ambulatory peritoneal dialysis. Clin Pharmacol Ther 1984; 35: 208–13.
362. Hodler JE, Galeazzi RL, Frey B, Rudhardt M, Seiler AJ. Pharmacokinetics of cefoperazone in patients undergoing chronic ambulatory peritoneal dialysis: clinical and pathophysiological implications. Eur J Clin Pharmacol 1984; 26: 609–12.
363. Johnson CA, Zimmerman SW, Reitberg DP, Whall TJ, Leggett JE, Craig WA. Pharmacokinetics and pharmacodynamics of Cefoperazone-Sulbactam in patients on continuous ambulatory peritoneal dialysis. Antimicrob Agents Chemother 1988; 32: 51–6.
364. Leehey DJ, Leid R, Chan AY, Ing TS. Cefoperazone in the treatment of peritonitis in continuous ambulatory peritoneal dialysis. Artif Organs 1988; 12: 482–3.
365. Alexander D, Bamertoglio J, Barriere S, Warnock D, Schoenfeld P. Cefotaxime pharmacokinetics during continuous ambulatory peritoneal dialysis. Clin Pharmacol Ther 1984; 35: 225 (abstract).
366. Matousovic K, Moravek J, Vitko S, Prat V, Horcickova M. Pharmacokinetics of intravenous and intraperitoneal cefotaxime in patients undergoing CAPD. Perit Dial Bull 1985; 5: 33–5.
367. Albin HC, Demotes-Mainrad FM, Bouchet JL, Vincon GA, Martin-Dupont C. Pharmacokinetics of intravenous and intraperitoneal cefotaxime in chronic ambulatory peritoneal dialysis. Clin Pharmacol Ther 1985; 38: 285–9.
368. Heim KL, Halstenson CE, Comty CM, Affrime MB, Matzke GR. Disposition of cefotaxime and desacetyl cefotaxime during continuous ambulatory peritoneal dialysis. Antimicrob Agents Chemother 1986; 30: 15–9.
369. Hasegawa H, Imada A, Horiuchi A, Nishii Y, Fukushima M, Kurokawa E. Pharmacokinetics of cefotaxime in patients undergoing hemodialysis and continuous ambulatory peritoneal dialysis. J Antimicrob Chemother 1984; 14 (suppl B): 135–42.
370. Petersen J, Stewart RDM, Catto GRD, Edward N. Pharmacokinetics of intraperitoneal cefotaxime treatment of peritonitis in patients on continuous ambulatory peritoneal dialysis. Nephron 1985; 40: 78–82.
371. Overgaard S, Lokkegaard N, Scroder S, Fugleberg S, Nielsen-Kudsk F. Cefotaxime disposition pharmacokinetics during peritoneal dialysis. Pharmacol & Toxicol 1987; 60: 321–4.
372. Raap CM, Nahata MC, Mentser MA, Mahan JD, Puri SK, Hubbard JA. Cefotaxime and metabolite disposition in two pediatric continuous ambulatory peritoneal dialysis patients. Ann Pharmacotherapy 1992; 26: 341–3.
373. Bald M, Rascher W, Bonzel KA, Muller-Wiefel DE. Pharmacokinetics of intraperitoneal cefotaxime in children with peritonitis undergoing

continuous ambulatory peritoneal dialysis. Perit Dial Int 1990; 10: 311–3.
374. Browning MJ, Holt HA, White LO, Chapman ST, Banks R, Reeves DS, Yates RA. Pharmacokinetics of cefotetam in patients with end-stage renal failure on maintenance dialysis. J Antimicrob Chemother 1986; 18: 103–6.
375. Greaves WL, Kreeft JH, Ogilvie RI, Richards GK. Cefoxitin disposition during peritoneal dialysis. Antimicrob Agents Chemother 1981; 253–5.
376. Arvidsson A, Alvan G, Tranaeus A, Malmborg AS. Pharmacokinetic studies of cefoxitin in continuous ambulatory peritoneal dialysis. Eur J Clin Pharmacol 1985; 28: 333–7.
377. Veys N, Lameire N, Malerczyk V, Lehr K, Rosenkranz B. Single dose pharmacokinetics of Cefpirome in hemodialysed patients and patients treated by CAPD. Clin Pharmacol Ther 1993; 54: 395–401.
378. Ryckelynck J Ph, Vergnaud M, Hurault de Ligny B, Allogche G, Malbruny B, Morel C. Pharmacocinétique de la ceftazidime par voie intrapéritonéale en dialyse péritonéale continue ambulatoire. Path Biol 1986; 34: 328–31.
379. Comstock TJ, Straughn B, Kraus AP, Meyer MC, Finn AL, Chubb JM. Ceftazidime pharmacokinetics during continuous peritoneal dialysis (CAPD) and intermittent peritoneal dialysis (IPD). Drug Intell Clin Pharmacy 1983; 17: 453 (abstract).
380. Gross ML, Somani P, Ribner BS, Raeader R, Freimer EH, Higgings Jr JT. Ceftizoxime elimination kinetics in continuous ambulatory peritoneal dialysis. Clin Pharmacol Ther 1983; 34: 673–80.
381. Burgess ED, Blair AD. Pharmacokinetics of ceftizoxime in patients undergoing continuous ambulatory peritoneal dialysis. Antimicrob Agents Chemother 1983; 24: 237–9.
382. Albin H, Ragnaud JM, Demotes-Mainard F, Vincon G, Couzineau M, Wone C. Pharmacokinetics of intravenous and intraperitoneal ceftriaxone in chronic ambulatory peritoneal dialysis. Eur J Clin Pharmacol 1986; 31: 479–83.
383. Favre H, Probst P. Pharmacokinetics of ceftriaxone after intravenous administration to CAPD patients with and without peritonitis. Chemoterapia 1987; 6 (suppl 2): 273–4.
384. Zaruba K, Rastorfer M, Probst PJ. Pharmacokinetics of Ceftriaxone in continuous ambulatory peritoneal dialysis patients after intraperitoneal administration. Chemoterapia 1987; 6 (suppl 6): 267–70.
385. Koup JR, Keller E, Neumann H, Stoeckel K. Ceftriaxone pharmacokinetics during peritoneal dialysis. Eur J Clin Pharmacol 1986; 30: 303–7.
386. Ti TY, Fortin L, Kreeft JH, East DS, Ogilvie RI, Somerville PJ. Kinetic disposition of intravenous ceftriaxone in normal subjects and patients with renal failure on hemodialysis or peritoneal dialysis. Antimicrob Agents Chemother 1984; 25: 83–7.
387. Dahl K, Walstad RA, Wideroe TE. The effect of peritonitis on the transperitoneal transport of cefuroxime in patients on CAPD treatment. Nephrol Dial Transpl 1990; 5: 272–81.
388. Davis GM, Forland SC, Cutler RE. Serum and dialysate concentrations of cephalexin following repeated dosing in CAPD patients. Am J Kid Dis 1985; 6: 177–80.
389. Munch R, Steurer J, Luthy R, Siegenthaler W, Kuhlmann U. Serum and dialysate concentrations of intraperitoneal cephalothin in patients undergoing chronic ambulatory peritoneal dialysis. Clin Nephrol 1983; 20: 40–3.
390. Johnson CA, Welling PG, Zimmerman SW. Pharmacokinetics of oral cephradine in continuous ambulatory peritoneal dialysis patients. Nephron 1984; 38: 57–61.
391. Singlas E, Boutron HF, Merdjan J, Brocard JF, Pocheville M, Fries D. Moxolactam kinetics during chronic ambulatory peritoneal dialysis. Clin Pharmacol Ther 1983; 34: 403–7.
392. Jones TE, Milne RW, Mudaliar Y, Sansom LN. Moxolactam kinetics during continuous ambulatory peritoneal dialysis after intraperitoneal administration. Antimicrob Agents Chemother 1985; 28: 293–8.
393. Morse G, Janicke D, Cafarell R, Piontek K, Apicella M, Jusko WJ, Walshe J. Moxolactam epimer disposition in patients undergoing continuous ambulatory peritoneal dialysis. Clin Pharmacol Ther 1985; 38: 150–6.
394. Albin H, Ragnaud JM, Demotes-Mainard F, Vincon G, Wone C. Pharmacokinetics of intravenous and intraperitoneal moxolactam in chronic ambulatory peritoneal dialysis. Eur J Clin Pharmacol 1986; 30: 299–302.
395. Pancorbo S, Compty C. Peritoneal transport of vancomycin in 4 patients undergoing continuous ambulatory peritoneal dialysis. Nephron 1982; 31: 37–9.
396. Bunke CM, Aronoff GR, Brier ME, Sloan RS, Luft FC. Vancomycin kinetics during continuous ambulatory peritoneal dialysis. Clin Pharmacol Ther 1983; 34: 631–7.
397. Blevins RD, Halstenson CE, Salem NG, Matzke GR. Pharmacokinetics of vancomycin in patients undergoing continuous ambulatory peritoneal dialysis. Antimicrob Agents chemother 1984; 25: 603–6.
398. Rogge MC, Johnson CA, Zimmerman SW, Welling PG. Vancomycin disposition during continuous ambulatory peritoneal dialysis: a pharmacokinetic analysis of peritoneal drug transport. Antimicrob Agents Chemother 1985; 27: 578–82.
399. Mounier M, Benevent D, Denis F. Pharmacocinétique de la vancomycine chez les patients insuffisants renaux chroniques en dialyse péritonéale continue ambulatoire (DPCA) après administration intra abdominale. Path Biol 1985; 33: 542–4.
400. Whitby M, Edwards R, Astan E, Finck RG. Pharmacokinetics of single dose intravenous vancomycin in CAPD peritonitis. J Antimicrob Chemother 1987; 19: 351–7.
401. Morse GD, Farolino DF, Apicella MA, Walshe JJ. Comparative study of intraperitoneal and intravenous pharmacokinetics of vancomycin during

CAPD. Antimicrob Agents Chemother 1987; 31: 173–7.
402. Neal D, Bailie GR. Clearance from dialysate and equilibration of intraperitoneal vancomycin in continuous ambulatory peritoneal dialysis. Clin Pharmacokinet 1990; 18: 485–90.
403. Rubin J. Vancomycin absorption from the peritoneal cavity during dialysis-related peritonitis. Perit Dial Int 1990; 10: 283–5.
404. Bailie GR, Eisele G, Venezia RA, Yoeum D, Hollister A. Prediction of serum vancomycin concentrations following intraperitoneal loading doses in continuous ambulatory peritoneal dialysis patients with peritonitis. Clin Pharmacokinet 1992; 22: 298–307.
405. Traina GL, Gentile MG, Fellin G, Rosina R, Cavenaghi L, Bruniva G, Nonati M. Pharmacokinetics of teicoplanin in patients on continuous ambulatory peritoneal dialysis. Eur J Clin Pharmacol 1986; 31: 501–4.
406. Jankneght R, Koelman HH, Nube MJ. Pharmacokinetics of rifampicin and teicoplanin during CAPD. Med Science Res 1987; 15: 171–2.
407. Guay DRP, Awni WM, Halstenson CE, Kenny MT, Keane WF, Matzkc ZGR. Teicoplanin pharmacokinetics in patients undergoing continuous ambulatory peritoneal dialysis after intravenous and intraperitoneal dosing. Antimicrob Agents Chemother 1989; 33: 2012–5.
408. Brouard RJ, Kapusnik JE, Gambertoglio JC, Schoenfeld PY, Sachdeva M, Freel K, Tozer TN. Teicoplanin pharmacokinetics and bioavailability during peritoneal dialysis. Clin Pharmacol Ther 1989; 45: 674–81.
409. Bonati M, Traina GL, Gentile MG, Fellin G, Rosina R, Cavenaghi L, Buniva G. Pharmacokinetics of intraperitoneal teicoplanin in patients with chronic renal failure on continuous ambulatory peritoneal dialysis. Brit J Clin Pharmacol 1988; 25: 761–6.
410. Keane WF, Everett ED, Golper TA, Gokal R, Halstenson C, Kawaguchi Y, Riella M, Vas S, Verbrugh HA. Peritoneal dialysis – related peritonitis treatment recommendations – update 1993. Perit Dial Bull 1993; 13: 14–28.
411. Boeschoten EW, Rietra PJGM, Krediet RT, Visser MJ, Arisz L. CAPD peritonitis: a prospective randomized trial of oral versus intraperitoneal treatment with cephradine. J Antimicrob Chemother 1985; 16: 789–97.
412. Knight KR, Polak A, Crump J, Mashell R. Laboratory diagnosis and treatment of CAPD peritonitis. Lancet 1982; 2: 1301–4.
413. Drew PJT, Casewell MW, Desai N, Houang ET, Simpson CN, Marsh FP. Cephalexin for the oral treatment of CAPD peritonitis. J Antimicrob Chemother 1984; 13: 153–9.
414. Ragnaud JM, Roche-Beziam MC, Marceau C, Demotes-Mainard F, Albin H, Prevost D, Wone C. Traitement des péritonites en dialyse péritonéale continue ambulatoire par une dose unique quotidienne de 1 g de céfotiam par voie intrapéritonéale. Path Biol 1986; 34: 512–6.
415. Fuiano G, Sepe V, Viscione M, Nani E, Conte G. Effectiveness of single dialy intraperitoneal administration of aztreonam and cefuroxime in the treatment of peritonitis in continuous ambulatory peritoneal dialysis (CAPD). Perit Dial Int 1989; 9: 273–5.
416. Mason NA, Johnson CE, O'Brien MA. Stability of ceftazidime and tobramycine sulfate in peritoneal dialysis solutions. Am J Hosp Pharm 1992; 49: 1139–42.
417. Chan MK, Chan PCK, Cheng IPK, Chan CY, Ng WSF. Pseudomonas peritonitis in CAPD patients: characteristics and outcome of treatment. Nephrol Dial Transpl 1989; 4: 814–7.
418. Gray HH, Goulding S, Eykyn SJ. Intraperitoneal vancomycin and ceftazidime in the treatment of CAPD peritonitis. Clin Nephrol 1985; 23: 81–4.
419. Beaman M, Solaro L, McGonigle RJS, Michael J, Adu D. Vancomycin and ceftazidime in the treatment of CAPD peritonitis. Nephron 1989; 51: 51–5.
420. Ragnaud JM, Roche-Bezian MC, Dupon M, Marceau C, Wone C. Traitement des péritonites en dialyse péritonéale continue ambulatoire par la ceftriaxone intrapéritonéale. Path Biol 1986; 36: 552–6.
421. Krothapalli RK, Senekjian HO, Ayus JC. Efficiency of intravenous vancomycin in the treatment of Gram-positive peritonitis in long-term peritoneal dialysis. Am J Med 1983; 75: 345–8.
422. Obermiller LE, Tzamaloukas AH, Leymon P, Avasthi PS. Intravenous vancomycin as initial treatment for Gram-positive peritonitis in patients on chronic peritoneal dialysis. Clin Nephrol 1985; 24: 256–60.
423. Johnson CA. Intraperitoneal vancomycin administration. Perit Dial Int 1991; 11: 9–11.
424. Gouge SF, Charney DI. Does intraperitoneal vancomycin cause chemical peritonitis? Perit Dial Int 1991; 11: 91 (letter).
425. Rowland M. Clinical pharmacokinetics of teicoplanin. Clin Pharmacokinet 1990; 18: 184–209.
426. Shalit I, Greenwood RB, Marks MI, Pederson JA, Frederick DL. Pharmacokinetics of single dose oral ciprofloxacin in patients undergoing CAPD. Antimicrob Agents Chemother 1986; 30: 152–6.
427. Golper TA, Hartstein AI, Morthland VH, Christensen JM. Effects of antacids and dialysate dwell times on multiple-dose pharmacokinetics of oral ciprofloxacin in patients on CAPD. Antimicrob Agents Chemother 1987; 31: 1787–90.
428. Stuck AE, Frey FJ, Heizmann P, Brandt R, Weiderkamm E. Pharmacokinetics and metabolism of intravenous and oral fleroxacin in subjects with normal and impaired renal function and in patients on CAPD. Antimicrob Agents Chemother 1989; 33: 373–81.
429. Lameire N, Rosenkranz B, Malerczyk V, Lehr KH, Veys N, Ringoir S. Ofloxacin pharmacokinetics in chronic renal failure and dialysis. Clin Pharmacokinet 1991; 21: 357–71.
430. Lode H, Hoffkin G, Prinzineg C, Glatzel P, Wiley

R, Obschewski P, Sievers B, Reimbitz D, Borner K, Koeppe P. Comparative pharmacokinetics of new quionolones. Drugs 1987; 34 (suppl I): 21–5.
432. Passlick J, Wonner R, Keller E, Essers L, Grabensee B. Single and multiple dose kinetics of ofloxacin in patients on CAPD. Perit Dial Int 1989; 9: 267–72.
433. Flor S. Pharmacokinetics of ofloxacin. Am J Med 1989; 87 (suppl 6C): 24–30.
434. Rosenkranz B, Malerczyk V, Zamba K, Jungbluth H, Lameire N. Pharmacokinetics of ofloxacin in CAPD. Kidney Int 1991; 39: 1329 (abstract).
435. Kampf D, Borner K, Hain H, Conrad W. Multiple-dose kinetics of ofloxacin after intraperitoneal application in CAPD patients. Perit Dial Int 1991; 11: 317–21.
436. Schmit JL, Hary L, Bou P, Renaud H, Westeel PF, Andrejak M, Fournier A. Pharmacokinetics of single-dose intravenous, oral and intraperitoneal pefloxacin in patients on chronic ambulatory peritoneal dialysis. Antimicrob Agents Chemotehr 1991; 35, 1492–4.
437. Nikolaidis P, Walker SE, Dombros N, Tourkantonis A, Paton TW, Oreopoulos DG. Single dose pefloxacin pharmacokinetics and metabolism in patients undergoing continuous ambulatory peritoneal dialysis (CAPD). Perit Dial Int 1991; 11: 59–63.
438. Gerig JS, Bolton ND, Swabb EA, Scheld WM, Bolton WK. Effect of hemodialysis and peritoneal dialysis on aztrenonam phrmacokinetics. Kidney Int 1984; 26: 308–18.
439. Nikolaidis P, Dombros N, Alexion P, Balaskas E, Tourkantonis A. Pharmacokinetics of aztreonam administered IP in continuous ambulatory peritoneal dialysis (CAPD) patients. Perit Dial Int 1989; 9: 57–9.
440. Brown J, Altmann P, Cunningham J, Shaw E, Marsh F. Pharmacokinetics of once daily intraperitoneal aztreonam and vancomycin in the treatment of CAPD peritonitis. J Antimicrob Chemother 1990; 25: 141–7.
441. Pancorbo S, Comty C. Pharmacokinetics of gentamicin in patients undergoing continuous ambulatory peritoneal dialysis. Antimicrob Agents Chemother 1981; 19: 605–7.
442. Paton TW, Manuel M, Walker SE. Tobramycin disposition in patients on continuous ambulatory peritoneal dialysis. Perit Dial Bull 1982; 2: 179–81.
443. Bunke CM, Aronoff GR, Brier ME, Sloan RS, Luft FC. Tobramycin kinetics during continuous ambulatory peritoneal dialysis. Clin Pharmacol Ther 1983; 34: 110–6.
444. Walshe JJ, Morse GD, Janicke DM, Apicella MA. Crossover pharmacokinetic analysis comparing intravenous and intraperitoneal administration of tobramycin. J Infect Dis 1986; 153: 796–9.
445. Halstenson CE, Matze GR, Comty CM. Intraperitoneal administration of tobraymcin during CAPD. Kidney Int 1984; 25: 256 (abstract).
446. Rubin J. Tobramycin absorption from the peritoneal cavity. Perit Dial Int 1990; 10: 295–7.
447. Sennesael JJ, Maes VA, Pierard D, Debeukelaer SH, Verbeelen DL. Streptomycin pharmacokinetics in relapsing mycobacterium xenopi peritonitis. Am J Nephrol 1990; 10: 422–5.
448. Smeltzer BD, Schwartzman MS, Bertino JS. Amikacin pharmacokinetics during continuous ambulatory peritoneal dialysis. Antimicrob Agents Chemother 1988; 32: 236–40.
449. Krediet RT, Boeschoten EW, Arisz L. Kanamycin as marker for middle-molecular solute transport in CAPD patients with and without peritonitis. Blood Purif 1987; 5: 291 (abstract).
450. Martea M, Hekster YA, Vree TB, Voets AJ, Berden JHM. Pharmacokinetics of cefradine, sulfamethosazole and trimethoprim and their metabolites in a patient with peritonitis undergoing continuous ambulatory peritoneal dialysis. Pharamceutisch Wkbl 1987; 9: 110–6.
451. Walker SE, Paton TW, Churchill DN, Ojo B, Manuel MA, Wright N. Trimethoprim-sulfamethoxazole pharmacokinetics during continuous ambulatory peritoneal dialysis (CAPD). Perit Dial Int 1989; 9: 51–5.
452. Rubin J, Planch A. Absorption of sulfamethoxazole and albumin from the peritoneal cavity. Trans Am Soc Artif Intern Organs 1990; 36: 834–7.
453. Bouchet JL, Albin H, Quentin CL, De Barbeyrac B, Vincon G, Martin-Dupont PH, Potaux L, Aparicio M. Pharmacokinetics of intravenous and intreaperitoneal fosfomycin in continuous ambulatory peritoneal dialysis. Clin Nephrol 1988; 29: 35–40.
454. Janknegt R. CAPD peritonitis and fluoroquinolones: a review. Perit Dial Int 1991; 11: 53–8.
455. De Fijter CWH, Biemond A, Oe LP, Moesker HL, Verhoef J, Donker AJM, Verbrugh HA. Pharmacokinetics of ciprofloxacin after intraperitoneal administration in uninfected patients undergoing CCPD. Adv in CAPD 1992; 8: 18–21.
456. Ludlam H, Barton I, White L, McMullin C, King A, Phillips I. Intraperitoneal ciprofloxacin for the treatment of peritonitis in patients receiving CAPD. J Antimicrob Chemother 1990; 25: 843–51.
457. Dratwa M, Glupczynski Y, Lameire N, Matthys D, Verschraegen G, van Eeckhoute M, Boelaert J, Schurgers M, van Landuyt H, Verbeelen D, Lauwers S. Aztreonam in CAPD peritonitis. Lancet 1987; 2: 213–4.
458. Dratwa M, Glupczynski Y, Lameire N, Matthys D, Verschraegen G, van Eeckhoute M, Boelaert J, Schurgers M, van Landuyt H, Verbeelen D, Lauwers S. Treatment of Gram-negative peritonitis with aztrenoam in patients undergoing continuous ambulatory peritoneal dialysis. Rev Infect Dis 1991; 13: S645–7.
459. Cheng IKP, Chan C-Y, Wong WT. A randomized prospective comparison of oral ofloxacin and intraperitoneal vancomycin plus aztreonam in the treatment of bacterial peritonitis complicating continuous ambulatory peritoneal dialysis (CAPD). Perit Dial Int 1991; 11: 27–30.
460. Chong TK, Piraino B, Bernardini J. Vestibular toxicity due to gentamicin in peritoneal dialysis patients. Perit Dial Int 1991; 11: 152–5.

461. Nikolaidis P, Vas S, Lawson V, Kennedy-Vosu L, Bernard A, Abraham G, Izatt S, Khanna S, Bargman JM, Oreopoulos DG. Is intraperitoneal tobramycin ototoxic in CAPD patients? Perit Dial Int 1991; 11: 156–61.
462. Glew RH, Pavuk RA. Stability of vancomycin and aminoglycoside antibiotics in peritoneal dialysis concentrate. Nephron 1981; 28: 241–3.
463. Konig U, Muller U, Binswanger U. Behandlung der peritonitis während kontinuerlicher ambulanter Peritonealdialyse (CAPD) mit Co-Trimoxazol, Cefazolin oder Vancomycin. Klin Wochenschrift 1987; 65: 562–70.
464. Seth SK, Visconti JA, Herbert LA, Krasny HC. Acyclovir pharmacokinetics in a patient on continuous ambulatory peritoneal dialysis. Clin Pharmacol 1985; 4: 320–2.
465. Shah GM, Winer RL, Krasny HC. Acyclovir pharmacokinetics in a patient on continuous ambulatory peritoneal dialysis. Am J Kidney Dis 1986; 7: 507–10.
466. Burgess ED, Gill MJ. Intraperitoneal administration of acyclovir in patients receiving continuous ambulatory peritoneal dialysis. J Clin Pharmacol 1990; 30: 997–1000.
467. Schwenk MH, Halstenson CE, Simpson ML, Pence TV, Reynolds DJ. Pharmacokinetics of zidovudine in an AIDS patient during continuous ambulatory peritoneal dialysis, American College Clinical Pharmacy, Kansas City, Missouri, 1990 (abstract 121).
468. Kremer D, Munar MY, Kohlhepp SJ, Swan SK, Stinnett EA, Gilbert DN, Young EW, Bennett WM. Zidovudine pharmacokinetics in five HIV seronegative patients undergoing continuous ambulatory peritoneal dialysis. Pharmacotherapy 1992; 12: 56–60.
469. Gallicano KD, Tobe S, Sahai J, McGilveray IJ, Cameron DW, Kriger F, Garber G. Pharmacokinetics of single and chronic dose zidovudine in two HIV positive patients undergoing continuous ambulatory peritoneal dialysis. J Acquir Immune Defic Syndr 1992; 5: 242–50.
470. Kerr CM, Perfect JR, Cran PC, Horgensen JH, Dutz DJ, Shelburne JD, Gallis HA, Gutman RA. Fungal peritonitis in patients on continuous ambulatory peritoneal dialysis. Ann Int Med 1983; 99: 334–7.
471. Fraser AK, O'Connor JP. Peritoneal penetration of amphotericin B. Perit Dial Bull 1984; 4: 264–5.
472. Debruyne D, Ryckelynck JP, Morelin M, Hurault de Ligney B, Lavaltier B, Bigot MC. Pharmacokinetics of fluconazole in patients undergoing continuous ambulatory peritoneal dialysis. Clin Pharmacokin 1990; 18: 491–8.
473. Debruyne D, Ryckelynck J Ph: Fluconazole serum, urine and dialysate levels in CAPD patients. Perit Dial Int 1992; 12: 328–9 (letter).
474. Cecchin E, Panarello G, de March IS. Fungal peritonitis in ambulatory peritoneal dialysis. Ann Int Med 1984; 100: 321 (letter).
475. Jones JM, Greenfeld RA. Administration of flucytosine to a patient on CAPD. Perit Dial Bull 1982; 2: 46–7.
476. Krediet RT, Boeschoten EW, Struijk DG, Arisz L. Pharmacokinetics of intraperitoneally administered 5-fluorocytosine in continuous ambulatory peritoneal dialysis. Nephrol Dial Transpl 1987; 2: 453 (abstract).
477. Eisenberg ES. Intraperitoneal flucytosine in the management of fungal peritonitis in patients on continuous ambulatory peritoneal dialysis. Am J Kidney Dis 1988; 11: 465–7.
478. Boelaert J, Schurgers M, Matthys E, Daneels R, van Peer A. Intraconazole pharmacokinetics in patients with renal dysfunction. Antimicrob. Agents and Chemother 1988; 32: 1595–7.
479. Doherty D, Seth S, Bay W. Fungal peritonitis and ketoconazole levels in a CAPD patient. Perit Dial Bull 1984; 4: S20 (abstract).
480. McGuire N, Port FK, Kauffman CA. Ketoconazole pharmacokinetics in continuous ambulatory peritoneal dialysis. Perit Dial Bull 1984; 4: 199–201.
481. Valainis GT, Morford DW. Ketoconazole levels in peritoneal fluid. Perit Dial Bull 1985; 5: 136 (letter).
482. Hedaya MA, Elmquist WF, Sawchuck RJ. Probenecid inhibits the metabolic and renal clearance of zidovudine (AZT) in human volunteers. Pharmacol Res 1990; 7: 411–7.
483. Collins JM, Unadkat JD. Clinical pharmacokinetics of zidovudine: an overview of current data. Clin Pharmacokin 1989; 17: 1–9.
484. Muther RS, Bennett WM. Clearance of amphotericin B and 5-fluorocytosine by peritoneal dialysis. Western J Med 1980; 133: 157–60.
485. Peterson LR, Hall WH, Kelty RH, Votava HJ. Therapy of candida peritonitis: penetration of amphotericin B into peritoneal fluid. Postgrad Med J 1978; 54: 340–2.
486. Kravitz SP, Berry PL. Successful treatment of aspergillus peritonitis in a child undergoing continuous ambulatory peritoneal dialysis. Arch Intern Med 1986; 146: 2061–2.
487. Khanna R, Oreopoulos DG, Vas S, McCready W, Dombros N. Fungal peritonitis in patients undergoing chronic intermittent or continuous peritoneal dialysis. Proc EDTA 1980; 17: 291–6.
488. Rault R. Candida peritonitis complicating chronic peritoneal dialysis. A report of five cases and review of the literature. Am J Kidney Dis 1983; 2: 544–7.
489. Levine JD, Bernard DB, Idelson BA, Farnham H, Saunders C, Sugar AM. Fungal peritonitis complicating continuous ambulatory peritoneal dialysis: successful treatment with fluconazole, a new orally active antifungal agent. Am J Med 1989; 86: 825–7.
490. Slingeneyer A, Laroche B, Steel F, Canaud B, Beraud JJ, Mion C. Oral ketoconazole plus IP 5 fluorocytosine as a sole treatment of fungal peritonitis in CAPD. Perit Dial Bull 1984; 4: S60 (abstract).
491. Paton TW, Manuel MA, Walker SE. Cimetidine disposition in patients on continuous ambulatory peritoneal dialysis. Perit Dial Bull 1982; 2: 73–6.
492. Kogan FJ, Sampliner RE, Myersohn M, Kazama

RM, Perrier D, Hones W, Michael UF. Cimetidine disposition in patients undergoing continuous ambulatory peritoneal dialysis. J Clin Pharmacol 1983; 20: 252–6.
493. Sica DA, Comstock T, Harford A, Eshelman F. Ranitidine pharmacokinetics in continuous ambulatory peritoneal dialysis. Eur J Clin Pharmacol 1987; 32: 587–91.
494. Gladziwa U, Klotz U, Krishna DR, Schmitt H, Glockner WM, Mann H. Pharmacokinetics and dynamics of famotidine in patients with renal failure. Brit J Clin Pharm 1988; 26: 315–21.
495. McCallum RW, Prakash C, Campoli-Richards DM, Goa KL. Cisapride: a preliminary review of its pharmacodynamic and pharmacokinetic properties and therapeutic use as a prokinetic agent in gastrointestinal motility disorders. Drugs 1988; 36: 652–81.
496. Jannsen Pharmaceutica: Data on file.
497. Lazarovitz AI, Page D. Intraperitoneal cisapride for the treatment of diabetes with gastroparesis and end-stage renal disease. Nephron 1990; 56: 107–9.
498. Gora ML, Visconti JA, Seth S, Shields B, Bay W. Pharmacokinetics of intraperitoneal metoclopramide in a patient with renal failure. Clin Pharmacol 1992; 11: 174–6.
499. Lameire N, Rosenkranz B, Brockmeier D. Pharmacokinetics of histamine (H_2)-receptor antagonists, including roxatidine, in chronic renal failure. Scand J Gastroenterol 1988; 23 (suppl. 146): 100–10.
500. Naesdal J, Anderson T, Bodemar G, Larrson R, Regardt CG. Pharmacokinetics of ^{14}C-Omeprazole in patients with impaired renal function. Clin Pharmacol Therapeutics 1986; 40: 344–51.
501. Howden CW, Payton CD, Meredith A, Hughes DMA, MacDougall AI, Reid JL, Forrest JAH. Antisecretory effect and oral pharmacokinetics of omeprazole in patients with chronic renal failure. Eur J Clin Pharmacol 1985; 28: 637–40.
502. Boelaert JR, Schurgers ML, Matthys EG, Belpaire FM, Daneels RF. Comparative pharmacokinetics of recombinant erythropoietin administration by the intravenous, subcutaneous and intraperitoneal routes in continuous ambulatory peritoneal dialysis patients. Perit Dial Int 1989; 9: 95–8.
503. Gahl GM, Passlick J, Pustelnik A, Kampf D, Grabensee B. Intraperitoneal versus intravenous recombinant human erythropoietin in stable CAPD patients. Proc 6th Congress EDTA – ERA Gotenburg 1990, 199 (abstract).
504. Hughes RT, Cotes PM, Oliver DO, Pippard MJ, Royston P. Correction of anemia of chronic renal failure with erythropoietin: pharmacokinetic studies on hemodialysis and CAPD. Contrib Nephrol 1989; 76: 122–30.
505. Kampf D, Kahl A, Passlick J, Pustelnik A, Eckardt KU. Single-dose kinetics of recombinant human erythropoietin after intravenous, subcutaneous and intraperitoneal administration. Contrib Nephrol 1989; 76: 106–11.
506. Kromer G, Solf A, Ehmer B, Kaufmann B, Quellhorst E. Single dose pharmacokinetics of recombinant human erythropoietin comparing intravenous, subcutaneous and intraperitoneal administration in IPD patients. Kidney Int 1990; 37: 311.
507. Macdougall IC, Roberts DE, Neubert P, Dharmasena AD, Coles GA, Williams JD. Pharmacokinetics of recombinant human erythropoietin in patients on continuous ambulatory peritoneal dialysis. Lancet 1989; 1: 425–7.
508. Stockenhuber F, Loibl U, Gottsauner-Wolf M, Jahn C, Manker W, Meisl THF, Balcke P. Pharmacokinetics and dose response after intravenous and subcutaneous administration of recombinant erythropoietin in patients on regular haemodialysis treatment or continuous ambulatory peritoneal dialysis. Nephron 1991; 59: 339–402.
509. Lui SF, Chung WWM, Leung CB, Chan K, Lai KN. Pharmacokinetics and pharmacodynamics of subcutaneous and intraperitoneal administration of recombinant human erythropoietin in patients on continuous ambulatory peritoneal dialysis. Clin Nephrol 1990; 33: 47–51.
510. Nissenson AR. Erythropoietin and peritoneal dialysis: the efficacy of intraperitoneal dosing. Perit Dial Int 1992; 12: 350–2.
511. Bargman J, Breborowicz Z, Rodela H, Sombolos K, Oreopoulos DG. Intraperitoneal administration of recombinant human erythropoietin in uremic animals. Perit Dial Int 1988; 8: 249–52.
512. Frenken LAM, Struijk DG, Coppens PJW, Tiggeler RGWL, Krediet RT, Koene RAP. Intraperitoneal administration of recombinant human erythropoietin. Perit Dial Int 1992; 12: 378–83.
513. Nasu T, Mitui H, Shinohara Y, Hayashida S, Ohtuka H. Effect of erythropoietin in CAPD patients: comparison between intravenous and intraperitoneal administration. Perit Dial Int 1992; 12: 373–7.
514. Schade DS, Eaton RP, Davis T, Akiya F, Phinney E, Kubica R, Vaughn EA, Day PW. The kinetics of peritoneal insulin absorption. Metabolism 1981; 30: 149–55.
516. Nelson JA, Stephen R, Landau ST, Wilson DE, Tyler FH. Intraperitoneal insulin administration produces a positive portal systemic blood insulin gradient in unanesthetized, unrestrained swine. Metabolism 1982; 31: 969–72.
517. Schade DS, Eaton RP, Friedman N, Spencer W. The intravenous, intraperitoneal and subcutaneous routes of insulin delivery in diabetic man. Diabetes 1979; 28: 1069–72.
518. Selam JJ, Slingeneyer A, Hedon B, Mares P, Berand JJ, Mirouze J. Long-term ambulatory peritoneal insulin infusion of brittle diabetes with portable pumps: comparison with intravenous and subcutaneous routes. Diabetes Care 1983; 6: 105–11.
519. Kritz J, Hagmuller H, Lovett R, Irsigler K. Implanted constant basal rate insulin infusion devices for type 1 (insulin-dependent) diabetic patients. Diabetologia 1983; 25: 78–81.
520. Micossi P, Bosi E, Cristallo M, Monti DL, Librenti

MC, Petrella G, Galimberti G, Spotti D, Guidici G, Vergani C, Dicarlo V, Pozza G. Chronic continuous intraperitoneal insulin infusion (CIPII) in type I diabetic patients non-satisfactorily responsive to continuous sub-cutaneous insulin infusion (CSII). Acta Diabetol Lat 1986; 23: 155–64.
521. Saudek CD, Selam JL, Pitt HA, Waxman K, Rubio M, Jeandidier N, Turner D, Fischell RE, Charles MA. A preliminary trial of the programmable implantable medication system for insulin delivery. N Engl J Med 1986; 31: 574–9.
522. Vaag A, Handberg A, Lauritzen M, Henriksen JE, Damgaard Pedersen K, Beck Nielsen H. Variation in absorption of NPH-insulin due to intramuscular injection. Diabetes Care 1990; 13: 74–6.
523. Wredling R, Liu D, Lins PE, Adamson U. Variation of insulin absorption during subcutaneous and in peritoneal infusion of insulin-dependent diabetic patients with unsatisfactory long-term glycemic response to continuous subcutaneous insulin infusion. Diabète & Métabolisme 1991; 17: 456–9.
524. Wideroe TE, Smeby LC, Berg KJ, Jorstad S, Svartas TM. Intraperitoneal (^{125}I) insulin absorption during intermittent and continuous peritoneal dialysis. Kidney Int 1983; 23: 22–8.
525. Peetoom JJ, Willekens FLA, Meinders AE. Absorption and biological effect of intraperitoneal insulin administration in patients with terminal renal failure treated by continuous ambulatory peritoneal dialysis. Neth J Med 1985; 28: 435–41.
526. Schade DS, Eaton RP. The peritoneum – a potential insulin delivery route for a mechanical pancreas. Diabetes Care 1980; 3: 229–34.
527. Shapiro DJ, Blumenkranz MJ, Levin SR. Coburn JW. Absorption and action of insulin added to peritoneal dialysate in dogs. Nephron 1979; 23: 174–80.
528. Rubin J, Bell AH, Andrews M, Jones Q, Planck A. Intraperitoneal insulin – a dose response curve. Trans Am Soc Artif Intern Organs 1989; 35: 17–21.
529. Beardsworth SF, Ahmad R, Terry E, Karim K. Intraperitoneal insulin: a protocol for administration during CAPD and review of published protocol. Perit Dial Bull 1988; 8: 145–51.
530. Brewer TE, Caldwell FT, Patterson RM, Flanigan WJ. Indwelling peritoneal (Tenckhoff) dialysis catheters – experience with 24 patients. Am J Med 1972; 219: 1011–5.
531. Heal MR, England AG, Goldsmith HJ. Four years experience with indwelling silastic cannulae for long-term peritoneal dialysis. Brit Med J 1973; 4: 596–600.
532. Lankisch PG, Tonnis JH, Fernandez-Redo E, Girndt J, Kramer P, Quellhorst E, Scheler F. Use of Tenckhoff catheter for peritoneal dialysis in terminal renal failure. Br Med J 1973; 4: 712–3.
533. Tenckhoff H. Catheter implantation. Dialysis and Transplantation 1972; 1: 18–21.
534. Tenckhoff H. Chronic peritoneal dialysis manual. Univ of Washington School of Medicine, Seattle, 1974.
535. Gotloib L, Crassweller P, Rodella H, Oreopoulos DG, Zellerman G, Ogilvie R, Hudson H, Brandes L, Vas S. Expermental models for studies of continuous peritoneal dialysis in uremic rabbits. Nephron 1982; 31: 254–9.
536. Takahashi S, Shimada A, Okada K, Kunto T, Nagura Y, Hatano M. Effect of intraperitoneal administration of heparin to patients on continuous ambulatory peritoneal dialysis. Perit Dial Internat 1991; 11: 81–3.
537. Schrader J, Tonnis HJ, Scheler F. Long-term intraperitoneal application of low molecular weight heparin in a continuous ambulatory peritoneal dialysis patient with deep vein thrombosis. Nephron 1986; 42: 83–4.
538. Tabata T, Shimada H, Emoto M, Morita A, Furumitsu Y, Fujita J, Inoue T, Miki T, Nishizawa Y, Morii H. Inhibitory effects of heparin and/or antithrombin III on intraperitoneal fibrin formation in continuous ambulatory peritoneal dialysis. Nephron 1990; 56: 391–5.
539. Allain P, Chalcil D, Mauras Y, Varin MC, Ang KS, Cam G, Simon P. Pharmacokinetics of desferrioxamine and of its iron and aluminum chelates in patients on peritoneal dialysis. Clin Chim Acta 1988; 173: 313–6.
540. Falk RJ, Mattern WD, Lamanna RW, Gitelman HJ, Parker NC, Cross RE, Rastall JR. Iron removal during continuous ambulatory peritoneal dialysis. Kidney Int 1983; 24: 110–2.
541. Payton D, Junor BJR, Fell GS. Successful treatment of aluminum encephalopathy by intraperitoneal desferrioxamine. Lancet 1984; 1: 1132–3.
542. Andreoli SP, Dunn D, Demyer W, Sherrard DJ, Bergstein JM. Intraperitoneal deferoxamine therapy for aluminum intoxication in a child undergoing continuous ambulatory peritoneal dialysis. J Pediatr 1985; 107: 760–3.
543. Hercz G, Salusky IB, Norris KC, Fine RN, Coburn JW. Aluminum removal by peritoneal dialysis: intravenous vs intraperitoneal deferoxamine. Kidney Int 1986; 30: 944–8.
544. O'Brien AAJ, McParland C, Keogh JAB. The use of intravenous and intraperitoneal desferrioxamine in aluminum ostemoalacia. Nephrol Dial Transplant 1987; 2: 117–9.
545. Guillot M, Lavocat C, Garabedian M, Sachs C, Balsan S, Gagnadoux MF, Broyer M. Evaluation of 25(OH)D loss in dialysate of children on continuous ambulatory peritoneal dialysis. Proc EDTA-ERA 1981; 18: 290–2.
546. Aloni Y, Shany S, Chaimovitz C. Losses of 25-hydroxy vitamin D in peritoneal fluid: possible mechanisms for bone disease in uremic patients treated with chronic ambulatory peritoneal dialysis. Mineral Electrolyte Metab 1983; 9: 82–6.
547. Shany S, Rapoport J, Goligorsky M, Yankowitz N, Zuili I, Chaimovitz C. Losses of 1, 25- and 24, 25-dihydroxy-cholecalciferol in the peritoneal fluid of patients treated with continuous ambulatory peritoneal dialysis. Nephron 1984; 36: 111–3.
548. Delmez JA, Dougan CS, Gearing BK, Rothstein M, Winders DW, Rapp N, Slatopolsky E. The effects

548. [continued] of intraperitoneal calcitriol on calcium and parathyroid hormone. Kidney Int 1987; 31: 795–9.
549. Salusky IB. Goodman WG, Horst R, Segre GV, Kim L, Nooris KC, Adams JS, Holloway M, fine RN, Coburn JW. Pharmacokinetics of calcitriol in continuous ambulatory peritoneal and cycling peritoneal dialysis patients. Am J Kidney Dis 1990; 16: 126–32.
550. Boeschoten EW, Schrijver J, Krediet RT, Schreuers WHP, Arisz L. Deficiencies of vitamins in CAPD patients: the effect of supplementation. Nephrol Dial Transplant 1988; 2: 187–93.
551. Marquardt ED, Ishisaka DY, Batra KK, Chin B. Removal of ethosuximide and phenobarbital by peritoneal dialysis in a child. Clin Pharmacy 1992; 11: 1030–1.
552. Guay DR, Meatherall RC, Baxter H, Jacyk WR, Penner B. Pharamcokinetics of metronidazole in patients undergoing continuous ambulatory peritoneal dialysis. Antimicrob Agents Chemother 1984; 25: 306–310.
553. Merdjan H, Beaumelou A, Diquet B, Chick O, Singlas E. Pharmacokinetics of ornidazole in patients with renal insufficiency: influence of hemodialysis and peritoneal dialysis. Br J Clin Pharmac 1985; 19: 211–7.
554. Hess B, Keusch G, Fluckiger J, Binswanger U. Zur Pharmakokinetik von Phenytoin bei kontinuerlicher ambulanter Peritonealdialyse. Schweiz Med Wschr 1984; 114: 16–9.
555. Leaky TEB, Elias-Jones AC, Coates PE, Smith KJ. Pharmacokinetics of theophylline and its metabolities during acute renal failure. Clin Pharmacokinet 1991; 21: 400–8.
556. Cefali EA, Poynor WJ, Sica D, Cox S. Pharmacokinetic comparison of flurbiprofen in end-stage renal disease subjects and subjects with normal renal function. J Clin Pharmacol 1991; 31: 808–14.
557. Schmith V, Piraino B, Smith RB, Kroboth PD. Alprazolam in end-stage renal disease. I. Pharmacokinetics. J Clin Pharmacol 1991; 31: 571–9.

8 CAPD systems and solutions

Mariano Feriani, Giuseppe La Greca, Frank L. Kriger, James F. Winchester

1. Introduction 233
2. Solutions (by Feriani M., La Greca G.) 233
3. Electrolytes 234
   3.1. Sodium 234
   3.2. Potassium 236
   3.3. Magnesium 236
   3.4. Calcium 237
4. Osmotic agents 238
   4.1. Low molecular weight agents 239
      4.1.1. Glucose 239
      4.1.2. Glycerol 241
      4.1.3. Xylitol 242
      4.1.4. Sorbitol 242
      4.1.5. Fructose 242
      4.1.6. Amino acids 242
   4.2. High molecular weight osmotic agents 245
      4.2.1. Albumin 245
      4.2.2. Synthetic polymers 246
      4.2.3. Plasma substitutes 246
      4.2.4. Glucose polymer 246
      4.2.5. Peptides 248
5. Acid base 248
   5.1. Acetate 249
   5.2. Lactate 249
   5.3. Bicarbonate 251
6. CAPD systems (by Kriger F. L., Winchester J.) 252
   6.1. Dialysis fluid containers 252
   6.2. Modern connection devices 253
   6.3. Simple connection methods 253
   6.4. The 'Y' systems 255
   6.5. Double bag systems 256
7. Connectology 256
8. The future 259
References 260

1. Introduction

This chapter will serve as a resource for the reader in the development of modern dialysis solutions for peritoneal dialysis, as well as an overview of systems used to deliver such dialysis solutions. Compositions of dialysis fluid vary widely in different counties, and readers are recommended to ascertain concentrations of solutes used in solutions prevalent in their own locale.

2. Solutions (by Feriani M., La Greca G.)

The basic principle of peritoneal dialysis is the solute composition of a solution infused in the peritoneal cavity tends to equilibrate with plasma water solute composition during the time. The different electrochemical concentration gradient is the driving force that allows such passive diffusion.

In addition, fluid movement across the peritoneal membrane occurs if different osmotic pressures are present in the infused solution and in plasma. Since fluid removal from the body is required in uremic patients, an osmotic agent is added to the dialysis solution to achieve a higher osmotic pressure thus leading to convective transport towards the peritoneal cavity.

Hence, the solute composition of the peritoneal fluid is the main tool for removing excess water and waste products, for supplying needed substances and of balancing disturbed solutes of uremic patients.

Several large pharmaceutical companies produce peritoneal dialysis solution, sterilized in varying volumes with different concentrations of glucose as the osmotic agent. The solutions for clinical use are now supplied in collapsible plastic containers. All the available solutions are similar in their constituent concentrations and up to a few years ago surprisingly similar to those used in the late 50's by Boen in Seattle [1] (Table 1).

Clinical evidence suggests some improvements in the solution composition and new developments are under clinical study.

In particular more physiological concentrations of calcium and magnesium have proved to be of clinical relevance, alternative substances to glucose (glycerol, amino acids and glucose polymers) as the osmotic agent have been clinically tested, acetate has been replaced by lactate as buffer, and the physiological buffer, bicarbonate, has been proposed.

The nephrology community has realized that peritoneal dialysis fluid has to be compatible with the living membrane and can be used not only for removing water and toxins but also for improving organic functions of uremic patients.

3. Electrolytes

End stage renal failure patients are not able to fully manage electrolyte balance. Unphysiological values of serum electrolytes can result in life threatening complications of the uremic syndrome. Sodium, potassium and magnesium have to be removed in order to maintain body homeostasis. Calcium uptake from the gastrointestinal tract is reduced and hypocalcemia is a common feature in the pre-dialysis phase if oral calcium and/or vitamin D are not supplemented.

Peritoneal dialysis fluid is tailored for correcting these imbalances and for restoring the normal electrolyte composition of the body.

3.1. Sodium

The sodium concentration in fresh peritoneal dialysis fluid ranged from 130 to 137 mmol/l among various manufacturing companies. In addition, different manufacturing procedures can lead to a 5% variation in declared sodium concentration.

It has been demonstrated in clinical studies [2] that different dialysate sodium concentrations (from 132 to 141 mmol/l) have no significant effect on serum sodium concentration. This could be explained by the peculiar characteristics of the electrolyte transport in CAPD.

Dialytic sodium balance is a function of both diffusion and convection [3]; net sodium movement by diffusion can result in net sodium uptake or removal depending on the concentration gradient between extracellular fluid and dialysis solution

Table 1. Composition of the peritoneal dialysis fluid.

		Boen Ref. [1]	Commercial CAPD
Na	mmol/l	135	132–134
K	mmol/l		0–2
Ca	mmol/l	1.5	1.25–1.75
Mg	mmol/l	0.75	0.25–0.75
Cl	mmol/l	107.5	95–106
Acetate	mmol/l	35	
Lactate	mmol/l		35–40
Glucose	g/dl	2.0 and higher	1.5–4.25

sodium concentration [4]. Peritoneal ultrafiltration removes sodium by convection. However, the net removal of sodium per liter of ultrafiltrate (about 70 mmol/l) is usually less than the extracellular fluid concentration of sodium because of a sieving effect [5–8].

Sodium removal is so markedly affected by ultrafiltration that over a wide range of drainage volume a significant influence of serum concentrations on total transport could not be seen [4]. However, since in a stable patient the daily drainage volume is fairly constant, Nolph et al. [4] have constructed nomograms to predict dialytic sodium balance in patients with different serum sodium values at a given dialysate sodium concentration (Fig. 1).

Variation in net sodium removal per day is a function of serum sodium concentration: an increase of dietary sodium intake will result in an increase in serum sodium that will lead to an increase in dialysate sodium removal. These changes in net daily removal with changes in serum concentration represent intrinsic autoregulatory mechanisms for adjustment of removal rates [4].

On the other hand, if expansion is isonatremic due to positive balances of both sodium and water, the correction will be done in two steps. First, the increase of ultrafiltration due to the increased number of hypertonic exchanges will result in a hyponatremic dialysate. Second, in this condition an increase in serum sodium concentration occurs leading to an increase in dialysate sodium removal.

A standard daily sodium intake of 150 mmol easily can be offset by 4 exchanges/day with about 1200 ml/day of ultrafiltration, if a 132 mmol/l sodium solution is used [4]. In addition residual renal function can substantially contribute to sodium removal. It has been reported that [9], if no major hormonal derangements exist, the urinary sodium content is rather constant at 70 mmol/l.

Since clinical studies have not reported specific side effects by using the currently available CAPD solutions with 132–134 mmol/l of sodium, few studies have dealt with a possible variation of the sodium content of the solutions. Colombi [9] using a 134 mmol/l sodium solution, at a 138 mmol/l serum sodium concentration, calculated the sodium removal at different urinary volume and at different daily ultrafiltration. In these conditions a daily ultrafiltration of 1100 ml and a urinary volume of 500 ml should maintain a constant serum sodium concentration if the sodium intake is about 150 mmol/day. Colombi [9] suggests that a reduction of dialysate sodium content to 130 mmol/l should

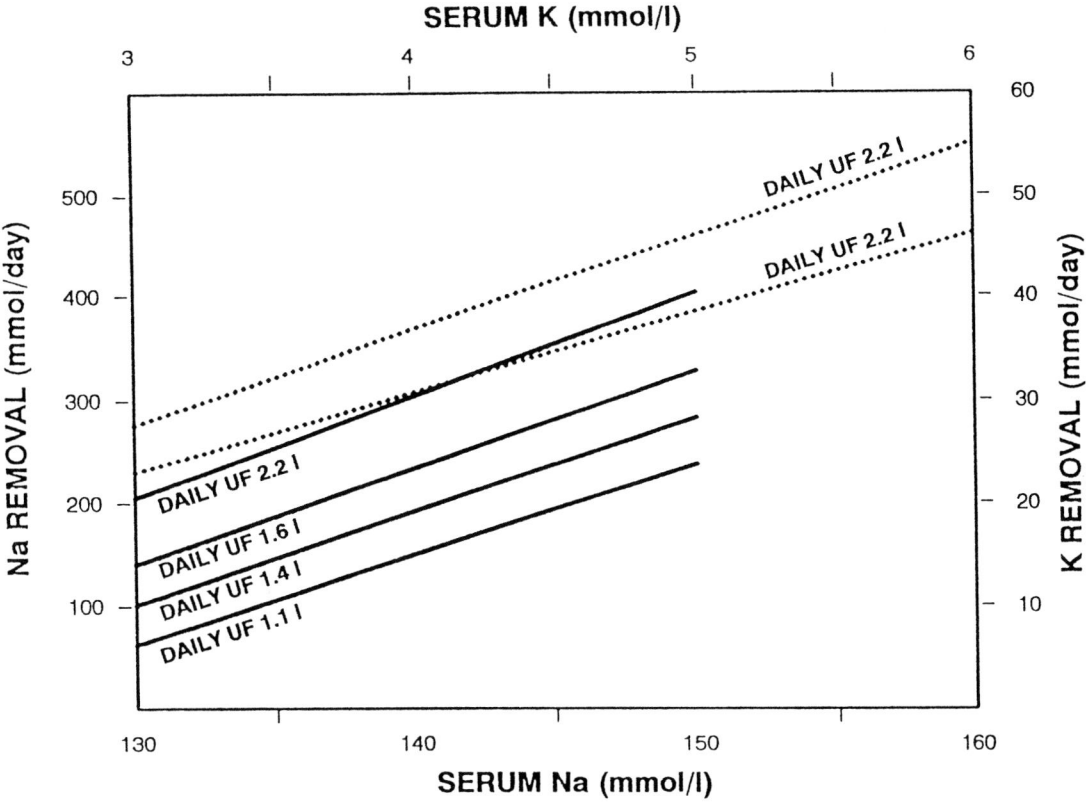

Figure 1. Relationship between daily sodium (solid line) and potassium (dotted line) removal and their respective serum concentrations at different daily ultrafiltration rates (modified from reference [4]).

be taken into account for patients without residual renal function. De Vecchi et al. [10], in order to correct orthostatic hypotension, reported to be common in CAPD patients, used a dialysate sodium concentration of 137 mmol/l in 38 unselected patients. Orthostatic systolic pressure increased in mean value from 129 to 139 mmHg (without statistical significance). Only 3 patients required an increase of previous antihypertensive therapy and in none of the patients was an increased sense of thirst or oedema recorded. In 3 hypotensive patients dialysate sodium concentration was increased to 142 mmol/l. One patient became hypertensive, one patient became normotensive while no changes were reported in the last patient. The authors concluded that a 137 mmol/l sodium solution enabled better control of hypotensive symptomatology, while a 142 mmol/l sodium concentration is not always effective in the treatment of severe hypotension in CAPD patients.

Recently an ultra low sodium (98 mmol/l) solution has been proposed [11] to correct fluid overload in patients with insufficient ultrafiltration. The use of this solution led to a reasonable body weight reduction without hypotension or fatigue. However, these data need to be confirmed in a larger study.

Since convection plays a prime role, the water removal rate is higher than the sodium removal rate and consequently, in rapid cycling techniques hypernatremia may occasionally occur [5–8]. The use of solutions with 140 mmol/l of sodium concentration resulted in severe thirst and poor blood pressure control [12] and hypernatremia over 160 mmol/l has been reported [13]. Raja et al. [6] suggested that the increase in serum sodium concentration could be avoided and an isonatremic ultrafiltrate achieved with a dialysate sodium concentration of 115–120 mmol/l in 7% dextrose dialysate and 125–130 mmol/l for a 4.25% dextrose dialysate. Similar results have been reported by Nolph et al. [8].

More recently Shen et al. [14] proposed a sodium concentration of 118 for 2.5% glucose solutions and 109 mmol/l for 4.25% glucose solutions. However solutions with the lower sodium concentrations have never been commercially available and tendencies to thirst and more difficult blood pressure control have been observed in patients on nightly intermittent peritoneal dialysis using dialysis solutions containing 132 mmol/l of sodium [15].

3.2. Potassium

Since hyperkalemia is one of the most harmful complications of end stage renal failure, dialysis treatment must contribute to potassium balance. Dialytic potassium removal is a function of the serum potassium concentration and of insulin bioavailability. The potassium concentration in commercially available CAPD fluids ranges from 0 to 2 mmol/l, 0 being the concentration most commonly used. Net potassium balance across the peritoneal membrane follows principles similar to those mentioned above for sodium. However, when potassium is absent in the dialysis solution and since potassium concentration in extracellular fluid is low, diffusion is the most important mechanism for net potassium removal [16].

Potassium should equilibrate slightly faster than sodium because of the lower nuclear charge density and the smaller hydration radius, but, even with long-dwell exchanges, dialysate potassium values are often below serum concentrations [3]. This is because cycle time may not have permitted complete equilibration and serum potassium concentrations are often artifactually high based on leaching of potassium from red cells during serum separation [4].

Nomograms to predict daily net potassium removal in relationship to serum potassium concentration have been published [4] (Fig. 1). It can be seen that convection minimally increases net potassium removal as was previously observed in IPD sessions with hypertonic dialysate [17].

Using a potassium-free solution for four 2 liter exchanges per day, about 30 mmol/day are lost with dialysate [18] and residual renal function could only add about 20 mmol per liter of urine to potassium removal [9]. This total amount is considerably lower than the usual daily intake of 70 to 80 mmol. In spite of this, most patients have a normal serum level, which can be explained by an increased faecal excretion of potassium [19]: it appears that the enhanced intestinal potassium excretion is particularly important at higher potassium intakes and is sensitive to changes in plasma concentration [20]. Insulin also promotes cellular uptake of potassium.

In an earlier report, 4 mmol/l potassium CAPD solution led to hyperkalemia in about 50% of patients thus requiring exchange resin treatment [21]. With the commonly used potassium free CAPD solutions, hypokalemia is found in 10–36% of patients [22–23], even though the muscle potassium [24] and total body potassium [25–26] contents have been reported to be slightly increased. It is not easy to understand whether the hypokalemia is a consequence of an anabolic state or reflects poor nutritional intake [27].

3.3. Magnesium

Magnesium is an important cation involved in several enzymatic reactions. The serum magnesium concentration in dialysis patients depends on the dietary intake and on dialysis fluid concentration.

Hypermagnesemia is a common finding in dialysis patients [28]. While it is almost impossible to show abnormalities related to modestly elevated magnesium concentrations, lowered serum magnesium has been associated with cardiac rhythm disturbances [29–30] and electrocardiographic abnormalities [31].

Commercially available CAPD solutions contain 0.25–0.75 mmol/l of magnesium. Since total serum magnesium normal values range from 0.65 to 0.98 mmol/l and the diffusible concentration is about 55%–60% of the total amount, when 0.75 mmol/l magnesium and 1.5% glucose solutions are used, a slight magnesium uptake from the dialysis solution usually occurs by diffusive gradient [32]. However, Kwong et al. with the same solution have reported a negative dialytic balance [33].

When ultrafiltration is increased with the 4.25% dextrose solution, convective removal counteracts diffusive uptake yielding negative magnesium mass transport [32]. In addition to being affected by convection and diffusive gradient, magnesium mass transfer is influenced by dwell time and peritoneal permeability because of its large hydration radius [32].

In most published reports [34–37], the use of 0.75 mmol/l magnesium solution resulted in an elevated serum magnesium. This high magnesium concentration may lead to an excessive body burden and potentially inhibit bone remodelling [38–39]. Others [40] underlined that hypermagnesemia does not appear to result in any clinical complications and, in addition, a possible protective role on arterial calcifications has been suggested. Despite hypermagnesemia [24], the muscle content of magnesium was not altered. Therefore the relationship of serum magnesium to intracellular magnesium concentration and total body magnesium in CAPD patients is not completely known. Since dietary magnesium intake is a function of protein intake, magnesium removal with standard 0.75 mmol/l magnesium solution is negligible and CAPD patients do not show a continuous increase in serum magnesium levels, stool magnesium losses probably play a certain role [2].

In order to correct hypermagnesemia Nolph et al. [34] have suggested lowering the magnesium dialysate concentration to 0.25 mmol/l. The use of this solution was not associated with hypomagnesemia and most serum magnesium concentrations fell into the normal range [34, 41].

A lower magnesium dialysis fluid might enable the treatment of hyperphosphatemia with magnesium salts as an additional, calcium free, phosphate binder [42]. Therefore the use of zero magnesium fluids have been investigated [43–44]. Magnesium salt supplementation may result in diarrhoea and monitoring of compliance and serum magnesium levels becomes mandatory in order to avoid the risk of hypomagnesemia.

3.4. Calcium

Standard CAPD solutions contain 1.75 mmol/l of calcium. Therefore since normal serum diffusible ionized calcium ranges from 1.15 to 1.29 mmol/l, calcium is absorbed from dialysate by diffusion [32]. A statistically significant correlation was found between positive calcium mass transfer and serum/dialysate gradient for ionized calcium [33]. Similarly, Blumenkrantz et al. [19] have reported that net dialysate calcium uptake correlates inversely with serum total calcium.

It is interesting to note that about 30% of the dialysate calcium is not ionized being "chelated" by lactate [33]. Ionic calcium probably crosses the peritoneum faster than chelated calcium and probably the serum to dialysate ionic calcium gradient is rapidly dissipated mainly because of the rapid increase in the dialysate pH that decreases dialysate calcium ionization [33].

When ultrafiltration occurs with the 4.25% glucose solution, calcium uptake has been reported to be decreased [32] or even negative [33, 45]. Different net ultrafiltrations could explain the discrepancies among different studies. Convective removal counteracts diffusive uptake and decreases serum to dialysate gradient by dilution [38].

While a negative calcium balance could result if the dialysis solution concentration is 1.5 mmol/l [46], the above mentioned kinetic studies [32, 33, 45] suggest that a 1.75 mmol/l calcium solution in clinical CAPD regimens (3 exchanges with 1.5% glucose and 1 exchange with 4.25% glucose) generally leads to peritoneal absorption of calcium and rapidly normalizes serum total and ionized calcium levels [37]. Some early reports suggested that this effect could be favourable for preventing the progression of renal osteodystrophy by avoiding the losses of bone calcium [36, 47]. However, other investigators did not confirm this improvement [46, 48–49].

The overall calcium mass-balance is also affected by gastrointestinal absorption. In CAPD patients an empirical relationship has been found between dietary intake and gastrointestinal absorption [19]. 720 mg/day of dietary calcium intake resulted in an estimated average gastrointestinal absorption of 25 mg [19]. If oral calcium carbonate is supplemented to reduce phosphate absorption, a significantly greater amount of calcium is reabsorbed from the gastrointestinal tract. Since the recommended dietary phosphorus intake for the CAPD patients is 1000 mg/day [50], it has been calculated that 700 mg/day of phosphorus are required to be bound in order to maintain neutral phosphorus balance [45]. This goal can be achieved by supplementation of 6.25 calcium carbonate (2500 mg of elemental calcium) [51], that leads to an average gastrointestinal absorption of 700 mg/day of calcium [52]. Hence, the total intestinal absorption from the diet and calcium carbonate is around 725 mg/day. This means that a number of patients have an increased risk of hypercalcemia and soft tissue calcification [53].

On the other hand aluminium-containing phosphate binders are the main source of aluminium in CAPD patients [54] and the dangers of aluminium toxicity, in the form of bone disease and encephalopathy are now well recognized [55–57].

A lower dialysate calcium concentration has been suggested to avoid the risk of calcium carbonate-related hypercalcemia [32]. Martis et al. [58] have calculated on a theoretical basis that a peritoneal dialysis fluid calcium concentration of 1.25 mmol/l would lead to a calcium removal of 160 mg/day when the serum ionized calcium is 1.3 mmol/l and to a greater loss during episodes of hypercalcemia. In a prospective clinical study, Hutchison et al. [41] have demonstrated that a 1.25 mmol/l calcium dialysate allowed the administration of larger doses of calcium carbonate to obtain good control of serum phosphate and maintained serum ionized calcium near to the upper limit of the normal range. Parathyroid hormone was suppressed in the majority of patients and bone history improved. Similar results have been achieved in a large multicentre study [59] in which 1 mmol/l calcium solution was used and low dose vitamin D and oral calcium carbonate as a phosphate binder were supplemented.

Reduced calcium fluids have been extensively studied by several investigators and the results confirm the benefit of this solution on uremic osteodystrophy [60–64]. Long-term usage of lower calcium dialysate by large numbers of patients raises the question of safety in cases of poor compliance to calcium carbonate supplementation. However, it has been shown in 12 patients that, with 1.5% glucose and 1.25 mmol/l calcium solution, there is a net gain of calcium from fluid to patient if the serum ionized calcium level is less than 1.25 mmol/l, thus a reduced risk of hypocalcemia could be expected [41]. Since with 4.25% glucose and low calcium solution there is a much greater tendency to lose calcium regardless of the serum ionized calcium, in CAPD patients using two or more hypertonic bags per day a careful surveillance of the mineral metabolism is needed.

Recently, rapid exacerbation of hyperparathyroidism in patients converted to low calcium dialysate without adequate calcium supplementation has been documented [65].

The commercially available solutions for intermittent treatment are essentially the same as for CAPD. Andersen [66] reported that a positive calcium transfer from dialysis fluid can be obtained with a 2.16 mmol/l calcium concentration in dialysate both during 1.5% and 4% glucose 30 minute dwell-time exchanges. A recent report suggests that, in automated peritoneal dialysis, the low calcium dialysis solution (1.25 mmol/l) could result in negative calcium balance [67].

In summary there is a recent tendency in clinical practice to use solutions with lower calcium content, especially when patients are treated with oral administration of calcium carbonate phosphate binding salts.

4. Osmotic agents

Since there is a clinical requirement to remove excess body water on a regular basis from patients with end stage renal failure, an osmotic agent has to be added to peritoneal dialysis fluid in order to achieve a difference in osmotic pressure between dialysis solution and blood. Net water removal is directly proportional to the osmolality gradient [68]. Since small molecular weight solutes generate greater osmolality per unit mass, these agents (crystalloids) were studied as osmotic agents in animals [69]. Only glucose appeared to be safe, effective and readily metabolized. The long-term safety of glucose was confirmed in the management of patients treated with intermittent peritoneal dialysis [70]. A rapid decline in osmotic gradient, as a consequence of glucose absorption, has been observed, mainly during the long dwell exchanges that are typical for CAPD treatment [71].

Several substances have been examined as alternative osmotic agents to glucose. Low molecular weight agents (glycerol, sorbitol, amino acids, xylitol and fructose) have been utilized to overcome some of the metabolic problems of glucose. The high molecular weight agents (glucose polymers, gelatin, polycations, dextrans and polypeptides) have been used because they would be less readily absorbed, yielding sustained ultrafiltration in the prolonged dwells and a reduced calorie load [72]. Since the osmotic driving force is dependent on the osmolality i.e. on the total number of osmotically active molecules in the solution, a much greater mass of high molecular weight agents is needed to obtain the equivalent osmolality gradient of small molecular weight substances [73]. At high concentration these large molecules are less soluble, hyperviscous, non physiological and can be allergenic. However, a high molar concentration of these substances is not needed in dialysis fluid because, since they are slowly reabsorbed, they provide a sustained slow ultrafiltration. This effect is very similar to that exerted by albumin in biological systems ("colloid" pressure) and could be exploited in peritoneal dialysis to achieve sustained ultrafiltration at low molar concentration using dialysis solution isosmotic with plasma [74].

A totally new approach to ultrafiltration in CAPD has been proposed by the group in Manchester [75]. If a small amount of a low molecular weight agent is added to a hypo-osmolar solution with a high molecular weight substance, a synergistic effect could be achieved. The crystalloid agent would initiate rapid ultrafiltration which would be maintained by the slower colloid effect. This bimodal ultrafiltration profile optimizes the net ultrafiltration for dwell time by adjusting the relative proportion of the two agents. It has been demonstrated that a 7.5% glucose polymer and

0.35% glucose solution provides ultrafiltration 40% greater than 7.5% glucose polymer solution alone over a 12 hour exchange [75].

In summary small solutes yield high osmolality, but cross the membrane very rapidly. Large solutes stay longer in the solution, but attract little water. While the smaller solutes should be favoured for short dwell time exchanges, the larger solutes should be suitable for exchanges with longer dwell times [73]. Estimated ultrafiltration patterns with several small and large solutes at the same percentage concentration are depicted in Fig. 2.

4.1. Low molecular weight osmotic agents

4.1.1. Glucose

Up to now, glucose is the only commercially available osmotic agent in peritoneal dialysis. Concentrations of glucose in the labels of commercial bags are expressed either as dextrose anhydrous concentration or as dextrose monohydrate concentration. Dextrose monohydrate concentrations of 1.5%, 2.5% and 4.25% correspond to 1.36%, 2.26% and 3.86% respectively of dextrose anhydrous. In the text, glucose concentrations are reported as dextrose monohydrate.

Since glucose is reabsorbed during dwell time, a progressive dissipation of osmotic gradient is recorded [3, 71, 73, 76–80]. This behaviour determines the characteristic curve of intraperitoneal volume (Fig. 3). Ultrafiltration rate is maximal at the beginning of the exchange and the peritoneal volume reaches the maximal peak after 2–3 hours of dwell when the equilibration between dialysate and plasma osmolality occurs. After this point absorption becomes evident with a progressive reduction of the amount of fluid in the peritoneal cavity. The rate of fluid absorption is mainly dependent on the lymphatic flux [81–82].

For intermittent peritoneal dialysis where short dwell times are used, glucose induces ultrafiltration throughout the exchange. However, for CAPD, where each exchange dwells for 4–8 hours, a high rate of glucose absorption can result in net fluid absorption. Some patients absorb glucose so rapidly that sufficient ultrafiltration cannot be achieved even with more concentrated glucose solutions [73]. Therefore, glucose absorption is a function of dialysate glucose concentration, length of exchange and membrane permeability of individual patients.

In clinical CAPD a significant correlation between the amount of glucose absorbed each day and the average concentration of glucose in dialysate has been found [83] and the net glucose daily uptake can be predicted from an empirical equation:

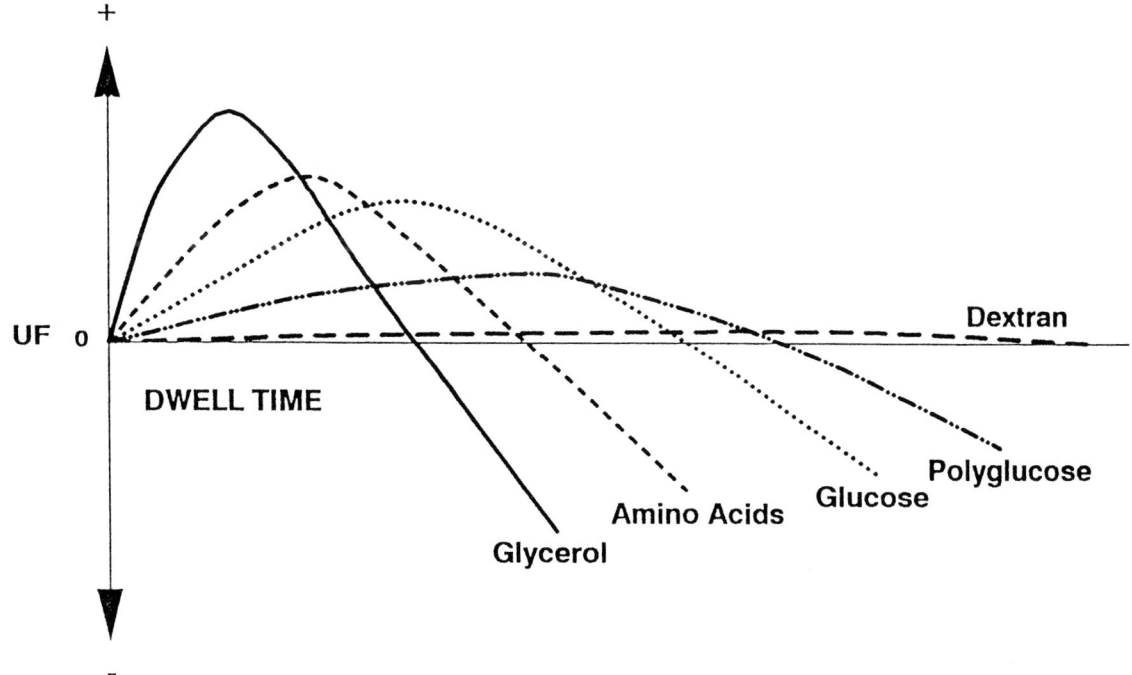

Figure 2. Estimated ultrafiltration patterns with different osmotic agents of various molecular weight at the same percentage concentration (modified from reference [73]) with permission of Karger AG, Basel).

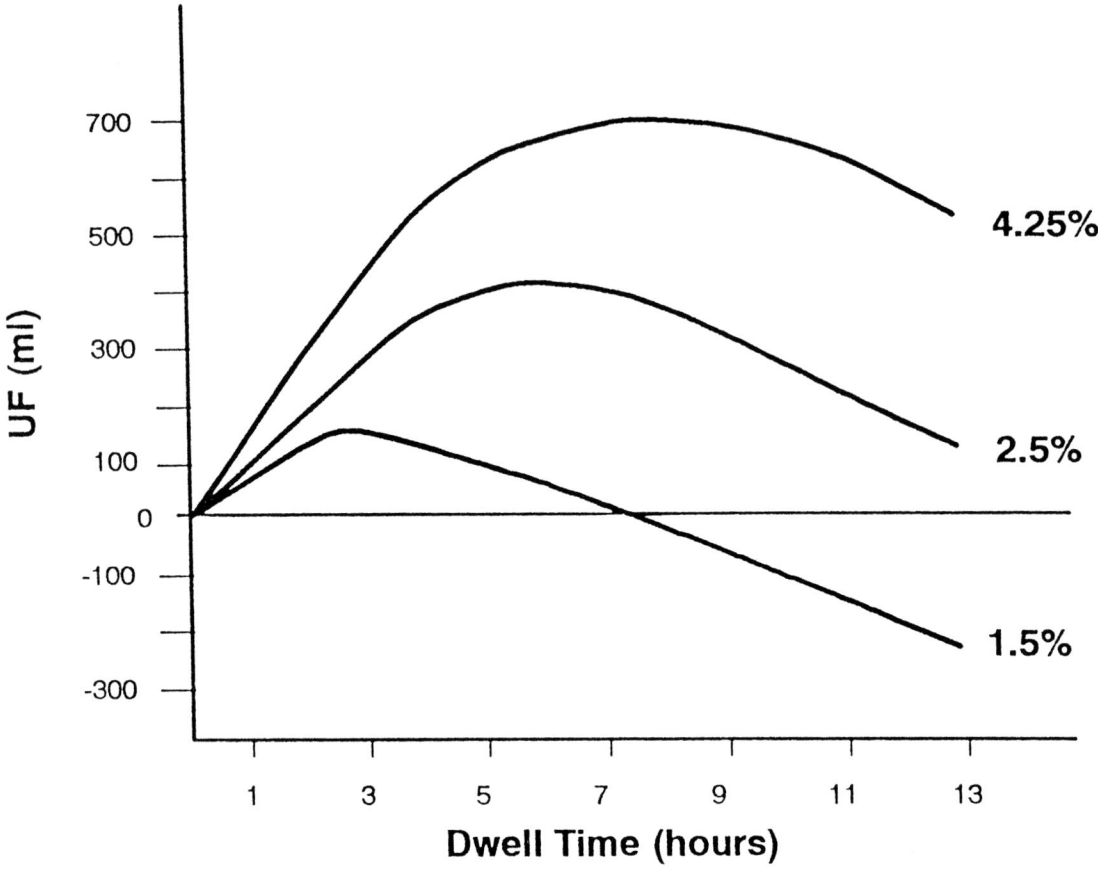

Figure 3. Approximate ultrafiltration volumes related to dwell time with solutions of 1.5%, 2.5%, and 4.25% dextrose concentration. (From reference [73] with permission of Karger AG, Basel).

grams of glucose absorbed/day = (11.3 × average dialysate glucose concentration − 10.9) × liters of inflow.

This relation has been confirmed by others [84]. Since about 60–80% of the glucose instilled into the peritoneal cavity is absorbed during a 6 hour dwell time, 45–60 g of glucose is absorbed from 4.25% solution, 24–40 g from 2.5% and 15–22 g from 1.5% [85]. Consequently the normal glucose uptake in CAPD patients ranges from 100 to 300 gr per day [83–88].

The amount of glucose absorbed contributed considerably to total energy intake (20.3%) and the added glucose calories from dialysate have been suggested to be beneficial for CAPD patients [83]. However, it has been highlighted that his amount of absorbed glucose can result in several disadvantages. Marked hyperglycemia has been observed in patients undergoing intermittent peritoneal dialysis [89–90]. Although CAPD exchanges with 1.5% glucose dialysate have only marginal effects on blood glucose and insulin levels [91–92], a constant tendency towards hyperglycemia and hyperinsulinemia has been reported [92–93]. During a hypertonic exchange (4.25% glucose), a blood glucose and plasma insulin peak occur after 45–90 minutes and glucagon levels decrease only slightly [84, 91–92, 94–95]. These changes are similar to those observed after an oral glucose load [95–96]. It has been reported that some patients on CAPD developed "de novo" diabetes mellitus due to the continuous hyperglycemic stress [85]. In addition, since sustained hyperinsulinemia may possibly increase atherogenesis, the elevated circulating insulin levels represent a potential risk factor for CAPD patients [85].

A hyperlipidemic effect of CAPD was demonstrated in several studies and it became apparent that hypertriglyceridemia and serum lipoprotein abnormalities were accentuated within the first months of the treatment [86–87, 97–102]. These effects were attributed to the continuous peritoneal absorption of glucose [103]. However, these changes were in part transitory [104], suggesting an adaptation to the peritoneal glucose load by spontaneous reduction of the oral carbohydrate intake [85, 88].

Recent investigations in the field of the peritoneal fluid biocompatibility have raised the question of the long term toxicity of solutions containing glucose on peritoneal resident cells. To prevent caramelization of glucose during heat sterilization, the pH of the solution is kept low (5–5.5). The high glucose concentration and the low pH of commercially available solutions have been demonstrated to affect peritoneal cellular host defense mechanisms and peritoneal mesothelial cell viability [105–112]. In addition, glucose is not entirely stable and some of its breakdown products can be detected in peritoneal dialysate especially when using fluids stored for long time. These degradation products of which 5-hydroxymethylfurfural (5-HMF) is the most easily measurable, have been found to be significantly elevated after 18 months of storage [113]. A marked reduction of peritoneal ultrafiltration has been associated with the use of solutions which have been stored for more than 18 months. 5-HMF is relatively non-toxic to biological tissues but combines readily with anions including lactate to form Schiff bases and thee compounds may alter the characteristics of many tissue components [114].

High intraperitoneal glucose concentration has been associated with a non-enzymatic glycosylation of proteins during severe peritonitis. Dobbie et al. [115] have demonstrated that repeated and severe episodes of peritonitis can remove the mesothelial layer, exposing the underlying stroma to highly concentrated glucose solutions. This condition can result in diabetiform reduplication of the basement membrane of mesothelium and stromal blood vessels and in irreversible changes in exposed proteins [116].

Biocompatibility problems of the solutions will be discussed in detail in Chapter 17.

4.1.2. Glycerol

Glycerol has been proposed as an alternative osmotic agent for CAPD solutions in order to overcome some metabolic effects of glucose mainly in diabetic patients [117–118]. In addition, glycerol containing solution has an initial pH higher than that of glucose and consequently it should be more biocompatible [117].

Glycerol is a small molecular weight sugar alcohol which does not require insulin for its metabolism. It is an essential part of neutral fat and enters the carbohydrate metabolic pathway [119]. Being a molecular smaller than glucose and therefore with higher osmolality per unit mass, it produces greater ultrafiltration than glucose during the early phase of dwell time. However, glycerol provides significantly lower total ultrafiltration than glucose since it diffuses very rapidly into the blood stream [73, 120–121]. Thus, the higher concentration of glycerol required to obtain an equal ultrafiltration to dextrose leads to an equivalent [122] or even increased [120] caloric load from CAPD solutions than glucose.

In non diabetic patients it was demonstrated that, in contrast to glucose, no rise in blood glucose and insulin concentrations occurred over a dialysis cycle [122]. However, a longer term study showed that the mean glucose and insulin concentrations rose steadily with the use of glycerol and a fall in fasting glucose on reverting to glucose-based solutions was observed [122].

In diabetic patients the use of glycerol was associated with an initial decreased requirement for insulin, but this favourable effect could not be maintained after 3–4 months [117]. Better control of glucose homeostasis and a better survival rate have been reported in these patients [119]. The use of glycerol-containing solutions inevitably leads to an accumulation of glycerol in the blood (normal value 0.12 mmol/l) [118, 123]. The mean blood peak values with the 1.4% and 2.5% glycerol solutions have been reported to be 0.62 and 11.65 mmol/l respectively [123]. These high glycerol levels have been associated with hyperosmolar symptoms in few cases. However the mean plasma osmolality in the studied population was similar to the value observed in CAPD patients using the standard glucose solution [123]. Long term studies have shown a dramatic increase of the blood fasting triglyceride concentrations after 6 months of treatment [119, 122]. Since glycerol is measured together with triglycerides by the standard methodology, when triglyceride concentrations were corrected for free glycerol concentrations, the measured triglyceride levels decreased [123].

In conclusion, until now there is a general agreement that glycerol solutions could have a finite use in diabetic CAPD patients, because of the better control of glucose homeostasis. However careful attention should be paid to the possible negative metabolic effects of glycerol [122–124]. In non diabetic CAPD patients the available evidence suggests that glycerol alone has little or no clinical advantage over glucose as an osmotic agent [73, 122, 125–126]. There may still be a role for the use of glycerol in combination with amino acids. Some recent experimental studies in rats have shown that this combination can be autoclaved and kept within a single solution without glucose caramelization [127–128]. The mixture of amino acids and glycerol can reduce carbohydrate absorption and improve the nutritional value of the CAPD solutions. The direct metabolism of both osmotic agents is independent of insulin which makes this solution particularly suitable for diabetic patients. In addition the solutions have a pH higher than that of currently available solutions, thus rendering them more physiological. Finally, formulations that assure the desired ultrafiltration can be selected [127]. Further studies in man are needed to confirm these findings.

4.1.3. Xylitol

Xylitol has been suggested for CAPD solutions instead of glucose as an osmotic agent in diabetic patients since its metabolism is insulin independent [129]. Preliminary data from a clinical study involving 4 diabetic CAPD patients treated for 6 months showed marked reduction in insulin requirement, better control of blood glucose levels and normalized levels of triglycerides, cholesterol and HDL-cholesterol. However an increase in lactic and uric acids has been recorded [129].

Since toxic effects occur at absorption rates over 150 g/day [38], in patients with fluid excess requiring frequent hyperosmolar exchanges the metabolic abnormalities induced by xylitol may be too dangerous [130].

4.1.4. Sorbitol

In the late 60's sorbitol was tried as substitute for glucose in dialysis fluids [131] in order to improve blood glucose control and to prevent hyperosmolar symptoms in diabetic patients undergoing intermittent peritoneal dialysis. However, since the rate of transperitoneal absorption exceeds the metabolic capacity, this substance accumulates in blood resulting in a hyperosmolar status leading to confusion, convulsion and coma [132–133].

For this reason the committee on choice of peritoneal dialysis solution did not recommend the use of sorbitol in dialysate in 1973 [134].

4.1.5. Fructose

Fructose has the same molecular weight as glucose and therefore has similar osmotic properties but its metabolism is predominantly hepatic and does not require insulin [135–136]. However it does not appear to provide any advantage over glucose and may be more potent than glucose in producing hypertriglyceridemia [124] and a hyperosmolar state [38].

4.1.6. Amino acids

In order to correct serum amino acid abnormalities and to prevent obligatory protein losses with dialysate, Gjessing [137] suggested supplementing peritoneal dialysis solutions with a mixture of amino acids in the late 60's.

More than 10 years later Oreopoulos *et al.* [138] described the osmotic properties of different concentrations of amino acids in solutions for peritoneal dialysis, in a uremic rabbit model. The dual goals, substitution of glucose in the solutions and nutritional improvement, were pointed out.

Osmotic efficacy. Molecular weights of amino acids range from 75 to 214 daltons. Since amino acid mixtures for peritoneal dialysis usually contain a higher proportion of smaller molecular weight compounds, the average molecular weight of these solutions approximate 100 daltons [73]. Even though the average molecular weight is smaller than glucose, the absorption rate is only slightly higher than glucose because, at neutral pH, amino acids are charged and consequently the absorption rate is lower than uncharged molecules with the equivalent molecular weight [73]. Several studies have been performed in order to evaluate the ultrafiltration capacity of amino acids solutions.

In an acute clinical study [139], a 2% amino acid based solution induced equivalent amounts of ultrafiltration and urea, creatinine and potassium removal compared to a 4.25% glucose solution over a 6 hour dwell time. The initial dialysate osmolality was similar for the two solutions and similar dialysate osmolality changes during dwell time were observed. At the end of the exchange, 90% of the administered amino acids were absorbed. The same group [140] later reported in a short term study that the ultrafiltration effect of the 1% amino acid solution (osmolality 364 mmOsm/kg) was intermediate between those of 1.5% (osmolality 346 mmOsm/kg) and 2.5% (396 mmOsm/kg) standard glucose solution. These data were substantially confirmed in a more recent study where Goodship *et al.* [141] found smaller but not statistically different ultrafiltrate volumes when comparing a 1% amino acid solution with a 1.5% glucose solution. A comparison of the ultrafiltration profile and solute mass transfer between 4.25% glucose (478 mmOsm/kg) and 2.76% amino acid (501 mmOsm/kg) solutions showed that intraperitoneal dialysate volume profiles were inseparable during the first 180 minutes of dwell although, during the latter part of the dwell, the volumes of the amino acid solution tended to decrease more rapidly than those of the glucose solution leading to decreased net ultrafiltration at the end of the 6 hour dwell time exchange [142]. These differences were not statistically significant. Dialysate sodium, potassium, urea and total protein levels as well a dialysate-to-plasma concentration ratios (D/P) for these solutes were similar with the two solutions during dwell, although D/P values after 360 minutes tended to be higher when using amino acids solutions. This difference was statistically significant for creatinine. In addition, the diffusive mass transport coefficient tended to be higher with amino acid solutions, but the difference was not statistically significant [142]. The conclusion was that the peritoneal permeability was not significantly altered by the use of amino acids instead of glucose [143].

In a more recent paper Young et al. [144] studied ultrafiltration and D/P ratios of several proteins in an 8 hour dwell time exchange using 1% amino acid solution in comparison with 1.5% glucose standard solution. Volumes of dialysate recovered at the end of the exchanges were significantly less after amino acid exchanges although the osmolality decreased comparably during the dwell time. At the end of the study period (12 weeks) amino acid absorption and protein losses were increased as compared to the beginning of the study. The clearances of the studied proteins expressed as D/P ratios were increased at the beginning of amino acid use by an average of 18% and after 12 weeks by 34%. D/P ratios for creatinine increased comparably by 7% and 10% but no differences were observed for urea. The increase in the peritoneal permeability during the use of amino acid based solution was attributed to an activation of complement by amino acids or their metabolites to produce C5a [145] and generation of prostaglandin E2 [146]. The increase in peritoneal permeability was reversed when standard glucose solutions were resumed [144].

Thus, there is clinical evidence that amino acid solutions can deliver ultrafiltration and small molecule clearances equivalent to those achieved with glucose solutions. The slight differences among various studies probably reflect the difference in concentration and composition of amino acids in the employed solutions. The osmotic power produced by different solutions is not only expressed by the osmolality, calculated or measured, but also depends on the degree of absorption and metabolism of each amino acid [147].

Nutritional efficacy, metabolic changes and clinical concerns. Several clinical studies have been performed to evaluate the nutritional value and changes in serum amino acids profile, lipids and glucose metabolism in CAPD patients treated with the amino acid solutions. Different fluid compositions and different patients, regarding nutritional status, have been taken into account.

In Table 2 the amino acid composition of the most used solutions is reported. In the first long term study [140], 1% amino acid fluid (solution A in Table 2) was alternated with glucose exchanges for four weeks in 6 patients. A slightly improved nutritional status and an increase in total body nitrogen and serum transferrin were detected. The mean dietary protein intake (0.96 to 0.93 g/kg/day), the energy intake (22 to 21.2 kcal/kg/day), the anthropometric indexes, the total body potassium and the serum albumin, insulin and glucagon levels did not change during the study. Plasma triglycerides tended to decrease and HDL cholesterol to increase but after 4 weeks these changes were not statistically significant. BUN levels increased sharply (59%) and serum bicarbonate dropped although 33 mmol/l of lactate, 7 mmol/l of acetate and 4.5 mmol/l of bicarbonate were present in the solution. The low plasma concentrations of branch-chained amino acids valine, isoleucine and leucine observed before treatment remained unchanged, while glycine increased and alanine decreased.

The same group [148] found rather discouraging results by using a daily 2% amino acid solution exchange over 5 to 6 months in 3 patients. Only one patient, who was severely malnourished with low total body nitrogen and daily protein intake, improved during the study. In the remaining 2 patients, who had a normal total body nitrogen and an adequate protein intake, the benefits of amino acid supplementation were neutralized by loss of appetite associated with the use of these solutions. The same results were obtained in a prospective randomized study [149] in which a 1% amino acid solution was evaluated for its ability to counteract the catabolic effect of peritonitis in CAPD patients. During 4 weeks 12 patients used the amino acid solution alternately with glucose solution, while 10 patients continued regular dialysis with glucose-based solutions only. There was no improvement of nitrogen balance, plasma amino acid pattern or nutritional status. BUN increased by 50% and nine out of twelve patients lost their appetite. The mean dietary protein and energy intakes decreased during peritonitis.

The most recent study with solution A of Table 2 was published by Dombros et al. [150]. 5 patients with low daily protein intake (<0.8 g/kg/bw) and low serum albumin (<35 g/l) received a 1% amino acid solution during the overnight exchange for 6 months, 3 patients, who received a 2% amino acid solution at the beginning of the study, developed symptoms of severe uremia such as anorexia, vomiting, malaise, pruritus, restlessness, abdominal cramps and a dramatic increase in BUN. The symptoms subsided upon reducing the amino acid concentrations from 2% to 1%. At the end of the study BUN slightly increased and total body nitrogen tended to decrease while oral total energy and protein intake, cholesterol, triglycerides, albumin, transferrin, skinfold thickness, total body potassium and plasma amino acid levels remained basically unchanged. The authors concluded that the ineffectiveness of the amino acid solution could be due to the amino acid composition of the fluid, the timing of administration or to a low caloric intake and/or that the patients were not severely malnourished.

These studies from the Toronto group used solutions not tailored to meet the needs of uremic patients (large amount of non-essential amino acids) and with an inadequate amount of buffer. Therefore they were not able to normalize the amino acid abnormalities in uremia and the solution itself contributed to acidosis. Furthermore the energy intake of the patients was low and consequently the intraperitoneal supply of amino acids was probably used as a source of energy [151]. These disadvantages are well recognized by the authors and stimulated the search for an amino acid composition solution more suitable for CAPD patients.

The new solutions contain an increased amount of essential amino acids while non-essential amino acid concentrations, namely glycine and alanine, were decreased. Pedersen et al. [152] studied 6 patients for 3 months with a 1% amino acid solution (solution B in Table 2) alternately with a 1.5% glucose solution. Patient protein intake at the beginning of treatment was 1.2–1.5 g/kg/day. During this study no detectable changes in the metabolism of glucose, fat and proteins occurred. In particular serum triglycerides, cholesterol, albumin and transferrin were not different from the pre-study values. Serum creatinine remained stable while serum BUN increased significantly during the study. Interestingly the serum branch-chained amino acids that

Table 2. Amino acid composition (mg/dl) of different studied solutions.

		A Ref. [140, 148, 149, 150]	B Ref. [152]	C Ref. [153, 155, 156, 157]	D Ref. [160]
EBCAA	Valine	46	67	126	139.3
EBCAA	Leucine	62	82.6	92	101.9
EBCAA	Isoleucine	48	60.8	77	84.9
EAA	Threonine	42	46.8	59	64.5
EAA	Tyrosine	4	7.8	6	30
EAA	Phenylalanine	62	–	75	57
EAA	Lysine	58	60.8	86	95.5
EAA	Hystidine	44	37.4	65	71.4
EAA	Tryptophan	18	15.6	25	27
EAA	Methionine	58	29.6	77	84.9
NEAA	Arginine	104	51.4	97	107.1
NEAA	Serine	–	116.9	46	50.9
NEAA	Proline	42	126.3	54	59.5
NEAA	Glycine	213	32.7	46	50.9
NEAA	Alanine	213	46.8	86	95.1
NEAA	Aspartic Acid	–	63.9	–	–
NEAA	Glutamic Acid	–	140.3	–	–

EBCAA Essential branch-chained amino acid.
EAA   Essential amino acid.
NEAA   Non essential amino acid.

were below the normal range in uremic patients, increased toward the normal values. The increased amount of BCAA in the solution could explain this effect. This solution contained 40 mmol/l of lactate and 5 mmol/l of bicarbonate were added to increase the pH of the fresh solution. However, no data was provided about acid base status of the patients.

Young et al. [153] studied 8 hypoalbuminemic CAPD patients using only a morning exchange with a different amino acid solution for 12 weeks (solution C in Table 2). A modest nutritional benefit was recorded. Transferrin significantly increased and cholesterol and apolipoprotein B tended to decrease. No significant changes occurred in mean dietary protein and energy intakes, fasting amino acids, albumin, prealbumin and apolipoprotein A. BUN increased by 36% and bicarbonate decreased by 13% without signs of uremia and clinical acidosis. As a part of the same study a more detailed analysis [154] showed a significant reduction of total and LDL cholesterol and apolipoprotein B. These parameters returned to baseline 2 weeks after the restoration of glucose fluid.

A more extended observation (6 months) in 6 non-malnourished patients with one exchange per day of the same solution [155] showed an improved estimated nitrogen balance and serum amino acid profile, an increase in dietary protein and energy intakes and a decrease in serum cholesterol and triglycerides. Plasma protein concentrations remained unchanged, BUN increased by 29%, blood bicarbonate and pH decreased (the employed solution contained 35 mmol/l of lactate). When this solution was used twice a day in 7 patients for 8 weeks [156] the plasma essential amino acid concentrations increased (in particular branch-chained amino acids) as well as serum albumin. However BUN rose by 63% and blood bicarbonate dropped by 31% and a significant acidosis developed in the patients. Other parameters such as anthropometry, total body potassium, dietary protein and caloric intakes, transferrin, insulin, glucagon, and lipids were unchanged.

The longest study available with the 1% amino acid solution describes 4 diabetic patients followed for more than 12 months [157]. Serum albumin and cholesterol increased as compared with a control group. In addition the amount of insulin administered was reduced in the group receiving amino acids. As expected azotemia increased by 68% and bicarbonate decreased.

In summary the above mentioned studies using the improved 1% amino acid solution demonstrated more beneficial effects than the previous solution if patients with signs of protein malnutrition and low dietary protein intake were included. Energy intake should be sufficient to prevent diversion of absorbed amino acids as an energy source [158].

Acidosis remained a common concern. This was most likely due to the acid load delivered by salts of basic amino acids (lysine hydrochloride) and that arising from metabolism of sulphur amino acids to sulphate (methionine) [159].

In order to further improve the clinical efficacy, a new formulation of the amino acid solution has been proposed and tested (solution D in Table 2). Essential amino acid concentrations were increased as well as lactate concentration (from 35 to 40 mmol/l). Total amino acid concentration was increased to 1.1% in order to provide the same osmotic effect as the 1.5% standard glucose solution. An international multicentre study in CAPD patients with signs of protein malnutrition has been performed [160]. The preliminary results [158–159] suggest that this solution improves nutritional status of CAPD patients who have a low protein intake. Mean nitrogen balance increased significantly during the treatment period. Statistically significant increases were also observed in serum transferrin, total proteins and midarm muscle circumference over the 20-day treatment period. The pre-exchange fasting amino acid pattern in plasma became more normal during the treatment phase.

In conclusion in malnourished CAPD patients dialysate with a more appropriate and recently introduced amino acid composition may improve their protein nutrition and metabolic status. However, increased BUN levels and the tendency toward acidosis remain problems to be solved and, finally, the cost of commercially available amino acid solutions, twice that of the standard glucose solution, has to be considered.

4.2. High molecular weight osmotic agents

4.2.1. Albumin

Almost one hundred years ago albumin was shown to delay peritoneal fluid absorption [161]. It is non toxic systemically and does not cause biochemical or metabolic derangements thus representing an ideal osmotic agent [162]. Because of its molecular weight (68,000 daltons) albumin is absorbed slowly from the peritoneal cavity and exerts a sustained oncotic effect as evaluated in a rat model [163].

However it is currently too expensive to be considered a substitute for glucose in clinical peritoneal dialysis and its use in humans has been restricted to study peritoneal fluid and solute transport [164].

4.2.2. Synthetic polymers

Polyacrylate, polyethylene-amine and dextran sulphate are the synthetic polymers which had been proposed and tried in an "in vitro" simulation of peritoneal dialysis, in rats and in rabbits [165–167]. Slow absorption and high osmotic driving forces in long dwell exchanges have been observed. However, polyacrylate induced intraperitoneal bleeding, damaged the peritoneal membrane and induced cardiovascular instability [167]. In addition, despite its high molecular weight (90,000 daltons) polyacrylate crossed the peritoneal membrane.

Dextran sodium sulphate with a molecular weight of 500,000 daltons exerts its osmotic effect by the sodium trapped in its glycosyl sulphate residue [166]. Dextran was supposed to be non toxic since, if absorbed, it should be metabolized. However in a rat and rabbit models intraperitoneal bleeding occurred leading to the death of animals [167]. Polyethylene-amine was even more toxic with the death of animals occurring in one hour [167]. Obviously the synthetic polymers are not suitable for clinical use.

4.2.3. Plasma substitutes

Gelatin, neutral dextran and hydroxyethyl starch are widely used in Europe as plasma substitutes and to treat severe hypotensive episodes in hemodialysis. Crude gelatine (5%) was first used in the late 40's as an osmotic agent during acute peritoneal dialysis [168]. More recently [167] a 9% gelatin solution was tested in a rat model and yielded higher and more sustained ultrafiltration during a 7 hour dwell time as compared with a 4.25% glucose solution. There were not untoward effects on rats and no alterations of the peritoneal membrane as evaluated with light and scanning electron microscopy.

High viscosity, gelation at room temperature and difficult sterilization, however, were major problems. In order to avoid these technical problems, a cross-linked gelatin, gelatin isocyanate (Hemaccel 20,000–35,000 daltons), was investigated [169] At 6 hour dwell time, the ultrafiltration volume of a 5.5% Hemaccel solution was similar to that of 4.25% glucose, while 10% Hemaccel yielded even higher ultrafiltration. Although gelatin is easily metabolized, the elimination half-life of Hemaccel is around 16 hours in hemodialyzed patients with minimal renal function and chronic toxicity is unknown [162]. In addition, when used as plasma substitute, Hemaccel has been associated with anaphylactoid reactions in 0.038% of the patients [170].

Neutral dextrans as osmotic agent in peritoneal dialysis were investigated in the late 60's [171]. Very low osmotic driving force was exerted by 6% dextran in saline and little ultrafiltration was achieved. These data were recently confirmed [172] while a 10% dextran solution showed a significant higher ultrafiltration [173]. However, despite its high molecular weight (40,000 or 70,000 daltons), 40% to 60% of dextran was absorbed over a six hour cycle [172]. Since accumulation of dextran in patients on maintenance hemodialysis has been demonstrated to yield reticuloendothelial system blockade, dextran does not seem to be a suitable alternative to glucose [174].

Hydroxyethyl starch (HES) is another synthetic substance in which starch has been modified by the introduction of a hydroxyethyl ether group and then hydrolyzed to yield a product with an average molecular weight of 480,000 daltons. Studies in a rat model with 10% and 6% concentration solutions have reported the same ultrafiltration profiles and absorption rates of those in which 6% and 10% dextran solutions were used [172–173]. In acute renal failure HES seemed to accumulate in liver in liver leading to a storage disease [175].

4.2.4. Glucose polymer

Glucose polymer (GP) or polyglucose is a mixture of polysaccharides consisting of linked glucose residues of varying chain length obtained by the hydrolysis of corn starch. More than 90% of the glucose bonds are α (1-4) glucosidic linkages, the remainder are α (1-6) linkages.

A preparation of fractioned glucose oligosaccharides with chain length ranging from 2 to 15 glucose units (average weight 710 daltons) was first acutely used in man in concentrations ranging from 3% to 8% GP mixture [176–177].

When compared to a 4.25% glucose solution, an 8% GP solution produced a similar ultrafiltration profile at 8 and 10 hour dwell times, despite a markedly lower initial osmolality (357 versus 485 mmOsm/kg). Solute clearances and D/P ratios for urea and creatinine were identical [177].

Fifty-seven percent and 77% of the glucose polymers were absorbed at 4 and 10 hours respectively. Although the solution was well tolerated by the patients, plasma oligosaccharide concentrations (in particular G2 and G5) sharply increased during the GP exchange and even higher concentrations were recorded during the subsequent exchange with the standard glucose solution, thus indicating a very slow metabolism and clearance of absorbed oligosaccharides in patients with renal insufficiency. The calculated half life was about 20 hours [177].

Serum free glucose concentrations changed little after the exchanges using the GP solutions. However the potential energy load from a single exchange of an 8% GP solution was approximately twice that of 4.25% glucose solution. The authors suggested that a combination of higher molecular weight glucose polymer would be more suitable for CAPD patients [178].

A new GP solution composition with average molecular weight 7,000 (67% low molecular weight fraction – G1 to G12 – and 33% high molecular weight fraction – G > 12 –, average length of polymers 5–6 units) was studied by Mistry et al. [179]. A 5% GP solution was compared to a 1.5% glucose solution, and a 10% GP to a 4.25% glucose solution. Both isotonic and hypertonic GP solutions showed significant increased net ultrafiltration as compared to the corresponding glucose solutions at 6 hour dwell time. Significant increases in creatinine, uric acid and phosphate D/P ratios were observed with GP solutions and similarly, average clearances of solutes were also significantly greater with GP solutions at both concentrations suggesting that GP solutions may alter peritoneal permeability. The GP absorption from dialysate at 6 hour dwell time was 42.5% and 59% respectively for the iso and hyperosmotic GP solutions. However the caloric load was greater than that provided by the absorption of glucose from standard solutions. Fractions with 5 to 9 glucose units showed the highest intraperitoneal disappearance without concomitant rise in serum levels, whereas maltose (G2) and maltotriose (G3) with a slightly lower disappearance, produced a substantial rise in serum levels, suggesting considerable breakdown of intermediate molecules to smaller units.

In subsequent studies [74, 180–181] a 5% solution of glucose polymer containing polymer fractions of variable chain length ranging from 4 to 300 glucose units with average molecular weight 16,800 was compared to a commercially available 1.5% glucose solution. Even though the standard glucose solution osmolality is slightly hypertonic (332 mmOsm/kg), a substantially greater net ultrafiltration was achieved at 6 hour dwell time with polymer. For glucose solution, a prolonged exchange time to 12 hours led to absorption of intraperitoneal volume resulting in a net deficit from the infused volume, while with GP solution ultrafiltration continued to increase without changes in dialysate osmolality throughout the 12 hour exchanges.

At 6 and 12 hours, 14.4% and 28.1% of glucose polymer had been absorbed. Thus in terms of total caloric load there was no difference between the two solutions, but GP solution provided less than 50% of the calorie load of the glucose dialysate per unit volume of ultrafiltrate. The previous finding regarding an enhanced peritoneal equilibration of solutes with a molecular size greater than that of urea was confirmed, and a 7–9 fold increase in serum maltose with GP solution was also recorded.

The group in Manchester started, in 1987, chronic clinical studies with a higher molecular weight (22,000) GP solution. Short term (7 days) study did not show any ill effects even with continuous use of 5% GP solutions over a 7 day period [182]. In 5 non diabetic patients 7.5% GP solution was used over a period of three months [183]. GP solution was substituted for the overnight glucose exchange. The overnight (12 hours) exchanges resulted in 500–1000 ml of net ultrafiltration and serum biochemistry remained stable during the study period. There was a steady-state accumulation of maltose and maltotriose at levels 30 times those in uremic sera. No side effects were recorded. A long term randomized multicentre study in over 200 patients (106 with one 7.5% GP solution exchange) recently demonstrated no side effects and similar morbid events in both study and control groups [184]. Serum osmolality remained in the normal range and 15 diabetic patients included in the study tolerated the GP solution without problems.

These studies indicate that GP solution can be used during the overnight exchange as a substitute for the hypertonic glucose solution, because of its sustained ultrafiltration over 12 hours. It could be also useful during the long diurnal exchange in patients undergoing automated PD. Moreover, GP solution could be beneficial for diabetic patients since it provides a caloric reduction per unit volume of ultrafiltration and does not generate an insulin response. Finally recent observation [185–186] have suggested that the GP solution is more biocompatible than glucose solution probably because of its lower osmolality.

The metabolism of the absorbed polymer is less than complete, resulting in increased levels of its breakdown products maltose and maltotriose, since the polymer is readily hydrolyzed by circulating amylase to disaccharide. Further metabolism from maltose to glucose is limited by the absence of maltase activity in the human circulation [187]. Even though substantial amounts of maltase have been demonstrated in a variety of extraintestinal tissues, the enzyme is most notably present in the kidneys. Therefore, in the absence of significant residual renal function, accumulation of maltose occurs [188]. Long term studies with GP solutions have demonstrated an increase in serum maltose during the first days of treatment, until transperitoneal elimination of maltose during the three glucose exchanges ensured a steady-state level. This sustained and elevated level was not associated with any serious adverse effects over 6 months and now over 2 years of therapy. However long term effects of these levels are not known. A storage disease is unlikely to occur. A number of non metabolizable substances, either because of congenital lack of a specific degradative enzyme (glycogenosis, mannosidosis etc.) or because they are synthetic (HES, dextrans, polyvinylpyrrolidone etc.) have been recognized to accumulate in tissues thus affecting several organ functions. Glucose polymers are metabolised by amylase to maltose, which accumulates in a steady state.

In addition, accumulation within the macrophages leading to impairment of the phagocytic function (defined as reticulo-endothelial system blockade) has been documented for dextrans, HES, PVP and gelatin in mice [189], but it is unlikely that glucose polymer could exert this effect since it is a natural product.

4.2.5. Peptides
The first use of a mixture of peptides as an osmotic agent in a rabbit model of peritoneal dialysis was described by Klein *et al.* in 1986 [190]. A 5% solution of milk whey protein was hydrolyzed using a combination of trypsin and chymotrypsin in order to prepare a peptide mixture 3 to 10 amino acids long. This preparation was found to have an average molecular weight of 857 daltons. Amino acid analysis of the mixture showed it to contain approximately 2% free amino acids; 46% essential amino acids comprised the peptides. As compared to 2.5% glucose solution, the peptide solution yielded twice the net ultrafiltration after one hour of dwell time; 25% of the glucose was absorbed from the dialysate compared to 3% peptides. No acute toxic effects were recorded.

Recently an acute study has been performed in CAPD patients [191] comparing a standard 2.5% glucose solution (osmolality 404 mmOsm/kg) to a peptide solution containing 1.5% glucose and 1% peptides (molecular weight 600–700) with a 381 mmOsm/kg osmolality. The peptide solution was well tolerated in all patients and no differences were found in clearances and mass transfer area coefficient for urea, creatinine and glucose indicating that no irritating effect of peptide solution was present. Despite a lower osmolality of the peptide solution, no significant changes in ultrafiltration at 4 and 8 hour dwell times were recorded. No differences in plasma amino acid profiles could be detected.

These preliminary data seems to indicate that peptide solutions could have potential use as osmotic agents in peritoneal dialysis. Possible additional effects on nutritional status should be further evaluated. The mixture has an allergenic potential and this needs to be guarded against.

5. Acid base

One of the major results achieved by CAPD is the better correction of metabolic acidosis and the maintenance of satisfactory acid-base status as compared to hemodialysis. This result appears to be stable over time and acid-base fluctuations, typical of intermittent treatments, are not observed. The steadiness of acid-base status depends on the continuous infusion of buffers in the absence of significant losses of bicarbonate into dialysate and permits stability of blood gases and ventilation [192].

In intermittent peritoneal dialysis treatment, the time course of blood acid base parameters follows the same rules as in hemodialysis. After a treatment session a rise in blood bicarbonate and pH is recorded while during the dialytic period a slow decrease in these parameter occurs until the start of the next session [193]. The actual correction of acid base imbalance depends on the quantity of buffer gained by the patient, on the patient's ability to metabolize the incoming buffer load and on the loss of bicarbonate and organic anions into the dialysate [193].

Bicarbonate was initially used in 1964 by Boen [194] in peritoneal dialysis fluid, but it was soon replaced by lactate when it was found that calcium carbonate precipitated and the solution became alkaline during autoclaving. However the sodium salts of several organic oxidizable anions (such as acetate, lactate, citrate, malate, pyruvate, succinate, etc.) are able to consume H+ derived from carbonic acid, causing the regeneration of bicarbonate [195]. Consequently, as alkaline agents lactate and acetate were introduced.

5.1. Acetate

Acetate was first described as buffer substance in peritoneal dialysis fluid by Boen in 1962 [196]. Acetate regenerates bicarbonate when acetate thiokinase activates the reaction between acetate and coenzyme A (CoA) to form acetylCoA, and one hydrogen ion is captured in this process. AcetylCoA may enter different metabolic pathways such as decarboxylation in the Krebs cycle, condensation in ketone bodies or fatty acids and glucose generation via gluconeogenesis [197]. The buffering effect is accomplished and hydrogen ion is transferred to the respiratory chain only when acetylCoA is decarboxylated.

Since only traces of acetate are normally produced by intermediate metabolism of fatty acids, the rate of the enzymatic reaction to acetylCoA is limited [192]. In uremic patients treated with hemodialysis this rate is further decreased to a value of about 3 mmol/min [198]. This acetate flux is far less than that provided by a dialysate containing 40 mmol/l of acetate infused in a IPD session at rate of 5 l/hour (0.94 mmol/min) [193]. However during the session a 4-fold increase in normal serum acetate levels has been recorded. These levels were fairly constant during each session and fell to normal values after the end of dialysis. During CAPD with a 38.5 mmol/l acetate solution, the acetate mass transfer rate was 0.3 mmol/min, and constantly high plasma levels were observed [199].

Acetate has been shown to correct uremic metabolic acidosis even better than lactate both in CAPD and in intermittent treatment.

However, these findings have today only historical relevance since acetate has been abandoned when it was associated with the peritoneal ultrafiltration loss and the development of sclerosing peritonitis [200–201].

5.2. Lactate

Lactate is the commonly used buffer in peritoneal dialysis.

In nature two stereoisomeric forms of lactate exist: D- and L-lactate. Commercially available peritoneal dialysis fluids contain either L-lactate or a mixture of L- and D-lactate. In humans, small quantities of D-lactate are normally generated in the methylglyoxal pathway, while the predominant form is L-lactate. D-lactate is slowly metabolized by an non-specific enzyme (D-2-hydroxyacid-dehydrogenase) NAD independent [202]. L-lactate, on the contrary, is easily metabolized to pyruvate by NAD dependent lactic dehydrogenase. The buffering effect of lactate is accomplished by its complete metabolism via the Krebs cycle as for acetate, or via gluconeogenesis. With incomplete metabolism of lactate, the buffering effect does not take place. Searle et al. [203] demonstrated that 80–85% of the lactate produced by normal metabolism is oxidized in the Krebs cycle, and only 15–20% is converted to glucose. While oxidation takes place in all cells with aerobic metabolism, gluconeogenesis is confined to the liver and renal cortex. L-lactate turnover in normal subjects ranges from 0.77 to 0.87 mmol/kg/hour [203]. In patients with hepatic disease the rate of metabolism may be lower with a consequent increase in serum lactate levels.

In CAPD patients the lactate infusion is about 0.19 mmol/kg/hour, i.e. 25% of endogenous metabolic production [204]. This lactate load does not represent a metabolic problem in patients with normal hepatic function as demonstrated by some studies reporting normal values of intermediate metabolites [205–206]. In IPD (5 l/hour) lactate infusion was 1 mmol/kg/hour [193] serum lactate levels only occasionally slightly increased during the season and these data were confirmed by others [206–207].

The lactate disappearance rate from dialysate is depicted in Fig. 4 [193, 208–209]. The rate of absorption is maximal in the first minutes of dwell, and subsequently approaches zero. This behaviour permits an adequate buffer transfer even when rapid exchanges are given. It must be noted that D-lactate and L-lactate may have different rates of transport. Rubin et al. [209] demonstrated that the peritoneal membrane can operate a stereospecific selection in the process of lactate transport. L-lactate has higher mass transfer rate and metabolism. D-lactate is very slowly metabolized, but the low mass transfer rate both in IPD and in CAPD seems to allow complete metabolism since D-lactic acidosis has never been documented [210]. Other studies have not confirmed different absorption rates of the two stereoisomers of lactate [206–207]. In CAPD, long dwell times enable an almost complete transfer of

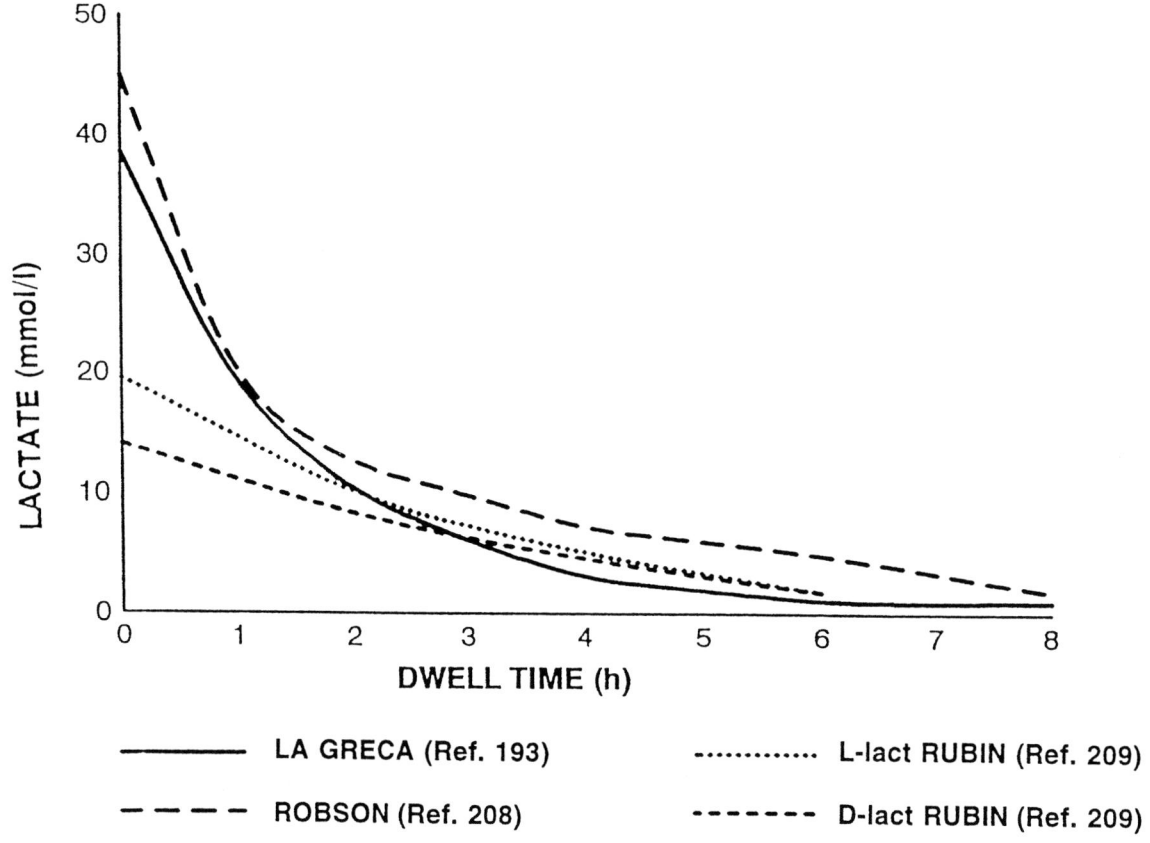

Figure 4. Disappearance of lactate from dialysate during dwell time (from reference [192]).

buffer from the dialysis solution, independently of the initial lactate solution concentration, and for this reason, this represents the major determinant of base gain.

During dwell time bicarbonate back diffuses into the dialysate. The major determinant of bicarbonate loss is the blood bicarbonate concentration. Several studies suggest a possible feed-back mechanism between blood bicarbonate concentration and the amount of bicarbonate lost in dialysate [205–206, 208, 211]. An increased blood bicarbonate level yields a parallel increase in bicarbonate loss that, in turn, results in a decrease in blood bicarbonate level. Inversely, in severe metabolic acidosis bicarbonate losses with dialysate are reduced, yielding a more favourable base balance.

Ultrafiltration also plays a role. It is evident that when dialysate/plasma equilibration occurs, an increase in drainage volume due to ultrafiltration, causes a greater loss of bicarbonate.

Finally organic anions, that are effective alkaline equivalent, are also lost in dialysate. Teehan *et al.* [205] have reported daily losses of 1 mmol of acetoacetate and 4.1 mmol of β hydroxybutyrate. Other substances are lost in the dialysate such as tricarboxylic anions, although they have never been quantified. A significant anion gap (36 ± 17 mmol/day) was observed in the effluent dialysate [205].

Commercially available CAPD solutions contain 35 or 40 mmol/l lactate. With a dialysis fluid lactate level of 35 mmol/l most patients display a chronic mild metabolic acidosis [18]. Teehan *et al.* [205] have demonstrated that lactate uptake from the peritoneal dialysis fluid was often exceeded by the bicarbonate loss and metabolic acid production. Out of 10 patients only two had a normal acid base status, the group having a mean arterial blood bicarbonate of 20.6 mmol/l and total CO2 (TCO2) of 22 mmol/l. Other clinical observations have confirmed these findings [212]. Nolph *et al.* [34] reported a mean venous TCO2 of 23.8 mmol/l in 163 determinations (78 patients), 38% of values being below 22 mmol/l. In order to correct the negative buffer balance and to improve acid base status, an increased lactate content to 40 mmol/l in CAPD solutions has been suggested [34]. Neither buffer balance studies nor serum lactate levels have been measured with this latter solution, however, significant better results on blood acid base status have been reported. Venous TCO2 increased to 27.4 mmol/l after four months of treatment (mean baseline value 23.4 mmol/l) while pH and pCO2 did not change [34]. It should be noted, however, that, since normal venous TCO2 ranges between 26.7 and 30.3 mmol/l (mean value 28.4 mmol/l) [213], in this study [34], 16% of patients had TCO2 values above the normal range, 52% under the normal range and 32% in the normal range, while the corresponding percentages in patients treated with the 35 mmol/l lactate solution were 3%, 75% and 22%. Moreover a recent observation [214] in 8 stable patients treated with a 40 mmol/l of lactate containing solution showed a mean arterial blood bicarbonate of 21.6 mmol/l and an increased anion gap of 21.4 mmol/l.

In summary the increased lactate content to 40 mmol/l in the CAPD solution has been shown to improve acid base status of a remarkable number of CAPD patients. However a significant percentage of patients still have metabolic acidosis, while metabolic alkalosis seems to occur in an increased number of patients. While the deleterious effects of metabolic acidosis on skeletal protein turnover is well known both in chronic renal failure rats and in patients [215–217], the long term effects of chronic metabolic alkalosis in CAPD patients is unknown.

Some metabolic side effects of infused lactate have been suggested, although there is no clear evidence that they have clinical relevance. Lactate is a powerful peripheral vasodilator, effects myocardial contractility, reduces blood pressure and could play a role in the blood lipid disorders of CAPD patients [218–219]. In addition, the administration of large amounts of L-lactate without proportionate amounts of its redox partner pyruvate results in a lowering of the cellular redox state and the linked phosphorylation potential. This effect could impair many vital cellular functions including the distribution of inorganic ions between intracellular and extracellular fluid [218, 220–221]. Unbalanced ratios of L-lactate to pyruvate also favour the so-called catabolic state associated with the action of corticosteroids and other hormones, potentiating the conversion of muscle protein into glucose [222].

The toxicity of D-lactate differs from that of L-lactate in that it is mainly observed in various forms of impaired cerebral function. Patients with blind loop syndrome and abnormal gut flora, producing enough of the D-isomer of lactic acid to elevate blood D-lactate to 3 mmol/l, developed clinically demonstrable encephalopathy [223]. The use of CAPD dialysate containing 40 mmol/l D, L-lactate has been reported to result in repeated episodes of cerebral dysfunction characterized clinically by agitated confusion, depression and hyperventilation resulting in life-threatening metabolic alkalosis [224].

Issues related to biocompatibility will be discussed in chapter 17.

5.3. Bicarbonate

The ideal buffer for peritoneal dialysis should be sodium bicarbonate since this substance is the physiological buffer for the body. However, solutions containing mixtures of bicarbonate, calcium, magnesium and glucose are difficult to prepare, sterilize, and store, since, during the autoclaving, calcium and magnesium precipitate as carbonate salts and glucose caramelizes, due to the high pH of the solution.

In single pass hemodialysis this problem has been solved by the so called "three-stream method" in which an acid and a basic (bicarbonate) solutions are continuously mixed with treated water. The acid solution which contains an organic acid, calcium, magnesium and glucose lowers the pH of the final solution. As a consequence carbonate ion concentration becomes so low that the solubility products of calcium and magnesium carbonate are not exceeded.

This concept was adapted to intermittent peritoneal dialysis by Ing et al. [225] and subsequently modified to a "two-stream method" in which equal volumes of an acid and basic (bicarbonate) solutions are simultaneously delivered by a roller pump to produce the final solution [226]. Later, these authors described [227] and used [228] during an IPD session a new method for producing bicarbonate solution. The bicarbonate content of a glass syringe is added to an acid solution placed in a second container to yield two liters of the final dialysate. No problems were encountered during the clinical IPD session.

Independently, a single container, which is divided into two compartments (one containing the acid and one containing the basic solutions) by a partition wall, was developed for CAPD solutions [229]. A breakable value in the partition wall is broken by external pressure just before use, thus allowing the mixing of the two solutions. The final dialysate pH value was around 7.4. One patient was treated for one week and three patients were treated for a few exchanges with this solution containing 35 mmol/l of bicarbonate [211]. The solution was well tolerated and no side effects occurred. The patient treated for one week had an increase in the blood bicarbonate content until a plateau was achieved at about 29 mmol/l after few days. In a subsequent study a solution containing 27 mmol/l of bicarbonate was employed in one patient for two months [230]. No biochemical changes were observed but blood bicarbonate remained stable at pre-study level (20 mmol/l).

In order to assess the safety and the better bicarbonate solution concentration for clinical use, "in vitro" stability tests, animal and kinetic studies have been performed. No calcium carbonate precipitation has been demonstrated for up to 40 mmol/l of bicarbonate and 2 mmol/l of calcium concentration solutions over a clinical use range of temperatures [231]. In a rat model, repeated intraperitoneal injections of 100 ml/kg were not associated with histological lesions, crystal formation and fibrosis [232]. Kinetic studies demonstrated that changes in dialysate bicarbonate concentration at different dwell times were correlated with serum bicarbonate levels independent of the bicarbonate content of the fresh solution, thus suggesting a self-limited bicarbonate absorption [233].

A recent short term clinical evaluation (4 weeks) with a 34 mmol/l bicarbonate solution in 6 patients was associated with an increase in blood bicarbonate, a slight but not statistically significant increase in ultrafiltration, a slight decrease in the creatinine D/P ratio and no changes in the principal biochemical parameters and dialysis adequacy, thus demonstrating that, at least in the short term, this solution is safe, well tolerated, does not affect peritoneal dialysis adequacy and is effective in the correction of uremic acidosis [234]. The authors suggested that slight changes in ultrafiltration and creatinine equilibration could reflect a better biocompatibility of this solution. These findings were confirmed in several "in vitro" observations.

The bicarbonate solution did not result in peritoneal vasodilatation as did lactate solution, showed less cytotoxic damage on mesothelial cells, did not affect phospholipid secretion of mesothelial cells [235] and eicosanoids and cytokines release from peripheral [186, 236] and peritoneal macrophages [237]. Moreover, in a recent study in a rabbit model, peritoneal membrane examination did not reveal microscopic or macroscopic differences among three groups of animals in which the control group was not dialyzed and the other two groups performed peritoneal dialysis by using either a standard lactate solution or a bicarbonate buffered solution [238].

An alternative approach to provide a stable bicarbonate solution has been described by Yatzidis [239]. A dipeptide, glycylglycine, has been added to a bicarbonate solution in order to stabilize the solution pH at about 7.35. This solution has been shown to be stable after 18 months in storage and has been tested in rabbits for up to 25 days with no pathological findings in the peritoneum. About 80% of glycylglycine were absorbed. In humans this substance is enzymatically degraded to glycine which is in turn metabolized to other non essential amino acids. The first clinical acute study demonstrated that glycylglycine-bicarbonate solution was well tolerated by patients and significantly increased next ultrafiltration as compared to a standard lactate solution [240]. In addition, since the solution must be cold sterilized by filtration in order to avoid glucose caramelization, the concentration of glucose by-products were considerably reduced [241].

6. CAPD systems (by Kriger F. L., Winchester J.)

6.1. Dialysis fluid containers

As pointed out above, commercially manufactured dialysis solutions are available in varied volumes, e.g., one or two litre glass bottles or rigid plastic bottles, 10 L plastic containers for cycling machines, and collapsible plastic bags in varying volumes from 300 ml to 3 L. The collapsible plastic bags can expand with fluid to allow for the volume of dialysate delivered, *plus* any ultrafiltrate transferred into it from the patient. The 10 L plastic containers are used solely with machinery for delivery of peritoneal dialysis fluid into and out of the peritoneum (i.e. CCPD, NIPD, TPD). Nearly all available bags have drug delivery port(s) adjacent to the dialysis fluid delivery port at the bottom of the bag, or on the side of the plastic bag. All drug delivery ports have resealable rubber covers. In addition to the above, solution concentrates, requiring a 20:1 dilution with water derived from reverse osmosis of tap water, are available in 2 L glass bottles or 2.5 L plastic bags. In the United States the transfer sets have a 'spike' (a rigid pointed hollow plastic tube), or luer lock, attached to the delivery line and connected to the Tenckhoff or other catheter, usually via an on-line plastic connector which screws onto a titanium connector on the catheter. The standard transfer sets are variable in length and have a check valve to stop and start the flow of dialysis fluid into and out of the patient. In the United Kingdom and Europe, and now in the United States, connection of the transfer set to the dialysis solution bag may be achieved through a luer lock system, with a protective povidone iodine laden clam shell (Baxter, Fresenius, Gambro), or a protective "cap" containing povidone iodine antiseptic (Baxter, Fresenius).

6.2. Modern connection devices (Fig. 5)

Man's ingenuity to prevent complications and to design unique devices and systems is no more evident than in the many variations in connector design, connector sterilization, and devices to simplify, automate and produce contaminant free delivery of dialysis fluid for peritoneal dialysis. The design changes and manufacturing methods go through many modifications and the reader would be advised to be current in the latest system available in the local area. Not all geographic locations have the "latest and best", due to governmental regulations and registration procedures which differ widely throughout the world.

6.3. Simple connection methods

The point of entry of the spike or luer lock system to the bag of dialysis fluid may be protected by a barrier consisting of two small sponges soaked in povidone iodine (Betadine) solution enclosed in a small plastic box (Fig. 6). Other manufacturers use the Safe-Lock system (of Saf-lok) (Fig. 7), or Safe-Lock 5"F" (Fresenius) (Fig. 8) which is sprayed with an antiseptic preparation principally consisting of an alcoholic solution containing phenol (in Europe), or other agent in the United States. Betadine solution may also be sprayed on to the luer lock connections to reduce the rate of peritonitis. Of historical interest is the Toronto Western Hospital peritoneal dialysis connector, which involved a needle from the dialysate delivery side passing through a zone of povidone iodine solution, thereby obtaining a disinfected connection [242]. Most recent attention has been in the advent of the "Y" system concept, and the growing penetration of disconnect systems which free the patient from carrying the empty dialysate bag during the long dwell period.

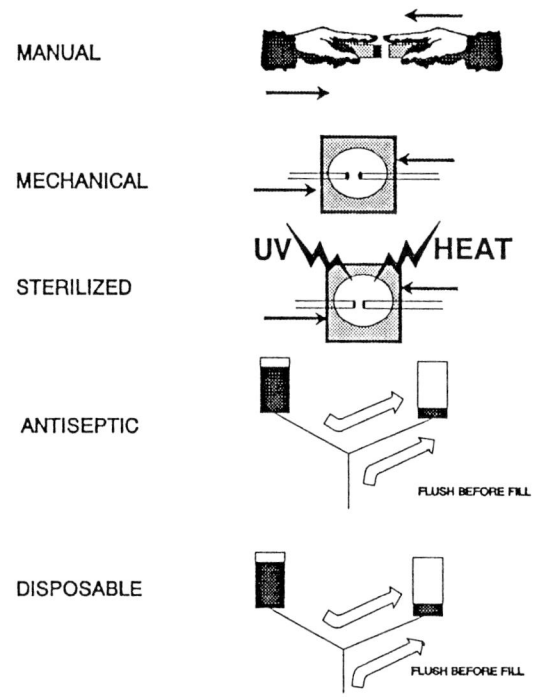

Figure 5. Connections and delivery systems.

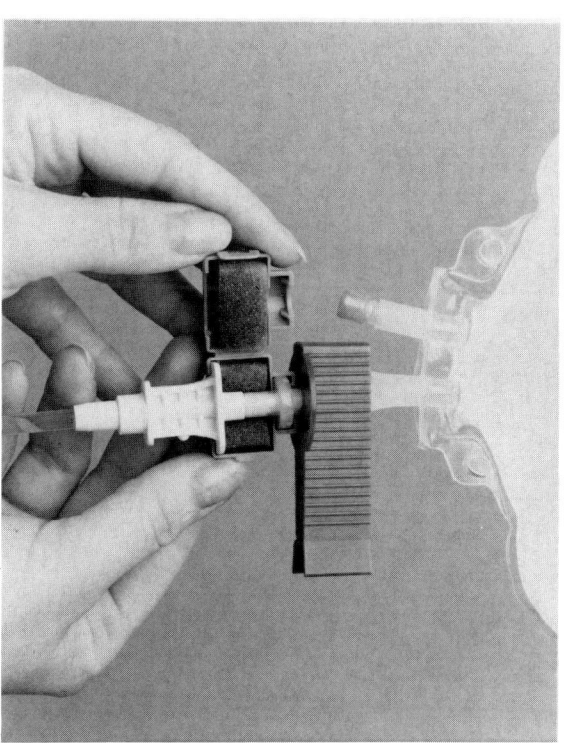

Figure 6. Povidone iodine containing connection shield.

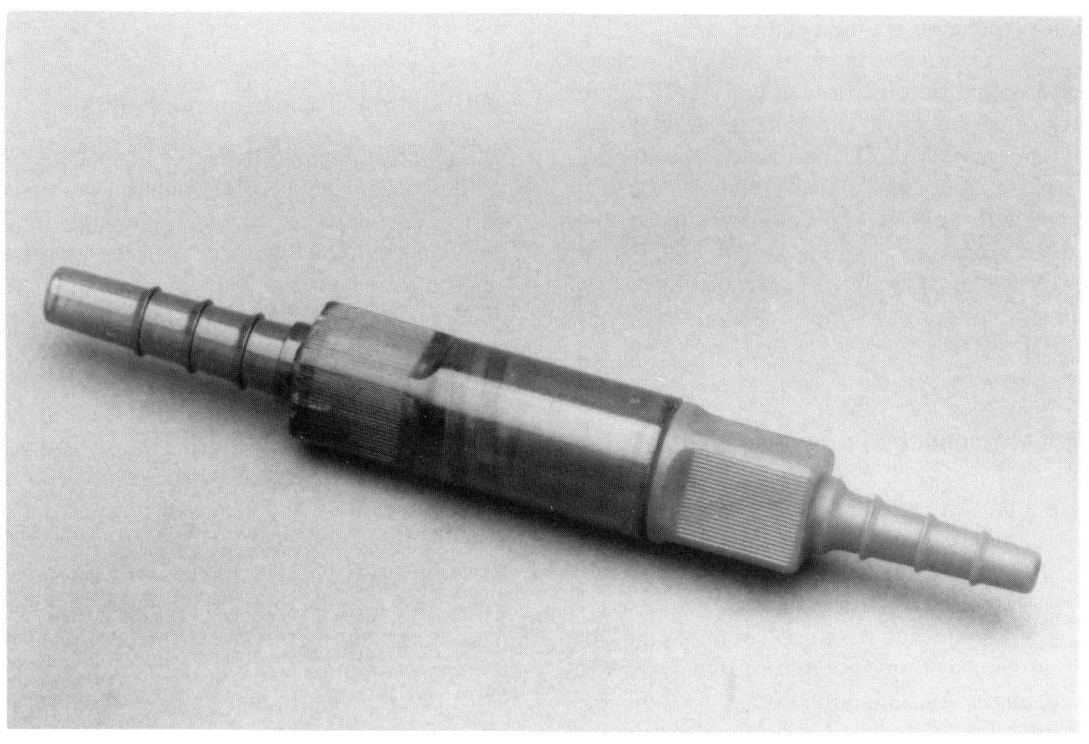

Figure 7. Safe Lock connector.

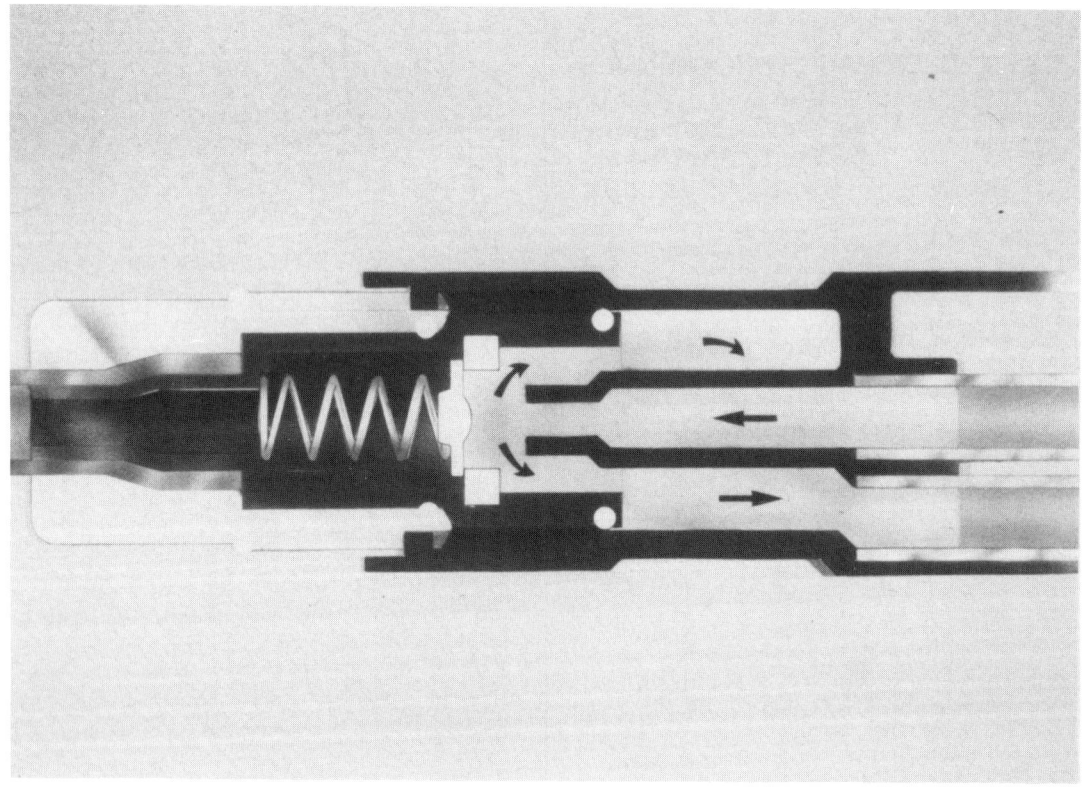

Figure 8. "5F" Safe lock connector.

CAPD SYSTEMS AND SOLUTIONS

6.4. The 'Y' systems (Fig. 9, Table 3 [243–266])

First described in Italy [267, 268] the dialysis fluid transfer set may be formed into a 'Y' shape, to which a full bag and an empty bag are placed at either end of the upper limbs of the 'Y' while the lower limb of the 'Y' is connected to the patient via a titanium connector or through a needle placed in a resealable rubber bung attached to the catheter [269]. The concept is that the delivery of dialysis fluid into the patient (the "fill"), is preceded by running out spent dialysate ("flush") into a waiting empty bag, carrying with it any contaminating bacteria, introduced by 'touch' contamination of the connection [270]. A second flush of the limbs of the "Y" is performed from the new bag, to carry bacterial into the spent dialysis fluid. After the spent dialysate is drained into the empty bag, instillation of fresh dialysis fluid follows. This concept of "flush" before "fill" is fundamental to "Y" systems, "O" systems and to disposable systems using two bags (one full and one empty to receive dialysis fluid), whether or not the patient may disconnect all bags from the 'Y', and become bag free. In general, it has been found that in vitro bacterial "washout" is sufficient that no antiseptic is required in-line [271], using disposable (one-time) systems, whereas the bacterial growth in reusable systems demands the use of antiseptics (mostly Amuchina, or Dakin's solutions, (sodium hypochlorite), or povidone iodine) in-line [272]. Early results with this system

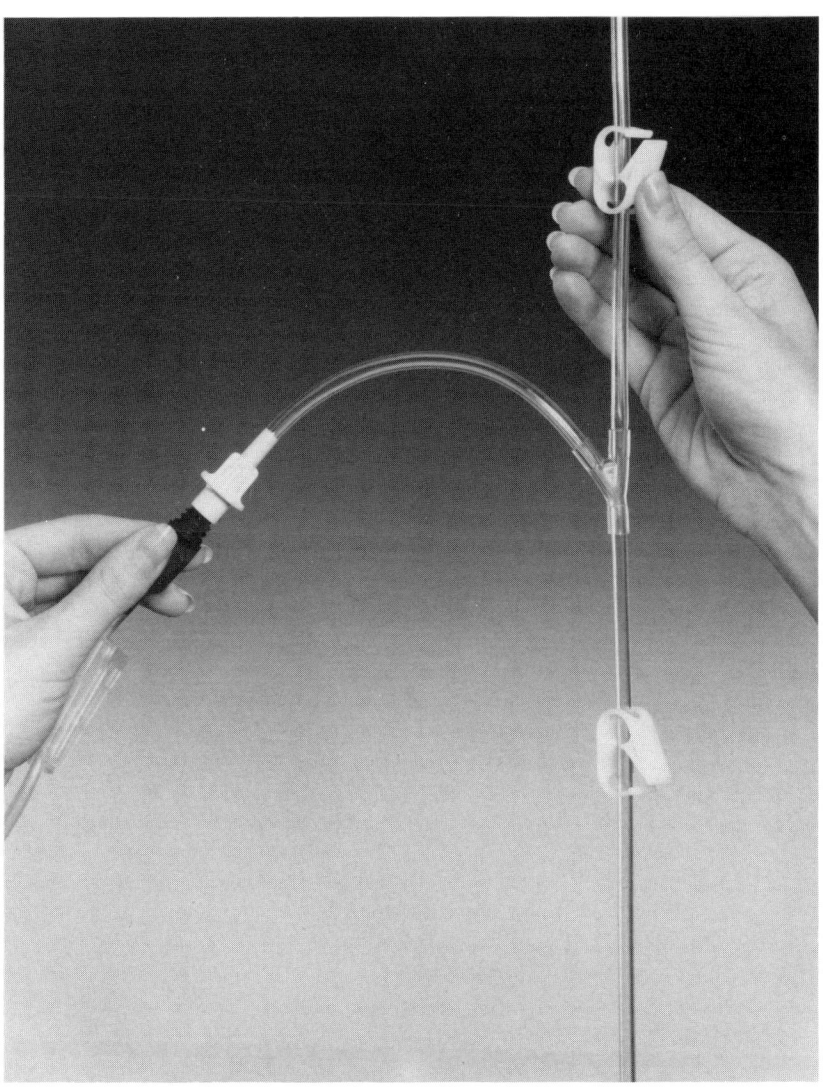

Figure 9. "Y" set.

which showed reduction in the frequency of peritonitis, compared to standard CAPD, have been confirmed using many variations on the "Y" (Table 3). The Baxter 'O' (reusable), and "Ultra" (disposable disconnect) systems are variations on the 'Y' system, as are "Freedom" (disposable disconnect, Fig. 10), or "ANDY" (non-disconnect) systems of Fresenius [273–275]. Many variations abound from different manufacturers (local or international) and the reader may wish to be familiar with them and their frequent design changes.

As can be seen from Table 3, results from the "Y" systems consistently give low peritonitis rates (when compared to controls using standard CAPD).

Disinfection is also a feature of the cap systems (Baxter, Fresenius), where a small reservoir of povidone-iodine solution is attached to the end of the transfer set, or to the end of the catheter after disconnection of the transfer set, at each dialysis fluid exchange.

6.5. Double bag systems (Fig. 11, Table 4 [269, 270, 276–280])

Double bag systems (one empty and the other filled with fresh dialysate) have been used since introduced by Bazzatto in 1980 [269, 270]. The original "Y" set and antiseptic in line, was replaced with a sterilized disposable completely integrated system [276–279], containing an empty bag, and a fresh dialysis containing bag (Baxter, Bieffe). The system still uses the "flush before fill" technique for exchanging fluids but no antiseptic is necessary. The results of such double bag systems, appear to be superior to the standard dialysis exchange procedure, and perhaps to the "Y" system. Comparative studies are awaited with interest, since the costs of manufacturing double bag systems are high compared to "Y" systems, although the savings in costs for the treatment of peritonitis may be considerable [281].

7. Connectology (Table 5 [282–292])

Approximately two-thirds of all episodes of peritonitis can be directly attributed to touch contamination of the connection between the transfer set and the dialysis bag containing fresh dialysis solutions [293]. This may be related to contamination of the spike or the luer-lock system, or inadequate

Table 3. "Y" set results.

References	Peritonitis (Control -PT MO)	Peritonitis (System -PT MO)	System
Nakamura '92 [243]	27.5	46.6	Ultra/solo
Strauss '90 [244]		31.5	"
Scalamogna '90 [245]	8.6	43.3	"
Burkart '90 [246]	7	18	"
Piraino '89 [247]	9	20	"
Swartz '89 [248]		18	"
Rottembourg '88 [249]	12.2	23	"
Bonnardeaux '92 [250]	9.6	29.4	"O"
Owen '92 [251]	4.9	13.4	"
Port '92 [252]	9	9.4	"
Bailie '90 [253]	8.83 (UV)	11.14	"
Junior '89 [254]		15.1	"
Villano '88 [255]		22.8	"
Ryckelynck '88 [256]		35.2	"
Lempert '86 [257]	12	16	"
Port '92 [252]	9	15	"Y"
Maiorca '90 [258]		43.3	"
Catizone '90 [259]	8.4	44.8	"
Churchill '89 [260]	9.9	21.5	"
Viglino '89 [261]		67	"
Maiorca '87 [262]		57	"
Maiorca '86 [263]	10.1	27.6	"
Cantaluppi '86 [264]	11.7	56.1	"
Maiorca '83 [265]	11	33	"
Buoncristiani '83 [266]		39.9	"

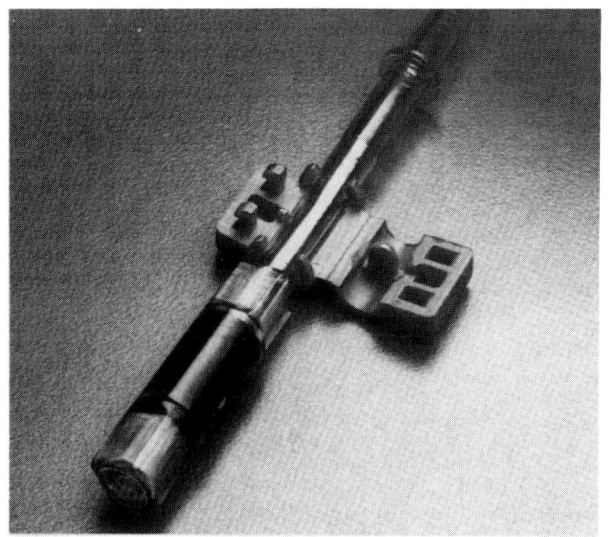

Figure 10. Prefilled disinfectant disconnect system (Fresenius).

sterilization by betadine, hypochlorite or alcoholic solutions and it has become clear that a fail-safe connection system is important to reduce the frequency of peritonitis. Several systems to prevent peritonitis based on connectology have been developed.

The first of these systems was the introduction of a microporous (0.22 um) bacterial filter, to filter inflowing fluid through a 270 cm^2 membrane area, between the connection to the dialysis fluid bag and the patient. This has been shown both in intermittent peritoneal dialysis [294] and in CAPD [295–297] to reduce the frequency of peritonitis, particularly in high risk subjects such as those with poor manual technique, history of frequent peritonitis, the elderly and also with long-term use [289, 290, 297]. These filters have largely been abandoned in favor of more convenient and cheaper systems and devices.

Mechanized devices, available from Baxter, and Fresenius (Fig. 12), facilitate, either automatically

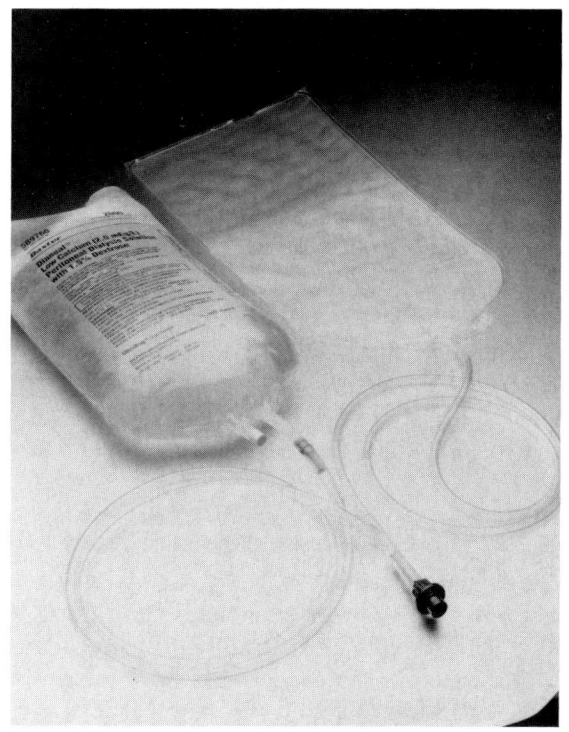

Figure 11. Double or twin bag.

or semi-automatically, connections of transfer set from spent dialysis fluid bags to fresh dialysis fluid bags (Fig. 5). One device the "Optum" also uses UV light sterilization (Fig. 13).

Other devices are available which attempt to sterilize the connection by either heat or ultraviolet radiation. The first device is the Terumo Flame-Lock system, which involves heating over a flame, ceramic connections at the bag and transfer set, after which a connection is made. Ota *et al.* have shown that the Flame-Lock device causes a reduction in the rate of peritonitis compared to standard connectology [288].

Another device employing heat sterilization is the "Thermoclave", Fresenius, which heats the con-

Table 4. Double/twin bag results.

References	PT months	Peritonitis* (System -PT MO)	Peritonitis* (Control -PT MO)
Lewis '92 [276]	890	37.1	25.8 (Y SET)
Balteau '91 [1977]	765	33.3	
Honkanen '91 [278]	300	27.3	11.3
Dryden '91 [279]	564	25	9.7
Bazzato '86 [280]	411	24.1	

* Mean patient months between episodes.

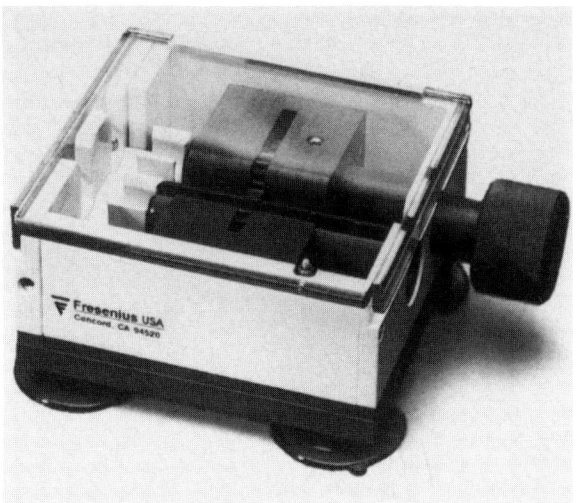

Figure 12. Manual connection device (Fresenius).

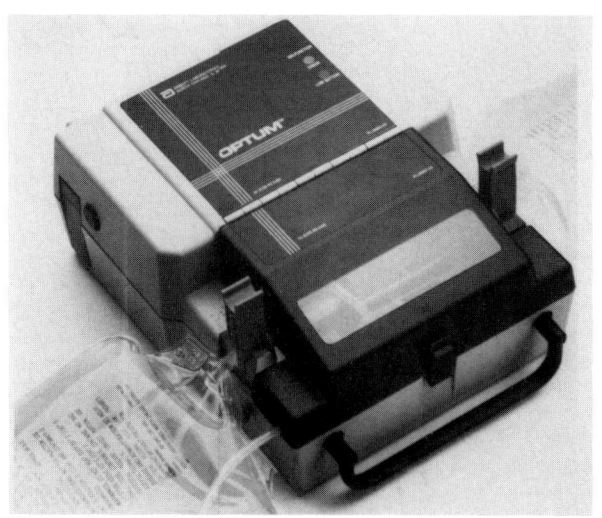

Figure 13. Fresenius "Optum" device.

nections to 80 °C for ten minutes: in vitro [300, 301], and in vivo [285, 286] utility have been demonstrated. Some concern has been raised that heat sterilization of dialysate may produce aldehydes which are potentially toxic [302].

Ultraviolet devices (Baxter, USA and Fresenius, USA), are apparati for the sterilization of the connecting surfaces before the connection is completed. This is performed inside a sealed box after which the connection is made (Figs. 13 and 14). The ultraviolet ray wave length is selected to kill common bacteria and fungi, and the device has been shown to reduce the incidence of positive cultures in vitro, and the device is effective in reducing the frequency of peritonitis, compared to standard systems.

Results are also similar to the peritonitis rate achieved with "Y" sets. The devices available either use full automation ("Optum", Fresenius, Fig. 13), or partial automation ("UVXD" and "UV Flash", Baxter, Fig. 14). The "UVXD" and "Optum" use mercury vapor derived UV light, which is effective in vitro at killing bacteria and fungi [298], although the xenon derived UV light (UV "Flash") would appear to be more effective for killing intraluminal organisms [299].

The Sterile Connection Device (SCD) of DuPont De Nemours and Company, marketed by Gambro in Europe (Figs. 15 and 16) is a device which uses a heated blade to cut through compressed parallel placed tubing from the used transfer set and the

Table 5. UV and sterilizing devices results.

References	Peritonitis* (Control -PT MO)	Peritonitis* (System -PT MO)	System
Nolph '85 [282]		13.7	UV
Tapson '87 [283]	3.6	6.8	"
Port '92 [252]	9	13.4	"
Boeschoten '87 [284]	4.8	5.9	"
Nakamura '92 [243]	27.5	46.6	"
Steinhauer '91 [285]	35.3 (Standard/UV)	41.9	Thermoclave
Olivas '91 [286]	9.5–9.8 (Standard/UV)	26.5–53	"
Hamilton '85 [287]	4.5	8.7 (High risk)	"
Ota '86 [288]	16.7	22.4	Flame-lock
Boeschoten '87 [284]	2.8	8.1	Filter
Slingeneyer '86 [289]		14.5–2.4	"
Rotellar '86 [290]	3.38	5.95	"
Slingeneyer '83 [291]		18	"
Winchester '83 [292]	2.8	10.3	"

* Mean patient months between episodes.

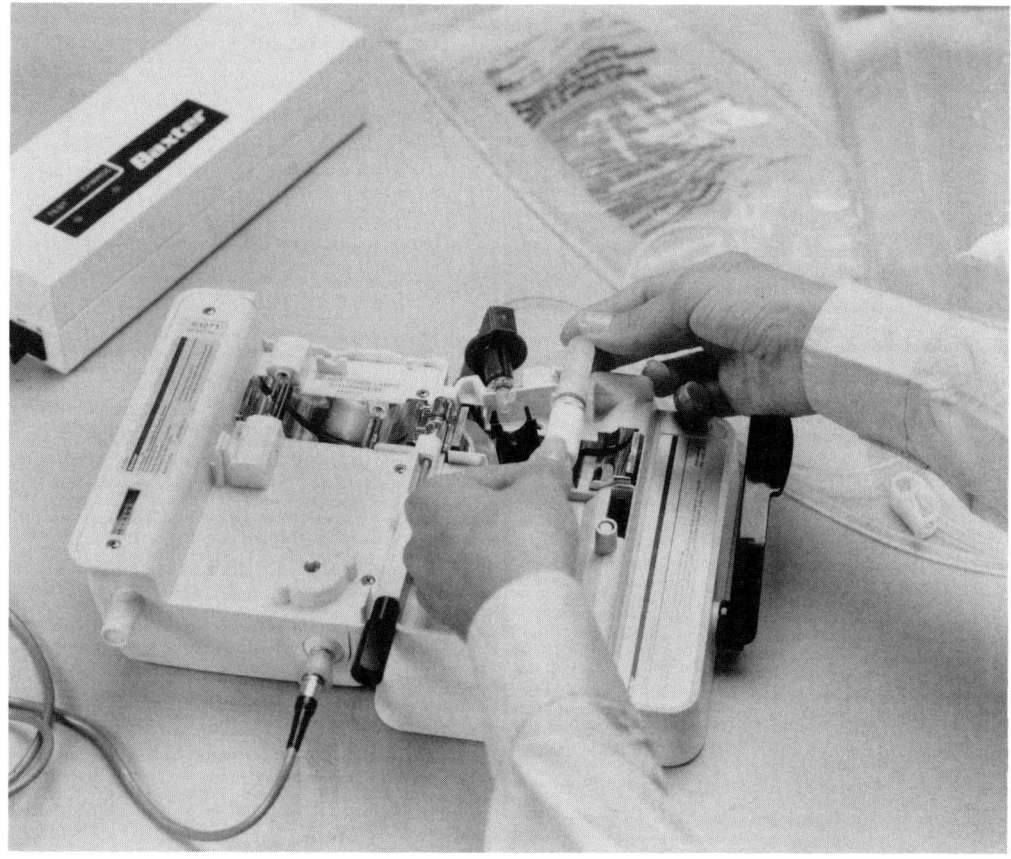

Figure 14. Baxter UV "Flash" device.

fresh dialysis bag. Thereafter the parallel tubing is rocked backwards aligning the fresh tubing with the transfer set. The melted plastic solidifies on cooling, leaving a patent line through which the dialysis fluid is transferred to the patient. Clinical experience with the SCD has demonstrated that there is high patient acceptance and a low incidence of touch contamination [287].

With the plethora of devices available, it is obvious that none of them is ideal, nor will they abolish all the episodes of peritonitis in CAPD patients, since about one third of the episodes of peritonitis may be related to hematogenous spread of bacteria, and the spread of bacteria along the subcutaneous tunnel along which the catheter enters the abdomen [293].

Catheters and cycling machines are outside the scope of this chapter, but the connection devices described here are also used to permit safe and effective exchanges for machine delivered peritoneal dialysis. A fuller discussion of catheters and their problems is presented in Chapters 9 and 10, and of cycler machines in Chapter 13.

7. The future

As can be appreciated from the foregoing, CAPD will continue to develop, particularly in the area of a search for solutions which have alternative osmotic agents to dextrose, are more physiologic in stabilizing pH, do not support bacterial growth and allow most efficient solute transfer, while at the same time preventing chemical and mineral loss or trace element intoxication. To date, no available solution fulfills all of these goals.

The CAPD patient at present is using disconnect systems more and more, and it is likely that the encumbrances of bag or transfer set will be a thing of the past. Devices that achieve sterile connections and disconnections are now a normal situation for many patients, and while they are expensive the advantages in keeping patients out of hospital for peritonitis may actually save money in the long run. Improvements in connectology have the potential to reduce the incidence of peritonitis by approximately two thirds. The ultimate goal in peritoneal dialysis is to develop a biocompatible catheter for

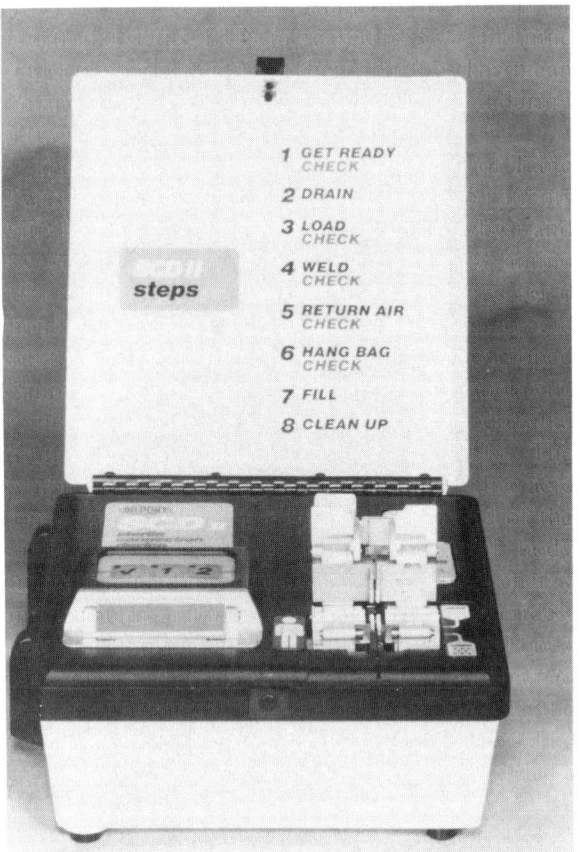

Figure 15. Dupont Sterile Connection Device (SCD). The two clamps at the lower right hand corner of the device are opened and the delivery lines from spent and fresh dialysis containers are placed in parallel over a heated blade which melts the plastic allowing a connection to be made between the spent and fresh delivery lines as seen in Figure 16.

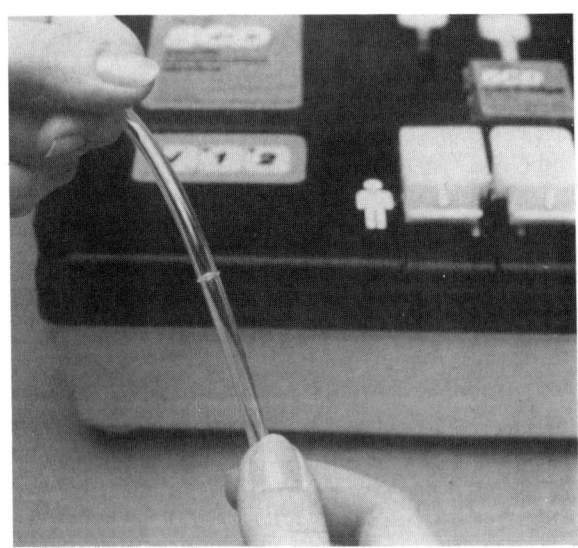

Figure 16. A strong patent seal between fresh and spent dialysis delivery tubing, made by the SCD.

peritoneal access, the single barrier to further increases in peritoneal dialysis usage world wide.

References

1. Boen ST. History of peritoneal dialysis. In: Nolph KD (ed), Peritoneal Dialysis. Dordrecht: Kluwer Academic Publishers 1989: 1–12.
2. Nolph KD, Parker A. The composition of dialysis solution for continuous ambulatory peritoneal dialysis. In: Legrain M (ed), Continuous ambulatory peritoneal dialysis. Amsterdam: Excerpta Medica 1980: 341–6.
3. Nolph KD, Twardowski ZJ, Popovich RP, Rubin J. Equilibration of peritoneal dialysis solutions during long dwell exchanges. J Lab Clin Med 1979; 93: 246–56.
4. Nolph KD, Sorkin MI, Moore H. Autoregulation of sodium and potassium removal during continuous ambulatory peritoneal dialysis. Trans Am Soc Artif Inter Organs 1980; 26: 334–7.
5. Nolph KD, Hano JE, Teschan PE. Peritoneal sodium transport during hypertonic peritoneal dialysis: physiologic mechanisms and clinical implications. Ann Intern Med 1969; 70: 931–41.
6. Raja RM, Cantor RE, Boreyco C, Bushchri H, Kramer MS, Rosenbaum JL. Sodium transport during ultrafiltration peritoneal dialysis. Trans Am Soc Artif Inter Organs 1972; 18: 429–35.
7. Raja RM, Kramer MS, Rosenbaum JL, Manchanda R, Lazaro N. Evaluation of hypertonic peritoneal dialysis solution with low sodium. Nephron 1973; 11: 342–53.
8. Ahearn DJ, Nolph KD. Controlled sodium removal with peritoneal dialysis. Trans Am Soc Artif Intern Organs 1972; 18: 423–8.
9. Colombi A. Fluid and electrolyte balance in CAPD patients. In: La Greca G, Chiaramonte S, Fabris A. Feriani M, Ronco C (eds), Peritoneal Dialysis: Proceedings of Third International Course on Peritoneal Dialysis. Milano: Wichtig Editore 1988: 265–7.
10. De Vecchi A, Paparella M, Scalamogna A, Guerra L, Casteinovo C. Effetti della variazione delle concentrazioni di sodio nel liquido di dialisi peritoneale. In: La Greca G, Petrella E, Cioni A (eds), I liquidi nella dialisi. Milano: Ghedini Editore 1991: 93–8.
11. Nakayama M, Yokoyama K, Kawaguchi Y, Sakai O. Effect of ultra low sodium concentration dialysate (ULNaD) in patients with UF loss. (abstract) Perit Dial Int 1991; (Suppl 1): 187.
12. Twardowski ZJ. New approaches to intermittent peritoneal dialysis therapies. In: Nolph KD (ed), Peritoneal Dialysis. Dordrecht: Kluwer Academic Publishers 1989: 133–51.
13. Gault MH, Ferguson EL, Sidhu JS, Corbin RP. Fluid and electrolyte complications of peritoneal dialysis. Choice of dialysis solutions. Ann Intern Med 1971; 75: 253–62.
14. Shen FH, Sherrard DJ, Scollard D, Merrit A, Curtis FK. Thist, relative hypernatremia and excessive

weight gain in maintenance peritoneal dialysis. Trans Am Soc Artif Intern Organ 1978; 24: 142–5.
15. Twardowski ZJ, Nolph KD, Khanna R, Gluck Z, Prowant BF, Ryan LP. Daily clearances with continuous ambulatory peritoneal dialysis and nightly peritoneal dialysis. Trans Am Soc Artif Intern Organs 1986; 32: 575–80.
16. Nolph KD. Kinetics of ultrafiltration and electrolyte transport during peritoneal dialysis. In: La Greca G, Chiaramonte S, Fabris A, Feriani M, Ronco C (eds), Peritoneal Dialysis: Proceedings of Second International Course on Peritoneal Dialysis. Milano: Wichtig Editore 1985: 47–50.
17. Brown ST, Ahearn DJ, Nolph KD. Potassium removal with peritoneal dialysis. Kidney Int 1973; 4: 67–9.
18. Gokal R. Continuous ambulatory peritoneal dialysis. In: Maher JF (ed), Replacement of Renal Function by Dialysis. Dordrecht: Kluwer Academic Publisher 1989: 590–615.
19. Blumenkrantz MJ, Kopple JD, Moran JK, Coburn JW. Metabolic balance studies and dietary protein requirements in patients undergoing continuous ambulatory peritoneal dialysis. Kidney Int 1982; 21: 849–61.
20. Sandle GI, Gaiger E, Tapster S, Goodship THJ. Evidence for large intestinal control of potassium homeostasis in uraemic patients undergoing CAPD. Clin Sci 1987; 73: 247–52.
21. Lameire N, Ringoir S. Introductory remarks: an overview of peritonitis and other complications of continuous ambulatory peritoneal dialysis. In: Legrain M (ed), Continuous ambulatory peritoneal dialysis. Amsterdam: Excerpta Medica 1980: 229–37.
22. Oreopoulos DG, Khanna R, William P et al. Continuous ambulatory peritoneal dialysis – 1981. Nephron 1982; 30: 293–303.
23. Spital A, Sterns RH. Potassium supplementation via the dialysate in continuous ambulatory peritoneal dialysis. Am J Kidney Dis 1985; 6: 173–6.
24. Lindholm B, Alvestrand A, Hultman F, Bergstrom J. Muscle water and electrolytes in patients undergoing continuous ambulatory peritoneal dialysis. Acta Med Scand 1986; 219: 323–30.
25. Heide B, Pierratos A, Khanna R et al. Nutritional status of patients undergoing continuous ambulatory peritoneal dialysis. Perit Dial Bull 1983; 3: 138–41.
26. Rubin J. Kirchner K, Barnes T, Teal N, Ray R, Bower JD. Evaluation of continuous ambulatory peritoneal dialysis. Am J Kidney Dis 1983; 3: 199–204.
27. Schilling H, Wu G, Petit J et al. Nutritional status of patients on long term CAPD. Perit Dial Bull 1985; 5: 12–18.
28. Randall RE, Cohen MD, Spray CC, Rossmeisl EC. Hypermagnesemia in renal failure: Etiology and toxic manifestation. Ann Intern Med 1964; 61: 73–8.
29. Whang R. Magnesium deficiency: pathogenesis, prevalence and clinical implications. Am J Med 1987; 82 (Suppl 3A): 24–9.
30. Hollifield J. Magnesium depletion, diuretics and arrhythmias. Am J Med 1987; 82 (Suppl #A): 30–7.
31. Selling M. Electrocardiographic patterns of magnesium depletion appearing in alcoholic heart disease. Ann NY Acad Sci 1969; 162: 906–17.
32. Parker A., Nolph KD. Magnesium and calcium mass transfer during continuous ambulatory peritoneal dialysis. Trans Am Soc Artif Intern Organs 1980; 26: 194–6.
33. Kwong MBL, Lee JSK, Chan MK. Transperitoneal calcium and magnesium transfer during an 8-hour dialysis. Perit Dial Bull 1987; 7: 85–9.
34. Nolph KD, Prowant B, Serkes KD et al. Multicentric evaluation of a new peritoneal dialysis solution with a high lactate and low magnesium concentration. Perit Dial Bull 1983; 3: 63–5.
35. Kohaut EC, Balfe JW, Potter D, Alexandre S, Lum G. Hypermagnesemia and mild hypocarbia in pediatric patients on CAPD. Perit Dial Bull 1983; 3: 41–2.
36. Rahman R, Heaton A, Goodship T et al. Renal osteodystrophy in patients on CAPD: a five year study Perit Dial Bull 1987; 7: 1–4.
37. Gokal R, Fryer R, McHugh M, Ward MK Kerr DNS. Calcium and phosphate control in patients on continuous ambulatory peritoneal dialysis. In: Legrain M (ed), Continuous ambulatory peritoneal dialysis. Amsterdam: Excerpta Medica 1980: 282–91.
38. Rubin J. Comments on dialysis solution, antibiotic transport poisonings and novel uses of peritoneal dialysis. In: Nolph KD (ed), Peritoneal Dialysis. Dordrecht: Kluwer Academic Publishers 1989: 199–229.
39. Gonella M. Plasma and tissue levels of magnesium in chronically hemodialyzed patients: effects of dialysate magnesium levels. Nephron 1983; 34: 141–5.
40. Meema HE, Oreopoulos DG, Rapoport A. Serum magnesium level and arterial calcification in end-stage renal disease. Kidney Int 1987; 32: 388–94.
41. Hutchison AJ, Freemont AJ, Boulton HF, Gokal R. Low-calcium dialysis fluid and oral calcium carbonate in CAPD. A method of controlling hyperphosphataemia whilst minimizing aluminium exposure and hypercalcaemia. Nephrol Dial Transpl 1992; 7: 1219–25.
42. Hutchison AJ, Gokal R. Improved solutions for peritoneal dialysis: physiological calcium solutions, osmotic agents and buffers. Kidney Int 1992; 42 (Suppl 38): S153–9.
43. Breuer J, Moniz C, Baldwin D, Parsons V. The effects of zero magnesium dialysate and magnesium supplements on ionized calcium concentration in patients on regular dialysis treatment. Nephrol Dial Transplant 1987; 2: 347–50.
44. Shan G, Winer R, Cutler R et al. Effects of a magnesium-free dialysate on magnesium metabolism during continuous ambulatory peritoneal dialysis. Am J Kidney Dis 1987; 10: 268–75.

45. Delmez JA, Slatopolsky E, Martin KJ, Gearing BN, Harter HR. Minerals, vitamin D, and parathyroid hormone in continuous ambulatory peritoneal dialysis. Kidney Int 1982; 21: 862–7.
46. Digenis G, Khanna R, Pierratos A et al. Renal osteodystrophy in patients maintained on CAPD for more than three years. Perit Dial Bull 1983; 3: 81–6.
47. Gokal R, Ramos JM, Ellis HA et al. Histological renal osteodystrophy and 25 hydroxycholecalciferol and aluminum levels in patients on continuous ambulatory peritoneal dialysis. Kidney Int 1983; 23: 15–21.
48. Delmez JA, Fallon M, Bergfeld M, Gearing BN, Dougan C, Teitelbaum S. Continuous ambulatory peritoneal dialysis and bone. Kidney Int 1986; 30: 379–84.
49. Bucciante G, Bianchi M, Valenti G. Progress of renal osteodystrophy during CAPD. Clin Nephrol 1984; 6: 279–83.
50. Lindholm B, Bergstrom J. Nutritional aspects of CAPD. In: Gokal R (ed), Continuous ambulatory peritoneal dialysis. Edinburgh: Churchill Livingstone 1986: 228–64.
51. Sheikh MS, Maguire JA, Emmett M et al. Reduction of dietary phosphorus absorption by phosphorus binders. A theoretical, in vitro, and in vivo study. J Clin Invest 1989; 83: 66–73.
52. Ramirez JA, Emmett M, White MG et al. The absorption of dietary phosphorus and calcium in hemodialysis patients. Kidney Int 1986; 30: 753–9.
53. Davenport A, Goel S, MacKenzie JC. Audit of the use of calcium carbonate as phosphate binder in 100 patients treated with continuous ambulatory peritoneal dialysis. Nephrol Dial Transplant 1992; 7: 632–5.
54. Joffe P, Olsen F. Heaf J. Gammelgaard B, Pondephant J. Aluminium concentrations in serum dialysate, urine and bone among patients undergoing continuous ambulatory peritoneal dialysis. Clin Nephrol 1989; 32: 133–8.
55. Andreoli S, Briggs J, Junior B. Aluminium intoxication from aluminium containing phosphate binders in children with azotemia not undergoing dialysis. N Engl J Med 1984; 310: 1074–9.
56. Ackrill P, Day J, Ahmed R. Aluminium and iron overload in chronic dialysis. Kidney Int 1988; 33 (Suppl 24): S163–7.
57. Altmann P, Dhanesha U, Hamon C, Cunningham J, Blair J, Marsch F. Disturbance of cerebral function by aluminium in hemodialysis patients without overt aluminium toxicity. Lancet 1989; ii: 7–12.
58. Martis L, Serkes KD, Nolph KD. Calcium as a phosphate binder: is there a need to adjust peritoneal dialysate calcium concentration for patients using CaCO3. Perit Dial Int 1989; 9: 325–8.
59. Weinreich, T, Passlick-Deetjen J, Ziegelmayer C, Ritz E. Experience with low D-Calcium concentration in CAPD (LCa 1 mM) – A randomized controlled multicenter trail. Perit Dial Int 1993; 13 (Suppl 1): S38.
60. Cunningham J, Beer J, Coldwell RD, Noonan K, Sawyer N, Makin HLJ. Dialysate calcium reduction in CAPD patients treated with calcium carbonate and alfacalcidol. Nephrol Dial Transplant 1992; 7: 63–8.
61. Ritz E, Weinreich T, Matthias S. It is necessary to readjust dialysis calcium concentration. J Nephrol 1992; 5: 70–4.
62. Brown CB, Hamdy NAT, Boletis J, Kanis JA. Rationale for the use of low calcium solution in CAPD. In: La Greca G, Ronco C, Feriani M, Chiaramonte S, Conz P (eds), Peritoneal Dialysis: Proceedings of Fourth International Course on Peritoneal Dialysis. Milano: Wichtig Editore 1991: 125–37.
63. Hutchison AJ, Gokal R. Towards tailored dialysis fluids in CAPD the role of reduced calcium and magnesium in dialysis solution. Perit Dial Int 1992; 12: 199–203.
64. Piraino B, Perlmutter JA, Holley JL, Johnston JR, Bernardini J. The use of dialysate containing 2.5 mEq/l calcium in peritoneal dialysis patients. Perit Dial Int 1992; 12: 75–6.
65. Beer J, Tailor D, Noonan K, Cunningham J. Rapid exacerbation of hyperparathyroidism in patients converted to low calcium dialysate without adequate calcium supplementation. Perit Dial Int 1993; 13 (Suppl 1): S30.
66. Andersen KEH. Calcium transfer during intermittent peritoneal dialysis. Nephron 1981; 29: 63–7.
67. Schmitt H, Ittel TH, Schafer L, Sieberth HG. Effect of a low calcium dialysis solution on serum parathyroid hormone in automated peritoneal dialysis. Perit Dial Int 1993; 13 (Suppl 1): S59.
68. Putman J. The living peritoneum as a dialysis membrane. Am J Physiol 1923; 63: 548–65.
69. Cunningham RS. Studies on absorption from serious cavities. III. The effect of dextrose upon the peritoneal mesothelium. Am J Physiol 1920; 53: 458–88.
70. Palmer RA, Quinton WE, Gray JF et al. Prolonged peritoneal dialysis for chronic renal failure. Lancet 1964; i: 700–2.
71. Rubin J, Nolph KD, Popovich RP, Moncrief JW. Drainage volumes during continuous ambulatory peritoneal dialysis. ASAIO J 1979; 2: 54–60.
72. Gokal R. Mistry CD. Glucose polymer as osmotic agent in CAPD. In: La Greca G, Ronco C, Feriani M. Chiaramonte S, Conz P (eds), Peritoneal Dialysis: Proceedings of Fourth International Course on Peritoneal Dialysis. Milano: Wichtig Editore 1991: 119–23.
73. Twardowski ZJ, Khanna R, Nolph KD. Osmotic agents and ultrafiltration in peritoneal dialysis. Nephron 1986; 42: 93–101.
74. Mistry CD, Mallick NP, Gokal R. Ultrafiltration with an isosmotic solution during long peritoneal dialysis exchanges. Lancet 1987; ii: 178–82.
75. Mistry CD, Gokal R. New osmotic agents for peritoneal dialysis: where we are and where we're going Semin Dial 1991; 4: 9–12.
76. Pyle WK, Moncrief JW, Popovich RP, Peritoneal transport evaluation in CAPD. In: Moncrief JW,

Popovich RP (eds), CAPD Update. New York: Masson Publishing USA Inc. 1981: 35–52.
77. Ronco C. Feriani M, Chiaramonte S et al. Pathophysiology of ultrafiltration in peritoneal dialysis. Perit Dial Int 1990; 10: 119–26.
78. Maher JF, Bennett RR, Hirszel P, Chakrabarti E. The mechanism of dextrose-enhanced transport rates. Kidney Int 1985; 28: 16–20.
79. Krediet RT, Boeschoten EW, Zuyderhoudt FMJ, Arisz L. The relationship between peritoneal glucose absorption and body fluid loss by ultrafiltration during continuous ambulatory peritoneal dialysis. Clin Nephrol 1987; 27: 51–5.
80. Maher JF. Peritoneal transport rate: mechanisms, limitation and methods for augmentation. Kidney Int 1980; 18: S117–21.
81. Nolph KD, Mactier RA, Khanna R, Twardowski ZJ, Moore H, McGary T. The kinetics of ultrafiltration during peritoneal dialysis: the role of lymphatics. Kidney Int 1987; 32: 219–26.
82. Mactier RA, Khanna R, Twardowski ZJ, Moore H, Nolph KD. Contribution of lymphatic absorption to loss of ultrafiltration and solute clearances in CAPD. J Clin Invest 1987; 80: 1311–6.
83. Grodstein GP, Blumenkrantz MJ, Kopple JD, Moran JK, Coburn JW. Glucose absorption during continuous ambulatory peritoneal dialysis. Kidney Int 1981; 19: 564–7.
84. DeSanto NG, Capodicasa G, Senatore R et al. Glucose utilization from dialysate in patients on continuous ambulatory peritoneal dialysis. Int J Artif Organs 1978; 2: 119–24.
85. Lindholm B, Bergstrom J. Nutritional management of patients undergoing peritoneal dialysis. In: Nolph KD (ed), Dordrecht: Kluwer Academic Publishers 1989: 230–60.
86. Kreusch G, Bammatter F, Mordasini R, Binswanger U. Serum lipoprotein concentrations during continuous ambulatory peritoneal dialysis. In: Gahl GM, Kessel M, Nolph KD (eds), Advances in peritoneal dialysis. Amsterdam, Excerpta Medica 1981: 427–9.
87. Lindholm B, Karlander SG, Norbek HE, Furst P, Bergstrom J. Carbohydrate and lipid metabolism in CAPD patients. In: Atkins R, Thomson N, Farrell P (eds), Peritoneal dialysis. Edinburgh: Churchill Livingstone 1981: 198–210.
88. Von Baeyer H, Gahl GM, Riedinger H et al. Adaptation of CAPD patients to the continuous peritoneal energy uptake. Kidney Int 1983; 23: 29–34.
89. Boyer J, Gill GN, Epstein FH. Hyperglycemia and hyperosmolality complicating peritoneal dialysis. Ann Intern Med 1967; 67: 568–72.
90. Nolph KD, Rosenfeld PS, Powell JT, Danforth JR. Peritoneal glucose transport and hyperglycemia during peritoneal dialysis. Am J Med Sci 1970; 259: 272–81.
91. Heaton A, Johnston DG, Burrin JM et al. Carbohydrate and lipid metabolism during continuous ambulatory peritoneal dialysis: the effect of a single dialysis cycle. Clin Sci 1983; 65: 539–45.
92. Amstrong VW, Creutzfeldt W, Ebert R, Fuchs C, Hilgers R, Scheler F. Effect of dialysis glucose load on plasma and glucoregulatory hormones in CAPD patients. Nephron 1985; 39: 141–5.
93. Amstrong VW, Buschamnn U, Ebert R, Fuchs C, Rieger J, Scheler F. Biochemical investigations of CAPD: plasma levels of trace elements and amino acids and impaired glucose tolerance during the course of treatment, Int J Artif Organs 1980; 3: 237–41.
94. Oreopoulos DG, Marliss E, Anderson et al. Nutritional aspects of CAPD and the potential use of amino acid containing dialysis solutions. Perit Dial Bull 1983; 3: 10–5.
95. Wideroe TE, Smeby LC, Myking OL. Plasma concentrations and transperitoneal transport of native insulin and C-peptide in patients on continuous ambulatory peritoneal dialysis. Kidney Int 1984; 25: 82–7.
96. Lindholm B, Bergstrom J, Karlander SG. Glucose metabolism in patients on continuous ambulatory peritoneal dialysis. Trans Am Soc Artif Intern Organs 1981; 17: 58–60.
97. Lindholm b, Bergstrom J, Norbek HE. Lipoprotein (LP) metabolism in patients on continuous ambulatory peritoneal dialysis. In: Gahl GM, Kessel M, Nolph KD (eds), Advances in peritoneal dialysis. Amsterdam: Excerpta Medica 1981: 434–6.
98. Lindholm B, Karlander SG, Norbek HE, Bergstrom J. Glucose and lipid metabolism in peritoneal dialysis. In: La Greca G, Biasioli S, Ronco C (eds), Peritoneal Dialysis: Proceedings of First International Course on Peritoneal Dialysis. Milano: Wichtig Editore 1982: 219–30.
99. Gokal R, Ramos JM, McGurk JG, Ward MK, Kerr DNS. Hyperlipidaemia in patients on continuous ambulatory peritoneal dialysis: In: Gahl GM, Kessel M, Nolph KD (eds), Advances in peritoneal dialysis. Amsterdam: Excerpta Medica 1981: 430–3.
100. Roncari DAK, Breckenridge WC, Khanna R, Oreopoulos DG. Rise in high-density lipoprotein-cholesterol in some patients treated with CAPD. Perit Dial Bull 1981; 1: 136–7.
101. Ramos JM, Heaton A, McGurk JG, Ward MK, Kerr DNS. Sequential changes in serum lipids and their subfractions in patients receiving continuous ambulatory peritoneal dialysis. Nephron 1983; 35: 20–3.
102. Nolph KD, Ryan KL, Prowant B, Twardowski ZJ. A cross sectional assessment of serum vitamin D an triglyceride concentration in a CAPD population. Perit Dial Bull 1984; 4: 232–7.
103. Lindholm B, Norbek, HE. Serum lipids and lipoproteins during continuous ambulatory peritoneal dialysis. Acta Med Scand 1986; 220: 143–51.
104. Khanna R, Breckenridge WC, Roncari DAK, Digenis G, Oreopoulos DG. Lipids abnormalities in patients undergoing continuous ambulatory peritoneal dialysis. Perit Dial Bull 1986; 3: S13–5.
105. Duwe AK, Vas SI, Weatherhead JW. Effect of composition of peritoneal dialysis fluid on

chemiluminescence, phagocytosis and bactericidal activity in vitro. Infect Immunity 1981; 33: 130–5.
106. Verbrugh HA, Verkooyen RP, Verhoef J, Oe PL, van der Meulen J. Defective complement-mediated opsonization and lysis of bacteria in commercial peritoneal dialysis solution. In: Maher JF, Winchester JF (eds), Frontiers in Peritoneal Dialysis. New York: Field, Rich and Associates Inc 1986: 559–64.
107. Gallimore B, Gagnon RF, Stevenson MM. Cytotoxicity of commercial peritoneal dialysis solutions towards peritoneal cells of chronically uremic mice. Nephron 1986; 43: 283–9.
108. Topley N, Alobaidi HM, Davies M et al. The effect of dialysate on peritoneal phagocyte oxidative metabolism. Kidney Int 1988: 34: 404–11.
109. Van Bronswijk H, Verbrugh HA, Bos HJ et al. Cytotoxic effects of commercial continuous ambulatory peritoneal dialysis (CAPD) fluids and of bacterial exoproducts on human mesothelial cells in vitro. Perit Dial Int 1989; 9: 197–202.
110. Manahan FJ, Ing BL, Chan JC et al. Effect of bicarbonate containing versus lactate containing peritoneal dialysis solutions on superoxide production by human neutrophils. Artif Organs 1989; 13: 495–7.
111. Topley N, Mackenzie R, Petersen MM et al. In vitro testing of a potentially biocompatible continuous ambulatory peritoneal dialysis fluid. Nephrol Dial Transplant 1991; 6: 574–81.
112. Jorres A, Jorres D, Topley N, Gahl GM, Mahiout A. Leukotriene release from peripheral and peritoneal leukocytes following exposure to solutions for peritoneal dialysis. Nephrol Dial Transplant 1991; 6: 495–501.
113. Henderson IS, Couper IA, Lumsden A. Potentially irritant glucose in unused CAPD fluid. In: Maher JF, Winchester JF (eds), Frontiers in Peritoneal Dialysis. New York: Field, Rich and Associates, Inc. 1986: 261–4.
114. Henderson IS, Couper IA, Lumsden A. The effect of shelf-life of peritoneal dialysis fluid on ultrafiltration in CAPD. In: La Greca G, Chiaramonte S, Fabris A, Feriani M, Ronco C (eds), Peritoneal Dialysis: Proceedings of Second International Course on Peritoneal Dialysis. Milano: Wichtig Editore 1986: 85–6.
115. Dobbie JW, Lloyd JK, Gall CA. Categorization of ultrastructural changes in peritoneal mesothelium, stroma and blood vessels in uremia and CAPD patients. In: Khanna R, Nolph KD, Prowant, P, Twardowski ZJ. Oreopoulos DG (eds), Advances in Continuous Ambulatory Peritoneal Dialysis. Toronto: Peritoneal Dialysis Bulletin Inc. 1990: 3–12.
116. Dobbie JW. Pathogenesis of peritoneal fibrosing syndromes (sclerosing peritonitis) in peritoneal dialysis. Perit Dial Int 1992; 12: 14–27.
117. De Paepe M, Matthijs E, Peluso F, Dolkart R, Lameire N. Experience with glycerol as the osmotic agent in peritoneal dialysis in diabetic and non-diabetic patients. In: Keen H, Legrain M (eds), Prevention and Treatment of Diabetic Nephropathy. Boston: MTP Press Limited 1983: 299–313.
118. Heaton A, Ward MK, Johnston DG, Nicholson DV, Alberti KGMM, Kerr DNS. Short-term studies on the use of glycerol as an osmotic agent in continuous ambulatory peritoneal dialysis. Clin Sci 1984; 67: 121–30.
119. Matthys E, Dolkart R, Lameire N. Extended use of a glycerol-containing dialysate in diabetic CAPD patients. Perit Dial Bull 1987; 7: 10–15.
120. Daniels FH, Leonard EF, Cortell S. Glucose and glycerol compared as osmotic agents for peritoneal dialysis. Kidney Int 1984; 25: 20–5.
121. Lindholm B, Werynski A, Bergstrom J. Kinetic of peritoneal dialysis with glycerol and glucose as osmotic agents. Trans Am Soc Artif Intern Organs 1987; 33: 19–27.
122. Heaton A, Ward MK, Johnston DG, Alberti KGMM, Kerr DNS. Evaluation of glycerol as an osmotic agent for continuous ambulatory peritoneal dialysis in end-stage renal failure. Clin Sci 1986; 70: 23–9.
123. Matthys E, Dolkart R, Lameire N. Potential hazards of glycerol dialysate in diabetic CAPD patients. Perit Dial Bull 1987; 7: 16–9.
124. Hain H, Kessel M. Aspects of new solutions for peritoneal dialysis. Nephrol Dial Transplant 1987; 2: 67–72.
125. Gokal R, Mistry C. Osmotic agents in continuous ambulatory peritoneal dialysis. In: La Greca G, Chiaramonte S, Fabris A, Feriani M, Ronco C (eds), Peritoneal Dialysis: Proceedings of Third International Course on Peritoneal Dialysis. Milano: Wichtig Editore 1988: 61–5.
126. Goodship THJ, Heaton A, Wilkinson R, Ward MK. The use of glycerol as an osmotic agent in continuous ambulatory peritoneal dialysis. In: Ota K, Maher J, Winchester J. Hirszel P (eds), Current Concepts in Peritoneal Dialysis. Amsterdam: Excerpta Medica 1992: 143–7.
127. Faict D, Lameire N, Kesteloot D, Peluso F. Evaluation of peritoneal dialysis solutions with amino acids and glycerol in a rat model. Nephrol Dial Transplant 1991; 6: 120–4.
128. Faict D, Hartman JP, Lameire N, Kesteloot D, Peluso F. The evaluation of a peritoneal dialysis solution with amino acids and glycerol in a new rat model. Perit Dial Int 1990; 10 (Suppl 1): S60.
129. Bazzato G, Coli U, Landini S et al. Xylitol and low dosages of insulin: new perspectives for diabetic uremic patients on CAPD. Perit Dial Bull 1982; 2: 161–4.
130. Wu G. Osmotic agents for peritoneal dialysis solutions. Perit Dial Bull 1982; 2: 151–4.
131. Yatuc W, Ward G, Shipetar G, Tenckhoff H. Substitution of sorbitol for dextrose in peritoneal irrigation fluid. A preliminary report. Trans Am Soc Artif Intern Organs 1976; 13: 168–71.
132. Raja RM, Moros JG, Kramer MS, Rosenbaum JL. Hyperosmolal coma complicating peritoneal dialysis with sorbitol dialysate. Ann Intern Med 1970; 73: 993–4.

133. Bischel MC, Barbour BH. Peritoneal dialysis with sorbitol versus dextrose dialysate: clinical findings and alterations of blood and cerebrospinal fluid. Nephron 1974; 12: 449–63.
134. Vidt DG. Recommendations on choice of peritoneal dialysis solutions. Ann Intern Med 1973; 78: 144–6.
135. Robson MD, Levi J, Rosenfeld JB. Hyperglycemia and hyperosmolality in peritoneal dialysis. Its prevention by the use of fructose. Proc EDTA 1969; 6: 300–6.
136. Raja RS, Kramer MS, Manchanda R, Lazaro N, Rosenbaum JL. Peritoneal dialysis with fructose dialysate. Prevention of hyperglycemia and hyperosmolality. Ann Inter Med 1973; 79: 511–7.
137. Gjessing J. Addition of amino acids to peritoneal dialysis fluid. Lancet 1968; ii: 82–3.
138. Oreopoulos DG, Crassweller P, Katirtzoglou A et al. Amino acids as an osmotic agent (instead of glucose) in continuous ambulatory peritoneal dialysis. In: Legrain M (ed), Continuous Ambulatory Peritoneal Dialysis. Amsterdam: Excerpta Medica 1980: 335–40.
139. Williams PF, Marliss EB, Harvey Anderson G et al. Effective use of amino acid dialysate over four weeks in CAPD patients. Perit Dial Bull 1983; 3: 66–73.
141. Goodship THJ, Lloyd S, McKenzie PW et al. Short-term studies on the use of amino acids as an osmotic agent in continuous ambulatory peritoneal dialysis. Clin Sci 1987; 73: 471–8.
142. Lindholm B, Werynsky A, Bergstrom J. Peritoneal dialysis with amino acid solutions: fluid and solute transport kinetics. Artif Organs 1988; 12: 2–10.
143. Lindholm B, Traneus A, Werynski A, Osterberg T, Bergstrom J. Amino acids for peritoneal dialysis: technical and metabolic implications. In: La Greca G, Chiaramonte S, Fabris A, Feriani M, Ronco C (eds), Peritoneal Dialysis: Proceedings of Second International Course on Peritoneal Dialysis. Milano: Wichtig Editore 1986: 149–54.
144. Young GA, Dibble JB, Taylor AE, Kendall S, Brownjohn AM. A longitudinal study of the effects of amino acid-based CAPD fluid on amino acid retention and protein losses. Nephrol Dial Transplant 1989; 4: 900–905.
145. Young GA, Dibble JB, Brownjohn AM. The use of amino acid based CAPD fluid in chronic renal failure. In: Lubec, Rosenthal (eds), Amino Acids, Chemistry, Biology and Medicine: 850–7.
146. Steinhauer HB, Lubrich-Birker I, Kluthe R, Horl WH, Schollmeyer P. Amino acid dialysate stimulates peritoneal prostaglandin E2 generation in human. In: Khanna R, Nolph KD, Prowant BF, Twardowski ZJ, Oreopoulos DG (eds), Advances in Peritoneal Dialysis. Toronto: Peritoneal Dialysis Bulletin Inc. 1988: 21–6.
147. Pedersen FB. Alternate use of amino acid and glucose solutions in CAPD. Contrib Nephrol 1991; 89: 147–54.
148. Schilling H, Wu G, Petit J et al. Effects of prolonged CAPD with amino acid containing solutions in three patients. In: Khanna R, Nolph KD, Prowant BF, Twardowski ZJ, Oreopoulos DG (eds), Advances in Continuous Ambulatory Peritoneal Dialysis. Toronto: University of Toronto Press 1985: 49–55.
149. Schilling H, Wu G, Pettit J et al. Use of amino acid containing solutions in continuous ambulatory peritoneal dialysis patients after peritonitis: results of a prospective controlled trial. Proc EDTA-ERA 1985; 22: 421–5.
150. Dombros NV, Prutis K, Tong M et al. Six-month overnight intraperitoneal amino-acid infusion in continuous ambulatory peritoneal dialysis (CAPD) patients. No effect on nutritional status. Perit Dial Int 1990; 10: 79–84.
151. Lindholm B, Bergstrom J. Amino acids in CAPD solutions: lights and shadows. In: La Greca G, Ronco C, Feriani M, Chiaramonte S, Conz P (eds), Peritoneal Dialysis: Proceedings of Fourth International Course on Peritoneal Dialysis. Milano: Wichtig Editore 1991: 139–43.
152. Pedersen FB, Dragsholt C, Laier E et al. Alternate use of amino acid and glucose solutions in CAPD.
153. Young GA, Dibble JB, Hobson SM et al. The use of an amino-acid-based CAPD fluid over 12 weeks. Nephrol Dial Transplant 1989; 4: 285–2.
154. Dibble JB, Young GA, Hobson SM, Brownjohn AM. Amino-acid-based continuous ambulatory peritoneal dialysis (CAPD) fluid over twelve weeks: effects on carbohydrate and lipid metabolism. Perit Dial Int 1990; 10: 71–7.
155. Bruno M, Bagins C, Marangella M et al. CAPD with an amino acid solution: a long-term, crossover study. Kidney Int 1989; 35: 1189–94.
156. Arfeen S, Goodship THJ, Kirkwood A, Ward MK. The nutritional/metabolic and hormonal effects of 8 weeks of continuous ambulatory peritoneal dialysis with a 1% amino acid solution. Clin Nephrol 1990; 33: 192–9.
157. Scanziani R, Dozio B, Iacuitti G, CAPD in diabetics: use of amino acids. In: Ota K, Maher J, Winchester J, Hirszel P (eds), Current concepts in peritoneal dialysis. Amsterdam: Excerpta Medica 1993: 1992: 628–32.
158. Lindholm B, Bergstrom J. Nutritional aspects on peritoneal dialysis. Kidney Int 1992; 42 (Suppl 38): S165–71.
159. Jones MR, Martis L, Algrim CE et al. Amino acid solutions for CAPD: rationale and clinical experience. Miner Electrolyte Metab 1992; 18: 309–15.
160. Bernard D, Kopple JD, Brunori G et al. Nutritional benefit of intraperitoneal (IP) amino acids (AA) in CAPD patients. (abstract) 6th Int Congr on Nutrition and Metabolism in Renal Disease, Harrogate, UK, August 1991.
161. Lazarus-Barlow WAS. Observations upon the initial rates of osmosis of certain substances in water and in fluids containing albumen. J Physiol 1895-6; 19: 140–66.
162. Hain H, Ghal G. Osmotic agent. An update. Contrib Nephrol 1991; 89: 119–27.
163. Daniels FH, Nedev ND, Cataldo T, Leonard EF, Cortell S. The use of polyelectrolytes as osmotic

agent for peritoneal dialysis. Kidney Int 1988; 33: 925–9.
164. Struijk DG, Bakker JC, Krediet RT, Koomen GCM, Stekkinger P, Arisz L. Effect of intraperitoneal administration of two different batches of albumin solutions on peritoneal solute transport in CAPD patients. Nephrol Dial Transplant 1991; 6: 198–202.
165. Nolph KD, Hopkins C, Rubin J et al. Polymer induced ultrafiltration in dialysis: high osmotic pressure due to impermeant polymer sodium. Trans Am Soc Artif Intern Organs 1978: 24; 162–7.
166. Rubin J, Nolph KD, McGary TJ. Osmotic ultrafiltration with dextran sodium sulfate: potential for use in peritoneal dialysis. J Dialysis 1979; 3: 251–64.
167. Twardowski ZJ, Moore HL, McGary TJ, Poskuta M, Stathakis C, Hirszel P. Polymers as osmotic agent for peritoneal dialysis. Perit Dial Bull 1984; 4 (Suppl 3): S125–31.
168. Frank HA, Seligman AM, Fine J. Further experiences with peritoneal irrigation for acute renal failure. Ann Surg 1948; 128: 561–608.
169. Twardowski ZJ, Hain H, McGary TJ, Moore HL, Keller RS. Sustained UF with gelatin dialysis solution during long dwell dialysis exchanges in rats. In: Maher JF, Winchester JF (eds), Frontiers is in peritoneal dialysis. New York: Field, Rich and Associates, Inc. 1986: 249–54.
170. Ring J, Messmer K. Incidence and severity of anaphylactoid reactions to colloid substitutes. Lancet 1977; ii: 466–9.
171. Gjessing J. The use of dextran as a dialysing fluid in peritoneal dialysis. Acta Med Scand 1969; 1985: 237–9.
172. Hain H, Schutte W. Pustelnik A, Gahl G, Kessel M. Ultrafiltration and absorption characteristics of hydroxyethylstarch and dextran during long dwell peritoneal dialysis exchanges in rat. In: Khanna R, Nolph KD, Prowant BF, Twardowski ZJ, Oreopoulos DG (eds), Advances in peritoneal dialysis. Toronto: Peritoneal Dialysis Bulletin Inc. 1989: 28–30.
173. Hain H, Kempf D, Schnell P, Gahl G, Kessel M. Ultrafiltration patterns of dextran and hydroxyethylstarch during long dwell peritoneal dialysis exchanges in nonuremic rats. In: Avram MM, Giordano C (eds), Ambulatory Peritoneal Dialysis. New York: Plenum Publishing Corporation 1990: 83–6.
174. Bergonzi G, Paties C, Vassallo G et al. Dextran deposit in tissues of patients undergoing hemodialysis. Nephrol Dial Transplant 1990; 5: 54–8.
175. Dienes HP, Gerharz CD, Wagner R, Weber M, John HD. Accumulation of hydroxyethyl starch (HES) in the liver of patients with renal failure and portal hypertension. J Hepatol 1986; 3: 223–7.
176. Higgins JT, Gross ML, Somani P. Patient tolerance and dialysis effectiveness of a glucose polymer-containing peritoneal dialysis solution. Perit Dial Bull 1984; 4: S131–3.
177. Winchester JF, Stegink LD, Ahman S et al. A comparison of glucose polymer and dextrose as osmotic agents in CAPD. In: Maher JF, Winchester JF (eds), Frontiers in Peritoneal Analysis. New York: Field, Rich and Associates, Inc. 1986: 231–40.
178. Winchester JF. Alternative osmotic agents to dextrose for peritoneal dialysis. In: La Greca G, Chiaramonte S, Fabris A, Feriani M, Ronco C (eds), Peritoneal Dialysis: Proceedings of Second International Course on Peritoneal Dialysis. Milano: Wichtig Editore 1986: 135–42.
179. Mistry CD, Gokal R, Mallick NP. Glucose polymer as an osmotic agent in CAPD. In: Maher JF, Winchester JF (eds), Frontiers in Peritoneal Dialysis. New York: Field, Rich and Associates, Inc. 1986: 241–8.
180. Mistry CD, Mallick NP, Gokal R. The advantage of glucose polymer as an osmotic agent in continuous peritoneal dialysis. Proc Eur Dial Transpl Assoc 1985; 22: 415–20.
181. Mistry CD, Mallick NP, Gokal R. The use of large molecular weight polymer (MW 20,000) as an osmotic agent in continuous ambulatory peritoneal dialysis (CAPD). In: Khanna R, Nolph KD, Prowant BF, Twardowski ZJ, Oreopoulos DG (eds), Advances in Peritoneal Dialysis. Toronto: Peritoneal Dialysis Bulletin Inc. 1986: 7–11.
182. Mistry CD, Gokal R. The use of hyposmolar glucose polymer solution in continuous ambulatory peritoneal dialysis. In: Avram MM, Giordano C (eds), Ambulatory peritoneal dialysis. New York: Plenum Publishing Corporation 1990: 83–6.
183. Mistry CD, Gokal R. Single daily use (12 h dwell) of 7.5% glucose polymer (m wt 18,700; Mn 7,300) + 0.35% glucose solution: a 3 month study. Nephrol Dial Transplant 1993; 8: 443–7.
184. Mistry CD, Gokal R, Peers E. Midas Study group. Results of a randomized multicentre, prospective study of Dextran 20 in CAPD patients. Kidney Int (in press).
185. de Fijter CWH, Oe PL, Verbrugh HA et al. Glucose polymers as osmotic agent in CAPD fluid: a more favorable effect on peritoneal macrophage (PMO) function than glucose-based solutions. Kidney Int 1991; 40: 978.
186. Jorres A, Gahl GM, Ludat K. Passlick-Deetjen J. CAPD dialysate inhibit cytokine production in PBMC activated with Staph. Epidermidis (S.epi): partial restoration by alternative PD fluids. Perit Dial Int 1993; 13 (Suppl 1): S56.
187. Mistry CD, Gokal R. The use of glucose polymer in CAPD: essential physiological and clinical conclusions: In: Ota K, Maher J, Winchester J, Hirszel P (eds), Current Concepts in Peritoneal Dialysis. Amsterdam: Excerpta Medica 1992: 138–42.
188. Mistry CD, Fox JE, Mallick NP, Gokal R. Circulating maltose and isomaltose in chronic renal failure. Kidney Int 1987; 32 (Suppl 22): S210–4.
189. Schildt B, Bouveng R, Sollenberg M. Plasma substitute induced impairment of reticuloendothelial system function. Acta Chir Scand 1975; 141: 7–13.
190. Klein E, Ward RA, Williams TE, Feldhoff PW.

Peptides as substitute osmotic agent for glucose in peritoneal dialysis. Trans Am Soc Artif Intern Organs 1989; 32: 550–3.
191. Imholz ALT, Lameire N, Faict D, Koomen GCM, Krediet RT, Martis L. Evaluation of short-chain polypeptides as an osmotic agent in CAPD patients. Perit Dial Int 1993; 13 (Suppl 1): S62.
192. La Greca G, Fabris A, Feriani M, Chiaramonte S, Ronco C. Acid base homeostasis in clinical dialysis. In: Maher JF (ed), Replacement of Renal Function by Dialysis. Dordrecht: Kluwer Academic Publisher 1989: 807–26.
193. La Greca G, Biasioli S, Chiaramonte S et al. Acid base balance on peritoneal dialysis. Clin Nephrol 1981; 16: 1–7.
194. Boen ST. Kinetics of peritoneal dialysis. Medicine 1961; 40: 243–387.
195. Preuss HG. Biochemistry of bicarbonate, lactate and acetate in man. North Med Proc 1977; 1: 1–9.
196. Boen ST, Mulinari AS, Dillard DH, Scribner BH. Periodic peritoneal dialysis in the management of chronic uremia. Trans Am Soc Artif Intern Organs 1962; 8: 256–62.
197. Biasioli S, Feriani M, Chiaramonte S, La Greca G. Buffers in peritoneal dialysis. Int J Artif Organs 1987; 10: 3–8.
198. Kveim M, Nesbakken R. Utilization of exogenous acetate during hemodialysis. Trans Am Soc Artif Intern Organs 1975; 21: 138–42.
199. La Greca G, Biasioli S, Brendolan A et al. Buffer balance in peritoneal dialysis. In: La Greca G, Biasioli S, Ronco C (eds), Peritoneal Dialysis: Proceedings of First International Course on Peritoneal Dialysis. Milano: Wichtig Editore 1982: 177–87.
200. Faller B, Marichal JF. Loss of ultrafiltration in CAPD: a role for acetate. Perit Dial Bull 1984; 4: 10–3.
201. Slingeneyer A, Mion C, Mourad G et al. Progressive sclerosing peritonitis. A late and severe complication of maintenance peritoneal dialysis. Trans Am Soc Artif Intern Organs 1983; 29: 633–6.
202. Brin M. The synthesis and metabolism of lactic acid isomers. Ann NY Acad Sci 1965; 119: 942–56.
203. Searle GL, Cavalieri RR, Determination of lactate kinetics in the human analysis of data from single injection. Proc Soc Exp Biol Med 1972; 139: 1002–11.
204. Fabris A, Biasioli S, Chiaramonte S et al. Buffer metabolism in CAPD: relationship with respiratory dynamics. Trans Am Soc Artif Intern Organs 1982; 28: 270–5.
205. Teehan BP, Schleifer CR, Reichard GA, Cupit MC, Sigler MH, Haff AC. Acid base studies in continuous ambulatory peritoneal dialysis. In: Moncrief JW, Popovich RP (eds), CAPD Update. New York: Masson Publishing USA Inc. 1981: 95–102.
206. Richardson RMA, Roscoe JM. Bicarbonate, L-lactate and D-lactate balance in intermittent peritoneal dialysis. Perit Dial Bull 1986; 6: 178–85.
207. Nolph KD, Twardowski ZJ, Khanna R et al. Tidal peritoneal dialysis with racemic or L-lactate solutions. Perit Dial Int 1990; 10: 161–4.
208. Robson MD, Faivoseviz A, Malmoud H. Physiological transfer of acid base. In: Legrain M (ed), Continuous Ambulatory Peritoneal Dialysis. Amsterdam: Excerpta Medica 1980: 194–8.
209. Rubin J, Adair C, Johnson B, Bower JD. Stereospecific lactate absorption during peritoneal dialysis. Nephron 1982; 31: 224–8.
210. Fine A. Metabolism of D-lactate in the dog and in man. Perit Dial Int 1989; 9: 99–101.
211. Feriani M, Biasioli S, Borin D et al. Bicarbonate buffer for CAPD solution. Trans Am Soc Artif Intern Organs 1985; 31: 668–71.
212. Nissenson AR. Acid base homeostasis in peritoneal dialysis patients. Int J Artif Organs 1984; 7: 175–6.
213. Gennari FJ, Cohen JJ, Kassirer JP. Normal acid base values. In: Cohen JJ, Kassirer JP (eds), Acid/Base. Boston: Little, Brown and Company 1982: 107–10.
214. Yamamoto T, Sakakura T, Yamakawa M et al. Clinical effects of long-term use of neutralized dialysate for continuous ambulatory peritoneal dialysis. Nephron 1992; 60: 324–9.
215. May RC, Kelly RA, Mitch WE. Mechanisms for defects in muscle protein metabolism in rats with chronic uremia. J Clin Invest 1987; 79: 1099–103.
216. Williams B, Hattersley J, Layward E, Walls J. Metabolic acidosis and skeletal muscle adaptation to low protein diets in chronic uremia. Kidney Int 1991; 40: 779–86.
217. Papadoyannakis NJ, Stefanidis CJ, McGeown M. The effect of the correction of metabolic acidosis on nitrogen and potassium balance of patients with chronic renal failure. Am J Clin Nutr 1984; 40: 623–7.
218. Frohlich ED. Vascular effects of the Krebs intermediate metabolites. Am J Physiol 1965; 208: 149–56.
219. Kirkendol PL, Devia CJ, Bower JD et al. Comparison of the cardiovascular effects of sodium acetate, sodium bicarbonate and other potential sources of fixed base in hemodialysis solutions. Trans Am Soc Artif Intern Organs 1977; 23: 399–404.
220. Veech RL. The untoward effects of the anions of dialysis fluid. Kidney Int 1988; 34: 587–97.
221. Veech RL. The toxic impact of parenteral solutions on the metabolism of cells: a hypothesis for physiological parenteral therapy: Am J Clin Nutr 1986; 44: 519–51.
222. Sistare FD, Haynes RC. The interaction between the cytosolic pyridine nucleotide redox potential and gluconeogensis from lactate/pyruvate in isolated rate hepatocytes. J Biol Chem 1985; 23: 12748–53.
223. Oh MS, Phelpo KR, Traube M et al. D-lactic acidosis in a man with the short bowel syndrome. N Engl J Med 1979; 301: 249–52.
224. Veech RL, Fowler RC. Cerebral dysfunction and respiratory alkalosis during peritoneal dialysis with D-lactate containing dialysis fluid. Am J Med 1986; 82: 572–3.

225. Ing TS, Quon MJ, Daugirdas JT, Ghandi VC, Epstain MB. Preparation of bicarbonate containing peritoneal dialysate using an automated dialysate delivery system. Int J Artif Organs 1981; 4: 148–9.
226. Ing TS, Quon MJ, Daugirdas JT, Liu P, Gandhi VC, Reid RR. On line preparation of bicarbonate containing dialysate for use in peritoneal dialysis. Int J Artif Organs 1981; 4: 308–9.
227. Ing TS, Humayun HM, Daugirdas JT et al. Preparation of bicarbonate-containing dialysate for peritoneal dialysis. Int J Artif Organs 1983; 6: 217–8.
228. Ing TS, Ghandi VC, Daugirdas JT, Reid RW, Hunt J, Popli S. Peritoneal dialysis using bicarbonate buffered dialysate. Int J Artif Organs 1984; 7: 166–8.
229. Feriani M, Biasioli S, Borin D et al. Bicarbonate solutions for peritoneal dialysis: a reality. Int J Artif Organs 1985; 8: 57–8.
230. Feriani M, La Greca G. CAPD with bicarbonate solution. In: Horl WH, Schollmeyer PJ (eds), New Perspectives in Hemodialysis, Peritoneal Dialysis, Arteriovenous Hemofiltration and Plasmapheresis. New York: Plenum Publishing Corporation 1989: 139–47.
231. Feriani M, Reinhard B, La Greca G. Calcium carbonate precipitation in oversatured bicarbonate containing CAPD solutions. In: La Greca G, Ronco C, Feriani M, Chiaramonte S, Conz P (eds), Peritoneal Dialysis: Proceedings of Fourth International Course on Peritoneal Dialysis. Milano: Wichtig Editore 1991: 145-51.
232. Gretz N, Kraft E, Meisinger E, Lasserre J, Strauch M. Calcium deposits due to bicarbonate containing CAPD solutions? In: Khanna R, Nolph KD, Prowant BF, Twardowski ZJ. Oreopoulos DG (eds), Advances in Peritoneal Dialysis. Toronto: Peritoneal Dialysis Bulletin Inc. 1988: 220–3.
233. Feriani M, Biasioli S, Barbacini S et al. Acid base correction in bicarbonate CAPD patients. In: Khanna R, Nolph KD, Prowant BF, Twardowski, ZJ. Oreopoulos DG (eds), Advances in Peritoneal Dialysis. Toronto: Peritoneal Dialysis Bulletin Inc. 1989: 191–4.
234. Feriani M, Dissegna D, La Greca G, Passlick-Deetjen J. Short term clinical study with bicarbonate containing peritoneal dialysis solution. Perit Dial Int 1994: (in press).
235. Di Paolo N, Grarosi G, Traversari L, Di Paolo M. Mesothelial biocompatibility of PD solutions. Perit Dial Int. 1993; 13 (Suppl 2): S109–12.
236. Jorres A, Gahl GM, Ludat K, Muller C, Passlick-Deetjen J. In vitro biocompatibility testing of a new bicarbonate buffered dialysis fluid for CAPD. Perit Dial Int 1992; 12: S26.
237. Andre A, Egle B, Dobos GH, Lubrich-Birkner I, Schollmeyer P, Steinhauer HB. Comparison of lactate and bicarbonate buffered peritoneal dialysate (PD) fluids: effect on human peritoneal macrophages (PMO). Perit Dial Int 1993; 13 (Suppl 1): S24.
238. Schambye HT, Flesner P, Pedersen RB et al. Bicarbonate-versus lactate-based CAPD fluids: a biocompatibility study in rabbits. Perit Dial Int 1992; 12: 281–6.
239. Yatzidis H. A new stable bicarbonate dialysis solution fr peritoneal dialysis: preliminary report. Perit Dial Int 1991; 11: 224–7.
240. Slingeneyer A, Faller B, Michel C, Przybylski C, Rolland R, Mion C. Increased ultrafiltration capacity using a new bicarbonate CAPD solution. Perit Dial Int 1993; 13 (Suppl 1): S57.
241. Slingeneyer A, Przybylski C, Rolland R, Mion C. A new bicarbonate buffered solution for CAPD. Perit Dial Int 1993; 13 (Suppl 1): S57.
242. Oreopoulos DG, Zellerman G, Izatt S. The Toronto ambulatory peritoneal dialysis connector. In: Legrain M (ed), Continuous Ambulatory Peritoneal Dialysis. Amsterdam: Excerpta Medica 1980: 73–8.
243. Nakamura Y, Hara Y, Ishida H, Morikawa K, Shigento K. A randomized trial to evaluate the effects of UV flash system on peritonitis rates in CAPD. In: Khanna R, Nolph KD, Prowant B, Twardowski ZJ, Oreopoulos DG (eds), Adv Perit Dial. Toronto: Peritoneal Dialysis Bulletin Inc. 1992; 8: 313–5.
244. Strauss FG, Holmes DL, Dennis RL, Nortman DF. Pre-spiking dialysate bags: improved peritonitis in patients on peritoneal dialysis. Adv Perit Dial 1991; 7: 193–5.
245. Scalamogna A, DeVecchi A, Castelnovo C et al. Long-term incidence of peritonitis in CAPD patients treated with the Y set technique: experience in a single center. Nephron 1990; 55: 24–7.
246. Burkart JM, Hylander B, Durnell-Figel T, Roberts D. Comparison of peritonitis rates during long-term use of standard spike versus ultraset in continuous ambulatory peritoneal dialysis. Perit Dial Int 1990; 10: 41–3.
247. Piraino B, Bernardini J, Sorkin MI. The effect of the Y-set on catheter infection rates in continuous ambulatory peritoneal dialysis patients. Am J Kidney Dis 1990; 16: 46–50.
248. Swartz R, Reynolds J, Lees P et al. Disconnect during continuous ambulatory peritoneal dialysis (CAPD): retrospective experience with three different systems. Perit Dial Int 1989; 9: 175–8.
249. Rottembourg J, Brouard R, Issad B, Allouache M, Nguyen J, Montassine MC, Kirstein E, Jacobs C. Prevention of peritonitis during continuous ambulatory peritoneal dialysis. Value of disconnect systems. Presse Med 1988; 17: 1349–53.
250. Bonnardeaux A, Ouimet D, Galarneau A et al. Peritonitis in continuous ambulatory peritoneal dialysis: impact of a compulsory switch from a standard to a y-connector system in a single North American Center. Am J Kidney Dis 1992; 19: 364–70.
251. Owen JE, Walker RG, Lemon J, Brett L, Mitrou D, Becker GJ. Randomized study of peritonitis with conventional versus O-Set techniques in continuous ambulatory peritoneal dialysis. Peritoneal Dial Int 1992; 12: 216–20.
252. Port FK, Held PJ, Nolph KD, Turenne MN, Wolfe

RA. Risk of peritonitis and technique failure by CAPD connection techniques. Kidney Int 1992, 42: 967–74.
253. Bailie GR, Rasmussen R, Hollister A, Eisele G. Incidence of CAPD peritonitis in patients using UVXD or O-set systems. Clin Nephrol 1990; 33: 252–4.
254. Junor BJR. CAPD disconnect systems. Blood Purif 1989; 7: 156–66.
255. Villano R. Multicenter registry of patients using the "O" set system for CAPD. In: Khanna R, Nolph KD, Prowant B, Twardowski ZJ, Oreopoulos DG (eds), Adv Perit Dial. Toronto: Peritoneal Dialysis Bulletin Inc. 1988: 304–7.
256. Ryckelynck JP, Verger C, Cam G, Faller B, Pierre D. Importance of the flush effect in disconnect systems. Adv Perit Dial, Proc 8th Annual CAPD Conf, Kansas City 1988; 4: 282–4.
257. Lempert KD, Kolb JA, Swartz RD, Campese V, Golper T, Winchester JF, Nolph KD, Husserl FE, Zimmerman SW, Kurtz SB, Mars R. A Multicenter Trial to Evaluate the Use of the CAPD "O" Set. Trans Am Soc Artif Intern Organs 1986; 32: 557–9.
258. Maiorca R, Cancarini GC. Experiences with the Y-system. In: Twardowski ZJ, Nolph KD, Khanna R (eds), Contemporary Issues in Nephrology: Peritoneal Dialysis 1990; 22: 167–73.
259. Catizone L, Zucchelli A, Gagliardini R, Zuccheli P. Long-term experience with the Y-connector in peritonitis prevention in continuous ambulatory peritoneal dialysis. In: Avram MM, Giordano C (eds), Ambulatory Peritoneal Dialysis. New York and London: Plenum Medical Book Co. 1990: 213–7.
260. Churchill DN, Taylor DW, Vas SI et al. Peritonitis in continuous ambulatory peritoneal dialysis (CAPD): a multicenter randomised clinical trial comparing the y-connector disinfectant system to standard systems. Perit Dial Int 1989; 9: 159–63.
261. Viglino G, Colombo A, Scalamonga A et al. Prospective randomized study of two Y devices in continuous ambulatory peritoneal dialysis (CAPD). Perit Dial Int 1989; 9: 165–8.
262. Maiorca R, Cancarini GC, Brasa S, Colombrita D, Manili L, Camerini C. Y-System with disinfectant in the prevention of peritonitis in CAPD. Contrib Nephrol 1987; 57: 178–84.
263. Maiorca R, Cancarini G, Manili L, Brasa S, Camerini C. Y-Connector with Amuchina in the prevention of peritonitis. In: La Greca G, Chiaramonte S, Fabris A, Feriani M, Ronco C (eds), Peritoneal Dialysis. Milano: Wichtig Editore 1986: 185–8.
264. Cantaluppi A, Scalamongna A, Guerra L, Casteinovo C, Graziani G, Ponticelli C. Peritonitis prevention in CAPD: efficacy of a Y-connector and disinfectant. In: Maher JF, Winchester JF (eds), Frontiers in Peritoneal Dialysis. New York: Field and Rich 1986: 198–202.
265. Maiorca R, Cantaluppi A, Cancarini GC, Scalamogna A, Broccoli R, Raziani Brasa S, Ponticelli C. Prospective controlled trial of a Y connector and disinfectant to prevent peritonitis in continuous ambulatory peritoneal dialysis. Lancet 1983; 2: 642–4.
266. Buoncristiani U, Carobi C, Cozzari M et al. Abatement of exogenous peritonitis risk using the Perugia CAPD system. Dial Transplant 1983 12: 14–25.
267. Buoncristiani U. Optimization of the "Y" set. In: La Greca G, Ronco C, Feriani M, Chiaramonte S, Conz P (eds), Peritoneal Dialysis. Milan: Wichtig Editore 1991: 279–93.
268. Viglino G, Cantaluppi, Gandolfo C, Peluso F, Cavalli PL. Y-Set evolution. In: La Greca G, Ronco C, Feriani M, Chiaramonte S, Conz P (eds), Peritoneal Dialysis. Milano: Wichtig Editore 1991: 281–93.
269. Bazzato G, Coli U, Landini S, Fracasso A, Morachiello P, Righetto F, Scanferia F. The double bag system for CAPD reduces the peritonitis rate. Trans Am Soc Artif Intern Organs 1984; 30: 690–2.
270. Bazzato G. CAPD by means of double bag, closed drainage infusion system. CAPD. Proc Int Symp Paris 1979. Amsterdam: Excerpta Medica 1980: 171–3.
271. Luzar MA, Slingeneyer A, Cantaluppi, Peluso F. In vitro study of flush effect of two reusable continuous ambulatory peritoneal dialysis (CAPD) disconnect systems. Perit Dial Bull 1989; 9: 169–72.
272. Verger C, Luzar MA. In vitro study of CAPD Y line systems. In: Khanna R, Nolph KD, Prowant B, Twardowski ZJ, Oreopoulos DG (eds), Adv Perit Dial. Toronto: Peritoneal Dialysis Bulletin Inc. 1986: 160–4.
273. Suki WN, Walshe J, Ashbrook DW et al. Multicenter evaluation of a bagless CAPD system. Trans Am Soc Artif Intern Organs 1986; 32: 572–4.
274. Diaz-Buxo JA, Walshe JJ, Flanigan M. Multicenter experience with Y-set CAPD system (Freedom set). Perit Dial Bull 1987; 7: S23.
275. Montenegro J, Gonzalez R, Martinez I, Saracho R. A new non-disconnect Y-system (ANDY) for CAPD. In: Ota K, Maher JF, Winchester JF, Hirszel P (eds), Current Concepts in Peritoneal Dialysis. Amsterdam: Excerpta Medica 1992: 205–8.
276. Lewis J, Abbott J, Crompton K, Fowler I, Smith B. CAPD disconnect systems UK peritonitis experience. In: Khanna R, Nolph KD, Prowant B, Twardowski ZJ, Oreopoulos DG (eds), Adv Perit Dial. Toronto: Peritoneal Dialysis Bulletin Inc. 1992; 8: 306–12.
277. Balteau PR, Peluso FP, Coles GA et al. Design and testing of the Baxter integrated disconnect system. Perit Dial Int 1991; 11: 131–6.
278. Honkanen E, Kala A-R, Gronhangen-Riska C. Divergent etiologies of CAPD peritonitis in double bag and traditional systems. In: Khanna R, Nolph KD, Prowant B, Twardowski ZJ, Oreopoulos DG (eds), Adv Perit Dial. Toronto: Peritoneal Dialysis Bulletin Inc. 1991: 129–32.

279. Dryden MS, McCann M, Wing AJ, Phillips L. Controlled trial of a Y-set delivery system to prevent peritonitis in patients receiving continuous ambulatory peritoneal dialysis. J Hosp Infect 1992; 20: 185–92.
280. Bazzatto G, Coli U, Landini S et al. Closter: a new connection for double-bag system to prevent peritonitis. Perit Dial Bull 1986; 7: 138–40.
282. Nolph KD, Prowant B, Serkes KD et al. A randomized multicenter trial to evaluate the effects of an ultraviolet germicidal system on peritonitis rate in continuous ambulatory peritoneal dialysis. Perit Dial Bull 1985; 5: 19–24.
283. Tapson JS, Hepplewhite PM, Wilkinson, R. Experience with the Travenol ultraviolet germicidal exchange system. Contrib Nephrol 1987; 57: 167–71.
284. Boeschoten EW, Southwood J, Struijk DG, Kredeit RT, Arisz L. Prevention of peritonitis: filter or UV system? Contrib Nephrol 1987; 57: 158–66.
285. Steinhauer HB, Keck I, Lubrich-Birkner I, Schollmeyer P. Randomized clinical trial comparing a heat sterilization system (Thermoclav) to standard connector systems in prevention of CAPD – associated peritonitis. In: La Greca G, Ronco C, Feriani M, Chiaramonte S, Conz P (eds), Peritoneal Dialysis. Milano: Wichtig Editore 1991: 275–81.
286. Olivas E, Jimenez C, Lopez A, Andres E, Sanchez Tarraga L. Reduction of the incidence of peritonitis in CAPD: effectiveness of heat sterilization of safelock connection. Contrib Nephrol 1991; 89: 62–7.
287. Hamilton R, Charytan C, Kurtz S, Ogden D, Rakowski T, Schreiber M, Sorkin M, Suki W, Winchester J, Adam P, Caruana R, Burkart J, Vidt D, Piraino, Silver M, Argy W. Reduction in peritonitis frequency by the Dupont sterile connection device. Trans Am Soc Artif Intern Organs 1985; 31: 651–4.
288. Ota K. Clinical experience in CAPD using Flamelock device: a group study. In: Maher JF, Winchester JF (eds), Frontiers in Peritoneal Dialysis. New York: Field and Rich 1986: 161–5.
289. Slingeneyer A, Mion C. Peritonitis prevention in CAPD. Seven years experience in Montpellier. In: La Greca G, Chiaramonte S, Fabris A, Feriani M, Ronco C (eds), Peritoneal Dialysis. Milano: Wichtig Editore 1986: 191–2.
290. Rotellar C, Winchester JF, Ash SR. Long term use of unidirectional bacteriologic filters to reduce peritonitis frequency in CAPD. In: Maher JF, Winchester JF (eds), Frontiers in Peritoneal Dialysis. New York: Field and Rich 1986: 203–6.
291. Slingeneyer A, Mion C. Peritonitis prevention in continuous ambulatory peritoneal dialysis: long-term efficacy of a bacteriologic filter. Proc Eur Dial Transplant Assoc 1983; 19: 388–95.
292. Winchester JF, Ash SR, Bousquet G, Rakowski TA, Barnard WF, Heeter E, Haley S. Successful peritonitis reduction with an unidirectional bacteriologic filter. Trans Am Soc Artif Intern Organs 1983; 29: 611–5.
293. Vas SI. Etiology and treatment of peritonitis. Trans Am Soc Artif Intern Organs 1984; 30: 682–4.
294. Sarles HE, Lindley JD, Fish JC et al. Peritoneal dialysis using a Millipore filter. Kidney Int 1976; 16: 54–6.
295. Mion C, Slingeneyer A, Liendo-Liendo C. Reduction in incidence of peritonitis associated with continuous ambulatory peritoneal dialysis. Proc Clin Dial Transplant Forum 1979; 9: 9–13.
296. Slingeneyer A, Mion C. Peritonitis prevention in CAPD. Long-term efficacy of a bacteriological filter. Proc Eur Dial Transplant Assoc 1983; 19: 388–95.
297. Ash SR, Winchester JF. Effect of the Peridex filter on peritonitis rates in an unselected CAPD population. Perit Dial Bull 1984; 4 (Suppl): S118–20.
298. Popovich RP, Moncrief JW, "P" Sorrels-Akar AJ, Mullins-Blackinson CV, Pyle K. The ultraviolet germicidal system: the elimination of distal contamination in CAPD. In: Maher JF, Winchester JF (eds), Frontiers in Peritoneal Dialysis. New York: Field and Rich 1986: 169–76.
299. Kubey W, Holmes CJ. The relationship between ultraviolet light absorbance of peritoneal dialysate and the effectiveness of mercury vapor and xenon flash disinfection devices for CAPD. In: Ota K, Maher JF, Winchester JF, Hirszel P (eds), Current Concepts in Peritoneal Dialysis. Amsterdam: Excerpta Medica 1992: 223–7.
300. Bielawa RJ, Carr KL, Bousquet GG. Intraluminal thermosterilization using a microwave autoclave. In: Maher JF, Winchester JF (eds), Frontiers in Peritoneal Dialysis. New York: Field and Rich 1986: 166–8.
301. Thomae U. Heat sterilisation of Safe-Lock®Connectors using the Thermocalve®. Contrib Nephrol 1987; 57: 172–7.
302. Nillson-Thorell CB, Wieslander AP, Muscalu N, Andren AHG, Kjellstrand PTT. Heat sterilization of fluids for peritoneal dialysis gives rise to aldehydes. Peritoneal Dial Int 1993; 13: 208–13.

9 Peritoneal dialysis access and exit site care

ZBYLUT J. TWARDOWSKI AND RAMESH KHANNA

1. Introduction 272
2. Historical perspective 272
3. Glossary 274
4. Factors influencing catheter complications 274
   4.1. Tissue reaction to a foreign body penetrating skin 275
   4.2. Tunnel morphology after healing process is completed 276
   4.3. Factors influencing healing and early infection 277
      4.3.1. Tissue perfusion 277
      4.3.2. Mechanical factors 277
      4.3.3. Microorganisms 277
      4.3.4. Epithelialization 278
      4.3.5. Cleansing agents 278
      4.3.6. Exit direction 278
      4.3.7. Systemic factors 278
   4.4. Factors influencing infection of healed catheter tunnel 278
      4.4.1. Bacterial colonization of the sinus 278
      4.4.2. *Staphylococcus aureus* nasal carriage 279
      4.4.3. Catheter skin-exit direction 279
      4.4.4. Sinus tract length 279
      4.4.5. Number of cuffs 280
      4.4.6. Material for the external cuff and tubing in the sinus 281
   4.5. External cuff extrusion 281
   4.6. Catheter tip migration 282
   4.7. Pericatheter leak 282
   4.8. Infusion/pressure pain 283
5. Frequently used catheters 283
   5.1. Straight and coiled Tenckhoff catheters 283
   5.2. Toronto Western Hospital catheters 283
   5.3. Swan neck catheters 284
      5.3.1. Swan neck Tenckhoff straight and coiled 284
      5.3.2. Swan neck Toronto 284
      5.3.3. Swan neck Missouri straight 285
      5.3.4. Swan neck Missouri coiled 285
      5.3.5. Swan neck presternal 285
      5.3.6. Radiopaque stripe 288
6. Accessories for implantation of catheters 288
   6.1. Stencils 288
   6.2. Stiffening stilette 288
   6.3. Tunneling devices 288
      6.3.1. Tenckhoff trocar 288
      6.3.2. Scanlan tunneler 288
      6.3.3. Exit trocar 288
   6.4. Peritoneoscopic equipment 289
   6.5. Seldinger (guide wire) with peel-away sheath equipment 289
   6.6. Nyton ties and a tension tool 290
7. Rigid catheter 290
   7.1. Pre-insertion patient assessment and preparation 290
   7.2. Insertion 290
   7.3. Complications 291
8. Soft catheter 293
   8.1. Patient preparation 293
      8.1.1. Acute dialysis 293
      8.1.2. Chronic dialysis 293
   8.2. Catheter preparation 293
   8.3. Implantation method 294
      8.3.1. Blind (Tenckhoff trocar) 294
      8.3.2. Peritoneoscopic 294
      8.3.3. Seldinger (guide wire) and peel-away sheath 294
      8.3.4. Surgical (by dissection) 294
9. Catheter break-in and catheter care 295
   9.1. Immediate intraperitoneal segment care 295
   9.2. Peritoneal dialysis 295
   9.3. Exit care 295
10. Early soft catheter complications 296
11. Late soft catheter complications 297
    11.1. Exit site infection 297
        11.1.1. Classification of exit site appearance 298
        11.1.2. Care and treatment recommendations 298
    11.2. External cuff extrusion 299
    11.3. Catheter obstruction 300
    11.4. Pericatheter leak 300
    11.5. Peritonitis 301
    11.6. Infusion or pressure pain 301
    11.7. Unusual complications 302
        11.7.1. Organ erosion 302
        11.7.2. Mechanical accidents 302
        11.7.3. Material breakdown 302
        11.7.4. Allergic reaction 302
12. Indications for catheter removal 302
    12.1. Malfunction 303
    12.2. Functioning catheter with a complication 303
    12.3. Functioning catheter that is no longer needed 303
13. Long term results 303
    13.1. Tenckhoff catheters 303
    13.2. Toronto Western Hospital catheters 304
    13.3. Column disc catheter 304
    13.4. National CAPD Registry survey 304
    13.5. Swan neck catheters 305
    13.4. United States Renal Data System report 1992 306
14. Concluding remarks 306
References 307

1. Introduction

One of the most important components of the peritoneal dialysis system is a permanent and trouble free access to the peritoneal cavity. The double cuff Tenckhoff catheter, developed in 1968 for treatment of patients with intermittent peritoneal dialysis [1], is also widely used for continuous ambulatory peritoneal dialysis (CAPD); however, CAPD increases catheter related complications due to higher intraabdominal pressure and numerous daily manipulations. These complications, such as catheter tip migration, dialysate leaks, and exit site infections are frequently encountered and often related to improper insertion and postimplantation care. Catheter exit site and tunnel infections are frequent in CAPD patients leading to morbidity, prolonged treatment, recurrent peritonitis, and catheter failure. Recent improvement in peritonitis rates due to wide-spread use of the Y-set has shifted the focus of attention to peritoneal access [2, 3, 4]. According to the National CAPD Registry, the overall three year survival of the various peritoneal catheters was 13–36% in the 1981–1987 period [5].

2. Historical perspective

In the early years of peritoneal dialysis the access was not specifically designed for the peritoneal dialysis, rather the available equipment used for other purposes was adapted. Ganter [6] used a metal trocar, Rosenak and Siwon [7] adjusted a glass cannula with multiple side holes used for surgical drains. Desider Engel [8] from Prague used a glass catheter with a mushroom like opening inside the peritoneum to maximize fluid distribution and prevent obstruction. Reid, Penfold and Jones [9] used a Foley catheter. Major problems in these years were leakage, infection and catheter occlusion by clot or omental fat sucked into the catheter lumen. Fine, Frank and Seligman [10] created a subcutaneous tunnel to hamper periluminal bacterial migration into the peritoneal cavity. They adapted a stainless steel sump drain for dialysate outflow and a rubber mushroom catheter for dialysis solution inflow. Although these innovations showed some improvement in infection rate and drainage, the overall results were not satisfactory and pericatheter leaks were frequent. Some unusual problems that we do not see these days were: rigidity of the tube with resulting pressure to viscera, suction of contaminated air into the peritoneal cavity, and difficulties of proper aseptic fixation of the tube to the abdominal wall.

Stephen Rosenak, a Hungarian physician, who became interested in continuous flow peritoneal dialysis in his medical student years in the 1920s [7], while working with Oppenheimer at the Mt. Sinai Hospital in New York, for the first time developed an access specifically for peritoneal dialysis [11]. Rosenak and Oppenheimer access consisted of a stainless steel flexible coil attached to a rubber drain and was suitable for continuous flow dialysis with inflow through the outer tube and outflow through the inner tube. This device did not gain popularity because all the major problems were not solved.

A major advance was the introduction of less rigid materials by French physicians. Derot et al. [12] and Marcel Legrain, while working with John Merril [13] in New York used polyvinyl tubes for peritoneal dialysis in acute renal failure. The next major progress was made in late 1950s when Maxwell, Rockney, Kleeman and Twiss [14] introduced a nylon catheter with multiple tiny distal perforations. The small diameter of perforations prevented particles of omentum from entering the catheter. At the same time, Doolan and co-workers [15] developed a polyvinyl catheter with multiple ridges to prevent omental wrapping. Both catheters were inserted into the peritoneal cavity with the help of a paracentesis trocar. Smooth, plastic materials were much less irritating to the peritoneum than previously used glass, rubber or steel, thereby omental occlusion became less frequent. The drainage of fluid from the peritoneal cavity was markedly improved, but leakage and pericatheter infections continued.

In the early 1960s, Dr. Belding Scribner from Seattle invited Dr. Boen from the Netherlands to continue his peritoneal dialysis research. Boen implanted a teflon button in the abdominal wall. Through this button a long catheter was inserted into the peritoneal cavity. After each dialysis the catheter was removed and the button was capped; thus, periodic peritoneal dialysis for chronic renal failure was introduced [16], to be followed by the repeated puncture method [17]. For each dialysis a new catheter had to be inserted. The insertion procedure required penetration of the abdominal wall with a paracentesis trocar. The resulting abdominal opening was of greater diameter than the catheter and pericatheter leaks were frequent.

To circumvent the dialysate leakage problem, Weston and Roberts [18] invented a stylet catheter, which was inserted without a trocar. A sharp stainless steel stylet inserted through the catheter was used to penetrate the abdominal wall. As a result, the abdominal opening fitted snugly around the catheter, thereby preventing leakage. This type of catheter is still being used for acute renal failure.

Other approaches to facilitate repeated puncture were a subcutaneous button [19], a Teflon® rod [20] and a plexiglass disc and polyvinyl balloon instead of a metal plate for the transabdominal cannula [21]. The necessity of repeated puncture or catheter insertion through the permanent opening has not gained popularity because this was impractical, especially for the home peritoneal dialysis. These catheters were also plagued with infections, dialysate leaks, and obstructions.

A major step forward in creating a permanent peritoneal access was made in 1964. Gutch [22] noticed lower protein losses with silicon rubber catheters as compared to those with polyvinyl ones, which suggested less irritation of the peritoneum with a new material. About the same time, Russel Palmer, a physician at the Canadian Army Medical Corps was developing a peritoneal access made of polyethylene, polypropylene, and nylon [23]. These catheters were relatively rigid, and not better than the other available at that time. He was looking for a better material, softer, and more biocompatible. With the help of Wayne Quinton, already successful in manufacturing silicon rubber shunts for hemodialysis, they developed a catheter which is a prototype of currently used coiled catheters [24]. The catheter was made of silicon rubber, the intraperitoneal end was coiled and had numerous perforations extending 23 centimeters from the tip; a long subcutaneous tunnel was supposed to hinder periluminal infection. To impede further infection and leakage, a tri-flanged step was created for securing the catheter in the deep abdominal fascia.

In 1965, Henry Tenckhoff, at the University of Washington, was beginning to treat patients on chronic peritoneal dialysis [25]. After an initial few dialyses in the hospital, the patients would be trained for home dialysis. On the weekends Tenckhoff would go to the patient's home, insert the catheter and begin dialysis. After the appropriate time on dialysis, the patient would remove the catheter and cover the exit wound with a dressing. Although the method was successful in Tenckhoff's hands, the technique was cumbersome, and Tenckhoff recognized its limitations. He was thinking of a more practical solution.

In 1968, McDonald and co-workers [26] developed an external seal composed of a polyester (Dacron®) sleeve and a polytetrafluoroethylene (Teflon®) skirt. Tissue ingrowth into these elements created a firm external seal to prevent leakage and microorganism migration. No subcutaneous tunnel was created, the catheter was inserted straight through the abdominal wall.

In the same year, Tenckhoff and Schechter published the results of their studies on a new catheter [1]. Their catheter was an improved version of the Palmer catheter. An intra-abdominal flange was replaced by a Dacron® cuff, a subcutaneous tunnel was shortened and the second, external cuff was used to decrease the length of the catheter sinus tract. Ultimately, the coiled intraperitoneal portion was replaced by a straight segment resembling the Gutch catheter. The intraperitoneal segment was kept open ended and the size of the side holes was optimized to 0.5 mm to prevent tissue suction. A shorter subcutaneous tunnel and straight intraperitoneal segment facilitated catheter implantation at the bedside with the aid of a specially designed trocar (Fig. 1). To avoid excessive bleeding the catheter was inserted through the midline. The Tenckhoff catheter has become the gold standard of peritoneal access. Few complications were reported in patients treated by periodic peritoneal dialysis. Twenty six years later, even today, the Tenckhoff

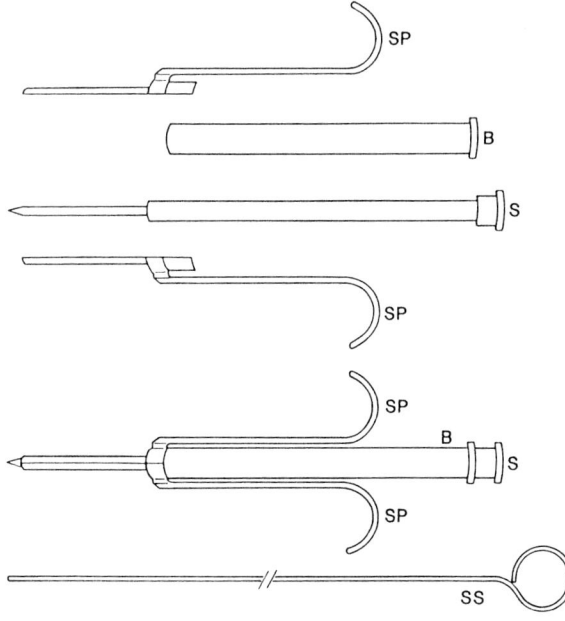

Figure 1. Tenckhoff trocar – assembled (below) and disassembled (above). SP – side pieces; S – pointed stylet; B – barrel; SS – stiffening stilette.

catheter in its original form is the most widely used catheter type. Some of the original recommendations for catheter insertion such as arcuate subcutaneous tunnels with downward directions of both intraperitoneal and external exits are still considered very important elements of catheter implantation.

To prevent exit infection, a subcutaneous catheter was developed by the Utah group [27]. The catheter had 2 tubes in the peritoneal cavity, and a subcutaneous container. The container was to be punctured for each dialysis. Another subcutaneous catheter was developed by Gotloib et al. [28]. Yet another approach to decrease exit site infection rates was to position the subcutaneous cuff at the skin level [29]. Unfortunately, contrary to expectations, such a position tends to increase infection rates [30].

To decrease catheter migration and omental wrapping the intraperitoneal segment of the catheter was provided with a saline inflatable balloon [31] or discs [32]. Valli et al. [33, 34] revived an idea of Goldberg et al. [31] and made a silicon rubber catheter with a balloon shaped intraperitoneal segment surrounding the catheter tip. Ash et al. [35] replaced the intraperitoneal tubing with a disc located immediately beneath the abdominal wall. Such a catheter cannot migrate but still may be obstructed by bowels or omentum.

Several new or improved catheters have been developed in recent years. Twardowski et al. [36] designed silicon rubber "swan neck" catheters that are permanently bent between two cuffs. These catheters may be implanted in an arcuate tunnel with their shape undistorted. A similar principle was applied by Cruz to polyurethane catheters [37].

This chapter will describe in detail some of those catheters which are in current use, their insertion technique, postimplantation care, and long term results. New, emerging techniques will be briefly reviewed.

3. Glossary

There are numerous catheter designs and implantation techniques. To avoid confusion we will briefly review terminology pertinent to the currently used peritoneal catheters [38]. After implantation the typical double cuff Tenckhoff catheter has three segments (Fig. 2): *Intraperitoneal* located intraperitoneally, *intramural* contained within the abdominal wall tunnel, and *external* situated outside of the skin exit. The *peritoneal catheter tunnel* is the passageway through the abdominal wall within which the peritoneal catheter is contained. Figure 3 depicts tissue structures in relation to cuff position in healed tunnels. Simple anchorless catheters, create peritoneal fistulas and predispose to fluid leaks and peritoneal infections. Such catheters were abandoned after introduction of Tenckhoff catheters in 1968. Tenckhoff catheters consist of the body or tubing and cuffs which are the bands of fabric affixed to the tubing for fibrous tissue ingrowth. After implantation of a single, deep cuff catheter the tunnel is composed of three parts: 1) the sinus tract located between the skin exit and the cuff, 2) the peritoneal tunnel recess, which is a peritoneal pocket covered with the mesothelium from the internal tunnel exit to the collagen mesothelial interface at the cuff, and 3) the tunnel proper comprising the tissue ingrown into the cuff. Another type of single cuff catheter is provided only with a superficial cuff, has a short sinus tract, but a long peritoneal recess. A properly implanted double cuff peritoneal catheter, designed by Tenckhoff for treatment of chronic renal failure creates a tunnel with a short sinus tract, a shallow peritoneal recess, and a 5–7 cm long tunnel proper, which consists of tissue ingrown into the cuffs and a fibrous sheath covering the intercuff tunnel segment.

4. Factors influencing catheter complications

The common complications of peritoneal dialysis catheters include (Table 1): exit/tunnel infection; external cuff extrusion; obstruction, which is usually a sequela of catheter tip migration out of the true pelvis with subsequent omental wrapping or tip entrapment in peritoneal adhesions; dialysate leaks; peritonitis; and infusion or pressure pain. This section of the chapter will describe factors that influence these complications. A video illustrating these factors has been recently produced [39].

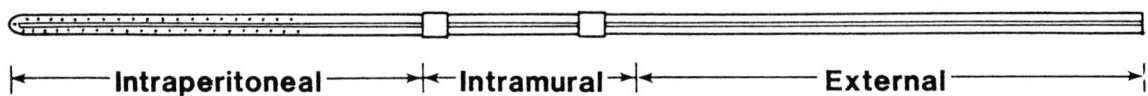

Figure 2. Diagram of double cuff Tenckhoff catheter showing three segments created after implantation.

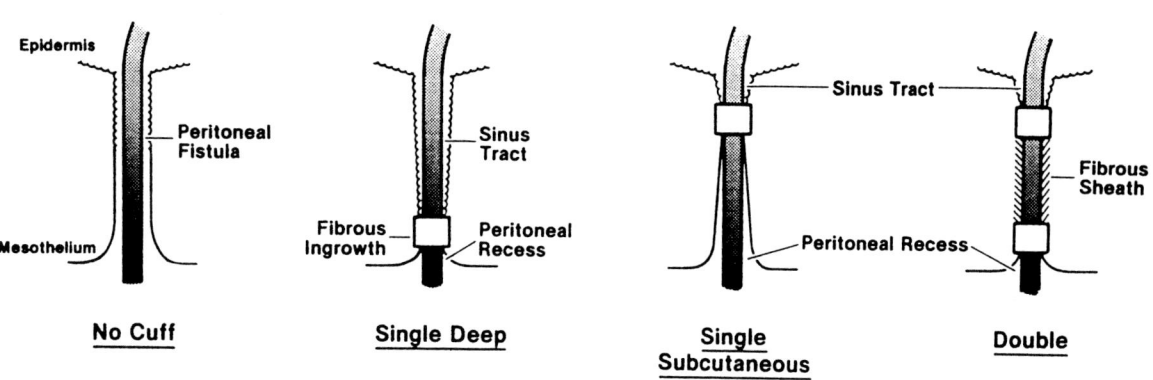

Figure 3. Tissue structures in relation to cuff position in healed tunnels. In catheters without cuffs a peritoneal fistula is formed. A single deep cuff creates a shallow peritoneal recess and a deep sinus tract predisposing to exit infection. A single subcutaneous cuff generates a shallow sinus tract and a deep peritoneal recess predisposing to pseudoherniae. Property positioned two cuffs limit the depth of both structures. Reproduced with permission from reference [53].

4.1. Tissue reaction to a foreign body penetrating skin

The tissue reaction begins immediately after a break in the integument occurs. Bleeding from capillaries and body fluids form a coagulum of a hydrophilic fibrin-fibronectin gel and cellular debris. Various cytokines coordinate the subsequent entry of inflammatory cells and fibroblasts and the formation of new blood vessels [40]. Polymorphonuclear neutrophil leukocytes phagocytize local bacteria and together with the coagulum form a scab. The polyester cuff is also filled with clotted blood. Gradually neutrophils, macrophages, fibroblasts, and new capillaries penetrate between the polyester fibers. Macrophages coalesce into giant cells completely or partially surrounding the polyester fibers and fibroblasts produce collagen fibers which intertwine with the polyester fibers. The formation of the strong fibrous tissue is completed after approximately six weeks. Healing of the sinus starts with the production, beneath the scab, of granulation tissue composed of new vessels and fibroblasts. Gradually neutrophils are replaced with mononuclear leukocytes, fibroblasts produce collagen fibers and a mature granulation tissue is formed. Upon this tissue, there is a peripheral ingrowth of new epidermal cells.

Epidermal cells spread over the granulation tissue beneath the scab. Based on animal experiments it has been widely accepted that epithelial cells spread over granulation tissue until they meet epithelial cells from the opposite "shore" or until they encounter dense collagen fibers [41–49]. Winter [49] postulated that in naturally occurring percutaneous organs such as teeth, the inhibition of epithelial migration is achieved by a periodontal membrane which consists of bundles of collagen fibers embedded in the cementum of the tooth. In his view, other situations where epidermal cell migration is inhibited include macroporous implants and skin autographs. Finally he assumed that the basement membrane, a collagenous structure, also inhibits basal cell invasion of the dermis.

The hypothesis that collagen fibers play a paramount role in inhibiting epithelial cell spreading [43] led to the development of several devices of porous material to encourage dermal ingrowth and to prevent epithelialization of the tunnel ("marsupialization") [29, 44, 45, 50]. It has been suggested that the epithelium adjacent to a silicone catheter

Table 1. Catheter related common complications.

Exit/tunnel infection
External cuff extrusion
Catheter obstruction
Pericatheter leak
Peritonitis
Infusion or pressure plan

tends to migrate toward and beyond the subcutaneous cuff, creating a sinus between the tubing and the skin that is prone to bacterial colonization with subsequent infection [45].

The development of an epithelialized tract seemed well supported in animal models [29, 44, 50] and in our previous reviews we cited these data as relevant also in human peritoneal catheter sinus tracts [51–53]. However; our recent study of catheter tunnels removed from patients showed that in almost all human peritoneal catheter tunnels the epithelium does not reach to the cuff but stops a few millimeters from the exit in the sinus tract [54]. These observations lead us to believe that granulation tissue *per se* can also inhibit epidermal cell spreading. This observation also has an important influence on catheter design and implantation, particularly the material for the superficial cuff and its distance from the exit.

In humans, unlike animals, the spreading of epidermis is slow. This discrepancy should not be surprising because the epidermal turnover rate in animals is about six to seven times faster than in humans [55]. We found that in fast healing catheter exits in humans the epidermis starts entering into the sinus after 2–3 weeks; in slow healing exits the epidermis starts entering into the sinus after 4–6 weeks [56]. The healing process is complete after about 4–8 weeks, when the epidermis covers approximately half of a visible sinus tract with the remaining half covered with granulation tissue [57].

4.2. Tunnel morphology after healing process is completed

A detailed description of peritoneal catheter tunnel morphology has been published elsewhere [54]. A well healed tunnel of a double cuff swan neck Missouri catheter removed electively (Fig. 4) consists of tissue ingrown to the flange and internal cuff, tissue surrounding the intercuff segment, tissue ingrown into the external cuff, and the sinus tract. The most external part (0.5–1 cm) of the sinus tract and the skin surrounding the skin exit of the tunnel constitute the exit site. In majority of humans the epidermal cells penetrate only a few millimeters from the skin exit and may reach the cuff located less than 15 mm from the exit [54, 58]. Although unusual, a single instance of keratinized epithelium penetration to the cuff located 45 mm from the exit has been reported [59]. Close to the exit the surface of the sinus tract is covered with wrinkled epidermis, containing all layers of epidermis including a horny layer. Deeper, epidermis loses the horny layer and becomes similar to the mucosal epithelium, hence the surface becomes glistening and

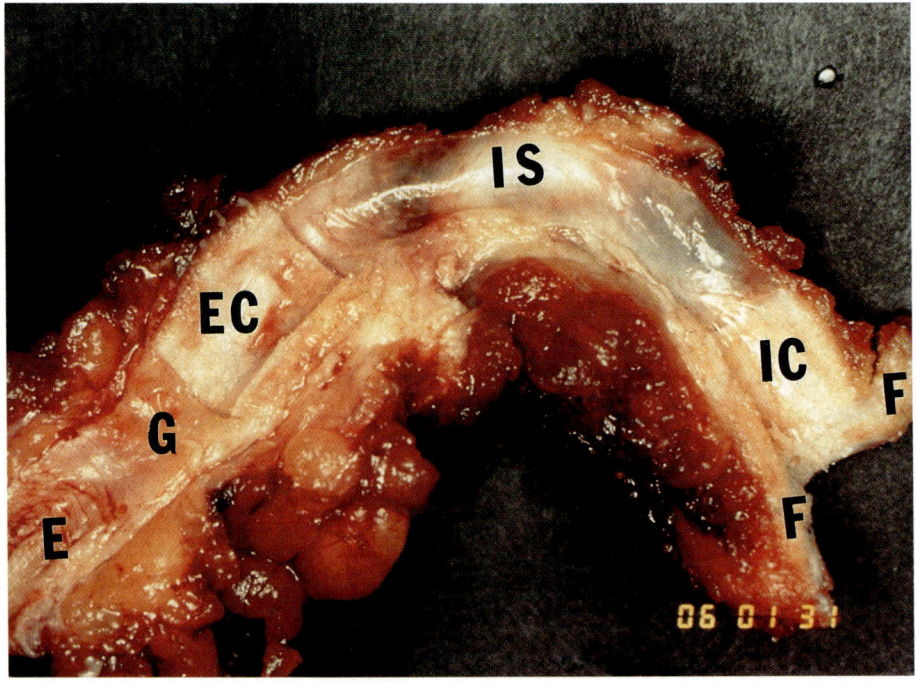

Figure 4. A well healed tunnel of a double cuff swan neck Missouri catheter removed electively. From the left: E – epithelium; G – granulation tissue; EC – external cuff; IS – intercuff segment; IC – internal cuff; F – flange.

white. The rest of the sinus tract is covered by the granulation tissue that is yellowish in appearance. A thick layer of collagen fibers surround the sinus. The granulation tissue contains numerous multinucleated giant cells, capillaries, cellular infiltrate composed mostly of mononuclear cells, and scant collagen fibers. The collagen fibers do not attach to the smooth surface of the silicone rubber, the material from which most peritoneal dialysis catheters are made.

The junction between the granulation tissue in the sinus and the cuff is well defined. The cuff is surrounded by a dense fibrous capsule that contains numerous capillaries. About 80% of the polyester fibers are surrounded completely or partially by multinucleated giant cells. Spaces between the polyester fibers are filled with mature collagen and fibroblasts. No neutrophils are seen in an uninfected cuff.

The junction between the cuff and the intercuff segment shows a smooth surface without granulation tissue. The glistening, shiny intercuff tunnel segment resembles a tendon sheath and contains numerous micropits. The absence of any cellular reaction indicates that bacteria do not reach this part of the tunnel. The surface is covered with an amorphous, mucinous substance on top of a modified layer of fibroblasts forming pseudo-synovium. There are not giant cells in this segment because silicon rubber *per se* does not induce giant cell formation.

The transition between the intercuff segment and the deep cuff is abrupt due to change from an avascular, acellular, fibrous sheath to a highly vascular and cellular tissue ingrown into the cuff. If the deep cuff is implanted into the muscle, the fibrous capsule surrounding the cuff and the cuff tissue itself are highly vascularized, otherwise the tissue ingrown into the cuff is similar to that of the external cuff.

4.3. Factors influencing healing and early infection

The most important factors influencing the healing process and early infections are (Table 2): tissue perfusion; mechanical factors; sinus bacterial colonization; epithelialization; local cleansing agent; exit direction; and systemic factors.

4.3.1. *Tissue perfusion*
The coagulum and necrotic tissue are gradually removed from the tunnel. Part of the necrotic tissue is absorbed, part is drained out of the tunnel. The tunnel should not be too tight, to allow free drainage of necrotic tissue and to prevent tissue edema; these decrease local perfusion and oxygen tension [60], which are critical for the wound healing process. On the other hand too large an incision prolongs healing by the shear volume of needed repair and the movement of loose tubing in the tunnel.

4.3.2. *Mechanical factors*
Mechanical stress slows the healing process [41]; thus the catheter should be relatively tightly anchored in the tunnel and also well immobilized outside the tunnel, especially during the break-in period. Frequent dressing changes, always associated with catheter manipulation, should be avoided during the healing period. Constricting sutures can cause pressure necrosis with skin sloughing and facilitate bacterial penetration into the tissue [61]; they must not be used.

4.3.3. *Microorganisms*
The presence of microorganisms in the wound is the major cause of impaired healing [62, 63]. Antibiotic penetration into the coagulum is poor, therefore, antibiotics should be present in sufficient concentrations in blood and tissue fluids before the coagulum is formed. This may be achieved if antibiotics are given prior to implantation. The humoral tissue reaction to the foreign implants is to coat them with various proteins, such as fibronectin, laminin, fibrin, collagen, and immunoglobulins. Some of these substances serve as receptors for colonizing organisms. A receptor site for binding *Staphylococcus aureus* has been identified within the 27-kilodalton amino-terminal fragment of fibronectin [64]. *Staphylococcus aureus* was found to have several receptor sites for soluble and solid-phase fibronectin [65, 66]. *Staphylococcus epidermidis* binding to fibronectin seems to be less extensive than that of *Staphylococcus aureus* [67]. Similar receptors to laminin were found in

Table 2. Factors influencing healing process and infection.

Tissue perfusion
Mechanical factors
Microorganisms
Epithelialization
Cleansing agents
Exit direction
Systemic factors

Staphylococcus aureus but not in *Staphylococcus epidermidis* [68]. Type IV collagen, vitronectin (S protein), and fibrin may also participate in bacterial adherence, but their role in foreign body colonization has not been clarified [69, 70].

Bacteria themselves, even without participation of specific protein receptors, may adhere to the foreign body by electrostatic attachment or by London-van der Waal's forces [71]. Adhered bacteria synthesize and excrete a variety of complex polysaccharides (biofilm) which serve to protect them from host mechanisms [72, 73]. It is not surprising that almost all peritoneal catheter exits and sinus tracts, even without signs of infection, are colonized by bacteria [57].

Maintaining sterility of the exit and sinus in the initial healing period is of utmost importance. Antibiotic penetration into the coagulum is poor, therefore, antibiotics should be present in sufficient concentration in blood and tissue fluids before the coagulum is formed. This may be achieved if antibiotics are given prior to implantation.

4.3.4. Epithelialization
Epidermal cells grow over the granulation tissue beneath the scab. If the scab is forcibly removed during cleansing, the epidermal layer is broken, thus prolonging the process of epidermization. Sinus epithelialization is supported by sterile and undisturbed conditions at the exit. Again, frequent dressing changes facilitate exit contamination; on the other hand, liquid serous or sanguinous exudate at the exit promote bacterial growth. Therefore, the exit should be kept dry but dressing changes should not be too frequent.

4.3.5. Cleansing agents
Cleansing agents should not only decrease the number of bacteria, but also be harmless to the body defenses. Strong oxidants like Povidone-iodine and hydrogen peroxide are cytotoxic to mammalian cells and should not be used [74, 75]. Non-ionic, amphophilic, non-toxic surfactants, widely used in burn wound care, facilitate necrotic tissue removal without jeopardizing body defense mechanisms [76]. In agreement with experience of others [77] we found 20% Poloxamer 188 (Shur-Clens®; Calgon Vestal Laboratories, St. Louis, MO, USA) to be innocuous, yet excellent in cleansing the exit from contaminants.

4.3.6. Exit direction
Exit direction is also important. Immediate post-implantation drainage of necrotic tissue is facilitated by gravity when the exit is directed downward.

4.3.7. Systemic factors
During the healing process part of the granulation tissue is gradually resorbed and replaced by fibrous tissue. The fibrous tissue and part of the granulation tissue is covered with the epidermis [54]. Impaired nutrition, diabetes mellitus, uremia, and corticosteroids are all known factors decreasing wound healing by decreasing fibrosis [78]. It is prudent to avoid permanent catheter implantation while the patient is severely uremic, malnourished or taking glucocorticoids. In Asia, asiatic acid, an extract of *Centella asiatica*, has been used for the treatment of skin wounds. The active ingredient of this extract (which also has mineralocorticoid properties) increases both collagen synthesis in cultured fibroblasts of human skin and tensile strength of skin wounds [79, 80]. Mineralocorticoids may also promote wound healing by increasing fibrosis, though controlled studies on wound healing acceleration in humans have not been performed yet.

4.4. Factors influencing infection of healed catheter tunnels

Design of the catheter and its location in the created tunnel influence exit and/or tunnel infection. Other factors which may influence infection rate include (Table 3): bacterial colonization of the sinus; *Staphylococcus aureus* nasal carriage status; catheter skin-exit direction; sinus tract length; number off cuffs; and materials for the external cuff and the tubing in the sinus.

4.4.1. Bacterial colonization of the sinus
Almost all healed catheter sinuses are colonized by bacteria [56]. It has been well established in the surgical literature that wound infection is the result of major disturbance in the balance between host defense and bacteria [63]. The number of bacteria as a critical factor in wound infection was already

Table 3. Factors influencing infection of healed catheter tunnels.

Bacterial colonization of the sinus
Staphylococcus aureus nasal carriage
Catheter skin-exit direction
Sinus tract length
Number off cuffs
Material for the external cuff and tubing in the sinus

recognized in World War I [62]. Elek [61] demonstrated that it requires 7.5×10^6 Staphylococcal organisms to produce a pustule in normal human skin but the number of bacteria necessary to cause infection was reduced 10,000-fold in the presence of a single suture. Bacterial virulence is also important; *Staphylococcus aureus* or *Pseudomonas aeruginosa* are more likely to induce an inflammatory response than is *Staphylococcus epidermidis*.

It appears that there is a constant struggle between the colonizing bacteria and defense mechanisms of the sinus tract. The part of the sinus tract covered with epidermis seems to respond to bacteria in the same way as the rest of the body integument but the part covered with granulation tissue appears to respond by constant exudation of serum with white blood cells to suppress bacterial proliferation and curb their penetration deeper into the sinus. If the number of bacteria increases, then the amount of exudate increases, granulation tissue proliferates and becomes more vascularized. The number of bacteria entering deeper into the sinus depends on the number and species of bacteria at the exit site, exit direction, as well as sinus tract length, the latter an important contributing factor in the amplitude of catheter movement in the sinus. Defense mechanisms, after the sinus is healed, are best in undamaged epidermis and granulation tissue; trauma to these structures may tilt the balance toward attacking microorganisms and allow their rapid multiplication.

4.4.2. *Staphylococcus aureus nasal carriage*
The importance of *Staphylococcus aureus* as an etiologic agent of peritoneal catheter exit site infection has been well established [81, 82]. Nasal carriage status of *Staphylococcus aureus* is reported to be common in patients undergoing hemodialysis [83], and peritoneal dialysis [84, 85]. A recent multicenter study found an increased incidence of exit site infections in nasal carriers of *Staphylococcus aureus*; in 85% of these infections the strain from the nares and the strain causing the infection were similar in phage type and antibiotic profile [86]. However, in our study we found that, by antibiotic profile, the strain causing exit infection and the strain cultured from nares are different [87]. Judging by our study, there is an increased probability of *Staphylococcus aureus* exit infection in patients who carry *Staphylococcus aureus* in nares, but the strain is not the same. A multicenter study currently underway in Europe will, it is hoped, settle the controversy. In this randomized, placebo controlled study the influence of intranasal mupirocin ointment on nasal carriage and incidence of exit site infection is to be assessed.

4.4.3. *Catheter skin-exit direction*
Tenckhoff's original recommendation of a downward pointing exit [1] received support in our retrospective analysis which found that, compared to upward directed exits, the exits directed downwards tended to be infected less frequently and, once infected, were significantly less resistant to treatment [36]. This should not be surprising since upward directed tunnels facilitate exit contamination by down flowing sweat, water, and dirt (Fig. 5). Once the exit is infected it is resistant to treatment because of poor external drainage; rather the pus tends to penetrate deeper into the tunnel. Also, downward drainage of necrotic tissue immediately post implantation is easier than drainage against gravity.

The advantage of caudal exit direction in preventing and treating infections has support in several other clinical conditions. Periodontitis, which may be considered as a naturally occurring "foreign" body exit site infection, inflicts most frequently the lower incisors ("exits" directed upward) [88]. The influence of exit position on the frequency and tenacity of paranasal sinus infections was postulated by Zuckerkandl in 19th century. The relatively frequent infections of the maxillary sinus are believed to be due to unfavorable conditions for discharge because the *ostium maxillare* (in the upright position of the body) is located at the highest point of the cavity; the cavity must be completely filled with secretions before the discharge may escape [89]. All of the other cavities are more favorably constructed for drainage and less likely to be infected [89]. Exit infections of long-term jugular and/or subclavian catheters are less frequent than those of peritoneal catheters. Using catheters with downward directed tunnels So *et al.* [90] reported 1 exit infection per 998 catheter days, Raaf [91] reported 16 exit site infections with 698 catheters in cancer patients.

4.4.4. *Sinus tract length*
The epidermis covering the sinus tract undergoes a turnover probably similar to the normal epidermis with cell maturation and desquamation; granulation tissue produces exudate. All these contents, if not expelled, create a conducive milieu for bacterial growth. With a long sinus tract the chances of infection are higher [41–43]; therefore, the sinus

UPWARD AND DOWNWARD TUNNEL DIRECTION – EXIT SITE INFECTION

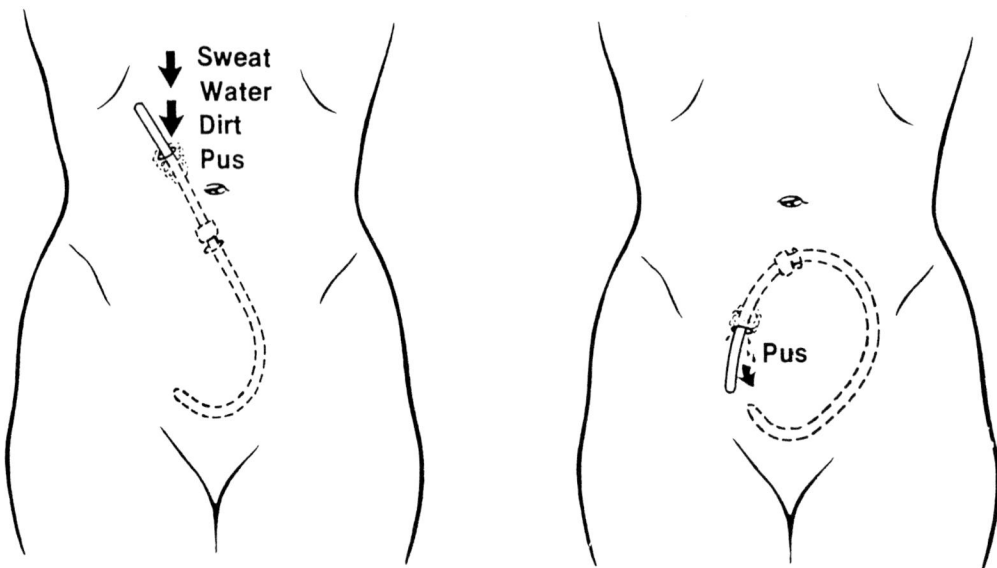

Figure 5. (Left) Exit easily contaminated with down flowing sweat, water, and dirt; difficult pus drainage prolongs treatment. (Right) Good pus drainage facilitates recovery. (Reproduced from reference [36] with permission.)

tract should be as short as possible; one to two centimeter length is appropriate. Tenckhoff recommended that "the subcutaneous Dacron® felt cuff should be located immediately beneath the skin exit" [92]. Such a localization of the cuff, however, predisposes to its extrusion. Indeed, in some centers the rate of extrusion reaches 100% [93]. In other centers the rate, although lower, was high enough to question the wisdom of using the superficial cuff at all.

4.4.5. Number of cuffs

Single (only external) cuff catheters were used by Tenckhoff for treatment of acute renal failure. This type of catheter used in patients undergoing chronic intermittent peritoneal dialysis yielded similar results to those of a double cuff catheter; however, with continuous ambulatory peritoneal dialysis, double cuff catheter survival was better than that of single cuff catheters [94]. The major complication of these single cuff catheters was a development of pseudoherniae due to high intraabdominal pressure with constant presence of fluid in the peritoneal cavity.

Another type of single cuff catheter is provided with only a deep cuff. This type of catheter has been used because of problems with external cuff extrusion and the questionable value of the external cuff. Exit site infections were found to be similar with single and double cuff catheters in some reports [95]; however, in a retrospective survey of catheter results in 395 patients, tunnel infections were almost 3 times more frequent with single cuff than with double cuffs [93]. In our institution we found that exit infections tended to be more frequent and were significantly more resistant to treatment with single cuff catheters compared to double cuff ones [36]. Also a recently published national study of the United States Renal Data System (USRDS) revealed an increased relative risk for a first peritonitis episode with a single cuff versus a double cuff catheter [96].

The discrepancy in the results may be due to the length of the sinus tract with different implantation techniques [53]. Usually, but not always, a longer sinus tract is created with a single cuff catheter than with a double cuff catheter. If a short sinus tract is present the results regarding exit infections should be similar irrespective of which cuff limits the depth of the sinus tract. Another reason for the inconsistency in the results may stem from the difference in the deep cuff position. Location of the deep cuff in the muscle provides better vascularization compared to the cuff located in the subcutaneous tissue. Fibrous tissue ingrowth is markedly stronger if the deep cuff is located in the belly of the rectus muscle rather than in the midline, because the muscle is much better vascularized. The location of the deep cuff in the rectus muscle may have an advantage in peritonitis prevention. The USRDS study [96] also revealed a reduced relative risk of a first peritonitis episode for lateral catheter placement versus midline insertion.

4.4.6. *Material for the external cuff and tubing in the sinus*

It has been postulated that the external cuff should provide a strong attachment of collagen fibers to limit the epidermal cell spreading [42]. As an example of a perfect arrangement, the anatomy of the tooth/gingival interface was cited [45]. The periodontal ligament attaches to the cementum creating an extremely strong bond. The cementum is com-posed of hydroxyapatite crystals, collagen fibers, proteoglycans and mucopolysaccharides [97]. Such a living material is unlikely to be used for the external cuff.

Dasse *et al.* [45] and Poirier *et al.* [50] evaluated collagen attachment to various materials on their elaborate external seal for the percutaneous energy transmission systems. In experiments on miniature pigs the Dacron® velour, especially wetted with saline before implantation, provided the strongest collagen attachment with an excellent inhibition of epidermal downgrowth. Preliminary experience with this device in CAPD patients was encouraging [45]; however, long term experience has not been published yet. Others have had very poor results. All catheters were ultimately removed due to exit/tunnel infection (Oreopoulos DG – personal communication).

Favorable experiences gained with Alumina ceramic in orthopedic surgery, otorhinolaryngology, and dentistry inspired Amano *et al.* [98] to use Alumina ceramic for a peritoneal catheter. Dog experiments with this material revealed only minimal skin downgrowth. Odgen et al. [30] and Boss et al. [99] found a very high rate of chronic exit site infections with Right Angle Gore-Tex® catheters, whose use has been abandoned.

As mentioned previously, the tissue ingrown into the cuff does into seem to constitute *per se* a critical barrier for infection spreading [54]. It seems that the basic beneficial role of the external cuff in infection prevention is by anchoring of the catheter resulting in restriction of its piston like movements, thus decreasing transport of bacteria into the sinus. Favorable results with a "wing" instead of cuff appear to give clinical support to this hypothesis [100].

Consistently poor results with cuffs implanted very close to the exit and the results of our study on catheter tunnel morphology [54] lead us to believe that it is not favorable to have epidermis attached to the cuff. The whole premise of the paramount importance of epidermal downgrowth inhibition to prevent exit/tunnel infection with transcutaneous devices based on animal experiments does not seem to be relevant for the transcutaneous devices in humans. One of the important difference between animals and humans is the fact that the epidermis in humans enters only a few millimeters into the sinus tract in majority of patients.

4.5. External cuff extrusion

Localization of the cuff close to the exit predisposes to its extrusion. There are at least 2 forces favoring cuff extrusion (Table 4): 1) the pushing force of catheter resilience and 2) pulling and tugging on the catheter. The resilience of the straight catheter implanted in an arcuate tunnel plays the most important role in cuff extrusion (Fig. 6). Pulling on the catheter with frequent CAPD exchanges contributes to this complication. There is a possibility that the high pressure in the abdomen with the constant presence of fluid in the peritoneal cavity while the patient is ambulatory also tends to push out the external cuff.

At present we think that the cuff should be implanted approximately 1–2 cm beneath the skin as a compromise between the requirement of a short sinus tract to prevent infections but not so short to favor cuff extrusions. Also, resilience forces should be eliminated by creating the tunnel in a shape similar to the shape of catheter, and tugging on the catheter should be avoided. It is extremely important to avoid resilience forces pushing on the cuff by implanting it relatively close to the skin exit. The catheter should not be implanted in an edematous region to avoid cuff extrusion once the edema is resolved.

Table 4. Causes of cuff extrusion.

Catheter resilence
Pulling and tugging
Intraabdominal pressure?

DOUBLE CUFF TENCKHOFF CATHETER

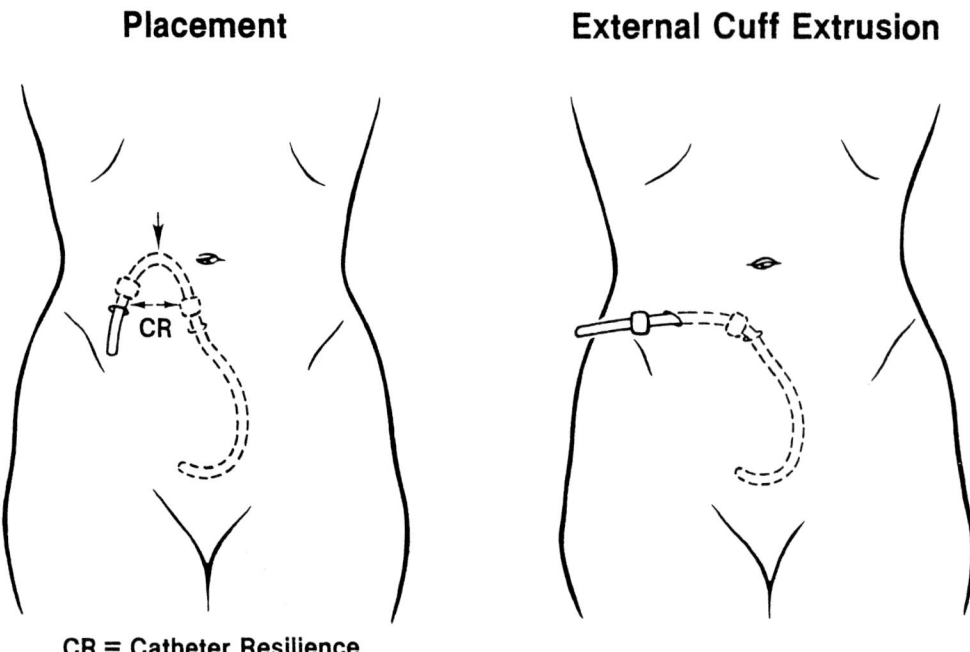

Figure 6. Double-cuff Tenckhoff catheter placed as proposed by Tenckhoff (left). Natural resilience of the straight catheter ("shape memory") forced into an arcuate tunnel tends to extrude the external cuff because the deep cuff cannot move (right). (Reproduced from reference [36] with permission.)

4.6. Catheter tip migration

One way or two way catheter obstruction is usually the result of catheter wrapping by the omentum. The best conditions for dialysate drainage are created with the catheter tip in the true pelvis because, in the majority of people, the omentum does not reach to the true pelvis. Tenckhoff recommended a caudal direction of the intraperitoneal catheter segment to prevent the catheter tip migration out of the true pelvis [92]. If the exit is directed caudally and a straight tunnel points cephalad the catheter must have an intraperitoneal bend to place the tip near the true pelvis and the tip easily translocates out of the true pelvis due to the silastic "shape memory". The internal cuff operates like a fulcrum on which resilience forces turn the catheter tip into the upper abdomen (Fig. 7). If the tip translocates to the left upper abdomen, the peristalsis of the descending colon may restore proper position of the tip; however, a tip translocated to the right upper abdomen usually does not return to the proper position because the forces of both catheter resilience and ascending colon peristalsis push the tip upwards. In support of this hypothesis are observations that when a catheter is implanted with a straight subcutaneous tunnel, with the external exit directed downward, and the intraperitoneal entrance directed upward, even if catheter tip is placed into the true pelvis during insertion, it migrates out to the upper abdomen significantly more frequently compared to the opposite tunnel direction [36, 101]. Our experience indicates that the dominant factor in catheter tip position is the resilience force of the catheter. To avoid the unfavorable influence of resilience forces on the intra-abdominal catheter segment, the catheter needs to be molded in the shape it is to be implanted in the tunnel.

4.7. Pericatheter leak

To avoid excessive bleeding the catheters are frequently inserted through the midline. In patients treated by intermittent peritoneal dialysis, dialysate leaks are rare because the intraabdominal pressure is low in the supine position. In CAPD patients, pericatheter leaks are frequent due to the continuous presence of dialysate in the upright position where

CATHETER TIP MIGRATION

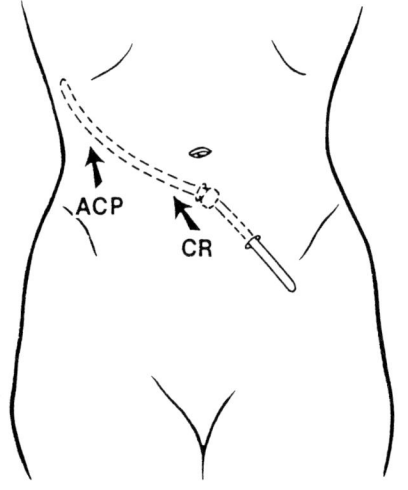
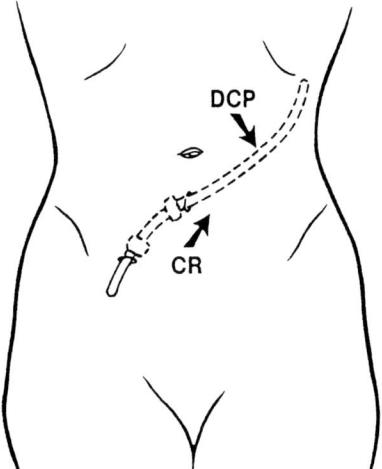

Figure 7. Straight catheter insertion: catheter tip migration out of true pelvis with external exit directed downward and intraperitoneal entrance directed upward either pointing to liver or spleen. Note the tendency of catheter to assume its original shape. ACP = ascending colon peristalsis. (Reproduced from reference [53] with permission.)

the intraabdominal pressure is high. Insertion of the deep cuff into the belly of the rectus muscle as recommended by Helfrich *et al.* [102] markedly reduces chances of pericatheter leak.

4.8. Infusion/pressure pain

Some patients experience pain at the tip of a catheter with a straight intraperitoneal segment. This pain is partly related to a "jet effect" of the rapidly flowing dialysis solution. Catheters with a coiled intraperitoneal segment are less likely to induce abdominal pain because more of the solution flows shower-like through side holes with only part of it through the main lumen that is not in direct contact with the peritoneal membrane. Moreover, the poking force of the coiled catheter is smaller than that of the straight one because the coiled intraperitoneal segment is more flexible. Finally, the larger contact area of the coiled catheter with the parietal peritoneum further reduces the pressure compared to the straight catheter tip.

5. Frequently used catheters

5.1. Straight and coiled Tenckhoff catheters

The catheter consists of the silicon rubber tubing with a 2.6 mm internal diameter and 5 mm external diameter. The catheter is provided with one or two polyester (Dacron®), 1 cm long cuffs. The overall length of the adult straight double cuff catheter is about 40 cm. The lengths of segments vary and are available in various lengths. The intraperitoneal segment has an open end and multiple 0.5 mm perforations over a distance of 11 cm from the tip. The coiled Tenckhoff catheter differs from the straight in having a coiled, 18.5 cm long perforated distal end. All Tenckhoff catheters are provided with a barium impregnated radiopaque stripe to assist in radiological visualization of the catheter.

5.2. Toronto Western Hospital catheters

The Toronto Western Hospital catheter was designed by Oreopoulos and Zellerman in 1976 [32]. Its main distinguishing feature is two flat silicon rubber discs on the intraperitoneal segment of the catheter (Fig. 8). These discs are to prevent

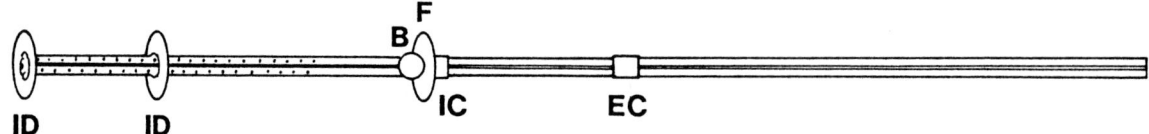

Figure 8. Toronto Western Hospital catheter. ID – intraperitoneal discs; B – bead; F – flange; IC – internal cuff; EC – external cuff.

the free movement of the catheter tip in the peritoneal cavity and thereby help the catheter tip remain in the true pelvis.

Further modifications that have been made since 1976 include the addition of a Dacron® flange, one centimeter in diameter, on the base of the peritoneal cuff and a Silastic® bead one millimeter distal to the Dacron® flange to provide a groove between them, in which the surgeon ties the peritoneum tightly.

Except for the absence of a subcutaneous cuff, the Toronto Western single cuff catheter is identical in design to the Toronto Western double cuff catheter. At the level of the Dacron® cuff, tissue fibrosis in and around the peritoneum forms an effective seal preventing fluid leak from occurring. This design affords a good barrier against early or late dialysate leaks and later incisional hernias.

The intraperitoneal segment of this catheter is 15 cm long and provided with two flat silicone rubber disks which are 1 mm thick and 28 mm in diameter and 5 cm apart. Because of their shape and design, two discs prevent the free mobility of intra-abdominal section of the catheter in the peritoneal cavity.

5.3. Swan neck catheters

The swan neck catheter design is based on a retrospective analysis of complication rates with Tenckhoff and Toronto Western Hospital catheters. The analysis showed that the lowest complication rates were with double cuff catheters implanted through the belly of the rectus muscle and with both internal and skin exits of the tunnel directed downward; however, the resulting arcuate tunnel led to frequent external cuff extrusion [36]. Swan neck catheters feature a permanent bend between cuffs (Table 5) [103]. The catheter was dubbed "swan neck" because of its shape. As a result of this design, catheters can be placed in an arcuate tunnel in an unstressed condition with both external and internal segments of the tunnel directed downward. Table 5 lists features preventing catheter complications.

Swan neck prototypes (Fig. 9) were designed in 1985 and used from August, 1985, to April, 1986. These catheters were made of 80° arc angle tubing and were inserted in a reversed U-shape tunnel with the incision at the top of the tunnel [104]. Only 27 of these catheters were inserted because we noted a tendency to cuff extrusions, which were confirmed by further experiences [105], and we have not used them since April, 1986 [105, 106]. Based on this observation the catheters were modified; the distance between cuffs was shortened from 8.5 cm to 5 cm in swan neck 2 and to 3 cm in swan neck 3 catheters and the bend was increased from 80° to 170–180° arc angle. The catheters were provided with short or long intraperitoneal segments, selected according to the patient size and insertion site, to secure the catheter tip position in the true pelvis [103, 105]. The intraperitoneal segment of the catheters, was changed to a coiled one (swan neck coiled).

5.3.1. *Swan neck Tenckhoff straight and coiled*

The Tenckhoff type of the swan neck peritoneal dialysis catheter is provided with two Dacron® cuffs. It differs from the double cuff Tenckhoff catheter only by being permanently bent between cuffs [103]. A subcutaneous tunnel has to be created in the same way as for other swan neck catheters.

5.3.2. *Swan neck Toronto*

The Toronto type of the swan neck catheter, a modification of the Toronto Western Hospital (TWH) catheter has a flange and bead circumferentially surrounding the catheter just below the internal cuff. Unlike the TWH catheter, the flange and bead are slanted approximately 45° relative to the axis of the catheter. Like TWH catheters these catheters are also provided with two intraperitoneal discs [103].

Table 5. Swan neck catheter features preventing complications.

Exit/tunnel infection	Downward exit, double cuff, short sinus
External cuff extrusion	Permanent bend between cuffs
Intraperitoneal tip migration	Downward intraperitoneal entrance
Pericatheter leak	Insertion through the rectus muscle
Peritonitis	Decreased tunnel infections
Infusion/pressure pain	Coiled intraperitoneal tip

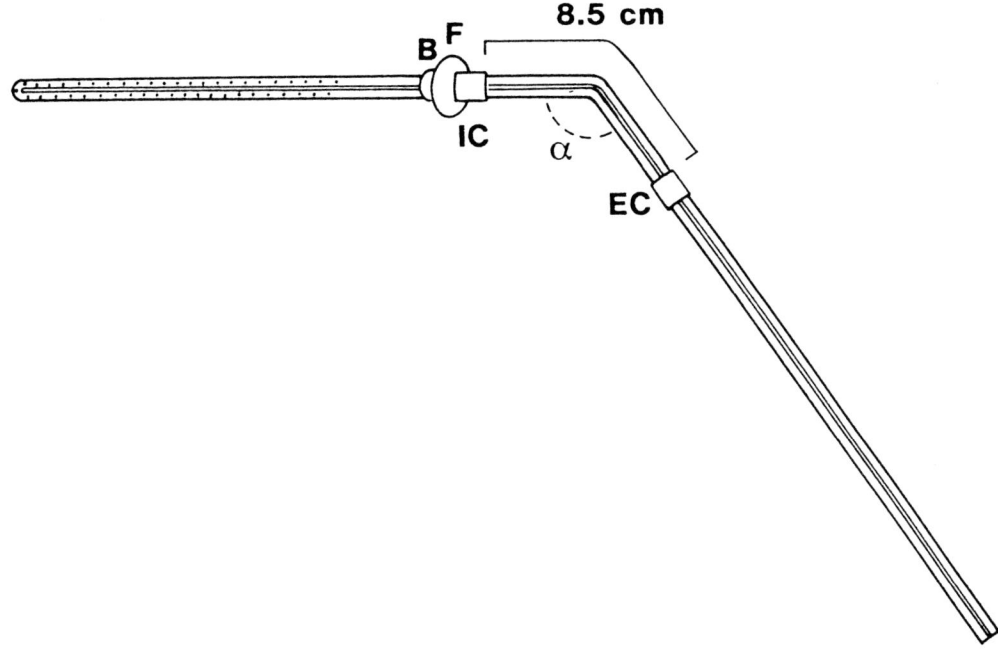

Figure 9. Swan neck Missouri prototype catheter. Arc angle = 180° − α = 80°. Cuff extrusions were common with these catheters because of insufficient bend and too long a distance between cuffs. We consider these catheters as suboptimal and we have not used them since April, 1986.

5.3.3. *Swan neck Missouri straight*

The swan neck Missouri catheter is identical to the swan neck Toronto catheter with the exception that it does not have intraperitoneal discs. The openings in the fascia and the peritoneum may be smaller for the tubing without discs, thus decreasing chances of pericatheter leaks.

5.3.4. *Swan neck Missouri coiled*

Swan neck Missouri 2 coiled catheters with the 5 cm intercuff distance (Fig. 10) are used in average to obese people. Swan neck Missouri 3 coiled catheters (Fig. 11) with 3 cm intercuff distance are used in lean to average persons. The catheters for left and right tunnels are mirror images of each other [103]. The overall survivals of straight and coiled swan neck Missouri catheters are not significantly different.

5.3.5. *Swan neck presternal*

Potential advantages of exit location in the chest instead of in the abdomen are shown in Table 6. The chest is a sturdy structure with minimal wall motion; the catheter exit located on the chest wall is subjected to minimal movements decreasing chances of trauma and contamination. Also, in patients with abdominal ostomies and in children with diapers, a chest exit location decreases chances of contamination. Clinical surgical experience indicates that wounds heal better after thoracic surgery than after abdominal surgery; this may be related to less chest mobility. All these favorable factors significantly reduce exit site infections. The catheter is also advantageous for psychosocial reasons. A long catheter tunnel combined with three cuffs, may curtail pericatheter bacterial penetration into the peritoneal cavity, thus reducing the incidence of peritonitis [39, 107, 108].

To accommodate these principles, we modified the swan neck peritoneal catheter to have an exit on the chest but preserving all advantages of the swan neck Missouri coiled catheters; minimizing catheter obstruction, cuff extrusion, pericatheter dialysate leak and infusion pain. A major difference from the swan neck Missouri catheter is in the length of the subcutaneous tunnel. The catheter (Fig. 12) is composed of two silicon rubber tubes, which are to be connected end to end at the time of implantation [107, 108]. The implanted lower (abdominal) tube constitutes the intraperitoneal catheter segment and a part of the intramural segment. The upper or chest tube constitutes the remaining part of the intramural segment and the external catheter segment. The lower tube is identical to the swan neck Missouri catheter, with the exception that it is not bent and does not have a second cuff. The

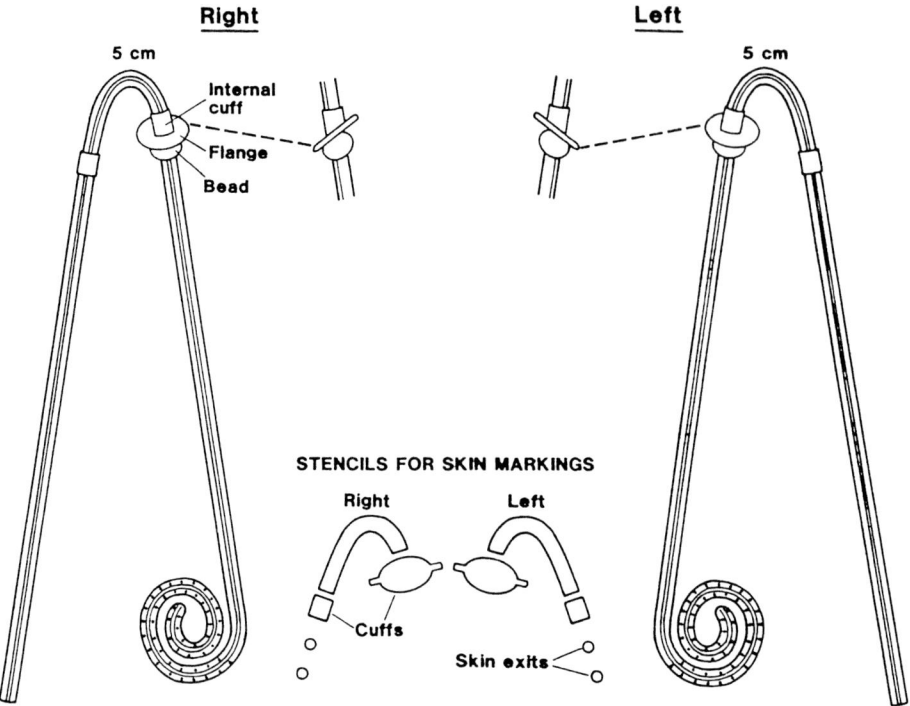

Figure 10. Swan neck Missouri 2 coiled (curled) catheters and stencils. Swan neck Missouri 2 catheters have 5 cm intercuff distance and intraperitoneal length of 32 cm from the bead to the tip. The flange and bead are slanted approximately 45° relative to the tubing axis. The catheters for left and right tunnels are mirror images of each other. The stencil follows exactly the shape of the intramural segment. The stencil can be flipped to be used for right or left catheter. The holes for exit site markings are located 2 cm and 1 cm from the cuff. A 2 cm mark is used for average or obese persons, a 1 cm mark is suitable for lean or average persons.

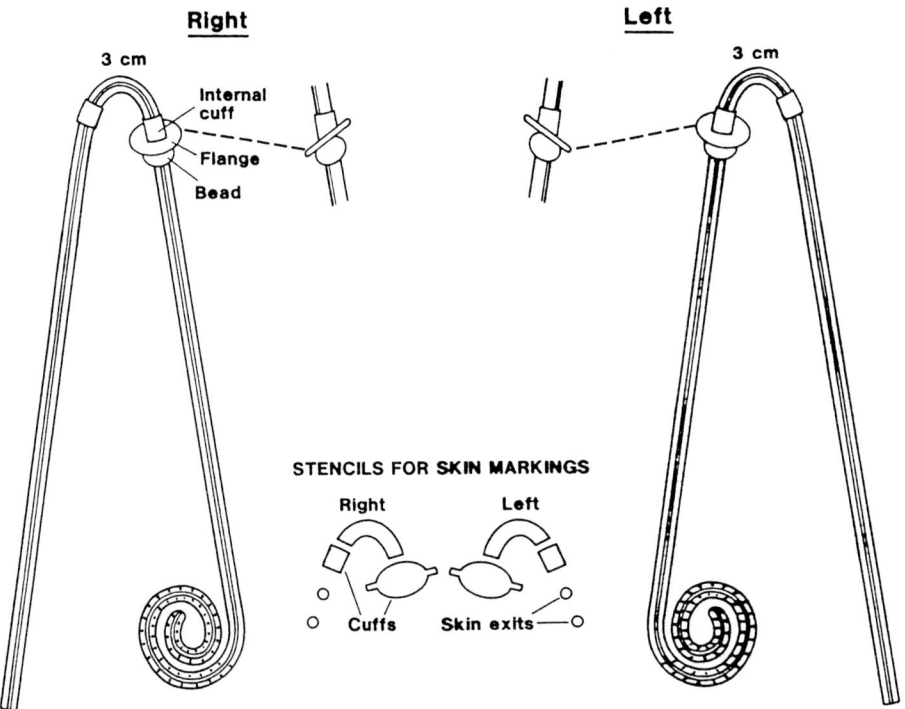

Figure 11. Swan neck Missouri 3 coiled catheters and stencils. It differs from the Swan neck Missouri 2 catheter only in the distance between cuffs, which is 3 cm. These catheters are used in lean or average persons.

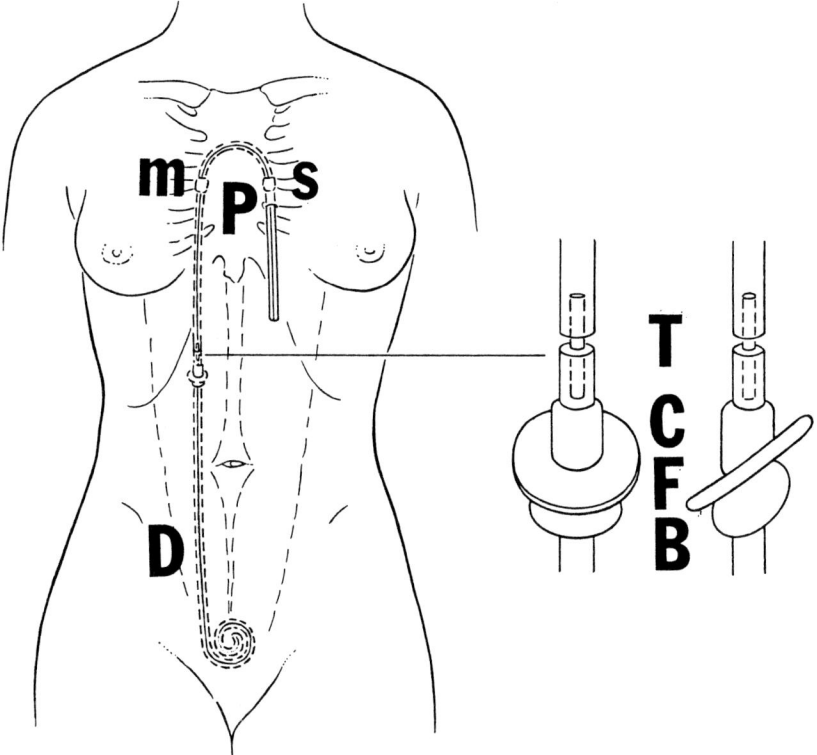

Figure 12. Swan neck presternal catheter in relation to the torso after implantation. D = distal tube; C = distal (deep) cuff located in the rectus muscle; F = flange; B = bead; T = titanium connector; P = proximal tube; m = medial (center) cuff; s = superficial cuff.

proximal end of the lower tube is straight and with a redundant length to be trimmed to the patient's size at the time of implantation. A titanium connector, provided in a package, is to be coupled with the distal part of the upper or chest part at the time of implantation.

The upper tube carries two porous cuffs, a superficial and a middle or central spaced 5 cm apart. The tube between the cuffs has a permanently bent section defining an arc angle of 180°. The distal lumen of the upper tube communicates with the proximal lumen of the lower tube through the titanium connector. The tubing grip of the titanium connector is so strong that the two parts of the catheter, especially after connection reinforcement with a prolene suture, practically cannot separate

Table 6. Potential advantages of the swan neck presternal catheter compared to the swan neck Missouri catheter.

Attribute	Advantage	Explanation
Exit on the chest	Decreased risk of exit infection	Good immobilization Good wound healing Loose gament/less pressure Easy exit site care Less fat thickness Far from ostomies Far from wet diapers (in small children) Less trauma with creeping (in small children)
	Psychosocial	Better body image for some patients Easy exit site care May take tub bath without risk of exit contamination
Three cuffs,	Decreased risk of peritonitis	Strong (triple) barrier, long tunnel distance for bacterial penetration

spontaneously in the tunnel [109]. The swan neck presternal catheter is available for children and infants. Tubing diameter is smaller for pediatric patients.

We have implanted seven of such catheters, mostly in patients with ostomies and extreme obesity. As predicted, clinical results in all patients have been satisfactory even though presternal catheters were implanted in patients in whom regular catheters with the exit on the abdomen would be difficult or impossible to implant. The exits healed well, the catheters were easy to immobilize and did not become infected for a cumulative observation period of 27 patient-months [110]. Patient acceptance of the exit position was excellent. Also in children preliminary results were excellent as reported by Sieniawska et al. [111].

5.3.6. Radiopaque stripe

The slanted flange and bead, and bent tunnel segment require that the swan neck Missouri and Toronto catheters for right and left tunnels be mirror images of each other. To facilitate recognition of right and left Toronto and Missouri catheters, each tubing has a radiopaque stripe in front of the catheter (Figs 10 and 11). In swan neck presternal catheters, the stripe facilitates also proper alignment of the lower and upper tubes. The stripe is also useful during insertion and post-implantation care, facilitating recognition of catheter twisting. Because of this last feature Tenckhoff type catheters are also provided with the stripe. Right and left swan neck Tenckhoff catheters differ only with respect to the position of the stripe. Unlike swan neck Toronto and Missouri catheters the swan neck Tenckhoff catheter intended for right or left tunnel may be implanted with an opposite tunnel. In this case the stripe should be kept in back of the catheter. Nevertheless, to retain uniformity of the stripe position it is recommended that swan neck Tenckhoff catheters be inserted with the corresponding tunnel direction (right tunnel with right catheter, left tunnel with left catheter).

6. Accessories for implantation of catheters

6.1. Stencils

Stencils have been developed for skin markings to facilitate creation of proper tunnels for swan neck catheters [103]. (Figs 10, 11). The stencils follow exactly the shape of the intramural segments of the catheters and the catheter tunnels must follow the shape of the catheters exactly as designed to maximize the advantages of this design. The stencils can be flipped to be used for right or left catheters. The holes for exit site markings are located 2 cm and 1 cm from the cuff. A 2 cm mark is used for average or obese persons, a 1 cm mark is suitable for lean or average persons.

6.2. Stiffening stilette

A 62 cm long stiffening stilette is used to facilitate catheter insertion into the true pelvis. During insertion, about 1 cm of catheter is left beyond the tip of the stilette to protect the bowels. The catheter resumes its natural shape after the stilette is removed [103].

6.3. Tunneling devices

6.3.1. Tenckhoff trocar (Fig. 1)
The trocar consists of: a sharp, stainless steel stylet; a solid, wide, open ended barrel; and two side pieces with handles [92], and can be used at the bedside.

6.3.2. Scanlan tunneler
A Scanlan tunneler is used during swan neck presternal catheter implantation to create a tunnel extending from the abdominal wall to the presternal or parasternal area. A tunneler to accommodate grafts up to 8 mm is suitable for presternal catheter implantation. The tunneler, developed for tunneling vascular grafts, consists of an outside sheath, a blunt tip, and a spring clamp. Depending on the size of the patient either a green (51 cm long) or an orange (30 cm long) tunneler may be used. A spring clamp serves to stiffen the tunneler as it is pushed through the subcutaneous tissue and to grasp and pull an upper tube through the sheath [107].

6.3.3. Exit trocar
The catheter tunnel extending from the cuff to the skin exit should have a diameter close to that of catheter tubing. Thus, the last portion of the tunnel (from external cuff to the exit) should be made with a piercing trocar (e.g., the Faller trocar) of external diameter similar to that of the catheter tubing [103, 107].

6.4. Peritoneoscopic equipment

The basic equipment (Fig. 13) required for this type of insertion includes a 2.2-mm diameter, 15-cm long Y-TEC peritoneoscope with a 2.5-mm steel cannula with an internal trocar and a spiral-wound Quill catheter guide surrounding the cannula [112].

6.5. Seldinger (guide wire) with peel-away sheath equipment

The essentials (Fig. 14) for this technique include a guide needle, attached to a syringe, a Seldinger guide wire, and a tapered dilator with surrounding scored peel-away sheath [113–117].

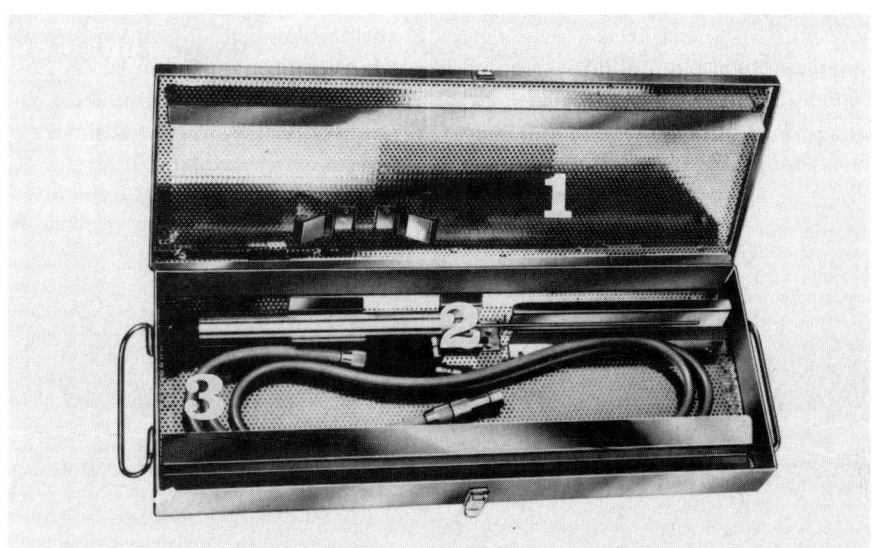

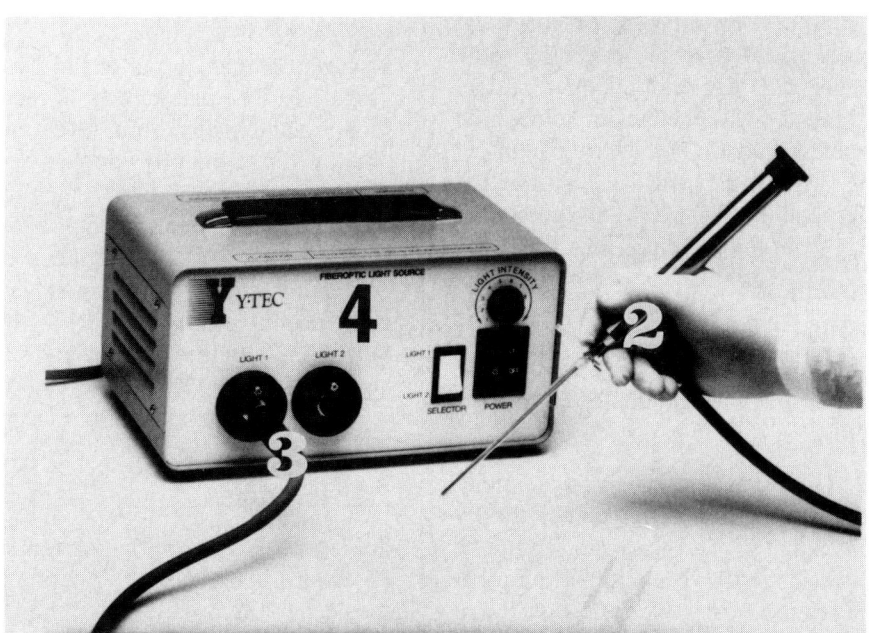

Figure 13. Components for the peritoneoscopic catheter insertion. Above: the sterilization tray (1); the Y-TEC® scope (2); and the light guide (3). Below is the Y-TEC® light source (4), with the scope (2), and light guide (3). This figure was kindly provided by John Navis, Medigroup, North Aurora, IL, USA.

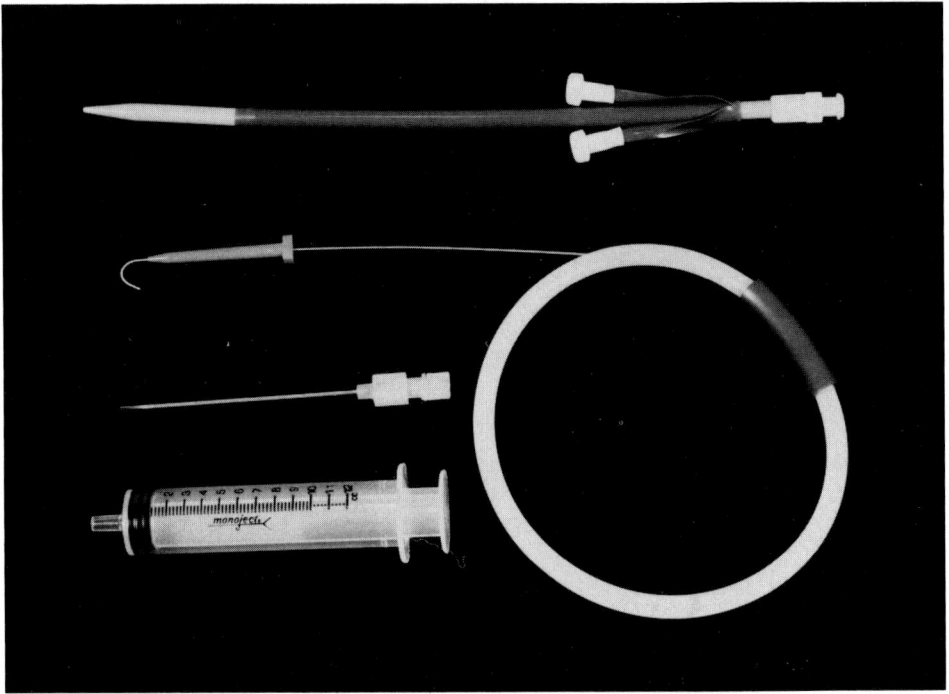

Figure 14. Equipment for guide-wire insertion method. From the top: peel-away sheath with dilator, guide-wire, needle, and syringe.

6.6. Nyton ties and a tension tool

Nyton ties and a tension tool are used to prevent disconnection of the titanium adaptor from the tubing. Care is taken to place the 4-inch tie in the groove between adapter ridges and not over a ridge. Then the tie is tightened with the tension tool which also trims the excess length. The locking segment is located at the stripe which will be positioned at the front of the patient (Fig. 15). This keeps the added bulk away from the patient [103, 107, 118].

7. Rigid catheter

7.1. Pre-insertion patient assessment and preparation

When the need to start peritoneal dialysis is urgent, one may elect to access the peritoneal cavity through a rigid catheter. This catheter could be inserted at the bedside, with very minimal preparation. Equipment required for paracentesis is all that is needed.

Bedside insertion should not be offered to patients who are extremely obese, or have had previous abdominal surgery, since abdominal adhesions increase the risk of inadvertent viscus perforation. In addition, this approach should not be done in children except by an experienced pediatric nephrologist or nephrologist with a pediatrician in attendance. If a nephrologist implants the catheter a surgeon should be on stand by, in case of complications. The patient should receive preoperative sedation and have nothing to eat or drink at least 12 hours prior to the procedure.

All observers and persons in the immediate area, including the patient, should wear surgical masks. Those patients who experience discomfort while completely supine should raise their heads slightly. If the patient is conscious, it may be useful to familiarize him with the Valsalva maneuver. The operator and assistant(s) should "scrub, gown and glove." A "circulating" nurse should be present to assist.

7.2. Insertion

Taking all sterile precautions, a small stab wound (2–3 mm) is made in the midline under local anesthesia, 2–3 cm below the umbilicus. The stab wound should be small so that the abdominal wall holds the catheter firmly and thus, minimizes dialysis solution leak.

With the stylet in place, the catheter is forced through the abdominal wall by a short thrust or

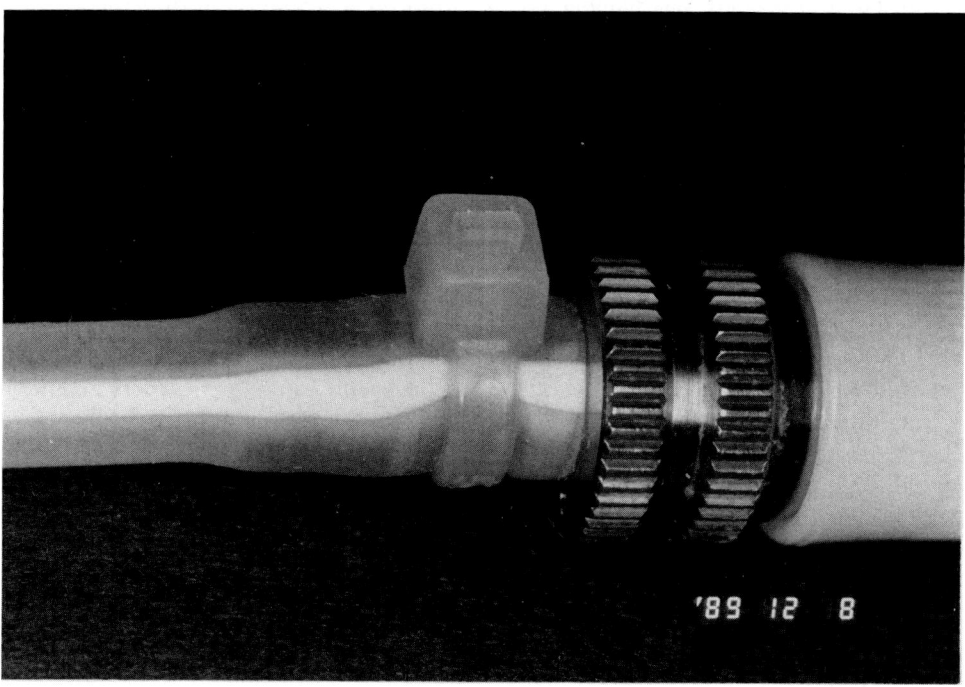

Figure 15. The nylon tie is placed over the catheter/adapter junction. The locking segment is over the stripe and will be away from the patient's skin.

preferably with a rotary motion. The operator will recognize the loss or resistance as a "pop" as soon as the peritoneal cavity is entered. While the catheter is being thrust through the abdominal wall, its tip is directed towards the coccyx. Because successful perforation of the abdominal wall for introduction of the catheter requires a sensitive "feel" for the pressure applied, infusion of 2–3 liters of dialysate with distend the abdomen which in turn will facilitate this maneuver. Some infuse 2 liters of dialysis fluid via a small gauge needle prior to stylet puncture. A co-operative patient can also assist successful penetration by voluntarily contracting the abdominal musculature.

Once the peritoneal cavity has been entered the stylet is withdrawn a few cm and the catheter is advanced deep into the pelvis. If the operator encounters resistance while the catheter is being advanced or if the patient complains of pain, the advance in this direction should be stopped and another direction tried. If this is still not possible, two or three liters of dialysis solution may be infused into the peritoneal cavity if this has not been done. It can be via the catheter if the holes in the distal end are in the cavity. This infusion accomplishes two important objectives; first, it facilitates recognition of the "true" intraperitoneal space; second, dialysis solution in the peritoneal cavity reduces the likelihood of viscus perforation by moving the intraabdominal contents away from the advancing catheter.

After one or two good in-and-out exchanges, the catheter is firmly secured to the skin with the aid of a metal disc.

7.3. Complications

Table 7 shows complications of rigid catheter insertion. After catheter implantation bloody effluent appears after the first exchange in approximately 30% of cases [119, 120]. This bleeding (usually minor) comes from the small vessels in the abdominal wall. After three to four exchanges, bleeding

Table 7. Complications of rigid catheter insertion.

Bleeding
Dialysis solution leak
Poor drainage
Extra-peritoneal space penetration
Viscus perforation
Peritonitis
Abdominal pain
Loss of rigid catheter in the peritoneum

usually stops unless the procedure has damaged a major vessel or the patient has a bleeding disorder. Pressure applied over the catheter insertion site usually controls minor bleeding. If the bleeding is copious, it may obstruct the catheter; in this event, it is a common practice to add 1000 units of heparin to each liter of dialysate to minimize the risk of obstruction. If bleeding persists, exploration may be necessary.

Dialysis solution leak is encountered in 14% to 36% of patients after rigid catheter insertion [119–121]. Frequent manipulation of the catheter to improve drainage increases the risk of dialysis solution leak from the catheter-exit site. Such leaks may also occur when the catheter is not properly secured to the skin. The risk of external leak is higher in elderly or debilitated patient who have lax abdominal walls. The presence of a large intra-abdominal mass, such as a polycystic kidney(s) may raise the intra-abdominal pressure to high levels and promote an external dialysis solution leak after the standard 2-liter volume has been instilled.

Fluid may extravasate into the abdominal wall, particularly in patients who have had a previous abdominal operation or multiple catheter insertion. This complication usually results from tears in the peritoneum or represents an infusion of dialysate into the potential space between the layers of abdominal wall. Uncommonly dialysis fluid may enter the pleural cavity [122–133]. In such cases, peritoneal dialysis is usually discontinued and the patients are switched to hemodialysis. Acute hydrothorax results from either a traumatic or a congenital defect in the diaphragm.

Inadequate drainage is frequent during initial dialysis, and may be due to one or more of the following factor; loss of siphon effect, one-way obstruction, and/or incorrect placement of the catheter. One-way (outflow) catheter obstruction may have multiple causes. Fibrin or blood clots may be trapped in the catheter and block the terminal holes, especially when dialysis is complicated by major hemorrhage or peritonitis. Poor outflow may also reflect extrinsic pressure on the catheter from adjacent organs such as a sigmoid colon full of feces or a distended bladder. Omental wrapping is likely if the catheter is misplaced into the upper abdomen.

Occasionally, accidental penetration of the extraperitoneal space by the catheter may cause poor drainage. In such a situation, continued infusion produces further dissection, and the fluid may become trapped and is no longer available for drainage. Loculation of fluid, another cause of poor drainage, is encountered in patients who have had previous intra-abdominal operations or peritonitis. Such loculation not only diminishes the surface area available for dialysis but may seriously reduce ultrafiltration capacity. The incidence of this complication is low, varying between 0.5% and 1.3% [121, 134, 135].

Perforation or laceration of internal organs during bedside insertion of catheter has been frequently reported. Lacerated or perforated organs include the bowel, bladder, liver, a polycystic kidney, aorta, mesenteric artery and hernia sac [131, 134–146]. Abdominal distention due to paralytic ileus or bowel obstruction may predispose the patient to bowel perforation. Those who are unconscious, cachectic or heavily sedated are also at high risk. Clinical evidence of bowel perforation includes sudden, sharp or severe abdominal pain followed by watery diarrhea, and poor drainage of dialysis solution, which may be cloudy, foul-smelling or mixed with fecal material. Such a situation requires prompt removal of the catheter, and allowing the perforation to seal off completely in about 12–24 hours.

The incidence of peritonitis when the stylet catheter was used, was 2.5% of all the dialyses [148]. The incidence of peritonitis almost doubled when the duration of dialysis was longer than 60 hours.

Abdominal pain may be encountered in as many as 56–75% of patients with the first use of the catheter [119]. There are many causes of abdominal pain, but catheter related pain occurs when it impinges on any of the viscera. Pain may occur during inflow and outflow of dialysis solution and also when the solution is dwelling. Outflow pain is due to entrapment of omentum in the catheter during the siphoning action of fluid drainage. Constant pain during the dialysis indicates pressure effects on intra-abdominal organs and often produces continuous rectal or low back pain. This complaint calls for an adjustment in catheter position.

Loss of a part or all of the rigid catheter has been reported following its manipulation with the trocar in place [119, 137, 139, 147, 148]. Its distal end may be amputated after intraabdominal kinking of the catheter, followed by manipulation. However, the presence of broken catheters within the abdominal cavity does not cause symptoms or ill effects. During laparoscopy, broken catheters have been found lying freely in the peritoneal cavity without causing a peritoneal reaction or have been found walled off by mesentery without an inflammatory reaction. On routine postmortem examination, Stein [149] discovered such a catheter in a patient who had had previous peritoneal dialysis. Exploration to retrieve the catheter is unnecessary because laparotomy is more hazardous than leaving the catheter in a severely ill patient. The incidence of catheter loss into the peritoneal cavity has been greatly reduced since the introduction of a design which incorporates a metal disc with a central hole; this not only allows the catheter to pass through the wall but also holds the catheter snugly to the skin of the abdominal wall.

8. Soft catheter

Because of the high frequency of dialysis solution leak, and poor drainage necessitating frequent catheter manipulation and resultant peritonitis with the use of rigid catheters, some centers prefer to insert single or double cuff Tenckhoff catheter for treatment of acute renal failure. Tenckhoff recommended use of single cuff catheters for acute cases [1]. For treatment of chronic renal failure only soft catheters are used.

8.1. Patient preparation

8.1.1. *Acute dialysis*
Patient assessment and preparation before soft catheter implantation for treatment of acute renal failure is the same as that before rigid catheter insertion.

8.1.2. *Chronic dialysis*
Patient preparation before catheter implantation for treatment of chronic renal failure is more elaborate [103, 107, 150–152]. Usually one day prior to surgery, chest and/or abdominal hair should be removed with an electric shaver.

8.1.2.1. *Abdominal exit* The belt line of the patient is identified, preferably in the sitting position, with slacks or pants as usually worn [103]. Depending on the size and shape of the abdomen, presence of previous scars, right or left handedness, and patient's preference, the tunnel is marked using the stencil (available with swan neck catheters) in such a way that the exit hole would be created at least 2 cm from the belt line. Skin markings may be made with any good surgical marker.

Women usually wear a belt above the umbilicus, hence stencils are marked below the belt line in female patients. The catheter should not be subjected to excessive motion with patient activities, and there should not be pressure on the tunnel when the patient bends forward. In obese people with pendulous abdomens, it is mandatory to insert the catheter above the skin fold as they can see the exit for its care. Men usually prefer a belt line below the umbilicus and there may not be enough space below the belt line; therefore a stencil is frequently marked above the belt line in male patients. The label of the chosen catheter type is written on the belly of the patient. A band with the catheter label is also attached to the patient's left wrist.

One gram of Vancomycin is given by slow intravenous infusion within 24 hours prior to surgery. In the evening preceding the surgery, a tap water enema is administered and the patient takes a shower. Skin markings may require correction if they become faint after the shower. Cephalosporins (1.0 g IV 1 hr preoperatively repeated 12 hr postoperatively) also constitute appropriate prophylactic therapy [151, 152].

8.1.2.2. *Presternal exit* Depending on the size of the patient, the abdominal cuff and flange location is marked over the rectus muscle [107]. To secure the catheter tip position in the true pelvis but without an excessive pressure on the pelvic peritoneum, the position of the cuff should be above the umbilicus in small persons and at the level of or slightly below the umbilicus in tall persons. To determine a preferable position of the deep cuff, a coiled catheter tip is placed on the public bone and the cuff position is marked. On the chest a superficial cuff is marked at the second or third intercostal spaces and the exit 1–2 cm from the cuff in the presternal or parasternal area. It is preferable not to cross the midline in patients likely to have heart surgery. Care is taken to avoid an exit site too close to a bras in females. Prophylactic antibiotics, shower, and enema are used in the same way as for abdominal exit [107].

8.2. Catheter preparation

Immediately before implantation the catheter is removed from the sterile peel back and immersed in sterile saline. Dacron® cuffs and the flange are gently squeezed to remove air [103, 107]. Thoroughly wetted cuffs provide markedly better tissue ingrowth compared to unwetted, air containing cuffs [50].

8.3. Implantation method

8.3.1. *Blind (Tenckhoff trocar)*
The detailed insertion is described in Chapter 10 and uses the equipment shown in Fig. 1.

8.3.2. *Peritoneoscopic*
The use of peritoneoscopy for peritoneal catheter placement was developed by Ash at Lafayette, Indiana [112, 153]. Tenckhoff and swan neck Tenckhoff (straight and coiled) catheters may be implanted with this technique. Like blind insertion, it is performed through a single abdominal puncture. Details of the insertion technique are given in Chapter 10.

8.3.3. *Seldinger (guide wire) and peel-away sheath*
This technique may be used for a straight and coiled Tenckhoff catheters as well as of swan neck Tenckhoff straight and coiled catheters. The pre-insertion patient preparation is similar to the one described for rigid catheter insertion. The procedure may be done with [113] or without [114–117] pre-filling the abdomen with dialysis solution. Prefilling of the abdomen is accomplished through a temporary peritoneal catheter. The technique is detailed in Chapter .

8.3.4. *Surgical (by dissection)*
Dissective placement is required for catheters with stabilizing devices at the parietal surfaces (swan neck Missouri, Toronto Western Hospital, and swan neck presternal) or large intraperitoneal discs (Lifecath® column disc). The paramedian approach through the rectus muscle is recommended [53, 103, 107]. Details of the surgical (by dissection) technique is given in Chapter 10. What follows here relates to details of other techniques, presternal insertion and the Moncrief/Popovich catheter insertion.

8.3.4.1. *Swan neck presternal*
A vertical 3–4 cm incision is made over the sternum at the level of the second and third rib [107, 108]. Using a combination of sharp and blunt dissection, two small subcutaneous pockets are made on both sides of the incision to accommodate the bent section of the upper (chest) tube of the catheter. The pockets are dissected enough to accommodate the middle and superficial cuffs. Careful hemostasis is essential.

To join the upper and lower tube a Scanlan tunneling device is pushed from the abdominal incision to the sternal one. The tunnel path is carefully guided. The blunt tip of the outside sheath is removed. Keeping the stripe in front as a guide, the abdominal end of the upper tube is grasped with the spring clamp and pulled caudally through the sheath and the sheath is removed by pulling in the caudal direction.

The middle cuff of the upper tube is carefully placed under the stencil mark. When the catheter is appropriately positioned the desired lengths of the tubes are measured and the tubes are trimmed. Enough lengths on both tubes should be left to facilitate connection. The titanium connector is inserted into the upper tube and secured with a Zero-Prolene suture placed over the groove. Then the connector is inserted into the lower tube. The stripes on both tubes are facing up. The tie is now placed on the lower tube over the groove of the titanium connector. Both sutures are tied together and the titanium connector is positioned in the subcutaneous tissue approximately 2–6 cm above the rectus sheath incision.

A trocar of the same size as the catheter tubing is attached and carefully passed through the pocket and the external exit indicated by the stencil mark. The stripe is facing front. The trocar is disconnected. The bent portion of the catheter is carefully positioned in the subcutaneous pocket. The titanium luer lock connector is attached. One liter of normal saline is infused through the infusion set and drained immediately. Outflow should be approximately 200 ml in one min. The wounds are checked for leaks, irrigated, and inspected for hemostasis. The transverse incision in the anterior rectus sheath is sewn with 2–0 monofilament nonabsorbable suture. Skin incisions are again inspected for hemostasis. Any bleeding vessels are cauterized and the incisions are closed with absorbable subcuticular sutures. The operative site is covered with several layers of high absorbency gauze dressings and secured with Tegaderm® which also immobilizes the catheter. The dressing is to be left in place for a week.

8.3.4.2. *Moncrief/Popovich technique*
This is a new technique which allows tissue ingrowth into the cuff material without exposure to the skin surface area. Unlike any other technique the distal (external segment) of the catheter is completely buried and remains in the subcutaneous tunnel until exteriorized after three to eight weeks post catheter insertion [155]. A video [156] demonstrating the technique is available from the Austin Biomedical Research Institute, 4211 Medical Parkway, Austin,

TX 78756, USA. Using swan neck catheters with this technique Moncrief and co-workers reported a significant reduction in peritonitis incidence [155].

9. Catheter break-in and catheter care

9.1. Immediate intraperitoneal segment care

In the recovery room the position of the catheter is checked by a plain X-ray of the abdomen. No catheter kink in the tunnel and the catheter tip in the true pelvis usually predict an excellent catheter function [103]. Plain X-ray of the Lifecath® column disc catheter is of little value in its function prediction.

9.2. Peritoneal dialysis

In the ward the patient is attached to the cycler to perform additional exchanges. Each liter of dialysis solution contains 1000 units of heparin. One half or one liter volumes of dialysis solutions are used for the first supine peritoneal dialysis. Usual cycler settings are: 10 min fill time, 0 min dwell, and 12 min outflow. In spite of clear dialysate in the first post-implantation washout, the dialysate is usually blood tinged during the first cycler exchange. No dwell exchanges are continued until the dialysate is clear. If immediate peritoneal dialysis is needed the patient continues on a cycler in the strict supine position with dwell time prolonged to 30–40 min. We do not commence peritoneal dialysis in the vertical position sooner than 10 days post implantation; thus CAPD or a last bag CCPD are not used for 10 days. The patient may be maintained on hemodialysis through temporary access for logistical reasons before peritoneal dialysis training can be started or may require hemodialysis because of the catheter malfunction (see below).

9.3. Exit care

To delay bacterial colonization of the exit site and minimize trauma, the dressing should not be changed frequently. The surgical dressing is gently removed after one week. Nonionic surfactant is used to help gauze removal if it is attached to the scab. If the scab is forcibly removed the epidermal layer is broken, a new scab has to be made and the epidermization is prolonged. Care is taken to avoid catheter pulling or twisting. The exit and skin surrounding the catheter are cleansed with nonionic surfactant (Shur Clens®), patted dry with sterile gauze, covered with several layers of gauze dressings, and secured with air-permeable tape. The dressing is changed after another week. Weekly dressing changes are continued until the healing process is completed, which takes 4–8 weeks. The patient may shower only before the dressing change otherwise must take sponge baths and avoid exit wetting.

Protecting the catheter from mechanical stress seems to be extremely important, especially during break-in. Catheters should be anchored in such a way that the patient's movements are only minimally transmitted to the exit. The method of catheter immobilization is individualized, depending on exit location and shape of the abdomen. We believe that better exit protection prevents infections in most patients.

The exit should be carefully evaluated every week for quality of healing. Unless a large hematoma in the wound is present, all exits look the same a week after implantation. The exit is painless or minimally tender with light pink color of less than 13 mm in diameter from border to border (including the width of the catheter). Blood clot or serosanguinous drainage is visible in the sinus. No epidermis is visible in the sinus and the granulation tissue is white and plain. Signs of good healing include a decrease in color saturation and diameter around the exit, change of drainage to serous, decreased drainage amount, decreased tenderness, and progression of epidermis into the sinus. An increase in color diameter or saturation around the exit, change of drainage to yellow, change of granulation tissue color to mottled, pink or red, change of granulation tissue into slightly exuberant or exuberant are signs of poor healing. Our exit site study [56] revealed two categories of healing exits: fast (or well) and slow (or poorly) healing. In fast healing exits, tenderness of the exit abates, pink color around the exit remains the same, granulation tissue in the sinus remains white and plain, the sinus becomes damp or dry two weeks after implantation. Epidermis starts to enter into the sinus within 2–4 weeks. Four to 6 weeks after implantation the epidermis covers at least half of the visible sinus achieving feature of a healed, good exit. In slow healing exits, the tenderness and serous drainage persist longer than one week, peri-exit color diameter and saturation increases, granulation tissue in the sinus becomes mottled, red or frankly exuberant. Epidermis does not enter into the sinus until 5–6 weeks post implantation. Serious drainage changes to yellow, purulent drainage. A slow healing exit is essentially tantamount to an early acutely infected exit and requires use of systemic antibiotics.

Late care, after the healing process is completed, is simpler. The results of a prospective study indicate that cleaning with soap and water is the least expensive and tends to prevent infections better than povidone-iodine painting and hydrogen peroxide cleaning [157]. It is worth realizing that the cleansing agent should not only decrease the number of bacteria, but also be harmless to the body defenses. Povidone-iodine is cytotoxic to mammalian cells in bacteriocidal concentrations [74, 75] and is harmful to granulation tissue if it enters the sinus. After cleansing, the exit has to be patted dry with sterile gauze, dried out additionally with a hot air blower for about 15–30 seconds until air is felt as warm. Then the catheter is well immobilized. Most of our patients use a dressing cover for 6–12 months after implantation. One year after implantation patients are allowed to omit use of a cover dressing, if desired. We could not find any reason why in some patients an uncovered exit seems to do better, in others worse.

We recommend that our patients use only a shower and avoid submersion in water, particularly in a jacuzzi, hot tub, or public pool, unless water tight exit protection can be implemented. Prolonged submersion in water containing high concentrations of bacteria frequently leads to severe infection with consequent loss of catheter. Swimming in the ocean, and well sterilized private pools is less dangerous. Exit care must be performed immediately after a shower or water submersion, with particular attention to obtaining a well dried exit. The surrounding skin is coated with a skin protector and secured with Tegaderm. Patients with the swan neck presternal catheter may take a hot tub bath without exit site submersion. Because of this feature this catheter was dubbed the "bath tub" catheter [108].

10. Early soft catheter complications

Early complications post soft catheter insertion are similar to those after implantation of the rigid catheter (Table 8), but their frequency is lower, particularly with surgical and peritoneoscopic insertion. Blood tinged dialysate is common post implantation but severe bleeding occurs very rarely with surgical insertion. Dialysate leaks are unlikely if ambulatory peritoneal dialysis is postponed for at least 10 days after implantation [158]. This complication is particularly rare with the Toronto Western Hospital, swan neck Missouri, swan neck presternal, and Lifecath® column disc catheters. Early leak is unusually external and may be confused with serous drainage from the exit. A diagnosis of a leak is supported by the drainage glucose concentration higher than the simultaneously measured blood glucose concentration.

Poor dialysate return is usually due to catheter obstruction if loss of siphon or tubing occlusion is ruled out. The most common reason of catheter obstruction is occlusion of the tip by bowel and/or bladder or intraluminal formation of clot (Table 8). Emptying the bladder and using laxatives may restore catheter function if there is occlusion by bladder or bowel. Clot may be prevented by rinsing out blood from the peritoneal cavity and using heparin and/or dislodged by pushing into the peritoneal cavity or pulling by suction using a syringe filled with heparinized saline. If these maneuvers are unsuccessful the catheter may be filled with urokinase (Abbokinase) 5,000 I.U. diluted in normal saline. Urokinase may open the obstruction in 10–15% of cases [159]. Catheter kinking in the tunnel usually is associated with two way obstruction, is recognizable on abdominal X-ray in two views, and requires surgical correction as soon as diagnosis is made. If the catheter is not kinked but does not function for 2 weeks, omental wrapping or multiple adhesions are most likely and omentectomy or adhesiolysis through laparoscopy may be required.

Another reason of obstruction may be catheter adherence to the peritoneum. This complication was found in children who have undergone partial omentectomy at the time of insertion of a single cuff, straight Tenckhoff catheter. Relocation of such catheters may be attempted with a so called

Table 8. Early catheter obstruction.

Cause	Prevention/treatment
Occlusion by bowel	Laxatives
Occlusion by bladder	Empty bladder
Clot	Rinse out blood, Heparin, urokinase, Dislodge
Omental wrap	Partial omentectomy
Multiple adhesions	Adhesiolysis
Kink in the tunnel	Surgical correction

"whiplash" technique [160]. After localization of the catheter adherence site, using a strict sterile technique, a blunted steel trocar is inserted into the catheter and gently advanced until the trocar is 5–7 cm proximal to the tip of the catheter. Using a deep cuff as a fulcrum and using short and rapid whiplash motions, the catheter is then freed from the adherence point. The catheter tip is then, under fluoroscopy, relocated to a new site. A modification of this method using a pliable copper thread was successfully used in adults [161]. A catheter migrated to the upper abdomen may be relocated using a guide wire [101, 162]. Although these methods may obviate the need for surgery, they are not without a risk. The guide wire may break during manipulations, perforate the catheter and lead to recurrent peritonitis. We do not use them in our institution considering them as too risky procedures.

Catheter migration out of the true pelvis is seen frequently on abdominal X-Rays done for various reasons in patients with functioning catheters [163]. While about 20% of X-rays showed the catheter tip translocated to the upper abdomen, only 20% of these translocated catheters (4% of the total) were obstructed. The remaining functioning malpositioned catheters were either permanently translocated or repositioned spontaneously to the true pelvis. About 3% of catheters in our series were obstructed with the tip in the true pelvis [164].

While the great majority of malpositioned catheters are not obstructed, a catheter with its tip in the upper abdomen is still about six times more likely to be obstructed than a normally positioned catheter. The migration of the catheter tip may, however, be the result of the obstruction rather than its cause; omentum entangling the catheter tip may be responsible for its translocation.

Relocation of the catheter is best done surgically using a laparoscopic method. In our experience if this method fails to restore catheter function, the peritoneum is not usable for peritoneal dialysis because of massive adhesions and replacement of the catheter in such a situation is worthless. The patient has to be transferred to hemodialysis.

Viscus perforation is unheard of with surgical catheter insertion. Early peritonitis with a soft catheter is half of that reported with a rigid catheter, even in the treatment of acute renal failure [147]. Abdominal pain is more likely with straight catheters due to a "jet effect" and tip pressure as discussed in the section 4.8.

11. Late soft catheter complications

Factors influencing catheter complications have been discussed in the section 4. (Table 1). Complications are not randomly distributed throughout the life of the catheter. Whereas leaks and malfunctions occur shortly after catheter implantation, infectious complications lead to catheter failure later [106].

11.1. Exit site infection

There is no single definition of exit-site infection that has achieved universal approval. The most widely accepted is that published by Pierratos in 1984 [165], which was agreed upon by the vast majority of Peritoneal Dialysis Bulletin Editorial Board members. Pierratos defined exit-site infection as: "Redness or skin induration or purulent discharge from the exit-site. Formation of the crust around the exit may not indicate infection. Positive cultures from the exit site in the absence of inflammation do not indicate infection". The definition implies the presence of infection in the instances where laboratory cultures are negative and rejects the existence of infection based on a positive culture without inflammation.

Several recent publications used similar criteria [166–168]. This definition, however, is not sufficiently precise to delineate infected from noninfected exits in many instances. Many other definitions used in the literature were recently reviewed [57]. It is inferred that an exit without signs of infection is healthy, thus only two categories (infected or not infected) are assumed. Descriptions of a normal exit site and various degrees of infections are rare [57, 169, 170]. The rates of exit infections and the outcome of treatment are astonishingly discrepant in the literature. Rates as low as 0.05 or 0.1 per patient per year [171, 172], or as high as 1.02 per patient per year [166], have been reported. It is likely that this discrepancy in infection rates does not reveal a real variation but reflects disagreement regarding exit site infection definition [169].

Attempts to classify exit appearance into two categories (infected and not infected) is difficult, if not impossible, because infected and uninfected exit appearances overlap. This overlap is due to the peculiarity of tissue reaction to the foreign body penetrating the skin and stems from the delicate balance between bacteria in the sinus and host defenses as described above. The presence of a small amount of exudate causing crust formation does not indicate infection but if the bacterial attack is more severe then the amount of exudate increases; granulation tissue proliferates, becomes more vascularized, epithelium regresses and signs of infection become obvious. Low grade exit infection may abate without systemic antibiotics.

11.1.1. Classification of exit site appearance

For the last 3 years we have been evaluating exit site appearance in the immediate post implantation period and later, after the exit is healed [56, 57, 170]. The classification is based on the cardinal signs of inflammation as proposed by Aulus Cornelius Celsus in his treatise, *De Medicina*, written in the 1st century AD. These are well known: *calor* (heat), *rubor* (redness), *turgor* (swelling), and *dolor* (pain). Additional features, specific for an exit of any skin penetrating foreign body, are: drainage, regression of epidermis, and exuberance (profuse overgrowth) of granulation tissue ("proud flesh"). Granulation tissue is defined as exuberant if it is significantly elevated above the epidermis level. Culture results did not influence exit classification. Positive cultures in exits not inflamed indicate colonization, not infection. Cultures were commonly negative from infected exits on antibiotic therapy. However, inflammation in almost all cases is caused by infection, regardless of culture results. Inflammatory response to tubing itself or local irritants is rare.

Improvement or deterioration of inflammation is associated with respective decreases or increases of pain, induration, drainage, and/or exuberant granulation tissue, and/or regression or progression of epithelium in the sinus. Increased lightness (pink, pale pink) or darkness (deep black, brown) and decrease in color diameter indicate improvement, increase in red color saturation and diameter indicate deterioration. Ultimately 5 categories of exit appearance have been established: acutely inflamed, chronically inflamed, equivocal, good, and perfect.

An acutely inflamed exit has the following features in various combinations: pain, induration, redness with diameter (border to border, including the width of the catheter) ≥ 13 mm, liquid external drainage, exuberant granulation tissue around exit and/or in the sinus, and duration of inflammation less than 4 weeks.

In a chronically inflamed exit the following features are typically present: liquid external drainage, exuberant granulation tissue around the exit and/or in the sinus, and duration of inflammation more than 4 weeks. The following features are typically absent: pain, induration, and redness.

In an equivocal exit the following features are commonly present: liquid drainage in the sinus only and slightly exuberant granulation tissue around the exit and/or in the sinus. External drainage is thick, if present; crust forms daily or dried exudate is seen on the dressing. External drainage may be expressed by applying pressure on the sinus. The following features are commonly absent: pain, induration, redness with diameter ≥ 13 mm, and distinctly exuberant granulation tissue.

A good exit is characterized by the presence of plain (not exuberant) granulation tissue in the sinus with visible epithelium in the sinus at least partly mucosal (fragile, not keratinized), and thick drainage or dampness in the sinus. Crust forms no more frequently than every 2 days; specks of crust (but not dried exudate) may be seen on the dressing. The following features are absent: pain, induration, redness (any diameter), any external drainage, liquid drainage in the sinus, exuberant (even slight) granulation tissue. The exit may be pale pink.

In a perfect exit the following features are usually present: the exit is mature, six months or older; strong, mature epithelium is present in the sinus; the sinus tract is usually dry but may be damp or may contain thick drainage; crust forms no more frequently than every 7 days, specks of crust may be seen on the dressing; exit color is natural or dark; pale pink color occasionally may be present. The following features are absent: pain, induration, pink or red color around exit, any external drainage, liquid drainage in the sinus, any visible granulation tissue.

Exit trauma is an important cause of exit site infection. Features of a traumatized exit depend on the intensity of trauma and time of examination. Common features of trauma are pain, bleeding, formation of scab, and deterioration of exit appearance: a perfect exit may transform to a good, equivocal or acutely infected one.

11.1.2. Care and treatment of recommendations

11.1.2.1. Acutely inflamed exit Systemic antibiotics for Gram positive organisms should be started before culture results are available. Excessive crust should be removed with Shur-Clens®. Dressing changes are to be performed twice or once daily depending on the amount of drainage. Catheter immobilization and protection from trauma (if not already implemented) are essential. Antibiotics should be adjusted as indicated by sensitivity tests when available, but antibiotics have to be changed, if there is no improvement, regardless of culture results. Treatment should be continued for seven days after criteria for a good exit are fulfilled. The catheter should be removed in cases of accompanying refractory peritonitis. Surgical intervention, such as sinus deroofing and/or cuff shaving in tunnel infections, needs to be considered. Our recent experience indicates that such procedures prolong catheter life only moderately.

Exuberant granulation tissue ("proud flesh") should be cauterized with a silver nitrate stick. In our experience such cauterization markedly expedites treatment and facilitates epithelialization. It is important to apply silver nitrate only to the granulation tissue and avoid touching epithelium; thus only a physician or nurse, not a patient, should apply the cautery. We use a 4.5 times magnifying loupe to facilitate precise application of silver nitrate. Surgical excision of the "proud flesh" is usually not needed.

Excision and/or cauterization of exuberant granulation tissue in wound care have been used for centuries. It was mentioned, probably for the first time, by Paul of Aegina (Paulus Aegineta – b.c. 625, d.c. 690, Alexandrian physician and surgeon) in *Epitomes iatrikes biblio hepta* (Medical Compendium in Seven Books) which contained nearly everything known about medical arts in that time. Through Persian master physician ar-Rāzī (Rhazes) in *Kitāb al-Mansūrī* (Book to al-Mansūr) and Abū al-Qāsim (Albucasis) one of Islam's foremost surgeons in *at-Taṣrīf* (The Method) it was adopted by Western medicine. Now this method is widely used in surgical practice, both human and veterinary [173].

11.1.2.2. *Chronically inflamed exit* Treatment is similar to that of acute inflammation; however, whereas one cauterization is usually sufficient in acute inflammation, several cauterizations once or twice weekly may be needed in chronic inflammation. Species of bacterial flora or antibiotic sensitivity usually changes during the course of therapy and antibiotics have to be changed accordingly. Features of a good exit may not be obtained for a long time; if features of an equivocal exit persist for several weeks, systemic antibiotics may be stopped and local antibiotics may be used.

11.1.2.3. *Equivocal exit* Treatment of equivocal exit stems from two observations: 1) an equivocal exit if untreated is likely to become explicitly inflamed, and 2) systemic antibiotics usually prevent development of acute infection. Cauterization of slightly exuberant granulation tissue may be sufficient. Local therapy with mupirocin (Bactroban®) ointment (for Gram positive organisms) or Neosporin® cream, ointment or ophthalmic solution for a variety of organisms including S. aureus and Pseudomonas may be successful.

11.1.2.4. *Good and perfect exit* Catheter immobilization, protection from trauma, use of liquid soap and water for daily care, and use of Shur-Clens® to remove large, irritating crust are appropriate measures to prevent infection. In our experience a perfect exit is unlikely to become infected unless severely traumatized or grossly contaminated after submersion in water loaded with bacteria.

11.1.2.5. *Traumatized exit* For severe trauma prophylactic antibiotics should be used. Mild trauma of a perfect exit with change of appearance to good does not require antibiotics. If the exit assumes an equivocal or acutely inflamed appearance, the treatment is the same as described above. It is prudent to administer systemic antibiotics if a patient's exit cannot be evaluated within two or three days after trauma.

11.1.2.6. *Local and systemic use of antibiotics for prophylaxis and treatment of exit infection* There is no evidence to support the use of prophylactic antibiotics to reduce the incidence or frequency of exit site tunnel infections [174, 175]. An exception may be a rare case with frequent recurrence of acute infection [176]. Local antibiotics in acute or chronic infection are of little value because they cannot achieve proper local concentrations before being washed away with large drainage; antibiotics administered systemically provide therapeutic concentrations locally by being excreted into the drainage. Local antibiotics can achieve high concentrations in the sinus in equivocal, good, or perfect exits but may be useful only in equivocal exits.

11.2. External cuff extrusion

As discussed in the section 4.5, the main cause of cuff extrusion is placement of the external segment of the catheter in any shape other than its natural design with the cuff too close to the exit. Due to the resilience force of the silicon rubber, the catheter tends to slowly assume its original shape and may push the cuff out of the sinus. If the cuff is not infected, it is left alone; however, the cuff usually becomes infected during this process and requires systemic antibiotics or even surgical intervention. If there is no peritonitis or deep cuff infection then the catheter may be saved, at least for some time, by shaving off the infected cuff [177]. Infection is another cause of cuff extrusion. In this instance the cuff becomes infected while still in the sinus and extruded by tissue retraction round the cuff. Two such extrusions were observed with swan neck Missouri catheters [106].

11.3. Catheter obstruction

"Capture" of the catheter by active omentum may cause outflow obstruction. Obstruction from this cause, in the absence of peritonitis, when it occurs is usually a postoperative event (related to a new catheter). We have never seen an obstruction (in the absence of peritonitis) due to omental "capture" as a late event. We believe that foreign body Silastic® is more prone to attract omentum very early. In time, with or without use, a proteinaceous (not bacterial) biofilm catheter coating may make the Silastic® less "foreign" to omental tissue. Slow drainage due to catheter translocation, occlusion by bowel or fibrin clot formation occurs from time to time in some patients. Laxatives and/or addition of heparin 500 U/L of dialysis solution are usually successful in restoring good catheter function. Some patients have a permanently translocated catheter out of the true pelvis. If the catheter functions (even with slower drainage) we do not attempt to reposition the catheter.

An unusual cause of Cruz catheter blockage, which occurred for weeks after initiation of dialysis as a result of the tip wrapping by a fallopian tube, was recently reported [178]. The fimbriae of the oviduct penetrated through the side holes of the catheter and occluded the central lumen. Catheter function was restored surgically. A high dialysis flow and bigger side holes of the polyurethane device (the Cruz™ catheter) as compared to silicon rubber catheters might have contributed to this complication.

11.4. Pericatheter leak

Dialysis solution leaks may occur months or even years after starting CAPD. Management of late leak is similar to the one described for early leak. However, most cases of late leak are refractory to conservative therapy and require surgical repair. As discussed earlier, pericatheter leaks are more likely with the midline catheter insertion than with the insertion through the rectus muscle [36, 102]. Similar to the acute leak, this complication is rarely seen with the catheters provided with a bead and polyester flange at the deep cuff (Toronto Western Hospital, swan neck Missouri, swan neck presternal). We have not observed a single late pericatheter leak with 181 swan neck Missouri catheters [106].

Contrary to the early leaks which are usually external, the late leaks infiltrate the abdominal wall (Table 9). The acute leak causes a sudden drop of ultrafiltration and usually occurs after sudden increase in intraabdominal pressure (heavy lifting, coughing or straining). The leak may be mild and intermittent. Such a leak may be difficult to localize. Immediately after leak occurrence the patient may be in good fluid balance without edema on the lower extremities. Abdominal wall edema reveals a dimpling of the skin that gives it the appearance of the skin of an orange (*peau d'orange*) and spongy feeling on palpation. Chronic leak is usually a sequela of the acute leak but may occur gradually. The patient is usually fluid overloaded due to poor drain volume, confirmed by a repeat peritoneal equilibration test which shows unchanged solute transport characteristics [179].

The best method of leak localization is CT scan with intraperitoneal contrast [180, 181]. Prior to the study the peritoneal cavity is drained completely. A fresh bag of 2 L 2.5% dextrose dialysis solution is prepared, 100 ml of 60% diatriazoate meglumine is injected into the dialysis solution bag through the

Table 9. Late dialysate leak

Acute	Chronic
After heavy lifting, coughing, or straining	Usually a sequela of acute leak
Sudden drop of ultrafiltration	Poor ultrafiltration
May be mild and intermittent	Fluid overload
Abdominal wall edema	Localized abdominal edema
Peau d'orange	Usually without thigh edema
Spongy feeling	

injection port, the solution is mixed and infused into the peritoneal cavity. No oral or intravenous contrast material is needed. To increase intra-abdominal pressure [154] the patients should stand up, walk, strain, cough and bend over for at least 30 minutes, then assume the supine position on the CT table. The images are taken every 6 mm with 6 mm slice thickness in the region of suspected leak, in other regions 12 mm slice thickness every 12 or 24 mm are used. An example of the leak around the Tenckhoff catheter implanted through the midline is shown in Fig. 16.

11.5. Peritonitis

Bacteria causing peritonitis, or migrated around the catheter may colonize the intraperitoneal segment. As discussed in the section 4.3.3. these bacteria synthesize biofilm, which protects them from host mechanisms and antibiotics. It is believed that such colonization may lead to recurrent peritonitis with the same organism [73].

Recurrent peritonitis may be also the result of deep cuff infection with formation of microabscesses [182]. Finally, bowel trauma by the catheter may lead to peritonitis [183]. This mechanism may explain higher removal rates due to peritonitis of the Toronto Western Hospital catheters found in the CAPD Registry Special Survey [5].

11.6. Infusion or pressure pain

The mechanism of this complication was discussed in the section 4.8. Coiled catheters are less likely than the straight ones to induce infusion pain. The pain is usually most intense at the beginning of infusion and at the end of drainage. In the majority of cases the pain is transient and disappears within a few weeks. Table 10 shows the maneuvers, which we use to alleviate the pain. If all these maneuvers are ineffective the catheter has to be replaced. The replacement catheter should be a coiled one and the catheter should be implanted in such a way that no undue pressure is exerted at the tip. Outflow pain

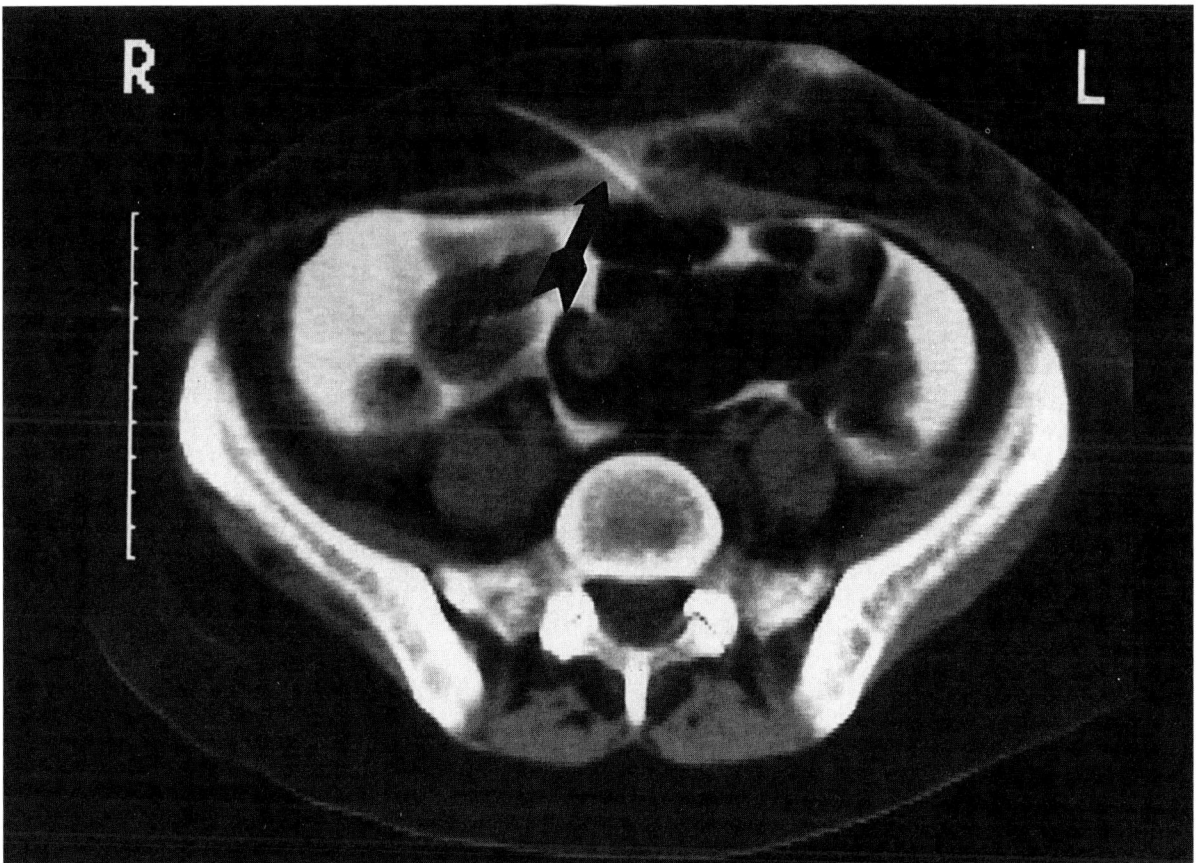

Figure 16. Contrast enhanced dialysate extravasating around the Tenckhoff catheter (arrow) implanted through the midline. Reproduced from reference [181] with permission.

is usually secondary to a negative pressure exerted on the peritoneum.

11.7. Unusual complications

11.7.1. *Organ erosion*
Damage of the internal organ leading to intraabdominal bleeding and/or peritonitis, as well as genital edema due to peritoneal laceration, have been reported as late catheter complications of straight Tenckhoff and Toronto Western Hospital catheters [183–193]. These complications are most likely due to the pressure exerted by "soft" but resilient tubing. In most instances the catheters had not been used for 1–12 weeks before the complication was diagnosed [184, 189–193]. No such complications have been reported with coiled (curled) catheters.

11.7.2. *Mechanical accidents*
Golper and Carpenter [194] reported two instances of catheters being accidentally cut with scissors. We have observed several such instances despite our teaching that scissors should not be used during dressing changes. Silicon rubber will not self-seal if punctured and such instances occur during implantation procedure and shaving of the cuff.

To avoid system contamination the catheter should be clamped immediately. If the damage is at least 15 mm from the exit the catheter may be saved using a peritoneal catheter repair kit available from the Quinton Instrument Co. While repairing the catheter, a sterile procedure must be strictly followed. The operator should "scrub, mask, and glove." A "circulating" nurse should be present to assist. The operating field has to be well protected with sterile towels, the catheter should be wrapped with Betadine® soaked gauze for 5 minutes. The catheter is transversely cut with a sterile blade proximal to the damaged site. The catheter clamp is released and the catheter is squeezed with fingers. The patient is asked to strain to allow dialysate flow from the peritoneal cavity. The flowing dialysate will flush eventual contaminants. While the fluid is still flowing, the teflon tubing of the repair kit is inserted into the catheter as far as possible. Then the silicon rubber tubing of the repair kit is clamped to stop dialysate flow. The connection is dried with gauze. A mold is positioned over the connection and filled with sterile silicon glue. The extension tubing is connected to the catheter in the usual way. The glue cures for 24 hours. Using this method we have been able to save seven catheters over a ten year period.

11.7.3. *Material breakdown*
There are reports of problems arising from the physical properties of the catheter material. The inclusion of barium sulphate throughout the entire catheter to render it radio-opaque has been reported to make the catheter brittle [195]. Currently the catheters contain only a strip of barium sulfate and seem to be less prone to this mode of failure. Silicon rubber catheters have been observed to stretch, crack or become brittle with age or after repeated exposure to Betadine® [195]. We have observed four such instances.

Polyurethane is even more likely to be damaged with aging because of so called *environmental stress cracking (ESC)*. As it name suggest, ESC leads to microcracks in the surface materials of a device, the result of corrosive forces of the living organisms. Once the process begins, ultimate failure is inevitable [196].

11.7.4. *Allergic reaction*
Eosinophilic peritonitis occurs most frequently in the postimplantation period. Although there are many possible causes of this entity, such as blood, air, antibiotics, one cannot exclude reaction to Silastic® tubing. As discussed in the section 10.2.3., gradually the Silastic® tubing is covered with proteinaceous biofilm. The coated catheter is less likely to cause allergic reaction. Allergic eosinophilic dermatitis due to silicon rubber has been reported [197, 198].

12. Indications for catheter removal

The need for catheter removal occurs under various conditions. These may be broadly categorized under two headings: catheter malfunction and complicating medical conditions with a functioning catheter. Finally the catheter may be removed electively because it is not needed.

Table 10. Maneuvers to alleviate infusion pain.

Slower infusion rate
Incomplete drainage
Tidal mode for nightly peritoneal dialysis
Solution alkalization (Na bicarbonate: 2–5 mEq/L)
1% Lidocaine – 2.5 ml/L (50 mg/exchange)
Catheter replacement

12.1. Malfunction

The decision to remove the catheter is usually made only when conservative measures (described in sections 10. and 11.3.) to restore function have failed. Catheter malfunction requiring catheter removal may be seen in the following conditions: 1) intraluminal obstruction with blood or fibrin clot or omental tissue incarceration. 2) catheter tip migration out of the pelvis with poor drainage, 3) a catheter kink along its course, 4) catheter tip caught in adhesions following severe peritonitis. In these situations, there usually are both inflow and outflow draining problems.

12.2. Functioning catheter with a complication

Under the following conditions catheters may have to be removed: 1) recurrent peritonitis with no identifiable cause, 2) peritonitis due to exit site and/or tunnel infection, 3) catheter with persistent exit site infection, 4) tunnel infection and abscess, 5) late recurrent dialysate leak through the exit site or into the layers of the abdominal wall, 6) unusual peritonitis i.e. tuberculosis, fungal, etc. 7) bowel perforation with multiple organism peritonitis, 8) refractory peritonitis of other causes, 9) severe abdominal pain either due to the catheter impinging on internal organs or during solution inflow, 10) catheter cuff extrusion with infection, and 11) accidental break in the continuity of the catheter.

12.3. Functioning catheter that is no longer needed:

This situation is encountered after a successful renal transplantation or peritoneal dialysis is discontinued because dialysis is no longer needed or the patient transfers to another form of dialysis.

13. Long term results

13.1. Tenckhoff catheters: A composite metaanalysis is reported in Chapter 10

Slingeneyer et al. [199] reported their early experience with 315 straight Tenckhoff catheters in 247 patients maintained mainly on IPD between September 1973 and September 1980. The cumulative duration of treatment was 410 patient-years. They observed the following catheter complications: bleeding into the subcutaneous tissue or peritoneum 1.9%, dialysate leak in 3.5%, and skin exit site infection in 10.5%. Skin exit site infection was more frequent in diabetic than in non-diabetic patients. They reported a 5.3% incidence of one-way obstruction requiring either catheter revision or replacement. Subcutaneous cuff extrusion necessitating cuff repositioning or catheter replacement occurred in 2.2%. Fifteen patients (4.7%) had persistent localized abdominal pain resulting in either replacement or revision (10 catheters). Incisional hernias were observed in five patients. Cumulative catheter survival was 79.9% at one year and 69.6% at two years. From this large experience they concluded that, despite limitations due to exit site infections and one-way obstruction, the Tenckhoff catheter provides adequate access for peritoneal dialysis. Most of Slingeneyer's patients were on IPD treatment. During intermittent peritoneal dialysis, the peritoneal cavity is empty most of the time, whereas during CAPD, this cavity is full nearly all the time. Therefore, catheter tip displacement is seen more frequently in CAPD.

Rubin and Adair [200] prospectively evaluated the complications encountered with the Tenckhoff catheter in CAPD patients between August 1981 and May 1983. They inserted 97 single cuff catheters into 90 patients, and 118 double-cuff catheters into 92 patients. Within 40 days of insertion of the single-cuff catheters, 25% had an associated complication that did not require catheter removal for correction, and 19 had a complication that required catheter removal. With the double-cuff catheters, 24% had an associated complication that did not require catheter removal, while 28% had catheter-related problems that required removal. In their long-term patients, the primary reason for catheter removal was failure of peritonitis to resolve. The catheter life span was 38% at 22 months for both single- and double-cuff catheters.

Rottembourg et al. [201] described their large experience with curled Tenckhoff catheters. Between August 1978 and January 1980, they inserted 48 straight Tenckhoff catheters; these they compared with 95 curled catheters inserted between February 1980 and April 1983. The most important difference between the two groups was the incidence of outflow obstruction: of the straight Tenckhoff catheters, 41.6% became dislodged and 85% of these had to be replaced; on the other hand only 10% of the curled catheters became dislodged and, of these, only 20% had to be replaced. Except for peri-operative pain, which was higher with the curled catheters, the frequency of other complications such as infection, dialysate leakage, exit site and tunnel infection and cuff extrusion, were similar in the two groups. For the straight Tenckhoff catheters, the cumulative catheter survival was 65% at one year and 60% at two years; for the curled catheters, these rates were 83% at one year and 78% at two years.

Swartz et al. [202] reported their experience with 213 curled (coiled) catheters implanted between January 1985 and December 1988, 134 percutaneously and 79 surgically. Overall probability of survival was 88%, 71%, and 61% at 1, 2, and 3 years respectively. Early external leaking developed in 29 catheters implanted percutaneously and 8 catheters inserted surgically. Outer cuff extrusions occurred in 19 catheters, but none of them led to the catheter loss. The authors considered coiled catheters superior to the straight catheters, mostly because of less drainage problems.

13.2. Toronto Western Hospital catheters

Hogg et al. [203] used the Toronto Western catheter with considerable success in children on long term CAPD. Six of the Toronto Western catheters were inserted in children who previously had either obstruction or leakage with one to four Tenckhoff catheters. Overall, they used 15 Toronto Western Hospital catheters in 12 children and compared the results with those of 23 Tenckhoff catheters in 9 children. The rate of obstruction with Toronto Western catheters (7%) was much lower than with Tenckhoff catheters (45%).

A retrospective analysis of single and double cuff Tenckhoff catheters and Toronto Western Hospital catheters by Flanigan et al. [204] showed that drainage failure occurred less frequently with Toronto catheters (9.4%) compared to single cuff (11.3%) and double cuff (20.6%) Tenckhoff catheters. However, in contrast to the experience of most centers with the use of Toronto Western Hospital catheters, Flanigan et al. observed a significantly lower survival for Toronto Western Hospital type I catheters. They attributed the lower survival of Toronto catheters to a higher incidence of unresponsive peritonitis in their patients using such catheters.

Grefberg from Sweden [205] in 1984 reported his comparative experience with the Tenckhoff and Toronto Western Hospital catheters. Catheters were randomly selected and both were surgically inserted. 59 Tenckhoff catheters were observed for 592 treatment months and 24 Toronto Western catheters for 220 treatment months. At 18 months, the cumulative life span of both catheters were similar at 80%. With regards to complications, 11 of the 59 Tenckhoff catheters became obstructed as opposed to one of 24 Toronto Western catheters. Swedish workers believe this high incidence of Tenckhoff catheter blockage was due to inexperience and that this complication would disappear with experience. With regard to exit site infection, tunnel abscess and dialysis leak, there was no difference between the two groups. Despite the advantages of Toronto Western catheters regarding catheter obstruction, they abandoned its use because laparotomy was needed whenever the catheter was removed, and the bowel was perforated during the removal of two Toronto Western catheters.

13.3. Column disc catheter

A multicenter experience reported using 89 column disc catheters [206]. Twenty catheters were placed in patients with previous failures of Tenckhoff catheters. Outflow failure was the most common cause of early failure and was less frequent after one month. Subcutaneous leak and herniation occurred rarely. Life table analysis revealed that compared to Tenckhoff catheters, the column disc catheter is more likely to fail in the early months but over the long-term is much less likely to fail.

13.4. National CAPD Registry survey

In 1987, the National CAPD Registry of the National Institute of Health reported the results of a survey that attempted to determine the natural history of implanted peritoneal catheters and to estimate the survival distribution of different types of catheters [5]. The survey also estimated frequency of catheter complications as well as reasons for catheter removal. Standard straight ($n = 957$; 64%) and curled ($n = 330$; 22%) Tenckhoff catheters, and Toronto Western Hospital catheters ($n = 94$; 6%), column-disc ($n = 49$; 3%), Gore-tex ($n = 28$; 2%), and others ($n = 2$; 0.1%) comprised the catheters reported for the survey. The survey did not clearly show major differences in catheter survival among various types of catheters. The probability of catheter survival at 6, 12, 18, 24, and 36 months for double cuff standard straight Tenckhoff catheter was 80, 70, 60, 51, and 33%, for standard curled Tenckhoff catheters was 85, 69, 51, 43 and 34%, and for double cuff Toronto Western catheter was 80, 69, 52, 35, and 22%, respectively.

The probability of survival at 6, 12, 18, and 24 months for column-disc catheter was 81, 71, 59, 47%, respectively. Table 11 presents the reasons of catheter failure. None of the Toronto Western Hospital catheters was removed because of drainage problem; however, they were most likely to be removed due to peritonitis. The reason for high failure rate due to peritonitis is unclear, but probably is related to the presence of intraperitoneal discs. Column-disc catheters had a high rate of failure due to peritonitis and obstruction (!) but the lowest rate of failure due to exit/tunnel infections. This survey also found exit site infection and peritonitis to be disproportionately distributed among the cuff types. Exit site infections were reported in proportionately more patients using a single subcutaneously placed cuff (13%) than for patients using a double cuff (7%). Gore-Tex catheters, which were designed to lower exit site infections had extremely high failure rate due to infections.

13.5. Swan neck catheters

At the University of Missouri, Columbia, between August, 1985 and September 1991, 181 swan neck catheters were implanted in 3 Columbia hospitals and cared for by the technique described above. Survival and complications were monitored prospectively. The prospectively collected data with the swan neck catheters, and retrospectively collected data with Tenckhoff and Toronto Western Hospital catheters were compared [105, 106].

There were 148 Tenckhoff and Toronto Western Hospital catheters, 27 swan neck prototypes, 105 swan neck Missouri 2 and 3 straight, and 49 swan neck Missouri 2 and 3 coiled (curled). The overall observation periods of Tenckhoff and Toronto Western Hospital catheters, swan neck prototypes, swan neck Missouri 2 and 3 straight, and swan neck Missouri 2 and 3 coiled were 1,859; 427; 1,487; and 305 catheter-months. The probability of catheter survival at 6, 12, 18, 24, and 36 months for Tenckhoff and Toronto Western Hospital catheters was 75, 61, 52, 48, 29%, similar to that reported by the CAPD Registry Special Survey [5], for swan neck prototypes was 100, 83, 67, 51, 31%, for swan neck Missouri 2 and 3 straight was 93, 85, 79, 68, and 61%, and for swan neck Missouri 2 and 3 curled was 88, and 88% at 6 and 12 months respectively.

The survival probability of swan neck Missouri straight and coiled catheters was significantly higher than that of Tenckhoff and Toronto Western Hospital catheters. Table 12 presents data regarding reasons of catheter failure leading to their removal. Compared to the CAPD Registry Special Survey [5], in our series more Tenckhoff and Toronto Western catheters were removed due to obstruction, but less due to peritonitis. Overall removal percentage was similar.

No malfunction or leak occurred with swan neck prototypes but a high cuff extrusion rate (as discussed in the section 5.3.) led to increased removals due to exit infections. Initial excellent results with these catheters because of elimination of leaks and malfunctions were obviated later by high infection rates.

Swan neck Missouri 2 and 3 with straight intraperitoneal segments yielded markedly better results. The estimated survival probability at three years doubled compared to previously used Tenckhoff and Toronto Western Hospital catheters. Improvement was noted in malfunctions, leaks, cuff extrusions, and exit/tunnel infections. Cuff extrusion occurred only in two swan neck straight catheters, in both instances after exit site infection, not due to catheter resilience. This was a notable reversal of the event sequence compared to previously used catheters, where cuff extrusion usually preceded exit/tunnel infection.

The results regarding survival and removal rates with swan neck coiled catheters were not signifi-

Table 11. Percent of catheters removed due to complications.*

Catheter	Exit/tunnel infection	Peritonitis	Leak	Obstruction
Straight	13	19	3	6
Coiled	12	21	5	5
Toronto WH	10	30	2	0
Column-disc	8	24	4	8
Gore-Tex	39	21	7	7

* Modified from Lindblad AS, et al. [5].

cantly different from that of the swan neck Missouri 2 and 3 straight catheters. Nevertheless, there are two major advantages of these catheters, the same as of other coiled catheters: a decrease in the incidence of infusion pain due to a "jet effect" and pain related to straight catheter tip pressure on the peritoneum experienced by some patients.

Low complication rates and higher probability of survival with swan neck catheters compared to other catheters have been reported also by others [207, 208]. A prospective comparison by life table analysis of 25 double cuff Tenckhoff and 25 swan neck catheters showed no statistically significant difference in survival and complications [209]. Preliminary experiences with swan neck presternal catheters in adults and in children are very encouraging [108, 109].

13.6. United States Renal Data System report 1992

In a national study of all patients starting CAPD therapy in the United States during January through June 1989, the prevailing catheter practices were appraised and the peritonitis risk was assessed by catheter related factors in 2,807 patients followed for up to 21 months [96]. Of these patients, 44 percent used a straight intraperitoneal segment with no bend, 40 percent used a curled (coiled) catheter with no bend, 12 percent used a catheter with "a preformed bend" [swan neck] with either a straight or curled intraperitoneal segment. Four percent of patients used "other (Lifecath and unspecified) catheters. Double cuff catheters were used in 78%, single deep cuff in 13%, single superficial in 5%, and data were not available in 10% of patients. Surgeons and nephrologists implanted 88% and 10% of catheters respectively (data for 2 percent unavailable). Surgical dissection was used in 74% of cases, peritoneoscopy in 6%, and blind (trocar of guide wire) in 8%. Midline insertion was used in 20%, paramedian in 33% and lateral in 14% of cases. Prophylactic antibiotics were used in 43% of insertions; data were not available in 28% and antibiotics were not used in 29% of cases. This study did not assess catheter survival; only the relative risk of a first peritonitis episode was analyzed using the Cox proportional hazards model. The relative risk of peritonitis was essentially identical for straight, curled, and bent catheters; the risk was significantly higher for "other" catheters. When the analysis was repeated with adjustment for possible center effect, the peritonitis risk was significantly lower among patients having catheters with "a permanent bend" [swan neck]. Compared to double cuff catheters, the risk of peritonitis was 16 and 31% higher for single deep cuff and single superficial cuff catheters respectively. Insertion by a nephrologist was associated with 15% higher peritonitis risk as compared to the insertion by a surgeon.

14. Concluding remarks

There are three essential prerequisites of peritoneal catheter performance: catheter design, implantation technique, and postimplantation care. Silicon rubber tubing with double polyester cuffs still is the best design. A permanent bend between cuffs (swan neck) offers an advantage because it allows implantation of the catheter in an unstressed condition in an arcuate tunnel with both internal and external exists directed downward. Surgical implantation virtually eliminated such complications as bowel perforation or massive bleeding. Other complications, such as obstruction, pericatheter leaks, and superficial cuff extrusions have been markedly reduced in recent years, particularly with the use of swan neck catheters and insertion through the rectus muscle instead of the midline.

The exit should be located in a place only minimally subjected to pressure and movement. Prophylactic antibiotics prior to implantation, and a meticulous sterile surgical technique with perfect

Table 12. Percent of catheters removed due to complications, University of Missouri 1982–1991.

Catheter	Exit/tunnel infection	Peritonitis	Leak	Obstruction
T/TWH*	13	14	3	14
Swan neck prototype	22	11	0	0
Swan neck straight	6	8	1	5
Swan neck coiled	8	2	0	2

* Tenckhoff and Toronto Western Hospital catheters.

hemostasis prevent early infection. Healing of the exit lasts 4–8 weeks. During this time a non-occlusive (air-permeable) dressing changed weekly is recommended. After the exit is healed the simplest and best method of care is protection from trauma, cleansing with water and liquid soap containing mild disinfectant, and avoidance of gross exit contamination. Early antibiotics with mild infection prevent severe infection leading to catheter loss. Whereas supine peritoneal dialysis may be started immediately post implantation, ambulatory peritoneal dialysis should be postponed for at least 10 days after implantation to avoid early leaks. The success of the catheter depends on the meticulous adherence to the details of catheter insertion and postimplantation care.

Exit site, tunnel infections, and catheter related peritonitis, although reduced, are still the most troublesome complications. Future research will concentrate on these problems. New humoral factors capable of accelerating healing, delayed exteriorization of external segment of the catheter, and use of a new exit location on the chest, instead of abdomen, may improve the results.

References

1. Tenckhoff J, Schechter H. A bacteriologically safe peritoneal access device. Trans Am Soc Artif Intern Organs 1968; 14: 181–7.
2. Buoncristiani U, Cozzari M, Quintaliani G, Carobi C. Abatement of exogenous peritonitis risk using the Perugia system. Dial Transplant 1983; 12: 14–25.
3. Maiorca R, Cantaluppi A, Cancarini GC, Scalamogna A, Broccoli R, Graziani G, Brasa S, Ponticelli C. Prospective controlled trial of a Y connector and disinfectant to prevent peritonitis in continuous ambulatory peritoneal dialysis. Lancet 1983; 2: 642–4.
4. Churchill DN, Taylor DW, Vas SI, Oreopoulos DG, Bettcher KB, Fenton SSA, Fine A, Lavoie S, Page D, Wu G, Beecroft ML, Pemberton R, Wilczynski NL, de Veber GA. Peritonitis in continuous ambulatory peritoneal dialysis (CAPD): a multicenter randomized clinical trial comparing the Y connector disinfectant system to standard system. Perit Dial Int 1989; 9: 159–63.
5. Lindblad AS, Hamilton RW, Novak JW. Complications of peritoneal catheters. In: Lindblad AS, Novak JW, Nolph KD (eds), Continuous Ambulatory Peritoneal Dialysis in the USA – Final Report of the National CAPD Registry. Kluwer Academic Publishers, Dordrecht 1989, pp 157–66.
6. Ganter G. Ueber die Beseitigung giftiger Stoffe aus dem Blute durch Dialyse. Munch Med Wschr 1923; 70: 1478–80.
7. Rosenak S, Siwon P. Experimentelle Untersuchungen über die peritoneale Ausscheidung harnpflichtiger Substanzen aus dem Blute. Mitt Grenzgeb Med Chir 1925; 39: 391–408.
8. Engel D, Kerkes A. Beitrage zum permeabilitats Problem: Entgiftungsstudien mittels des lebenden Peritoneums als "Dialysator". Ztschr f D ges Exp Med 1927; 55: 574–601.
9. Reid R, Penfold JB, Jones RN. Anuria treated by renal decapsulation and peritoneal dialysis. Lancet 1946; 2: 749–53.
10. Fine J, Frank HA, Seligman AM. The treatment of acute renal failure by peritoneal irrigation. Ann Surg 1946; 124: 857–78.
11. Rosenak SS, Oppenheimer GD. An improved drain for peritoneal lavage. Surgery 1948; 23: 832–33.
12. Derot M, Tanzet P, Roussilon J, Bernier JJ. La dialyse peritoneale dans le traitment de l'uremie aigue. J Urol 1949; 55: 113–21.
13. Legrain M, Merril JP. Short term continuous peritoneal dialysis. NEJM 1953; 248: 125–29.
14. Maxwell MH, Rockney RE, Kleeman CR, Twiss MR. Peritoneal dialysis. JAMA 1959; 170: 917–24.
15. Doolan PD, Murphy WP, Wiggins RA, Carter NW, Cooper WC, Watten RH, Alpen EL. An evaluation of intermittent peritoneal lavage. Am J Med 1959; 26: 831–44.
16. Boen ST, Mulinari AS, Dillard DH, Scribner BH. Periodic peritoneal dialysis in the management of chronic uremia. Trans Amer Soc Artif Intern Organs 1962; 8: 256–65.
17. Boen ST, Mion CM, Curtis FK, Shilipetar G. Periodic peritoneal dialysis using the repeated puncture technique and an automated cycling machine. Trans Am Soc Art Intern Organs 1964; 10: 409–13.
18. Weston RE, Roberts M. Clinical use of stylet catheter for peritoneal dialysis. Arch Int Med 1965; 115: 659–62.
19. Mallette WG, McPhaul JJ, Bledsoe F, McIntosh DA, Koegel E. A clinically successful subcutaneous peritoneal access button for repeated peritoneal dialysis. Trans Amer Soc Artif Intern Organs 1964; 10: 396–98.
20. Jacob GB, Deane N. Repeated peritoneal dialysis by the catheter replacement method: description of technique and a replaceable prosthesis for chronic access to the peritoneal cavity. Proc Eur Dial Transpl Assoc 1967; 4: 136–40.
21. Barry KG, Shambaugh GE, Goler D. A new flexible cannula and seal to provide prolonged access for peritoneal drainage and other procedures. J Urol 1963; 90: 125–28.
22. Gutch CF. Peritoneal dialysis. Trans Am Soc Artif Intern Organs 1964; 10: 406–7.
23. Palmer RA, Maybee TK, Henry EW, Eden J. Peritoneal dialysis in acute and chronic renal failure. Can Med Assoc J 1963; 88: 920–27.
24. Palmer RA, Quinton WE, Gray JE. Prolonged peritoneal dialysis for chronic renal failure. Lancet 1964; 1: 700–2.
25. Tenckhoff H, Schechter H, Boen ST. One year experience with home peritoneal dialysis. Trans Am Soc Artif Intern Organs 1965; 11: 11–4.

26. McDonald HP Jr, Gerber N, Mischra D, Wolm L, Peng B, Waterhouse K. Subcutaneous Dacron® and Teflon® cloth adjuncts for arterio venous shunts and peritoneal dialysis catheters. Trans Am Soc Artif Intern Organs 1968; 14: 176–80.
27. Stephen RI, Atkin-Thor E, Kolff WJ. Recirculating peritoneal dialysis with subcutaneous catheter. Trans Am Soc Artif Inter Organs 1976; 22: 575–84.
28. Gotloib L, Nisencorn I, Garmizo AL, Galili N, Servadio C, Sudarsky M. Subcutaneous intraperitoneal prosthesis for maintenance of peritoneal dialysis. Lancet 1975; 1: 1318–20.
29. Daly BDT, Dasse KA, Haudenschild CC, Clay W, Szycher M, Ober NS, Cleveland RJ. Percutaneous energy transmission systems: long-term survival. Trans Amer Soc Artif Intern Organs 1983; 29: 526–30.
30. Ogden DA, Benavente G, Wheeler D, Zukoski CF. Experience with the right angle Gore-Tex® peritoneal dialysis catheter. In: Khanna R, Nolph KD, Prowant BF, Twardowski ZJ, Oreopoulos GD (eds), Advances in Continuous Ambulatory Peritoneal Dialysis. Selected Papers from the Sixth Annual CAPD Conference, Kansas City, Missouri, February 1986. Peritoneal Dialysis Bulletin Inc., Toronto 1986; pp 155–9.
31. Goldberg EM, Hill W. A new peritoneal access prosthesis. Proc Clin Dial Transpl Forum 1973; 3: 122–25.
32. Oreopoulos DG, Izatt S, Zellerman G, Karanicolas S, Mathews RE. A prospective study of the effectiveness of three permanent peritoneal catheters. Proc Clin Dial Transplant Forum 1976; 6: 96–100.
33. Valli A, Comotti C, Torelli D, Crescimanno U, Valentini A, Riegler P, Huber W, Borghi M, Gruttadauria C, Scavoranat P, Pecchini F. A new catheter for peritoneal dialysis. Trans Am Soc Am Inter Organs 1983; 29: 629–32.
34. Valli A, Andreotti C, Degetto P, Midiri R, Mazzon M, Rovati C, Valentini A, Crescimanno U, Depaoli Vitali E, Manili L, Camerini C. 48-months' experience with Valli-2 catheter. In: Khanna R, Nolph KD, Prowant BF, Twardowski ZJ, Oreopoulos DG (eds), Advances in Continuous Ambulatory Peritoneal Dialysis, Selected Papers from the Eight Annual CAPD Conference, Kansas City, Missouri, February 1988. Peritoneal Dialysis Bulletin, Inc., Toronto 1988; pp 292–7.
35. Ash SR, Johnson H, Hartman J, Granger J, Koszuta J, Sell L, Dhein C, Blevins W, Thornhill JA. The column disc peritoneal catheter. A peritoneal access device with improved drainage. ASAIO J 1980; 3: 109–15.
36. Twardowski ZJ, Nolph KD, Khanna R, Prowant BF, Ryan LP. The need for a "Swan Neck" permanently bent, arcuate peritoneal dialysis catheter. Perit Dial Bull 1985; 5: 219–23.
37. Cruz C. Clinical experience with a new peritoneal access device (the Cruz™ catheter). In: Ota K, Maher J, Winchester J, Hirszel P, Ito K, Suzuki T (eds), Current Concepts in Peritoneal Dialysis: Proceedings of the Fifth Congress of the International Society for Peritoneal Dialysis, Kyoto, July 21–24, 1990. Amsterdam, London, New York. Excerpta Medica, Tokyo 1992, pp 164–9.
38. Twardowski ZJ. Peritoneal dialysis glossary. II. Perit Dial Int 1988; 8: 15–7.
39. Twardowski ZJ, Khanna R, Nolph KD, Nichols WK. Peritoneal dialysis catheter: principles of design, implantation, and early care. Video produced by the Academic Support Center, University of Missouri, Columbia, MO, USA, 1993.
40. Blistein-Willinger E. The role of growth factors in wound healing. Skin Pharmacol 1991; 4: 175–82.
41. Kantrowitz A, Freed PS, Ciarkowski AA, Hayashi I, Vaughan FL, VeShancey JI, Gray RH, Brabec RK, Bernstein IA. Development of a percutaneous access device. Trans Am Soc Artif Intern Organs 1980; 26: 444–9.
42. Hall CW, Adams LM, Ghidoni JJ. Development of skin interfacing cannula. Trans Amer Soc Artif Intern Organs 1975; 21: 281–7.
43. Yaffe A, Ahoshan S. Cessation of epithelial cell movement at native type I collagen-epithelial interface in vitro. Collagen Res Rel 1985; 5: 533–40.
44. Bar-Lev A, Freed PS, Mandell G, et al. Long-term percutaneous access device. In: Khanna R, Nolph KD, Prowant BF, Twardowski ZJ, Oreopoulos GD (eds), Advances in Continuous Ambulatory Peritoneal Dialysis. Selected Papers from the Seventh Annual CAPD Conference, Kansas City, Missouri, February 1987. Peritoneal Dialysis Bulletin Inc., Toronto 1987; pp 81–7.
45. Dasse KA, Daly BDT, Bousquet G, King D, Smith T, Mondou R, Poirier VL. A polyurethane percutaneous access device for peritoneal dialysis. In: Khanna R, Nolph KD, Prowant BF, Twardowski ZJ, Oreopoulos GD (eds), Advances in Continuous Ambulatory Peritoneal Dialysis. Selected Papers from the Eighth Annual CAPD Conference, Kansas City, Missouri, February 1988. Peritoneal Dialysis Bulletin Inc., Tokyo 1988; pp 245–52.
46. Krawczyk WAS. Some ultrastructural aspects of epidermal repair in two model wound healing systems. In: Maibach HI, Rovee DT (eds), Epidermal Wound Healing. Year Book Medical Publishers, Chicago 1972; pp 123–31.
47. Winter GD. Movement of epidermal cells over the wound surface. In: Montagna W, Billingham RE, (eds), Advances in Biology of Skin – Vol. 5, Wound Healing. Pergamon Press, Oxford 1964; pp 113–27.
48. Winter GD. Epidermal regeneration studied in the domestic pig. In: Maibach HI, Rovee DT (eds), Epidermal Wound Healing. Year Book Medical Publishers, Chicago 1972; pp 71–112.
49. Winter GD. Transcutaneous implants: reactions of the skin-implant interface. J Biomed Mater Res 1974; 8: 99–113.
50. Poirier VL, Daly BDT, Dasse KA, Haudenschild CC, Fine RE. Elimination of tunnel infection. In: Maher JF, Winchester JF (eds), Frontiers in

Peritoneal Dialysis. Proceedings of the III International Symposium on Peritoneal Dialysis, Washington, D.C., 1984. Published by Field, Rich & Assoc. Inc., New York 1986; pp 210–7.
51. Twardowski ZJ, Prowant BF. Can new catheter design eliminate exit site and tunnel infections? Perspectives in Peritoneal Dialysis 1986; 4(2): 5–9.
52. Khanna R, Twardowski ZJ. Peritoneal catheter exit site. Perit Dial Int 1988; 8: 119–23.
53. Twardowski ZJ, Khanna R. Swan neck peritoneal dialysis catheter. In: Andreucci VE (ed), Vascular and Peritoneal Access for Dialysis. Published by Kluwer Academic Publishers B.V., Boston/Dordrecht/London 1989; pp 271–89.
54. Twardowski ZJ, Dobbie JW, Moore HL, Nichols WK, DeSpain JD, Anderson PC, Khanna R, Nolph KD, Loy TS. Morphology of peritoneal dialysis catheter tunnels. Macroscopy and light microscopy. Perit Dial Int 1991; 11: 237–51.
55. Wright NA. The cell proliferation kinetics of the epidermis. In: Goldsmith LA (ed), Biochemistry and Physiology of the Skin. Oxford University Press, New York 1983; pp 203–29.
56. Twardowski ZJ, Prowant BF, Nolph KD, Khanna R, Moore HL. Peritoneal catheter (PC) exit site (ES): appearance, and factors influencing healing. Abstracts of the XIIth International Congress of Nephrology, Jerusalem, Israel, June 13–19, 1993, Abstracts, p 311.
57. Twardowski ZJ. Exit site infection. In: La Greca G, Ronco C, Feriani M, Chiaramonte S, Conz P (ed), Peritoneal Dialysis. Proceedings of Fourth International Course on Peritoneal Dialysis, Vicenza, Italy, May 21–24, 1991. Milano: Wichtig Editore 1991: 241–5.
58. Stricker GE, Tenckhoff HAM. A transcutaneous prosthesis for prolonged access to the peritoneal cavity. Surgery 1971; 69: 70–4.
59. Pru CP, Barriola JA, Garcia V. Pathological evaluation of one cuff peritoneal dialysis catheter tunnel (OCPDCT). (Abstract) Perit Dial Int 1993; 13 (suppl 1): S24.
60. Heppenstall RB, Littooy FN, Fuchs R, Sheldon GF, Hunt TK. Gas tensions in healing tissues of traumatized patients. Surgery 1974; 75: 874–80.
61. Elek SD. Experimental Staphylococcal infections in the skin of man. Ann New York Acad Sci 1956; 54: 85–90.
62. Hepburn H. Delayed primary suture of wounds. Br Med J 1919; 1: 181–3.
63. Krizek TJ, Robson MC. Biology of surgical infection. Surg Clin North Am 1975; 55: 1261–7.
64. Mosher DF, Proctor RA. Binding and factor XIIIa-mediated cross-linking of a 27 kilodalton fragment of fibronectin to *Staphylococcus aureus*. Science 1980; 209: 927–9.
65. Maxe I, Rydén C, Wadström T, Rubin K. Specific attachment of *Staphylococcus aureus* to immobilized fibronectin. Infect Immun 1986; 54: 695–704.
66. Proctor RA. The Staphylococcal fibronectin receptor: evidence for its importance in invasive infections. Rev Infect Dis 1987; 9 (suppl): S335–40.
67. Russel PB, Kline J, Yoder MC, Polin RA. Staphylococcal adherence to polyvinyl chloride and heparin-bonded polyurethane catheters is species dependent and enhanced by fibronectin. J Clin Microbiol 1987; 25: 1083–7.
68. Lopes JD, dos Reis M, Brentani RR. Presence of laminin receptors in *Staphylococcus aureus*. Science 1985; 229: 275–7.
69. Vercelotti GM, McCarthy JB, Lindholm P, Peterson PK, Jacob HS, Furcht LT. Extracellular matrix proteins (fibronectin, laminin, and type IV collagen) bind and aggregate bacteria. Am J Pathol 1985; 120: 13–21.
70. Dickinson GM, Bisno AL. Infections associated with indwelling devices: concepts of pathogenesis; infections associated with intravascular devices. Antimicrob Agents Chemother 1989; 33: 597–601.
71. Marshall KC. Mechanism of bacterial adhesion at solid water interfaces. In: Savage DC, Fletcher M, eds. Bacterial Adhesion: Mechanisms and Physiological Significance. New York: Plenum Publishing Corp. 1985: 133–61.
72. Costerton JW, Watkins L. Adherence of bacteria to foreign bodies: the role of biofilm. In: Root RK, Trunkey DD, Sande MA (ed), New Surgical and Medical Approaches in Infectious Diseases. Churchill Livingstone Inc., New York 1987; pp 17–30.
73. Dasgupta MK, Bettcher KB, Ulan RA, Burns V, Lam K, Dossetor JB, Costerton JW. Relationship of adherent bacterial biofilms to peritonitis in chronic ambulatory peritoneal dialysis. Perit Dial Bull 1987; 7: 168–73.
74. Van den Broek PJ, Buys LF, Van Furth R. Interaction of povidone-iodine compounds, phagocytic cells, and macroorganisms. Antimicrob Agents Chemother 1982; 22: 593–7.
75. Iwasaki N, Kamoi K, Bae RD, Tsutsui T. Cytotoxicity of povidone-iodine on cultured mammalian cells. J Jap Assoc Periodont 1989; 31: 836–42.
76. Laufman H. Current use of skin and wound cleansers and antiseptics. Amer J Surg 1989; 157: 359–65.
77. Bryant CA, Rodeheaver GT, Reem EM, Nitcher LS, Kennedy JC, Edlich RF. Search for a nontoxic surgical scrub solution for periorbital lacerations. Ann Emerg Med 1984; 13: 317–9.
78. Orgill D, Demling R. Current concepts and approaches to wound healing. Critical Care Medicine 1988; 16: 899–908.
79. Rosen H, Blumenthal A, McCallum J. Effect of asiaticoside on wound healing in the rat. Proc Soc Exp Biol Med 1967; 125: 279–80.
80. Maquart FX, Bellon G, Gillery P, Wegrowski Y, Borel JP. Stimulation of collagen synthesis in fibroblast cultures by a triterpene extracted from *Centella asiatica*. Connect Tissue Res 1990; 24: 107–20.
81. Zimmerman SW, O'Brien M, Wiedenhoeft FA, Johnson CA: *Staphylococcus aureus* peritoneal catheter-related infections: a cause of catheter loss and peritonitis. Perit Dial Int 1988; 8: 191–94.

82. Abraham G, Savin E, Ayiomamitis A, Izatt S, Vas SI, Mathews RE, Oreopoulos DG. Natural history of exit-site infection (ESI) in patients on continuous ambulatory peritoneal dialysis (CAPD). Perit Dial Int 1988; 8: 211–6.
83. Yu VL, Goetz A, Wagener M, Smith PB, Rihs JD, Hanchett J, Zuravleff JJ. *Staphylococcus aureus* nasal carriage and infection in patients on hemodialysis. N Engl J Med 1986; 315: 91–6.
84. Davies SJ, Ogg CS, Cameron JS, Poston S, Nobble WC: *Staphylococcus aureus* nasal carriage, exit-site infection and catheter loss in patients treated with continuous ambulatory peritoneal dialysis. Perit Dial Int 1989; 9: 61–4.
85. Sewell CM, Clarrige J, Lacke C, Weinman EJ, Young EJ. Staphylococcal nasal carriage and subsequent infection in peritoneal dialysis patients. JAMA 1982; 248: 1493–5.
86. Luzar MA, Coles GA, Faller B, Slingeneyer A, Dah GD, Briat C, Wone C, Knefati Y, Kessler M, Peluso F. *Staphylococcus aureus* nasal carriage and infection in patients on continuous ambulatory peritoneal dialysis. N Engl J Med 1990; 322: 505–9.
87. Twardowski ZJ, Prowant BF. *Staphylococcus aureus* nasal carriage is not associated with an increased incidence of exit site infection with the same organism. Proceedings of the ISPD Meeting, Thessaloniki, Greece, October 1–4, 1992. Perit Dial Int 1993; 13 (suppl): S306–9.
88. Bossert WA, Marks HH. Prevalence and characteristics of periodontal disease on 12,800 persons under periodic dental observation. J Am Dent Assoc 1956; 52: 429–42.
89. Hajek M. Pathology and Treatment of the Inflammatory Diseases of the Nasal Accessory Sinuses. Translated and edited by Heitger JD, Hansel FK, 5th ed. St. Louis, The Mosby Co. 1926: 100.
90. So SKS, Mahan JD Jr, Mauer SM, Sutherland DER, Nevins TE. Hickman catheter for pediatric hemodialysis: a 3-year experience. Trans Am Soc Artif Intern Organs 1984; 30: 619–23.
91. Raaf JH. Results from use of 826 vascular access devices in cancer patients. Cancer 1985; 55: 1312–21.
92. Tenckhoff H. Home peritoneal dialysis. In: Massry SG, Sellers AL (eds), Clinical Aspects of Uremia and Dialysis. Charles C Thomas Publ., Springfield, IL 1976: 583–615.
93. Smith C. CAPD: one cuff vs two cuff catheters in reference to incidence of infection. In: Maher JF, Winchester JF (eds), Frontiers in Peritoneal Dialysis: Proceedings of the III International Symposium on Peritoneal Dialysis, Washington, D.C., 1984. Published by Field, Rich & Assoc. Inc., New York 1986; pp 181–2.
94. Diaz-Buxo JA, Geissinger WT. Single cuff versus double cuff Tenckhoff catheter. Perit Dial Bull 1984; 4 (suppl 3): S100–2.
95. Kim D, Burke D, Izatt S, Mathews R, Wu G, Khanna R, Vas S, Oreopoulos DG. Single- or double-cuff peritoneal catheters? A prospective comparison. Trans Am Soc Artif Intern Organs 1984; 30: 232–5.
96. U.S. Renal Data System, USRDS 1992 Annual Data Report, VI. Catheter-Related Factors and Peritonitis Risk in CAPD Patients. Am J Kidney Dis 1992; 5 (suppl 2): 48–54.
97. Schroeder HE, Page RC. The normal periodontium. In: Schluger S, Youdelis RA, Page RC (eds), Periodontal Disease. Philadelphia: Lea & Febiger 1978: 7–55.
98. Amano I, Katoh T, Inagaki Y. Clinical experience with Alumina ceramic transcutaneous connector to prevent skin-exit infection around CAPD catheter. In: Khanna R, Nolph KD, Prowant BF, Twardowski ZJ, Oreopoulos GD (eds), Advances in Continuous Ambulatory Peritoneal Dialysis. Selected Papers from the Tenth Annual Conference on Peritoneal Dialysis, Dallas, Texas, February 1990. Toronto: Peritoneal Dialysis Bulletin, Inc. 1990: 150–4.
99. Boss HP, Ganger KH, Gluck Z: Gore-tex versus Oreopoulos peritoneal catheters: a clinical evaluation and comparison (letter). Perit Dial Bull 1987; 7: 209.
100. Rottembourg J, Quinton W, Durande JP, Brouard R. Wings as subcutaneous cuff in prevention of exit-site infection in CAPD patients. Abstracts of the IV International Symposium on Peritoneal Dialysis, Vicenza, Italy, June 29–July 2, 1987. Peritoneal Dial Bull 1987; 7 (suppl): S63.
101. Schleifer CR, Ziemek H, Teehan BP, Benz RL, Sigler MH, Gilgore GS. Migration of peritoneal catheters: personal experience and a survey of 72 other units. Perit Dial Bull 1987; 7: 189–93.
102. Helfrich GB, Pechan BW, Alijani MR, Bernard WF, Rakowski TA, Winchester JF. Reduced catheter complications with lateral placement. Perit Dial Bull 1983; 3 (suppl 4): S2–4.
103. Twardowski ZJ, Nichols WK, Khanna R, Nolph KS. Swan neck Missouri peritoneal dialysis catheters: design, insertion, and break-in. Video produced by the Academic Support Center, University of Missouri, Columbia, MO, USA, 1993.
104. Twardowski ZJ, Khanna R, Nolph KD, Nichols WK, Ryan LP. Preliminary experience with the Swan Neck peritoneal dialysis catheter. Trans Am Soc Artif Intern Organs 1986; 32: 64–7.
105. Twardowski ZJ, Prowant BF, Khanna R, Nichols WK, Nolph KD. Long-term experience with Swan Neck Missouri catheters. ASAIO Transactions 1990; 36: M491–4.
106. Twardowski ZJ, Prowant BF, Nichols WK, Nolph KD, Khanna R. Six year experience with swan neck catheter. Perit Dial Int 1992; 12: 384–9.
107. Twardowski ZJ, Nichols WK, Khanna R, Nolph KD. Swan neck presternal peritoneal dialysis catheter: design, insertion, and break-in. Video produced by the Academic Support Center, University of Missouri, Columbia, MO, USA, 1993.
108. Twardowski ZJ, Nichols WK, Nolph KD, Khanna R. Swan neck presternal ("bath tub") catheter for

peritoneal dialysis. In: Khanna R, Nolph KD, Prowant BF, Twardowski ZJ, Oreopoulos DG, eds. Advances in Peritoneal Dialysis. Selected Papers from the Twelve Annual Conference on Peritoneal Dialysis, Seattle, Washington, February 1992. Toronto: Edited by Peritoneal Dialysis Bulletin, Inc. 1992; 8: 316–24.
109. Twardowski ZJ, Nichols WK, Nolph KD, Khanna R. Swan neck presternal peritoneal dialysis catheter. Proceedings of the ISPD Meeting, Thessaloniki, Greece, October 1–4, 1992. Perit Dial Int 1993; 13 (suppl): S130-2.
110. Twardowski ZJ, Nichols WK, Nolph KD, Khanna R. Swan neck presternal catheter for peritoneal dialysis – eighteen month experience in adults. Abstracts. The XIIth International Congress of Nephrology, Jerusalem, Israel, June 13–19, 1993, p 335.
111. Sieniawska M, Blaim M, Warchol S. Swan neck presternal catheter (SNPC) for CAPD in children. Perit Dial Int 1993; 13 (suppl 1): S22.
112. Ash SR, Daugirdas JT. Peritoneal access devices. In: Daugirdas JT, Ing TS (eds), Handbook of Dialysis. Boston: Little Brown and Company 1988: 194–218.
113. Gonzales AR, Goltz GM, Eaton CL, Ratajeski G, Olin JW. The peel away method for insertion of Tenckhoff cathcter. (Abstracts) Amer Soc Nephrol 1983; 16: 119A.
114. Updike S, O'Brien M, Peterson W, Zimmerman S. Placement of catheter using pacemaker-like introducer with peel-away sleeve. Abstracts, Amer Soc Nephrol 1984; 17: 87A.
115. Updike S, Zimmerman S, O'Brien M, Peterson W. Peel-Away® sheath technique for placing peritoneal dialysis catheters. Video produced by Television Studio, School of Nursing, University of Wisconsin, Madison, WI, USA, 1984.
116. Zappacosta AR, Perras ST, Closkey GM. Seldinger technique for Tenckhoff catheter placement. ASAIO Trans 1991; 37: 13–5.
117. Zappacosta AR: Seldinger technique for placement of the Tenckhoff catheter. Video produced by the Bryn Mawr Hospital, 1984.
118. Schmidt LM, Craig PC, Prowant BF, Twardowski ZJ. A simple method of preventing accidental disconnection at the peritoneal catheter adapter junction. Perit Dial Int 1990; 10: 309–10.
119. Vaamonde CA, Michael VF, Metzger RA, Carrol KE. Complications of acute peritoneal dialysis. J Chron Dis 1975; 28: 637–59.
120. Valk TW, Swartz RD, Hsu CH. Peritoneal dialysis in acute renal failure: analysis of outcome and complications. Dial Transpl 1980; 9: 48–54.
121. Maher JF, Schreiner GE. Hazards and complications of dialysis. N Engl J Med 1965; 273: 370–7.
122. Anderson G, Bergquist-Poppen M, Bergstrom J. Collste LG, Huttman E. Glucose absorption from the dialysis fluid during peritoneal dialysis. Scand J. Urol Nephrol 1971; 5: 77.
123. Firmat J, Zucchini A. Peritoneal dialysis in acute renal failure. Contrib Nephrol (Karger, Basel) 1979; 17: 33–8.
124. Edward SR, Unger AM. Acute hydrothorax a new complication of peritoneal dialysis. JAMA 1967; 199: 853–5.
125. Finn R, Jowett EW: Acute hydrothorax: complication of peritoneal dialysis. Br Med J 1970; 2: 94.
126. Holm J, Lieden B, Lindgrist B. Unilateral effusion – a rare complication of peritoneal dialysis. Scand J Urol Nephrol 1971; 5: 84–5.
127. Haberli R, Stucki P. Akuter hydro-thorax als komplikation bei peritonealdialyse. Praxis 1971; 60: 13–4.
128. Fehmirling E, Christensen E. Hydrothorax under peritonealidalyse. Ugeskr Laeg 1975; 137: 1650–1.
129. Alquier Ph, Achard J, Bonhomme R. Hydrothorax aign au loure de dialyses péritoneales. A propose de 5 cas. La Nouv Presse Med 1975; 4: 192.
130. Rudnick MR, Coyle, JF, Beck H, McCurdy DK. Acute massive hydrothorax complicating peritoneal dialysis, report of 2 cases and a review of the literature. Clin Nephrol 1980; 12: 38–44.
131. Milutinovic J, Wu W-S, Lindholm DD, LeRoy Lapp N. Acute massive unilateral hydrothorax: a rare complication of chronic peritoneal dialysis. South Med J 1980; 73: 827–8.
132. Grefberg N, Danielson BG, Benson L, Pitkanen P. Right sided hydrothorax complicating peritoneal dialysis. Nephron 1983; 34: 130–4.
133. Kennedy JM: Procedures used to demonstrate a pleuroperitoneal communication: a review. Perit Dial Bull 1985; 5: 168–70.
134. Ribot S, Jacobs MG, Frankel HJ, Bernstein A. Complications of peritoneal dialysis. Am J Med Sci 1966; 252: 505–17.
135. Mion CM, Boen ST. Analysis of factors responsible for the formation of adhesions during chronic peritoneal dialysis. Am J Med Sci 1965; 250: 675–9.
136. Matalon R, Levine S, Eisinger RP. Hazards in routine use of peritoneal dialysis. NY State J Med 1971; 71: 219–24.
137. Henderson LW. Peritoneal dialysis. In: Massry SG, Sellers AL (eds), Clinical Aspects of Uremia and Dialysis. Charles C Thomas, Springfield, IL 1976; p 574.
138. Simkin EP, Wright FK. Perforating injuries of the bowel complicating peritoneal catheter insertion. Lancet 1968; 1: 61–7.
139. Chugh KS, Bhattacharya K, Amaresan MS, Sharma BK, Bansal VK. Peritoneal dialysis our experience based on 550 dialyses. J Assoc Physicians India 1972; 20: 215–21.
140. Nienhuis LI. Clinical peritoneal dialysis. Arch Surg 1966; 93: 643–53.
141. Pauli HG, Billikofer E, Vorburger C. Clinical experience with peritoneal dialysis. Helv Med Acta 1966; 33: 51–8.
142. Krebs RA, Burtiss BB. Bowel perforation. JAMA 1966; 198: 486–7.
143. Denovales EL, Avendano LN. Risks of peritoneal catheter insertion (letter). Lancet 1968; 1: 473.
144. Dunea G. Peritoneal dialysis and hemodialysis. Med Clin North Am 1971; 55: 155–75.
145. Rigalosi RS, Maher JF, Schreiner GE. Intestinal

perforation during peritoneal dialysis. Ann Intern Med 1964; 70: 1013–5.
146. Edwards DH, Gardner RD, Williams DG. Rupture of a hernial sac: a complication of peritoneal dialysis. J Urol 1972; 108: 255–6.
147. Goldsmith HJ, Edwards EC, Moorhead PJ, Wright FK. Difficulties encountered in intermittent dialysis for chronic renal failure. Br J Urol 1966; 38: 625–34.
148. Smith E, Chamberlain MJ. Complications of peritoneal dialysis. Br Med J 1965; 1: 126–7.
149. Stein MF Jr. Intraperitoneal loss of dialysis catheter. Ann Intern Med 1969; 71: 869–70.
150. Oreopoulos DG, Helfrich GB, Khanna R, Lum GM, Matthews R, Paulsen K, Twardowski ZJ, Vas SI. Peritoneal dialysis catheter implantation. Video developed by Baxter's Catheter and Exit Site Advisory Committee, Baxter Healthcare Corporation, 1988.
151. Oreopoulos DG, Helfrich GB, Khanna R, Lum GM, Matthews R, Paulsen K, Twardowski ZJ, Vas SI. Peritoneal catheters and exit-site practices: current recommendations. Perit Dial Bull 1987; 7: 130–8.
152. Gokal R, Ash SR, Helfrich GB, Holmes CJ, Joffe P, Nichols WK, Oreopoulos DG, Riella MC, Slingeneyer A, Twardowski ZJ, Vas SI. Peritoneal catheters and exit-site practices: toward optimum peritoneal access. Perit Dial Int 1992; 13: 29–39.
153. Ash S. Y-TEC peritoneoscopic implantation of the peritoneal dialysis catheter. Video produced by Medigroup Inc., North Aurora, IL, USA, 1993.
154. Twardowski ZJ, Khanna R, Nolph KD, Scalamogna A, Metzler MH, Schneider TW, Prowant BF, Ryan LP. Intraabdominal pressure during natural activities in patients treated with continuous ambulatory peritoneal dialysis. Nephron 1986; 44: 129–35.
155. Moncrief JW, Popovich RP, Broadrick LJ, He ZZ, Simmons EE, Tate RA. Moncrief-Popovich catheter: a new peritoneal access technique for patients on peritoneal dialysis. ASAIO J 1993; 39: 62–5.
156. Moncrief-Popovich catheter. A video produced by Austin Biomedical Research Institute Austin, TX USA.
157. Prowant BF, Schmidt LM, Twardowski ZJ, Griebel CK, Burrows L, Ryan LP, Satalowich RJ. Peritoneal dialysis catheter exit site care. Amer Nephr Nurs Assoc J 1988; 15: 219–22.
158. Twardowski ZJ, Ryan LP, Kennedy JM. Catheter break-in for continuous ambulatory peritoneal dialysis-University of Missouri experience. Perit Dial Bull 1984; 4 (suppl 3): S110–1.
159. Ash SR, Carr DJ, Diaz-Buxo JA. Peritoneal access devices: hydraulic function and compatibility. In: Nissenson AR, Fine RN, Gentile DE (eds), Clinical Dialysis, Second Edition. Norwalk, Connecticut: Published by Appleton & Lange 1990; pp 212–239.
160. O'Regan S, Garel L, Patriquin H, Yazbeck S. Outflow obstruction: whiplash technique for catheter mobilization. Perit Dial Int 1988; 8: 265–8.
161. Honkanen E, Eklund B, Laasonen L, Ylinen K, Grönhagen-Riska C. Reposition of a displaced peritoneal catheter: the Helsinki whiplash method. In: Khanna R, Nolph KD, Prowant BF, Twardowski ZJ, Oreopoulos DG (eds), Advances in Peritoneal Dialysis. Selected Papers from the Tenth Annual Conference on Peritoneal Dialysis, Dallas, Texas, February 1990. Peritoneal Dialysis Bulletin Inc., Toronto 1990; 6: 159–64.
162. Yoshihara K, Yoshi S, Miyagi S. The α replacement method for the displacement of the swan neck catheter. (Abstract) Perit Dial Int 1993: 13 (suppl 1): S17.
163. Erosy FF, Twardowski ZJ, Satalowich RJ, Ketchersid T. A retrospective analysis of peritoneal catheter (PDC) position and function in 91 patients. Abstracts of the VIth Congress of the International Society for Peritoneal Dialysis, Thessaloniki, Greece, October 1–4, 1992. Perit Dial Int 1992; 12 (suppl 2): S49.
164. Twardowski ZJ. Malposition and poor drainage of peritoneal catheters. Seminars in Dialysis (Dialysis Clinic section) 1990; 3: 57.
165. Pierratos A. Peritoneal dialysis glossary. Perit Dial Bull 1984; 4: 2–3.
166. Keane WF, Everett ED, Fine RN, Golper TA, Vas SI, Peterson PK. CAPD related peritonitis management and antibiotic therapy recommendations. Perit Dial bull 1987; 7: 55–68.
167. Piraino B, Bernardini J, Sorkin M. Catheter infections as a factor in the transfer of continuous ambulatory peritoneal dialysis patients to hemodialysis. Am J Kidney Dis 1989; 13: 365–9.
168. Luzar MA, Brown CB, Balf D, Hill L, Issad B, Monnier B, Moulard J, Sabatier JC, Wauquier JP, Peluso F. Exit-site care and exit-site infection in continuous ambulatory peritoneal dialysis (CAPD): results of a randomized multicenter trial. Perit Dial Int 1990; 10: 25–29.
169. Copley JB. Prevention of peritoneal dialysis catheter-related infections. Am J Kidney Dis 1987; 10: 401–7.
170. Twardowski ZJ. peritoneal catheter exit site infections: prevention, diagnosis, treatment, and future directions. Seminars in Dialysis 1992; 5: 305–15.
171. Gloor HJ, Nichols WK, Sorkin MI, Prowant BF, Kennedy JM, Baker B, Nolph KD. Peritoneal access and related complications in continuous ambulatory peritoneal dialysis. Am J Med 1983; 74: 593–8.
172. Vogt K, Binswanger U, Buchmann P, Baumgartner D, Keusch G, Largiadèr F. Catheter-related complications during continuous ambulatory peritoneal dialysis (CAPD): a retrospective study on sixty-two double cuff Tenckhoff catheters. Am J Kidney Dis 1987; 10: 47–51.
173. Bertone AL. Management of exuberant granulation tissue. Vet Clin North Am: Equine Pract 1989; 5: 551–62.
174. Low DE, Bas SI, Oreopoulos DG, Manuel RA, Saiphoo CS, Finer C, Dombros N. Randomized clinical trial of prophylactic cephalexin in CAPD. Lancet 1980; 2: 753–4.
175. Chruchill DN, Oreopoulos DG, Taylor DW, Vas

SI, Manuel MA, Wu G. Peritonitis in CAPD patients – a randomized clinical trial of trimethoprim-sulfamethoxazole prophylaxis. (Abstracts) Amer Soc Nephrol 1987; 20: 97A.
176. Twardowski ZJ. Management of recurrent catheter exit site infection. Seminars in Dialysis 1993; 6: 406–8.
177. Nichols WK, Nolph KD. A technique for managing exit site and cuff infection in Tenckhoff catheters. Perit Dial Bull 1983; 3 (suppl 4): S4–5.
178. Aboujloud MS, Cruz C, Dow RD, Mozes MF. Peritoneal catheter obstruction by a fallopian tube: a case report. Perit Dial Int 1992; 12: 257–8.
179. Twardowski ZJ. Clinical value of standardized equilibration tests in CAPD patients. Blood Purif 1989; 7: 95–108.
180. Twardowski ZJ, Tully RJ, Nichols WK, Sunderrajan S. Computerized tomography in the diagnosis of subcutaneous leak sites during continuous ambulatory peritoneal dialysis (CAPD). Perit Dial Bull 1984; 4: 163–6.
181. Twardowski ZJ, Tully RJ, Ersoy FF, Dedhia NM. Computerized tomography with and without intraperitoneal contrast for determination of intraabdominal fluid distribution and diagnosis of complications in peritoneal dialysis patients. ASAIO Transactions 1990; 36: 95–103.
182. Dimitriadis A, Antoniou S, Toliou T, Papadopoulos C. Tissue reaction to deep cuff of Tenckhoff catheter and peritonitis. In: Khanna R, Nolph KD, Prowant BF, Twardowski ZJ, Oreopoulos DG (eds), Advances in Peritoneal Dialysis. Selected papers from the Tenth Annual Conference on Peritoneal Dialysis, Dallas, Texas, February 1990. Peritoneal Dialysis Bulletin Inc., Toronto 1990; 6: 155–158.
183. Grefberg N, Danielson BG, Nilsson P, Wahlberg J. An unusual complication of the Toronto Western Hospital catheter (letter). Perit Dial Bull 1983; 3: 219.
184. della Volpe M, Iberti M, Ortensia A, Veronesi GV. Erosion of the sigmoid by a permanent peritoneal catheter (letter). Perit Dial Bull 1984; 4: 108.
185. Watson LC, Thompson JC. Erosion of the colon by a long dwelling peritoneal catheter. JAMA 1980; 243: 2155–7.
186. Valles M, Cantarell C, Vila J, Tovar JL. Delayed perforation of the colon by a Tenckhoff catheter. Perit Dial Bull 1982; 2: 190.
187. Shohat J, Shapira Z, Yussim A, Boner G. An unusual cause of massive intraperitoneal bleeding in CAPD (letter). Perit Dial Bull 1984; 4: 257–8.
188. de los Santos AC, von Eye O, d'Avila D, Mottin CC. Rupture of the spleen: a complication of continuous ambulatory peritoneal dialysis. Perit Dial Bull 1986; 6: 203–4.
189. Braden GL, Germain MJ, Guardione VA, Fitzgibbons JP. Infected intraabdominal hematoma associated with an indwelling Tenckhoff catheter. Perit Dial Bull 1984; 4: 248–50.
190. Jamison MH, Fleming SJ, Ackrill P, Schofield PF. Erosion of rectum by Tenckhoff catheter. Br J Surg 1988; 75: 360.
191. Brady HR, Abraham G, Oreopoulos DG, Cardella CJ. Bowel erosion due to a dormant peritoneal catheter in immunosupressed renal transplant recipients. Perit Dial Int 1988; 8: 163–5.
192. Kourie TB, Botha JR. Erosion of caecum by a Tenckhoff catheter. A case report. S Afr J Surg 1985; 23: 117–8.
193. Shröder CH, Rieu P, De Jong MCWJ, Monnens LAH. Peritoneal laceration: a rare cause of scrotal edema in a 2-year old boy. (Abstract) Perit Dial Int 1993; 13: S27.
194. Golper TA, Carpenter J. Accidents with Tenckhoff catheters. Ann Intern Med 1981; 95: 121–2.
195. Ward RA, Klein E, Wathen R (eds), Peritoneal catheters. In: Investigation of the Risks and Hazards with Devices Associated with Peritoneal Dialysis and Sorbent Regenerated Dialysate Delivery Systems. Perit Dial Bull 1983; 3 (suppl 3): S9–17.
196. Szycher M, Siciliano AA, Reed AM. Polyurethane in medical devices. Medical Design and Material 1991: 18–25.
197. Kurihara S, Tani Y, Tateishi K, Yuri T, Kitada H, Sugishita N, Fukuda Y, Ishikawa I, Shinoda A, Hayakawa Y. Allergic eosinophilic dermatitis due to silicone rubber: a rare but troublesome complication of the Tenckhoff catheter. Perit Dial Bull 1985; 5: 65–7.
198. Prowant BF, Schmidt LM, Twardowski ZJ, Taylor HM, Ryan LP, Satalowich RJ, Burrows L, Griebel CK, Burrows LM. Use of exudate smears for diagnosis of peritoneal catheter exit site infection. In: Avram MM, Giordano C (eds), Ambulatory Peritoneal Dialysis: Proceedings of the IVth Congress of the International Society for Peritoneal Dialysis, Venice, Italy, June 29–July 2, 1987. New York: Plenum Publishing Company 1990: 220–2.
199. Slingeneyer A, Balmes M, Mion C. Surgical implantation of the Tenckhoff catheter in peritoneal dialysis. In: La Greca G, Biasioli S, Ronco C, eds. Peritoneal Dialysis. Milano: Wichtig Editore 1983: 133–6.
200. Rubin J, Adair C. Peritoneal access using the Tenckhoff catheter. Perspective in Peritoneal Dialysis 1983; 1: 2–3.
201. Rottembourg J, De Groc F: Peritoneal access using the curled Tenckhoff catheter. Perspectives in Peritoneal Dialysis 1983; 1: 7–9.
202. Swartz R, Messana J, Rocher L, Reynolds J, Starmann B, Lees P. The curled catheter: dependable device for percutaneous peritoneal access. Perit Dial Int 1990; 10: 231–5.
203. Hogg RJ, Coln D, Chang J, Arant BS, Houser M. The Toronto Western Hospital catheter in a pediatric dialysis program. Am J Kidney Disease 1983; 3: 219–23.
204. Flanigan MJ, Ngheim DD, Schulack JA, Ullrich GE, Freeman RM. The use and complications of three peritoneal dialysis catheter designs: a retrospective analysis. Trans Am Soc Artif Intern Organs 1987; 33: 33–8.
205. Grefberg N. Clinical aspects of continuous ambu-

latory peritoneal dialysis. Scan J Urol and Nephrology 1983; (suppl 72): 1–46.
206. Ash SR, Slingeneyer A, Scchardin KE. Peritoneal access using the column-disc catheter. Perspective in Peritoneal Dialysis 1983; 1: 9–11.
207. Bozkurt F, Keller E, Schollmeyer P. Swan Neck peritoneal dialysis catheter can reduce complications in CAPD patients. Abstracts of the IVth Congress of the International Society for Peritoneal Dialysis, Venice, Italy, June 29–July 2, 1987. Peritoneal Dialysis Bulletin, Supplement 1987: 7 (suppl 2): S9.
208. Gucek A, Bren FA, Lindic J, Premru V, Kveder R. CAPD catheter survival: our 9-year experience. (Abstract) Perit Dial Int 1992; 12 (suppl 2): S49.
209. Ahlmén J, Brunes L, Schönborg C. A randomized comparison of two peritoneal dialysis catheters. ASAIO 1993 Abstracts. 39th Annual Meeting, New Orleans Hilton Hotel, New Orleans, Louisiana, April 29–30 & May 1, 1993: 110.

10 Placement, repair, and removal of chronic peritoneal catheters

STEPHEN R. ASH AND W. KIRT NICHOLS

1. Designs of chronic peritoneal dialysis catheters — 315
2. Proper position of peritoneal dialysis catheter components — 317
3. Materials of peritoneal catheter construction — 318
4. Placement techniques for peritoneal catheters — 319
   - 4.1. Dissective (surgical) technique — 319
   - 4.2. Blind techniques — 322
   - 4.3. Peritoneoscopic technique — 322
5. Complications of peritoneal catheters: relation to catheter type and implantation method — 322
6. Prophylactic antibiotics — 323
7. Break-in techniques/burying catheters — 326
8. Removal of subcutaneous cuff — 326
9. Repair of pericatheter hernias and leaks — 330
10. Repositioning intraperitoneal catheters; removing omental attachments — 330
11. Removal of peritoneal dialysis catheters — 330
References — 331

1. Designs of chronic peritoneal dialysis catheters

Chronic peritoneal dialysis catheters are constructed of soft materials like silicone rubber or polyurethane. The intraperitoneal portion may contain 1 mm side holes like acute peritoneal dialysis catheters, but may also have slots or larger holes for passage of the peritoneal fluid, and shapes or protrusions to prevent omentum from enveloping the catheter [1]. Some chronic catheters have discs, bubbles (beads) or flanges at the parietal peritoneum to fix the catheter position. Almost all have two extraperitoneal Dacron® cuffs, which promote a local inflammatory response, producing a fibrous plug to fix the catheter in position, prevent fluid leaks, and prevent bacterial migration along the catheter [2, 3, 4]. Finally, some chronic catheters have pre-formed angles in the subcutaneous tubing to create a caudally-directed exit site without strain between the deep and superficial cuffs [1, 2].

As shown in Fig. 1, chronic peritoneal dialysis catheters have a variety of IP or intraperitoneal designs physically combined with a number of EP or extraperitoneal designs [2, 5].

Intraperitoneal designs of chronic catheters include the following:

- straight Tenckhoff: 15 cm of tubing with 1 mm diameter side holes over the innermost 10 cm.
- curled Tenckhoff: short straight section leading to a curled portion with side holes.
- Oreopoulos-Zellerman (Toronto-Western™): sim-ilar to the straight Tenckhoff but with two intraperitoneal perpendicular discs, designed to hold visceral peritoneum and omentum away from the side holes.
- Lifecath® (column disc): two 7 cm diameter discs separated by perpendicular columns, which create thin slots through which peritoneal fluid is directed along the parietal peritoneal surface.

Extraperitoneal designs of chronic catheters include the following:

- single cuff: a single Dacron cuff, usually placed within or adjacent to the musculature.
- disc-bubble 1 cuff (1 cuff Toronto™): a single Dacron cuff attached to a perpendicular Dacron disc, adjacent to a solid silicone bubble (bead); the parietal peritoneum and posterior rectus sheath are closed between the bead the disk.
- dual cuff: two Dacron cuffs, the deep cuff within or adjacent to the musculature and the subcutaneous cuff 2 cm from the skin surface, with the outer-cuff tubing straight or slightly curved.
- disc-bubble 2 cuff (2 cuff Toronto): the perpendicular disc-bubble at the parietal peritoneum, with a second subcutaneous cuff.
- arcuate (Swan Neck™): dual cuffs, with a preformed 150 degree bend in the inter-cuff tubing, to provide a caudally directed exit site without strain on the cuffs, and to balance the extrusion forces on the deep cuff with those of the subcutaneous cuff.

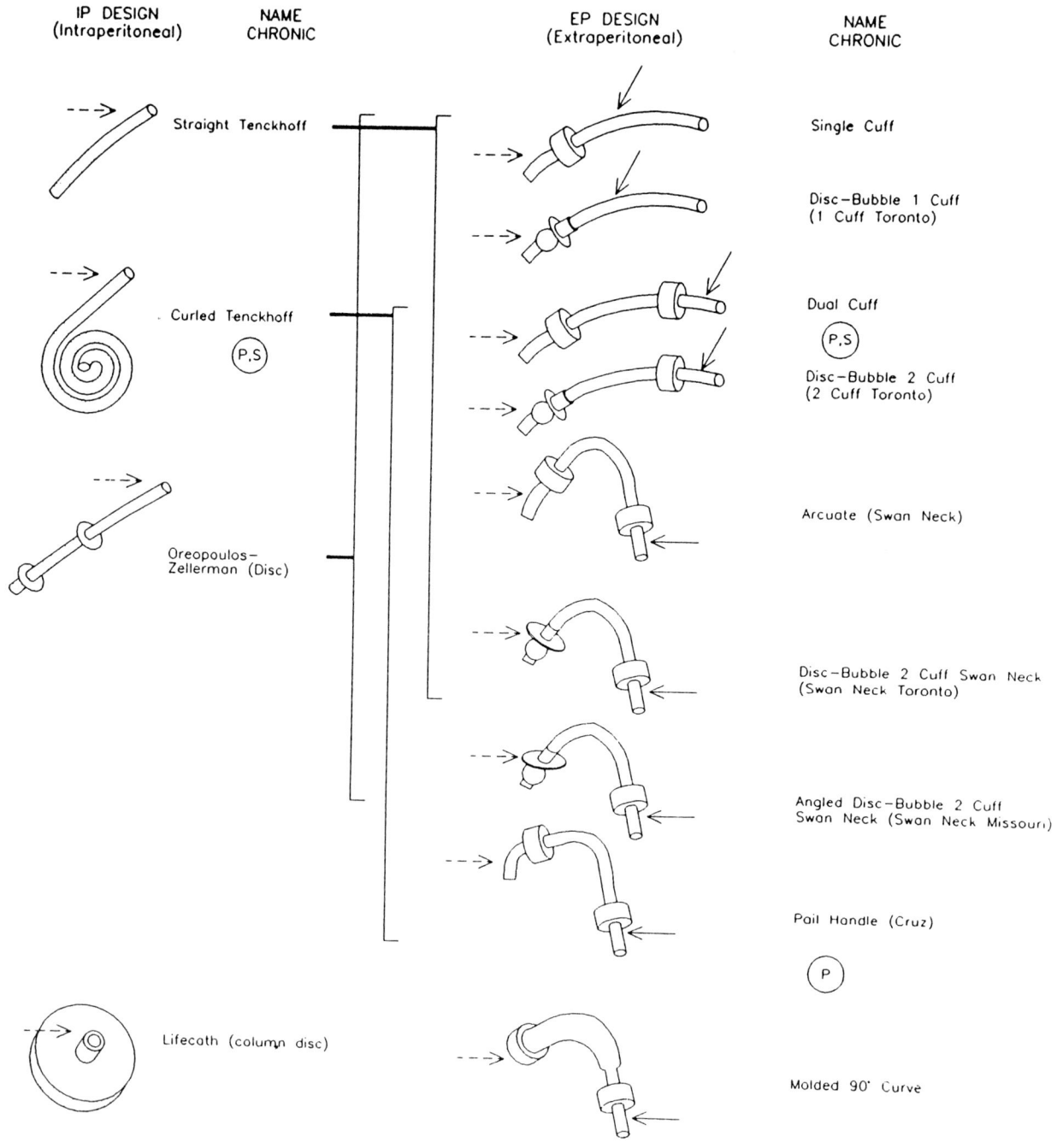

Figure 1. Combinations of intraperitoneal and extraperitoneal designs in currently available peritoneal catheters. Intraperitoneal (IP) designs are on the left side, and extraperitoneal (EP) designs on the right. The letters in circles indicate materials of construction: P = polyurethane; P,S = polyurethane or silicone; no letter = only in silicone. The **dotted** arrow indicates the location of the parietal peritoneum, and the **solid** arrow the location of the skin surface.

- disc-bubble 2 cuff Swan Neck (Swan Neck Toronto): the perpendicular disc-bubble at the parietal peritoneum, a preformed 150 degree bend in subcutaneous tubing, and a subcutaneous cuff.
- angled disc-bubble 2 cuff Swan Neck (Swan Neck Missouri): a disc-bubble mounted at 45 degree angle to the tubing at the parietal peritoneal surface, a 150 degree bend in the inter-cuff tunnel, and a subcutaneous cuff.
- Cruz™ (pail-handle): similar to the arcuate catheter but with two 90 degree bends, one to direct the intraperitoneal portion parallel to the parietal peritoneum, and one to direct the inter-cuff portion downward towards the subcutaneous cuff and skin exit site.
- molded 90 degree curve: for the Lifecath, a molded portion directing the inter-cuff tubing downward towards the subcutaneous cuff and skin exit site.

2. Proper position of peritoneal dialysis catheter components

There is general consensus regarding proper location of intraperitoneal and extracorporeal components of chronic peritoneal catheters [1, 2, 5]. As shown in Fig. 2, the intraperitoneal portion of a Tenckhoff-type catheter should be directed between the visceral and parietal peritoneum, towards the left or right lower quadrant (because omentum is less here than in the upper abdomen). The deep cuff should be placed within the abdominal wall musculature, to assure rapid tissue ingrowth to the cuff. Since the parietal peritoneum surrounds the catheter and extends to the deep cuff, having the deep cuff outside the abdominal wall creates a potential hernial sac. The superficial cuff should be located 1–2 cm from the skin exit site. Stratified squamous epithelium of the skin migrates along the catheter track to grow toward the superficial cuff, converting to granulomatous tissue at about this level. The tubing at the exit site may be directed caudally or laterally, but a cranial direction will result in a high incidence of exit infections [6].

During the placement of a peritoneal catheter it is best to choose a deep cuff location which minimises the chance of involving major vessels. Figure 3 demonstrates the major vessels and landmarks of the anterior abdominal wall. The superficial epigastric arteries course from the femoral artery and ligament towards the umbilicus, anterior to the rectus sheath. The inferior epigastric arteries lie behind the rectus muscles, roughly in the middle of the rectus sheath. Considering the position of arteries, the safest locations for placing the deep cuff are at the medial or lateral borders of the rectus muscles. For procedures using a trocar or needle,

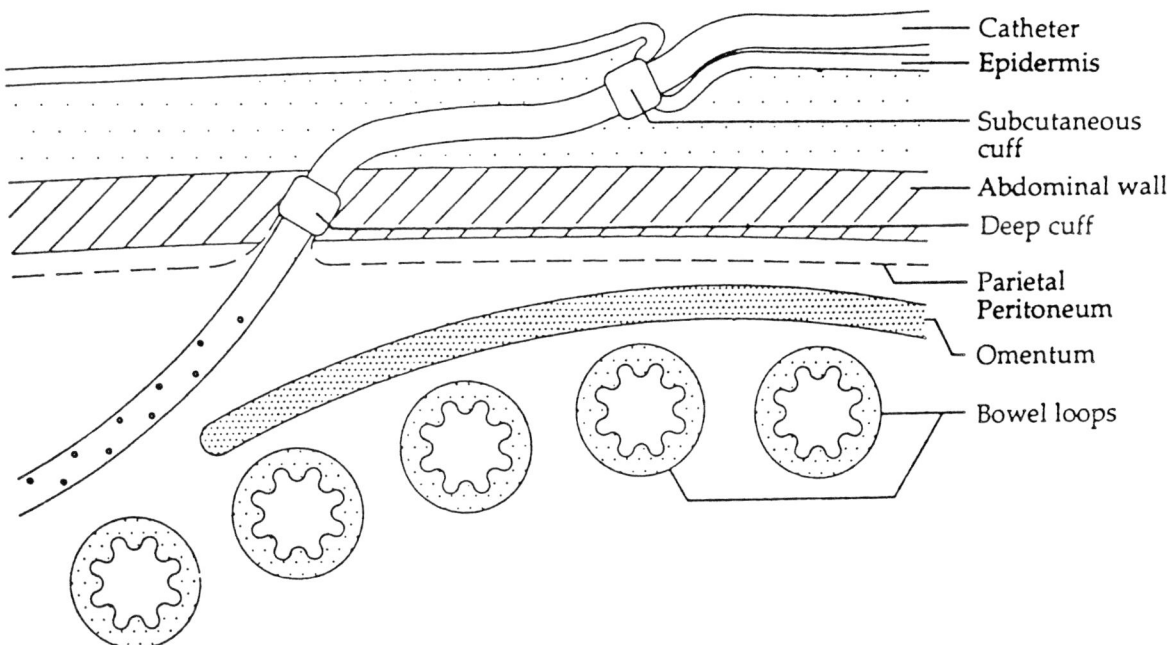

Figure 2. Cross section of the abdominal wall with a dual cuff Tenckhoff catheter in position, showing preferred location of intraperitoneal portion, deep cuff, and subcutaneous cuff.

the preferred insertion point is half-way between the anterior superior iliac spine and the midline (through the outer border of the rectus sheath). The alternative insertion point is at the midline 2 cm below the umbilicus [1]. In either location, the insertion point is at the level of or cranial to the anterior superior iliac spine; with a cannula or needle directed towards the coccyx, there is minimal risk of puncturing the bladder or iliac vessels (solid squares, Fig. 3). In dissective placement, the deep cuff can be placed more towards the center of the rectus and more caudally, using care to identify and avoid any major vessels (open squares, Fig. 3).

3. Materials of peritoneal catheter construction

Historically, chronic peritoneal catheters have been constructed from hydrophobic silicone. These catheters suffer from a variety of problems: growth of biofilm on the catheter leading to recurrent peritonitis, omental attachment to the catheter side holes leading to outflow obstruction, and mechanical failure leading to catheter breakage and detachment of connectors. Recently, curled peritoneal catheters have been introduced which are constructed of hydrophilic polyurethane, having thinner walls and either a small outer diameter or larger internal diameter than silicone catheters. Polyurethane is smoother and stronger than silicone, but bonding of Dacron cuffs requires more care. Polyurethane catheters have not yet been proven to have a lower incidence of recurrent peritonitis, outflow obstruction, or mechanical failure (see the Cruz articles, Table 1). However, the catheters have been shown to allow more rapid infusion and drainage of dialysate [7]. If a patient develops one of the above

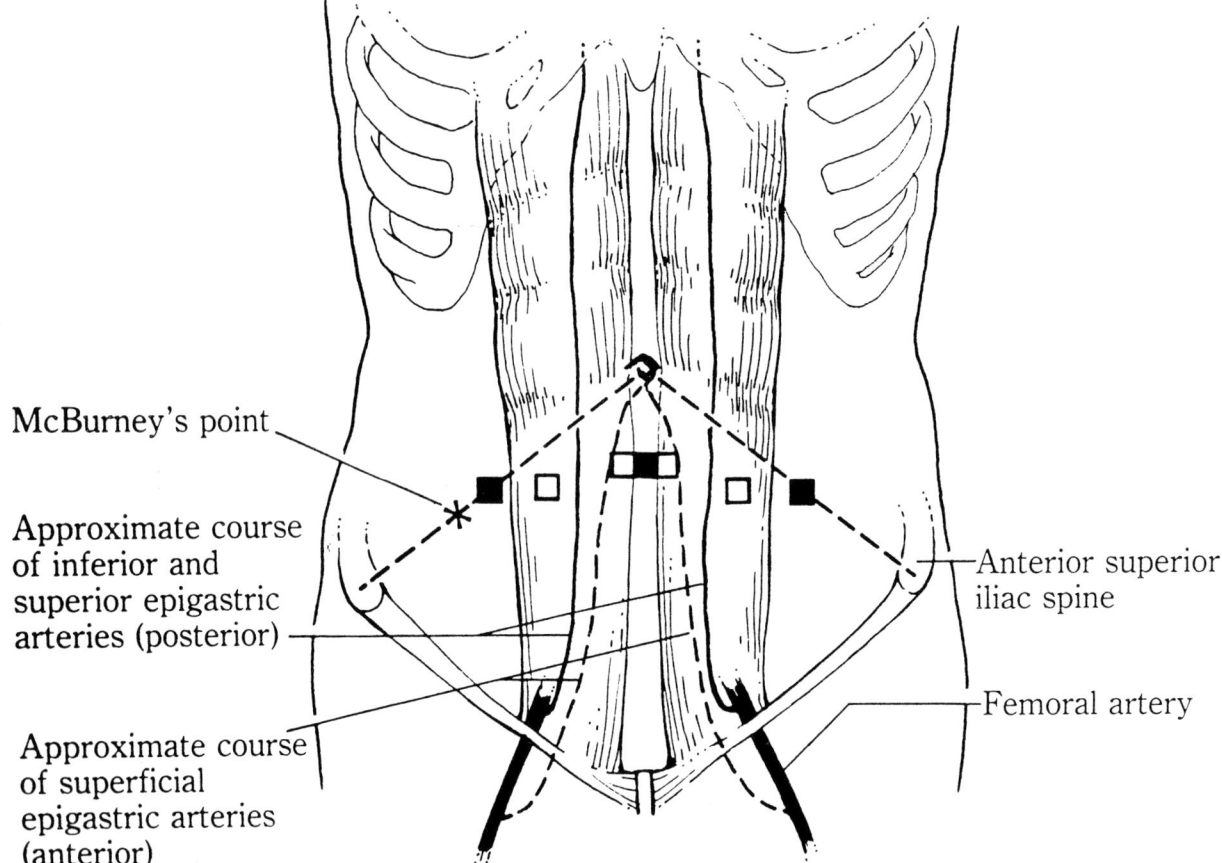

Figure 3. Major blood vessels and landmarks of the abdominal cavity, indication preferred points for location of the deep cuff of a chronic peritoneal catheter. Solid squares indicate points of penetration by cannula and trocar during peritoneoscopic catheter placement, and by needle during blind placement, and subsequent location of deep cuff. Open squares represent the points of entry during dissective (Surgical) placement, and subsequent location of deep cuff. (Originally published in Daugridaz, JT. Handbook of Dialysis. Boston: Little Brown, p. 198. Reproduced with permission).

complications of a silicone peritoneal catheter, it is reasonable to use a polyurethane catheter as the next peritoneal access device. Placement techniques are the same for both types of catheters.

4. Placement techniques for peritoneal catheters

Peritoneal dialysis catheters must be placed with strict attention to asepsis, whether the procedure is within a surgical suite, outpatient procedure room, or intensive care unit. The patient's bladder is emptied. Everyone in the room wears a cap and mask (including the patient), and the physician and assistant wear sterile gowns and gloves. The abdomen is scrubbed with povidone-iodine soap and solution, and carefully draped. A plastic "sticky" drape affords an effective skin barrier. Local anesthetic is injected into the skin and abdominal wall (unless general anesthesia is given).

Chronic peritoneal catheters are placed by one of three techniques: dissective (surgical), blind, and peritoneoscopic. Since surgeons and nephrologists use all of these techniques in a variety of hospital settings, classifying placement techniques as merely "surgical" or "medical" is imprecise.

4.1. Dissective (surgical) techniques

The steps of placement of a permanent peritoneal dialysis catheter (a Swan Neck Missouri™ catheter) are depicted in Figs. 4(a–l). Placement by dissection begins with a 3–5 cm skin incision usually placed over the rectus muscle. In the case of the Swan Neck Missouri catheter, a stencil is available and the location is marked preoperatively by the peritoneal dialysis nurse. A combination of blunt and sharp dissection is used to reach the level of the anterior rectus sheath. Bleeding is carefully and precisely controlled with electrocautery. A 2–3 cm incision is made in the anterior rectus sheath and the muscle fibers are separated by blunt dissection in a vertical direction. A self retaining retractor aids in maintaining exposure. A "purse string" suture (1.5 cm diameter) is then placed in the posterior rectus fascia and a small (0.5 cm) incision is made through the posterior rectus fascia and peritoneum using care to avoid bowel injury. The peritoneal and fascial edges are elevated to create an air pocket between the abdominal wall and the underlying viscera. The catheter is prepared on the "back table" by soaking in and flushing with sterile saline. The cuffs are squeezed under saline to expel air from the interstices of the Dacron material. A stiffening stylet is moistened with saline and inserted into the catheter leaving about 1 cm of soft catheter beyond the tip of the stylet. The catheter is directed by feel into the lower abdomen/pelvis. If any obstruction to passage is encountered, the catheter should be pulled back and redirected. When the majority of the intraperitoneal portion of the catheter is in the abdomen the stiffening stylet is removed. For the Lifecath or the Toronto-Western catheters a slightly larger peritoneal incision is necessary. The Lifecath disc is folded in half, held with a blunt hemostat, inserted through the incision into the peritoneal cavity and released. The perpendicular discs of the Toronto-Western catheter are advanced through the peritoneal opening with the catheter.

The peritoneum and posterior rectus fascia are closed snugly around the catheter (below the cuff or between the bead and cuff in the Toronto-Western or Missouri catheters) by tying the purse string suture or by closing the larger incision used for the Toronto Western or Lifecath catheter.

A "stab" wound is made in the anterior rectus fascia approximately 1.5 cm above the transverse incision and the catheter carefully pulled through. The position of the exit site is determined and the catheter is attached to a sharp trocar. A subcutaneous tunnel is then constructed by passing the trochar from "inside" the wound "out" positioning the subcutaneous cuff (if present) approximately 2 cm from the skin exit site. Care must be used to avoid sharp angulation of the catheter in the subcutaneous tunnel. Placement of the exit site is greatly facilitated by premarking the patient with the stencil provided with the Swan Neck Missouri catheter. Since the Swan Neck catheter has a preformed bend in the subcutaneous tunnel, a small pocket must be made with blunt dissection to accommodate the bend. At this time, the catheter is connected to dialysate tubing and tested for acceptable inflow, outflow and the absence of leak by infusing and draining 1000 cc of fluid. The anterior rectus fascia is then closed with a permanent monofilament suture, leaving the deep cuff buried in the rectus muscle.

The skin incision is carefully closed in layers after performing meticulous hemostasis with an electrocautery pencil. The skin is closed with an absorbable subcuticular closure. *No sutures are used at the exit site.*

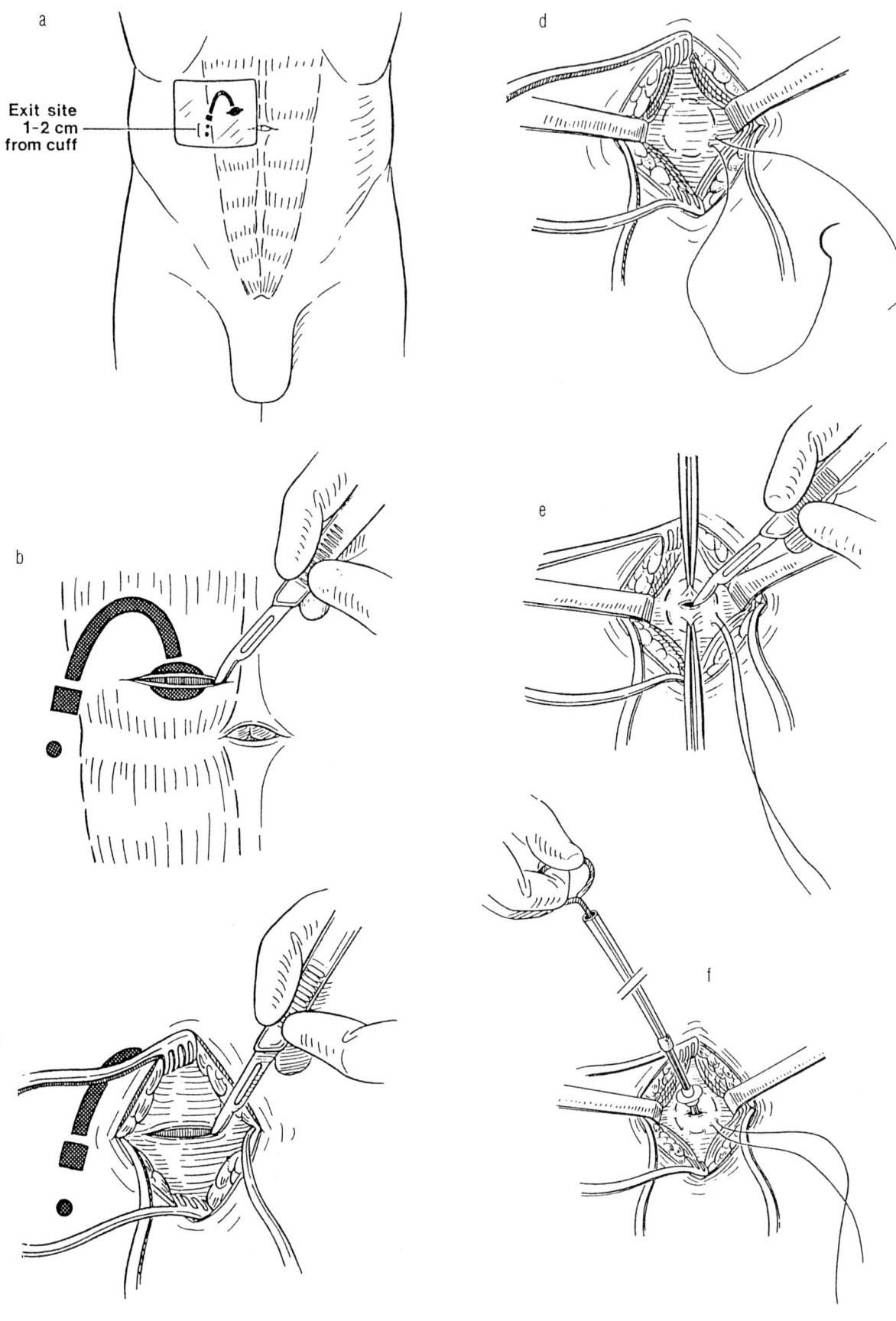

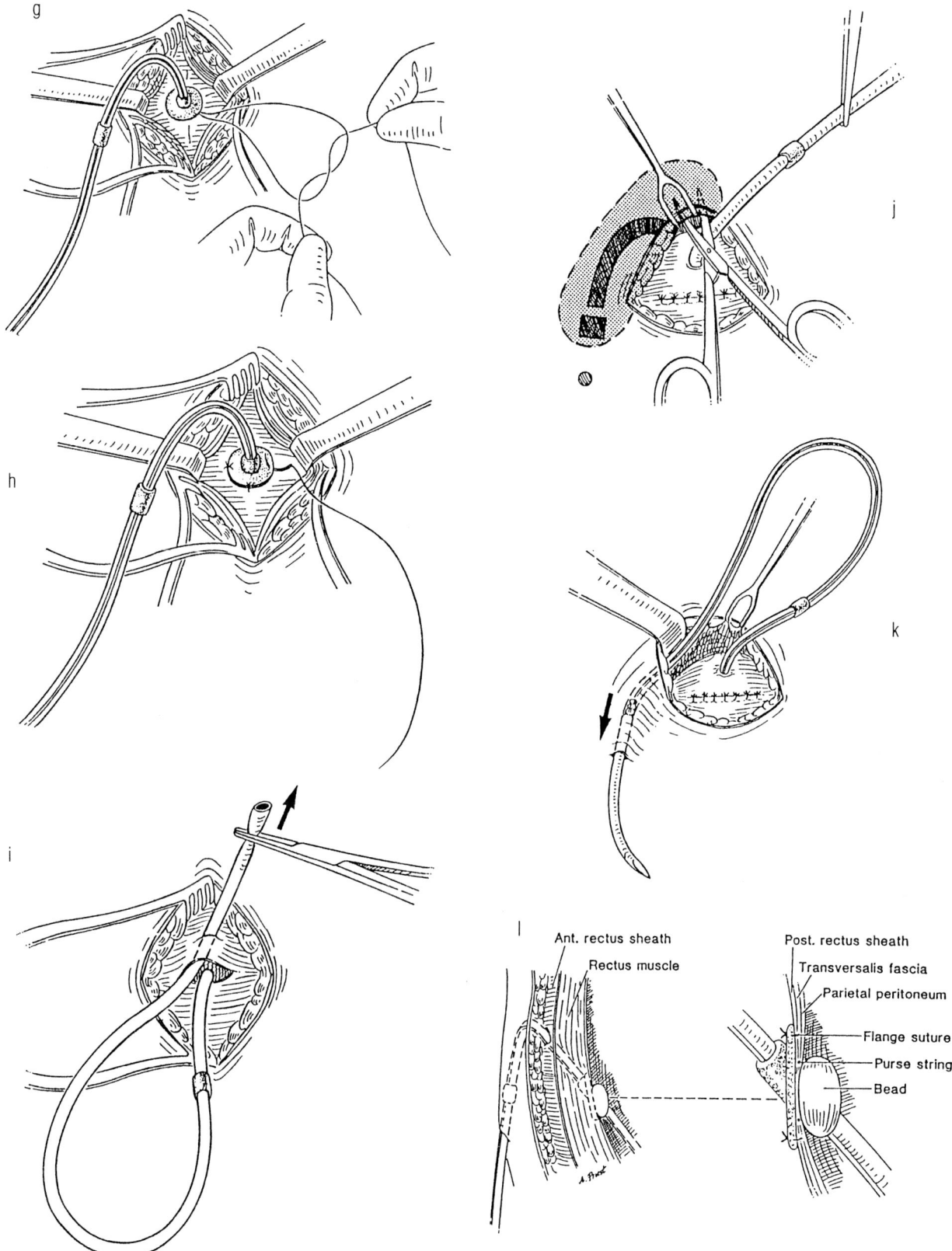

Figure 4(a–l). Steps of placement of a Swan Neck Missouri catheter by dissection. For discussion see text. *4(l):* Relation of disc-bubble portion to peritoneum and rectus muscle.

4.2. Blind techniques

There are two methods of blind insertion of Tenckhoff-type peritoneal dialysis catheters: the Tenckhoff trocar method and the guidewire/split-sheath method. Both begin with a 2–3 cm incision in the skin and blunt dissection to the abdominal musculature, as with acute catheters. A Verres needle or over-the-needle catheter is inserted to the abdomen and two liters of dialysate infused. Next, a large bore steel tube with internal trocar, or split-sheath with internal dilator, is inserted into the abdomen. The catheter is then advanced through the tube or split-sheath, the deep cuff eventually reaching the outer fascia of the abdominal musculature. If desired, and if exposure is adequate, the deep cuff can be advanced into the musculature by compressing it with hemostats and rotating while advancing the hemostats.

With the Tenckhoff trocar method, the cylinder is assembled from two half-cylinders, an internal trocar is inserted, and the tube and trocar are advanced into the abdomen. The trocar is removed and the catheter (with internal stylet) is advanced into the tube until the cuff stops at a narrowing portion of the cylinder. The half cylinders and stylet are removed, leaving the cuff at the outer fascia of the abdominal musculature. The subcutaneous tunnel is created exactly as in dissective placement.

With the guidewire split-sheath technique, after the abdomen is filled with fluid by a small needle or catheter, a guidewire is inserted through the needle or IV-type catheter, and the needle removed. A tapered dilator enlarges the hole through the abdominal wall, then a cylindrical split-sheath (separable to two halves) is inserted into the abdomen over an internal dilator. The guidewire and dilator are removed, and the Tenckhoff catheter with internal stylet is directed into the sheath. As the cuff enters the sheath, the sheath is split to allow the cuff to advance and stop at the outer fascia of the abdominal musculature. The sheath is removed over the catheter and advanced into the abdominal musculature. The subcutaneous tunnel is created exactly as in dissective placement.

4.3. Peritoneoscopic technique

The basic components required for peritoneoscopic implantation of Tenckhoff-type catheters are shown in Fig. 5. Peritoneoscopic placement of Tenckhoff-type catheters with the Y-TEC® system, like some blind techniques, is performed through a single abdominal puncture [5, 6]. Figure 6 demonstrates the consecutive steps used to place Tenckhoff-type catheters with the peritoneoscopic approach. Peritoneoscopic placement differs from both blind and dissective techniques in several ways:

(1) The intraperitoneal position of the first object inserted to the abdomen (a cannula) is confirmed with the 2.2 mm diameter Y-TEC peritoneoscope, before any fluid is infused to the abdomen.
(2) Gas, not liquid, is used to inflate the abdomen (about 600 cc), which effectively separates visceral and parietal peritoneal surfaces (since gas is less dense than any of the viscera.)
(3) The entire anterior peritoneal space is inspected, and the catheter location is selected by directing the peritoneoscope between visceral and parietal omentum, avoiding adhesions and loops of bowel.
(4) A spiral-wound Quill® catheter guide is left in the abdomen to direct the full length of the catheter into the previously-inspected tract.
(5) The cuff is advanced within the Quill guide to reach the abdominal musculature (using the Cuff-Implantation™ tool); the Quill guide expands the musculature to accept the cuff. Suturing the anterior rectus sheath is not necessary unless the catheter is to be used for immediate full-volume exchanges in patients with thin abdominal musculature. The 2–3 cm primary incision allows one or two sutures to be placed in most patients; obese patients will require a larger incision to allow visualization of the musculature.

5. Complications of peritoneal catheters: relation to catheter type and implantation method

The complications of peritoneal dialysis catheters are those expected of a transcutaneous catheter which leads into an abdomen filled with bowel loops, mobile omentum, and fluid: peritonitis, catheter infection, outflow failure, and subcutaneous leak. Each of the catheter placement methods are generally successful, but each has certain advantages.

Table 1 presents a meta-analysis of the incidence of complications of peritoneal catheters in numerous studies, organized by type of catheter, method of placement, and the average length of

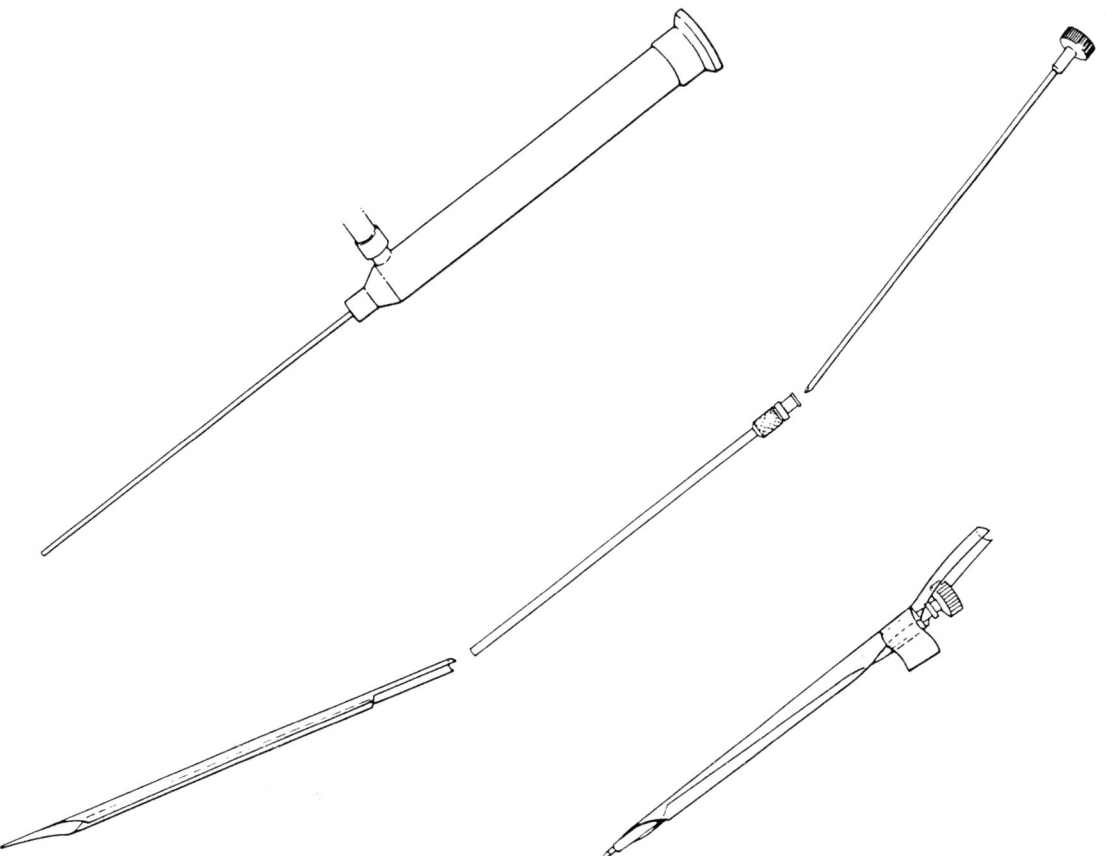

Figure 5. The basic components required for peritoneoscopic implantation of a Tenckhoff-type peritoneal catheter by Y-Tec® technique: the stylet, 2.5 mm diameter cannula, coiled Quill® catheter guide, and the Y-Tec® peritoneoscope (© Mediagroup Inc. N. Aurora, IL).

catheter follow-up. Listed are all catheter-related complications, not merely those leading to catheter removal. Infectious complications are defined as all infections except intermittent peritonitis with varying organisms. For standard dual-cuff straight Tenckhoff catheters, which can be placed by many methods, Table 1 indicates that catheters placed peritoneoscopically have the lowest incidence of all complications (3%, 3%, and 2% for infection, outflow, and leak problems respectively). Blind placement of dual-cuff Tenckhoffs results in a higher average complication rate (13%, 24%, 5%) as does surgical placement (31%, 13%, 11%). Results are similar for curled dual-cuff Tenckhoff catheters. Some studies of blind and surgical techniques report much better success, as do studies of peritoneoscopy by physicians with considerable experience. Thus, the advantages of peritoneoscopic placement in all centers may not be as great as in the published studies of Table 1.

Table 1 also demonstrates that some types of peritoneal catheters have low rates of certain complications, especially those with a catheter fixation device at the parietal peritoneum. The Missouri coiled catheter, with a bubble (bead) within the peritoneum and a Dacron disc outside the peritoneum and deep fascia, has a relatively low rate of infection (16%), and a low rate of outflow failure (4%) and subcutaneous leak (0%). The Lifecath, with a 2″ diameter disc at the parietal peritoneal surface also has a low infection rate (9%), and a low rate of outflow failure (7%) and subcutaneous leak (3%). These two catheters must be placed by surgical dissection, limiting their general use. Furthermore, removal is somewhat more difficult, requiring dissection to the parietal peritoneum instead of merely to a deep cuff within the abdominal musculature as with Tenckhoff-type catheters.

6. Prophylactic antibiotics

Chronic peritoneal dialysis catheters are foreign bodies which will remain in place for a long period of time, similar to aortic grafts, AV grafts for

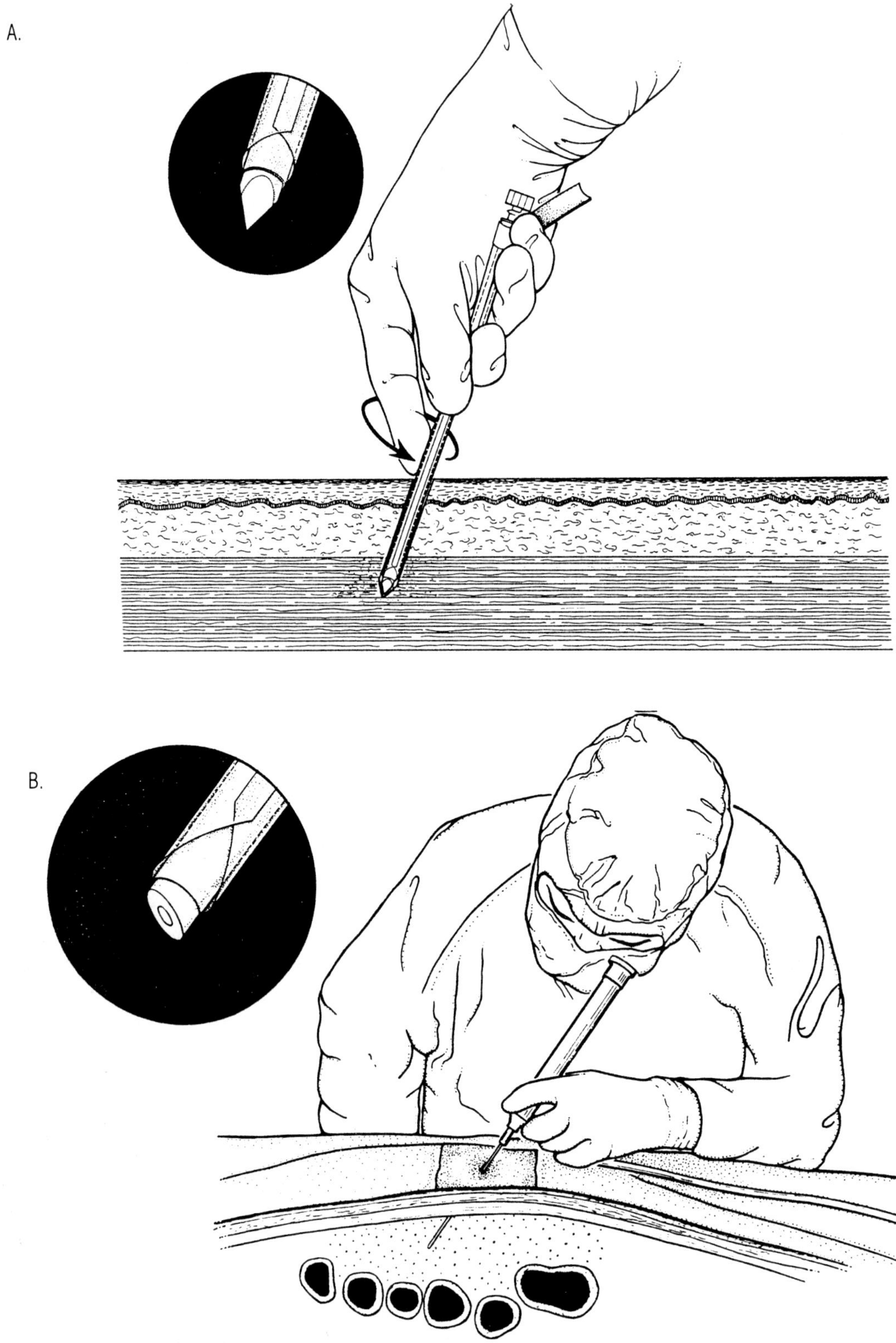

Figure 6. Steps of implantation of a Tenckhoff-type catheter using the Y-Tec® systems and peritoneoscope:
A. Insertion of the trocar, 2.5 mm cannula and coiled Quill® guide through the abdominal wall.
B. After removal of the trocar, visual inspection confirms intraperitoneal location of the cannula; subsequent air insufflation creates a space through which the cannula and Quill guide are advanced, between visceral and parietal peritoneum.

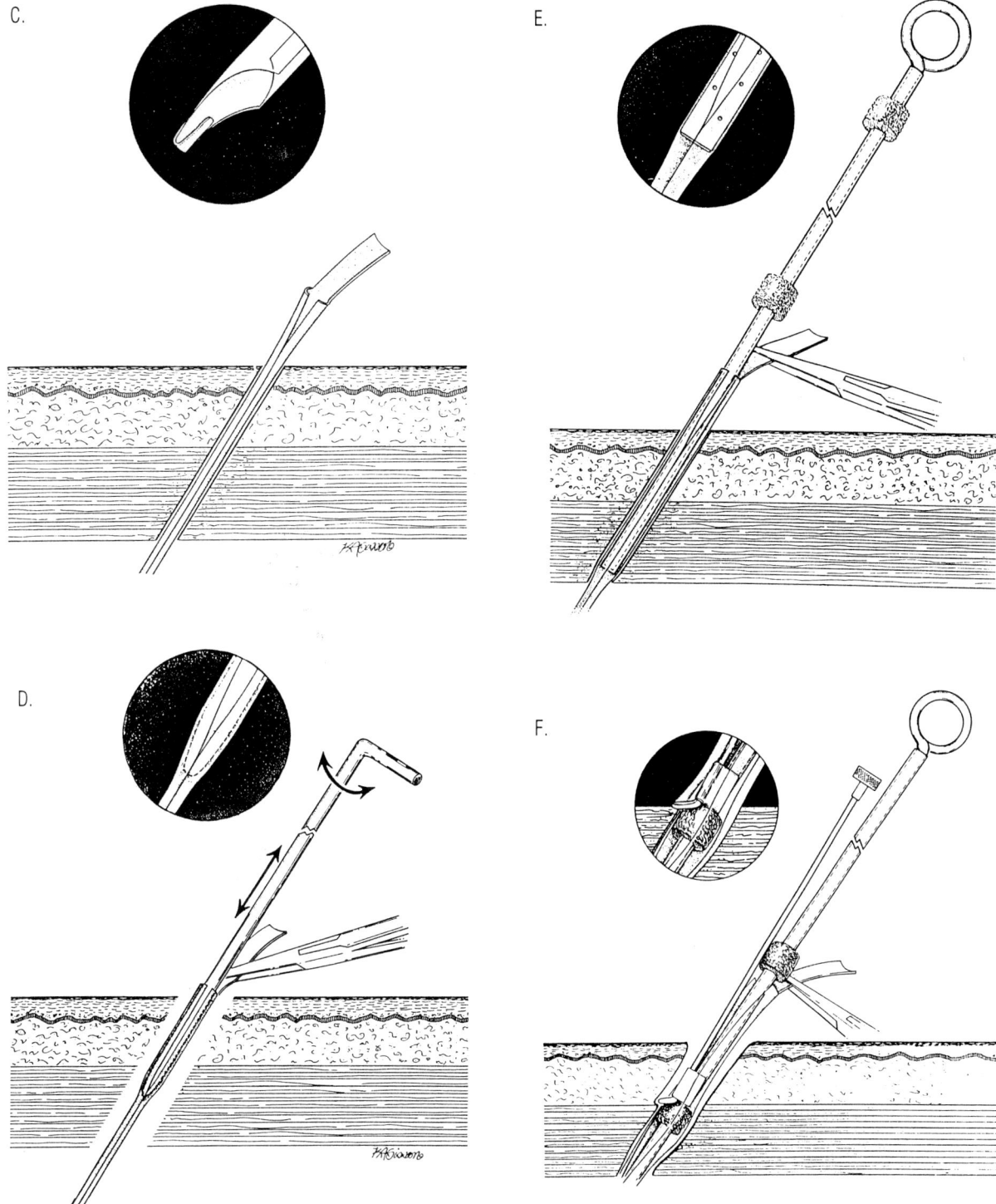

Figure 6. Steps of implantation of a Tenckhoff-type catheter using the Y-Tec peritoneoscope:
C. The Quill guide, left in the desired catheter location.
D. Radial dilation of the coiled Quill guide to 6 mm diameter.
E. Insertion of the Tenckhoff catheter (with internal stylet) through the dilated Quill guide; the deep cuff will stop at the outer fascia.
F. With the Cuff-Implanter™ tool, the deep cuff is advanced through the Quill guide into the abdominal musculature.
G. The Quill guide is removed while holding the catheter stationary. After the stylet is removed, the free end of the catheter is then tunneled subcutaneously to place the superficial cuff 2 cm from the exit site (© Mediagroup, Inc., N. Aurora, IL).

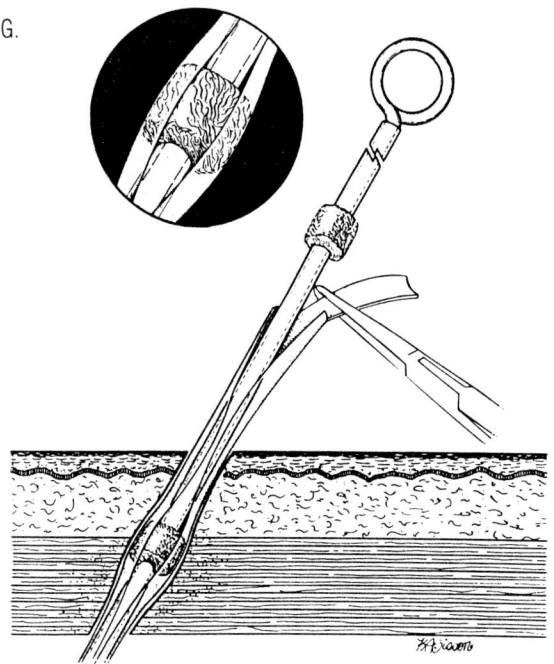

Figure 6. (G).

dialysis, and artificial hips. Since prophylactic (especially anti-staphylococcal) antibiotics are effective in diminishing post-operative infections of these other foreign bodies and there is little risk, it makes sense to administer them before placement of chronic peritoneal dialysis catheters [9]. Some studies have indicated that prophylactic antibiotics do not decrease the incidence of exit infection or peritonitis [8], and other studies show diminution in peritonitis for carriers of S. Aureus [9]. According to the 1992 USRDS study, 30% or more of centers do not routinely use prophylactic antibiotics for catheter placement. The study showed no difference in rate of early peritonitis between patients having antibiotic prophylactics and those not having them [4].

7. Break-in techniques/burying catheters

If possible, peritoneal dialysis catheters should be placed several weeks before they are needed for treatment of uremia. This allows time for ingrowth of tissue into the cuffs before the abdomen is filled with fluid while the patient is ambulatory. During this time, infusion of fluid into and out of the catheter will confirm that the catheter is patent and that it will effectively drain the abdomen. These infusions are performed on a variety of schedules, some of which can be used to treat uremia [10]. There are several common themes of catheter break in technique, all designed to diminish intraperitoneal pressure and to minimize pericatheter leaks:

- heparinized saline or dialysis solution (from 50 cc to 2000 cc) are infused to the abdomen at least three times weekly; the larger volumes are drained.
- part of each day, the abdomen is left dry.
- activity is limited when the fluid is in place, or else volume is limited to 1 liter or less.
- the patient is instructed to cough as little as possible.
- full volume exchanges with the patient active when full (CAPD) are delayed for 2–4 wks.

These schedules of break-in have always seemed sensible, but they may not be necessary. Peritoneal dialysis catheters have been left in place without use for up to 3 months after successful renal transplant, without any untoward complications except a rare spontaneous bowel perforation (with straight Tenckhoff catheters, usually). Peritoneal dialysate is not perfectly "physiologic," eliciting outpouring of interferon, interleukins, leukotrienes, etc. from the peritoneum; normal saline is somewhat more physiologic, having less acidity and no lactate. Any chronic peritoneal catheter placed has a risk of bacterial migration from the skin along the catheter to seed the cuffs, especially before the cuffs are well grown in.

Drs Moncrief and Popovich recently described a technique in which the transcutaneous portion of the catheter (external segment) is buried below the skin in a tunnel, and the skin incisions closed over the catheter. Approximately 3–5 weeks later, the exit site is opened, the external segment brought through the skin, and dialysis is begun. Outside of 1000 units of heparin in 10 cc saline infused into the catheter before skin closure, there is no fluid infused to the catheter. Each of the catheters placed in this manner have functioned well hydraulically when exteriorized. The benefit of this technique is a decrease in peritonitis rate, presumably by decreasing bacterial seeding of the catheter before the fibrous tissue has grown into the cuffs [11, 12].

8. Removal of subcutaneous cuff

If the subcutaneous (superficial) cuff of a peritoneal catheter begins to extrude through the skin, this

Table 1. Compliations of peritoneal catheters by type and plaement technique.

Catheter type: IP, SQ Placement Method					(FRACTION OF CATHETERS)		
Ref. no.	Year	Principal Investigator	No. of Catheters	Mean Follow-up (months)	Infectious Complications	Outflow Failures	Subcutaneous Leak
1. Tenckhoff straight, dual-cuff							
Blind							
18	1968	Tenckhoff	4	7.8	0.25	0.50	0.00
27	1984	Diaz-Buxo (IPD)	29	48.0	−a	0.15	0.05
		(CAPD)	31	24.0	−	0.05	0.00
29	1985	Bierman	222	24.0	0.12	0.36	0.03
39	1985	Valenti	30	13.7	−	−	0.26
32	1986	Slingeneyer	428	21.0	0.12	0.06	0.03
55	1991	Nebel	49	9.6	0.05	0.30	0.02
				21.16	0.13	0.24	0.05
Surgical							
19	1972	Brewer	24	1.14	0.10	0.40	−
20	1973	Thomas	16	4.11	−	−	0.16
21	1975	Giordano	10	10.0	0.41	−	0.58
22	1977	Karanikolas	91	8.3	0.07	0.05	001
23	1981	Khanna	132	13.3	0.19	0.07	0.07
24	1981	Rottembourg	48	12.0	−	−	0.30
25	1982	Ponce	94	24.0	−	0.17	0.18
30	1985	Odor	150	6.1	0.10	0.33	0.00
31	1985	Twardowski	83	18.0	0.50	0.11	−
33	1987	Flanigan	63	9.8	0.20	0.20	0.00
47	1989	Gibel	49	14.5	0.44	−	0.02
43	1989	Baker	1322	pt-month	0.09	−	−
45	1989	Davis	220	47.0	−	0.04	0.06
49	1990	Stegmayr	30	5.4	0.13	−	0.00
50	1990	Akyol	20	13.1	1.20	0.20	0.00
52	1991	Piraino	228	36.0	1.00	0.04	0.06
56	1990	Shah	44	19.0	0.09	0.05	0.09
60	1990	Rabin					
		(midline)	24	2.0	0.08	0.05	0.16
		(lateral)	26	2.0	0.11	0.00	0.08
				13.0	0.31	0.13	0.11
Peritoneoscopic							
26	1983	Ash	61	10.0	0.02	0.04	0.05
28	1984	Handt	98	27.0	0.15	0.00	0.00
42	1987	Cruz	10	6.5	0.00	0.01	0.01
58	1992	Adamson	100	10.0	0.01	0.04	0.09
61	1993	Donate (w/o scope)	27	7.0	0.00	0.07	0.00
62	1993	Swartz (10 mm scope)	38	7.0	0.00	0.03	0.00
				11.25	0.03	0.03	0.02
General							
46	1988	Nolph/Registry	1128	24.0	0.31	0.06	0.02
Teckhoff straight, dual-cuff, arcuate							
Blind							
55	1991	Nebel	23	14.5	0.22	0.17	0.43
Surgical							
40	1987	Bozkurt	3	12.0	0.00	0.00	0.00
41	1988	Ishizak	31	8.5	0.16	0.00	0.03
				10.2	0.08	0.00	0.01

Table 1 (Continued)

Catheter type: IP, SQ Placement Method					(FRACTION OF CATHETERS)		
Ref. no.	Year	Principal Investigator	No. of Catheters	Mean Follow-up (months)	Infectious Complications	Outflow Failures	Subcutaneous Leak
General							
63	1991	Multic. (Spain)	92	7.0	0.49	0.90	0.16
Tenckhoff straight, dual cuff w/peritoneal flange, arcuate (Missouri straight catheter)							
Surgical							
48	1987	Twardowski	17	4.5	0.23	0.05	0.00
43	1989	Baker	226	pt-months	0.09	—	—
54	1991	Twardowski	103	9.0	0.10	0.05	0.01
8	1992	Twardowski	105	24.0	0.47	0.06	0.01
				12.5	0.22	0.05	0.01
Tenckhoff straight, single-cuff							
Blind/Trocar							
27	1984	Diaz-Buxo (IPD)	240	48.0	—	0.10	0.02
		(CCPD)	134	24.0	—	0.03	0.05
33	1987	Flanigan	79	9.8	—	0.12	0.00
57	1991	Zappacosta	101	36.0	0.15	0.07	0.03
				29.4	0.15	0.08	0.02
General							
46	1988	Nolph/Registry	308	24.0	0.33	0.02	0.05
Surgical							
66	1988	Copley (a few peritoneoscopic)	95	1.0	0.00	—	—
2. Tenckhoff curled, dual-cuff							
Blind							
18	1968	Tenckhoff	2	7.0	0.50	0.00	0.00
24	1981	Rottenbourg	12	12.0	0.02	0.04	—
38	1989	Swartz	134	24.0	0.75	0.11	0.28
51	1990	Swartz	134	12.3	0.75	0.11	0.22
				13.8	0.50	0.06	0.17
Surgical							
29	1985	Bierman	43	24.0	0.12	0.30	0.02
38	1989	Swartz	79	24.0	0.88	0.11	0.14
44	1989	Cruz	118	13.0	0.26	0.10	0.10
50	1990	Akyol	20	12.8	1.00	0.10	0.10
51	1990	Swartz	79	12.1	0.88	0.14	0.10
53	1991	Pastan	42	3.4	0.26	—	0.26
60	1990	Rubin					
		(midline)	24	2.0	0.16	0.16	0.16
		(lateral)	17	2.0	0.06	0.11	0.06
13	1991	Scalamonga	163	30.0	0.58	—	—
65	1991	Dryden	108	12.0	0.04	—	—
64	1992	Scabardi (short)	132	24.0	—	0.09	—
				14.5	0.42	0.14	0.12
Peritoneoscopic							
42	1988	Cruz	80	6.5	0.00	0.01	0.01
44	1989	Cruz	150	12.0	0.01	0.01	0.01
53	1991	Pastan	46	8.4	0.22	—	0.26
				8.9	0.08	0.01	0.09

Table 1 (Continued)

Catheter type: IP, SQ Placement Method					(FRACTION OF CATHETERS)		
Ref. no.	Year	Principal Investigator	No. of Catheters	Mean Follow-up (months)	Infectious Complications	Outflow Failures	Subcutaneous Leak
General							
46	1988	Nolph/Registry	330	24.0	0.26	0.05	0.05
Tenchkoff curled, dual cuff, arcuate							
Surgical/Buried							
11	1993	Moncreif	74	3.0	0.07	–	–
12	1992	Han	74	7.0	0.63	–	–
				5.0	0.35	–	–
Surgical							
59	1992	Wadhwa	78	13.0	0.43	–	–
General							
63	1991	Multic. (Spain)	45	7.0	0.49	0.30	0.16
Tenckhoff curled, dual cuff w/peritoneal flange, arcuate (Missouri coiled catheter)							
Surgical							
8	1992	Twardowski	49	12.0	0.16	0.04	0.00
3. *Perpendicular disc*, dual-cuff (Toronto western)							
Surgical							
25	1982	Ponce 2cuff	90	1.0	0.12	0.09	0.00
	1982	Ponce 3cuff	83	4.0	0.10	0.15	–
34	1984	Kim 1cuff	37	6.5	0.33	0.00	0.00
	1984	Kim 2cuff	38	5.7	0.45	0.03	0.00
33	1987	Flanigan 2cuff	53	9.2	0.15	0.10	0.00
				5.3	0.23	0.07	0.00
General							
46	1988	Nolph/Registry	94	24.0	0.40	0.00	0.00
4. *Column-disc*, dual-cuff (Lifecath)							
Surgical							
35	1980	Ash	1	32.0	0.00	0.00	0.00
36	1984	Thornhill	46	8.0	0.05	0.00	0.00
37	1983	Ash	87	12.0	0.09	0.02	0.00
32	1986	Slingeneyer	66	12.0	0.12	0.12	0.14
46	1988	Nolph/Registry	49	24.0	*0.32	0.08	0.02
56	1990	Shah	23	20.0	0.00	0.22	0.00
				18.0	0.09	0.07	0.03

[a] Dash, – indicates no data reported.
* Exit Infections = 0.04.

sometimes results in a persistent exit site infection. Some exit site infections are resistant to all therapy even if the subcutaneous cuff is not extruding. If there are no signs of tunnel or deep cuff infection, and no unresolved peritonitis in a functioning dual-cuff catheter, removing the subcutaneous cuff merely converts the dual-cuff catheter to a single-cuff catheter. Removing the subcutaneous cuff allows the exit infection to resolve in half of cases unresponsive to other treatments [13].

In the presence of exit infection, removing the subcutaneous cuff is an easy procedure. Submerge the head of a disposable safety razor (such as a BIC®) in 70% alcohol solution. Swab the exit site with povidone-iodine solution. Pull on the catheter to expose the cuff through the exit site, and apply the razor blade to the surface of the cuff, near the skin. Pull the blade in direction parallel to the catheter. Swirl the razor in the alcohol solution to release fragments of Dacron. Repeat these steps, with the razor blade each time contacting a different sector of the cuff. Continue removing the Dacron material until the underlying surface is relatively smooth and the same radius as the catheter material. Release the catheter and swab the exit site with povidone-iodine.

9. Repair of pericatheter hernias and leaks

Typically, pericatheter leaks are best managed by returning to a "break in" schedule for several weeks. This means maintaining the patient's abdomen in a dry state for day or night or both. During this period, the patient may need to be maintained on hemodialysis. IPD or supine dialysis may provide adequate dialysis and still avoid leaks. If a leak cannot be corrected by these techniques the catheter should be removed and a new catheter placed. Surgical techniques used to salvage a catheter with a pericatheter leak are for the most part anecdotal.

In a similar fashion, pericatheter hernias are difficult problems to manage without removing the offending peritoneal dialysis catheter. Any attempt to repair a pericatheter hernia leaving the catheter intact will likely either compromise the hernia repair or catheter function. Pericatheter hernia and pericatheter leaks are problems that are best avoided by meticulous attention to placement of the catheter initially.

10. Repositioning intraperitoneal catheters; removing omental attachments

If the intraperitoneal segment of a peritoneal dialysis catheter has developed outflow failure and has migrated, omental attachment is the likely reason for the outflow failure. One benefit of using peritoneoscopic placement for a second peritoneal dialysis catheter is that the procedure can confirm omental attachment to the first catheter. The cannula of the Y-Tec peritoneoscope, with the surrounding Quill guide, is placed into the abdomen at a location suitable for the deep cuff of a second catheter. Peritoneoscopy is begun as usual, and air is infused through the cannula. The site of peritoneal entry of the current catheter is viewed through the peritoneoscope. The portion of the catheter with side-holes is usually not visible at this time, being buried in omentum and viscera. The scope is passed underneath the exposed portion of the catheter (under vision) and then rotated 90–120 degrees, towards the contralateral pelvis, dragging the catheter with the scope. When the scope is retracted, the new position of the catheter can be inspected. The side-holes of catheter will not be visible if there is still omental attachment. A second catheter can be placed at this time, using the Quill guide already in position, and then the first catheter can be removed. Alternatively, a number of endoscopic techniques have been developed to strip the omentum from the catheter. These can be performed by removing the small peritoneoscope and cannula, and placing a larger laparoscope through the Quill guide, then separating the omentum from the catheter. Some radiographic techniques with guide wires have been able to reposition catheters [14]. None of these repositioning techniques are completely effective. In one study, only 25% of repositioned catheters were functional one month later [15]. Placement of a second catheter and removal of the first catheter, or surgical repositioning with local omentectomy (through an incision near the deep cuff) are more effective [16].

11. Removal of peritoneal dialysis catheters

All chronic peritoneal dialysis catheters have either one or two Dacron cuffs attached to the tubing. These cuffs are placed in the musculature of the abdominal wall and subcutaneous tissue. Within weeks, tissue ingrowth into the Dacron cuffs occurs in the subcutaneous position and in the intramuscular location. For this reason, these catheters must be removed by careful dissection. Catheters are typically removed for one of four reasons; recurrent peritonitis, exit or tunnel infection, a successful renal transplant, or outflow failure.

The procedure is begun by prepping with povidone iodine solution. A plastic "sticky" barrier drape is applied to the patient's abdominal wall and the remainder of wound is sterilely draped. A local or general anesthetic may be used. The catheter is approached by reopening the old primary incision (over the deep cuff). Careful attention to hemostasis is important. Using sharp dissection, the Dacron cuffs are freed from the surrounding tissue. It is important to remove *all portions of the Dacron cuffs.* Residual Dacron cuff may serve as a nidus for chronic infection. Careful attention must be used when removing the catheter from the peritoneal cavity to avoid bowel injury. Generally there is a small opening in the posterior fascia and peritoneum following the removal of a peritoneal dialysis catheter. Depending upon the extent of tissue ingrowth, the hole may measure 1–2 cm. Careful closure of this fascial wound with a permanent suture is important to prevent the patient from developing an incisional hernia in the future. The remainder of the fascial layers are then closed. The skin incision may be closed primarily or packed open for secondary closure if exit site or tunnel infection is present.

References

1. Ash SR. Peritoneal access devices and placement techniques. In: Nissenson AR and Fine RN (ed), Dialysis Therapy, 2nd ed, Hanley & Belfus, Inc. Publishers, 1993; pp 23–30.
2. Ash SR. Chronical peritoneal dialysis catheters: effects of catheter design, materials, and location. Sem in Dial 1990; 3: 39–46.
3. Twardowski ZJ. Periontoneal dialysis catheter exit site infections: prevention, diagnosis, treatment, and future directions. Sem in Dial 1992; 5: 305–15.
4. U.S. Renal Data System 1992 Annual Data Report. Chapter VI: Catheter-related factors and peritoneal risk in CAPD patients. Am J Kidney Dis 1992; 20 (Suppl 2): 40–54.
5. Ash SR, Daugirdas JT. Peritoneal Access Devices. In: Daugirdas JT and Ing TS (eds), Handbook of Dialysis, Little, Brown and Company, Boston 1988; pp 194–218.
6. Twardowski ZJ et al. Preliminary experience with the swan neck peritoneal dialysis catheter. Trans Am Soc Artif Intern Organs 1986; 32: 64.
7. Cruz C, Bonilla H, Melendez A, Faber MD, Dumler F. Flow dynamics in peritoneal dialysis; the search for optimal CAPD systems. (Abstract) Perit Dial Int 1991; 11 (Suppl 1): 54.
8. Twardowski ZJ, Prowant BF, Nichols WK, Nolph KD, Khanna R. Six-year experience with swan neck catheters. Perit Dial Intl 1992; 12: 384–9.
9. Swartz R, Messana J, Starmann B, Weber M, Reynolds J. Preventing Staphylococcus aureus infection during chronic peritoneal dialysis. J of Amer Soc of Neph 1991; 2: 1085–91.
10. Gokal R, Ash SR, Helfrich GB et al. Peritoneal catheters and exit-site practices: toward optimum peritoneal access. Perit Dial Int 1993; 3: 29–39
11. Moncrief JW, Popovich RP, Broadrick LJ, He ZZ, Simmons EE, Tate RA. The Moncrief-Popovich catheter: a new peritoneal access technique for patients on peritoneal dialysis. ASAIO Trans 1993; 39: 62–5.
12. Han DC, Cha HK, So IN, Chung SH et al. Subcutaneously implanted catheters reduce the incidence of peritonitis during CAPD by eliminating infection by periluminal route. Advances in Perit Dial 1992; 8: 298–300.
13. Scalamogna A, Castelnovo C, De Vechhi A, Ponticelli C. Exit-site and tunnel infections in continous ambulatory peritoneal dialysis patients. Am J Kidney Dis 1991; 6: 674–7.
14. Honkanen E, Eklund B, Laasonen L, Ylinen K, Gronhagen-Riska C. Reposition of a displaced peritoneal catheter: the Heisinki whiplash method. Advances in Perit Dial 1990; 6: 159–64.
15. Shah GM, Sabo A, Nguyen T, Juler GL. Peritoneal catheters: a comparative study of column disc and Tenckhoff catheters. Int J of Artif Organs 1990; 13: 267–72.
16. Swartz R, Messana J, Reynolds J, Ranjit U. Simultaneous catheter replacement and removal in refractory peritoneal dialysis infections. Kidney Intl 1991; 40: 1160–5.
17. Diaz-Buxo JA. Mechanical complications of chronic peritoneal dialysis catheters. Sem in Dial 1991; 4: 106–11.
18. Tenckhoff H, Schechter H. A bacteriologically safe peritoneal access device. Trans Am Soc Artif Intern Organs 1968; 14: 181–5.
19. Brewer TE, Caldwell FT, Patterson RM, Flanigan WJ. Indwelling peritoneal (Tenckhoff) dialysis catheter: experience with 24 patients. JAMA 1972; 219: 1011–5.
20. Thomas C, Mahoney JF, Darlison P, Storey BG, Steward JH. Peritoneal dialysis using a semi-permanent intro-abdominal catheter. Med J Aust 1973; 2: 1037–9.
21. Giordano C, Desanto NG, Papa A et al. Short daily peritoneal dialysis. Kidney Int 1975; 7: 425–403
22. Karanicolas S, Oreopoulos DG, Pylychuk G et al. Home peritoneal dialysis: three years experience in Toronto. Can Med Assoc J 1977; 116: 266–9.
23. Khanna R, Oreopoulos DB, Dombros N et al. CAPD after three years: still promising treatment. Perit Dial Bull 1981; 1: 24–34.
24. Rottembourg J, Dominque J, Von Lantehen M, Issad B, Shahat YE. Straight or curled Tenckhoff peritoneal catheter for continuous ambulatory peritoneal dialysis (CAPD). Perit Dial Bull 1981; 1: 123–4.
25. Ponce SP, Pierratos A, Izatt S et al. Comparison of the survival and complications of three permanent peritoneal dialysis catheters. Perit Dial Bull 1982; 2: 82–5.
26. Ash SR, Handt AE, Block R. Peritoneoscopic Placement of the Tenckhoff catheter: further clinical experience. Perit Dial Bull 1983; 3: 8–12.
27. Diaz-Buxo JA, Geissinger. Single cuff versus double cuff Tenckhoff catheter. Perit Dial Bull 1984; 4: 100–2.
28. Handt AE, Ash SR. Longevity of Tenckhoff catheters placed by the Vitec® Peritoneoscopic technique. Perspect Peritoneal Dial 1984; 2: 30–3
29. Bierman M, Kasperbauer J, Kisek A et al. Peritoneal catheter survival and complications in end stage renal disease. Perit Dial Bull 1985; 5: 229–33.
30. Odor A, Alessio-Robles L, Leuchter J et al. Experience with 150 consecutive peritoneal catheters in

patients on CAPD. Perit Dial Bull 1985; 5: 226–9.
31. Twardowski ZJ, Nolph KD, Khanna R, Prowant BF, Ryan LP, Nichols WK. The need for a "swan neck" permanently bent, arcuate peritoneal dialysis catheter. Perit Dial Bull 1985; 5: 219–223.
32. Slingeneyer A, Mion C. Peritoneal catheters: update 1985. In: LaGreca et al. (ed), Peritoneal Dialysis (Proceedings of 2nd International Vicenza Conference), Wichting Editore Publishers, Milano, 1986; pp 171–3.
33. Flanigan MJ, Hgheim DD, Schulak JA, Ullrich GE, Freeman RM. The use and complications of three peritoneal dialysis catheter designs – a retrospective analysis. Trans Am Soc Artif Intern Organs 1987; 33: 33–38.
34. Kim D, Burke D, Izatt S et al. Single- or double-cuff peritoneal catheters? A prospective comparison. Trans Am Soc Artif Intern Organs 1984; 30: 232–5.
35. Ash SR, Johnson H, Hartman J et al. The column disc peritoneal catheter: a peritoneal access device with improved drainage. Trans Am Soc Artif Intern Organs 1980; 3: 109–13.
36. Thornhill JA, Ash SR, Dhein CR, Polzin DJ, Osborne CA. Peritoneal dialysis with the purdue column disc catheter. Min Vet 1980; 20: 27–33.
37. Ash SR, Slingeneyer A, Schardin KE. Further clinical experience with the Lifecath peritoneal implant. Perspect Peritoneal Dialysis 1983; 1: 9–11.
38. Swartz R, Rocher L, Messana J, Reynolds J, Lees P, Starmann B. The curled catheter: optimal access choice for chronic peritoneal dialysis (CPD). ASAIO Abstracts 1989; 18: 77.
38. Valenti G, Cresseri D, Bianchi ML, Corghi E, Lorenz M, Buccianti G. Surgical complications during continuous ambulatory peritoneal dialysis. Perit Dial Bull 1985; 5: 39–42.
40. Bozhurt F, Keller E, Schollmeyer. Swan neck peritoneal dialysis catheter can reduce catheter complications in CAPD patients. Perit Dial Bull 1987; 7: S9.
41. Ishizaki M, Suzuki K, Kurosawa K, Shishido Y, Takahashi H: Swan neck Sendai catheter: a modification of the swan neck Tenckhoff catheter. Peritoneal Dial Int 1988; 8: 221–2.
42. Cruz C, Melendez A, Faber M, Provenzano R, Sawaya P. Can the incidence of peritoneal catheter tunnel infections be reduced? (Abstract) Peritoneal Dial Int 1988; 8: 72.
43. Baker WB, Pratt J, Stone K, Hall J, Moore M, Startling J. Peritonitis and exit site infection rates using single-cuff Tenckhoff Missouri swan-neck peritoneal catheters (Abstract). Peritoneal Dial Int 1989; 9: 51.
44. Cruz C, Faber M, Melendez A. Peritoneoscopic implantation of Tenckhoff catheters for CAPD: effect on catheter function, survival and tunnel infection (Abstract). Peritoneal Dial Int 1989; 9: S1.
45. Davis DS, McMorrow RG. The importance of surgical expertise in preventing peritoneal catheter complications (Abstract). Peritoneal Dial Int 1989; 9: S1.
46. Lindblad AS, Novak JS, Nolph KD et al. Final report of the national CAPD Registry. NIADDK July 1988; pp 7–67.
47. Gibel LJ, Quintana BJ, Tzamaloukas AH. Soft tissue complications of Tenckhoff catheters (Ab-stract). Peritoneal Dial Int 1989; 9: S1.
48. Twardowski ZJ, Khanna R, Nichols WK et al. Low complication rates with swan neck short tunnel peritoneal catheter. Perit Dial Bull 1987; 7 (Suppl): 80.
49. Stegmayr V, Hedberg B, Sandzen B, Wikdahl AM. Absence of leakage by insertion of peritoneal dialysis catheter through the rectus muscle. Peritoneal Dial Int 1990; 10: 53–5.
50. Akyol AM, Porteous C, Brown MW. A comparison of two types of catheters for continuous ambulatory peritoneal dialysis (CAPD). Peritoneal Dial Int 1990; 10: 63–6.
51. Swartz R, Messana J, Rocher L, Reynolds J, Starmann B, Lees P. The curled catheter: dependable device for percutanoneous peritoneal access. Peritoneal Dial Int 1990; 10: 231–5.
52. Piraino B, Bernardini J, Centa PK, Johnston JR, Sorkin MI. The effect of body weight on CAPD related infections and catheter loss. Peritoneal Dial Int 1991; 11: 64–8.
53. Pastan S, Gassensmith C, Manatunga AK, Copley JB, Smith EJ, Hamburger RJ. Prospective comparison of peritoneoscopic and surgical implantation of CAPD catheters. Trans Am Soc Artif Intern Organs 1991; 37: M154–6.
54. Twardowski ZJ, Prowant BF, Khanna R, Nichols WK, Nolph KD. Long-term experience with Swan Neck Missouri catheters. Trans Am Soc Artif Organs 1991; 36: M154–6.
55. Nebel M, Marczewski K, Finke K. Three years of experience with the Swan-Neck Tenckhoff catheter. Advances in Peritoneal Dial 1991; 7: 208–13.
56. Shah GM, Sabo A, Nguyen T, Juler GL. Peritoneal catheters: a comparative study of column disc and Tenckhoff catheters. Int J of Art Organs 1990; 13: 267–72.
57. Zappacosta AR, Perras ST, Closkey GM. Seldinger technique for Tenckhoff catheter placement. Trans Am Soc for Artif Organs 1991; 37: 13–5.
58. Adamson AS, Kelleher JP, Snell ME, Hulme B. Endoscopic placement of CAPD catheters: a review of one hundred procedures. Nephrol Dial Transplant 1992; 7: 855–7.
59. Wadhawa NK, Cabralda T, Suh H, Kwilekval K, Mason R. Exit-site/tunnel infection and catheter outcome in peritoneal dialysis patients. Advances in Perit Dial 1992; 8: 325–7.
60. Rubin J, Didlake R, Raju S, Hsu H. A prospective randomized evaluation of chronic peritoneal catheters. ASAIO Trans 1990; 36: M497–500.
61. Donate T et al. Peritoneal catheter (PC) implantation through Y-Tec system. (Abstract) Perit Dial Intl 1993; 13 (Suppl 1): S39.

62. Swartz DA, Sandroni SE, Moles KA. Laparoscopic Tenckhoff catheter placement: A single center's experience. (Abstract) Perit Dial Intl 1993; 13 (Suppl 1): S31.
63. Multicentric group of study of Continuous Ambulatory Peritoneal Dialysis (Spain). Multicentric prospective study of swan neck peritoneal catheters with intraperitoneal (IP) segment straight of coiled. (Abstract) Perit Dial Int 1991; 11 (Suppl 1), 203.
64. Scabardi M, Ronco C, Chiaramonte S, Feriani M, Agostini F, La Greca G. Dynamic catheterography in the early diagnosis of peritoneal catheter malfunction. Int J of Artif Organs 1992; 15: 358–64.
65. Dryden MS, Ludlam HA, Wing AJ, Phillips I. Active intervention dramatically reduces CAPD-associated infection. Advances in Perit Dial 1991; 7: 125–8.
66. Copley JB, Smith BJ, Koger DM, Rodgers DJ, Folwar M. Prevention of postoperative peritoneal catheter catheter-related infections. Perit Dial Int 1988; 8: 195–7.

11 Organization of the peritoneal dialysis program – the nurses' role

L. UTTLEY AND B. PROWANT

1. Requirements of a PD program — 335
2. Establishing a PD program — 336
3. Training area — 336
4. Team interactions — 337
5. Head nurse/senior clinical manager — 337
6. Qualities of a PD nurse — 337
    6.1. Broad renal and nursing background — 337
    6.2. Teaching skills — 337
    6.3. Patience — 337
    6.4. Consistency — 338
    6.5. Flexibility — 338
    6.6. Sense of humour — 338
    6.7. Ability to comunicate — 338
    6.8 Judgement — 338
7. Nursing staff numbers — 338
    7.1. Staff recruitment — 339
    7.2. Staff orientation — 339
    7.3. Staff stress — 340
    7.4. Method of nursing — 340
8. Call systems — 341
9. Legal issues — 341
10. Cost effectiveness — 341
11. Quality improvement — 342
12. Standards — 342
13. Protocols — 342
14. Teaching — 342
15. Problem solving — 344
16. Follow-up care — 344
    16.1. Clinics — 344
    16.2. Home visits — 344
    16.3. Telephone calls — 346
    16.4. Nursing home follow-up — 346
    16.5. Limited follow-up at general hospital — 346
    16.6. Hospitalized patients — 346
17. Catheter break in — 346
18. Exit site care — 347
19. The nurse and peritonitis — 347
    19.1. Nursing procedure following diagnosis of peritonitis — 347
20. Administration of erythropoietin — 348
21. Special problems for patients with diabetes — 348
    21.1. Training — 348
    21.2. Follow up care — 348
22. Special problems of the elderly — 349
23. PET testing/adequacy — 349
24. Tidal peritoneal dialysis (TPD) — 350
25. Miscellaneous information — 351
    25.1. Holidays — 351
    25.2. Swimming — 351
    25.3. Showering, bathing — 351
    25.4. Warming of solutions — 351
    25.5. Body image — 352
    25.6. Compliance/non compliance — 352
        25.6.1. Culture — 352
        25.6.2. Depression — 352
        25.6.3. Social support — 352
        25.6.4. Amount of treatment — 352
        25.6.5. Knowledge — 352
    25.7. Infection control procedures — 353
    25.8. Disaster preparedness — 353
26. Research — 353
References — 354

The organization of a peritoneal dialysis (PD) program requires time, thought and careful planning. Managing a patient on PD embraces thorough technical instruction and motivation, carried out in a proper environment conductive for training. In most PD units the cornerstone of this approach is invariably the nurse whose responsibility it is to supply both instruction and motivation, by precept, by example, and encouragement [1]. This chapter reviews the essential elements required, the role and qualities of a PD nurse, protocols and teaching plans, all of which are crucial to the success of any PD program.

1. Requirements of a PD program

Although PD is a simple technique, it is now generally accepted that it should ideally be performed in the right setting, with appropriate staff and facilities and be integrated into a renal replacement program [2, 3]. Doctors, nurses and paramedical staff need to work together to form a cohesive multi-disciplinary team. A teaching plan needs to be established and step by step protocols formulated, prior to the admittance of any patient. The temptation to open a PD unit without guidelines or experienced personnel should be avoided. The major requirements are outlined in Table 1. Using these broad guidelines, it is possible to deliver to the patient the care required for his continued long-term well being.

2. Establishing a PD program

If PD is to be a success it is essential that it is integrated with haemodialysis and transplantation [4, 5]. Temporary haemodialysis is often necessary due to catheter removal, peritonitis, hernia repair or other medical and surgical related problems [6]. In an integrated program patients can transfer back and forth between therapies with ease and continuity of care can be achieved over many years.

A PD head nurse should be appointed to spearhead the program [7]. It is imperative that she has total commitment to the treatment and believes that patients can dialyze safely and effectively at home; indeed this should be the philosophy for all PD personnel including the medical director whose main task is to monitor both patients and dialysis process [8]. If a PD program is to obtain adequate space, personnel and equipment it is crucial that the finance to support the program and allow it to flourish is agreed at the outset. Little will be achieved if there are staffing shortages, inflexibility with dialysis systems and inadequate space for training and follow-up care. PD can be a revenue producing treatment but in order to profit one has to invest. Severe budget restrictions can lead to inadequate patient care and low staff morale, "a noose around the neck" in the running of any PD program.

The effectiveness of the PD program as a whole should be monitored [9]. Evaluation of rates of infection, hospitalization and mortality should take place annually and such quality assurance reviews can ensure periodic revision to protocols and procedures. Keeping the multi-disciplinary term enthusiastic and creative about program innovations can ensure that the patients receive the highest standard of dialysis and rehabilitation.

3. Training area

All PD programs should have an area that is conducive to learning and free from through traffic. The training area should be calm and peaceful providing the privacy necessary for learning whilst reducing the risk of cross-infection. Depending on the catchment population a program may be training two or three patients at any one time. Whilst some of the teaching sessions will need to be on an individual basis, some group sessions may be appropriate and the accomodation should befit both types. It is desirable that part of the training area should mimic closely the conditions a patient would have in their own home, to avoid confusion and disorientation after discharge. The area needs to be light and airy with ample space for free movement. Good artificial lighting especially for the poorly sighted is essential. A resource area with comfortable seating where patients can make use of visual aids, computers and practice equipment can double as a rest area for patients training on an out-patient basis. It may be necessary in some cases for patients to be admitted whilst training therefore bedroom and en suite facilities should be provided. The overall area will accommodate all procedures and personnel (Table 2) whilst the individual training rooms require essential equipment (Table 3).

Table 1. Essential requirement for PD programs.

Place	Suitable location Single rooms or purpose built PD area for training Out-patient follow-up care facilities Back up HD; in-patient beds
Staff	Adequate experienced medical and nursing staff 24 hour on-call Multidisciplinary team approach
Training	Teaching plan and training manual Established protocols Continuing education Commitment to teaching PD
Equipment	Reliable equipment suitable for all patients Storage space Home delivery system
Finance	Adequate funding for patient population Compliance with statutory regulations

Table 2. Rooms required in PD unit.

Resource room	– group training area visual aids, teaching equipment rest area
Single rooms	– CCPD exchange, CAPD

Store room
Toilet/showers
Nurses office
Doctors office
Clean utility room
Dirty utility room
Clerical and Administration offices – computer base
Access to emergency beds and haemodialysis
Clinic area

For patients who are severely disabled or blind it is often a good idea to perform whole or part of the training program in the patient's own home. Adaptations may already have been made to accommodate the disability and the patient will inevitably feel more at ease [10]. The patient will then avoid the unnecessary upheaval of learning the procedures in hospital and adapting them to the home situation which may be quite different.

4. Team interactions

The necessity of interdisciplinary collaboration and a team approach to PD patient care has been emphasized [11]. The team typically includes physicians, nurses, dietitian and social worker, but is often expanded to include others such as the surgeon responsible for catheter placement, a microbiologist, a psychologist, a physiotherapist, or rehabilitation specialist. PD programs may also encourage the patient and family to participate in the team's discussion and decision making processes.

At least some formal structure is required to promote optimal function of the team. Definition of roles and job responsibilities is essential. Shared goals and philosophy regarding home peritoneal dialysis therapy will promote cohesion and reduce conflict among members. Regularly scheduled team meetings and/or patient care conferences give the entire team opportunity for interaction and collaborative decision making. PD clinics that are structured so two or three team members see the patient together also facilitate communication among team members.

5. Head nurse/senior clinical manager

When planning a PD program a senior nurse should be appointed before the unit is opened for patient care. She should have a broad background in dialysis theory and be familiar and experienced in

Table 3. Equipment requirements in PD training room.

Comfortable chair/bed
Washbasin
Surface/Trolley
Weighing scales
Dripstand/hook
Shelving for consumables
Bag warming equipment
APD machine

dealing with all types of dialysis and complications. She should have leadership potential, be an independent worker, innovative, creative and empathic [12]. It is very desirable that the nurse should possess a recognized qualification in nephrology nursing such as the English National Board 136 Certificate (United Kingdom) or the Certified Nephrology Nurse credential (CNN) (United States). A survey undertaken by Brennan for the American Association of Nephrology Nurses (ANNA) showed that 68% of head nurses (N = 625) had 6–15 years experience in nephrology nursing practice with 19% holding associate degrees, 36% bachelor's degrees and 40% were diploma graduates [13]. The senior nurse becomes the key member of the nursing staff and will liaise with other members of the team, co-ordinate nursing duties and ensure continuing nursing care (Table 4).

6. Qualities of a PD nurse

A PD nurse must have total commitment and belief in the treatment and possess several important qualities [14].

6.1. Broad renal and nursing background

The nurse should be familiar with other forms of renal replacement therapies especially since PD patients may have had, or are likely to have; haemodialysis or transplantation. She should also have a broad background in general medical and surgical nursing.

6.2. Teaching skills

It is a common but erroneous belief that anyone can teach PD. It requires special skills and the success depends upon the approach adopted. Many nurses are not familiar with self care and do not believe that patients can perform nursing duties with the same accuracy. The nurse must want the patient to succeed, and be able to impart her knowledge to make the patient independent and confident at home. The ability to communicate with people of all walks of life and backgrounds is crucial.

6.3. Patience

This must be in evidence at all times, particularly during teaching sessions. It is of no value to unnecessarily speed up the training. Procedures may have to be repeated many times until the patient is able to perform them correctly. A patient should not be belittled for making mistakes. Encouragement at all times is highly desirable.

6.4. Consistency

The nurse needs to remember that a less than rigid technique may lead to an episode of infection.

Table 4. Duties of the senior nurse.

Patient care
1. Accountable for basic nursing practise
2. Responsible for continuity of care in the home
3. Assessment of patients – pre dialysis
4. Communication with physicians and other team members regarding patient problems
5. Collaboration with ward/floor staff for in-patient care
6. Responsible for control of infection
7. Communication with patient's family, assessment of coping strategies
8. Recognition and management of peritonitis and other PD complications

Administration
1. Organization and administration of nursing services
2. Responsibility for nursing budget and compliance with reimbursement regulations
3. Organization of follow-up clinics
4. Evaluation of new equipment
5. Participation in renal committees, multidisciplinary team meetings
6. Co-ordination of teaching including securing resources and teaching aids
7. Responsible for data-collection and computing services
8. Implementation of quality assurance programme

Educator
1. Development and implementation of a patient training programme
2. Assessor and teacher of nurses in training, licensed, practical nurses (LPN's) and technicians
3. Assist in patient teaching
4. Teaches at in-service sessions
5. Presents papers at local, regional, national and international meetings

Staff care
1. Responsible for staff well being and morale
2. Duty rotas and holiday administration
3. Counselling of staff – to prevent "burn-out"
4. Responsible for continuing education programmes

Research
1. Implementation of research projects into PD
2. Attends and encourages staff to participate in professional organisations
3. Evaluation of nursing practice
4. Collaboration with physicians and research fellows in PD research

Therefore consistency in teaching various procedures must be of prime importance to avoid patient confusion. Consistency is akin to a life support system for a PD patient and all members of the nursing team should work together to avoid disaster.

6.5. Flexibility

Every patient is different and each is their own person. Therefore a degree of flexibility is called for in the approach to patient training and follow up. Using innovation and ingenuity the nurse needs to cover every aspect of patient care without jeopardising the consistency and routine that PD requires.

6.6. Sense of humour

This is an essential component of the PD nurse's make-up. Stress is a common factor amongst staff and patients [15] and a sense of humour can diffuse a difficult and tense situation. This is particularly important when dealing with patients and families in their own homes.

6.7. Ability to communicate

Better patient care and training will only result with good communication. The PD nurse must establish a rapport with patients and families as well as other members of the multi-disciplinary team.

6.8. Judgement

Good judgement, the ability to lead and make decisions are desirable attributes for any PD nurse.

7. Nursing staff numbers

It is the head nurse who will assess the projected work load based on patient population increases and give advice to higher authorities on the staffing levels required. The most important changes and development affecting nephrology nursing during the 1980's have been the switch from task orientated to primary nursing, the increase in the number of patients, and changing case mix to include more elderly and diabetic patients [16]. The high risk patient requires more nursing supervision and this will inevitably affect staffing levels [17]. Other important factors to consider when determining adequate staffing levels are the amount of non-nursing duties performed by nurses, extensive haemodialysis and/or transplantation responsibilities, in-patient peritoneal dialysis responsibilities and follow-up care including home visiting.

Studies suggest that the desirable staff-patient ratio for adequate cover is one nurse per 15 patients [8, 17, 18]. However, this ratio is becoming increasingly more difficult to achieve and there are various reasons for this. Firstly, financial restrictions brought about by changes in the health service in the UK [19] and the reduction in the reimbursement regulations in the USA [20] have had a serious effect on the staffing of dialysis units. Staff salaries usually represent the largest portion of operating expenses, which have had to be reduced. More units are replacing registered nurses with licenced practical nurses (LPN's), licenced vocational nurses (LVN's) and technicians [21]. Salaries in some units have been frozen and on call and overtime payment reduced or eliminated. Staff education programs have also been decreased.

These cutbacks have resulted in low staff morale, increased sickness, rapid staff turnover and burnout [22]. This is on top of an already established shortage of nurses throughout the western world. Renal units will in the future have to look closely at the effectiveness of direct patient care by professional registered nurses versus LPN/LVN's. However, organizational outcomes such as job satisfaction of the professional nurse should also be taken into consideration [23]. Many nurses are now leaving the hospital environment to work in industry where they are offered better working conditions and higher salaries and the recruitment and retention of professional nurses for PD units has become a formidable task.

7.1. Staff recruitment

Peritoneal dialysis is a home therapy, that requires the patient and family to accept the responsibility for self care. The focus of nursing care is initially to teach the patient to perform dialysis and manage renal disease at home, and subsequently to provide ongoing guidance and support. It is, therefore, important to recruit nurses who not only believe in the concept that patients can care for themselves effectively but who are also willing to assist patients to become independent; nurses should also enjoy teaching and chronic care. It is often very difficult for acute care nurses used to working with high technology and a fast pace, to adjust to a position in home dialysis therapy.

7.2. Staff orientation

Because few nursing schools offer formal education in dialysis, on-the-job orientation, in-service and continuing education are critical prerequisites to quality care. Peritoneal dialysis orientation is extensive and may last 6–8 weeks. Topics unique to peritoneal dialysis are listed in Table 5. Nurses with haemodialysis or other nephrology nursing experience may complete orientation more quickly because they already have knowledge of renal anatomy and physiology, renal diseases, and chronic renal failure. It is imperative that all nurses review principles of patient and adult education. The nurse orientee is frequently assigned a mentor to work with to observe procedures, patient education, and clinical care. The mentor then serves as a consultant to advise and assist the new nurse as she begins

Table 5. Staff orientation topics specific to peritoneal dialysis.

1. Program philosophy
2. Brief history of PD
3. Anatomy of the peritoneum
4. PD kinetics
5. Factors affecting PD efficiency
6. Types of peritoneal dialysis
7. PD catheters
8. Catheter insertion
    Preoperative nursing care
    Postoperative catheter care
9. Catheter Break-in
10. Catheter exit site care
    Postoperative care
    Chronic care
    Care of the inflamed/infected exit
11. Dialysis prescriptions
    Solutions
    Exchange volumes
    Dextrose concentrations
    Evaluation of membrane characteristics
    Assessment of adequacy
12. Procedures
    CAPD exchanges
    Intraperitoneal medications
    Cycler dialysis
    Tubing changes
    Catheter repair
13. Patient education
14. Nursing follow-up and management
15. Dietary recommendations for PD patients
16. Routine medications
17. Acceptable blood chemistries
18. Infectious complications of PD
19. Non-infectious complications of PD
    Early complications (post catheter insertion)
    Late complications
20. Technical problems
21. Options for back up dialysis

providing direct patient care. Because the emphasis is on understanding the dialysis process and nursing management of PD patients, it may be several months before new staff members are entirely comfortable with the role.

In-service education can be used to update staff on new products, drugs, policies and procedures, and essentials such as cardio-pulmonary resuscitation and disaster drills. In-service education meetings can also be used to review various nephrology nursing topics in preparation for certification examinations, to present data from clinical research projects, and as a forum for nurses to share what they have learned at national or international meetings.

7.3. Staff stress

Burnout, has been described as a syndrome of emotion, exhaustion, depersonalization, and reduced personal accomplishment. A recent survey of nephrology nurses in the USA found that scores for burnout were higher than in previously reported studies of nurses and physicians [24]. The same study identifies the workload, patient interactions, death and dying issues, and a lack of staff support as the most frequent work related stresses. Another survey supports the concept that patient interactions are stressful, indicating that nephrology nurses view the typical patient as old, chronically ill, dependent, noncompliant and often in a negative mood [25]. Nurses working more than 40 hours per week had significantly higher levels of burnout than their counterparts. Strategies to reduce job related stress include maintaining adequate staffing, flexible scheduling and providing assistance and emotional support for nurses with a heavy caseload. A more global and proactive strategy is to encourage staff members to recognize and appreciate the expertise and talents of their colleagues and to develop an environment where they support and complement one another.

A focused plan for job enrichment and professional enhancement can contribute to improved morale, motivation, job satisfaction and reduced staff turnover. Nurses may be assigned specific projects that will challenge them to learn new information or enable them to develop new skills. Such projects could include developing patient education modules or materials, responsibility for peritonitis data, participation in quality improvement projects, reviewing and revising policies and procedures, and responsibility for an in-service education program.

Clinical nurses should also be encouraged to develop clinical expertise in relevant specialties such as geriatric nursing and management of diabetic patients.

Opportunities to attend continuing education meetings outside the institution will give staff members a broader perspective of nephrology nursing and state of the art information. These meetings also help develop a network with other nurse colleagues, to discuss problems and impart information. Participation in continuing education meetings often stimulates staff members to try new approaches in clinical care, to initiate new projects, to become involved in research, or to learn more about a particular area of interest.

Nurses and managers alike can achieve intellectual and professional advancement by participating in research projects, presenting at professional meetings and serving on institutional committees.

7.4. Method of nursing

The head nurse and higher nursing authorities will be responsible for establishing the method of nursing that will best suit the patient needs. PD is a continuous process, leading from hospital to home and lends itself to assigned patient care or the primary nursing system [26]. A primary nurse is assigned specific patients and assumes the responsibility for providing total nursing care. According to Marram et al., there are five components to this: continuity, accountability, autonomy, authority and personalised patient-centred care [27]. These can be simplified into the nurse's role, nurse-patient relationships and the structure in which the nurse works [28]. In this type of care assigned patients will be trained and looked after following discharge by the same nurse. The nurse teaches the patient on a one to one basis giving general nursing care, assessing progress and discussing problems. Following discharge the same nurse will follow patients at the out-patient clinic and visit them in their homes. In this way, a good relationship and rapport is established with patients and their families. The nursing process then becomes complete and continuous. During 'off duty' and holidays, patient care is handed over to a deputy or associate nurse. This method of nursing is common throughout the USA and Van Waeleghan et al. state that 50% of units throughout Europe now employ primary nursing [16].

In Europe, but particularly in the UK where home visiting is more extensive, separate home visiting nurses who work with the primary nurse have been employed. The home PD nurse is an invaluable member of the team whose aim is to reduce morbidity, increase support, and help in achieving rehabilitation, especially in the high risk group of patients such as the elderly and diabetic [29]. Starmann et al. noted that 93% of nurses stated that the high risk groups of patients required 2–3 hours per week per patient post-training nursing care [17]. One may then conclude that having separate home visiting nurses to deliver care will reduce the workload and responsibilities on the already overstretched unit staff while giving home patients quality care in their own homes. The aim and role of a home visiting nurse are outlined in Table 6.

8. Call systems

Most peritoneal dialysis programs provide both physician and nursing back up support for home patients. In some programs rotating call is considered part of the job description and nursing staff do not receive additional payment. In our experience, patients rarely abuse the call system and most calls are made to report a new problem or complication.

The primary disincentive for a nursing on-call system is the expense. The assumption has been made that the on-call physician can and will intervene appropriately for all types of problems. Yet nurses working in PD programs without continuous backup nursing support report that patients are much more reluctant to call physicians, and that physicians aren't always effective in assisting patients with nursing related problems. Therefore, these problems often worsen over the weekend and ultimately require excessive nursing time on Monday or even result in emergency room visits or hospitalization.

9. Legal issues

Expanded nursing practice has resulted in part from increasing nursing knowledge and specialization. Many PD nurses operate in expanded roles. Key issues to consider are whether the functions performed by the PD nursing staff are within the legal definition of nursing and whether the dialysis unit policies and procedures are specific as to the role of the PD nurse. Policies and procedures must be periodically reviewed to ensure that they are complete, accurate and current. Medication procedures should specifically address antibiotic administration. Job descriptions and responsibilities of unlicensed nurses and technicians must not place either these individuals or the supervising professional nurses in legal jeopardy. Rosario [30] has recommended a number of strategies that can reduce the risk of legal complications (Table 7).

10. Cost effectiveness

Nursing time and dialysis supplies are the most costly components of a chronic peritoneal dialysis program. Appropriate use of non-nursing personnel

Table 6. Aim and roles of home visiting nurse.

Aims
1. To reduce hospital visits and in-patient stays to a minimum
2. Prevent peritonitis
3. Continue and reinforce learning process
4. Encourage a return to previous or improved social status
5. Nurturing a close link between home and hospital
6. Giving moral support to the patient and his family

Roles
1. Assessing patients home pre-dialysis
2. Establishing home PD in newly discharged patients
3. Observations of exchange procedures at home
4. Performing transfer set changes at home
5. Routine visits
6. Initiation of therapy for peritonitis and other infections
7. Record keeping
8. Trouble shooting re problems connected with employment, holidays etc
9. Counselling and support of both family and patient

Table 7. Strategies to reduce legal complications.

1. Obtain voluntary consent for dialysis treatment from a competent person
2. Document that recommendations for treatment were made without pressure and that consent was not coerced
3. Do not treat any patient without physician orders
4. Do not dispense prescription medications to the patient for home use
5. Document the client's response to education. (Training or education check lists do not serve as documentation of the patient's response)
6. Update patient education materials periodically
7. Review dialysis procedures with the patient at specific intervals
8. Review discharge instructions with the patient and give a written copy of instructions
9. Each nurse should stay well within the area of individual competence
10. Communicate with the client in a caring and professional manner and foster a good nurse-patient relationship.

can greatly enhance the efficiency of a PD program with significant cost savings. Secretarial/clerical personnel or technicians can be used for scheduling, inventory, ordering and stocking supplies, assembling medical records, transient patient arrangements, medical record request, monthly charges, routine computer entry and data collection, machine setup and tear-down, machine maintenance, blood sampling, nonsterile dialysate sampling, and other technical procedures.

Inventory control for the out-patient clinic, in-patient unit and home patient supplies is also a very effective method of controlling costs. Anticipating an appropriate distribution of dextrose concentrations and avoiding excessive waste associated with prescription changes can dramatically reduce the amount of unused and outdated dialysis solution in the patient's home. Reuse of cycler tubing has been demonstrated to be both safe and cost effective [31].

11. Quality improvement

A continuing evaluation of quality is recommended. Whether such a program is called Quality Assurance, or Quality Improvement, the overall goals are to continuously enhance the level of care and improve clinical outcomes. The most important aspects of PD care for quality assurance can be divided under 4 headings: recruitment, training and education, infection control, and follow up monitoring. There are several aspects of peritoneal dialysis which should be reviewed annually. These include peritonitis rates, catheter complications, and technique survival. The effectiveness of education and the patient's self-care should also be evaluated. Fluid control, calcium and phosphorus balance and blood pressure management may be used as indicators of self-care. Other areas for quality assessment in chronic peritoneal dialysis programs are listed in Table 8.

The continuous quality process should involve several members of the team and may also include patients. Once problems are identified, efforts are directed at determining the source and contributing factors. Then an action plan can be developed and implemented. Continued monitoring or re-evaluation documents the effectiveness of the interventions.

12. Standards

A set of standards of clinical practice is a basic requirement to ensure quality care and successfully trained patients. Mason states that nursing standards define unequivocally what quality care is and provide specific criteria that can be used to determine whether quality care has been provided [32]. A standard describes what should be done and how the patient will benefit from the care. The American Nephrology Nurses Association has published standards of clinical practice for nephrology nurses [33]. These standards can be adapted to suit any dialysis unit.

13. Protocols

Each unit needs to have protocols for various procedures eg. peritonitis to ensure safe consistent care. It is essential that all members of the team are aware of those and any amendments that are made. Protocols are developed by the nursing staff and the medical director and should be reviewed on a regular basis. Table 9 outlines the protocols required for a peritoneal dialysis program.

14. Teaching

Initial learning is only part of the process of patient education. The second part is that of retaining the information and the ability to adapt techniques and

Table 8. Areas for quality improvement projects in peritoneal dialysis.

1. Adequacy of dialysis
2. Catheters
    Incidence of catheter complications
    Catheter survival
3. Dialysis policies, procedures and protocols
4. Documentation
5. Fluid balance and blood pressure control
6. Glucose control in diabetic patients
7. Haematocrit levels
8. Hospitalization rate for dialysis related problems
9. Infection control practices
10. Infectious complications
    Overall peritonitis incidence
    Etiology of peritonitis episodes
    Proportion of recurrent peritonitis episodes
    Exit site infection incidence
11. Management of dialysis, fluid balance during hospital admission
12. Nutritional status
13. Patient satisfaction
14. Phosphorus control
15. Technique survival
    Reasons for transfer to haemodialysis
        Inadequate ultrafiltration
        Inadequate solute clearance

procedures to the home environment. The PD nurse must remember that renal failure patients may be uraemic at the beginning of a training period. They have short attention spans and decreased levels of concentration thus requiring more repitition of information, clarification, positive reinforcement and reassurance [34]. The planning phase of the teaching process is critical to achieving a successful outcome. Unless an individual is ready to learn, learning will not take place despite the fact that teaching occurs [35]. Therefore the patient's ability and readiness to learn should be assessed and the equipment and teaching tools best suited to that patient selected. Each patient will be different and will require varying teaching strategies. The PD system and teaching aids used will depend upon the patient's age, intelligence, disability and cognitive state.

A teaching plan (Table 10) will encourage consistency but needs to be flexible and adaptable to patient needs. The plan is set in separate stages, each stage having several modules. These modules will define the objectives and discuss teaching methods. The primary nurse will follow these modules, utilizing such aids as videos, practise equipment, dummy torso, books and computer assisted learning packages [36]. Lecture and discussion are the primary modes of patient teaching along with demonstration and simulation problem solving.

A training manual should be available for patient use. This manual encompasses all the information a patient is likely to need, eg information regarding supplies, record keeping, patient support groups, holidays, together with an outline of all essential procedures and protocols. These need to be written in a simple form and be easy to follow and read

[35]. The manual should be translated into other languages if there are significant ethnic patient groups. Illiterate patients should be provided with step by step photographs or videos where possible while blind patients may be given audio tapes or information in Braille.

Table 10. Example of teaching plan.

Stage 1
a) Acceptance of need for treatment
b) Introduction to renal disease
c) Principles of peritoneal dialysis
d) Introduction to CAPD, APD
e) Personal hygiene

Stage 2
a) Asceptic technique – handwashing
b) Steps in exchange procedure – setting up cycler

Stage 3
a) Emergency procedures for contamination
b) Exit site care

State 4
a) Addition of medication to bags

Stage 5
a) Complications
   1. Peritonitis   7. Pain
   2. Exit site infection   8. Bleeding
   3. Fluid balance   9. Machine faults
   4. Fibrin   10. Constipation
   5. Drainage-inflow   11. Itching
   6. Leaks

Stage 6
a) Record keeping
b) Weight, blood pressure control
c) Diet

Stage 7
a) Home adaptations
b) Bag warming
c) Supplies of equipment

Stage 8
a) Clinic
b) Home visiting
c) Communication with hospital
d) Employment, hobbies, sports
e) Psycho-social, counselling]
f) Holidays
g) Patient Association
h) Transplantation

Stage 9
a) Overall evaluation

Table 9. Protocols.

1. CAPD exchange procedure (for each system)
2. Cycler set up procedure (including re-use of lines)
3. Intermittent PD regimes, e.g. IPD, CCPD
4. Exit site care
5. Administration of intraperitoneal medication
6. Transfer set change procedure
7. Peritoneal equilibration test
8. Treatment of infections –   peritonitis
                                          exit site
9. Managing complications e.g. poor inflow – outflow
                                             crack in catheter
10. Holiday dialysis
11. Discharge to home
12. EPO usage

Evaluation is an integral part of patient training and should take place throughout the teaching process. Refresher classes are required regularly once the patient is home particularly if they develop a problem such as peritonitis or if procedures are changed [37]. The training period varies in length depending upon the patient's ability to learn but on average takes between 5–10 days. However the greatest challenge in teaching peritoneal dialysis is the relatively short time available for staff to facilitate a patient's positive adjustment to what may be a lifelong treatment. It may be necessary for the training period to be lengthened beyond the necessary mastery of dialysis procedures because the patient may need additional support [38]. A patient should not be discharged to self care until everyone including the patient feels they are ready.

15. Problem solving

Problem solving is an integral and important part of any home PD program. Patients must be able to recognise, assess and correct common PD problems. A problem solving guide (Table 11) should be included in the patient manual or the patient should receive information which is now available, some of which is from commercial sources [39].

16. Follow-up care

PD patients require frequent monitoring, guidance and support after discharge home.

16.1. Clinics

Clinic visits are required on a regular basis, the first visit is typically scheduled a week post discharge. Thereafter the frequency is adjusted depending on how well the patient is coping and how often he is visited by the nursing team. Most units require the patient to attend clinic at least every 8–12 weeks once home dialysis is established. A clinic visit will allow the patient to query problems that have arisen and also express his anxieties. The medical team will assess blood pressure control, fluid balance, exit site status, blood chemistry, medication and dietary control. X-rays, ECG, lipids and PTH levels may be done as appropriate. The visit will give the nursing team an opportunity to re-inforce procedures and perform transfer set changes. Dietitians and social workers should be made available to the patient when necessary [12].

16.2. Home visits

Regular home visits are an important part of follow up care, as the family and patient need to realize that continuing support is available. Visiting the patient at home provides valuable insight about family interactions. Often problems regarding the patient's health are of a personal nature eg. psychosexual problems, and a couple may be too embarrassed to discuss these issues at the hospital. In familiar surroundings when there is an atmosphere of rapport and trust, these topics can be more easily aired.

It is advisable that the first exchange after discharge from hospital is in the presence of a nurse,

Table 11. Problem solving guide.

Problem	Treatment
Difficulty with draining in	
• Check roller clamp open	
• Bag snap seal broken	
• Twisted or kinked tube	• Attempt to untwist or remove kink
• Blockage caused by air or fibrin	• Squeeze bag. Add Heparin to next bag if fibrin
If these measures fail to produce inflow, call the hospital	
Difficulty with draining out	
• Check roller clamp open	
• Bag lower than abdomen	
• Twisted or kinked tube	• Attempt to untwist or remove kink
• Blockage caused by fibrin	• Milk tubing to remove fibrin Add Heparin to next bag
• Constipation	• Take laxative

Table 11 (Continued)

Problem	Treatment
Disconnection of tubing	
• Disconnection at catheter	• Clamp catheter Go to hospital
• Disconnection at bag	• Clamp line, reconnect using clean technique. DO NOT drain in Go to hospital

When a disconnection occurs it is important to commence antibiotic therapy as soon as possible

Fluid related
- Cloudy effluent
- Blood in effluent
- Deep yellow or orange effluent

- Inform hospital immediately
- Do an exchange. If it does not clear inform hospital
- Ensure it is not cloudy
  Colour may be caused by antibiotics, excessive dwell time, jaundice

Equipment related
- Breakage of roller clamp
- Hole in line

- Clamp line, will require line change
- Clamp at junction with catheter, will require line change and antibiotics
  Go to hospital

Symptom related

Abdominal pain
- Constipation
- Dialysis fluid cold or hot
- Hypertonic Bags
- Peritonitis

- Inflow – outflow
- Dragging cramp-like pain on complete drainage

- Take mild laxative
- Check bag temperature

- Drain out, if cloudy
  Inform hospital
- Slow down rate of inflow-outflow
- Stop drainage towards the end of drain phase

Shoulder pain
- Caused by pressure in abdomen or air under diaphragm

- Take analgesic
- Drain in knee chest position

Headaches
- High blood pressure

- Check blood pressure
  Inform hospital

Cramps
- Dehydration

- Replace fluid and salt as instructed

Itching

- Comply with medication regimes
  Inform hospital

Dizziness
- Low blood pressure

- Check blood pressure, weight
  Inform hospital

Swollen ankles
- Fluid overload

- Check weight. Reduce fluid, salt, intake.
  Use stronger solution

Shortness of breath
- Fluid overload

- Check weight
  Inform hospital

High temperature

- Check clarity of effluent
  Check exit site
  Inform hospital

she can reassure the patient and help him to adapt the procedure to the home environment. Thereafter the home visiting nurse will continue to make routine calls to those patients with perceived problems (eg. high risk groups) as well as to those doing well. Dialysis problems, medical, social and supply problems will all need discussion [40]. Close liason will be kept with other members of the multi-disciplinary team including local community nurses, social workers and family doctors. Early recognition and management of problems will assist in keeping the patient healthy, well rehabilitated and will hopefully reduce hospital visits and in-patient stays.

16.3. Telephone calls

After discharge to home, telephone communication becomes an important part of follow-up care. Patients should be given telephone numbers where PD trained nurses can be contacted 24 hours a day. They should be encouraged to contact the staff with problems and should not be made to feel a nuisance when doing so. Any instructions or information given over the telephone should be clear and precise, if possible in the patient's own language and should only be given by experienced nurses. Telephone calls can be extremely time consuming for the nursing staff and this factor should be taken into account when staffing levels are negotiated.

16.4. Nursing home follow-up

Nursing homes can provide a much needed haven for some PD patients particularly the elderly and disabled [41]. Care must be taken by the training nurses to co-ordinate with the nursing home staff all that is entailed in managing PD therapy. PD nurses have successfully taught the staff at nursing homes in a similar way to that used for a patient and his family. It is important at the initial contact to address all their problems and encourage a mutually co-operative relationship. Education and in-servicing of staff is initiated before the patient is placed, and regular refresher courses, visits and telephone contact help to foster a team approach [42].

16.5. Limited follow-up at general hospital

PD programs can share follow up care successfully with affiliated hospitals, particularly when patients live a long distance away from the main center [43]. This has the advantage not only of reducing travel but also cost. Clinics can be held and will follow the same practices and protocols as the parent clinic. Infections and minor problems can also be treated on an on call basis. Nursing staff may require some training into PD procedures and it is imperative that the hospital has supplies and follows procedures compatible with those the patients use at home. Goodwill and co-operation will be required by both parties but expert local care would be welcomed by the patient.

16.6. Hospitalized patients

Patients may have to be admitted for dialysis or other problems into a hospital ward. During this time it is possible that exchanges may have to be performed by nursing staff. It is essential that only trained staff are involved in any PD procedures to avoid contamination and infection. If the hospital cannot provide such nurses then nurses from the parent unit must perform the PD procedures until members of staff can be trained. If this is impossible the patient will have to be transferred to a hospital with a PD program. In any event liaison should be maintained between staff at both nursing and medical levels.

17. Catheter break in

Increased intra abdominal pressure (IAP) in patients on peritoneal dialysis has been implicated as a cause of dialysate leaks, which interferes with tissue ingrowth after catheter insertion and increases the risk of infection [44]. The goal of catheter break in protocols is to keep intra abdominal pressure as low as possible. One way to do this is to delay using the catheter for peritoneal dialysis for 10–14 days. The catheter is rinsed with heparinized saline or dialysis solution post operatively until bleeding is resolved and the effluent is clear. Following complete drainage of the peritoneal cavity 50 to 100 ml of heparinized solution may be infused to cushion the catheter.

If peritoneal dialysis is initiated shortly after catheter insertion, dialyzing with small exchange volumes with the patient supine will reduce intra abdominal pressure. It is also important to avoid constipation and straining and control coughing or vomiting, as these activities have been shown to dramatically increase intra abdominal pressure in patients receiving PD [45].

18. Exit site care

Exit site and tunnel infections are all to frequent complications of peritoneal dialysis and often necessitate catheter removal.

Peritoneal catheter exit site care has two primary goals: to prevent exit site infection and to identify problems promptly. There are three essential components of care: (i) cleansing the exit site to remove dirt and decrease bacteria, (ii) securing the catheter to prevent pressure, movement or accidental trauma (iii) and examining the exit site and catheter tunnel for signs of infection [46]. Several common elements emerge from studies of post insertion catheter care [47, 48, 49]. These include prophylactic antibiotic coverage, restricting dressing changes to PD staff, strict aseptic technique, catheter immobilization and povidone iodine as a cleansing agent alone or in combination with hydrogen peroxide, exit dried after cleansing and procedures continued for ≥ 7 days.

A 1991 international survey of exit site care practices in 535 PD programs (mostly North American and Europe) provided information regarding the prevalence of specific components of exit site care [50] The most common practices include prophylactic antibiotic therapy at catheter insertion [62%] with postoperative dressing changes limited to specially trained staff (86.9%); the use of sterile technique (63.7%); povidone iodine (83.4%) and gauze dressings (75.3%). The post operative procedure was followed from less than 7 days to as long as 6 weeks. Centres in the USA were more likely than those in other countries to use povidone iodine and hydrogen peroxide for post operative dressing changes.

The consensus in the literature is not as great for chronic care; however, a few common elements emerge: the exit site is cleansed daily to several times weekly with soap or medical disinfectant, dried and the catheter is secured.

These views are reflected in data from the international survey [50]. The most frequent components of chronic exit site care procedures were daily care done with shower or bathing (85.8%), antibacterial or pure soap for catheter cleansing (70%), hydrogen peroxide only as needed (59.3%), catheter stabilization (84.7%), dressings optional (63%), and gauze dressings when used (80.9%). Twice daily exit care, change in cleansing agent and topical antibiotics were recommended for inflamed or infected exits. European centres were more likely than those in North America to recommend exit site care separate from bathing. They were less likely to use povidone iodine or hydrogen peroxide and were more likely to use a variety of other cleansing agents. Canadian and European centres were twice as likely to require dressings, and the Canadian centres used more semipermeable and occlusive dressings.

19. The nurse and peritonitis

Peritonitis continues to be the major cause of morbidity in PD patients. Although there is a multitude of factors directly or indirectly related in the causation, the prevention to some extent depends upon the compliance of the patient and his ability to adhere to a strict routine [51]. The tedium and monotony of repeated exchanges day in day out can easily lead to mistakes.

A strict, aseptic exchange technique remains the cornerstone of prevention of peritonitis in the majority of patients, however, since the introduction of the Y disconnect systems infection rates have decreased [52]. Infection rates of patients utilizing cyclers and ultraviolet light are also less than those using standard PD systems [53, 54].

To prevent peritonitis the nurses should ensure that the dialysis system chosen matches the patient's abilities. Regular re-evaluation of the technique procedure can help in identifying and eliminating problem areas, however, it may be prudent to change a patient's system to a Y set or UV system if peritonitis occurs frequently.

Effective teaching to identify and treat contamination and disconnection will reduce the incidence of infection. Prophylactic antibiotics for such calamities are recommended [55].

19.1. Nursing procedure following diagnosis of peritonitis

1. The patient must attend a PD Unit or an associated centre versed in the handling of PD fluid and culture technique.

2. The diagnosis is confirmed from a freshly drained effluent, which is sent for cell count and a full bacteriological analysis.

3. Appropriate first line antibiotics [56] are injected into the next bag. The procedure for drawing up the antibiotics, dose and injection into the bag should be reviewed with the patient, if he has to administer antibiotics at home.

4. It is advisable to give heparin with the antibiotic to prevent fibrin clots.

5. There is usually a need to review fluid balance as there is invariably a loss of ultrafiltration during a peritonitis episode.

6. Following the cure of the infection the nurse needs to review the exchange procedure and elicit a cause if possible. The nurse can take this opportunity to reassure the patient and his family while ensuring that short cuts in procedures are not being taken. Patients and relatives will require help and understanding during an infection to overcome the guilt and depression that may result.

20. Administration of erythropoietin

The ability of recombinant human erythropoietin (EPO) to correct the anaemia of renal failure has dramatically improved the lives of patients with endstage renal disease (57–58). As its use becomes more widespread, PD nurses will need to know how to administer the drug and monitor the patients receiving it for progress and side effects. Various studies have taken place to discuss the feasibility of giving EPO either by subcutaneous injection or intraperitoneally in the dialysis solution [59, 60]. Intraperitoneal administration limits drug absorbtion and the higher cost of achieving an adequate haemoglobin level rules out this method [61]. Subcutaneous administration has proven to be effective using low doses and the slower absorption produced by this method of injection mimics the production of endogenous EPO more closely than the peaks and troughs that result from IV administration [60]. PD patients are uniquely suited to self administration of EPO because they are experienced with home procedures and can usually be taught the injection procedure in one session [62].

Most PD patients will already be familiar with injection techniques but will require further education in aseptic technique, selection of injection site, storage of EPO and potential problems. Nursing and patient education care plans such as the one by Prowant et al. [63] should be used so that both nurses and patients understand the rationale for EPO usage, can identify the side effects and make appropriate interventions.

Regular clinic attendance is necessary and nurses should be alert for causes of reduced response to EPO such as infection, bleeding, iron deficiency, aluminium overload and severe hyperparathyroidism [64]. Monthly monitoring of blood counts and serum ferritin, should take place and in addition nurses should also monitor the blood pressure, vascular access and the patient's well being to minimize side effects [65].

21. Special problems for patients with diabetes

The number of patients with diabetes treated by PD continues to grow. The advantages of PD for this group of patients include the maintenance of a residual renal function, use of intraperitoneal insulin, better blood pressure control and a less rigid fluid and dietary regimen [66]. Unfortunately, most dialysis patients with diabetes have other complications including retinopathy, coronary artery and peripheral vascular disease, autonomic neuropathy, and in addition suffer from malnutrition [67]. It is a challenge to all PD nurses to assist these patients to manage and adapt to two chronic illnesses and hopefully to enhance their quality of life.

21.1. Training

When selecting the type of equipment best suited to the patient's needs visual acuity, mobility, manual dexterity and the use of a partner should be taken into account. For blind patients devices such as exchange and UV devices can assist the patient with the exchange procedure while click syringes, injection aids and Novopens® can help with the insulin injections. If a partner is needed it may be less tedious to have the patient dialysed overnight using a cycler.

The PD training nurse may have to displace bad habits that have accumulated over a number of years [68]. Careless regard for insulin dose, diet and foot care must now be replaced with good technique and careful monitoring. Sterile technique is now vital if insulin is to be injected into dialysis bags and the nurse must motivate the patient to high standards. A change from subcutaneous injection to intraperitoneal injection may aid compliance. Initially the patient may have to monitor blood glucose levels several times a day and make adjustments to insulin dosage when using hypertonic solutions.

21.2. Follow up care

A multidisciplinary approach to care is used to the best advantage when treating patients with diabetes and renal failure. Specialist help from dietitians, opthalmologists, diabetologists and foot care nurses will assist the patient to achieve good rehabilitation.

At Manchester Royal Infirmary PD patients with diabetes attend a joint Renal/Diabetic clinic where access to all these specialities are found under one roof. This not only reduces the number of clinics the patient has to visit but also ensures that all possible complications are seen at an early stage and are monitored thoroughly [69]. The importance of support from the patient's family cannot be over emphasized. Anderson et al. observed that when the courage and strength of family members has been drained the patient may be unable to continue alone [70]. The family burden is often beyond the limits of tolerance, therefore when necessary families should be offered respite care, support and encouragement so that they do not surrender their own optimism and determination [71].

22. Special problems of the elderly

Among the most common problems of elderly populations are visual and hearing losses. Compensating for these losses is important, especially during patient education. Working in an environment free from background noise is recommended for the hearing impaired. Sitting at the same level, establishing eye contact, speaking slowly, clearly and not too loudly all improve comprehension.

Good vision in elderly patients is dependent on good light, good contrast and adequate size [72]. Written instructions for the elderly should be in large print in a simple, bold typeface. Good lighting and a contrasting background are essential for the work area where PD exchanges or cycler connections will be done.

A number of factors contribute to poor nutrition in the elderly PD population. Taste and smell perception diminish with age and dysgeusia is a common symptom of uraemia and inadequate dialysis. Elderly patients with lack of dentition or poorly fitting dentures may compensate by changing to soft foods which limits protein intake. Furthermore, individuals on a limited income may not be able to afford protein rich foods. Finally, the added anorexia of ESRD compounds the problem of obtaining adequate protein, and calories from dialysis glucose absorption may blunt the appetite. Correcting dental problems, liberalizing the dietary recommendations and identifying sources of supplemental income may improve both caloric and protein intake.

Safety is also a major concern for elderly patients. A list of aging changes that predispose to falls includes 10 items [73]. Six of the ten conditions are common in the elderly endstage renal disease population: diabetes mellitus, visual impairment, gait changes, reduced postural control, postural hypotension and reduced cerebral functioning. Excessive fluid removal and resulting dehydration further increases the risk of falls in PD patients. Because tripping causes many falls, it is important that both the clinic and patient home do not have loose mats, and slippery floors. Good lighting also reduces the risk of falls. The temperature of dialysis solutions should also be carefully monitored in elderly patients.

23. PET testing/adequacy

The peritoneal equilibration test (PET) is a diagnostic procedure to assess an individual patient's peritoneal membrane characteristic [74]. For haemodialysis therapy the characteristics for each type of dialyser are well defined and are used in determining the dialysis prescription. Data from the PET is analogous to the package insert that gives the performance characteristics of each dialyser.

The PET consists of one dialysis exchange using a standardised volume (2L), dextrose concentration (2.5%) and dwell time (4 hours), with a single blood sample and 2 and 4 hour dialysate samples [75]. Results are presented as dialysate to plasma ratios for creatinine and the ratio of glucose at 2 and 4 hours to glucose at time 0. These data give information as to how the patients peritoneal transport characteristics compare to the "average". An initial PET done shortly after initiating PD gives the physician information upon which to base the optimal dialysis prescription.

Patients with low transport rates have slow glucose absorption and slow solute transport. This results in excellent ultrafiltration, but often inadequate solute removal. These patients do best on a continuous dialysis therapy with more than four exchanges or more than 2.0 litre exchange volumes [76].

Patients with high transport rates have rapid glucose absorption with poor ultrafiltration and are likely to have problems with fluid removal. This group has good solute removal, but these patients benefit from shorter dialysis exchanges that are drained at or before the peak ultrafiltration volume. Intermittent cycler dialysis is often prescribed for these patients [76].

Repeat peritoneal equilibration tests may be used

to document changes in membrane characteristics, to aid in the diagnosis of internal leaks and to help confirm or rule out the likelihood that a patient is not performing exchanges as reported [77] and even predict or confirm membrane failure associated with sclerosing encapsulating peritonitis [78]. The chronic dialysis program associated with the University of Missouri recommends that all patients have an initial PET and that repeat equilibration tests be done only as clinically indicated.

It is important that each dialysis unit has a detailed procedure for performing the peritoneal equilibration test. This helps maintain consistency from one test to the next, so that data can be analysed for changes and trends. If an individual patient does not tolerate 2L exchanges and the equilibration test is done with a 1.5L volume, this should be clearly documented so that subsequent tests for the same patient will be performed in the same manner.

A fast equilibration test [79] has been proposed. The patient initiates the equilibration test exchange at home and comes to the clinic for sampling of dialysate and blood at the four hour dwell time; therefore this test is less expensive and less time consuming. In a clinical study comparing fast PET to standard PET results [80] 2 of 15 patients did not complete the fast PET as instructed and 1 patient had dramatically different drain volumes between the two tests. In fact, she had not used a 2L fill volume. The authors recommended the initial PET use the standardized technique, but that the fast PET may be used for subsequent clinical screening.

Common errors in performing the peritoneal equilibration test are incomplete draining of the previous exchange or equilibration test exchange, poor mixing of dialysate for 0 and 2 hour samples, allowing fresh dialysis solution to infuse into the equilibration test drain bag when using a Y system, incorrect labelling of the dialysate samples and mathematical errors (when calculations are done by hand).

It is important to note that the peritoneal equilibration test is not an indicator of the adequacy of dialysis. Twentyfour hour clearances and kinetic modelling are used to assess dialysis adequacy. Both require simultaneous 24 hour urine and dialysate collections. Common errors in these collections are patients bringing too many or too few bags to the unit, not collecting the urine and dialysate on the same day, inadequate clamping of the bags so dialysate is lost, not recording the exchange times (actual time may be slightly less than, or greater than, 24 hours) or urine collection time, and leaving the clinic without having blood drawn. We have found that the incidence of such errors can be reduced by giving the patients detailed verbal and written instructions and by giving them a form to record exchange times and voidings. Both staff and patients may make errors during dialysate sampling.

Evaluation of adequacy is discussed in another chapter; however, it is worth emphasising that the resulting data represent the dialysis the patient has done only for the 24 hour collection period and this may or may not represent the dialysis the patient routinely receives.

24. Tidal peritoneal dialysis (TPD)

Tidal peritoneal dialysis has been shown to improve clearances in intermittent peritoneal dialysis [81]. Prior to initiating TPD Craig and Kuharcik recommended that a) a peritoneal equilibration test be performed, b) residual renal clearance be determined, c) body surface area be estimated and the amount of required creatinine clearance and ultrafiltration be estimated and d) the dialysate volume (L) per treatment be determined [82]. The tidal volume is approximately 1/2 of the total exchange volume tolerated in a supine position. When determining the amount of solution to hang, add the initial fill volume, plus the tidal fill volume x number of exchanges minus one, and add an additional 300–500 ml to prime and purge tubing. Cycle time is determined by subtracting the initial fill and final drain times and the length of one dwell from the total dialysis time and dividing the remaining time by the total number of exchanges minus one. The tidal ultrafiltration volume is determined by dividing the total UF by the number of cycles. If the final drain volume is less than the initial fill plus cycle UF, the cycle UF should be reduced; if it is higher, the cycle UF should be increased accordingly. The patient will need to change the cycle UF setting depending on the dialysis solution dextrose concentration. Written instructions for the tidal UF volume for each prescribed combination of dextrose dialysis solutions provides the patient with a reference and reduces errors. Tidal dialysis is somewhat more complex than regular IPD, and patients may require somewhat longer training time and more detailed home records. TPD is also relatively more expensive because of the larger volume of dialysis solution that is used.

25. Miscellaneous information

25.1. Holidays

The ability to perform exchanges almost anywhere has always been one of the big advantages of CAPD and there are some cycler machines which can be dismantled and be transported by car, allowing APD patients some flexibility with holiday arrangements. Certain steps must be taken to ensure the procedure remains consistent and all eventualities are covered if a crisis occurs.

Firstly the patient should inform the unit when and where the holiday will take place. If the holiday is of short duration and within a short distance, the patient may transport the dialysis equipment himself. If the holiday is abroad or some distance away, arrangements should be made for delivery of the equipment to the holiday destination. Most manufacturers are happy to make these arrangements. Several weeks notice is often necessary and it is helpful if patients are reminded of this by the nursing staff at clinics or home visits.

Holiday insurance should be arranged by the patient who should be aware that pre existing medical conditions may not be covered. Certain countries have reciprocal arrangements as for example countries within the European Community. Before departure, the patient should receive from the unit:

1. A letter giving medical and dialysis details.
2. Name and address of nearest dialysis facility to holiday accommodation.
3. Antibiotic therapy for use in the event of peritonitis if this cannot be obtained at the holiday destination.

At Manchester Royal Infirmary the patients now benefit from an annual holiday organized and accompanied by two of the experienced PD nursing staff. This enables the elderly, disabled patients, patients who live alone and new patients who are not yet confident, a chance to take a holiday without the worry of organization and fear of inability to cope with a crisis while away from home. Families and spouses are also encouraged to take a holiday with the patient group or are given this opportunity to take a break separately. The accompanying nurses organize the travel arrangements, accommodation, social activities and will perform the dialysis for patients who normally require help. The benefits of this holiday to the patients outweigh the obvious hard work involved for the nurses and such holidays can only be recommended.

25.2. Swimming

Submersion of exit sites which have not completely healed or have recently been traumatized or infected may be a risk factor for infection. Yet many patients find swimming beneficial both physically and psychologically and PD should not be an absolute contra-indication [39, 83], however, swimming in dirty water should be avoided. To ensure that the water does not contaminate the PD equipment the following procedure should be carried out.

1. Tightly fold the bag and tubing
2. Place in a water proof bag (freezer bag)
3. Seal waterproof bag with adhesive or twist ties
4. Conceal inside bathing costume (full costume for females, boxer type shorts for males)
5. Following swimming the exit site should be cleansed and redressed and the connection shield should if used be replaced.

Stoma care dressings have been used with some success in PD patients while swimming [84]. These can provide a watertight seal for several days. Patients who have a disconnect system will have little problem in disguising their cannula and will only require a waterproof dressing.

25.3. Showering, bathing

PD patients must be encouraged to have high standards of personal hygiene. It is preferable that they take a shower every day however, if desirable they can take a bath. Bathwater should be shallow and should not cover the exit site. During bathing the bag and tubing should be kept as dry as possible, so should be hung over the side of the bath or placed outside the shower. Following bathing the exit site should be inspected, cleansed, dried and redressed.

25.4. Warming of solutions

It is not essential to warm PD fluid but some patients experience discomfort when infusing cold solutions. APD machines have an inbuilt warming mechanism which is temperature controlled. CAPD patients have various ways of warming the fluid in the home, the most common ones are:

1. Airing cupboards.
2. Hot water bottles – used in conjunction with insulated bags.
3. Heating pads specially manufactured for this purpose.
4. Radiators.
5. Microwave ovens.

Microwave warming of solutions is not acceptable in all countries due to legal safety measures brought about by the potential risk for patient burns, resulting from hot spots within the dialysis fluid when warmed by this method. A recent study by Armstrong and Zalatan [85] in the USA suggests microwave warming is a safe procedure in the hospital setting. Following warming, the dialysis fluid should be agitated to even out the temperature of the fluid in the bag; however, it should be noted that microwave ovens vary in wattage and size and this could produce a difference in heating factors.

25.5. Body image

The specific changes brought about to introduce peritoneal dialysis are essential and necessary evils to sustain life, yet patient acceptance of these intrusions can take a considerable period of time. Not surprisingly PD patients are often shocked when told that the insertion of a Tenckhoff catheter into the abdomen will be necessary to facilitate the exchange procedure. They fear that they may look different and more noticeable even though the bag and tubing can be concealed under the clothing [86]. Randerson and Farrel reported that the peritoneal catheter and bag inhibited sexual activity in approximately 20% of patients [87] whilst Paris states 76% of female CAPD patients and 47% males are worried about their body image [88]. She also reported that 50% of patients expressed negative changes regarding body image and sex life. The large volumes of fluid in the abdomen plus obesity due to absorption of glucose from dialysis fluids can also cause negative feelings and anxiety.

Pre dialysis counselling and careful psychological preparation can often alleviate the stress and tensions associated with body image misconceptions. The exit site placement and patient lifestyle should be discussed between surgeon and patient before operation. Practical issues such as concealment of tubing and bag and reassurance regarding attractive clothing should be discussed early as disillusionment at this stage could mean total rejection of the procedure. Patients could be introduced to others who are established on PD and who can discuss problems at first hand. With the advent of disconnect systems body image problems have been greatly improved [89]. Patients now report that they have more freedom of movement, are no longer afraid the catheter will be displaced and are more confident. The nurse should try to understand the needs of her patients whose lives and psyche are affected by body image problems and time should be spent helping the patients come to terms and explore their feelings.

25.6. Compliance/non compliance

Non compliance is an age old problem dating back to the time of Hippocrates but still remains a significant threat to morbidity and mortality in the PD population [90]. There are several factors which lead to the patient's inability to follow dietary, fluid and medication regimes and should be considered by the health care team when trying to convince patients to comply.

25.6.1. *Culture*

Culturally related habits may affect a patient's beliefs and behaviour about his illness and treatment. Dietary restrictions which tear apart his traditional eating habits may simply impose too great a strain to be followed [91].

25.6.2. *Depression*

Depression with symptoms of loss of interest and motivation, feelings of helplessness and loss of control may result in patients ignoring restrictions.

25.6.3. *Social support*

Healthcare teams often underestimate the part that a stable relationship, employment and an active social life has on compliance with tedious regimes. Hartman and Becker found less compliance when patients had little social support; however, increased compliance was associated with marriage [92].

25.6.4. *Amount of treatment*

The compliance rate declines with an increase in treatment and procedures. PD patients have several strict regimens to follow at any one time and may find the burden of compliance too great.

25.6.5. *Knowledge*

It is essential that PD patients understand their illness and treatment regimes. Sadly, it is not always the case that adequate knowledge will enhance patient compliance. In a study of 136 home dialysis patients Uttley *et al.* showed that 87% of patients studied (n = 120) had adequate knowledge of bone disease and phosphate control; however, 79% admitted to non-compliance with drug regimens [93].

The health care team should always assess a patient's psychological, social and medical situation when determining possible causes for non compliance. Practical reasons such as finance and ability to shop and cook should also be explored and assistance given where necessary. On-going educational programs will be more productive and encouragement should be given when compliance is achieved. The patient has a right to know everything about the treatment regime including what will happen if the plan is not followed. When the team has ascertained that the patient is neither ignorant nor misinformed, the responsibility of complying with therapy then rests with the patient. It is unrealistic for the team to assume that they can control patient behaviour, as most of the events that determine compliance are connected with ordinary everyday living, which ultimately is most subject to influence by the patient alone.

25.7. Infection control procedures

Universal body substance precautions recommended in 1987 treat all body substances from all patients as potentially infectious [94]. Infection control procedures specific to dialysis [95] and peritoneal dialysis have also be recommended [96]. Staff are required to wear gloves to handle and transport dialysate bags. Bags are to be kept in a covered container in the disposal area until the end of each day. The individual disposing the dialysate must wear gloves, a plastic apron and face shield and avoid splashing when emptying bags. Empty bags and tubing must be disposed of in plastic rubbish bags labelled "infectious waste". 1:10 bleach solution is poured into the disposal sinks and allowed to remain for 30 minutes.

Guidelines for home patients specify that the patient should dispose of dialysate in the toilet and empty bags should be placed in a plastic bag, secured with a knot and placed in the refuse. If another person disposes the dialysate they should wear gloves and avoid splashing [94–97].

25.8. Disaster preparedness

Disaster plans recommend that home dialysis patients keep a 2 week supply of medications and 2–4 weeks of dialysis supplies. Alternative methods of warming solutions should be reviewed in preparation for power shortages. Patients using electric or battery operated devices for dialysis exchanges need to keep batteries charged and/or be prepared to switch to a manual system. Likewise, cycler patients may be cross trained to perform manual CAPD exchanges, but need to have appropriate solution volumes for CAPD exchanges. Patients should wear medical information emblems which identify them as dialysis recipients at all times. Patients should also receive information regarding the length of time they can safely go without dialysis exchanges, an emergency diet plan, and emergency communications with the dialysis unit.

26. Research

Stetler, a nurse researcher, identified several levels of involvement in nursing research [98]. The most basic level of using the scientific process for clinical problem solving. A second level is research utilization incorporating pertinent research findings in clinical practice. The next level is to facilitate and/or participate in the research projects directed by others. All PD nurses can participate in research at these three levels.

Because continuous peritoneal dialysis is a relatively new form of therapy, clinical research provides information, regarding intervention strategies and outcomes. Research activities, like clinical care, are often undertaken by the inter-disciplinary team and this provides nurses with opportunities to participate in clinical research directed by others and to learn research related skills.

Well defined clinical research inevitably improves the quality of care in chronic dialysis programs, enhanced care may result from a) increased knowledge, b) improved assessment skills, c) more effective patient education, d) improved documentation and communication among team members, e) alternative methods of managing problems, f) identification for risk factors for specific complications and g) development of new procedures, dialysis regimes or delivery systems.

References

1. Oreopoulos DG. Nurses from yesterday's handmaidens to todays knowledgeable colleagues. Perit Dial Bull 1983; 4: 171–2.
2. Clayton S. The organization and implementation of a peritoneal dialysis program. Perit Dial Bull 1981; 1: 134–6.
3. Marsden A, Uttley L, Moon J. A successful CAPD program – what are the essential requirements. Proc EDTNA 1985; 14: 80–5.
4. Boen ST. Integration of CAPD into endstage renal failure programs: Present and future. In: Atkins RC, Thomson NM, Farrell PC (eds), Peritoneal Dialysis. Churchill Livingstone, Edinburgh 1981; pp 424–9.
5. Gokal R. CAPD. In: Parson FM, Ogg CS (eds), Renal failure who cares. MTP Press, Lancaster 1982; pp 137–50.
6. Eaton A, Penn A, Bungey M, Ogg, LS. HD Support for a CAPD program. In: Monkhouse P, Stevens E (eds), Aspects of Renal Care 1. Bailliere, Tindall, Eastbourne 1986; pp 87–92.
7. Oreopoulos DG. Requirements for the organization of a continuous ambulatory peritoneal dialysis program. Nephron 1979; 24: 261–3.
8. Holley JL et al. Initiating a PD program: Personnel administrative requirements. Patient Recruitment and Training Seminars in Dialysis 1990; 3: 123–6.
9. Holley JL, Piraino BM. Operating a peritoneal dialysis program, patient and program monitoring. Seminars in Dialysis 1990; 3: 182–6.
10. Jerrum C. CAPD: The state of the art. Nursing 1991; 4(30): 28–30.
11. Nolph KD, Prowant BF, Webb J. National conference of continuous ambulatory peritoneal dialysis. Perit Dial Bull 1981; 1: 65–6.
12. Green M. The nuts and bolts of establishing a home training program. AANNT J 1983; 10(5): 42–5.
13. Brennan DT. Impact of prospective payment regulations. Results of head nurse survey. ANNA J 1984; 11(7): 49–52.
14. Oreopoulos DG. The peritoneal dialysis nurse. The key to success. Perit Dial Bull 1981; 1: 113–4.
15. Morris B. Nursing intervention to prevent CAPD burnout. Contemporary Dialysis and Nephrology. July, 1990; pp 23–4.
16. Van Waeleghem JP, Gammer N, Lambert, MC et al. Development of nephrology nursing care in Europe 1978–1988. ANNA J 1989; 16: 233–5.
17. Starmann B, Lees P, Reynolds J. University of Michigan national CAPD survey. Dialysis Transplantation 1988; 17: 475–7.
18. Ray R, Samar D. CAPD nursing follow up: How much time does it take? J Am Assoc Nephrol Nurses Technicians 1981; 8(3): 26–7.
19. Gokal R. Who's for CAPD? BMJ 1993; 306: 1559–60.
20. Public Law (PL) October 1972, 92-603. Public Law (PL) June 1978, 95-292. Omnibus Budget Reconciliation Act (PL) 1981, 97-35.
21. Jordon P. 1988 nursing shortage survey. ANNA J 1988; 15: 253–5.
22. Muthny FA. Job strains and job satisfaction of dialysis nurses. Psychotherapy and psychosomatics 1989; 51: 150–5.
23. Parker J. Reduction in ESRD reimbursement rate: Identifying research priorities and quality indicators. ANNA J 1990; 17: 147–50.
24. Lewis SL, Campbell MA, Becktell PJ et al. Work stress, burnout, and sense of coherence among dialysis nurses. ANNA J 1992; 19: 545–53.
25. Taylor S, Breckenridge D, Butera E. Images of nephrology nursing practice: Report of a survey. ANNA J 1992; 19: 361–6.
26. Zappacosta AR, Perras ST. CAPD, Lippincott, Philadelphia 1984; pp 24–65.
27. Marram GD, Barrett MW, Brevis EO. Primary nursing; A model for individualized care. 2nd ed. C.V. Mosby Company, St. Louis 1979.
28. Perras S, Mattern M, Hugues C et al. Primary nursing is the key to success in an out-patient CAPD teaching program. Nephrology Nurse 1983; 5(4): 8–11.
29. Moon J, Uttley L, Manos J et al. Home CAPD nurse, an asset to a CAPD program. In: Maher JF, Winchester JF (eds), Frontiers in Peritoneal Dialysis. Field Rich, New York 1986; pp 360–3.
30. Rosario M. Nursing management of a PD program: Legal issues. Syllabus, 11th annual conference on peritoneal dialysis, Nashville, Tennessee 1991; pp 179–201.
31. Frederick GA. Re-use with continuous cyclic peritoneal dialysis. ANNA J 1986; 13(2): 80–2.
32. Mason EJ. How to write meaningful nursing standards, 2nd ed John Wiley & Son, New York 1984.
33. Brennan DT, Burrows-Hudson S, Day C, Libonate J. Standards of practice for nephrology nursing. A.J. Jannetti Inc. Pitman, New Jersey 1988.
34. Lancaster LE (ed). Core curriculum for nephrology nursing. A.J. Jannetti Inc. Pitman, New Jersey 1991.
35. Jeffrey JE, Burton HJ, Meidenheim, AP, Lindsay RM. A comparison of home training and problems encountered with initial home dialysis. Hemodialysis versus CAPD. ANNTJ 1982; 9(4): 56–62.
36. Luker KA, Caress AL. Rethinking patient education. Journal of Advanced Nursing 1989; 14: 711–8.
37. Hanson PC. Teaching CAPD. Nephrology Nurse, May/June, 1980; pp 41–2.
38. Guzman VM, Atherton E, Roy C. Training for peritoneal self care options. CAPD IPD CCPD AANNT 1983; 10(5): 33–7.
39. Coles GA. Manual of peritoneal dialysis. Practical procedures for medical and nursing staff. Kluwer Academic Publishers, Lancaster 1990.
40. Peterson L. Clark M. Assessment of the role of the community renal nurse. AANNT J 1981; 8(3): 20–3.
41. Uttley L. CAPD in the elderly, follow up care. In: Ota K et al. (eds), Current concepts in peritoneal dialysis. Excerpta Medica, Amsterdam 1992; pp 932–6.
42. Schleifer CR. Peritoneal dialysis in nursing homes. In: Nissenson AR (ed), Peritoneal dialysis in the geriatric patient. Perit Dial Bull 1990; 6 (supp): 86–90.
43. Manos J, Uttley L, Moon J et al. Successful joint care of CAPD patients with two district general hos-

pitals. In: Avram M et al. (eds), Ambulatory peritoneal dialysis. Plenum Medical, New York 1990; pp 272-3.
44. Tenckhoff H, 1974 Chronic peritoneal dialysis: A manual for patients, dialysis personnel and physicians. Seattle: University of Washington.
45. Twardowski ZJ, Khanna R, Nolph KD et al. Intra abdominal pressure during natural activities in patients treated with continuous ambulatory peritoneal dialysis. Nephron 1986; 44: 129-35.
46. Khanna R, Twadowski, ZJ. Peritoneal catheter exit site (editorial). Perit Dial Int 1988; 8: 119-23.
47. Copley JB, Smith BJ, Koger DM, Rodgers DJ, Fowler M. Prevention of postoperative peritoneal dialysis catheter related infections. Perit Dial Int 1988; 8: 195-7.
48. Jenson SR, Pomeroy M, Davidson M, Cox M, McMurray SD. Evaluation of dressing protocols that reduce peritoneal dialysis catheter exit site infections. ANNA J 1989; 16: 425-31.
49. Gokal R, Ash SR, Helfrich GB et al. Peritoneal catheter and exit site practices: Toward optimum peritoneal access. Perit Dial Int 1993; 13: 29-39.
50. Prowant BF, Warady, BA, Nolph KD. Peritoneal dialysis catheter exit site care: Results of an international survey. Perit Dial Int 1993; 13: 149-54.
51. Oreopoulos DG, Vas S, Khanna R. Prevention of peritonitis during CAPD. Perit Dial Bull 1981; 5: 518-20.
52. Maiorca R, Cantaluppi A, Cancarini GC et al. Prospective controlled trial of a Y-connector and disinfectant to prevent peritonitis in continuous ambulatory peritoneal dialysis. Lancet 1983; 2: 642-4.
53. Diaz-Buxo JA. Does CCPD lower the peritonitis rate? Contributions to Nephrology 1987; 57: 191-6.
54. Zappacosta AR, Perras ST. Reduction of CAPD peritonitis rate by ultraviolet light with dialysate exchange assist device. Dialysis Transplant 1988; 17: 483-5.
55. Baxter Health Care Corporation. The Best Demonstrated Practices Program: Peritonitis management and antibiotic therapy practices. Deerfield IL 1987.
56. Keane WF, Everett ED, Golper TA et al. PD related peritonitis treatment recommendations 1993 update, Perit Dial Bull 1993; 13: 14-28.
57. Winearls CG, Oliver DO, Pippard MJ et al. Effect of human erythropoietin derived from recombinant DNA on the anaemia of patients maintained by chronic haemodialysis. Lancet 1986; 2: 1175-8.
58. Cotton SL, Holechek MJ. Management of anemia using RHuEPO in patients on chronic haemodialysis. ANNA J 1989; 16: 463-8.
59. Boelaert JR, Schurgers ML, Matthys EG et al. Comparative pharmacokinetics of RHuEPO administered by IV SC IP routes in CAPD patients. Perit Dial Int 1989; 9: 95-8.
60. Lui SF, Chung WW, Leung CB et al. Pharmacokinetics and pharmacodynamics of SC and IP administration of RHuEPO in patients on CAPD. Clinical Nephrology 1990; 33: 47-51.
61. Frenken LA, Coppens PJ et al. Intraperitoneal erythropoeitin. Lancet 1988; 2: 1495.
62. York S, Kinney R, Taber T. Self-administration of epoetin beta by PD patients. ANNA J 1991; 18: 549-52.
63. Prowant BF, Gallagher NM, Binkley LS et al. Nephrology nursing care plan and patient education plan for the patient receiving Epogen. ANNA J 1991; 18: 188-94.
64. Oliver DO. Treatment of anaemia in CRF with RHuEPO. In: PM Monkhouse (ed), Aspects of renal care, 3. Bailliere Tindall, London 1989; pp 21-7.
65. Linderstrom A, Birany P, Bergstrom K. Dialysis nurses responsibilities regarding the side effects of RHuEPO. EDTNA ERCA J 1990; 13: 24-5.
66. Gokal R, Friedman EA, Rottembourg J et al. PD in diabetic ESRD patients. Dialysis Transplantation 1991; 20: 59, 63, 66, 88.
67. Haas LB. Chronic complications of diabetes mellitus: peritoneal dialysis. ANNA J 1992; 19: 439-46.
68. Clayton S. Training the diabetic patient on CAPD. Perit Dial Bull 1982; 2 (suppl): S38-9.
69. Bouton AJM, Gokal R, Masson EA. The formation of a diabetic nephropathy clinic. Report of the first six months experience. Postgraduate Medical Journal 1988; 64 (suppl 3): 84.
70. Anderson RB, Conway PA, Piening S et al. Was it worth it? Significant others' view of diabetic renal failure Dialysis Transplantation 1986; 15: 315-20.
71. Piening S. Family stress in diabetic renal failure. Health and Social Work 1984; 9(2): 134-41.
72. Cullinan TR. Sight. In: Redfern SJ (ed). Nursing elderly people, 2nd ed. Churchill Livingstone, Edinburgh 1991; pp 91-8.
73. Ham RJ, Pattee J, Marcy ML. Accidents in the elderly. In: Hamm RJ, Holtzman JM, Marcy ML, Smith RM (eds), Primary care geriatrics. John Wright, Boston 1983; pp 235-57.
74. Twardowski ZJ, Nolph KD, Khanna R et al. Peritoneal equilibration test. Perit Dial Bull 1987; 7: 138-47.
75. Schmidt LM, Prowant BF. How to do a peritoneal equilibration test. ANNA J 1991; 18: 368-70.
76. Twardowski ZJ. Clinical value of standardized equilibration tests in CAPD patients. Blood Purification 1989; 7: 95-108.
77. Prowant BF, Schmidt LM. The peritoneal equilibration test: A nursing discussion. ANNA J 1991; 18: 361-6.
78. Verger C, Larpent L, Dumontet M. Prognostic value of peritoneal equilibration curves in CAPD patients. In: Maher JF, Winchester JF (eds), Frontiers in peritoneal dialysis. Field, Rich and Associates, New York 1986; pp 88-93.
79. Twardowski ZJ. The fast peritoneal equilibration test. Seminars in Dialysis 1990; 3: 141-2.
80. Adcock A, Fox K, Walker P et al. Clinical experience and comparative analysis of the standard and fast peritoneal equilibration tests (PET). In: Khanna R, Nolph KD, Prowant BF, Twardowski ZJ, Oreopoulos DG (eds), Advances in peritoneal dialysis, Vol 8. Toronto: Perit Dial Bull, pp 59-61.
81. Twardowski ZJ, Nolph KD, Khanna R et al. Daily clearances with continuous ambulatory peritoneal

dialysis and nightly peritoneal dialysis. Trans Am Soc Artif Int Organs 1986; 32: 575–80.
82. Craig C, Kuharcik C. Tidal peritoneal dialysis. Syllabus, 13th annual conference on peritoneal dialysis, San Diego, California 1993; pp 186–99.
83. Vigneux A, Steele BT. CAPD is not a contraindication for swimming in children. Perit Dial Bull 1982; 2: 99.
84. Sandahl LL, Owens EL. Use of ostomy pouch for pediatric CAPD swimmers. ANNA J 1989; 16: 274–7.
85. Armstong S, Zalatan SJ. Microwave warming of PD fluid. ANNA J 1992; 19: 535–40.
86. Uttley L, Gokal R. Organisation of a CAPD Program: The nurses, role in CAPD. In: Gokal R, (ed), CAPD. Churchill Livingstone, Edinburgh 1986; pp 145–62.
87. Randerson DH, Farrell PC. Subjective assessment of CAPD patients. In: Gahl GH, Kessel M, Nolph KD (eds), Advances in Peritoneal Dialysis. Excerta Medica, Amsterdam 1981; pp 236–9.
88. Paris V. CAPD body image and sexuality, are they compatible. EDTNA/ERCA journal 1992; 28: 33–4.
89. Verger C, Dumont M, Misrahi B et al. CAPD without wearing bags, less peritonitis more freedom. EDTNA J 1983; 12: 38–43.
90. King K. Noncompliance in the chronic dialysis population. Dialysis Transplant 1991; 20(2): 67–8.
91. Berg J, Berg BL. Compliance, diet and cultural factors among black Americans with ESRD, Journal of the Black National Nurses Association 1989; 13: 16–28.
92. Hartman PE, Becker MH. Non-compliance with prescribed regimen among chronic hemodialysis patients. Dialysis Transplant 1978; 7(10): 978–89.
93. Uttley L, Fawcett J, Hutchinson A. Phosphate control -what do our patients know? EDTNA Journal 1993; in press.
94. Recommendations for prevention of HIV transmission in health-care settings, 1987; MMWR 36(2S): 3S–18S.
95. Recommendations for providing dialysis treatment to patients infected with human T-lymphotrophic virus type III/lymphadenopathy-associated virus, 1986 MMWR 35(23): 376–8, 383.
96. Schoenfeld P. Renal Disease and HIV infection: Clinical course, treatment outcome, and infection control. ANNA J 1990; 17: 21–28.
97. Baldasseroni A. The HIV positive patient on peritoneal dialysis: Nursing Issues. Syllabus, 12th annual conference on peritoneal dialysis, Seattle, Washington 1992; pp 361–7.
98. Stetler CB. Nurses and research, responsibility and involvement. NITA 1983; p 207.

12 Continuous ambulatory peritoneal dialysis

J. W. MONCRIEF, R. P. POPOVICH, N. V. DOMBROS, G. E. DIGENIS AND
D. G. OREOPOULOS

1. Introduction 357
2. History 357
3. Principles and concepts of CAPD 358
4. CAPD compared to IPD/CCPD 360
5. CAPD compared to hemodialysis 361
6. Technique 362
   6.1. Larger molecules 362
   6.2. Ultrafiltration 363
7. Management of a CAPD program 364
   7.1. Program development 364
   7.2. Site of training 364
   7.3. Hospital back-up 364
   7.4. Training 364
   7.5. Patient management 365
   7.6. Telephone contact 365
   7.7. Laboratory tests 365
   7.8. Medications 366
8. Complications 366
   8.1. Catheter related complications 366
      8.1.1. Early (during training) catheter related complications 366
      8.1.2. Late (or chronic) catheter related complications 368
   8.2. Complications related to the presence of dialysate in the peritoneal cavity 370
      8.2.1. Hernias 370
      8.2.2. Abdominal wall and genital edema 370
      8.2.3. Hemoperitoneum 371
      8.2.4. Hydrothorax 371
      8.2.5. Respiratory dysfunction 372
      8.2.6. Back pain 372
   8.3. Failure of ultrafiltration in CAPD 372
   8.4. Sclerosing encapsulating peritonitis and peritoneal calcification 372
   8.5. Nutritional and metabolic complications 373
      8.5.1. Carbohydrate metabolism 373
      8.5.2. Lipid abnormalities 373
      8.5.3. Malnutrition 374
      8.5.4. Vitamins 376
   8.6. Cardiovascular complications and blood pressure control 376
   8.7. Anemia 376
   8.8. Gastrointestinal complications 377
   8.9. Skeletoarticular complications 377
   8.10. Amyloidosis-related disorders 378
   8.11. Urinary stones 378
   8.12. Pruritus 378
9. Patient and technique survival 379
   9.1. CAPD versus HD 379
      9.1.1. Patient survival 379
      9.1.2. Causes of death 380
      9.1.3. Technique survival 380
      9.1.4. Reasons for drop-out 381
   9.2. Morbidity on CAPD 381
      9.2.1. Cardiovascular morbidity 381
      9.2.2. Infections 381
      9.2.3. Skeleto-articular disorders 381
10. Psychosocial aspects of CAPD 381
11. Long term results 382
12. Future developments 383
13. Conclusions 384
References 384

1. Introduction

The therapeutic, clinical and economic success of Continuous Ambulatory Peritoneal Dialysis (CAPD) has spawned an entirely new industry. Peritoneal dialysis is now offered in most chronic dialysis programs throughout the world [1]. In many countries where dialysis in performed, a substantial minority and in many cases a majority of patients undergo chronic support of their end stage renal disease with this modality (Fig. 1). Many national and international symposia are dedicated to the research projects associated with this broad, expanding therapeutic system [2–6]. Technological and product developments have created a new industry to manufacture and distribute the materials required to safely deliver CAPD. In the past decade, a new society, (International Society for Peritoneal Dialysis), dedicated to the study of peritoneal dialysis has been organized and a new international journal, (Peritoneal Dialysis International), has been developed for the dissemination of scientific information.

2. History

In the 1970's, intermittent peritoneal dialysis (IPD) performed 30–40 hours weekly was considered a marginal to unacceptable alternative to hemodialysis in the management of chronic end-stage renal

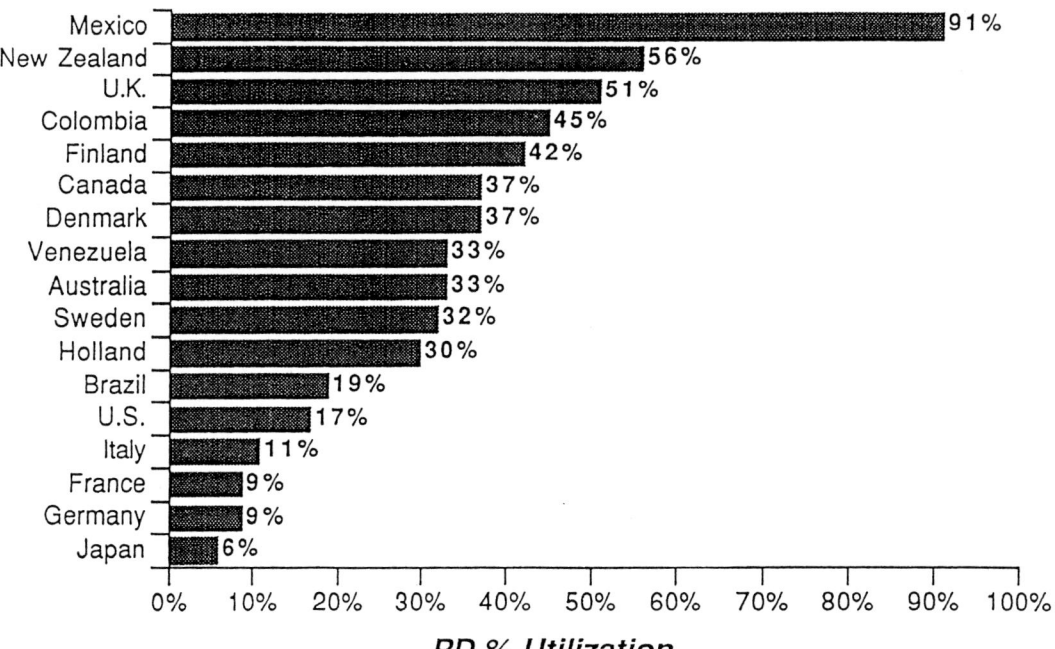

Figure 1. Global PD utilization.

disease. A publication from the National Institutes of Health documented that fewer than three percent of the population of patients managed with dialysis were on IPD [7].

The fundamental problem of intermittent dialysis procedures is that they require delivery in a specific place. The use of large quantities of dialysate solution delivered from a fixed location requires a substantial time commitment by staff and patients. Access and infection are also problem areas.

The thrust of research in intermittent dialysis had been to improve efficiency. This effort was present in both the technique of hemodialysis (HD) and IPD. The increase in dialysate flow rate and the increased size of the surface area, as well as the increased blood flow rate in the hemodialysis procedure, allowed improvement in the clearance of small and medium sized molecules. Small molecule clearance (urea) could be achieved at a range of 150–180 ml/min with a 1 sq meter dialyzer. This allowed the patient to undergo adequate dialysis (prevent uremia) if applied 3–5 hours three times per week. Efforts had been made to increase the efficiency of peritoneal dialysis by increasing dialysis flow rate [8]. Peritoneal clearances however, proved to be primarily either mass transfer or blood flow limited. The maximum urea clearance achievable was approximately 35 ml/min with a dialysis flow rate of 70–80 ml/min (Fig. 2). Under usual operating conditions (one or two 2-liter exchanges per hour), the clearance is in the range of only 20 ml/min or less. Because of this low clearance, IPD required more hours (30–50) of dialysis time commitment on a weekly basis to achieve the same results as twelve hours per week with hemodialysis. Neither of the procedures was portable, but the much shorter time commitment of hemodialysis proved so crucial that it became the dominant therapy of choice for staff assisted and home dialysis prior to the introduction of CAPD by Popovich and Moncrief in 1976 [9, 10].

3. Principles and concepts of CAPD

The clinical protocol for CAPD was derived from a simplified kinetic analysis of the patient CAPD system. For low dialysis clearance systems such as urea removal via CAPD, Popovich and Moncrief [11], have demonstrated that body fluids may be considered as a single well mixed pool. With this simplification, the blood urea concentration level (C_B) in the body will be determined by the solution of the macroscopic mass balance equation (12).

$$\frac{d}{dt}(V_B C_B) = G - K_R C_B - K_D C_B \qquad (1)$$

| Accumu-
tion
rate | Genera-
tion
rate | Renal
removal
rate | Dialysis
removal
rate |

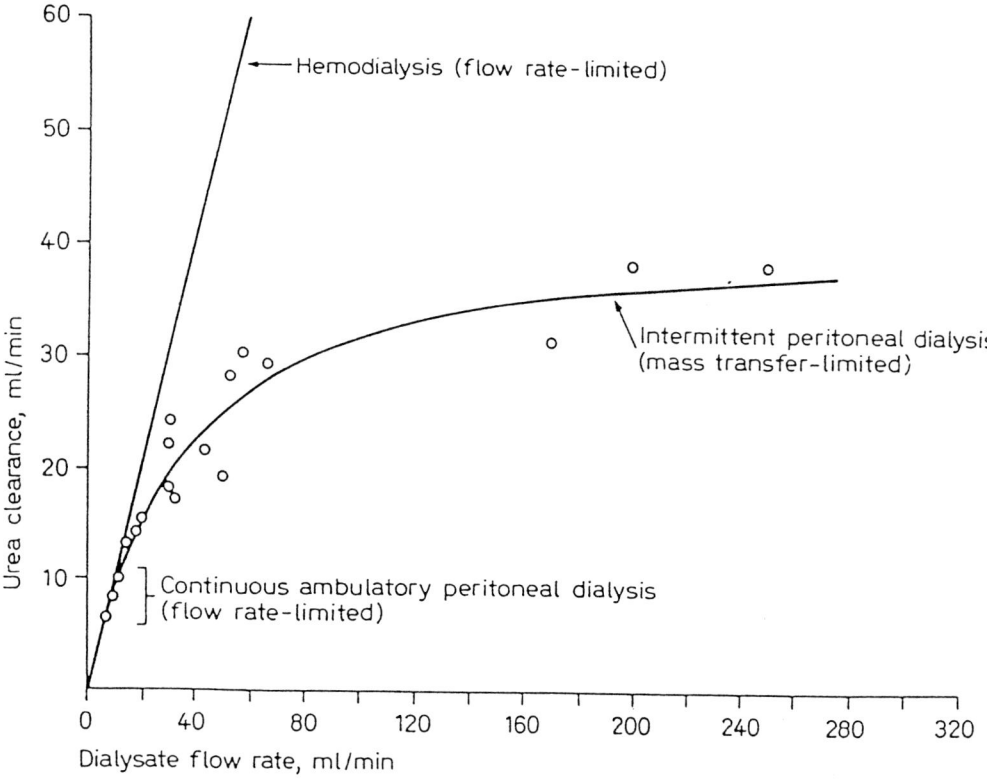

Figure 2. Urea clearance as a function of dialysate flow rate: Hemodialysis, IPD, CAPD.

In Equation (1) V_B is the volume of distribution, G is the net generation rate, K_R is the residual renal clearance and K_D is the dialysis clearance. The accumulation term is the time derivative of the total urea mass in the system. This term is equal to zero if the dialysis treatment is continuous, i.e., the urea concentration and volume of distribution are constant. Setting the accumulation term equal to zero and solving the resulting algebraic equation for the steady state urea concentration level yields:

$$C_B = \frac{G}{K_R + K_D} = \frac{G}{K} \qquad (2)$$

where K is the total system clearance. Note that the clearances are additive.

In the worst case basis residual renal clearance, K_R, is equal to zero. We employed a typical blood urea BUN nitrogen generation rate of 5.7 mg/min [13] and established 80 mg/dl as a reasonable upper limit for the BUN of a patient. Using this data, equation (2) was solved for the required dialysis clearance.

$$K_D = \frac{G}{C_B} = \frac{5.7 \text{ mg/min}}{0.8 \text{ mg/ml}} = 7.1 \text{ ml/min} \qquad (3)$$

or

$$KD = 7.1 \text{ ml/min} \times 1440 \text{ min/day}$$
$$= 10,200 \text{ ml/day}. \qquad (3)$$

This simplified kinetic analysis predicted that about 10 liters/day is required to maintain the average 70 kilogram anephric patient with a BUN of about 80 mg/dl. Since these equations are completely general, this dialysis clearance can be obtained using any dialysis technique. In the case of peritoneal dialysis, the clearance is defined by:

$$K_D = \frac{V_D C_D}{T C_B} \qquad (5)$$

where V_D is the drained dialysate volume with a mean BUN concentration C_D over a total time period T.

Two liter infusions were typically employed with intermittent peritoneal dialysis. This suggested a dwell time of approximately five hours (10 L/day ÷ 2 L/exchange = 5 exchanges/day). We assumed that equilibrium would occur between the concentration of urea in the dialysate, C_D, and blood, C_B

over such a prolonged dwell period. With $C_D = C_B$, Equation (5) reduces to:

$$K_D = \frac{V_D}{T} = Q_D = \text{dialysate flow rate.} \quad (6)$$

Thus, this simplified model leads directly to the CAPD clinical protocol. The theory predicts that an anephric patient will maintain a steady BUN level of approximately 80 mg/dl if 10L of dialysate are allowed to equilibrate with body fluids on a daily basis. Given the normal infusion volume of 2.0L, four infusions will result in a total of 8.0L. To remove accumulated body fluids, approximately 2 L/day are ultrafiltrated. This yields a total drained volume of 10 L/day as predicted above and has evolved into the standard CAPD clinical protocol.

4. CAPD compared to IPD/CCPD

Numerous models of peritoneal dialysis have subsequently evolved. Most of these are complex [14] and are beyond the scope of this chapter. However, the models demonstrate that BUN clearance is a complex function of three dominant parameters [15]: the peritoneal blood flow rate, Q_B, the dialysate flow rate, Q_D, and the mass transfer-area coefficient (MTAC). Two conclusions can be deduced from the models. The clearance can never exceed the lowest value of these parameters and the clearance will be approximately equal to the value of one of the parameters if its value is significantly lower than the other two. For example, the MTAC for large solutes is very low. The clearance will be approximately equal to the MTAC for this case and is said to be *mass transfer limited*. Increasing the blood or dialysate flow rates will not significantly increase the clearance. On the other hand, the clearance is said to be *dialysate flow rate limited* if the value of the dialysate flow rate is much less than either Q_B or the MTAC. In this case, the clearance will essentially equal the value of the dialysate flow rate.

Figure 2 further illustrates these concepts. Blood urea nitrogen clearance is presented as a function of dialysate flow rate. In the case of hemodialysis, Q_B and the MTAC are much larger than the value of dialysate flow rate over the domain shown. Consequently, the clearance is essentially equal to Q_D (the straight line). The situation for peritoneal dialysis is more complex. Intermittent peritoneal dialysis is generally performed with dialysate flow rates in the range of 30–40 ml/min with a urea clearance of approximately 20 ml/min. At higher dialysate flow rates, the urea clearance approaches a maximum equal to the value of the MTAC (the *mass transfer limited* region). These clinical results demonstrate that the clearance of intermittent peritoneal dialysis is limited to some extent by a low mass transfer – area coefficient. This analysis assumes that the peritoneal capillary blood flow rate is sufficiently large to preclude it becoming a limiting parameter as suggested by Nolph et al. [16].

Mass transfer-area coefficients are known to vary considerably from patient to patient [17, 18]. Indeed, documented MTAC's in one patient were found to be only 20% of normal [19]. The effect of a low mass transfer-area coefficient can have serious consequences in intermittent techniques where efficiency must be maximized over shorter time periods to provide adequate therapy. Due to the low clearance obtained even under the best of circumstances, these patients are poor candidates for IPD. If treated with IPD, these patients may exhibit symptoms of under-dialysis or develop other serious complications. This may partly explain the poor survivability of some IPD patients [20].

To a large extent CAPD overcomes the problem of a low efficiency inherent in peritoneal dialysis caused by the low MTAC value by making continuous operation an integral part of the procedure. CAPD is performed continuously (168 hr/week) as opposed to only about 40 hr/week for IPD. This dramatically lowers the dialysate flow rate to the range 7 to 9 ml/min. Since the dialysate flow rate in CAPD is much less than the average MTAC, the flow rate becomes the dominant factor in determining solute clearance. The mass transfer-area coefficient would have to be significantly below normal before membrane properties would exert a significant effect on clearances. Thus, only those patients with significant loss or lack of transport ability will have problems associated with decreased clearances. In most circumstances, utilizing increased infusion volumes or adding an additional CAPD exchange per day can adequately compensate. With IPD, decreased transport ability may significantly affect clearance with the possibility of underdialysis.

These effects are also prevalent for other intermittent procedures such a nightly peritoneal dialysis (NIPD, 50–84 hours weekly) but to a lesser extent because of the increased treatment times relative to IPD. Patients being considered for peritoneal dialysis may be tested for peritoneal membrane transport properties. The most commonly utilized procedure is the peritoneal equilibration test (PET) described in Chapter 4. Those patients with enhanced transportability should be good candidates for either CAPD or the intermittent procedures. However, those patients who have impaired transport may fare better on CAPD.

5. CAPD compared to hemodialysis

High clearance intermittent therapies such as hemodialysis (HD) involve inherent peaks and valleys in the concentration of blood urea nitrogen during the course of the therapy. If control of the peak BUN is important in preventing uremic toxicity (the peak concentration hypothesis), it can be demonstrated [21] that any intermittent therapy requires a greater dose of therapy to maintain the peak concentration at the steady state value of CAPD (assuming the same BUN generation rate). Although the peak concentration hypothesis remains unproven, it is compatible with the observed clinical need for higher weekly clearances with intermittent therapies. For example, most centers strive for a weekly KT/V urea value (weekly urea clearance in L/total body water in L) for chronic hemodialysis at or above 3.0, whereas the typical weekly KT/V value for CAPD [21] varies between 1.5 and 1.8. Clearly, clearance indices such as KT/V urea with a continuous therapy such as CAPD differ in many ways from the same clearance indices when used to quantitate an intermittent therapy.

Nolph et al. [22] considered the comparison of KT/V urea for CAPD versus hemodialysis. Typical patient parameters were employed: a body weight of 70 kg, body water $V = 40L$ (57% of body weight), a urea nitrogen generation rate of 7 gm/day, and negligible residual renal function. The CAPD patient was assigned 4 exchanges of 2 liters each with 2 liters of ultrafiltrate per day, 7 days per week. Complete equilibration between serum and dialysate urea was assumed for simplicity.

Under steady state conditions, the blood urea nitrogen concentration is determined by Equation (2):

$$C_B = \frac{G}{K_D} = \frac{(7 \text{ gm/day})}{(10 \text{ L/day})} = 0.7 \text{ gm/L} = 70 \text{ mg/dl}.$$

Note that the clearance is equal to the drained dialysate volume as outlined in Equation (6). The corresponding KT/V value is given by:

$$(KT/V)_{day} = \frac{(10 \text{ L/day}) (1 \text{ day})}{(40L)} = 0.25$$

and

$$(KT/V)_{week} = 0.25 \times 7 = 1.75.$$

In the case of hemodialysis, the patient was assigned to thrice weekly treatments with a targeted KT/V of a 1.0 per treatment, or 3.0 for the week. Four liters of ultrafiltration were assumed with a dialyzer clearance of 167 ml/min for 240 minutes. A variable volume urea kinetic model was utilized to complete the BUN profile over the 3 weekly dialyses. The results are shown in Table 1. Urea removal is the greatest (18.6 gm) for the first dialysis of the week. This is a result of the highest pre-dialysis BUN following the longest interdialytic interval over the weekend. The total cumulative removal is 49 gm, being equal to the urea nitrogen on a weekly basis (7 gm/day × 7 days).

A comparison of the two prescribed therapies is revealing. It takes four days of CAPD to achieve the same KT/V as with 4 hours of hemodialysis. Alternately, the urea nitrogen removed in four days on CAPD (28 gm) is significantly greater than with 4 hours of hemodialysis (14.7 gm to 18.6 gm). This difference is explained by the fact that the urea nitrogen concentration declines rapidly with time during hemodialysis (a result of the high urea removal rate across the dialysis membrane compared to the generation rate). Urea is cleared in hemodialysis at a time-averaged BUN concentration of only 43 mg/dl compared to the steady state CAPD BUN of 70 mg/dl. From a clinical perspective, a KT/V per week ratio of 1.8 for HD/CAPD seems to yield comparable results. These

Table 1. BUN profile over 3 weekly HD.

Weekly $(KT/V)_{HD} = 3.0$

	BUN		Urea Nitrogen Removal
	Pre	Post	
Monday	67	30	18.6 gm
Wednesday	57	26	15.7 gm
Friday	53	24	14.7 gm
			49.0 gm

Time Avg. Conc. 43 mg/dl

observations were the genesis of the peak concentration hypothesis [21].

Popovich [22] presented a technique for adjusting the KT/V urea in CAPD to a hemodialysis equivalent. In its most simplified form (neglecting residual renal function, identical generation rates, evenly spaced HD treatments, etc.) the ratio between the predialysis BUN in hemodialysis (C_{HD}) and the steady state CAPD concentration (C_{CAPD}) can be approximated by the following equation:

$$\frac{C_{HD}}{C_{CAPD}} = \frac{(KT/V)_{CAPD}}{[1.0 - \exp(-KT/V)_{HD}]}. \quad (7)$$

The exponential term incorporating the hemodialysis KT/V term accounts for the effects of the decline in the metabolite concentration and concomitant mass transfer rate during the hemodialysis procedure.

For the clinical example outlined above:

$(KT/V)_{HD} = 1.0$
$(KT/V)_{CAPD} = 1.75$ per week ÷ 3 = 0.583.

Substitution into Equation (7) yields:

$$\frac{C_{HD}}{C_{CAPD}} = \frac{0.583}{[1.0 - \exp(-1.0)_{HD}]} = 0.92.$$

This predicts a predialysis BUN concentration for evenly spaced thrice weekly hemodialysis treatments of:

$C_{HD} = 0.92 \times 70$ mg/dl = 64 mg/dl.

This falls within the range illustrated in Table 1.

Support for the peak concentration hypothesis and the concept of adjusting the KT/V urea for CAPD and HD to kinetic equivalency has recently been reported by Gotch [23]. The relationships of protein catabolic rate to KT/V urea became essentially identical for CAPD and HD when KT/V urea values in CAPD patients were converted to the thrice weekly KT/V values. Thus, it is inappropriate to directly compare KT/V values between CAPD and HD. Peak concentrations of BUN on hemodialysis can be maintained at or below those of CAPD at the same urea nitrogen removal rates only if weekly KT/V values on HD approach 1.5 to 1.8 times those of CAPD.

6. Technique

Continuous Ambulatory Peritoneal Dialysis, as modeled, utilizes the smallest volume of dialysis fluid, i.e., the lowest dialysate flow rate to achieve the goal of preventing uremia [24, 25]. Continuous dialysis takes place during a prolonged dwell time of dialysis fluid in the peritoneal cavity while the patient is ambulatory. The procedure is thus portable.

If two liters of dialysate are placed in the peritoneal cavity and the dwell times extended so that equilibration of blood and dialysate urea occurs, the drained volume of dialysate will then equal the urea clearance. As outlined above, this requires a total of approximately 10 liters of drained volume per day. This can technically be done by the following steps:

1. Infuse 2 liters of dialysate into the peritoneal cavity.
2. Extend the dwell time to allow equilibration of urea nitrogen.
3. Drain this volume and reinfuse two more liters.
4. Exchange the volume 4 times a day at convenient intervals.
5. Adjust the dialysate tonicity to produce approximately 2 liters of ultrafiltrate (two-1.5% glucose, two 4.25% glucose), to achieve a total drained volume of 10 liters/day.

The procedure which will adequately remove small molecules (i.e., urea, mol wt 60) is, therefore, defined.

6.1. Larger molecules

As the molecules of interest increase in molecular weight, increasing efficiency is seen as a consequence of the prolonged dwell time. A molecule of 5200 daltons (inulin) will diffuse from the blood compartment into the dialysate very slowly, and the concentration gradient between the blood and the dialysate will be maintained for an extended period. A single exchange of 12 hours will produce excellent removal of this size molecule. Because of the rapid decrease in hemodialysis clearance with increasing molecular weight, CAPD is approximately six times better at removing inulin size molecules than is intermittent hemodialysis at 15 hours per week [24]. Table 2 shows ratios of peak solute concentrations using different dialysis therapies for solutes in the molecular weight ranges of urea, vitamin B_{12}, and inulin. Solute appearance rates are assumed constant and identical for all treatments. For molecules near 5200 daltons, peak serum concentrations with thrice weekly hemodialysis with standard cellulosic membranes would be 6.9 times steady state values of CAPD.

Table 2. Effect of molecular weight on membrane transport rate. Numbers are peak concentration ratios.

Solute	MW	HD/CAPD	IPD/HD	IPD/CAPD
Urea	60	0.99	1.4	1.4
Vitamin B12	1,355	3.2	0.79	2.4
Inulin	5,200	6.9	0.34	2.6

* CAPD with 4 exchanges/day, residual renal clearance = 0.

6.2. Ultrafiltration

Although many factors such as osmotic gradient between blood and dialysate, peritoneal membrane thickness, status of vasoconstriction, hydration of the peritoneal membrane and total infused volume effect ultrafiltration rates during peritoneal dialysis, the present clinically controllable factor is the dialysate tonicity. As dialysate tonicity increases, the ultrafiltration rate proportionately increases. Glucose is the osmotic agent in commercially available solutions and upon instillation of a hypertonic solution of 4.25% glucose, an immediate ultrafiltration rate of approximately 15 to 25 ml/min will occur (Fig. 3). As glucose is simultaneously diffusing from the dialysate to the blood, the tonicity will diminish and the ultrafiltration rate will fall proportionately. The glucose transport will occur at a gradually decreasing rate and is related to the concentration gradient between blood and dialysate. Net positive ultrafiltration (from blood to dialysate) will occur over approximately the first 3 to 4 hours. A similar but less dramatic ultrafiltration will occur with instillation of a 1.5% glucose solution. The total ultrafiltered volume with instillation of 2000 ml of a 1.5% glucose solution will approximate 300 ml. Roughly 1L of ultrafiltrate will occur with infusion of 2000 ml of 4.25% glucose solution. As isotonicity between blood and dialysate is achieved, the reverse flow of the isotonic fluid

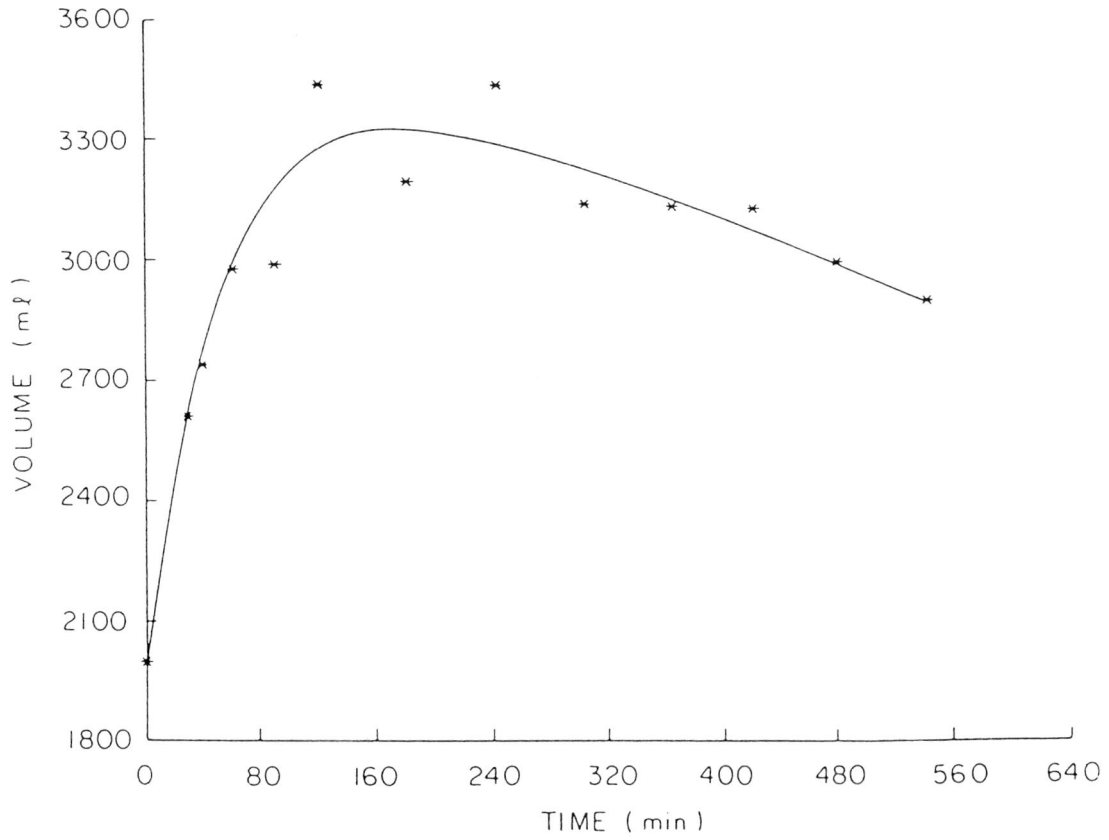

Figure 3. Volume and rate of ultrafiltration from the infusion of 4.25% glucose.

from the peritoneal cavity into the blood vascular space will occur at a rate of 1 ± 0.5 ml/min (Fig. 3) [14]. This reverse flow is important in evaluating the total ultrafiltration available and drained volume will be decreased by approximately 60 ml/hr after the first 3 to 4 hours of osmotically controlled ultrafiltration (Fig. 3).

Dialysate with a glucose concentration of 2.5% and 3.5% is available and produces ultrafiltration rates and volumes intermediate to that of the 1.5% glucose and the 4.25% glucose solutions. The advantage of these solution concentrations is the avoidance of the intermittent symptoms of distension (due to large ultrafiltration volume) occasionally created by the 4.25% glucose solution [25].

In 1976, CAPD was first delivered in the manner described utilizing glass containers [24]. Plastic containers were unavailable in the United States at that time but were available in Canada. Dr. Dimitrios Oreopoulos at Toronto Western Hospital adopted the procedure utilizing collapsable plastic containers which markedly reduced the connections and disconnections required with a concomitant decrease in the incidence of peritonitis [26–28]. This development allowed the procedure to be adopted as a standard dialysis delivery system. This technique has been thoroughly reviewed elsewhere [25, 26].

Subsequent development of the "drain before fill" concept from Italy [29–32] in which dialysate was drained immediately after connection cleared contaminating bacteria on the interior of the line at the connection site. This drain before fill technique reduced the incidence of peritonitis. Several adaptations to this technique are presently available in clinical practice. These include disposable or reusable tubing set, some of which contain sterilizing solutions. Adaptation of this drain before fill disconnect system has also "been adopted" with an ultraviolet light system (UVXD, Baxter International) which has also been demonstrated to reduce the incidence of peritonitis [33].

7. Management of a CAPD program

7.1. Program development

CAPD is truly self/home dialysis which allows improved freedom and self reliance by the individual patients. All training programs require the continuous commitment and ready availability of medical staff for training, support, and back-up. The commitment of the nephrologist and nursing personnel to sterile technique, chronic catheter care, and patient training methods will be necessary for a successful program. The technique is extremely simple. Problems may arise quickly, however, and be demanding on the medical and nursing staff. Thus, adequate personnel proportionate to the patient population is essential. One nurse to each 10 to 15 outpatients and a schedule for 24 hour a day coverage is required (Chapter 11).

The first week of training should be carried out on a one-to-one basis with a nurse dedicated to the education of each patient. By the end of the first week, the patient is usually performing the technique independently. At that point, trouble-shooting and observation can be done in small groups, but no more than one nurse to three patients is practical.

7.2. Site of training

In-hospital CAPD training is practiced in some centers. Outpatient training is preferable, however, because it decreases the cost and prevents the "ill patient" syndrome that may occur within hospital procedures. Little equipment is required and 100 to 120 square feet of training space per patient is adequate.

7.3. Hospital back-up

Although hospitalization has become less frequent, good hospital back-up and expert management of the patient is required. Most centers have found that specialized nursing personnel should manage both the outpatient training and follow up, as well as in hospital back-up and management.

7.4. Training

Day 1 to 4

Ten to fifteen training sessions are usually required to prepare a patient to manage CAPD. The training sessions are carried out on a daily basis. The sessions are begun after catheter break-in and each session is carried on for 6 to 8 hours as the patient's physical, emotional, and mental status allows. During the first few days, exchanges are made approximately each $1\frac{1}{2}$ to 2 hours. These rapid changes allow for better urea and small molecule control and avoid the need for backup dialysis [34]. It also increases patient learning by repetition and may be used to more rapidly control the expanded intravascular volumes so commonly present. This will bring blood pressure under control as antihypertensive medications are tapered. During these early training days, the patient is taught to make the exchanges using simulation models while the nurse makes the actual exchange. At the end of the training day two liters of dialysate are left in the abdomen overnight. If discomfort occurs during the night, the patient is instructed to drain enough solution until relief is achieved. One hundred to 300 ml drainage is usually adequate, but some patients may have to drain as much as 1 liter.

Day 4 to 6

After the first few days, as technical skills improve, the nurse allows the patient to make the exchanges with supervision. As this practice improves technique, the patient then makes exchanges in the unit without supervision and then makes his/her own exchange at night. When this is accomplished, the patient begins the CAPD regime of four exchanges per day. This degree of expertise can usually be reached within the first week of training so that the patient is ready to make all four exchanges in the absence of the staff.

Day 8 to 12

During the following week, continued exchange and theory training is undertaken. Repeated documentation of successful adherence to the rigid technique is observed by the staff. Question and answer sessions are carried out with a "trouble-shooting" format and, near the end of the second week, the patient is given a battery of tests to evaluate both the theoretical and practical aspects of accumulated knowledge. When these test are successfully completed, the patient is graduated from the CAPD training program and signs a release stating that CAPD training has included theoretical and practical aspects of the necessary information. The patient is then given supplies and sent home to perform the technique for two weeks.

7.5. Patient management

Within 2 to 3 days, contact is made by telephone. At the two week visit, re-evaluation of the technique is undertaken, and the nurse makes a home visit to evaluate the patient's home environment. Suggestions for change are made as clinically indicated. The patient is seen each two weeks for the first 3 months. With each visit, observation of a complete exchange is performed. After 3 months, the visits are reduced to one per month. During these visits, clinical evaluation by the physician is made and the catheter site is inspected. Documentation of compliance and discussion of potential theoretical problems is carried out by the staff.

7.6. Telephone contact

Close contact with and encouragement of the patient is done by a weekly telephone call which includes specific questions about blood pressure, dry weight, last scale weight, appetite, sense of well-being, catheter site evaluation, and dialysate flow characteristics. The calls serve to detect incipient and slowly developing problems and also keep the patient aware of the concern of the staff and reduce the reluctance to call if problems arise. The educational process is also continued by these calls.

7.7. Laboratory tests

During the training phase, laboratory evaluation is done on the first day and subsequently every other day unless unusual parameters are reported. Hyperkalemia or hypokalemia may require daily testing for serum potassium. If the BUN does not begin to fall or if the blood sugar starts to rise, more frequent evaluation may be necessary. A list of the routine laboratory tests is in Table 3. If the BUN and creatinine are not stable at acceptable levels or slowly declining during the first week, a transport evaluation using the dialysate and serum creatinine comparison (PET test) [35] is performed.

Table 3. Routine laboratory tests.

Every month:
BUN	Total protein
Creatinine	Albumin
Sodium	Alk. phosphatase
Potassium	Bilirubin
CO_2	SGOT
Calcium	Hct
Magnesium	Hgb

Every 6 months:
Residual renal function	Nerve conduction velocity
24 hour urine volume	Bone mineral density
Dialysate protein	Weekly KT/V urea and/or weekly
PET	Ccr

Yearly:
Chest X-ray	EKG
Parathyroid hormone (PTH)	

7.8. Medications

Medications taken by the patient before beginning dialysis are adjusted with the initiation of CAPD. These include diuretics, phosphate binding agents, and occasionally digitalis preparations. Patients are maintained on water soluble vitamins. Antihypertensive medications are generally tapered during the early phase of training. During this time, intravascular volume is contracted by ultrafiltration. Insulin dosage is adjusted to accommodate the increased glucose load. If the blood sugar is difficult to control or serum triglyceride levels climb over 500 mg/dl, initiation of insulin in the dialysis solution may be beneficial [36]. This latter route of administration increases the risk of contamination of the dialysate, and a specific and safe technique to add insulin to the bags is essential [33]. Rarely, a patient who is very compliant and lives a great distance from the center, will be instructed in the technique of adding antibiotics to the dialysis solution and the patient given a starter dose of cephalosporin. The patient is instructed to contact the unit by telephone before using this medication.

8. Complications

8.1. Catheter related complications

8.1.1. *Early (during training) catheter related complications*

8.1.1.1. *Surgical wound infection.* Although rare nowadays, infection of the incision is a serious complication, which could jeopardize the success of the catheter and/or the method. Usually, the responsible organisms are *staph aureus* and *pseudomonas* species. Contamination can be prevented by strict adherence to sterile precautions, control of bleeding and the use of prophylactic antibiotics.

8.1.1.2. *Visceral trauma or perforation.* Infrequently, operators have perforated or injured large and small bowel, mesenteric arteries, aorta, urinary bladder and other abdominal viscera during blind catheter insertion but rarely during the open surgical technique. One should avoid forceful insertion against intra-abdominal resistance.

8.1.1.3. *Bloody effluent.* This rare complication is due chiefly to incomplete hemostasis. The origin of bleeding is typically the anterior abdominal wall. In addition, lysed peritoneal adhesions from previous surgery could cause intra-abdominal bleeding. Intraperitoneal heparin (500–1000 u/L of dialysate) helps to prevent clot formation and subsequent catheter obstruction. Several in and out exchanges of unwarmed dialysis solution usually clear the dialysate of blood.

8.1.1.4. *Abdominal Pain.* Diffuse or local abdominal pain and tenderness around the incision area immediately after catheter implantation is of minor significance, and can be controlled with simple analgesics. Three to four per cent of patients have pain over the perineal area, in the rectum or the urinary bladder [37], which is due to pressure from the intra-abdominal segment of the catheter on the organs of the minor pelvis: usually, it passes off spontaneously 1–2 weeks after implantation. If the pain is severe or lasts longer, the attending physician should verify radiologically the position of the catheter and then move it by using a trocar or during laparotomy or peritoneoscopy. Localized outflow pain usually indicates that the catheter is trapped in the omentum. Low or high dialysate temperatures may induce diffuse abdominal pain; a temperature of 37°C is recommended.

Occasionally, the jetting of the fluid against an abdominal organ during inflow or low dialysate acidity may cause abdominal pain, which can be relieved by relocation of the catheter and elevation of the pH with sodium bicarbonate (5–25 mEq/L) [38].

8.1.1.5. *Reflex ileus.* Following catheter insertion, reflex ileus is common but rarely persists beyond 24 to 36 hours.

8.1.1.6. *Dialysate leakage (early).* Early pericatheter leakage of the dialysis fluid occurs in about 7% to 29% of catheters placed through the midline. The incidence is much lower (6.5%) with the more commonly used paramedian insertion [37–39]. Risk factors for leakage are obesity, diabetes mellitus, age over 60 years, multiparity, chronic use of steroids and previous abdominal operation including previous catheter insertion [37–41]. Clinically, leakage presents as a discharge of clear dialysate around the catheter at its exit-site or as a localized swelling secondary to infiltration of the subcutaneous tissue of the anterior abdominal wall, or as a genital swelling. Early leakage can be managed by temporary discontinuation of CAPD, substitution with IPD or NIPD with small volumes in the supine position, or temporary hemodialysis for 1 to 2 weeks [41].

8.1.1.7. *Wound hematoma.* The main reasons for the development of hematoma over the incision and in the subcutaneous tunnel are bleeding diathesis, hypertension and poor surgical technique. Hematomas predispose to delayed healing, infection and early dialysate leakage.

8.1.1.8. *Catheter malfunction (early and late).* Malfunction is common with chronic peritoneal catheters [37, 42–44] and it presents as a one-way or two-way obstruction. The former is present when peritoneal dialysis fluid flows easily into the peritoneal cavity, but its outflow is slow (partial obstruction) or absent. In two-way obstruction, peritoneal dialysis fluid does not flow in or out of the cavity (complete obstruction). The overall incidence of malfunction during and after catheter insertion (break-in period) is approximately 15–20% of implanted catheters [37, 42]. The main causes of such malfunction are a) obstruction and b) dislodgement (Table 4).

a) *Catheter obstruction.* Obstruction during the early postoperative period usually is due to blood or fibrin clots in the catheter lumen, which may resolve within a few days. Clots, mainly of fibrin, also are seen after the training period, particularly following episodes of peritonitis [45]. After peritonitis, tissue debris and adhesions may also obstruct the catheter. Adhesions alone are an infrequent cause of malfunction, but when they occur produce one-way obstruction and are usually seen in patients with previous abdominal operations. Frequently omentum wrapping itself around the intraperitoneal segment will produce catheter obstruction and dislodgement [43, 44]. This complication is seen more frequently with the straight type of Tenckhoff catheter than with the coiled and the Toronto Western types [46–48]. Because of this, some centers perform routine partial or total omentectomy when they insert straight Tenckhoff catheters [49]. A similar but unusual cause of partial or complete obstruction is the encasement of the catheter by the fallopian tube fimbriae [50–53]. Distention of a loop of the sigmoid colon, usually associated with constipation, frequently may cause slow or incomplete drainage.

Kinking of the intramural segment of the catheter commonly is due to poor insertion technique, particularly when the subcutaneous tunnel is directed downwards. However kinking occurs more frequently when the intra-abdominal segment of the catheter becomes involved with bowel or omentum. Finally, intraluminal lithiasis produced catheter obstruction in one patient [54].

b) *Catheter dislodgement.* Dislodgement of the catheter tip may reflect incorrect placement or most commonly pulling away secondary to omental wrapping [43, 47].

8.1.1.9. *Management of catheter malfunction.* The correct management of these malfunctions depends upon the cause, the timing in relation to catheter insertion and the mode of presentation i.e., one- or two-way obstruction. One should always exclude a functional cause of obstruction (constipation or bowel-loop distension) before looking for a mechanical cause [46]. Constipation responds readily to bowel stimulation by enema or an oral laxative. If such measures do not re-establish catheter function, the catheter position should be checked on a plain film of the abdomen (posterior-anterior and lateral views). If the catheter is in the true pelvis, do a cannulogram to determine the cause of the malfunction. Usually two-way obstruction is due to an intraluminal blood clot (early) or a fibrin clot (usually a late complication, particularly after peritonitis). Clots can be dislodged by forceful irrigation ("Flush") with a syringe containing 20 ml of normal saline with 500–1000 units of heparin [55]. Alternatively, one can apply manual pressure to a dialysis bag containing heparin, 500–1000 u/L [8]. Also fibrinolytic agents

Table 4. Causes of catheter malfunction.

A. Obstruction
   - blood clot
   - fibrin clot
   - kinking
   - tissue debris
   - adhesions
   - omentum
   - fallopian tube fimbriae
   - constipation
   - bowel loop
   - lithiasis
B. Dislodgement (migration, malposition, displacement)
   - incorrect placement including an insertion site that is disproportionally low in relation to catheter's IP segment length
   - resilience forces of silicone rubber
   - wrapping and pulling by omentum

such as streptokinase or urokinase [56–60] can be infused into the lumen. If irrigation fails, one may try to remove the clot using the Italian corkscrew [43] and/or the endoscopy brush [61]. If these measures fail, an open procedure is required.

Sudden two-way obstruction usually is due to kinking of the intramural or intra-abdominal segment of the catheter. Two-way obstruction of insidious onset after episodes of peritonitis may reflect loculation of the catheter by adhesions or omental wrapping. Irrespective of its ultimate position, malfunction associated with refractory catheter migration calls for surgical repositioning or replacement. Obviously, a malpositioned but well-functioning catheter requires no response.

8.1.2. *Late (or chronic) catheter related complications*

8.1.2.1. *Exit-site and tunnel infection.* "Tunnel" refers to the catheter's pathway from the skin through the subcutaneous fat and muscle to the peritoneal cuff. In double-cuff catheters, the tunnel is the area between the two cuffs. A non-infected (normal) exit-site should be clean, dry, painless and not inflamed.

To date, we do not have a universally accepted definition of exit-site infection (ESI). Most investigators define ESI by redness and/or skin induration or purulent discharge from the exit-site and the presence of exuberant granulation tissue (proud flesh) [46, 52–64, 67]. Formation of a crust around the exit-site may not indicate infection. Positive cultures from the exit site in the absence of inflammation do not indicate infection. The minimum (border to border) size of erythema constituting an infection is said to range from 4 to 13 mm [46, 64]. These infections are widely recognized as significant complications of peritoneal dialysis.

Exit-site infection is unpredictable and may develop at any time during CAPD and tends to be prolonged, chronic or recurrent. Both exit-site and tunnel infections are major causes of morbidity among CAPD patients because they lead to recurrent peritonitis, catheter failure and prolonged hospitalization.

According to the USA CAPD Registry the three-year catheter survival varies from 6 to 36%. Eight to 39% of catheters are removed because of exit or tunnel infection [65]. The proportion of PD patients transferred to HD each year parallels catheter loss rates, which in turn appear to be related to exit-site infection rather than to peritonitis rates [66]. A new implantation technique in which the external catheter segment is implanted under the skin for 4–8 weeks prior to exposure may allow better cuff healing and reduce tunnel infections [68]. Dasgupta reported the absence of bacterial biofilm on this catheter in opposition of the presence of this biofilm on other catheters.

With the recent reduction in peritonitis following the introduction of the various forms of the disconnect system, exit-site and tunnel infections have become the primary infectious complications of peritoneal dialysis [64, 67].

Some of the risk factors which may predispose to ESI include peritoneal dialysate leak, and excessive movement of the catheter such as pulling and twisting during bag exchange. Other factors include a tight tunnel and pressure necrosis caused by constricting sutures [64]. Also some workers have observed that nasal carriage of *staph aureus* is associated with a higher incidence of ESI [69–72]. A multicenter study in seven European hospitals showed that 77% of diabetics and 36% of non-diabetic patients on CAPD were persistent nasal carriers of *staph aureus* and that these carriers had a four fold higher risk of developing an ESI. Twenty-four of 34 ESIs were caused by *s. aureus* and 85% of these infections were caused by the same strain of *s. aureus* as that found at the nares [72]. Twardowski *et al.* [73] have disputed these findings. In a recent study Boelaert *et al.* [74] have found that nasal Mupirocin ointment decreases the incidence of *staph aureus* bacteraemias in hemodialysis patients. Regarding CAPD a large, randomized, placebo-controlled multicenter trial is underway in Europe to study the effect of intranasal mupirocin ointment on nasal carriage and the incidence of ESI. Until the results of this study become known, eradication of nasal *s. aureus* using naseptin or mupirocin ointments or oral quinolones and clindamycin remains empirical [46].

S. aureus is responsible for 25–85% of ESI while multiple organisms, including *s. aureus*, are isolated from 16–35% of the patients [67]. Other microorganisms that have been isolated include enteric gram negative (7–14%), s. epidermidis (5–14%), pseudomonas aeruginosa (8–12%) and fungi (1–3%). Finally, 7 to 11% of patients with ESI have negative exit-site cultures [67].

Exit-site infection rates vary widely from 0.05 episodes per patient year [75] to 1.02 episodes per patient year [76]. Apparently this discrepancy reflects mainly the disagreement on the definition of exit-site infection, and, to a lesser degree, a real variation in infection rates among the various centers and the applied protocols of exit-site care.

Exit-site infection is seen with all types of permanent peritoneal catheters in use today [63]. Three prospective studies by Kim [77], Diaz-Buxo [78] and Mitwalli [79] found no difference in infection rates between single- and double-cuff catheters. However, in a retrospective study in 395 patients, tunnel infections were almost three times more frequent with single-cuff than with double-cuff catheters [80]. According to the USRDS 1992 Annual Data Report [81] the relative peritonitis risk was significantly increased for single-cuff versus double-cuff catheters ($RR = 1.20$, $p = 0.01$). In a retrospective analysis of swan-neck catheters which are characterized by a downward directed exit, Twardowski et al. found these catheters to have a tendency for fewer infections than with other catheters [82].

In a retrospective study Burkart et al. found no overall difference in ESI rates in 96 patients on disconnect versus 60 patients on non-disconnect systems, despite a reduction in peritonitis rates with the disconnect systems [83].

Long-term exit-site care may be based upon cleansing with hydrogen peroxide in combination with soap or povidone iodine scrub [84], cleansing with povidone iodine alone [85, 86] and cleansing with soap and water [45, 87].

In a recent randomized multicenter trial Luzar et al. [88] found that the group of patients using povidone iodine and sterile nonocclusive dressing 2 to 3 times weekly, had a significantly lower rate of ESI than the group using nondisinfectant soap and water to cleanse the exit-site daily (0.27 episodes/patients year versus 0.71, $p \sim 0.0183$).

There is no agreement concerning when patients can start daily showering and cleaning of the exit-site. Some workers advocate two and others up to eight weeks after implantation. Usually swimming in the ocean or chlorinated swimming pools is permitted 4–8 weeks after catheter implantation [46].

Regarding treatment of an exit-site infection, erythema alone may be treated with topical chlorhexidine, mupirocin or dilute hydrogen peroxide. Purulent drainage with gram-positive organisms requires a first-generation oral cephalosporin, penicillinase- resistant penicillin or vancomycin IV or IP. Also oral rifampin could be given in persistent infections. For gram negative organisms, ciprofloxacin is recommended for adults and ceftazidime for children. Usually, the recommended duration of therapy is 2–4 weeks. In patients with chronic ESI without peritonitis, longer antibiotic treatment could be considered. For pseudomonas or fungal infections associated with peritonitis the treatment of choice is early catheter removal. The new catheter could be implanted in the opposite side of the abdomen at least two weeks following removal of the infected catheter. In the absence of peritonitis, one might consider simultaneous catheter replacement.

When ESI is associated with tunnel infection, consider deroofing of the tunnel and removal (shaving) of the external cuff, if other efforts are unsuccessful. However, in many cases infection progresses and ultimately the catheter must be replaced.

Currently we have no hard evidence that supports the use of prophylactic antibiotics to reduce ESI or tunnel infections. In one study, however, in 64 patients, who were assigned randomly to receive either rifampin (300 mg twice daily for five days every three months), or no treatment, the rifampin treated patients had a significantly lower ESI rate (0.26 versus 0.93 episodes per patient year) [89].

8.1.2.2. *Cuff extrusion.* A major cause of cuff extrusion is the resilience of the silicon rubber which directs the catheter to assume its original shape. Infection, another important cause of such extrusion is discussed under ESI (Chapter 9).

8.1.2.3. *Dialysate leakage (late).* While external leakage develops early after implantation, subcutaneous leakage may develop at any time. When the site of dialysate leakage is unknown, one may do computed tomography after infusion of 2L of dialysate containing a radio contrast material or isotope scanning, to identify the source of the leak [90, 91]. Management of the late leakage is similar to that described for early leakage. However most late leakages are refractory to conservative treatment and require surgical repair [43, 44].

8.1.2.4. *Various other abdominal events in CAPD patients.* In addition to catheter-related complications and to those related to the presence of dialysate in the peritoneal cavity, CAPD patients develop the same abdominal events as those encountered in the general population. Some clues to a surgical emergency in a CAPD patient with a typical "acute abdomen" are: localized abdominal pain and tenderness, bowel-loop dilatation and an unusual increase in free intraperitoneal air on x-ray; mixed flora on Gram stain or culture of dialysate;

refractory peritonitis high peritoneal fluid amylase; and hemoperitoneum with measurable hematocrit [92].

8.2. Complications related to the presence of dialysate in the peritoneal cavity

The pressure in the empty peritoneal cavity varies from 0.5 to 1.5 cm H_2O [93]. With the dialysate volumes used in current clinical practice, intra-abdominal pressures range between 2 to 10 cm H_2O. In patients using 3-liter exchanges, Twardowski et al. [94] have demonstrated pressures as high as 14 cm H_2O. Other factors affecting the intra-abdominal pressure are body weight, abdominal girth, body mass index and age. Also activities such as walking, coughing, straining and even simple postural changes increase intra-abdominal pressure; it is higher in the sitting position [94]. Hylander et al. [95] have found that elevated intra-abdominal pressures do not produce a significant increase in intragastric or lower-esophageal-sphincter pressures and peristalsis.

Many of the complications described in this section are consequences of increased intra-abdominal pressure.

8.2.1. Hernias

Many workers have estimated that between 10 and 25 percent of the CAPD population have hernias [96–99]. Predisposing factors for their development are old age, female sex, multiparity, obesity, previous hernia repair and early pericatheter dialysate leakage [96, 99]. The literature contains descriptions of many types of hernias. Bargman, in a recent review [100] reports the following types of hernias in patients on peritoneal dialysis: inguinal, umbilical, catheter incision and exit-site, ventral, epigastric, other incisional, cystocele, enterocele, foramen of Morgani, Richter's, Spigelian and obturator. The most common types of hernias are inquinal, catheter incision, and umbilical. These are followed by other incisional sites and ventral hernias. These all represent sites of structural weakness, particularly under the influence of constantly increased intra-abdominal pressure. Herniation is more common after a midline incision than after paramedian incision [101]. Bowel incarceration and strangulation, which can mimic peritonitis, is a risk in all hernias particularly the smaller ones.

If they are small, hernias should be repaired. Large hernias can be observed and are repaired if they are seen to be expanding. Following repair, patients can be started on CAPD after 2–4 weeks. In the interval they are managed on intermittent peritoneal dialysis with small volumes or on hemodialysis.

8.2.2. Abdominal wall and genital edema

This distressing complication which may develop in 10% of CAPD patients [100, 102, 103], has been attributed to two different mechanisms [103]. Firstly, through defects in the peritoneum as at the catheter insertion site or a previous incision or hernia, the dialysate, facilitated by the increased intra-abdominal pressure, may dissect into the soft tissues of the anterior abdominal wall. There it can produce abdominal wall edema and also track inferiorly to produce genital edema. Secondly, dialysate can flow through a patent *processus vaginalis* into the *tunica vaginalis* and present as hydrocele or, dissecting through the *tunica vaginalis* may appear as scrotal or labial edema.

Abdominal wall edema should be suspected in the presence of decreased effluent volume, increased abdominal girth and body weight especially in the absence of edema elsewhere. The differential diagnosis of genital edema includes hydrocele, indirect hernia and scrotal edema.

Nuclear medicine and radiologic imaging may be helpful in the diagnosis of abdominal wall and genital edema or subclinical hernias. After scintigraphy of the lower abdominal and genital areas following the intraperitoneal introduction of radioisotope, several investigators have succeeded in demonstrating inguinal and umbilical hernias [102, 104]. Computerized tomographic scanning using contrast medium (diatrizoate meglumine 100 ml) instilled into the peritoneal cavity with 2L of dialysate is more sensitive in identifying peritoneal leaks [105–109].

For small leaks the initial therapeutic approach should be conservative, that is bed rest and methods to lower intra-abdominal pressure. Several days of small-volume dialysis in the supine position may help to seal small tears or defects in the peritoneum. If not, or if the edema recurs, CAPD should be discontinued and the patient converted to temporary hemodialysis for 4 to 6 weeks. Persisting edema requires surgical correction. Abraham et al. described 18 patients with genital edema; in 13, the causes were repaired surgically and, in five, the edema responded to temporary cessation of CAPD [110]. With large hernias the initial approach should be surgical repair of the underlying defect.

8.2.3. *Hemoperitoneum*

Hemoperitoneum is an infrequent and usually benign and transient complication of CAPD [111, 112]. As little as 2 ml of blood can make 1L of dialysate appear "blood tinged" [113]. Thus, occult intraperitoneal bleeding is readily apparent in CAPD patients but is diagnosed rarely in those not on peritoneal dialysis [114].

Peritoneal bleeding has been noted after extracorporeal lithotripsy in a CAPD patient [115]. Hemoperitoneum may occur at any time during CAPD and the association of hemoperitoneum with menstruation is well known [111, 116]. In a recent review by Greenberg *et al.*, 64% of the episodes of hemoperitoneum in women of childbearing age were related to menses or ovulation [112]. The basic mechanisms of hemoperitoneum during menstruation, which is self-limited and of little clinical consequence, is retrograde menstruation and endometriosis [114]. Other causes of hemoperitoneum include colonoscopy [117] catheter repositioning, femoral hematoma, minor abdominal trauma and increased physical activity, idiopathic thrombocytopenic purpura, and pancytopenia [112]. Finally in a few cases no cause is found [112]. It should be emphasized that minor intraperitoneal bleeding may accompany any type of intra-abdominal lesion or a lesion in adjacent extraperitoneal structures, e.g., polycystic kidney disease with intracystic bleeding [118], renal angiomyolipoma [119], cholecystitis, pancreatitis and sclerosing peritonitis [112, 120]. Finally in rare cases significant bleeding may require immediate intervention in the presence of ruptured ovarian cyst [112], post pelvic irradiation [121] ruptured spleen [122], calcific peritonitis [120] renal carcinoma [123], iliopsoas hematoma [124] post-peritonitis, adhesions and post-catheter placement [112].

8.2.4. *Hydrothorax*

Large pleural effusions are a rare complication of CAPD. Its true incidence is unknown. Bargman [100] reviewed 70 cases from the literature up to 1993 but this number did not include 50 additional cases from Japan [125]. The latter a collaborative study of 161 Japanese centers, found the incidence of hydrothorax to be 1.6% (50 of 3195 patients). While, in most series [100], most of those who develop hydrothorax are women, only 23/50 (46%) of the Japanese patients were female. The interval between the onset of CAPD and development of hydrothorax ranges from the first dialysis exchange to 8 years later.

Clinical presentation of the hydrothorax varies from asymptomatic pleural effusion found accidentally on a chest radiograph to acute, life-threatening, respiratory failure. Thirty-seven of the 50 Japanese patients developed dyspnea but the remaining 13 (36%) had no symptoms. In a CAPD patient with hydrothorax, dyspnea may be misinterpreted as a symptom of congestive heart failure; then, it may be treated with more hypertonic solutions, which will aggravate the pleural effusion by increasing the ultrafiltration and thus the intraperitoneal volume and pressure [100].

Approximately 90% of hydrothoraces occur on the right side [100, 125–127], probably because the defects are found mainly in the tendinous part of the hemidiaphragm [128]. The heart and pericardium cover the left-sided defects [100].

Apparently the fluid traverses the diaphragm *via* the diaphragmatic lymphatics or through diaphragmatic defects. Also areas have been observed where the pleura is lifted off the diaphragm forming "bleds" or blisters [129]. Under increased intra-abdominal pressure, dialysate could cause these defects to rupture and allow fluid to enter the thoracic cavity [100].

Analysis of the pleural fluid reveals a transudate (protein < 3 g/dl) that has a low concentration of lactate dehydrogenase and a high concentration of glucose consistent with dialysate. Intraperitoneal instillation of methylene blue should be avoided because it is unreliable and also because it may produce chemical peritonitis [130]. For confirmation of the leak, technetium 99m-tagged macro-aggregated albumin, sulphur colloid or human albumin in small doses (3–5 mCi) is added to 2L dialysate bags and instilled in the peritoneal cavity. In the presence of a pleuroperitoneal communication, radioactivity will be detected in the thorax [131–133]. Experience with computed tomography is limited using the radiocontrast agent, iopamidol [134]. The attending physician also should rule out other causes of hydrothorax, such as cardiac failure, inflammatory, infectious and malignant disease.

Namoto *et al.* [125] reported that interruption of CAPD alone or in combination with pleurodesis was successful in resolving hydrothorax in over 50% of their patients; the remaining 23 (46%) were transferred to HD permanently.

In recurring cases of hydrothorax, pleurodesis with talc [127], tetracycline [127, 130], fibrin adhesive [135] or autologous blood [136] has been applied with varying success. Alternatively one may

8.2.5. Respiratory dysfunction

At the initiation of CAPD, elevation of the diaphragm by the dialysate leads, a) to a decrease in total lung capacity (TLC) and functional residual capacity (FRC) [138, 139], b) interferes with gas exchange leading to ventilation-perfusion mismatch and arterial hypoxemia [139, 140], c) theoretically can predispose to atelectasis and pneumonia [141], although these complications rarely are seen in clinical practice [139]. However, later in the course of CAPD some adjustment takes place such as redistribution of blood toward the better ventilated upper segments of the lungs. Whatever the cause, the FRC improves and the arterial saturation may return to normal with time [138, 142].

Rebuck [143] suggests that, in the presence of intraperitoneal fluid, diaphragmatic contractility may increase thus, compensating for the effect of diminished lung volumes.

Airways resistance is not affected in patients with chronic obstructive pulmonary disease undergoing CAPD. Peritoneal dialysis need not be withheld from these patients [139, 144].

8.2.6. Back pain

Low back pain in CAPD patients may be due to poor muscle tone, poor posture and low exercise tolerance, degenerative or metabolic bone disease of the spine, arthritis of the hip or knee, neuropathy, myopathy and abdominal hernias. Also dialysis fluid alters spinal mechanics by increasing the intra-abdominal volume, pulling forward the centre of gravity, and aggravating back strain by increasing lumbar lordosis [145]. Individually tailored exercise programs, back education and a special abdominal support may help in the management of low back pain. When these measures fail, the patient may have to convert to night-time peritoneal dialysis [100].

8.3. Ultrafiltration failure in CAPD

Ultrafiltration (UF) failure in PD Patients was first described in 1981 by Oreopoulos et al. [146] in Canada and by Faller and Marichal in Europe [147]. Usually when UF failure develops, solute transport is preserved [146]; however in a smaller percentage of patients, UF failure is accompanied by impairment of such transport due to extensive peritoneal adhesions or sclerosing encapsulating peritonitis [148]. Patients, who develop UF failure often exhibit high peritoneal solute permeability at the initiation of CAPD [149].

UF failure may be associated with the following clinical conditions:

(a) Peritonitis. A transient period of UF failure follows almost every episode of peritonitis due chiefly to rapid glucose absorption and an increase in lymphatic absorption [150–152].
(b) Sclerosing encapsulating peritonitis [153–155].
(c) Long-term CAPD. UF failure in long-term CAPD almost always is associated with high solute transport [156–160]. Failure of UF is responsible for 8–14% of those who fail CAPD [159, 160].

Manoeuvres to improve UF in PD include short dwell times and "peritoneal rest" with discontinuation of CAPD for 3–6 months [159, 160]. Also, phosphatidylcholine, Verapamil and Amphotericin B have been used experimentally in the treatment of UF failure in CAPD. Phosphatidylcholine is the main constituent of the surface active material found in the effluent of CAPD patients [161]. Probably its action is related to its surface-active properties and/or its cholinergic effect which decreases lymphatic absorption [162]. Intraperitoneal administration of phosphatidylcholine increases UF in patients with UF failure [163] and in those with normal UF [164, 165]. In some studies oral administration of this surfactant had no effect [166, 167] but it was effective in others [163, 168]. Chronic oral administration of verapamil is said to improve UF in CAPD patients [169]. Finally, amphotericin B intraperitoneally increases net UF in rabbits but it is rarely used in humans because it provokes chemical peritonitis [170].

8.4. Sclerosing encapsulating peritonitis and peritoneal calcification

Sclerosing encapsulating peritonitis (SEP) is a serious, infrequent, lethal complication of CAPD that is characterized by non-specific symptoms and signs such as anorexia, nausea, vomiting, malnutrition (cachexia) abdominal pain, intermittent bowel obstruction, decreased ultrafiltration and solute clearance and bloody ascites. "Sclerosing" implies formation of dense collagenous tissue. "Encapsulating" refers to the cocooning of the small bowel by a sheath of new fibrous tissue. "Peritonitis" implies mononuclear inflammatory infiltration of this new tissue [171].

This dramatic syndrome has been reported mainly from European centers [153, 154, 172–175] but clusters of cases also have been reported from Australia [176] and Hong Kong [177] and sporadic cases from the United States [178, 179]. Although a few workers have reported that SEP may regress after early discontinuation of CAPD [180], most believe that it is a diffuse, progressive condition that does not regress after such cessation. This complication has appeared several to many months after transfer to HD or renal transplantation [177].

The cause of sclerosing peritonitis is unknown but it seems that multiple causal agents, acting simultaneously or sequentially, trigger and perpetuate the inflammatory process that leads to peritoneal fibrosis [181]. Postulated cause of this syndrome include acetate containing dialysate, recurrent or severe peritonitis, formaldehyde, chlorhexidine, plastic particles, interleukin-1 production, hypertonic dialysate and beta-blockers [114]. The common denominator among these postulated causes is that they induce irritation of the mesothelial layer leading to serositis. Mesothelial loss and exposure of the fibroblasts to the constituents of the dialysis solution predisposes to fibrogenesis within the peritoneum [171]. The end result may be a spectrum of alterations ranging from peritoneal opacification through a "tanned peritoneum" syndrome to sclerosing encapsulating peritonitis [182].

The mortality of SEP is high ranging from 50% to over 90% [177, 178]. Current medical treatment and surgical release of small bowel obstruction have not been proved to be satisfactory [183]. Obviously prevention is more important than treatment. Even though the overall incidence of SEP is showing a marked decline during the last five years, the best prevention is still careful and sensible treatment of severe peritoneal damage [182]. The chief measures of prevention are, 1) early removal of catheter in severe peritonitis – a condition in which the mesothelium no longer can protect the peritoneal surface effectively, 2) reduction in the use of hypertonic dialysate to avoid exposure of the naked stroma to the effects of glucose and 3) resting the peritoneum, if feasible, to allow remesothelialization [182].

Peritoneal calcification is a rare complication of long-term CAPD; only six instances have been reported in the literature [122, 184, 185]. This complication which presents with persistent abdominal pain, irregular bowel movements, bloody effluent and decreased ultrafiltration, is identified by simple abdominal radiographs ("flat plates") and computed tomography. At laparotomy the parietal and visceral peritoneum is thickened, fibrosed and covered by numerous hard and brittle calcified plaques, densely adherent to the underlying tissues. This complication is associated with recurrent peritonitis [120, 184] hyperphosphatemia, hypercalcemia, acetate-containing dialysate [120], hyperparathyroidism [120, 184] and even the hypoparathyroid state [185].

8.5. Nutritional and metabolic complications

8.5.1. *Carbohydrate metabolism*

During CAPD the approximately 60–80% of dialysate glucose absorbed via the peritoneum accounts for an average 100–150 g/day (500–800 Kcal/day) or 30–40% of the total energy intake. Continuous absorption of glucose results in increased insulin secretion and increased plasma insulin levels. The last reflects peripheral insulin resistance – the hallmark of abnormal carbohydrate metabolism is chronic renal failure. During an oral glucose tolerance test in CAPD patients blood glucose, insulin and growth-hormone curves resemble those observed in a typical form of mild maturity onset diabetes [186]. Prospective studies show that this carbohydrate intolerance does not deteriorate over the first [187, 188] or six [189] years of CAPD therapy. However, after initiation of CAPD, a few patients (approximately 5%) will develop diabetes *de novo*.

8.5.2. *Lipid abnormalities*

Dyslipoproteinemia in CAPD, which arises against a background of "uremic dyslipoproteinemia", is aggravated by the continuous absorption of glucose through the peritoneum; it appears to be different in many ways from the dyslipoproteinemia of hemodialysis [190].

Several studies have demonstrated that CAPD induces hyperlipidemia which becomes apparent within the first few months of therapy [191–195]. Approximately 50–70% of CAPD patients will develop hypertriglyceridemia and about 30% have high total cholesterol levels [192, 194, 195].

Decreased HDL cholesterol, elevated LDL and VLDL cholesterol, and the hypertriglyceridemia observed in CAPD resemble Frederickson's types III and IV patterns on electrophoresis [191–193, 195]. Apolipoprotein A-I and A-II levels are low or normal [196–198] probably because their small size allows increased peritoneal loss. It is possible that such losses may contribute to the lower HDL levels found in CAPD. Apolipoprotein A-IV is elevated, indicating impaired reversed cholesterol transport mechanisms [199]. Also in many CAPD patients apolipoprotein-B is elevated [200–202] probably because of its high molecular weight and consequent low peritoneal clearance [188]. A further explanation of the hypertriglyceridemia of CAPD may be the decreased lipoprotein-lipase activity that decreases the removal of circulating triglycerides [203]. None has explained the association of hypertriglyceridemia and low serum carnitine levels in CAPD patients.

In many patients the aggravation of hyperlipoproteinemia in CAPD appears to be transitory but still it may induce or accelerate already-established atherosclerosis [193, 195]. However, we need further clarification concerning the long-term effects of CAPD dyslipoproteinemia on systemic atherosclerotic vascular disease and on peritoneal vasculature. Uremic dyslipoproteinemia can be managed by non-pharmacological or by pharmacological means. Non-pharmacological therapy includes dietary advice concerning both weight reduction and reduction of saturated fats and carbohydrates, regular physical exercise, cessation of smoking and restriction of alcohol intake [204]. The preservation of residual renal function and water restriction help to decrease the need for hypertonic solutions and thus avoid excessive glucose absorption.

Until recently older antihyperlipidemic agents have been unsuccessful but newer agents such as the HMG CoA reductase inhibitors are promising. However long-term studies are required to assess their impact on atherosclerosis.

8.5.3. Malnutrition

During the first year of therapy net anabolism in CAPD patients is indicated by several signs: namely true weight gain, slight improvement in anthropometric parameters, rise in serum protein levels and an increase in hemoglobin levels. However, a large proportion of CAPD patients on long-term CAPD demonstrate signs of protein-energy malnutrition. As early as 1981 Williams et al. [205] pointed out that daily dietary protein and caloric intake and total body nitrogen (TBN) decrease significantly, with time on CAPD. Subsequently two other studies from the same center [206, 207] have shown similar results. Other studies have shown suppressed energy and protein intakes in children undergoing CAPD [208], a significant nitrogen depletion – 88.2% of normal in men and 87.5% in women on CAPD [209], and in non diabetic women on CAPD considerably smaller anthropometric measurements [210].

Using "subjective global assessment", Fenton et al. [211] found malnutrition in 18.1% of patients on CAPD for less than three months, compared to 41.6% on CAPD for longer than three months. Using the same method in a multicenter study conducted in 224 patients in six centers in Europe and North America, Young et al. [212], found that 18 (8%) patients were severely malnourished, 73 (32.6%) were mildly to moderately malnourished and the remaining 133 (59.4%) showed no evidence of malnutrition. Diabetics had a higher incidence of malnutrition (mild to moderate) than non-diabetics and females had a higher incidence than males. Loss of residual renal function correlated with muscle wasting and months on CAPD. It should be noted that the prevalence of malnutrition is similar in CAPD and in HD patients. In a cross-sectional study, Marckman recorded malnutrition in 56% of CAPD (9/16) and in 53% of HD (17/32) patients [213]. In a multicenter study comparing 609 HD and 138 CAPD patients, Nelson et al. [210] found no differences between the nutritional status in the two groups.

One can group the main causes of malnutrition in CAPD under three headings: 1) inadequate energy intake, 2) increased losses, and 3) increased utilization [214].

1) In uremics on CAPD inadequate nutrient intake is further aggravated by inadequate dialysis, constipation, nausea, vomiting and loss of appetite. Oreopoulos et al. [215] have shown that glucose has an anorectic effect in nonuremic rabbits. The presence of dialysate in the abdominal cavity does not affect food intake in CAPD patients [216], probably because the presence of dialysate in the abdomen does not effect intragastric pressures [95]. Generally patients on CAPD have a lower protein intake than those on HD [217] but indirect evidence suggests that CAPD patients may have lower average protein requirements than HD patients [218].

2) In CAPD the average peritoneal protein loss varies between 5 and 15 g/day [219–222]; though constant in the same patient, there is a large interindividual variation [219, 220]. During peritonitis, this amount may be increased by 50–100% [219, 221]. The major fraction of total dialysate protein is albumin [48–65%] but IgG accounts for 15%. Albumin losses average 5–6 g/day while the

serum albumin levels are at 3.5 g/dl. Total daily amino acid losses average 2.5 g [223] and range from 1.2 to 3.4 g/day. Despite these relatively large losses, total serum proteins are maintained at low normal levels (6.5 g/dl) even after prolonged periods on CAPD [224, 225].

Protein catabolic factors in CAPD include physical inactivity, low energy intake, metabolic acidosis, loss of metabolizing renal tissue, infections and cytokine release [226].

Underdialyzed CAPD patients may enter a vicious cycle of low protein-energy intake and enhanced protein catabolism, leading to progressive malnutrition, muscle wasting and increased morbidity and mortality [218].

8.5.3.1. Prevention and treatment of malnutrition in CAPD patients

It is important for the attending physician to identify those CAPD patients who are at particular risk for malnutrition and to monitor them carefully so as to intervene promptly and appropriately. Vulnerable patients are the elderly, those with poor dietary protein intake, a metabolic primary renal disease such as diabetes mellitus or amyloidosis, severe or prolonged peritonitis or other intercurrent catabolic illness and finally those undergoing surgery. Serum albumin level is an excellent predictor of death, hospitalization days, and technique failure [227, 228]. Many investigators have described a significant positive correlation between PCR and amount of dialysis measured by the clearance of urea (KT/V) [227–234]. This observation suggests that, in CAPD patients, underdialysis may be a primary and most important cause of malnutrition.

To maintain good nutrition in well-dialysed CAPD patients, one must supply nutrients adequate for the daily requirements and to cover peritoneal losses. The recommended daily dietary requirements for steady CAPD patients are: 1.2–1.3 g/kg of protein and 35–42 Kcal/kg as total energy [235]. However a malnourished CAPD patient requires more aggressive management. When underdialysis is present or is suspected, it should be corrected by increasing the number of daily exchanges and/or the volume of dialysate or by a change to hemodialysis. Metabolic acidosis should be corrected with sodium bicarbonate per os. The malnourished CAPD patient should be offered oral protein supplementation and, if these measures are not effective one should try parenteral nutrition or intraperitoneal amino acids.

8.5.3.2. Use of intraperitoneal amino acids.

An amino-acid solution is viewed as an ideal osmotic alternative for CAPD because it provides nutrients, could treat, or at least prevent, protein depletion and at the same time avoid glucose-induced side effects [191].

Following experiments in rabbits, investigators at Toronto Western Hospital [236] were the first to administer amino acids as a dialysis solution to CAPD patients. They showed that amino-acid-containing dialysis solutions remove solutes and exert ultrafiltration in a manner similar to glucose-containing solutions.

To date a number of publications from several centers [237–248] have described the effects of amino acid solutions administered intraperitoneally in CAPD patients, for periods varying from one to six months. When used over short periods (4 weeks) in malnourished CAPD patients [237–241] amino acid containing solutions can increase total body nitrogen, and induce a positive nitrogen balance and minor changes in plasma amino acids [237, 239, 241]. However serum albumin and other indices of nutritional status do not change significantly. Furthermore these patients had an increase in blood urea, a decrease in serum bicarbonate levels and (in one study) significant gastrointestinal complications [240].

Overall, evidence suggests that 1% amino-acid solutions are well tolerated, provide adequate dialysis and ultrafiltration and when used for relatively short periods (3–4 weeks) could induce a positive nitrogen balance in malnourished CAPD patients. However, the patients still face such problems as increased serum urea levels and a tendency towards acidosis. Cost is also an additional problem. In most studies, intraperitoneal administration of amino acids over long periods [242–248] have provided insignificant improvement in nutritional status of CAPD patients (these are reviewed in detail elsewhere in this book).

We need further studies to identify the ideal conditions of intraperitoneal administration of amino acids in malnourished CAPD patients over long periods. Points that need clarification are: optimal composition, timing of administration, its relation to oral energy intake, the role of induced acidosis and finally proper patient selection i.e., mildly or severely malnourished, post-peritonitis, diabetes etc. Moreover, further studies are needed to establish whether improved nutritional status will reduce morbidity and mortality in CAPD patients.

8.5.4. Vitamins

Varying amounts of some of the water-soluble vitamins are lost in the dialysate and unless these are replaced, CAPD patients may develop severe depletion syndromes. On the other hand overcorrection of the low serum vitamin levels may lead to hypervitaminosis.

A review of studies on the vitamin supplementation in CAPD patients [249] recommends the following:

– Supplements of vitamin B1 in a dose of 30–40 mg/day.
– Vitamin B6 at a dose of 10–15 mg/day
– Vitamin B12 in small amounts in patients on long-term CAPD.
– Vitamin C in a dose of no more than 100 mg/day.
– Folic acid probably at small doses of 0.5–1 mg/day.

Supplements of lipid-soluble vitamins A and E are not needed because their blood levels in CAPD patients are high. Requirements for Vitamin D, which vary widely, are discussed elsewhere in this book (Chapter 18).

8.6. Cardiovascular complications and blood pressure control

Approximately 50% of the deaths in HD or CAPD patients are associated with cardiovascular events [250]. Although pre-existing cardiac disease and/or associated risk factors can explain the high cardiovascular mortality, we cannot discount the effect of dialysis per se [251]. Use of the two-liter exchanges do not seem to impair venous return or cardiac function to any significant extent [252].

Heart disease in CAPD includes left ventricular hypertrophy, left atrial dilatation and pericardial thickening conditions that are found in about onehalf of the patients [253]. Pericardial effusion develops in about 5% of CAPD patients, a much smaller fraction than the one seen in HD patients [254]. Pericarditis also may be the result of viral infection [251]. The main factors underlying heart disease in CAPD patients are: hypertension, anemia, coronary-artery disease, diabetes, hyperlipidemia, uremic toxins, electrolyte disorders, fluid overload, malnutrition, infection, old age and smoking [251].

Hypertension is the primary cause of renal insufficiency in about 25% of ESRD patients and contributes to renal failure.

Anemia aggravates cardiac disease because of decreased blood supply to the myocardium. The heart which has usually diminished wall thickness from atherosclerosis and has a weakened myocardium and dilated chambers, has to cope with hyperdynamic circulation [251].

Hypertension and anemia are the most important and most correctable causes of impaired cardiac function. Both are better controlled in CAPD than in HD patients [255].

Hyperlipidemia is common in patients with renal failure and is present before dialysis begins [256]. In CAPD, glucose absorption has been correlated with weight gain and the increased triglyceride levels [257] which may contribute to accelerated atherosclerosis and ischemic heart disease [258].

Ventricular ectopy in CAPD patients may be related to cardiac ischemia and/or electrolyte abnormalities that usually are caused by increased levels of potassium, calcium or magnesium [252].

Chronic hypotension usually combined with orthostatic hypotension is not infrequent especially in the elderly [255, 259]. Inadequate reactivity of sympathetic system in the upright position and underestimation of patient's "dry weight" seem to be the most important factors in the development of orthostatic hypotension [260]. Finally, some workers have reported exacerbation of peripheral vascular disease in diabetic CAPD patients with pre-existing atherosclerotic changes of the peripheral arteries [255].

8.7. Anemia

As in other ESRD patients anemia in individuals treated with CAPD is due chiefly to decreased production of erythropoietin (EPO). Other contributing factors [261–263] are decreased red-bloodcell survival and low response to endogenous EPO.

Several workers have reported significant increase in hemoglobin levels during the first 3 to 6 months of CAPD [264–267]. This increase may be due to such factors as improved volume control leading to a decrease in plasma volume [264], and increased red cell mass as a result of improved erythropoiesis probably because of increased clearance of middle molecules [265, 267]. As a result, CAPD patients require fewer blood transfusions (0.34 units per month) compared to those in HD (0.602 units per month) [268, 269].

Also CAPD patients require smaller and less frequent doses of rHEPO than HD patients. In a large clinical study that included 57 dialysis centers, 65% of 4940 HD patients were treated with EPO compared to only 34% of 2028 CAPD patients

[270]. rHEPO commonly is administered by the subcutaneous route [271, 272].

8.8. Gastrointestinal complications

Before the start of CAPD, patients may complain of epigastric distress, anorexia, nausea and vomiting, which subside within a few days of initiation. Later in the course of CAPD patients may present with GI symptoms or signs that may be related to CAPD itself. The most important of these complaints is acute pancreatitis. Some investigators believe that dialysate may irritate the pancreas by its increased glucose concentration or because of toxic substances originating from the dialysate, the CAPD bags or the tubing [273, 274]. Also high triglyceride levels may also predispose to pancreatitis in CAPD patients [275]. However, Gupta et al. [276] found that the prevalence of acute pancreatitis in CAPD was no higher than in HD, suggesting that peritoneal dialysis *per se* is not a risk factor for this complication. During CAPD, increase in effluent amylase is highly suggestive of acute pancreatitis and this enzyme should be measured in each patient with severe or persistent unexplained peritonitis [273–277].

Intestinal perforation (usually colonic) occurs in CAPD patients with diverticulitis [278–282]. About 1.3–1.6% of PD population will have such perforation and it will be accompanied by peritonitis caused by multiple organisms, especially gram-negative bacteria and anaerobes [283].

Gallstones and cholecystitis are common among CAPD population. In fact, Nelson et al. found that 26 out of 114 CAPD patients (23%) had evidence of gallstones (by ultrasound) or a history of cholecystectomy [284]. Cholecystectomy either laparoscopic or percutaneous may be performed without interruption of peritoneal dialysis. Patients may have to be treated with intermittent peritoneal dialysis for 2–3 weeks before returning to CAPD.

8.9. Skeletoarticular complications

Long-term CAPD patients frequently develop such skeletoarticular complications as renal osteodystrophy and amyloidosis related disorders, both of which produce morbidity.

In most CAPD patients, bone biopsies show a low turnover disorder (osteomalacia and adynamic bone disease), or a high turnover disorder (hyperparathyroid bone disease-osteitis fibrosa) or a mixture of these two conditions [285].

Low bone turnover reflects the inability of osteoid to mineralise efficiently (osteomalacia) or to form bone (adynamic bone lesion). While osteomalacia is characterized by an increase in osteoid volume, adynamic or aplastic bone is characterized by a significant decrease in bone turnover without osteoid excess. Usually, this relatively new histological entity is associated with hypercalcemia and normal or low plasma levels of parathyroid hormone [286].

In particular, Malluche and Monier-Faugere [286] described adynamic bone in chronic dialysis patients after they had reviewed all bone biopsies performed in 1803 patients during the decade 1982 to 1991. The incidence of this entity had increased steadily up to 1991. In a group of 602 patients in whom the mode of dialysis could be established, these authors observed adynamic bone lesion in 16.8% of CAPD and 10.4% of HD patients. This difference, though not statistically significant, could not be explained by a difference in age, the number of diabetics or aluminum deposition. It is interesting that despite the decrease in the use of aluminum containing phosphate binders over the last few years approximately 60% of the patients had a positive stain for aluminum in their biopsies. This percentage was even higher (76%) in patients with adynamic bone.

Factors known to be associated with adynamic bone include aluminum accumulation, increased age, increased vascular calcification, diabetes and increased use of calcium carbonate [285–291]. Its pathogenesis is obscure. Adynamic bone may be more frequent in chronic CAPD patients than in HD patients; in a 2-year prospective study of 445 dialysis patients, Pei et al. [287] found a significantly lower prevalence of high-turnover bone disease among CAPD than HD patients (13% vs 44%). Aluminum bone lesion was found in 33% of HD and 22% of PD patients. Interestingly, adynamic bone lesion was recognized in almost one-half of PD patients while in HD patients its prevalence was 18%.

It seems that, as a complication, adynamic bone lesion has replaced high-turnover osteodystrophy in CAPD patients [287, 290, 291]. The mechanism responsible for this abnormal state may be a suppression of parathyroid hormone by an increase in serum levels of ionized calcium, secondary to the increased use of calcium salts (usually carbonate) as a phosphate binder, and the administration of calcitriol [289, 292].

The clinical consequences of adynamic bone are

unknown. Pei and his collaborators [287] believe that patients with this form of bone lesion have less bone pain and fewer pathological fractures than those with high-turnover bone disease and osteomalacia secondary to aluminum. However, long term damage resulting from this entity is not known [286].

8.10. Amyloidosis-related disorders

We have much to learn about dialysis-related amyloidosis in long-term dialysis patients and its relationship to such "rheumatic" manifestations as carpal tunnel syndrome, chronic synovitis, formation of bone cysts (usually in the wrists, hips and shoulders), as well as destructive arthropathy, usually involving the cervical region of the vertebral column [293]. Systemic and visceral amyloid involvement has also been reported [294, 295].

The incidence of dialysis-related amyloidosis increases progressively with time on dialysis and affects almost 80% of patients dialyzed for more than 15 years [296]. Nevertheless not all long-term dialysis patients develop amyloidosis; in contrast, some of them develop such manifestations relatively early [297].

Beta-2-microglobulin (β_2m), a polypeptide with a molecular weight of about 12,000 daltons which is the common chain of the HLA class I antigens [298] has been considered to be the precursor protein in amyloid formation [299]. Because there is no correlation between serum β_2m levels and the development of amyloidosis [300, 301] amyloidogenesis seems to require some additional factor(s) [302]. These factors are poorly defined although interest has focussed on macrophages and plasma-proteinase inhibitors [303–305].

Serum β_2m levels tend to be lower in CAPD patients than in HD [306–310] probably because they have greater residual renal function and remove β_2m more efficiently *via* the effluent [311].

It should be noticed, however, that serum β_2m levels are much higher than normal in both dialysis groups. In fact, these patients generate β_2m in the range of 1000 to 1500 mg/week [312]. Mean weekly removal of β_2m by CAPD is 240 mg and by the residual renal function about 150 mg [311]. As a result, CAPD does not remove enough β_2m to compensate for the daily β_2m production [311, 313]. The same is true for high-flux hemodialysis filters while conventional hemodialysis, which uses cuprophan, does not remove β_2m [311].

Amyloid-related complications are not unusual in long-term CAPD patients [314]. Carpal tunnel syndrome is found with the same frequency in both HD and CAPD patients. A high prevalence of arthralgias and synovitis that Chalmers *et al.* described in IPD patients in Canada probably was the result of β_2m amyloidosis [315].

Destructive spondyloarthropathy, such as that first described by Kuntz *et al.* [316] among patients on long term hemodialysis, also has been reported in a woman treated exclusively by CAPD for 13 years [317].

8.11. Urinary stones

Urinary calculi and their consequences (renal colic and the passing of stones) are common in chronic (> 6 months) HD or PD patients who have no history of renal stone disease and maintain a daily urinary output of more than 100 ml [318–323]. Most of these stones contain a proteinaceous substance – a matrix that seems to be derived from β_2-microglobulin, and calcium oxalate in various proportions [320–322]. Acquired cystic disease of the kidney in chronic dialysis patients probably predisposes to stone formation [324]. Oren *et al.* [322] found that 5.4% (10 of 186) of CAPD patients passed stones over a four-year period. None of these patients had nephrolithiasis as a primary renal disease. Most of the stones consisted of calcium oxalate mixed with protein matrix. The mean daily urine output of these stone formers was 335 ml and the calcium-oxalate activity product was in the metastable region in which spontaneous precipitation occurs. These authors suggest that treatment with calcitriol contributes to stone formation in CAPD patients, because they found a highly significant correlation between the dosage of this vitamin and urinary calcium concentration. Ozasa and Ota [325] have also stressed the importance of urine calcium in dialysis related stone formation and proposed that the association of β_2 microglobulin, lysozyme, serum-amyloid P component and glycosaminoglycans induces kidney stone formation, but only through a calcium mediated mechanism.

8.12. Pruritus

Uremic pruritus is encountered in 25 to 59% of CAPD patients. This symptom is more frequent in hemodialysis patients and especially in uremic patients before dialysis [326]. Frequently pruritus resolves spontaneously, occurs in paroxysms and is generalized or localized to the trunk or extremities. While some patients find pruritus tolerable, others find it to be a continuous curse. The latter patients cannot sleep and occasionally may become depressed and suicidal [327]. The etiology of uremic pruritus remains obscure but several factors present in uremia may create an environment that predisposes to pruritus. These factors include xerosis, elevated plasma levels of vitamin A, calcium, magnesium, phosphorus and PTH, peripheral neuropathy, mast cell and histamine involvement and allergic reactions. Most of the usual therapeutic approaches to pruritus help only a few patients [326]. The most effective current treatment seems to be phototherapy with ultraviolet B radiation [326, 328].

9. Patient and technique survival

9.1. CAPD versus HD

9.1.1 Patient survival

The only scientifically correct way to compare CAPD with HD is to do a long-term, prospective, randomized study that includes a large number of unselected randomly allocated patients. Such a study could answer the questions regarding the relative effectiveness of each of these alternative therapies [329, 330]. However, because of objective and ethical obstacles such a study has not been done and probably will not be done in the future [331]. As a result our knowledge concerning the morbidity, and patient and technique survival in CAPD *vs* HD is based on comparative studies that usually are retrospective and uncontrolled. The disadvantages of such studies are partially overcome by the large number of patients who have been followed for several years [332–339]. However, because of differences in the criteria used to select patients for treatment, the results of these studies vary widely [331]. In most European studies, CAPD patients are older than those on HD and a greater proportion of them have diabetes and other comorbid conditions [333, 334, 339]. Data from USA however showed that in that country, CAPD patients are younger and more of them have diabetes, while HD patients have a greater number of comorbid conditions [332, 338].

One may distinguish the risk of death due to the therapeutic method from other risk factors by using the Cox model of regression analysis [340]. Recently Vonesh [341] has explained the meaning of the relative risk of death in this model. Using this model, several studies in Europe and USA have demonstrated that the risk of death due to the method of treatment did not differ significantly between CAPD and HD patients [331–335, 342–344] (Table 5).

The Michigan Registry Study of 1990 that included 2754 patients [344] showed a significant increase in annual death rate (6% per year) among in-center HD patients, who were treated between 1980 to 1987, while during the same period there was a small, though not statistically significant, decline in CAPD death rate (1% per year). The 1992 report of the same registry [345], which included 4288 patients, showed that young non-diabetic CAPD patients with glomerulonephritis as their primary renal disease had a lower mortality rate than those on HD. Those who had nephrosclerosis and other primary causes of ESRD displayed no difference in mortality on the two treatment modes.

Many European studies, when reporting on patient survival with both modalities, gave similar survival results up to the 6th year despite their preferential use of CAPD among high-risk patients [332, 337, 342, 343, 346]. Although elderly patients treated with CAPD have more comorbid conditions at the onset of therapy their survival is similar to those on HD [347–350]. Using the Cox model, Maiorca *et al.* [333, 339] observed that the adjusted relative risk of death was higher in HD patients older than 67 years but this difference was not statistically significant. On the contrary, data from the USRDS and the Michigan Kidney Registry Study [351–353] showed that the death rate was higher in elderly CAPD patients, especially in those with diabetes. These differences may reflect biases in patient selection or a different distribution of co-morbid conditions [355].

The risk of dying on any form of dialysis is 2 to 3-fold higher in diabetic patients than it is in those whose primary renal disease is glomerulonephritis [356]. However, no one has demonstrated a clear difference between the outcome of diabetics of HD and those on CAPD. According to the USRDS study [354] – the results of which are unadjusted for co-existing diseases, mortality rates tend to be higher for HD in younger diabetic patients (40 years or below) while these rates were higher for CAPD in older diabetic patients.

In the study of Michigan Kidney Registry of 1992 [345] diabetics treated by CAPD had a significantly lower mortality rate during the decade of 80's (change in risk per year – 9% p:0.001), while in the same period the mortality rates in diabetics on HD increased although the difference was not statistically significant (change in risk per year + 4%, $p > 0.05$).

A more recent report from the same registry [352] that used the Cox proportional hazards analysis showed that diabetics 20–59 years old who were treated with CAPD had a significantly lower relative risk of death compared to diabetics of the same age range treated with HD ($p < 0.01$). On the contrary, diabetics over 60 years had a higher risk of mortality on CAPD than on HD, although the difference was not statistically significant.

9.1.2. Causes of death

Worldwide, most dialysis registries report that the major causes of death in HD and PD patients are cardiovascular events and septicemia [339, 353, 354, 357–359]. Cardiovascular events account for about 50% of deaths in the CAPD population [353, 354].

Withdrawal from dialysis, the third most frequent primary cause of death in patients over 65 years, is much more common in white than in black patients [330, 356]. In diabetics, death due to withdrawal is almost 3-fold greater than among those who have glomerulonephritis or hypertensive ESRD.

It is interesting that sclerosing encapsulating peritonitis seems to have disappeared as a cause of death since the profession discontinued the use of chlorhexidine as a disinfectant and acetate as a buffer. In France where this complication was observed in the early 80's [153], the prevalence of sclerosing encapsulating peritonitis has been progressively reduced.

9.1.3. Technique survival

Usually, technique survival refers to the percentage of patients, calculated by actuarial analysis, who are still on the original mode of dialysis. In performing this analysis, many investigators ignore changes in the type of PD systems and most of them consider patients, who were transplanted or who recovered their renal function or died as "lost to follow-up" [360]. Moreover, in studies using heterogeneous populations, analysis should be based on Cox proportional hazards regression model to adjust for prognostic differences [340].

During the last 10 years, many studies have shown that HD has a better technique survival than CAPD [332, 333, 337, 350, 361, 362]. However Marishal et al. could demonstrate no statistically significant difference in technique survival between HD and CAPD [363].

The study of Maiorca et al. [333] which had the longest follow-up, showed that HD patients had a better technique survival than CAPD patients but after adjustment with the Cox model, the difference was not significant. It is interesting, however, that data from the various CAPD centers show significant difference probably because they use different patient selection criteria [331–333, 337].

One would expect that the recent decrease in peritonitis rates would improve technique survival.

Table 5. Relative risk of death.

Author	Ref.		# Pts.	HD	CAPD	P
Serkes KD (1990)	(332)	Diabetics Non-diabetics	187 480	1.00 1.00	0.90 0.62	NS NS
Burton PR (1987)	(335)		389	1.30	1.00	NS
Maiorca R (1988)	(342)		259	1.00	1.35	NS
Italian multicenter (1991)	(333)		853	1.00	1.34	NS
Wolfe RA (1990)	(344)		2,754	1.00	0.98	NS
Nelson CB (1992)	(345)	Diabetics Non-diabetics	1,458 2,830	1.00 1.00	0.4–0.7 0.73–1.05	< 0.05* NS**

Modified from Maiorca et al., Kidney Int. 1993 (331).
* For diabetics younger than 52 years
** Lower values correspond to patients with GN as primary renal disease.

Indeed, a special USRDS study showed that actuarial technique survival was 77.4% at one year in patients using the Y-set and 61% in patients using the standard spike technique. The corresponding peritonitis rates were one episode per 15 and 9 patient months respectively [333].

Overall improvements in CAPD technique also increased patient survival, as in the Michigan Kidney Registry data, discussed above [342, 345].

9.1.4. Reasons for drop-out

Patients on CAPD change their type of dialysis more often than do those on HD. In fact, 11–15% of CAPD patients and 3–7% of HD patients change the mode of dialysis [332, 336, 337].

The major reasons cited for discontinuing CAPD are peritonitis and catheter related complications [332, 333]. On the contrary, the main reasons for technique failure in HD are cardiovascular instability and loss of vascular access [160, 365].

About 1.7 to 2.5% of CAPD patients at risk discontinue CAPD because of "inadequate dialysis" and 5 to 7.2% because of peritonitis [331, 333, 337]. According to the data from several registries, discontinuation ("drop-out") from CAPD is due to peritonitis (27–52%), "other medical reasons" (21%), psychosocial factors (19%), catheter-related problems (14%) and loss of peritoneal function (8–14%) [160, 365].

Experience with CAPD has shown that most of the permanent transfers to HD occur during the first year of treatment. As time passes, the percentage of patients transferred permanently to HD decreases [366, 367].

9.2. Morbidity on CAPD

Morbidity in dialysis patients is due mainly to cardiovascular disease, infections and skeleto-articular disorders [354, 357]. In the absence of a prospective, randomized, controlled trial comparing HD and CAPD, our knowledge concerning morbidity is based on large cohorts of HD and CAPD patients.

9.2.1. Cardiovascular morbidity

CAPD patients seem to be at a lower risk for left ventricular hypertrophy because of better control of blood pressure, lack of arteriovenous communication and lower degree of anemia. On the other hand, in CAPD an elevation of low density lipoproteins (LDL) may increase the patient's susceptibility to antherosclerosis [225].

9.2.2. Infections

Uremia and malnutrition, which are frequent complications in CAPD and HD patients [226], impair neutrophilic phagocytic ability and thus increase susceptibility to infections [368, 369]. The most common infections are those of vascular access and pneumonia in HD patients, and peritonitis and exit-site infections in CAPD patients.

A recent study found that the probability of a local vascular access infection by 12 months in HD patient was 4.5% for fistulas and 19.7% for vascular grafts. Predominant organisms were staphylococcus aureus and coagulase-negative staphylococci [370].

In CAPD, multicenter controlled clinical studies have demonstrated that use of Y-set decreases the peritonitis rate due mainly to the prevention of coagulase-negative staphylococcal peritoneal infection [371, 372]. Nevertheless, peritonitis due to *staph aureus* remains a major problem [371]. In fact, the annual probability of developing this latter infection is almost 15% [371] and 20–30% of these episodes will require catheter removal [71].

9.2.3. Skeleto-articular disorders

Such disorders are the result of renal osteodystrophy and amyloidosis-related complications in long-term dialysis patients [255]. These are analyzed in the section of complications. It should be emphasized that among CAPD patients, those with higher residual renal function and fewer epeisodes of peritonitis may be at a lower risk of amyloidosis complications [255, 373].

10. Psychosocial aspects of CAPD

Although it is a life-saving procedure, dialysis produces a significant disruption of life style because it reduces a patient's autonomy and independence and causes a marked shift in family roles and responsibilities [375].

Because there are several different modalities, it is important to know the relative impact of each on patient's quality of life [330]. However, the accurate calculation of this multidimensional value depends on the efficiency of dialysis and also on coexisting morbidity. Furthermore dialysis patients have complaints and disabilities that may be the result of the primary disease.

Quality of life is greatly influenced by factors such as age, race, underlying disease (diabetes, cardiovascular disorder etc.), education, socio-economic status, nutritional status and dialysis technique.

Any difference in the quality of life outcome, may be attributed to pretreatment differences in demographic, medical, psychosocial of rehabilitative characteristics [375].

A common finding of many quality of life studies is that renal transplant recipients have better psychosocial function than those on dialysis [329, 376–379]. Kalman et al. [380] however, found no difference in psychiatric morbidity between dialysis and transplant patients, even though the former were older and had more serious medical illness. Correction of anemia by rHEPO produces a significant improvement in the quality of life of HD or CAPD patients even if they are aged or disabled [381, 382].

With respect to several quality of life criteria (lower illness, lower modality-related stress, higher employment and better cognitive function), usually CAPD holds a middle position between renal transplantation and in-center HD [378, 379, 383, 384]. Nevertheless, psychosexual problems are prominent in CAPD patients [379]. Concerning rehabilitation the existing evidence suggests that CAPD patients are marginally better rehabilitated than HD patients [358, 379, 385]. The outcome with home HD is similar to CAPD in terms of psychosocial function. Thus, these modalities should be considered as complementary rather than competing forms of home dialysis [386].

11. Long term results

Compared to HD, CAPD has only recently emerged as a long-term maintenance therapy for ESRD. Much progress has been made with the fundamental requirements of peritoneal access, delivery of dialysis and control of the infectious complications of CAPD. Now we must define the factors that may help to keep patients in a CAPD program, and help to predict the state of health to be anticipated after several years of such therapy.

If one takes into account comorbid conditions, patient survival on CAPD and HD are comparable [387]. In most large cohort studies, the major determinants of mortality in both HD and CAPD are age, diabetes and atherosclerosis [160, 331, 342–344, 361]. Additional factors that have been identified in other studies are: male gender, low level of physical activity, frequent episodes of peritonitis and amyloidosis [344–350]. Ataman et al. [388] reported that, among 34 patients who remained on CAPD for more than four years, the most frequent causes of death were myocardial infarction, sepsis and cardiac failure. Another study of 10 patients maintained on CAPD for more than seven years found that four died of or during peritonitis and one died of myocardial infarction [225].

During the past decade comparisons of technique survival on CAPD and HD usually favor HD. Peritonitis is the most frequent cause of hospitalization and also is the main cause of dropout; it accounts for approximately 30% of transfers from CAPD to HD [160, 389]. Peritonitis, severe or recurrent, can cause permanent damage to peritoneal membrane and significantly increases protein losses. The attendant physical and psychological suffering often discourages patient and family from continuing on CAPD. In most centers the use of disconnect devices has been associated with a decline in the rate of peritonitis and with improved technique survival [343, 389, 390]. Other causes of technique failure in CAPD include loss of peritoneal function, catheter-related problems, patients' preference for other modes and malnutrition.

Over time, many CAPD patients may need increasingly hypertonic exchanges. Dombros et al. [225] who studied 10 patients who had been on CAPD for seven to 11 years found that five required more hypertonic exchanges as time passed, whereas three remained on the same osmotic concentration and two were served by less tonic solutions. In another study, Lameire et al. [391] found that peritoneal ultrafiltration remained steady for five years in 16 patients. Long-term changes in peritoneal permeability may reflect mesothelial denudation [392, 390] but this process usually does not progress to severe peritoneal sclerosis. As noted earlier, the incidence of severe peritoneal sclerosis (encapsulating peritonitis) has declined following the avoidance of acetate-containing dialysate, immediate and effective treatment of peritonitis with early catheter removal in refractory cases and avoidance of chlorhexidine as an antiseptic.

Peritoneal transport characteristics may fluctuate over time in long-term CAPD patients; in 34 patients reported by Ataman et al. [388], serum creatinine increased significantly over a four-year period. In contrast, in the studies by Dombros et al. there was a gradual decrease in serum creatinine over 7–10 years. On the other hand, in a longitudinal, five-year study of 16 patients by Lameire et al. [391], the peritoneal clearance of urea and creatinine remained steady. In that study total weekly KT/V urea decreased with time from 0.96 ± 0.06 at the beginning to 0.55 ± 0.05 after five years of treatment. This decline was due primarily to decrease in residual renal function and also to an increase in body weight. Usually body weight is found to increase in most long-term CAPD studies, [225, 335, 394–398]. Several investigators have recommended total KT/V urea (the sum of peritoneal clearance and renal clearance) as an index of dialysis adequacy. Consequently, as patients lose residual renal function [228, 391] and suffer an increase in body weight [145, 228, 349, 342, 391] which affects the calculation of the urea distribution volume [228, 391], the supervising physician must adjust peritoneal dialysis prescription to maintain a weekly KT/V of 1.8 or a total weekly clearance in the range of 50–55 L of creatinine clearance per 1.73 m^2 body surface area [387].

Long-term follow-up of other prognostic parameters in CAPD patients show that serum total proteins and albumin remain in the low normal range [225, 331] and thus hypoalbuminemia does not appear to be a significant hazard [50]. Hemoglobin, after an initial increase, remains stable above 9 g/dl [225, 388, 394]. Serum cholesterol and triglyceride levels do not change significantly during long (5–7 years) periods on CAPD [225, 388]. The mean blood pressure shows a gradual decrease up to the fourth year, then it starts to increase again reaching statistical significance at the sixth year [225].

Biochemical, hormonal and radiological parameters of bone metabolism indicate persistent mild hyperparathyroidism and the presence of the low-turnover, "aplastic" bone state [225]. However, β_2-microglobulin-related amyloid bone disease is common and one patient, who had been maintained on CAPD for 15 years (the longest survivor to date) developed destructive spondyloarthropathy of the cervical spine that was managed successfully [317]. The above noted observations are in agreement with those from other studies that involve large numbers of patients but shorter (up to 5 years) periods of followup [331, 342, 388]. Thus, in some CAPD patients, at least it appears that, the delicate peritoneal membrane can maintain its dialysis and ultrafiltration capacity over many years, despite repeated exposure to acidic and hypertonic solutions and the insult of frequent peritonitis.

Although we have not proved it, it appears that CAPD therapy may be able to maintain large numbers of patients on CAPD therapy for 10 years or more [387].

12. Future developments

While CAPD has been established as a successful treatment of ESRD for periods of 5–10 years, we still do not know whether it is reliable for longer periods (> 10 years). The presence of a small number of patients, who have remained on CAPD for over 10 years (one up to 15 years), suggests that long term CAPD is possible, at least under certain circumstances that the nephrology community looking after those patients is called to identify. The main reasons for discontinuing CAPD are peritonitis, catheter/exit-site infections and psychological reasons. The main causes of death are cardio/cerebrovascular accidents.

Internationally, peritonitis seems to be decreasing since the introduction of the various disconnect systems. There is early evidence that these systems lower the CAPD drop-out rates.

Exit-site/tunnel infections remain a major challenge for the CAPD nephrologist and he/she should direct more efforts to the prevention of this complication. As a matter of urgency we should establish whether treatment of nasal-*staph aureus* carriers will prevent exit-site infections.

Cardio/cerebrovascular events are the main cause of deaths in all forms of dialysis and the contribution of lipid abnormalities to these complications in healthy people is well established. It remains to be determined whether CAPD patients, who have a slightly higher tendency to hypertriglyceridemia and hypercholesterolemia than HD patients, are more prone to those complications and whether these can be prevented by correction of abnormal blood lipid levels with medication or through dialysis with osmotic agents other than glucose.

Malnutrition remains a major complication of CAPD and during the last few years great interest has been shown in the relationship between protein catabolic rate, dietary protein/energy intake and the amount of dialysis. We expect that as this relationship becomes known and accepted by most nephrologists, they will prevent malnutrition in a large percentage of patients by providing adequate dialysis. In those patients who are adequately dialysed but for a variety of reasons cannot ingest adequate amounts of protein, malnutrition may be prevented by dialysis solutions containing amino acids.

We need studies to delineate the mechanisms responsible for damage to the mesothelial cells and the peritoneal membrane in general. Such knowledge will contribute to a reduction in the frequency of membrane failure (ultrafiltration and solute transport) and a reduction in the numbers of patients leaving CAPD because of these complications. Already we have evidence that peritoneal ultrastructure is more or less intact in those patients who have had only a few episodes of peritonitis. Other factors related to the hypertonicity and the acid pH of dialysis solution are the subject of intensive investigation. Once we elucidate the role of these factors on the integrity of the peritoneal membrane, use of dialysis solutions with the appropriate composition will help us keep intact the peritoneal membrane over long periods. In this connection preliminary experience with bicarbonate-containing neutral pH solutions and alternative osmotic agents offer promise.

We foresee that, to be maintained on this modality an increasing number of CAPD patients will require automated PD performed overnight for a variety of reasons such as ultrafiltration failure, back pain, recurrent hernias and preference. However, we are concerned about the high cost of such treatment especially if the patient requires more than 8L of solution to be adequately dialysed, as is in the majority of cases. We expect that new innovated methods will allow us to use large volumes of inexpensive dialysis solutions.

Finally, as the elderly make up an increasing fraction of new patients on dialysis, we must identify the exact place of CAPD in this population. Its use in a high percentage of elderly in countries such as the UK and Canada, suggests that this treatment may offer special advantages to elderly patients with ESRD.

13. Conclusions

The introduction of CAPD brought dramatic changes in the treatment of patients with ESRD especially children. In certain countries where hemodialysis facilities were not used extensively, CAPD enabled nephrologists to treat a large population of ESRD patients who otherwise would not have been treated.

During the last decade, we have gained important knowledge concerning peritoneal anatomy, physiology, peritoneal defences, lymphatics and simultaneously technological developments have made CAPD simple and safe. Undoubtedly, further research will help us to prevent the major complications and thus allow a larger percentage of our patients to start and remain on this treatment.

Contrary to the beliefs and attitudes of the early years following its introduction, CAPD is now accepted as a complementary treatment to HD and transplantation, which allows the physician to provide the ESRD patient with a wider spectrum of treatments and thus maintain them in a productive/high quality life over many years.

References

1. Nolph, KD. What's new in peritoneal dialysis – an overview. Kidney Int 1992; 42, 38: 2-148-1-162.
2. Legrain M (ed). Continuous Ambulatory Peritoneal Dialysis. Proceedings of an International Symposium: 1979 Nov 2–3; Paris, Excerpta Medica, Amsterdam 1980.
3. Moncrief JW, Popovich RP. CAPD Update, continuous ambulatory peritoneal dialysis, New York, Mason Publishing 1981.
4. Gahl GM, Kessel M, Nolph KD. Advances in peritoneal dialysis. Proceedings of the second international symposium on peritoneal dialysis: West Berlin, Excerpta Medica, Amsterdam, 1981.
5. La Greca G, Biasioli S, Ronco C. Peritoneal Dialysis. First international course on peritoneal dialysis, Vincenza, Italy, Wichtig Editore, Milano 1982.
6. Khanna R, Nolph KD, Prowant, B, Twardowski ZJ, Oreopoulos DG. Advances in continuous ambulatory peritoneal dialysis: Peritoneal Dialysis Bulletin Inc., Toronto, 1988.
7. Wineman RJ. End-stage renal disease, Dialysis Transpl 1978; 7: 1034.
8. Bomar JB, Jr. The transport of uremic metabolites in peritoneal dialysis, dissertation for PhD at the University of Texas at Austin, August 1975.
9. Popovich RP, Moncrief JW, Decherd JP, Bomar JB, Pyle WK. The definition of a novel portable/wearable equilibrium peritoneal dialysis technique. Trans Am Soc Artif Intern Organs (Abstract) 1976; 5: 64.
10. Popovich RP, Pyle WK, Moncrief JW, Dechard JF, Brooks S. Preliminary verification of the low dialysis clearance hypothesis via a novel equilibrium peritoneal dialysis technique. Trans Austral Conf Heat and Mass Transfer, Univ of Sidney Press, Sidney, Australia 1977; 2: 217.
11. Popovich RP, Hlavinka DJ, Bomar JB, Moncrief JW, Dechard JF: The Consequences of Physiological Resistances on Metabolite Removal from the Patient-Artificial Kidney System. Trans Am Soc Artif Intern Organs 1975; 21: 108–15.
12. Bird RB, Stewart WE, Lightfoot EN. Transport Phenomena, John Wiley and Sons, New York 1960.
13. Gotch FA, Sargent JA, Keen M, Prowitt M, Grady M. Solute Kinetics in Intermittent Dialysis Therapy, 9th Ann Rep – Contractors Conf 1976; pp 98–101.
14. Popovich RP, Moncrief JW. Transport Kinetics, In: K. Nolph (ed), Peritoneal Dialysis. Martinus Nijhoff, Boston 1985.

15. Popovich RP, Hiatt MP, Moncrief JW, Pyle WK. Mathematical modeling and minimum treatment requirements in peritoneal dialysis. In: Uremia, C. Giordano and E. Freidman (eds), Wichtig Editore, Milano 1981.
16. Nolph KD, Miller F, Rubin J. Popovich RP. New Directions in Peritoneal Dialysis Applications. Kidney Int 1980; 18(S10): S111–6.
17. Oreopoulos DG. Criteria for adequacy of peritoneal dialysis. Perit Dial Bull 1983; 3: 1–2.
18. Farrell PC. Long-term studies on the human peritoneum. In: La Greca (ed), Peritoneal Dialysis, Wichtig Editore, Milan 1988: pp 99–107.
19. Popovich RP, Pyle WK, Hiatt MP, Moncrief JW. Comparative Kinetic Studies of Dialysis. Proc Northeastern Physicians Conf, New York, Oct 20 1979.
20. Boen ST, Mion C, Slingeneyer A. The Past 15 Years – The role of peritoneal dialysis in the treatment of end stage renal disease. In: Uremia, Giordano C, Friedman E (eds), Wichtig Editore, Milano 1981.
21. Keshaviah PR, Nolph KD, Van Stone JC. The peak concentration hypothesis: A urea kinetic approach to comparing the adequacy of continuous ambulatory peritoneal dialysis (CAPD) and hemodialysis. Perit Dial Int 1989; 9: 257–60.
22. Nolph KD, Keshaviah P, Popovich PR. Problems in comparison of clearances prescriptions in hemodialysis and continuous ambulatory peritoneal dialysis. Perit Dial Int 1991; 11: 298–300.
23. Gotch FA. The application of urea kinetic modeling to CAPD. In: La Greca G, Ronco C, Feriani M, Chairamonte S, Conz P (eds), Perit Dial (Proceedings of the Fourth International Course on Peritoneal Dialysis). Wichtig Editore, Milano 1991; pp 47–51.
24. Moncrief JW, Popovich RP, Nolph KD. Additional experience with continuous ambulatory peritoneal dialysis (CAPD). Trans Am Soc Artif Intern Organs 1978; 24: 476–83.
25. Popovich RP, Moncrief JW, Nolph KD, Ghods AJ, Twardowski ZJ, Pyle WK. Continuous ambulatory peritoneal dialysis. Ann Intern Med 1978; 88-4: 449–56.
26. Oreopoulos DG, Robson M, Izatt S, Clayton SL, DeVeber GA. A simple and safe technique for continuous ambulatory peritoneal dialysis (CAPD). Trans Am Soc Artif Intern Organs 1979; 24: 484–8.
27. Oreopoulos DG. The coming of age of continuous ambulatory peritoneal dialysis (CAPD). Dial Transpl 1979; 8: 460–2.
28. Oreopoulos DG, Khanna R, Williams P, Vas SI. Continuous ambulatory peritoneal dialysis – 1981. Nephron 1982; 30: 293–303.
29. Bazzato G, Coli U, Landini S et al. Continuous ambulatory peritoneal dialysis without wearing a bag: complete freedom of patient and significant reduction of peritonitis. Proc EDTA 1980; 17: 266–75.
30. Buoncristiani U, Cozzari M, Quintiliani G et al. Abatement of exogenous peritonitis risk using the Perugia CAPD system. Dial Transpl 1983; 12: 14–25.
31. Bielawa RJ, Carr KL et al. Intraluminal thermosterilization using a microwave autoclave. Abstr. III International Symposium on Peritoneal Dialysis, Washington, June 1984; p S5.
32. Bazzato G, Coli U, Landini S et al. Double-bag system for handicapped CAPD patients. Abst Proc. EDTA 1984; p 53.
33. US Renal Data System, USRDS. Annual Report, the National Institutes of Health, National Institute of Diabetes and Digestive and Kidney Disease, Bethesda, MD 1992; p 42.
34. Moncrief JW. Continuous ambulatory peritoneal dialysis. Dial Transpl 1978; 7: 809–10.
35. Twardowski Z. New Approaches to Intermittent Peritoneal Dialysis Therapies. In: Nolph K (ed), Peritoneal Dialysis. Kluwer Academic Publishers, Dordrecht 1989, pp 133–48.
36. Moncrief JW, Pyle WK, Simon P, Popovich RP. Hypertrygliceridemia, diabetes mellitus, and insulin administration in patients undergoing continuous ambulatory peritoneal dialysis, In: Moncrief JW, Popovich PR (eds), CAPD Update: Continuous Ambulatory Peritoneal Dialysis, New York 1981; pp 143–65.
37. Ponce PE, Pierratos A, Izatt S et al. Comparison of the survival and complications of three permanent peritoneal dialysis catheters. Perit Dial Bull 1982; 2: 82–6.
38. Bunchman TE, Ballal SH. Treatment of inflow pain by pH adjustment of dialysate in peritoneal dialysis. Perit Dial Int 1991; 11: 179–80.
39. Lovinggood JP. Peritoneal catheter implantation for CAPD. Perit Dial Bull 1984; 4: S106.
40. Helfrich GB, Pechan BW, Alijani MR, Bernard WF, Rakowski TA, Winchester JF. Reduction of catheter complications with lateral placement. Perit Dial Bull 1983; 3 (suppl 4): S2–4.
41. Khanna R, Izatt S, Burke D, Mathews R, Vas S, Oreopoulos DG. Experience with the Toronto Western Hospital permanent peritoneal catheter. Perit Dial Bull 1984; 4: 95–8.
42. Gloor HJ, Nichols WK, Sorkin MI et al. Peritoneal access and related complications in continuous ambulatory peritoneal dialysis. Am J Med 1983; 74: 593–8.
43. Khanna R, Twardowski ZJ. Peritoneal access. In: Nolph KD (ed), Peritoneal Dialysis. Kluwer Academic Publishers, Dordrecht 1989; pp 319–42.
44. Veitch P. Surgical aspects of CAPD. In: Gokal R (ed), Continuous ambulatory peritoneal dialysis. Churchill Livingstone, Edinburgh 1986; pp 110–44.
45. Khanna R, Oreopoulos DG. Peritoneal Dialysis. In: Schrier RW, Gottschalk CW (eds), Diseases of the Kidney. Little, Brown and Company, Boston 1993: pp 2969–3030.
46. Gokal R, Ash SR, Helfrich GB et al. Peritoneal catheters and exit-site practices: Toward optimum peritoneal access. Perit Dial Int 1993; 13: 29–39.
47. Ash S. Chronic peritoneal dialysis catheters:

Effects of catheter design, materials and location. Semin Dial 1990; 3: 39–46.
48. Oreopoulos DG, Izatt S, Zellerman G, Karanikolaou S, Mathews RE. A prospective study of the effectiveness of three permanent peritoneal catheters. Proc Clin Dial Trans Forum 1976; 6: 96–100.
49. Nicholson ML, Burton PR, Donnelly PK, Veitch PS, Walls J. The role of omentectomy in continuous ambulatory peritoneal dialysis. Perit Dial Int 1991; 11: 330–2.
50. Harrison NA, Howell GP, Rainford DJ. Fallopian tube capture of a peritoneal catheter. Nephron 1988; 50: 258.
51. Abidin MR, Spector DA, Kittur DS. Peritoneal dialysis catheter outflow obstruction due to oviductal fimbriae: a case report. Am J. Kidney Dis 1990; 16: 256–8.
52. Aboujoud MS, Cruz C, Dow RW, Mozes MF. Peritoneal Dialysis catheter obstruction by a fallopian tube: a case report. Perit Dial Int 1992; 12: 257–8.
53. McAllister RJ, Morgan SH. Fallopian tube capture of chronic peritoneal dialysis catheters. Perit Dial Int 1993; 13: 74–6.
54. Antoniou S, Syreggelas D, Papadopoulos Ch, Dimitriadis A. Intraluminal lithiasis of a peritoneal catheter. Perit Dial Int 1991; 11: 358–60.
55. Khanna R, Oreopoulos DG, Dombros N et al. Continuous ambulatory peritoneal dialysis after three years: Still a promising treatment. Perit Dial Bull 1981; 1: 24–34.
56. Palacios M, Schley W, Dougherry JS. Use of streptokinase to clear peritoneal catheters. Dial Transpl 1982; 1: 172–4.
57. Block RA, Taylor B, Grederick G. Intraperitoneal infusion of streptokinase in the treatment of recurrent peritonitis. Perit Dial Bull 1983; 3: 162–3.
58. Scalamogna A, Castelnovo C, Cantaluppi A. Intraperitoneal infusion of streptokinase in the treatment of a total peritoneal catheter obstruction. Perit Dial Bull 1986; 6: 41.
59. Bergstein JM, Andreoli SP, West KW, Grosfeld JL. Streptokinase therapy for occluded Tenckhoff catheters in children on CAPD. Perit Dial Int 1988; 8: 137–9.
60. Benevent D, Peryonnet P, Brignon P. Urokinase infusion for obstructed catheters and peritonitis. Perit Dial Bull 1985; 5: 77.
61. Sharp J, Eastham EJ, Coulthard MG. Removal of a fibrin plug from within a silastic peritoneal dialysis catheter: the sheastard sweep. Perit Dial Int 1990; 10: 61–2.
62. Pierratos A. Peritoneal dialysis glossary. Perit Dial Bull 1984; 4: 2–3.
63. Khanna R and Twardowski ZJ. Peritoneal catheter exit site (editorial). Perit Dial Int 1988; 8: 119–23.
64. Twardowski ZJ. Peritoneal catheter exit-site infections: prevention diagnosis, treatment, and future directions. Semin Dial 1992; 5: 305–15.
65. Lindblad AS, Hamilton RW, Novak JW. Complications of peritoneal catheters. In: Lindblad AS, Novak JW, Nolph KD (eds), Continuous ambulatory peritoneal dialysis in the USA. Final report of the National CAPD registry. Kluwer Academic Publishers, Dordrecht 1989; pp 157–66.
66. Bernardini J, Holley JL, Johnston JR, Perlmutter JA, Piraino B. An analysis of ten-year trends in infections in adults on continuous ambulatory peritoneal dialysis. Clin Nephrol 1991; 36: 29–34.
67. Luzar MA. Exit-site infection in continuous ambulatory peritoneal dialysis: a review. Perit Dial Int 1991; 11: 333–40.
68. Moncrief JW, Popovich PR, Broadrick LJ, He ZZ, Simmon EE, Tates RA. The Moncrief-Popovich Catheter: A New Peritoneal Access Technique for Patients on Peritoneal Dialysis. ASAIO Journal 1993; 39: 62–5.
69. Sewell CM, Clarridge J, Lacke C, Weinman EJ, Young EJ. Staphylococcal nasal carriage and subsequent infection in peritoneal dialysis patients. JAMA 1982; 248: 1493–5.
70. Ahrens ER, Zimmerman SW, Leggett J et al. Increased incidence of exit-site infections in CAPD patients with nasal carriage of staphylococcus aureus (abstract). Kidney Int 1988; 33: 243.
71. Davies SJ, Ogg CS, Cameron JS et al. Staphylococcus aureus nasal carriage, exit-site infection and catheter loss in patients treated with continuous ambulatory peritoneal dialysis. Perit Dial Int 1989; 9: 61–4.
72. Luzar MA, Coles GA, Faller B et al. Staphylococcus aureus nasal carriage and infection in patients on continuous ambulatory peritoneal dialysis. N Engl J Med 1990; 322: 505–9.
73. Twardowski ZJ, Prowant BF, Nolph KD, Khanna R, Schmidt LM. Culture results in periexit smears and sinus tract washouts of peritoneal catheters and swabs from nares. Abstracts, Vth Congress of the International Society for Peritoneal Dialysis. Kyoto, Japan, July 21–24, 1990; p 60.
74. Boelaert JR, Van Landuyt HW, Godard CA et al. Nasal mupirocin ointment decreases the incidence of staphylococcus aureus bacteremias in hemodialysis patients. Nephrol Dial Transplant 1993; 8: 235–9.
75. Vogt K, Binswanger U, Buchman NP et al. Catheter related complications during continuous ambulatory peritoneal dialysis: A retrospective study on sixty-two double cuff Tenckhoff catheters. Am J Kidney Dis 1987; 10: 47–51.
76. Piraino B, Bernardini J, Sorkin M. A five year study of the microbiologic results of exit-site infections and peritonitis in continuous ambulatory peritoneal dialysis. Am J Kidney Dis 1987; 10: 281–6.
77. Kim D, Burke D, Izatt S et al. Single- or double-cuff peritoneal catheters? A prospective comparison. Trans Am Soc Artif Intern Organs 1984; 30: 232–5.
78. Diaz-Buxo JA, Geissinger WT. Single cuff versus double cuff Tenckchoff catheter. Perit Dial Bull 1984; 4: S100–2.
79. Mitwalli A, Kim D, Wu G et al. Single vs. double cuff peritoneal catheters: a prospective controlled trial. In: Khanna R, Nolph KD, Prowant BP,

Twardowski ZJ, Oreopoulos DG (eds), Advances in CAPD. Peritoneal Dialysis Bulletin Inc., Toronto 1985; pp 35–40.
80. Smith C. CAPD: One cuff vs two cuff catheters in reference to incidence of infection. In: Maher JF, Winchester JF (eds), Frontiers in peritoneal dialysis. Proceedings of the 3rd International Symposium on Peritoneal Dialysis. Washington DC, Field, Rich and Associates Inc., New York 1986; pp 181–6.
81. Catheter-related factors and peritonitis risk in CAPD patients. US Renal Data System, USRDS 1992 Annual Data Report, The National Institutes of Health, National Institute of Diabetes and Digestive and Kidney Diseases, Bethesda, MD, August 1992 and Am J Kidney Dis 1992; 20 (suppl 2): 48–54.
82. Twardowski ZJ, Prowant BF, Nichols WK, Nolph KD, Khanna R. Six-year experience with swan neck catheters. Perit Dial Int 1992; 12: 384–9.
83. Burkart JM, Jordan JR, Durnell TA, Case LD. Comparison of exit-site infections in disconnect versus nondisconnect systems for peritoneal dialysis. Perit Dial Int 1992; 12: 317–20.
84. Clayton S, Quinton C, Oreopoulos DG. Training technique for continuous ambulatory peritoneal dialysis. Perit Dial Bull 1981; 1: S23–4.
85. Starzomski RC. Three techniques for peritoneal catheter exit-site dressings. ANNA J 1984; 11: 9–16.
86. Piraino B, Bernardini J, Sorkin M. The influence of peritoneal catheter exit-site infections on peritonitis tunnel infections and catheter loss in patients on continuous ambulatory peritoneal dialysis. Am J Kidney Dis 1986; 8: 436–40.
87. Prowant BF, Schmidt LM, Twardowski ZJ et al. Peritoneal dialysis catheter exit-site care. ANNA J 1988; 15: 219–22.
88. Luzar MA, Brown C, Balf D et al. Exit-site care and exit-site infection in CAPD: results of a randomized multicenter trial. Perit Dial Int 1990; 10: 25–9.
89. Zimmerman SW, Ahrens E, Johnson CA et al. Randomized controlled trial of prophylactic rifampin for peritoneal dialysis related infections. Am J Kidney Dis 1991; 18: 225–31.
90. Twardowski ZJ, Tully RJ, Nicholas WK, Sunderjan S. Computerized tomography in the diagnosis of subcutaneous leak sites during CAPD. Perit Dial Bull 1984; 4: 163–6.
91. Mandel P, Faegenburg D, Imbriano L. The use of technitium-99m sulfur colloid in the detection of patent processus vaginalis in patients on continuous ambulatory peritoneal dialysis. Clin Nucl Med 1985; 10(8): 553–5.
92. Steiner RW and Halasz NA. Abdominal catastrophies and other unusual events in continuous ambulatory peritoneal dialysis patients. Am J Kidney Dis 1990; 15: 1–7.
93. Gotloib L, Mines M, Garmizo L, Varka I. Hemodynamic effects of increased intra-abdominal pressure in peritoneal dialysis. Perit Dial Bull 1981; 1: 41–3.
94. Twardowski ZJ, Khanna R, Nolph KD et al. Intra-abdominal pressure during natural activities in patients treated with continuous ambulatory peritoneal dialysis. Nephron 1986; 44: 129–35.
95. Hylander BI, Dalton CB, Castel DO, Burkart J, Rossner S. Effect of intraperitoneal fluid volume changes on esophageal pressures: Studies in patients on continuous ambulatory peritoneal dialysis. Am J Kidney Dis 1991; 17: 307–10.
96. Digenis GE, Khanna R, Mathews R, Oreopoulos DG. Abdominal hernias in patients undergoing continuous ambulatory peritoneal dialysis. Perit Dial Bull 1982; 2: 115–7.
97. Engeset J, Youngson G. Ambulatory peritoneal dialysis and hernias complications. Surg Clin N Am 1984; 64: 385–92.
98. Rocco MV, Stone WJ. Abdominal hernias in chronic peritoneal dialysis: A review. Perit Dial Bull 1985; 5: 171–4.
99. O'Connor JP, Rigby RJ, Hardie IR et al. Abdominal hernias complicating continuous ambulatory peritoneal dialysis. Am J Nephrol 1986; 6: 271–4.
100. Bargman JM. Complications of peritoneal dialysis related to increased intraabdominal pressure. Kidney Int 1993; 43 (suppl 40): S75–80.
101. Spence P, Mathews R, Khanna R, Oreopoulos DG. Improved results with a paramedian technique for the insertion of peritoneal dialysis catheters. Surg Gyn Obstet 1985; 161: 585–7.
102. Tzamaloukas AH, Gibel LJ, Eisenberg B et al. Scrotal edema in patients on CAPD: Causes, differential diagnosis and management. Dial Transplant 1992; 21: 581–90.
103. Kopecky R, Funk M, Kreitzer P. Localized genital edema in patients undergoing continuous ambulatory peritoneal dialysis. J Urol 1985; 134: 880–4.
104. Schurgers MLC, Boelaert JRO, Daneels RFS, Robbens EF, Vandelanottee MMJ. Open processus vaginalis. Perit Dial Bull 1983; 3: 30–1.
105. Schultz SG, Harmon TM, Nachtnebel KL. Computerized tomographic scanning with intraperitoneal contrast enhancement in a CAPD patient with localized edema. Perit Dial Bull 1984; 4: 253–4.
106. Singal K, Segel DP, Bruns FJ, Fraley DS, Adler S, Julian TB. Genital edema in patients on continuous ambulatory peritoneal dialysis: Report of 3 cases and review of the literature. Am J Nephrol 1986; 6: 471–5.
107. Brown DL, Johnson JB, Kraus AP, Duke RA, Barrett MR. Computed tomography with intraperitoneal contrast medium for localization of peritoneal dialysis leaks. J Comp Assist Tomography 1987; 11: 276–8.
108. Litherland J, Gibson M, Sambrook P, Lupton E, Beaman M, Ackrill P. Investigation and treatment of poor drains of dialysate fluid associated with anterior abdominal wall leaks in patients on chronic ambulatory peritoneal dialysis. Nephrol Dial Transplant 1992; 7: 1030–4.
109. Scanziani R, Dozio B, Caimi F, De Rossi N, Magri

F, Surian M. Peritoneography and peritoneal computerized tomography: a new approach to noninfectious complications of CAPD. Nephrol Dial Transplant 1992; 7: 1035–8.
110. Abraham G, Blake PG, Mathews RE, Bargman JM, Izatt S, Oreopoulos DG. Genital swelling as a surgical complication of continuous ambulatory peritoneal dialysis. Surgery Gyn Obstet 1990; 170: 306–8.
111. Oreopoulos DG, Khanna R, Williams P et al. Continuous ambulatory peritoneal dialysis – 1981. Nephron 1982; 20: 293–303.
112. Greenberg A, Bernardini J, Piraino BM, Johnston JR, Perlmutter JA. Hemoperitoneum complicating chronic peritoneal dialysis: Single-center experience and literature review. Am J Kidney Dis 1992; 19: 252–6.
113. Nace GS, George AL Jr, Stone WJ. Hemoperitoneum: a red flag in CAPD. Perit Dial Bull 1985; 5: 42–4.
114. Bargman JM, Oreopoulos DG. Complications other than peritonitis or those related to the catheter and the fate of uremic organ dysfunction in patients receiving peritoneal dialysis. In: Nolph KD (ed), Peritoneal Dialysis. Kluwer Academic Publishers, Dordrecht 1989; pp 289–318.
115. Husserl F, Tapia N. Peritoneal bleeding in a CAPD patient after extracorporeal lithotripsy (letter). Perit Dial Bull 1987; 7: 262.
116. Blumenkrantz M, Gallagher N, Bashore R et al. Retrograde menstruation in women undergoing chronic peritoneal dialysis. Obstet Gynecol 1981; 57: 667–70.
117. Walshe JJ, Lee JB, Gerbasi JR. Continuous ambulatory peritoneal dialysis complicated by massive hemoperitoneum after colonoscopy. Gastrointest Endosc 1987; 33: 468–9.
118. Blake P, Abraham G. Bloody effluent during CAPD in a patient with polycystic kidneys. Perit Dial Int 1988; 8: 167.
119. Ramon G, Miguel A, Caridad A, Colomer B. Bloody peritoneal fluid in a patient with tuberous sclerosis in a CAPD program. Perit Dial Int 1989; 9: 353.
120. Francis DMA, Busmanis I, Becker G. Peritoneal calcification in a peritoneal dialysis patient: A case report. Perit Dial Int 1990; 10: 237–40.
121. Hassell LH, Moore J Jr, Conklin JJ. Hemoperitoneum during continuous ambulatory peritoneal dialysis: A possible complication of radiation induced peritoneal injury. Clin Nephrol 1984; 21: 241–3.
122. Abaete de los Santos C, von Eye O, D'Avila D, Mottin CC. Rupture of the spleen: A complication of continuous ambulatory peritoneal dialysis. Perit Dial Bull 1986; 6: 203–4.
123. Twardowski ZJ (Discussant), Schreiber MJ Jr (Presentor). A 55 year-old man with hematuria and blood-tinged dialysate. In peritoneal dialysis case forum (Twardowski ZJ (ed), Schreiber MJ Jr, Burkart JM, associate eds). Perit Dial Int 1992; 12: 61–6.
124. Campisi S, Cavatorta F, De Lucia E. Iliopsoas spontaneous hematoma: An unusual cause of hemoperitoneum in CAPD patients. Perit Dial Int 1992; 12: 78.
125. Namoto Y, Suga T, Nakajima K et al. Acute hydrothorax in continuous ambulatory peritoneal dialysis – A collaborative study of 161 centers. Am J Nephrol 1989; 9: 363–7.
126. Chow CC, Sung JY, Cheung CK, Hamilton-Wood C, Lai KN. Massive hydrothorax in continuous ambulatory peritoneal dialysis: diagnosis, management and review of the literature. NZ Med J 1988; 101(850): 475–7.
127. Abraham G, Shokker A, Blake P, Oreopoulos DG. Massive hydrothorax in patients on peritoneal dialysis: a literature review. In: Khanna R, Nolph KD, Prowant B, Twardowski ZJ, Oreopoulos DG (eds), Advances in Continuous Ambulatory Peritoneal Dialysis, Peritoneal Dialysis Bulletin Inc, Toronto 1988; pp 121–5.
128. Boeschoten EW, Krediet RT, Roos CM, Kloek JJ, Schipper MEI, Arisz L. Leakage of dialysate across the diaphragm: An important complication of continuous ambulatory peritoneal dialysis. Neth J Med 1986; 29: 242–6.
129. Lieberman FL, Hidemura R, Peters RL, Reynolds TB. Pathogenesis and treatment of hydrothorax complicating cirrhosis with ascites. Ann Int Med 1966; 64: 341–51.
130. Benz R, Schleifer C. Hydrothorax in CAPD. Successful treatment with intraperitoneal tetracycline and a review of the literature. Am J Kidney 1985; 2: 136–40.
131. Kennedy J. Procedures used to demonstrate a pleuroperitoneal communication: A review. Perit Dial Bull 1985; 5: 168–70.
132. Adam WR, Arkles LB, Gill G, Meagher EJ, Thomas GW. Hydrothorax with peritoneal dialysis: Radionuclide detection of a pleuroperitoneal connection. Aust NZ J Med 1980; 10: 330–2.
133. Gibbons G, Baumert J. Unilateral hydrothorax complicating peritoneal dialysis. Use of radionuclide imaging. Clin Nucl Med 1983; 3: 83–4.
134. Walker F, McAllister C, McKee P, McNulty J. Intraperitoneal Iopamidol, a new radio contrast agent in the diagnosis of a pleuroperitoneal communication (letter). Perit Dial Bull 1986; 6: 108–9.
135. Vlachojannis J, Boettcher I, Brandt L, Schoeppe W. A new treatment for unilateral recurrent hyrothorax during CAPD. Perit Dial Bull 1985; 5: 180–1.
136. Hidai H, Takatsu S, Chiba T. Intrathoracic instillation of autologous blood in treating massive hydrothorax following CAPD. Perit Dial Int 1989; 9: 221–4.
137. Pattison CW, Rodger RSG, Adu D, Michael J, Mathews HR. Surgical treatment of hydrothorax complicating continuous ambulatory peritoneal dialysis. Clin Nephrol 1984; 21: 191–3.
138. Taveira da Silva AM, Davis WB, Winchester JF, Coleman DE, Weir CW. Peritoneal dialysate infusion and lung function in continuous ambulatory peritoneal dialysis. Clin Nephrol 1985; 24: 79–83.

139. O'Brien AAJ, Power J, O'Brien L, Clancy L, Keogh JAB. The effect of peritoneal dialysate on pulmonary function and blood gases in CAPD patients. Irish J Med Sci 1990; 159: 215–6.
140. Goggin MJ, Joekes AM. Gas exchange in renal failure. Pulmonary gas exchange during peritoneal dialysis. Br Med J 1981; 2: 247–8.
141. Berlyne GM, Lee HA, Ralston AJ, Woolcock JA. Pulmonary complications of peritoneal dialysis. Lancet 1966; 2: 75–8.
142. Singh S, Dale A, Morgan B, Sahebjami H. Serial studies of pulmonary function in continuous ambulatory peritoneal dialysis. Chest 1984; 86: 874–7.
143. Rebuck AS. Peritoneal dialysis and the mechanics of the diaphragm. Perit Dial Bull 1982; 2: 109–10.
144. Oreopoulos DG, Rebuck AS. Risks and benefits of peritoneal dialysis. Chest 1985; 88: 6742.
145. Hamodraka-Mailis A. Pathogenesis and treatment of back pain in peritoneal dialysis patients. Perit Dial Bull 1983; 3 (suppl 3): S41–3.
146. Oreopoulos DG, Gotloib L, Calderaro V et al. For how long can peritoneal dialysis be continued? Can Med Assoc J 1981; 124: 12–3.
147. Faller B, Marichal J. F. Loss of ultrafiltration in continuous ambulatory peritoneal dialysis: clinical data. In: Gahl G, Kessel M, Nolph KD (eds), Advances in Peritoneal Dialysis. Excerpta Medica, Amsterdam 1981; pp 227–32.
148. Slingeneyer A, Canard B, Mion C. Permanent loss of ultrafiltration capacity of the peritoneum in long-term peritoneal dialysis: an epidemiological study. Nephron 1983; 33: 133–8.
149. Wideroe TE, Smeby L, Mjaland S et al. Long-term changes in transperitoneal water transport during continuous ambulatory peritoneal dialysis. Nephron 1984; 38: 238–47.
150. Krediet RT, Zuijderhandt FMJ, Boeschoten EW, Arisz L. Alternations in the peritoneal transport of water and solutes during peritonitis in continuous ambulatory peritoneal dialysis patients. Eur J Clin Invest 1987; 17: 43–52.
151. Raja RM, Kramer MS, Barber K. Solute transport and ultrafiltration during peritonitis in CAPD patients. ASAIO J 1984; 7: 8–11.
152. Krediet RT, Arisz L. Fluid and solute transport across the peritoneum during continuous ambulatory peritoneal dialysis. Perit Dial Int 1989; 9: 15–25.
153. Slingeneyer A, Mion C, Mourad G et al. Progressive sclerosing peritonitis: a late and severe complication of maintenance peritoneal dialysis. Trans Am Soc Art Int Organs 1983; 29: 633–40.
154. Rottembourg J, Gahl GM, Poignet JL et al. Severe abdominal complication in patients undergoing continuous ambulatory peritoneal dialysis. Proc Eur Dial Transplant Ass 1983; 20: 236–42.
155. Verger C, Celicaut B. Peritoneal permeability and encapsulating peritonitis. Lancet 1985; 1: 986–7.
156. Blake PG, Abraham G, Sombolos K et al. Changes in peritoneal membrane transport rates in patients on long-term CAPD. Adv Perit Dial 1989; 5: 3–7.
157. Selgas R, Munoz J, Cigarran S et al. Peritoneal functional parameters after five years on continuous ambulatory peritoneal dialysis: the effect of late peritonitis. Perit Dial Int 1989; 9: 329–32.
158. Park MS, Lee J, Lee SM et al. Peritoneal solute clearances after four years of continuous ambulatory peritoneal dialysis. Perit Dial Int 1989; 9: 75–8.
159. Cantaluppi A, Castelnovo C, Moriggi M, Scalamogna A. Ultrafiltration failure in continuous ambulatory peritoneal dialysis. In: Khanna R, Nolph KD, Prowant BF, Twardowski ZJ, Oreopoulos DG (eds), Advances in CAPD Perit Dial Bull Inc 1986; pp 12–5.
160. Nolph HK. Clinical results with peritoneal dialysis. Registry experiences. In: Twardowski ZJ, Nolph KD, Khanna R, Stein JH (eds), Peritoneal Dialysis. Contemporary Issues in Nephrology. Churchill Livinstone, New York 1991; 22: 127–44.
161. Grahame GR, Torchia M, Dankenich KA, Ferguson IA. Surface active material in peritoneal effluent of CAPD patients. Perit Dial Bull 1985; 5: 109–11.
162. Mactier RA, Khanna R, Twardowski ZJ, Moore H, Nolph KD. Influence of phosphatidylcholine on peritoneal transport and lymphatic absorption during peritoneal dialysis in the rat. Perit Dial Int 1988; 8: 179–86.
163. Di Paolo N, Buoncristiani U, Capotondo L et al. Phosphatidylcholine and peritoneal transport during peritoneal dialysis. Nephron 1986; 44: 365–70.
164. Dombros N, Balaskas E. Savidis N, Tourkantonis A, Sombolos K. Phosphatidylcholine increases ultrafiltration in continuous ambulatory peritoneal dialysis patients. In: Avram MM, Giordano C (eds), Ambulatory Peritoneal Dialysis. Plenum, New York 1990; pp 39–41.
165. Krack G, Viglino G, Cavalli PL et al. Intraperitoneal administration of phosphatidylcholine improves ultrafiltration in continuous ambulatory peritoneal dialysis patients. Perit Dial Int 1992; 12: 359–64.
166. Chan PCK, Tam SCF, Robinson JD et al. Effect of phosphatidylcholine on ultrafiltration in patients on continuous ambulatory peritoneal dialysis. Nephron 1991; 59: 100–3.
167. De Vecchi A, Castelnovo C, Guerra L, Scalamogna A. Phosphatidylcholine administration in continuous ambulatory peritoneal dialysis patients with reduced ultrafiltration. Perit Dial Int 1989; 9: 207–10.
168. Chan H, Abraham G, Oreopoulos DG. Oral lecithin improves ultrafiltration in patients on peritoneal dialysis. Perit Dial Int 1989; 9: 203–5.
169. Lamperi S, Carozzi S, Nasini MG. Calcium antagonists improve ultrafiltration in patients on continuous ambulatory peritoneal dialysis. ASAIO Trans 1987; 33: 657–63.
170. Maher JF, Hirszel P, Chakrabati E, Bennett RR. Contrasting effects of amphotericin B and the solvent desoxycholate on peritoneal transport. Nephron 1986; 43: 38–42.
171. Dobbie JW. Pathology of the peritoneum. In:

Bengmark S (ed), The peritoneum and peritoneal access. Wright, London 1989; pp 42–52.
172. Bradley JA, McWhinnie DL, Hamilton DNH et al. Sclerosing obstructive peritonitis after continuous ambulatory peritoneal dialysis. Lancet 1983; 2: 113–4.
173. Hauglustaine D, Van Meerbeek J, Monballyn J, Goddeeris P, Lauwerijns J, Michielsen P. Sclerosing peritonitis with mural bowel fibrosis in a patient on long term CAPD. Clin Nephrol 1984; 22: 158–62.
174. Junor BJR, Rriggs JD, Forwell MA et al. Sclerosing peritonitis – the contribution of chlorhexidine in alcohol. Perit Dial Bull 1985; 5: 101–4.
175. Verger C, Celicout B, Larpent L et al. Sclerosing encapsulating peritonitis during continuous ambulatory peritoneal dialysis. La Presse Medical 1986; 15: 1311–4.
176. Heale WF, Letch KA, Dawborn JK, Evans SM. Long term complications of peritonitis in peritoneal dialysis. In: Atkins RC, Thomson NM, Farrell PC (eds), Peritoneal Dialysis. Churchill Livingstone, Edinburgh 1981; pp 284–90.
177. Lo WK, Chan KT, Leung ACT, Pang SW, Tse CY. Sclerosing peritonitis complicating prolonged use of chlorhexidine in alcohol in the connection procedure for continuous ambulatory peritoneal dialysis. Perit Dial Int 1991; 11: 166–72.
178. Pusateri R, Ross R, Marshall O et al. Sclerosing encapsulating peritonitis: report of a case with small bowel obstruction managed by long-term home parenteral hyperalimentation and a review of the literature. Am J Kidney Dis 1986; 8: 56–60.
179. Daugirdas J, Gandhi VC, McShane et al. Peritoneal sclerosis in continuous ambulatory peritoneal dialysis patients dialyzed exclusively with lactate – buffered dialysate. Int J Artif Organs 1986; 9: 413–6.
180. Korzets A, Korzets Z, Peer G et al. Sclerosing peritonitis – possible early diagnosis by computerized tomography of the abdomen. Am J Nephrol 1988; 8: 143–6.
181. Mion C, Slingeneyer A. Sclerosing peritonitis: What is it? In: LaGreca G, Chiaramonte S, Fabris A, Feriani M, Ronco C (eds), Peritoneal Dialysis. Wichtig Editore, Milano 1986; pp 215–22.
182. Dobbie JW. Pathogenesis of peritoneal fibrosing syndromes (sclerosing peritonitis) in Peritoneal Dialysis. Perit Dial Int 1992; 12: 14–27.
183. Jackson BT. Surgical treatment of sclerosing peritonitis caused by practolol. Br J Surg 1977; 64: 225–57.
184. Marichal JF, Faller B, Brignon P, Wagner D, Straub P. Progressive calcifying peritonitis: A new complication of CAPD? Nephron 1987; 45: 229–32.
185. Wakabayashi Y, Kawaguchi Y, Shigematsu T et al. Three cases of extensive peritoneal calcification in patients with long-term CAPD (Abstract). Perit Dial Int 1993; 13(1): 99.
186. Von Baeyer H, Gahl GM, Riedinger H et al. Adaptation of CAPD patients to the continuous peritoneal energy intake. Kidney Int 1983; 23: 29–34.
187. Lindholm B, Karlander SG. Glucose tolerance in patients undergoing continuous ambulatory peritoneal dialysis. Acta Med Scand 1986; 220: 477–83.
188. Wideroe TE. Smeby LC, Myking OL. Plasma concentrations and transperitoneal transport of native insulin and C-peptide in patients on continuous ambulatory peritoneal dialysis. Kidney Int 1984; 25: 82–7.
189. Lameire N, Matthys D, Matthys E, Beheydt R. Effects of long-term CAPD on carbohydrate and lipid metabolism. Clin Nephrol 1988; 30 (suppl 1): S53–8.
190. Thomas ME, Moorhead JF. Lipids in CAPD: A review. In: Coles GA, Davies M, Williams JD (eds), CAPD: Host defence, Nutrition and Ultrafiltration. Contrib Nephrol. Karger, Basel 1990; 85: 92–9.
191. Oreopoulos DG, Crassweller P, Katirtzoglou A et al. Amino acids as an osmotic agent (instead of glucose) in continuous ambulatory peritoneal dialysis. In: Legrain M (ed), Continuous ambulatory peritoneal dialysis. Excerpta Medica, Amsterdam 1979; pp 335–40.
192. Oreopoulos DG, Clayton S, Dombros N et al. Nineteen months' experience with continuous ambulatory peritoneal dialysis. Proc Eur Dial Transplant Assoc 1979; 11: 178–83.
193. Norbeck HE. Lipid abnormalities in continuous ambulatory peritoneal dialysis patients. In: Legrain M (ed), Continuous Ambulatory Peritoneal Dialysis. Excerpta Medica, Amsterdam 1979; 298–301.
194. Chan MK, Varghese Z, Persaud JW et al. Hyperlipidemia in patients on maintenance hemo- and peritoneal dialysis: The relative pathogenic roles of triglyceride production and triglyceride removal. Clin Nephrol 1982; 17: 183–90.
195. Lindholm B, Norbeck HE. Serum lipids and lipoproteins during continuous ambulatory peritoneal dialysis. Acta Med Scand 1986; 220: 143–51.
196. Steele J, Billington J, Janus E, Moran J. Lipids, lipoproteins and apolipoproteins A-I and B and apolipoprotein losses in continuous ambulatory peritoneal dialysis. Atherosclerosis 1989; 79: 47–50.
197. Saku K, Sasaki J, Naito S, Arakawa K. Lipoprotein and apolipoprotein losses during continuous ambularoty peritoneal dialysis. Nephron 1989; 51: 220–4.
198. Chan MK, Yeung CK. Lipid metabolism in 31 Chinese patients on three 2-liter exchanges of CAPD. Perit Dial Bull 1986; 6: 12–6.
199. Dieplinger H, Lobentanz EM, Konig P et al. Plasma apolipoprotein A-IV metabolism in patients with chronic renal disease. Europ J Clin Invest 1992; 22: 166–74.
200. Sniderman A, Cianflone K, Kwitezovich PO Jr, Hutchinson T, Barre P, Prichard S. Hyperapobetalipoproteinemia: The major dyslipoproteinemia in patients with chronic renal

201. Fein PA, Fletcher D, Antignani A et al. Variability of peritoneal clearances for apolipoprotein and its relationship to susceptibility for atherosclerotic changes in CAPD. In: Khanna R, Nolph KD, Prowant BF, Twardowski ZJ, Oreopoulos DG (eds), Advances in Peritoneal Dialysis. Peritoneal Dialysis Bulletin Inc, Toronto 1989; pp 185–9.
202. Shoji T, Nishizawa Y, Nishitani, Yamakawa M, Morii H. Role of hypoalbuminemia and lipoprotein lipase on hyperlipoproteinemia in continuous ambulatory peritoneal dialysis. Metabolism 1991; 40: 1002–8.
203. Wessel-Aas T, Blomhoff JP, Wideroe TE. The effect of systemic heparinization on plasma lipoproteins and toxicity in patients on hemodialysis and continuous ambulatory peritoneal dialysis. Acta Med Scand 1984; 216: 85–92.
204. Atkins RC, Wood C. Hyperlipidemia in continuous ambulatory peritoneal dialysis patients should be treated. In: Dombros NV, Tourkantonis A (guest eds), "Peritoneal Dialysis in the Nineties". Perit Dial Int 1993: 13 (suppl 2): 415–7.
205. Williams P. Kay R, Harrison J et al. Nutritional and anthropometric assessment of patients on CAPD over one year: Contrasting changes in total body nitrogen and potassium. Perit Dial Bull 1981; 1: 82–7.
206. Heide B, Pierratos A, Khanna R et al. Nutritional status of patients undergoing continuous ambulatory peritoneal dialysis. Perit Dial Bull 1983; 3: 138–41.
207. Schilling H, Wu G, Petit J et al. Nutritional status of patients on long-term CAPD. Perit Dial Bull 1985; 5: 12–8.
208. Salusky IB, Fine RN, Nelson D et al. Nutritional status of children undergoing continuous ambulatory peritoneal dialysis. Am J Clin Nutr 1983; 38: 599–611.
209. Pollock CA, Allen BJ, Warden RA et al. Total body nitrogen by neutron activation in maintenance dialysis. Am J Kidney Dis 1990; 16: 38–45.
210. Nelson EE, Hong CD, Pesce AL, Peterson DW, Singh S, Pollak VE. Anthropometric norms in dialysis population. Am J Kidney Dis 1990; 16: 32–7.
211. Fenton SSA, Johnston N, Delmore T et al. Nutritional assessment of continuous ambulatory peritoneal dialysis patients. Trans Am Soc Artif Intern Irgans 1987; 33: 969–72.
212. Young GA, Kopple JD, Lindholm B et al. Nutritional assessment of CAPD patients. An international study. Am J Kidney Dis 1991; 17: 462–71.
213. Marckman P. Nutritional status of patients on hemodialysis and peritoneal dialysis. Clin Nephrol 1988; 29: 75–8.
214. Dombros NV, Digenis GE, Oreopoulos DG. Malnutrition in continuous ambulatory peritoneal dialysis and use of intraperitoneal amino acids. In: Berlyne GM (ed) The Kidney Today: Selected Topics in Renal Science. Contrib Nephrol. Karger, Basel 1992; 100: 188–206.
215. Oreopoulos DG, Marliss EB, Anderson GH et al. Nutritional aspects of CAPD and the potential use of amino acid containing dialysis solutions. Perit Dial Bull 1983; 3: S10–2.
216. Torrington J, Jenkins JH, Coles GA. The effect of the dialysate on food consumption by continuous ambulatory peritoneal dialysis. J Renal Nutr 1992; 2: 113–6.
217. Hylander B, Barkelling B, Rossner S. Eating behaviour in continuous ambulatory peritoneal dialysis patients. Am J Kidney Dis 1992; 20: 592–7.
218. Lindholm B, Bergstrom J. Nutritional aspects on peritoneal dialysis. Kidney Int 1992; 42 (suppl 38): S165–71.
219. Blumenkrantz MJ, Gahl GM, Kopple JD et al. Protein losses during peritoneal dialysis. Kidney Int 1981; 19: 593–602.
220. Lindholm B, Bergstrom J. Protein and amino acid metabolism in patients undergoing continuous ambulatory peritoneal dialysis. Clin Nephrol 1988; 30: S59–63.
221. Rubin J, Nolph KD, Arfania D et al. Protein losses in continuous ambulatory peritoneal dialysis. Nephrol 1981; 28: 218–21.
222. Dulaney JT, Hatch FE. Peritoneal dialysis and loss of proteins. A review. Kidney Int 1984; 26: 253–62.
223. Dombros N, Oren A, Marliss EB et al. Plasma amino acid profiles and amino acid losses in patients undergoing CAPD. Perit Dial Bull 1982; 2: 27–32.
224. Dombros N, Digenis GE, Abraham G, Oreopoulos DG. Long-term (> 5 years) experience with CAPD (Abstract). Perit Dial Int 1988; 8: 76.
225. Dombros N, Digenis GE, Sombolos K, Abraham G, Balaskas E, Oreopoulos DG. Long-term continuous ambulatory peritoneal dialysis. Clin Nephrol 1993; 39: 70–4.
226. Bergstrom J, Lindholm B. Nutrition and adequacy of dialysis. How do hemodialysis and CAPD compare: Kidney Int 1993; 43 (suppl 40): S39–50.
227. Teehan BP, Schleifer CR, Brown JM, Sigler MH, Raimondo J. Urea kinetic analysis and clinical outcome on CAPD: A five year longitudinal study. In: Khanna R, Nolph KD, Prowant BF, Twardowski ZJ, Oreopoulos DG (eds), Advances in Peritoneal Dialysis. Peritoneal Dialysis Bulletin Inc., Toronto 1990; pp 181–5.
228. Blake PG, Sombolos K, Abraham G et al. Lack of correlation between urea kinetic indices and clinical outcomes in CAPD patients. Kidney Int 1991; 39: 700–6.
229. Schoenfeld PY, Henry RR, Laird NM, Roxe DM. Assessment of nutritional status of the National Cooperative Study population. Kidney Int 1983; 23 (suppl 13): 80–8.
230. Lysaght MJ, Pollock CA, Hallet MD, Ibles LS. Farrel PC. The relevance of urea kinetic modeling to CAPD. Trans Am Soc Artif Intern Organs 1989; 35: 784–90.
231. Lindsay RM, Spanner E. A hypothesis: The protein catabolic rate is dependent upon the type and

amount of treatment in dialyzed uremic patients. Am J Kidney Dis 1989; 13: 382–9.
232. Keshaviah PR, Nolph KD, Van Stone JC. The peak concentration hypothesis: A urea kinetic approach to comparing the adequacy of continuous ambulatory peritoneal dialysis and hemodialysis. Perit Dial Int 1989; 9: 257–60.
233. Keshaviah PR, Nolph KD, Prowant BF et al. Defining adequacy of CAPD with urea kinetics. In: Khanna R, Nolph KD, Prowant BF, Twardowski ZJ, Oreopoulos DG (eds), Advances in Peritoneal Dialysis. Peritoneal Dialysis Bulletin Inc, Toronto 1990; 6: 173–8.
234. Bergstrom J, Alvestrand A, Lindholm B, Tranaeus A. Relationship between KT/V and protein catabolic rate is different in continuous peritoneal dialysis and haemodialysis patients (Abstract). J Am Soc Nephrol 1991; 2: 358.
235. Blumenkrantz MJ, Kopple JD, Moran JK, Coburn JW. Metabolic balance studies and dietary protein requirements in patients undergoing CAPD. Kidney Int 1982; 21: 849–61.
236. Williams, P, Marliss EB, Anderson GH et al. Amino acid absorpotion following intraperitoneal administration in CAPD patients. Perit Dial Bull 1982; 2: 124–30.
237. Oren A. Wu G, Anderson GH et al. Effective use of amino acid dialysate over four weeks in CAPD patients. Perit Dial Bull 1983; 3: 66–73.
238. Okamura K, Yamauchi J, Nakahama H et al. The effects of adding essential amino acids to the dialysis solution of continuous ambulatory peritoneal dialysis patients. In: Maekawa M, Nolph KD, Kishimoto T, Moncrief JM (eds), Machine Free Dialysis for Patient Convenience. The Fourth ISAO official Satellite Symposium on CAPD. ISAO Press, Cleveland 1984; pp 103–7.
239. Bernard D, Kopple JD, Brunori G et al. Nutritional benefits of interperitoneal amino acids in CAPD patients (Abstract). 6th Int Cong on Nutrition and Metabolism in Renal Diseases, Harrogate, Aug 1991.
240. Fenton S, Cummings A, Richardson R et al. Low protein catabolic rate: Can it be corrected with intraperitoneal amino acid supplements (Abstract). Perit Dial Int 1991; 11 (suppl 1): 79.
241. Jones M, Martis L, Algrim C et al. Intraperitoneal amino acids: results of a clinical trial (Abstract). Perit Dial Int 1992; 12 (suppl 2): S26.
242. Pedersen FB, Dragsholt C, Laier E et al. Alternate use of amino acid and glucose solutions in CAPD. Perit Dial Bull 1985; 5: 215–8.
243. Young GA, Dibble JB, Hobson SM et al. The use of an amino acid-based CAPD fluid over 12 weeks. Nephrol Dial Transplant 1989; 4: 285–92.
244. Arfeen S, Goodship TH, Kirkwood A, Ward MK. The nutritional/metabolic and hormonal effects of 8 weeks of continuous ambulatory peritoneal dialysis with a 1% amino acid solution. Clin Nephrol 1990; 33: 192–9.
245. Schilling H, Wu G, Petit J et al. Effects of prolonged CAPD amino acid containing solutions in three patients. In: Khanna R, Nolph KD, Prowant BF, Twardowski ZJ, Oreopoulos DG (eds), Advances in CAPD. Peritoneal Dialysis Bulletin Inc, Toronto 1985; pp 49–55.
246. Bruno M, Bagnis C, Marangella M et al. CAPD with an amino acid dialysis solution: A long-term, cross-over study. Kidney Int 1989; 35: 1189–94.
247. Dombros N, Prutis K, Tong M et al. Six-month overnight intraperitoneal amino acid infusion in CAPD patients: No effect on nutritional status. Perit Dial Int 1990; 10: 79–84.
248. Scanziani R, Dozio B, Iacuitti G. CAPD in Diabetics: Use of amino acids. In: Khanna R, Nolph KD, Prowant BF, Twardowski ZJ, Oreopoulos DG (eds), Advances in Peritoneal Dialysis 1990. Peritoneal Dialysis Bulletin Inc, Toronto 1990; 6: 53–5.
249. Digenis GE, Dombros N, Charytan C, Oreopoulos DG. Supplements for the CAPD patient (vitamins, folic acid, zinc, iron and anabolic steroids). Perit Dial Bull 1987; 7: 219–23.
250. Held PJ, Port FK, Webb RL et al. Excerpts from United States Renal Data System 1991. Annual data report. Am J Kidney Dis 1991; 181 (suppl 2): 1–127.
251. Maher JF. Cardiovascular disease and risk factors in patients treated by continuous ambulatory peritoneal dialysis. Dombros NV, Tourkantonis A (guest eds) "Peritoneal Dialysis in the Nineties". Perit Dial Int 1993; 13 (suppl 2): 389–93.
252. Giangrande A. Cardiovascular system in continuous ambulatory peritoneal peritoneal dialysis. Contrib Nephrol 1990; 84: 52–9.
253. Huting J, Kramer W, Reitinger J et al. Cardiac structure and function in continuous ambulatory peritoneal dialysis: influence of blood purification and hypercirculation. Am Heart J 1990; 119: 344–52.
254. Alpert MA, Van Stone J, Twardowski ZJ et al. Comparative cardiac effects of hemodialysis and continuous ambulatory peritoneal dialysis. Clin Cardiol 1986; 9: 52–60.
255. Churchill DN. Comparative morbidity among hemodialysis and continuous ambulatory peritoneal dialysis patients. Kidney Int 1993; 43 (suppl 40): S16–22.
256. Attman PD, Alanporic P. Lipid abnormalities in chronic renal insufficiency. Kidney Int 1991; 39 (suppl 31): 516–23.
257. Boeschoten EW, Znyderhandt FMJ, Krediet RT, Arisz L. Changes in weight and lipid concentrations during CAPD treatment. Perit Dial Int 1988; 8: 19–24.
258. Wu G, and the University of Toronto Collaborative Dialysis Group: Cardiovascular deaths among CAPD patients. Perit Dial Bull 1983; 3: 523–6.
259. Kurtz SB, Wong G, Anderson CF et al. Continuous ambulatory peritoneal dialysis: Three years' experience at the Mayo Clinic. Mayo Clin Proc 1983; 58: 633–8.
260. Leenen FHH, Shah P, Boer WH, Khanna R, Oreopoulos DG. Hypotension on CAPD: An approach to treatment. Perit Dial Bull 1983; 3: S33–5.

261. Eschbach JW, Funk D, Adamson JW et al. Erythropoiesis, in patients with renal failure undergoing chronic dialysis. N Engl J Med 1967; 276: 653–8.
262. Eschbach JW, Adamson JW. Anemia of end-stage renal disease. Kidney Int 1985; 28: 1–5.
263. McGonigle RJS, Wallin JD, Shadduck RK, Fisher JW. Erythropoietin deficiency and inhibition of erythropoiesis in renal insufficiency. Kidney Int 1984; 25: 437–44.
264. DePaepe M, Schelstratte K. Ringoir S, Lameire NH. Influence of continuous ambulatory peritoneal dialysis on the anemia of endstage renal disease. Kidney Int 1983; 23: 744–8.
265. Zappocosta AR, Caro J, Erslev A. Normalization of hematocrit in patients with end-stage renal disease on continuous ambulatory peritoneal dialysis: The role of erythropoietin. Am J Med 1982; 72: 53–7.
266. Lindblad AS, Nolph KD. Hematocrit values in the CAPD/CCPD population: A report of the National CAPD Registry. Perit Dial Int 1990; 10: 275–8.
267. Saltissi D, Coles GA, Napier AF, Bentley P. The hematologic response to continuous ambulatory peritoneal dialysis. Clin Nephrol 1984; 22: 21–7.
268. Mohini R. Clinical efficacy of recombinant human erythropoietin in hemodialysis patients. Semin Nephrol 1989; 9 (suppl 1): 16–21.
269. Nissenson AR, Swartz R, Zimmerman S et al. A double-blind, placebo-controlled study of recombinant human erythropoietin in peritoneal dialysis patients (abstract). J Am Soc Nephrol 1990; 1: 405.
270. Parthasarathy R, Johnson CA, Zimmerman SW. Iron dextran use in dialysis patients on erythropoietin (abstract). J Am Soc Nephrol 1990; 1: 405.
271. Lui SF, Chung WWM, Leung CB, Chan K, Lai KN. Pharmacokinetics and pharmacodynamics of subcutaneous and intraperitoneal administration of recombinant human erythropoietin in patients on CAPD. Clin Nephrol 1990; 33: 47–51.
272. Eisele G, Bailie GR, Clement C, Wong E. Erythropoietin in continuous ambulatory peritoneal dialysis: Experience with subcutaneous administration. Perit Dial Int 1992; 12: 34–6.
273. Caruana R, Wolfman N, Karstaedt N et al. Pancreatitis: an important cause of abdominal symptoms in patients on peritoneal dialysis. Am J Kidney Dis 1986; 7: 135–40.
274. Rutsky E, Robards M, Van Dyke J et al. Acute pancreatitis in patients with end-stage renal disease without transplantation. Arch Intern Mid 1986; 146: 1741–5.
275. deBoer B, Agar J. The role of hyperlipidemia in the etiology of pancreatitis in CAPD (letter). Perit Dial Bull 1987; 7: 264.
276. Gupta A, Yuan ZY, Balaskas EV, Khanna R, Oreopoulos DG. CAPD and Pancreatitis: No correlation. Perit Dial Int 1992; 12: 309–16.
277. Burkart JM (Discussant), Khanna R (Presenter). A 69-year old male, with elevated amylase in blood and cloudy dialysate. In: Twardowski ZJ (ed), Schreiber MJ, Burkart JM (assoc eds), Peritoneal dialysis case forum. Perit Dial Int 1993; 13: 142–8.
278. Rotellar C, Black J, Winchester JF et al. Ten years experience with continuous ambulatory peritoneal dialysis. Am J Kidney Dis 1991; 17: 158–64.
279. Vallos M, Cantavell C, Vila J et al. Delayed perforation of the colon by Tenckhoff catheter. Perit Dial Bull 1982; 2: 190.
280. Haj M, Kristal B, Shasha SM. Delayed laceration of intestinal wall by the permanent Tenckhoff peritoneal catheter. Perit Dial Int 1988; 8: 25.
281. Rotellar C, Sivarajan SD, Mazzoni MJ et al. Bowel perforation in CAPD patients. Perit Dial Int 1992; 12: 396–8.
282. Korzets Z, Golan E, Ben-Dahan J, Neufeld D, Bernheim J. Decubitus small-bowel perforation in ongoing continuous ambulatory peritoneal dialysis. Nephrol Dial Transplant 1992; 7: 79–81.
283. Brady HR, Abraham G, Oreopoulos DG, Cardella CJ. Bowel erosion due to a dormant peritoneal catheter in immunosuppressed renal transplant recipient. Perit Dial Int 1988; 8: 163.
284. Nelson W, Khanna R, Mathews R et al. Gallbladder stones, cholecystitis and cholecystectomy in patients on continuous ambulatory peritoneal dialysis. Perit Dial Bull 1984; 4: 245–8.
285. Malluche HH, Faugere MC. Renal bone disease 1990: An unmet challenge for the nephrologist. Kidney Int 1990; 38: 193–211.
286. Malluche HH, Monier-Faugere MC. Risk of adynamic bone disease in dialyzed patients. Kidney Int 1992; 42 (suppl 38): S62–7.
287. Pei Y, Hercz G, Greenwood C et al. Non-invasive prediction of aluminum bone disease in hemo and peritoneal dialysis patients. Kidney Int 1992; 41: 1374–82.
288. Hutchison AJ, Whitehouse RW, Boulton HF et al. Characteristics and natural history of the adynamic bone (AB) lesion in CAPD patients. (Abstract) Perit Dial Int 1992; 12 (suppl 2): S79.
289. Sherrard DJ, Hercz G, Pei Y et al. The spectrum of bone disease in end-stage renal failure. An evolving disorder. Kidney Int 1993; 43: 436–42.
290. Delmez JA, Fallon MD, Bergferd MA et al. Continuous ambulatory peritoneal dialysis and bone. Kidney Int 1986; 30: 379–84.
291. Rahman R, Heaton A, Goodship THJ. Renal osteodystrophy in patients on continuous ambulatory peritoneal dialysis: a five-year study. Perit Dial Bull 1987; 7: 20–6.
292. Delmez JA, Duggan CS, Gearing BK et al. The effects of intraperitoneal calcitriol on calcium and parathyroid hormone. Kidney Int 1987; 31: 795–9.
293. Bardin T, Zingraff J, Kuntz D, Drueke T. Dialysis related amyloidosis. Nephrol Dial Transplant 1986; 1: 151–4.
294. Ogawa H, Saito A, Hirabayashi N, Hara K. Amyloid deposition in systemic organs in long-term hemodialysis patients. Clin Nephrol 1987; 28: 199–204.
295. Campistol JM, Sole M, Munoz-Gomez J, Lopez-Pedret J, Revert L. Systemic involvement of dialysis-amyloidosis. Am J Nephrol 1990; 10: 389–96.
296. Stone WJ, Hakim RM. Beta-2-microglobulin

amyloidosis in long-term dialysis patients. Am J Nephrol 1989; 9: 177–83.
297. Ogawa H, Saito A, Oda D, Nakajima M, Chung TG. Detection of novel β_2-microglobulin in the serum of hemodialysis patients and its amyloidogenic predisposition. Clin Nephrol 1988; 30: 158–63.
298. Cummingham BA, Wang JL, Bergard I, Peterson PA. The complete amino acid sequence of β_2-microglobulin. Biochemistry 1973; 12: 4811–21.
299. Gorevic PD, Casey TT, Stone WJ et al. β_2-microglobulin is an amyloidogenic protein in man. J Clin Invest 1985; 76: 2425–9.
300. Hurst NP, VanderBerg R, Disney A et al. Dialysis related arthropathy: a survey of 95 patients receiving chronic hemodialysis with special reference to β_2-microglobulin related amyloidosis. An Rheum Dis 1989; 48: 409–20.
301. Gejyo F, Homma N, Suzuki Y, Arakawa M. Serum levels of β_2-microglobulin as a new form of amyloid protein in patients undergoing long-term hemodialysis. N Engl J Med 1986; 314: 585–6.
302. Woo P, O-Brien J, Robson M, Ansell BM. A genetic marker for systemic amyloidosis in juvenile arthritis. Lancet 1987; 2: 767–9.
303. Gejyo F, Arakawa M. Dialysis amyloidosis: current disease concepts and new perspectives for its treatment. Contrib Nephrol 1990; 78; 47–60.
304. Shirahama T, Miura K, Ju ST et al. Amyloid enhancing factor-loaded macrophages in amyloid filbril formation. Lab Invest 1990; 62: 61–8.
305. Campistol JM, Shirahama T, Abraham C et al. Demonstration of plasma proteinase inhibitors in β_2-microglobulin amyloid deposits. Kidney Int 1992; 42: 915–23.
306. Jadoul M, Noel H, VanYpersele de Strihou C. β_2-microglobulin amyloidosis in a patient treated exclusively by continuous ambulatory peritoneal dialysis. Am J Kidney Dis 1990, 15: 86–8.
307. Cruz A, Gonzalez T, Balsa A, Miguel JL, Gijon J. Destructive spondyloarthropathy in long-term CAPD and hemodialysis. J Rheumatol 1989; 16: 1169–70.
308. Canaud B, Assougna A, Falvier JL et al. β_2-microglobulin serum levels in maintenance dialysis. ASAIO Trans 1988; 34: 923–9.
309. Blumberg A, Burgi W. Behavior of β_2-microglobulin in patients with chronic renal failure undergoing hemodialysis, hemofiltration and continuous ambulatory peritoneal dialysis. Clin Nephrol 1987; 27: 245–9.
310. Lysaght MJ, Pollack CA, Moran JE, Ibels LS, Farrell PC. β_2-microglobulin removal during continuous ambulatory peritoneal dialysis. Perit Dial Int 1989; 9: 29–35.
311. Lysaght MJ, Vonesh EF, Gotch F et al. The influence of dialysis treatment modality on the decline of remaining renal function. ASAIO trans 1991; 37: 598–604.
312. Karlson FA, Wibell L, Ervin PE. β_2-microglobulin in clinical medicine. Scand J Clin Lab Invest 1980; 40 (suppl): 293–9.
313. Sethi D, Murphy CMB, Brown EA, Muller BR, Gower PE. Clearance of β_2-microglobulin using continuous ambulatory peritoneal dialysis. Nephron 1989; 52: 352–5.
314. Colombi A, Wegmann W. β_2-microglobulin amyloidosis in a patient on long-term continuous ambulatory peritoneal dialysis. Perit Dial Int 1989; 9: 321–4.
315. Chalmers A, Reynolds WJ, Oreopoulos DG et al. The arthropathy of maintenance intermittent peritoneal dialysis. Can Med Assoc J 1980; 123: 635–8.
316. Kuntz D, Naveau B, Bardin T et al. Destructive spondyloarthropathy in hemodialyzed patients: a new syndrome. Arthritis Rheum 1984; 27: 369–75.
317. Digenis GE, Davidson G, Dombros N et al. Destructive spondyloarthropathy in a patient on CAPD for 13 years. Perit Dial Int 1994; 13: 228–31.
318. Oreopoulos DG, Silverberg S. Calcium oxalate urinary tract stones in patients on maintenance dialysis. N Engl J Med 1974; 290: 1438–9.
319. Caralps A, Lioveras J, Andreu J et al. Urinary calculi in chronic dialysis patients. Lancet 1979; 2: 1024–5.
320. Bommer J, Ritz E, Tschope W et al. Urinary matrix calculi consisting of microfibrilar protein in patients on maintenance hemodialysis. Kidney Int 1979; 16: 722–8.
321. Ozasa H, Suzuki T, Takahashi K, Ota K. Protein components of amyloid like kidney stones of chronic hemodialysis patients. Nephron 1989; 53: 257–60.
322. Oren A, Husdan H, Cheng P et al. Calcium oxalate kidney stones in patients on continuous ambulatory peritoneal dialysis. Kidney Int 1984, 25: 534–8.
323. Digenis GE, Dombros NV, Orepoulos DG. Kidney stones in chronic dialysis patients. Sem Dial 1992; 5: 11–2.
324. Waldherr R, Michisch O, Bommer J, Ritz F. Clinical expression and impact of acquired cysts in progressive renal disease. In: Davison AM (ed), Proceedings of the Xth Int Congress of Nephrology 1988; pp 1126–37.
325. Ozasa H, Ota K. Mechanism of kidney stones formation in chronic hemodialysis patients. Nephron 1991; 58: 242–3.
326. Balaskas EV, Oreopoulos DG. Uremic pruritus. Dial Transpl 1992; 21: 192–244.
327. Francos GC. Uremic pruritus. Semin Dial 1988; 1: 209–12.
328. Gilchrest BA, Rowe JW, Brown RS et al. Ultraviolet phototherapy of uremic pruritus: long-term results and possible mechanisms of action. Ann Int Med 1979; 91: 17–21.
329. Evans RW, Manninen DL, Garrison LP et al. The quality of life of patients with end-stage renal failure. N Engl J Med 1985; 312: 553–9.
330. Simmons RG, Abress L. Quality of life issues for end-stage renal disease patients. Am J Kidney Dis 1990; 15: 201–8.
331. Maiorca R, Cancarini GC, Brunori G, Camerini C, Manili L. Morbidity and mortality of CAPD and

hemodialysis. Kidney Int 1993; 43 (suupl 40); S4-15.
332. Serkes KD, Blagg CR, Nolph KD, Vonesh EF, Shapiro F. Comparison of patients and technique survival in continuous ambulatory peritoneal dialysis (CAPD) and hemodialysis: a multicenter study. Perit Dial Int 1990; 10: 15-9.
333. Maiorca R, Vonesh EF, Cavalli P et al. A multi-center, selection-adjusted comparison of patient and technqiue survivals on CAPD and hemodialysis. Perit Dial Int 1991; 11: 118-27.
334. Gentil MA, Carriazo A, Pavon MI et al. Comparison of survival in continuous ambulatory peritoneal dialysis and hospital hemodialysis: a multicentric study. Nephrol Dial Transplant 1991; 6: 444-51.
335. Burton PR, Walls J. Selection-adjusted comparison of life expectancy of patients on continuous ambulatory peritoneal dialysis hemodialysis and renal transplantation. Lancet 1987; 2: 1115-9.
336. Firanek CA, Vonesh EF, Korbet SM. Patient and technique survival among an urban population of peritoneal dialysis patients. An 8-year experience. Am J Kidney Dis 1991; 18: 91-6.
337. Gokal R, Jakubowski C, King J et al. Outcome in patients on continuous ambulatory peritoneal dialysis and hemodialysis: 4-year analysis of a prospective multi-center study. Lancet 1987; 2: 1105-9.
338. US Renal Data System (USRDS) 1992. Annual report. The National Institutes of Health, National Institute of Diabetes and Digestive and Kidney Disease. Patient selection to peritoneal dialysis versus hemodialysis according to comorbid conditions 1992; pp 7-11.
339. Bruner FP, Broyer M, Brynger H et al. Survival on renal replacement therapy: data from the EDTA Registry. Nephrol Dial Transplant 1988; 3: 109-22.
340. Cox DR. Regression models and life-tables (with discussion). J R Stat Soc Series B 1972; 34: 197-220.
341. Vonesh EF. Relative risks can be risky. Perit Dial Int 1993; 13: 5-9.
342. Maiorca R, Vonesh EF, Cancarini GC et al. A six-year comparison of patient and technique survivals in CAPD and HD. Kidney Int 1988; 34: 518-24.
343. Maiorca R, Cancarini GC, Camerini C et al. Is CAPD competitive with haemodialysis for long-term treatment of uraemic patients? Nephrol Dial Transplant 1989; 4: 244-53.
344. Wolfe RA, Port FK, Hawthorne VM, Guire KE. A comparison of survival among dialytic therapies of choice: In-center hemodialysis versus continuous ambulatory peritoneal dialysis at home. Am J Kidney Dis 1990; 15: 433-40.
345. Nelson CB, Port FK, Wolfe RA, Guire KE. Comparison of continuous ambulatory peritoneal dialysis and hemodialysis patient survival with evaluation of trends during the 1980s. J Am Soc Nephrol 1992; 3: 1147-55.
346. Piccoli G, Segoloni GP, Quarello F et al. CAPD in Italy: data from two registries. In: La Greca G, Chiaramonte S, Fabris A et al (eds), Peritoneal Dialysis, Wichtig Editore, Milano 1988; pp 217-21.
347. Nolph KD, Lindblad AS, Novak JW, Steinberg SM. Experiences with the elderly in the National CAPD Registry. In: Nissenson AR (ed), Peritoneal Dialysis in the Geriatric Patient. Advances Peritoneal Dialysis. Peritoneal Dialysis Publication Inc, Toronto 1990; 6 (suppl): 33-7.
348. Gokal R. CAPD in the elderly European and UK experience. In: Nissenson AR (ed), Peritoneal Dialysis in the Geriatric Patient. Advances in Peritoneal Dialysis. Peritoneal Dialysis Publications Inc, Toronto 1990; 6 (suppl): 38-40.
349. Posen GA, Fenton SSA, Arbus GS, Churchill DN, Jeffery JR. The Canadian experience with peritoneal dialysis in the elderly. In: Nissenson AR (ed), Peritoneal Dialysis in the Geriatric Patient. Advances in Peritoneal Dialysis. Peritoneal Dialysis Publications Inc, Toronto 1990; 6 (suppl): 47-50.
350. Mallinsen WJW, Fleming SJ, Shaw JEH, Baker LRI, Cattell WR. Survival in elderly patients presenting with uremia. Q J Med (New Series) 1984; 53: 301-7.
351. Nissenson AR. Chronic peritoneal dialysis in the elderly. Ger Nephrol Urol 1991; 1: 3-12.
352. Nelson CB, Port FK, Wolfe RA, Guire KE. Dialysis patient survival. Evaluation of CAPD versus HD using 3 techniques (abstract). Perit Dial Int 1992; 12 (suppl): 144.
353. US Renal Data System: USRDS 1991. Annual Report. The National Institutes of Health. National Institute of Diabetes and Digestive and Kidney Disease. Survival probability and causes of death. Bethesda, MD, August 1 1991; pp 31-40.
354. Raine AEG, Margreiter R, Brunner FP et al. Report on management of Renal Failure in Europe, XXII 1991. Nephrol Dial Transplant 1992; 7 (suppl 2): 7-35.
355. Nissenson AR. Dialysis therapy in the elderly patient. Kidney Int 1993; 43 (suppl 40): S51-7.
356. Port FK. Mortality and causes of death in patients with end-stage renal failure. Am J Kidney Dis 1990; 15: 215-7.
357. Canadian Organ Replacement Registry, 1989 Annual Report. Don Mills, Ontario, Hospital Medical Records Institute, March 1991.
358. Fourteenth report of the Australia and New Zealand Dialysis and Transplant Registry (ANZDATA) Disney APS (ed) Oct 1991; pp 34-40.
359. Brunner FP, Ehrich JHH, Fassbinder W et al. Combined report on regular dialysis and transplantation in Europe. 1990, Nephrol Dial Transpl 1991; 6 (suppl. 4): 5-29.
360. Nolph KD. What's new in peritoneal dialysis – an overview. Kidney Int 1992; 42 (suppl 38): S148-52.
361. Twelfth report of the Australia and New Zealand combined Dialysis and transplant registry. Disney APS (eds), Woodville, South Australia, Queen Elizabeth Hospital, 1989.
362. Gokal R, Baillod R, Bogle S et al. Multi-center

study on outcome of treatment in patients on continuous ambulatory peritoneal dilaysis and haemodialysis. Nephrol Dial Trans 1987; 2: 172–8.
363. Marichal JF, Cordier B, Faller B, Brignon P. Continuous ambulatory peritoneal dialysis or center haemodialysis? Retrospective evaluation of the success of both methods. Perit Dial Int 1990; 10; 205–8.
364. Port FK, Held PJ, Nolph KD, Turenne MN, Wolfe RA. Risk of peritonitis and technique failure by CAPD connection technique: A national study. Kidney Int 1992; 42: 967–74.
365. Finkelstein FD, Sorkin M, Cramton CW, Nolph KD. Initiatives in Peritoneal Dialysis: Where do we go from here? Perit Dial Int 1991; 11: 274–8.
366. Steinberg SM, Cutler SJ, Nolph KD et al. A comprehensive Report on the experience of patients on continuous ambulatory peritoneal dialysis for the treatment of end-stage renal disease. Am J. Kidney Dis 1984; 4: 233–41.
367. Piraino B, Bernardini J, Sorkin M. Catheter infections as a factor in the transfer of continuous ambulatory peritoneal dialysis patients to hemodialysis. Am J Kidney Dis 1989; 13: 365–9.
368. Goldman M, Vanherweghem JL. Bacterial infection in chronic hemodialysis patients; epidemiologic and pathophysiologic aspects. Adv Nephrol 1990; 19: 315–32.
369. Douglas SD, Schopfer K. Phagocyte function in protein-calorie malnutrition. Clin Exp Immunol 1974; 17: 121–8.
370. Chruchill DN, Taylor DW, Cook RJ et al. Canadian hemodialysis morbidity study. Am J Kidney Dis 1992; 19: 214–34.
371. Canadian CAPD Clinical Trials Group. Peritonitis in continuous ambulatory peritoneal dialysis; a multicenter randomized clinical trial comparing the Y connector disinfectant system to standard systems. Perit Dial Int 1989; 9: 159–63.
372. Dryden MS, McCann M, Wing AJ, Phillips I. Controlled trial of a Y-set dialysis delivery system to prevent peritonitis in patients receiving continuous ambulatory peritoneal dialysis. J. Hosp Infect 1992; 20: 185–92.
373. Carozzi S, Nasini MG, Schelotto C et al. Peritoneal macrophages beta-2 microglobulin production and bacterial peritonitis in CAPD patients. ASAIO Trans 1990; 36: M369–71.
374. Binik YM, Denis GM, Orme CM. Psychological stress and coping in end-stage renal disease. In: Neufeld RWJ (ed), Advances in Investigation of Psychological Stress. Wiley, New York 1989; pp 305–42.
375. Levenson JL, Glocheski S. Psychological factors affecting end-stage renal disease. A review. Psychosomatics 1991; 32: 382–9.
376. Petrie K. Psychological well-being and psychiatric disturbance in dialysis and renal transplant patients. Br J Med Psychol 1989; 62: 91–6.
377. Morris PL, Jones B. Life satisfaction across treatment methods for patients with end-stage renal failure. Med J Aust 1989; 150: 428–32.
378. Koch U, Muthny FA. Quality of life in patients with end-stage renal disease in relation to the method of treatment. Psychother Psychosom 1990; 54: 161–71.
379. Simmons RG, Anderson CR, Abress LK. Quality of life and rehabilitation differences among four ESRD therapy groups. Scand J Urol Nephrol 1990; (suppl 131): 7–22.
380. Kalman TP, Wilson PG, Kalman CM. Psychiatric morbidity in long-term renal transplant recipients and patients undergoing dialysis. JAMA 1983; 250: 55–8.
381. Evans RW, Rader B, Manninen D. The quality of life of hemodialysis recipients treated with recombinant human erythropoietin. JAMA 1990; 263: 825–30.
382. Auer J, Simon G, Stevens J et al. Quality of life improvements in CAPD patients treated with subcutaneously administered erythropoietin for anemia. Perit Dial Int 1992; 12: 40–2.
383. Wolcott DL, Wellish DK, Marsh JT et al. Relationship of dialysis modality and other factors to cognitive function in chronic dialysis patients. Am J Kidney Dis 1988; 12: 275–84.
384. Wolcott DL. Nissenson AR. Quality of life in chronic dialysis patients: A critical comparison of CAPD and hemodialysis. Am J Kidney Dis 1988; 11: 402–12.
385. Gokal R. Quality of life in patients undergoing renal replacement therapy. Kidney Int 1993; 43 (suppl 40): 523–7.
386. Grant AC, Rodger RSC, Howie CA et al. Dialysis at home in the West of Scotland: a comparison of hemodialysis and continuous ambulatory peritoneal dialysis in age- and sex-matched controls. Perit Dial Int 1992; 12: 365–8.
387. Nolph KD. Continuous ambulatory peritoneal dialysis as a long-term treatment for end stage renal disease (editorial). Am J Kidney Dis 1991; 17: 154–7.
388. Ataman R, Burton PR, Gokal R, Brown CB, Marsh FP, Walls J. Long-term CAPD – some UK experience. Clin Nephrol 1988; 30: S71–5.
389. Lindblad AS, Novak JW, Nolph KD. Continuous ambulatory peritoneal dialysis in the USA – Final report of the National CAPD registry 1981–1988. Kluwer Academic, Dordrecht 1989.
390. Holden AL, Gaumer G. Best demonstrated practices program promoting CAPD patient retention in the United States. In: Khanna R, Nolph KD, Prowant B, Twardowski ZJ, Oreopoulos DG (eds), Advances in CAPD. Peritoneal Dialysis Bulletin Inc, Toronto 1987; pp 186–91.
391. Lameire NH, Vanholder R, Veyt D. Lambert MC, Ringoir S. A longitudinal five year survey of urea kinetic paramaters in CAPD patients. Kidney Int 1992; 42: 426–32.
392. Dobbie JW. Monitoring peritoneal histopathology in peritoneal dialysis: The role of biopsy registry. Dial Transplant 1989; 18: 319–25.
393. Pollock CA, Ibels LS, Eckstein RP et al. Peritoneal morphology on maintenance dialysis. Am J Nephrol 1989; 9: 198–203.

394. Gilmour J, Wu G, Khanna R, Schilling H, Mitwalli A, Oreopoulos DG. Long-term continuous ambulatory peritoneal dialysis. Perit Dial Bull 1985; 5: 112–8.
395. Nolph KD, Gutler S, Steinberg S, Novak JW. Special Studies from the NIH USA CAPD registry. Perit Dial Bull 1986; 6: 39–45.
396. Heaton A, Roger RSC, Sellars L et al. Continuous ambulatory peritoneal dialysis after the honeymoon: review of experience in Newcastle 1979–1984. Brit Med J 1986; pp 938–41.
397. Faller B, Pierre D, Verger C et al. One thousand years treatment of CAPD. A French multicenter cooperative study on drop-out rate (Abstract). Perit Dial Bull 1986; 6 (suppl 4): S6.
398. Gokal R. Continuous ambulatory peritoneal dialysis. Ten years on. Q J Med 1987; 63: 465–72.

13 Automated peritoneal dialysis

JOSE A. DIAZ-BUXO AND WADI N. SUKI

1. 1.1. Introduction 399
   1.2. History 399
2. 2.1. Technique 400
   2.2 Peritoneal dialysis cyclers 401
3. Peritoneal dialysis solutions 403
4. Physiologic considerations 403
   4.1. Ultrafiltration 403
   4.2. Solute removal 403
   4.3. Contributions of the diurnal cycles 404
   4.4. Relative efficiency of different modalities of APD 405
   4.5. Relationship between intraperitoneal volume and intra-abdominal pressure 406
   4.6. Effect of posture on peritoneal solute transport 406
   4.7. Steady physiologic state 407
   4.8. Selection of APD modality 407
   4.9. Formulation of adequate prescription for APD 407
5. Clinical experience with CCPD 408
   5.1. Hematologic and biochemical paramters 408
      5.1.1. Hematological parameters 408
      5.1.2. Nitrogenous waste-products 409
      5.1.3. Calcium, phosphorus, and renal osteodystrophy 409
      5.1.4. Nutritional status 409
   5.2. Blood pressure control 410
   5.3. Selected complications of CCPD 410
      5.3.1. Peritonitis 410
      5.3.2. Exit site infections and catheter replacements 411
      5.3.3. Hernias and other complications due to increased intra-abdominal pressure 412
      5.3.4. Catheter related complications 412
   5.4. Morbidity and mortality 412
6. Treatment of diabetics with CCPD 413
7. Treatment of children with CCPD 413
8. CCPD in the treatment of acute renal failure 413
9. Renal transplantation in CCPD patients 414
10. Conclusions 414
References 414

1.1. Introduction

Automated peritoneal dialysis (APD) is a broad term that is used to refer to all forms of peritoneal dialysis (PD) employing a mechanical device to assist in the delivery and drainage of the dialysate [1]. Among the therapeutic regimens encompassed by APD are continuous cyclic peritoneal dialysis (CCPD), intermittent peritoneal dialysis (IPD), nightly intermittent peritoneal dialysis (NIPD) and tidal peritoneal dialysis (TPD). Automating the delivery of PD has many obvious benefits and some that are not so obvious.

The most obvious advantage of APD is that it eliminates the need for intensive human manual involvement, reducing the PD process to two procedures per day: setting up the dialysis machine and connecting the patient, and disconnecting the patient and dismantling the machine. In addition to its simplicity and this minimalistic aspect of APD, added advantages include the ability to receive treatment at home, carried out by the patient or by a helper, and in the latter case without overburdening the helper. Furthermore, the fact that the treatment can be carried out during the night, enables the patient and the helper, where applicable, to rest during the night and affords all parties involved freedom from all procedures during most of the daytime hours.

A less obvious advantage of automated dialysis is a reduction in the rate of peritonitis. It is not surprising therefore, that recent data indicate that as many as 33% of all new patients going on PD in the United States are being treated with APD. In fact, in the past five years, APD has been the fastest growing modality of renal replacement therapy in the United States. In 1992 the number of patients being treated with APD was almost 5800 and this number is expected to grow to 9500 in 1994.

1.2. History

In the early 1960's the first attempts were made to automate the delivery of PD. One of the earliest attempts was by Fred S. T. Boen who, while at the University of Washington, developed an automated unit which could be operated during the night and consisted of a 40 liter 'carboy' container, filled with sterilized peritoneal dialysate which was delivered through an automatic solenoid device that would open and close a switch allowing a present amount of fluid in and out of the peritoneal cavity [2]. This device was used for treating patients suffering from renal failure in their homes. In 1961, Norman Lasker developed a simple gravity-fed device which used sterilized 2-liter bottles of dialysate and had a flexible, plastic reservoir bag [3]. This device had the advantage of measuring the volume of fluid to be instilled into the peritoneal cavity and warming the solution before it was instilled. The Lasker 'cycler' was the forerunner of the subsequent generation of cyclers; one of the earliest to become commercially available was the cycler manufactured by American Medical Products (AMP).

Cyclers were initially used for the performance of IPD. Patients would undergo PD in cycles lasting 1 or more hours, for as long as 24 hours once a week, 12 hours two or more times a week, or even shorter treatments lasting 6 to 8 hours performed as many as five times a week. With the introduction in 1976 of the concept of equilibrium PD by Popovich and Moncrief, and the subsequent development of the treatment modality which came to be called continuous ambulatory peritoneal dialysis (CAPD) [4], interest in PD as a viable treatment modality for end-stage renal disease was revived. This revival was facilitated by the development of collapsible plastic bag containers for peritoneal dialysate. It quickly became clear to several groups who flocked to CAPD that this modality was not suited for the manually or visually impaired nor for the very young. Thus, children, elderly patients with tremors, Parkinsonism or strokes, and diabetics with blindness and neuropathy, strokes and limb amputations could not avail themselves of this technique.

In the late 1970's two groups, that of Diaz-Buxo in Charlotte, North Carolina and that of Suki in Houston, Texas began to experiment with the adaptation of automated cyclers to equilibrium dialysis. Both groups reported their experience simultaneously in 1981 [5–7], and the technique they developed came to be known as continuous cyclic peritoneal dialysis or CCPD. An automated form of equilibrium PD, CCPD, consisted of a reversal of the usual rhythm of CAPD, so that 3 or 4 exchanges are automatically carried out during the patient's sleeping hours and another exchange is instilled into the patient's peritoneal cavity in the morning before the patient is disconnected from the cycler. This exchange remains in the patient's abdomen until automated dialysis is resumed the following evening. Each treatment, therefore, begins with the patient emptying out the fluid that dwelled in the peritoneal cavity during the day before initiating the filling cycle. This sequence of fluid movement, perhaps was responsible for the reduced peritonitis rate observed in some facilities using this technique.

A variation of CCPD is TPD. This technique uses a reserve volume and a rapidly exchanged tidal volume designed to improve the efficiency of dialysis. This technique was first introduced under the name of reciprocating PD and revived by Twardowski as tidal PD [8, 9, 10]. Newer modifications of this latter system have recently been presented by Baxter investigators employing an air driven displacement system which delivers pulses of dialysate [11]. This pulsed system offers the theoretic advantage of providing a measure of stirring, thereby minimizing or eliminating unstirred layers of dialysate, and improving solute transport.

2.1. Technique

APD is suitable for use with any type of peritoneal catheter, whether of the straight or curled Tenckhoff variety, or the column-disk type. The central requirement is that of an automated cycler of the volume-regulated and/or time-regulated variety. To meet the needs of APD, a cycler must be able to deliver a variety of preset volumes, at a preset time. Through appropriate connectology the cycler is connected to the dialysis catheter before the patient retires for the night. The cycler is programmed to deliver 3 or more cycles during the night, of a volume previously determined to be well tolerated by the patient. Patients tolerate larger volumes of fluid during recumbency than they do in the upright posture. Furthermore, dialysis efficiency increases with larger volumes. Thus, volumes of 2–3 liters could be attempted in order to provide the greatest dose of dialysis attainable. In the morning prior to disconnecting, a final exchange of 1–2 liters is introduced and allowed to remain until it is time for the nightly cycles, or a total of approximately 14–15 hours. It is desirable that this exchange be of 2.5 or 4.25% dextrose solution in order to maximize the volume of dialysate recovered at the end of this period in the face of continued absorption of dialysate from the peritoneal cavity.

With the availability of 3 and 5 liter dialysate bags only 2 or 3 bag spikings may be necessary for a treatment. Furthermore, the availability of manifolds with multiple prongs for spiking dialysate bottles and a single prong leading to the patient's catheter, the number of connections and, therefore, the chance for touch contamination is greatly diminished. In addition, the setup time is considerably minimized much to the advantage of the patient and/or helper. A number of modifications of this system have been introduced and used with considerable success. These include disconnect systems which use the principle of external occlusion and allow clamping followed by severing the line for simplification of disconnection [12]. The system is never open at the time of disconnection and sterility is preserved until the next CCPD session (Fig. 1). Other modifications include the multiple tubing set (MTS^{TM}) which allows set up on bags and tubing for as many as 3 consecutive days of dialysis, thereby greatly reducing the total setup time [13]. These modifications have been shown to be safe without an increased risk of peritonitis.

NPD uses the same basic technology as described for CCPD, while eliminating the diurnal cycle. TPD requires the use of a volume regulated cycler. The cycler is programmed to maintain a reserve volume and to cycle a tidal volume. The dialysate flow patterns for CAPD, CCPD, NPD and TPD are graphically presented in Fig. 2.

2.2. Peritoneal dialysis cyclers

The spectrum of cyclers that has been introduced over the past 30 years has varied widely from the very simple to the very elaborate and sophisticated. They range from the traditional gravity-driven system, to the partially pump-driven system, on to the totally pump-driven system. The partially pump dependent systems rely on a pump to propel the dialysate from a large dialysate bag to a smaller dialysate bag, laying on a heated cradle which may also serve as a scale which determines the volume to be infused into the patient. Virtually all recent cyclers preheat the solution before instillation into the patient to avoid hypothermia, patient discomfort, arrhythmias, or vasoconstriction of the splanchnic circulation. It should be pointed out, however, that considering the dwell times for 3 or 4 exchanges in CCPD being of the order of 3 hours each, it is most unlikely that such complications

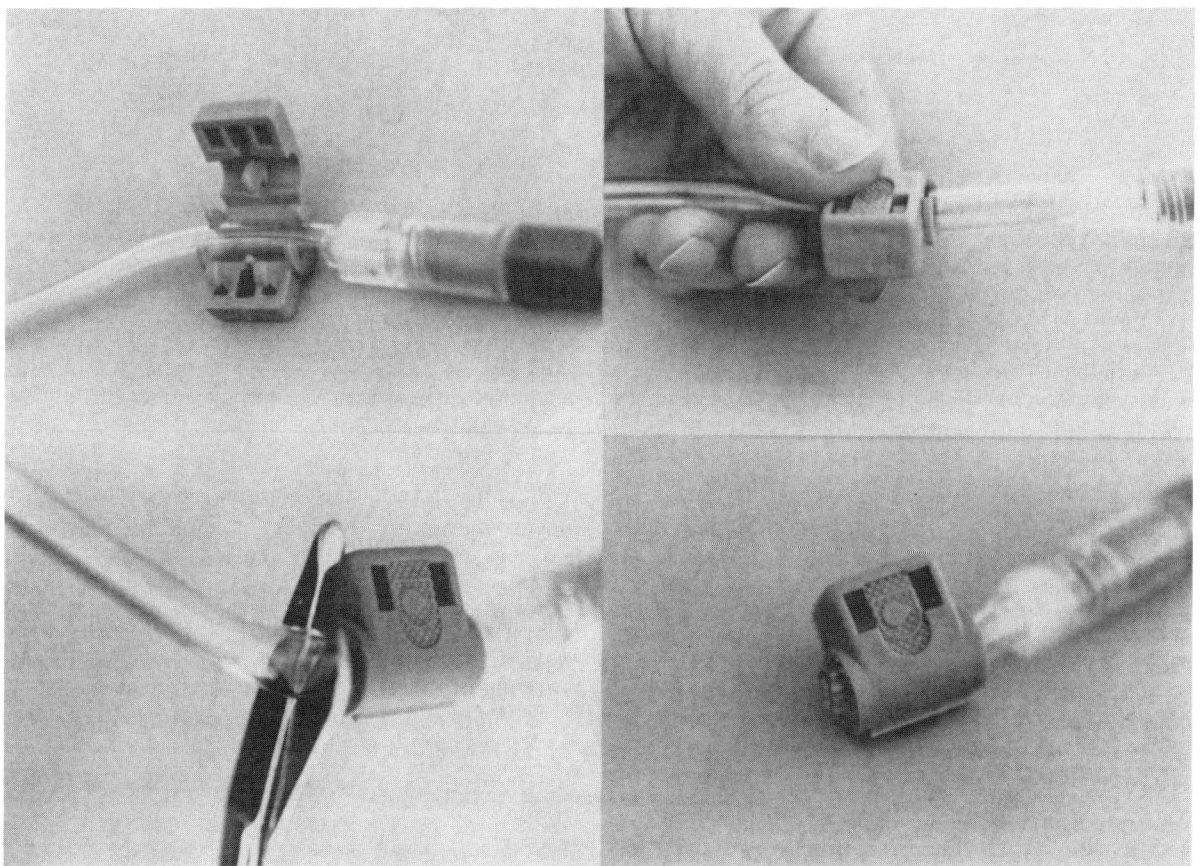

Figure 1. Disposable clamp for disconnection after nocturnal cycle of CCPD using external occlusion.

DIALYSATE FLOW PATTERNS

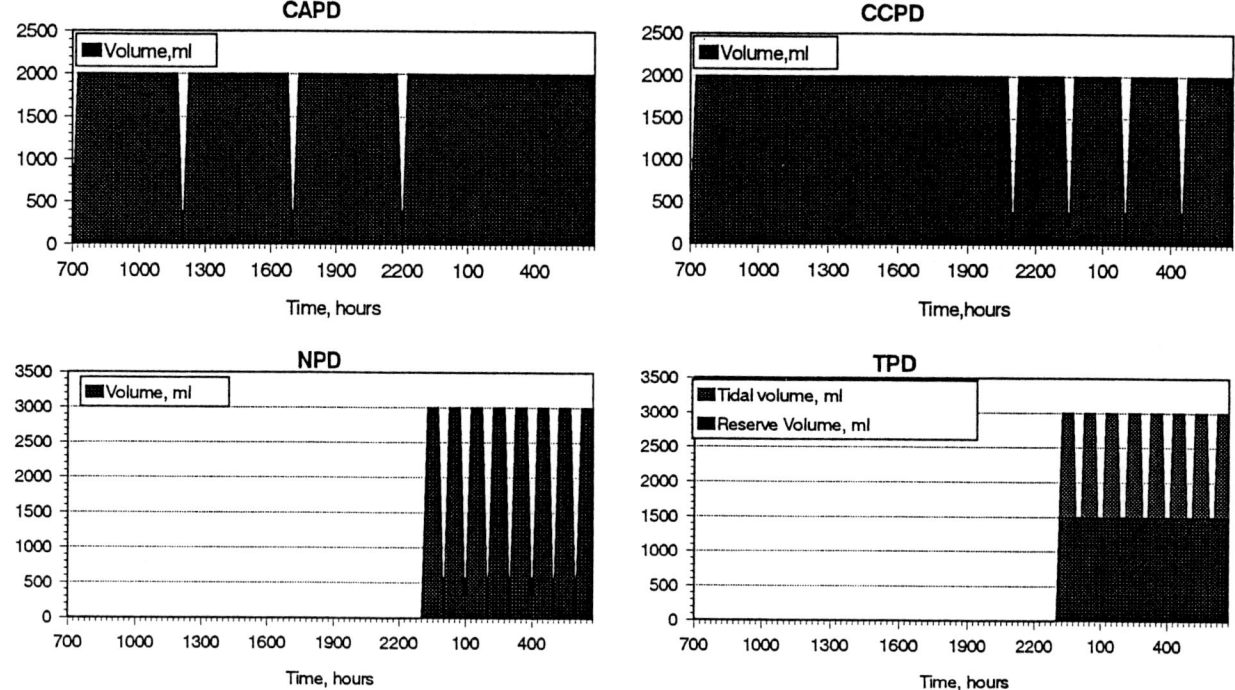

Figure 2.

would ensue. Other features of peritoneal cyclers include the capacity to deliver a predetermined volume of dialysate and the measurement, usually through weighing with built-in scales, of the spent dialysate volume, thereby affording the opportunity to maintain a record, which can be stored in the memory of the cycler, and report the instantaneous as well as cumulative ultrafiltration (UF) rate. The ability to monitor UF is most useful in the hospital setting where patients may require close monitoring of fluid shifts and UF volume, or where patients may be too sick or incapacitated to be weighed at frequent intervals or to be weighed at all.

An advantage of the partially pump-driven system is that it allows the use of less expensive large volume dialysate bags such as a 5 liter bag. A large volume of fluid does not have to be carried overhead in order to utilize gravity for the fill cycle. Instead, the high capacity bag can be suspended on built-in hooks at waist level, and a roller pump is used to pump dialysate from this reservoir to a smaller bag laying on the heater cradle which is approximately 20 cm above the level of the patient's abdominal cavity, thereby using gravity for dialysate inflow.

Totally pump-driven systems use pumps, both to instill dialysate into the patient and to drain spent dialysate. Such systems may be most suited for TPD wherein the volume of dialysate instilled and withdrawn is smaller than the total volume of dialysate in the peritoneal cavity. This is less likely to be associated with overdistention of the abdomen or with the accidental application of excessive negative pressure. Besides, the strategic placement of positive and negative pressure monitors could render such a system very safe. The advantage of such a system could be that the instillation of small pulsed volumes of dialysate may provide sufficient stirring of the fluid in the peritoneal cavity to overcome the effect of unstirred layers and to improve dialysis efficiency. Such cyclers are now under development and nearing release for clinical trials.

3. Peritoneal dialysis solutions

With one exception, the solutions used for APD are the same as those used for CAPD. These solutions have fixed concentrations of sodium, magnesium and lactate and are free of potassium. The variables available are in dextrose and in calcium concentrations. Three general types of solutions are used: 1.5%, 2.5% and 4.25% with respect to dextrose, providing increasing degrees of hypertonicity and increased UF potential. The solution used for the daytime exchange should be of the 2.5% or 4.25% strength in order to minimize the total volume of dialysate absorbed during this long dwell time. The other variable is the concentration of calcium. With the adoption of calcium salts, particularly the carbonate and the acetate, as phosphate binders, significant degrees of hypercalcemia have been observed necessitating the development of dialysate solutions containing only 2.5 mEq/l of calcium instead of the usual 3.5 meq/l (Table 1).

The one exception to the similarity in solutions used in APD versus CAPD is the situation in which frequent short-dwell exchanges are used for the purpose of effecting significant UF. Because of the sieving effect of the peritoneal membrane, the ultrafiltrate removed has a lower concentration of sodium than that of the patient, contributing to the development of hypernatremia and hyperosmolarity. For such purposes, therefore, the use of lower sodium concentrations may be necessary [14, 15].

4. Physiologic considerations

The physiological principles governing solute and water transport across the peritoneal membrane were described in Chapters 4, 5 and 6. A good understanding of these principles is essential in the manipulation of UF and solute removal with APD and in the optimization of prescription. The main physiologic difference between CAPD and most APD techniques is the marked variation in cycle duration with APD. While most exchanges of CAPD are long enough to allow virtual equilibration of small molecules, APD uses shorter, more frequent exchanges, and often a higher total dialysate flow (Fig. 2).

A second significant difference is the possible use of larger exchange volumes that may affect clearance and UF. Larger volumes during the night are usually better tolerated with the patient in the supine position. Combining a high dialysate flow and a high intraperitoneal volume can be effectively used to enhance PD.

4.1. Ultrafiltration

Ultrafiltration is achieved by creating a transperitoneal osmotic gradient using hypertonic dialysis solutions. Commercially available dialysate contains 1.5 to 4.25% dextrose. The peritoneal UF rate curve exhibits an exponential decay configuration, paralleling glucose disappearance (absorption) from dialysate and the dilutional effect contributed by UF. It follows that maximum net UF can be achieved by shortening the dwell time, thus using the region of maximum gradient, or by increasing the exchange volume, which also increases the osmotic gradient. Patients with extraordinary UF requirements may also benefit from additional, shorter exchanges. This maneuver results in higher UF per gram of absorbed glucose, an important consideration in the treatment of patients with diabetes, obesity or hyperlipidemia [16].

For practical purposes most of the net UF takes place during the nocturnal exchanges of CCPD. Even with the use of 4.25% dextrose solutions, most patients will absorb 12–20% of the volume infused for the diurnal cycle after 14 hours of dwell.

4.2. Solute removal

The clearances for small molecules are highly dependent on dialysate flow. Full equilibration between dialysate and plasma for urea is attained within 4 hours of dialysate dwell for most patients. The early portion of the cycle is characterized by a faster rate of equilibration with eventual flattening of the curve.

The influence of intraperitoneal volume (Vip) on solute removal (peritoneal clearance, Kp) and overall peritoneal permeability-area product (KoA) has not been fully characterized. However, it is well accepted that the plasma to dialysate (D/P) gradient is the diffusive driving force for solute transfer. This diffusive gradient is maximized by increasing dialysate flow by either higher flow rates with equal

Table 1. Composition of standard solutions for APD.

Dextrose	(%)	1.5–4.25
Sodium	(mEq/L)	132
Potassium	(mEq/L)	0
Calcium	(mEq/L)	2.5–3.5
Magnesium	(mEq/L)	0.5–1.5
Lactate	(mEq/L)	35–40

Vip or by increasing the Vip. The former is associated with a reduction in effective dialysis time as the flow increases due to an increasing ratio of inflow + outflow time to total cycle time. The latter, however, increases the diffusive gradient without effect on dialysis time. Kp is a function of dialysate flow rate and KoA. Data are also accumulating to suggest the KoA is strongly dependent on Vip [17–19].

Analysis of the data reported by Twardowski *et al.* with various Vip's suggests that KoA is nearly proportional to Vip [19]. Similarly, Brandes *et al.* have reported a strong correlation between Vip and normalized mass transfer area coefficient (MTAC) [17]. This relationship is linear in the range of 0.5 to 2.0 L and plateaus at higher Vip. Our own recent observations show that KoA is highly dependent on Vip and essentially doubles by increasing the Vip from 1.0 to 3.0 L in adult patients [18].

Use of this knowledge, combined with the fact that patients undergoing APD usually tolerate higher Vip's, can serve to enhance small solute removal in a convenient and effective manner whenever necessary. Further analysis of the contribution of higher peritoneal dialysate flow rates and increments in Vip is essential in our quest for more efficient PD.

The equilibration of middle molecules is significantly slower. Even at the end of the long diurnal exchanges of CCPD equilibration is incomplete for molecules such as inulin and Vitamin B_{12}. KoA is inversely proportional to solute molecular weight. Thus, maximal efficiency for larger solutes peaks at lower dialysate flow rates. Continuous PD modalities generally provide superior middle molecule clearances than intermittent dialysis, regardless of peritoneal dialysate flow rates.

4.3. Contributions of the diurnal cycles

The recognition of a causal relationship between intra-abdominal pressure (IAP), body position and certain complications of PD, has stimulated modifications in the CCPD protocol. The most common modifications are the reduction in the diurnal Vip or total elimination of the diurnal cycle and an increase in the total dialysate flow of the nocturnal cycles to partially compensate for the loss in total clearance of small solutes. The elimination of the diurnal cycle of CCPD results in IPD or NPD and has a significant impact on solute removal in patients with normal peritoneal transport rates.

Diaz-Buxo *et al.* studied the contributions of the diurnal cycle of CCPD to urea and creatinine clearance and protein losses in 12 patients with normal solute transport rates [20]. Peritoneal transport rates were assessed by standard peritoneal equilibration tests (PET). The ratio of dialysate glucose concentration at 4 hours to the initial glucose concentration (D4/Do) ranged between 0.33 and 0.42 for the 12 patients studied (Fig. 3). Three study protocols were used. The nocturnal exchanges lasted 10 hours and used 1.5% dextrose dialysate. The diurnal exchange lasted 14 hours and used 4.5% dextrose dialysate. Protocol I consisted of three, 2 L nocturnal exchanges and the diurnal exchange. Protocol II used four, 2 L exchanges and totally eliminated the diurnal exchange and Protocol III used three, 2 L nocturnal exchanges and also eliminated the diurnal cycle. The sequence of the studies was randomized. Figure 4 summarizes the urea and creatinine clearances for the different protocols. Significantly greater clearances were obtained for both urea and creatinine with Protocol I (CCPD)

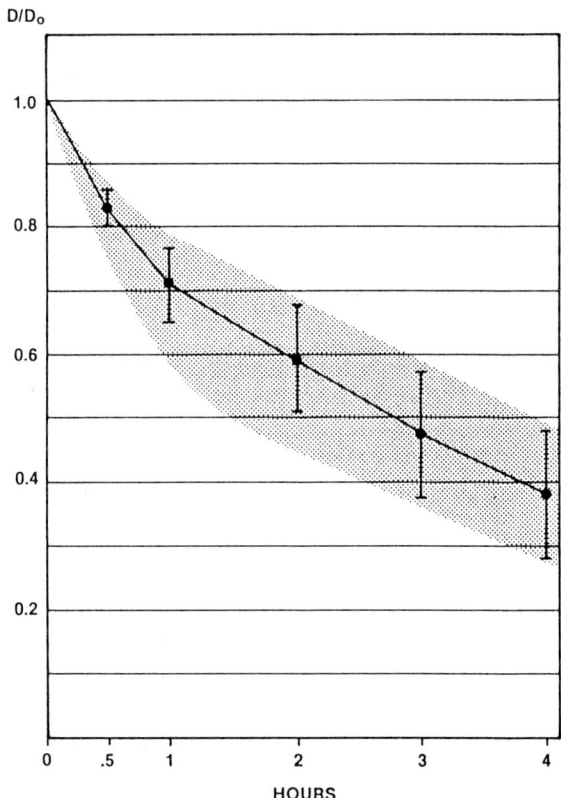

Figure 3. Equilibration curve for glucose for the study population using 2 l of 2.5% dextrose dialysate. D/D_0 refers to glucose concentration in dialysate at time t/glucose concentration in dialysate immediately after instillation. The shaded area represents mean ± 1SD for our total populaton [16].

than with II or III that eliminated the diurnal cycles (NPD). No differences in protein losses were observed among the three protocols. These data suggest that an increase in nocturnal dialysate flow of this magnitude only partially compensates for the loss in clearance otherwise provided by the diurnal cycle. The difference should be even larger for larger solutes. This experience is consistent with that of Twardowski *et al.* who showed that NPD required three times the dialysate flow to provide the same urea clearance as CAPD and that creatinine clearance with CAPD was superior to that of NPD using 26 L of dialysate over 8 hours for patients with normal peritoneal transport rates [16].

Although reductions in diurnal Vip may be necessary in some patients due to intolerance or to the development of complications associated with increased IAP (vide infra), most patients on CCPD can tolerate a diurnal Vip 50–75% of the nocturnal exchange volume. Patients with high peritoneal transport rates benefit from complete elimination of the diurnal cycle and transfer to NPD or TPD. The long-term effects of a 10–20% reduction in the efficiency of solute removal may have significant clinical consequences, particularly in patients with little or no residual renal function [21, 22].

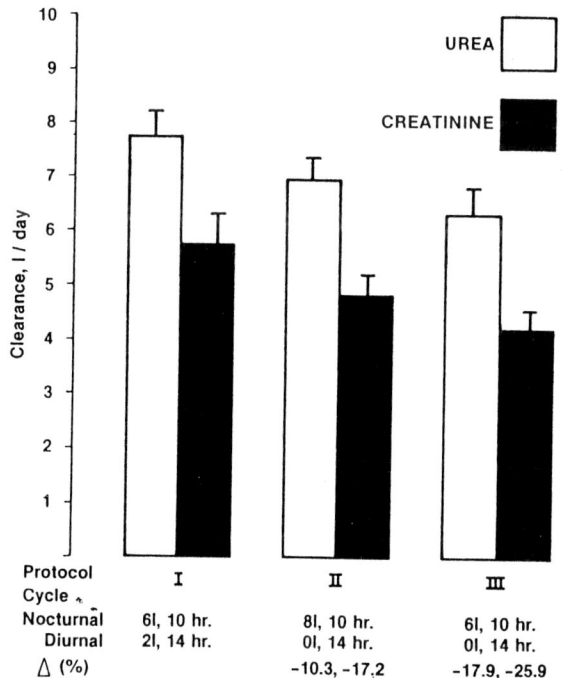

Figure 4. Daily urea and creatinine clearance with different dialysis protocols [16].

4.4. Relative efficiency of different modalities of APD

Based on the aforementioned principles, it is evident that the efficiency of the different modalities of PD will be affected by total effective dialysis time, peritoneal dialysate flow, Vip, the patient's specific solute transport rate and the magnitude of the convective component (net UF). Less clear is the influence of the specific technique (i.e., TPD or NPD).

The most common modalities of PD use a well defined inflow-dwell-outflow fluid pattern, rather than a continuous inflow-outflow pattern. The first method is effective only during the periods of dialysate contact with the peritoneum, but is interrupted by the periods required for inflow and drainage. For practical purposes, these periods are short and of little clinical consequences, as with CAPD and CCPD. However, during high flow APD, with dialysate flow rates exceeding 2 L per hour, the non-dialytic period becomes significant. This problem is worse in patients with slow peritoneal drainage. The continuous method eliminates the non-dialytic period, but requires two catheters or a double catheter. It also has the disadvantage of possible mixing or recirculation of spent dialysate if the two catheters are too close to each other.

An alternative approach is TPD [8, 9, 23]. This technique periodically injects a certain volume of dialysate (tidal volume or TV), maintains a constant intraperitoneal volume (residual volume or RV) and periodically drains a volume similar to the TV plus UF. The major potential advantage of this system is the improved mixing of fluid layers, thus enhancing solute transport. However, the early experiences did not confirm this notion and suggested that the improved clearances were only the result of elimination of the wasted periods of non-dialysis required for inflow and outflow at high dialysate flow rates, or, due to an increase in effective peritoneal area when a larger Vip was used for reciprocating PD.

More recently, Twardowski *et al.* have reported their experience with TPD [10, 19, 24]. Analysis of their data initially suggested that TPD was 20–30% more efficient than NPD in clearing urea [19]. However, the authors compared patients undergoing NPD using a Vip = 2 L and those undergoing TPD with a Vip = 3 L. The differences in magnitude of Vip fully account for the improved urea clearances in TPD.

Shah et al. measured urea and creatinine clearances in the same patient during IPD and TPD using the same dialysate flow rate and isovolumic (Vip = 1.5 L) exchanges [25]. No differences in clearance were observed among the studies. They concluded that, if duration of dwell and Vip are kept constant, TPD offers no advantage over IPD. Notwithstanding the attractiveness of the mixing theory, the present state of knowledge does not prove an advantage of TPD over high flow NPD within a certain range of dialysate flow rate.

Table 2 summarizes the typical clearances obtained with various modalities of APD and with CAPD. These figures are approximations assuming an ideal patient with average solute transport rates, adequate catheter function and stable metabolic status.

4.5. Relationship between intraperitoneal volume and intra-abdominal pressure

A positive linear relationship between Vip and IAP has been established [26–28]. This relationship is maintained regardless of the patient's position, but the slope of the curve shifts with changes in position (Fig. 5). Increments in pressure with a given volume are higher in the upright than in the supine positions and further increase in the sitting position [27, 28]. Therefore, the same or even larger volumes of dialysate are better tolerated while the patient is supine than during periods of activity. Larger Vip's are generally possible during the nocturnal cycles of APD.

The effects of Vip and position on IAP should be kept in mind when prescribing APD. Since net UF peaks in most patients approximately three hours after infusion of hypertonic dialysate for the diurnal cycle of CCPD, and since this time often coincides

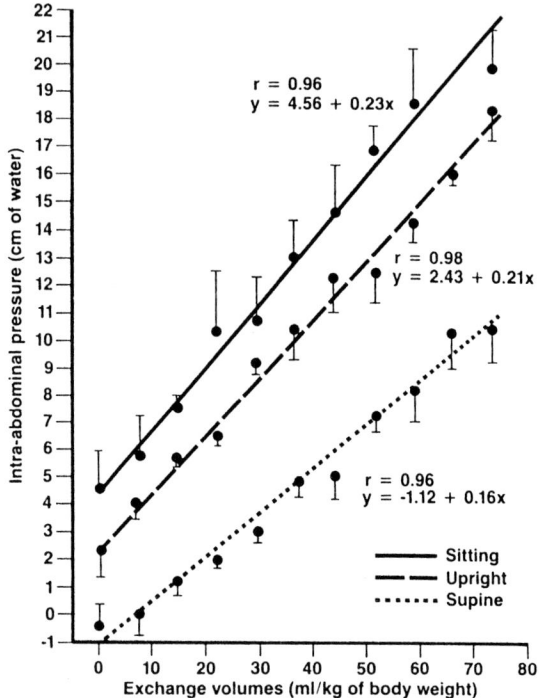

Figure 5. Comparative effect of dialysate volume and patient position on intra-abdominal pressure. Means ± SEM [14].

with the ingestion of food, further increasing IAP, it is wise to reduce the volume of the diurnal exchange if abdominal discomfort is observed. The appropriate reduction in diurnal Vip has resulted in a significant decrease in the incidence of complications related to IAP.

4.6. Effect of posture on peritoneal solute transport

Curatola et al. found that both urea and creatinine clearance decreased in the sitting position in comparison with those obtained in the supine position [29]. More recently, Fukudome et al. evaluated the effect of posture on peritoneal blood flow with the use of color flow-Doppler ultrasound (CFDU) [30]. The authors measured portal blood flow in CAPD patients as an indicator of peritoneal blood flow. The velocity of flow was significantly increased in the supine position. Their results suggest a higher efficacy of CAPD in the supine position. If indeed solute transport is accelerated in the supine position, the various modalities of APD should offer an additional advantage over CAPD. Conversely, Otero et al. have failed to verify any influence of posture on solute transport or UF [31]. This problem requires further analysis with controlled studies.

Table 2. Weekly clearance (L/wk) for various PD prescriptions.

	Prescription	Kp urea	Kp creatinine
CAPD	2L × 4; 24 hr	59.5	44.1
CCPD	2L × 5; 10 hr 2L × 1; 14 hr	57	43
IPD	4L/hr; 40 hr/wk	58	34
NPD	Vip = 2L; 24L/8 hr Vip = 3L; 24L/8kr	57.9 64.0	36.9 43
TPD	Vip = 2L; 24L/8 hr TV = 1.0l, RV = 1.0L	58	37
TPD	Vip = 3L; 24L/8 hr TV = 1.5L, RV = 1.5L	65.8	44.1

4.7. Steady physiologic state

One of the most desirable features of continuous PD (CPD) is the maintenance of a steady physiological state as reflected by minimal fluctuations in body chemistries. CCPD is the only modality of APD that preserves this continuous characteristic. Although the bulk of solute removal and UF occurs at night, the clearance of middle molecules remains constant. The minor variations in small solute concentration and osmolality in blood are not clinically significant. However, the use of high flow APD (i.e., TPD, NPD) should result in larger fluctuations in blood concentrations of solutes due to their higher rate of solute removal and UF during the brief periods of dialysis. In practice, these fluctuations should not represent a significant limitation since most patients on three times weekly hemodialysis (HD) tolerate therapy for many years without obvious evidence of disequilibrium. However, consideration to these interruptions must be given in the formulation of optimal prescriptions using urea kinetic modeling (UKM) since equivalency of dialysis between HD and PD is based on the Peak Concentration Hypothesis (vide infra).

4.8. Selection of APD modality

Approximately 17% of patients undergoing chronic PD in the USA use a modality of APD [32]. The vast majority are on CCPD. The selection of APD versus CAPD is mostly influenced by the patient's preference, the physician's biases and predilections and the availability of equipment and supplies [33–36]. More than 75% of children who require chronic dialysis are treated with various forms of PD [37], with CCPD as the dominant form of therapy. This preference is due to the adaptability of CCPD to the parents and patient schedule and the freedom it allows for work and recreation [35]. APD is instrumental when a partner is required due to patient's visual or neuromuscular impairments. Viglino et al. have called attention to this problem and reported that among their home PD patients 41.7% were in need of a partner [38]. In the USA more than 20% of all patients undergoing CAPD are helped by a partner to effect their exchanges [39]. The percentage is much higher (33.3%) among the elderly [39].

An important consideration in the selection of APD is the individual's peritoneal solute transport rate. Patients with high solute transport rates require more frequent cycles of short duration in order to accomplish proper UF. NPD is the therapy of choice in these instances. Large patients and those with high dietary protein intake require higher clearance of small solutes. High flow APD is recommended in their treatment. Unless a state of fast peritoneal solute transport dictates otherwise, CPD is preferable. CCPD with high PD flow at night, CCPD with an additional manual diurnal exchange, TPD with diurnal exchanges or CAPD with additional nocturnal automated cycles are the available choices for high flow continuous APD [34, 40].

CCPD has been proposed for patients with high peritonitis rates. The experience during the past 12 years with CCPD has been most favorable in this regard. A transfer to CCPD or other forms of APD may reduce the rate of peritonitis in these patients by virtue of the inherent qualities of these techniques, or more likely, by engaging the help of a more capable operator – the partner.

APD is also beneficial in the treatment of patients with complications related to increased IAP (vide supra). In attempting to reduce IAP it is imperative that the prescription is not altered to the extent of sacrificing clearance and compromising adequacy of therapy.

The main deterrent in selecting APD for these and other conditions is the additional expense associated with automated equipment and larger dialysate volumes. Nonetheless, we should consider the potential benefits to the patient and society and the *total* cost of therapy. King et al. compared the efficacy, cost and complication rates among patients on APD and CAPD over a two year period [41]. When consideration was given to the total cost of therapy for these patients, APD was found to be a cost-effective alternative to CAPD with considerable advantages for some patients.

4.9. Formulation of adequate prescription for APD

Adequacy of PD is discussed in Chapter 14. The same general principles apply to CAPD as to APD. However, a few differences between these therapies must be considered in the formulation and understanding of an adequate prescription.

Many recent studies have used UKM for the prescription of PD [22, 42–51]. The reasons for selecting this solute relate to the extensive experience accumulated during the past decade with UKM in HD patients, the fact that urea is a surrogate of protein metabolism and should provide good correlation between dialysis dose and nutrition, and the simplicity of measuring urea in blood and dialysate. The majority of the initial reports on the application of UKM to CAPD have shown good correlation between dialysis dose and clinical outcome.

It has also become evident that the magnitude of normalized urea clearance (KT/V) required in HD is much larger than that required in CAPD to provide equivalent clinical results. Several possibilities have been proposed to explain this difference, the most popular being: that CAPD provides better middle molecule clearance which compensates for its limited urea clearance; and that HD is an intermittent therapy while CAPD maintains a steady state concentration of BUN. At the same KT/V both CAPD and HD will have the same time average concentration of urea (TACurea), but in HD BUN concentrations will exceed TACurea approximately 50% of the time. Keshaviah *et al.* have suggested the Peak Concentration Hypothesis that postulates that uremic toxicity is associated with the peak urea concentration rather than the TACurea [52]. This hypothesis explains why a significantly higher KT/V is required in HD to maintain a peak BUN concentration similar to the steady BUN concentration of CAPD.

Based on this hypothesis, Gotch has transformed the relationship between BUN, normalized protein catabolic rate (NPCR) and KT/V in HD to CAPD and has mapped the "domain of adequate dialysis for CAPD" [48, 51]. Preliminary studies to validate these mathematical relationships have been most promising [22, 46, 53–56]. However, two basic differences between CAPD and APD must be considered before directly applying these mathematical analyses to APD. First, as dialysate flow rate increases in intermittent therapies (IPD and NPD) the ratio of non-dialytic period required for inflow and outflow/dialytic period (dwell) increases, thus reducing efficiency.

Second, certain forms of APD are truly intermittent and allow peak concentrations of BUN similar to HD (i.e., IPD thrice weekly). Therefore, a straightforward application of the equivalency concept is inappropriate. Although, these considerations may be of little clinical consequence for patients undergoing CCPD, adjustments are necessary for intermittent modalities. Theoretical and clinical studies are underway to resolve this issue.

5. Clinical experience with CCPD

5.1. Hematologic and biochemical parameters

A number of publications have reported on the hematologic and biochemical profiles of patients of different age groups undergoing CCPD [5–7, 57, 58]. While the results are similar to those of patients undergoing CAPD, certain selected features of patients undergoing CCPD are worthy of mention.

5.1.1. *Hematological parameters*

Several reports have pointed to an improvement in hemoglobin concentrations among patients undergoing CCPD, as was previously reported for patients undergoing treatment with CAPD [59–61]. These reports describe a pattern of rapid improvement in hemoglobin and hematocrit during the first 3 months of therapy followed by slower increase in the subsequent 6 months. These changes are accompanied by an initial drop in weight upon initiation of dialysis, reflecting a contraction of plasma volume as edema fluid is removed [61]. The subsequent increase, however, most likely represents an increase in the red cell mass. Actual measurement of the plasma volume and red cell mass has confirmed these predictions [61]. Another study has shown an increase in reticulocyte count correlating with recovery of the erythroid cell proliferative activity in patients undergoing CAPD, but without a change in serum level of erythropoietin, suggesting that CAPD may improve bone marrow function perhaps by removal of substances which inhibit erythropoiesis [62].

It is of interest, however, that the data of the National CAPD Registry as published in its Final Report [63] do not support these earlier observations. In this report the mean hematocrit level for 608 patients undergoing CAPD or CCPD was 29.4%. A significant rise in hematocrit level was not seen during the early months of CAPD/CCPD therapy, the hematocrits being 28.1% at less than 3 months of treatment, 30.2% at 3–6 months, 29.9% at 6–9 months and 29.2% at 9–12 months. There were, however, factors identified to be associated with lower hematocrit levels which included: female sex, non-white race, absence of kidney tissue or a report of transfusion within the past 60 days. Polycystic kidneys were associated with elevated hematocrit levels. In this report there were no comparisons with the hematocrit levels prior to initiation of dialysis and thus, an early increase in hematocrit could not be discerned. Nevertheless, the previously reported progressive increase in hematocrit was not observed.

At present, recombinant human erythropoietin has become widely used. Patients undergoing PD respond briskly to doses given subcutaneously once every 1 to 2 weeks [64].

5.1.2. Nitrogenous waste-products

The levels of BUN and creatinine vary widely among patients [5, 7, 57, 58]. Although increases in BUN and/or creatinine concentrations have been observed among CCPD patients when compared to CAPD patients, using similar dialysate flows it would be important to strictly control the dialysis dose delivered and the time of blood sampling relative to the dialysis cycles before a firm conclusion can be reached.

5.1.3. Calcium, phosphorus, and renal osteodystrophy

There are no data pointing to any differences between CAPD and CCPD with regard to the serum calcium and phosphorus concentrations, the dosage of phosphate binders consumed or the need for supplementation with active vitamin D analogs. With the almost exclusive reliance on calcium salts as phosphate binders in recent years, however, more and more patients have had to use the lower calcium concentration of 2.5 mEq/l than in previous years. The percent of patients using lower concentrations in different programs varies between 25 and 50%.

With the almost complete replacement of aluminum compounds with calcium salts as phosphate binders, aluminum-related osteomalacia has become a vanishing disorder. In addition, there are data in patients undergoing CAPD pointing to reductions in serum PTH levels and enhancement of the mineralizing capacity of osteoblasts, resulting in improvements in the skeleton [65, 66]. The data in this area, however, are fragmentary. Any future studies attempting to delineate mineral and bone metabolism in CCPD patients must exercise caution in design since the inclusion of such groups as diabetics, who are known to have a lower incidence of hyperparathyroidism, could bias the results [67].

In addition to the foregoing, improvement of acid-base balance with a more constant maintenance of a normal acid-base status may have contributed to the improvement in renal osteodystrophy when compared to HD.

5.1.4. Nutritional status

As for CAPD, patients undergoing CCPD tend to maintain serum albumin levels in the low-normal or mildly depressed range. To a significant degree, the low albumin concentration is the result of suboptimal consumption of protein in the diet. Although an intake level of 1.2 gm of protein/kg body weight per day has been estimated to be required for patients undergoing PD to maintain a neutral nitrogen balance, most patients fail to meet that target.

One factor involved in the decreased protein intake may be the satiety induced by the constant load of glucose absorbed from the peritoneal dialysate [68]. In this regard, CCPD has an advantage over CAPD in that it provides a greater net UF per gram of glucose absorbed during the shorter nocturnal cycles. However, the prolonged daytime cycle, generally of high glucose concentration, does result in considerable glucose absorption during the daytime.

Another factor in the pathogenesis of lower serum albumin levels may be the increased intra-abdominal pressure generated by intraperitoneal dialysate which also interferes with food intake by causing early satiety or by aggravating symptoms of gastrointestinal reflux. When these symptoms are severe, one may need to resort to reduction in the volume of the diurnal exchange.

A third factor involved in the pathogenesis of the hypoalbuminemia may be protein loss into the peritoneal fluid. Protein losses for non-infected patients vary between 6 and 12 gm/day [69]. The loss of protein in the peritoneal fluid does not seem to vary with the number or length of exchanges [70], although greater losses can be observed in patients using more hypertonic dextrose solutions. Peritonitis, however, can cause major increases in protein loss [69], and the effect may be persistent. In one study [71], protein losses in patients who had never experienced peritonitis averaged only 5.69 gm/day as compared with 9.7 gm/day in patients who had at least one prior episode of peritonitis.

The increased glucose absorption during PD may result in hyperglycemia, hypertriglyceridemia and obesity. Hypercholesterolemia, however, has not been a significant problem in most patients. In diabetics with hypertriglyceridemia, significant reductions in the triglyceride levels can be achieved with the addition of insulin in doses of 5–15 units per liter of peritoneal dialysate [72]. In non-diabetic patients, however, there is no effect of intraperitoneal insulin instillation on any lipid parameters [73].

5.2. Blood pressure control

Whereas approximately 80% of renal failure patients are hypertensive, requiring multiple anti-hypertensive drugs for blood pressure control prior to the initiation of dialysis, only some 10% continue to require anti-hypertensive agents after 6 months of treatment on CCPD. Hypotension is infrequent among non-diabetic patients, but it does occur in as many as 30% of diabetics, most likely consequent to autonomic neuropathy caused by diabetics. Orthostatic hypotension may be present in these patients, even when their intravascular volume is normal or even increased.

5.3. Selected complications of CCPD

Qualitatively, the complications of CCPD are similar to those encountered with CAPD. However, quantitative differences may exist in the incidence of these complications in the two modalities.

5.3.1. Peritonitis

Peritonitis is the most frequent complication of chronic PD and a frequent cause of hospitalization and discontinuation of PD treatment. As early as 1981, when the technique of CCPD was first introduced, however, CCPD was reported by Price and Suki [7] to be associated with a lower peritonitis incidence than CAPD. They reported that whereas the incidence in CAPD patients was 1 episode every 7.2 patient-months, or 1.67 episodes per patient-year, the incidence in CCPD patients was 1 episode per 18.2 patient-months, or 0.66 episodes per patient-year. Subsequently, a number of workers have reported lower incidence of peritonitis in CCPD as opposed to CAPD [74–76].

Unlike these early observations, the National CAPD Registry in its Final Report published in 1988 [77] failed to show any significant differences between CAPD and CCPD. Overall, peritonitis incidence in CAPD was 1.4 episodes per patient year of observation, whereas it was 1.3 for CCPD. This lack of difference was observed whether in patients who had never been treated with dialysis before and were undergoing PD for the first time, or whether they had been on HD and have transferred to PD, or had both, PD and HD in the past. The probability of patients new to dialysis of experiencing the first episode of peritonitis for CCPD and for CAPD were 37% vs 40% at 6 months, 56% vs 60% at 1 year, 78% vs 80% at 2 years and 84% vs 89% at 3 years. These differences are small and probably insignificant.

Unlike this negative observation, a number of recent reports have continued to show a lower peritonitis rate in CCPD than in CAPD. Rottembourg and coworkers [78] reported 1 episode of peritonitis every 24 patient-months in CCPD vs 11.7 patient-months in CAPD. Holley et al. [79] reported a peritonitis rate of 0.3 episodes per year for CCPD vs 0.5 for CAPD using the Y-set, and 1.3 episodes for CAPD employing the spike system. De Fijter and coworkers [80] carried out a prospective randomized trial in which all new patients were randomized to either CAPD, using the Y connector, or to CCPD. They observed that CCPD patients have remained peritonitis-free significantly longer than those on CAPD-Y. The quartile time to first peritonitis episode was greater than 12 months in CCPD vs 3 months in CAPD-Y; and also observed a significantly lower peritonitis incidence with a median time to the second peritonitis episode being 18 months for CCPD and 6 months for CAPD. In the pediatric age group whereas most reports describe no difference in peritonitis incidence or rate between CAPD and CCPD [81–84], a difference in favor of CCPD is occasionally reported [85].

Multiple factors may be invoked to explain a lower peritonitis incidence rate in patients undergoing CCPD. Some of these factors are self evident and are a function of the technique employed, whether for CCPD or for CAPD. One obvious difference between CCPD and CAPD is the number of connections needed to be made between the peritoneal catheter and the dialysis delivery system, that being 1 for CCPD and 4 or more for CAPD. Although the number of spikes into the dialysate bags may be similar in CAPD and CCPD when using 2 liter bags, this would not overcome the advantage of CCPD since the spiking of the bags is made between two sterile components. Besides, the introduction of 3 and 5 liter bags, which have become more widely used in CCPD in recent years, further reduces the number of spikes necessary and diminishes the chance of contamination.

Another favorable factor in CCPD, as compared to CAPD, is the initial direction of flow upon connecting the patient's catheter to the delivery system. After emptying the spent fluid, patients on CAPD disconnect and reconnect to a new bag and fill. This sequence poses a risk of flushing into the peritoneum organisms which may have entered the tubing at the time of making the connection. In CCPD on the other hand, the patient always empties after making the connection, before dialysate is infused into the peritoneal cavity.

Any contamination that may have resulted from the connection process will have been flushed outward with the initial emptying. The introduction in CAPD of bagless PD systems as the freedom set, O-set and the Y-set has resulted in a significant reduction in the incidence of peritonitis [86–89]. These systems share with CCPD the flush before fill dialysate flow pattern. It has been shown experimentally that lines precontaminated with microorganisms of low adhesiveness, such as Staph epidermidis, clear with flushing so long as the contact time of the bacteria with the line has been brief [90, 91], as would be the case in making a connection.

Other less obvious factors involved in reducing the incidence of peritonitis in CCPD have been brought to light by recent investigations. Two such factors appear to be peritoneal macrophage phagocytic activity and the opsonic activity of the effluent as affected by the prolonged dwell time of the daytime cycle in CCPD and by the dextrose concentration. In a series of studies, de Fijter and coworkers [92, 93], have reported an increase in peritoneal macrophage phagocytic capacity with increased dwell time. These changes were accompanied by an increase in the peritoneal macrophage peak chemoluminescence response and effluent opsonic activity. The increase in opsonic activity with prolonged dwell times was associated with an increase in IgG levels [93]. Furthermore, not only did phagocyte function improve, but the number of phagocytes was also observed to increase with prolonged dwell times. Another factor that influences macrophage phagocytic activity is the dextrose concentration which is an indirect function of dwell time. De Fijter and coworkers demonstrated a depression of peritoneal macrophage phagocytic function with higher glucose concentrations [94]. These macrophages exposed to higher glucose concentrations were also less able to mount a respiratory burst. Since during the prolonged daytime dwell, the glucose concentrations in the peritoneal fluid fall to lower levels in CCPD than during the shorter dwells of CAPD, it is conceivable that macrophage function would be better preserved.

As pointed out in the section on Peritoneal Dialysis Solutions, the use of dialysates with lower calcium concentration has been on the rise in recent years. Piraino et al. [95] have recently pointed out an increase in the risk of peritonitis from 0.58 episodes per patient-year when using 3.5 mEq/l calcium to 0.82 episodes per patient-year when using 2.5 mEq/l calcium; the proportion of peritonitis episodes due to Staph epidermidis increased from 20 to 61% after conversion to the lower calcium containing dialysate. These findings have not been substantiated by other more carefully conducted studies; Hutchison et al. [123] found no such increase in peritonitis rate in a controlled series of patients using the 2.5 mEq/l solution as compared to those using a 3.5 mEq/l calcium in the fluid. This observation raises an important consideration in the analysis and comparison of peritonitis rates.

5.3.2. Exit site infections and catheter replacements

The Final Report of the National CAPD Registry [77] showed an equal incidence of exit site/tunnel infections in CAPD and in CCPD of 0.6 episodes per patient-year of observation. An essentially equal rate of catheter replacement in the two modalities was also reported (0.2 episodes per patient-year for CAPD and 0.3 episodes per patient-year for CCPD). In patients who were new to dialysis, the cumulative probability of experiencing the first exit site/tunnel infection for CAPD and CCPD respectively, was 22% and 21% at 6 months, 33% and 30% at 12 months, 49% and 48% at 24 months and 59% and 63% at 36 months. For catheter replacement, the corresponding rates were 10% and 11% at 6 months, 25% and 21% at 12 months, 32% and 30% at 24 months and 43% and 45% at 36 months. The equal rates of exit site/tunnel infections between the two modalities suggest that this could not be a factor in the lower peritonitis rate in CCPD discussed above.

In a study by Burkart et al. [96] comparing disconnect technologies, which include CAPD with the Y-set and APD, vs non-disconnect technologies, which consist of spike and ultraviolet connection, a lower peritonitis rate was observed in the disconnect group (0.6 vs 0.99 episodes per patient-year) but no difference was observed in exit site infection rates, being 0.35 and 0.38 per patient-year respectively. Also, there was no difference in the time to the first exit site infection or the time to the first catheter removal. In another study by Holley and coworkers [79], however, catheter infections were lowest among CCPD patients (0.5 episodes per patient-year or 1 episode every 25 patient-months), followed by CAPD patients using the Y-set (0.8 episodes per patient-year or 1 episode every 14 patient-months), followed by CAPD patients using the spike system who had the highest rates of catheter infections (1.2 episodes per patient-year or 1 episode every 10 patient-months). These differences in exit site/tunnel infection catheter infections were associated with corresponding differences in peritonitis rates. The reason for the differences in rates between disconnect and non-disconnect technologies is not immediately apparent.

5.3.3. *Hernias and other complications due to increased intra-abdominal pressure*

The increase in intra-abdominal pressure caused by distention of the peritoneal cavity with dialysate plays an important role in the development or aggravation of certain complications of CAPD and CCPD. Limiting the volume of fluid employed in the diurnal cycle to less than 2 liters, or 28 ml/kg/body weight, has resulted in a decline in the incidence of these complications [97]. A 25-35% reduction in the diurnal volume is recommended for patients who are at risk for developing these complications or who are symptomatic at the initiation of therapy. Umbilical, inguinal, abdominal and diaphragmatic hernias have been reported to be higher in CAPD than in APD modalities [97-101]. They have been reported to develop in 9-24% of patients undergoing CAPD, but in only 2-3% of patients on IPD or on reduced diurnal volume CCPD [97]. The incidence was 9% in CCPD prior to reduction of diurnal volume. The further increase in intraperitoneal pressure caused by contraction of the abdominal musculature in the erect posture must contribute to this difference between CAPD and APD. Most patients who developed hernias were multiparous, elderly females with weakened abdominal walls. Following surgical repair of the hernias, patients returned to CCPD, using reduced dialysate volumes for the diurnal exchange (1000-1500 ml) without recurrence of hernias.

Dialysate leaks may be the consequence of increased intra-abdominal pressure. Depending on the location, leaks can manifest as genital edema, anterior wall edema, or a pericatheter pseudohernia. The latter is a dilated structure of fibrous tissue and muscle, not lined by peritoneum, which occurs around or in proximity to the catheter exit site and is easily reducible and collapses when the abdominal cavity is empty. Using radiocontrast material, entry of peritoneal fluid around the catheter and into the hernial sac can be demonstrated [102]. This complication has been encountered more often with single-cuff peritoneal catheters than with double-cuff catheters [97]. Replacing the catheter with a double cuff catheter, waiting 10-14 days before reinitiating PD, and using volumes up to 2 liters at night and 1-1/2 liters during the day, allowed resumption of CCPD without recurrence of this complication.

Low back pain, gastro-esophageal reflux and other complications resulting from increased intra-abdominal pressure have been similarly managed with reduced diurnal volume. Patients may be transferred to NPD to manage these complications, since patients tolerate higher intra-abdominal volumes during recumbency at night, thereby compensating for the reduction in daytime dialysate flow.

5.3.4. *Catheter related complications*

The incidence of complications related to the dialysis catheter has been the same in CCPD and in CAPD. Catheter outflow obstruction, which is most often due to omentum wrapping around the intraperitoneal segment of the catheter, or to catheter migration, occurs less frequently in CAPD and in CCPD than with IPD. Exercise and enemas are among the conservative measures which may correct the problem in the majority of patients.

Loss of UF ability caused by increased peritoneal solute transport rates has been seen with both CAPD and CCPD and the underlying cause can be identified with the PET done on all patients at the time of commencing dialysis, and repeated at intervals especially in patients whose UF ability appears to be changing. Other factors which may interface with the ability to effectively remove fluid include: 1) increased sodium intake, 2) increased sodium concentration of the dialysate, 3) decreased residual renal function, 4) decreased surface area available for transperitoneal exchange caused by catheter problems, 5) uncontrolled hyperglycemia in diabetics which reduces the transperitoneal osmotic gradient, and 6) severe hypoalbuminemia resulting in edema and difficulty with mobilization of fluid from the interstitial spaces. Patients exhibiting difficulty in fluid removal must be evaluated carefully to discern loss of UF from other factors.

5.4. Morbidity and mortality

Data on specific morbidity and mortality rates for APD is lacking. The United States Renal Data System has reported the combined result of CAPD and CCPD [103]. Most of the available data derive from individual centers and consist of small series. The interpretation of the data is also difficult due to selection bias. Possible selection factors that may affect outcome include: 1) age, which has been characterized as a risk factor for peritonitis among younger patients and a high risk factor for cardiovascular disease among the elderly [104]; 2) high rates of peritonitis; 3) need for partner assistance; 4) abnormal peritoneal solute transport rates with impaired UF; 5) complications related to increased IAP; and 6) need for more efficient solute removal in patients who have lost residual renal function.

The 1987 NIH CAPD Registry reported hospitalization rates for CCPD similar to those for CAPD [105]. Technique and patient survival have also been comparable to CAPD. Diaz-Buxo et al. have observed a cumulative probability of transfer to HD, IPD, CAPD or off dialysis without return of renal function of 18 and 25% at 1 and 2 years respectively. The annual mortality rate for the first three years was 10% [106]. Suki et al. have reviewed the outcome of their CCPD population for seven years and the causes of dropout in these patients [107]. They identified three high risk factors for termination of therapy: 1) age (50% of the patients were >50 years of age); 2) comorbid factors which rendered 56% of the patients dependent upon a partner and; 3) diabetes mellitus, which affected one third of the patients. Only 12.5% of the patients transferred to HD. The major causes of dropout were death and transplantation. The survival rates for CAPD and CCPD have also been reported to be similar by the CAPD Registry and by individual series [105, 108].

6. Treatment of diabetics with CCPD

In this volume an entire chapter is devoted to the treatment of diabetics with PD. Discussion of this subject, save for aspects of intraperitoneal insulin dosing in CCPD, will be very limited.

In a study by Aujla et al. [109] intraperitoneal insulin requirements were evaluated in patients switched from CAPD to CCPD. The authors found that the mean total daily intraperitoneal insulin dose on CCPD was 85% of the mean dose on CAPD with comparable glycemic control. Of the total daily intraperitoneal insulin 25–58% (mean of 41%) was administered in the diurnal exchange of patients on CCPD. The total intraperitoneal insulin dose on CCPD was between 1.2 and 2.4 (mean 1.9) fold the subcutaneous insulin dose used predialysis. Based on these observations, the authors proposed guidelines for converting intraperitoneal insulin doses for patients switched from CAPD to CCPD recommending a reduction in the total daily insulin dose by 15%, and administering approximately 40% of the total dose in the diurnal exchange.

7. Treatment of children with CCPD

Children comprise a significant portion of patients being treated with CCPD. Several features of CCPD make it particularly useful for the therapy of children: 1) it offers adequate dialysis with minimal medical contact, 2) increases the amount of free time for recreation and study during the day, and 3) allows the use of a partner, usually a parent, without significant restriction of their productive time. In this volume an entire chapter is devoted to this subject, and therefore no further discussion will be undertaken here.

8. CCPD in the treatment of acute renal failure

Peritoneal dialysis offers many advantages for the treatment of patients suffering from acute renal failure: 1) it is a continuous therapy offering stable blood biochemical profile without the wide fluctuations associated with HD; 2) the ease of continuous UF without the wide hemodynamic fluctuations caused by rapid UF during HD; 3) the lack of a need for heparinization in post-surgical and post-traumatic patients; 4) the minimum personnel effort needed in conducting the treatment when CCPD is used; 5) the flexibility of variations in frequency and volume of exchanges and of their dwell time, and in the concentration of glucose in order to manage hypercatabolic patients and/or patients with volume overload; 7) the peritoneal cavity may serve as a source for delivery of nutrients, in that the glucose present in the solution provides a source of calories, and amino acids can be added to the PD fluid as a source of essential nitrogen compounds. A number of reports describing the successful use of PD in treating this group of patients have been published [110, 111].

9. Renal transplantation in CCPD patients

Transplantation is a major cause for drop-out from PD. There are two concerns relating to transplantation in patients undergoing CCPD treatments: the immune competence of these patients and the potential for peritoneal and catheter-related complications post-transplantation.

The basis for concern regarding the patients' immune competence rests on clinical investigations showing enhanced immunologic responsiveness in patients undergoing PD when compared to patients undergoing HD [112, 113], and the laboratory evidence suggesting improved cellular immunity among CAPD patients [114, 115]. A less marked effect of pre-transplant blood transfusions in PD patients [112, 113, 116] and the reports of increased ratio of helper to suppressor T-cells among patients in association with lower 1-year graft survival rates [112, 113] have contributed to the concern. However, current data show no evidence for an effect on outcome of renal transplantation related to the pre-transplant dialysis modality [117–122].

The presence of a catheter in the peritoneal cavity is a potential source for peritonitis and septicemia following transplantation. Special precautions must be exercised, therefore, whenever patients undergoing PD come for transplantation. The following recommendations are designed to maintain the peritoneal access until adequate allograft function has been established and to prevent septic complications: 1) the abdomen should be drained prior to transplantation surgery, 2) a peritoneal fluid sample should be tested for cell count and differential, and for culture, 3) the exit site should be inspected and cleaned daily, 4) the catheter should be irrigated every 48 hours to ensure patency, 5) the catheter should be removed within 2 weeks after surgery or as soon as adequate graft function is established. If these guidelines are adhered to the transition from PD to transplantation should proceed smoothly.

10. Conclusions

APD modalities have provided important options for patients to choose from for the treatment of end-stage renal disease. In addition, they offer the advantages of automated nightly dialysis with freedom from treatment chores in the daytime; relative ease of administration of therapy by a partner or a helper in cases where the patient may suffer a mental, physical or visual impairment; the potential for lower peritonitis rates and the potential for application to patients with high solute transport rates requiring rapid, short-dwell exchanges to effect net UF of salt and water. The relative ease of performing CCPD, the daytime freedom and the low complication rates may be important factors contributing to improved quality of life and a higher level of rehabilitation.

References

1. Twardowski ZJ. Peritoneal dialysis glossary II. Perit Dial Int 1988; 8: 15–7.
2. Boen ST, Mulinari AS, Dillar DH, Scribner BH. Periodic peritoneal dialysis in the management of chronic uremia. Trans Am Soc Artif Intern Organs 1962; 8: 256–62.
3. Lasker N, McCauley EP, Passerotti CT. Chronic peritoneal dialysis. Trans Am Soc Artif Intern Organs 1966; 12: 94–7.
4. Popovich RP, Moncrief JW, Nolph KD, Ghods AJ, Twardowski ZJ, Pyle WK. Continuous ambulatory peritoneal dialysis. Ann Intern Med 1978; 88: 449–56.
5. Diaz-Buxo JA, Walker PJ, Farmer CD, Chandler JT, Holt KL, Cox P. Continuous cyclic peritoneal dialysis. Trans Am Soc Artif Intern Organs 1981; 27: 51–3.
6. Nakagawa D, Price C, Stinebaugh B, Suki W. Continuous cyclic peritoneal dialysis: a viable option in the treatment of chronic renal failure. Trans Am Soc Artif Intern Organs 1981; 27: 55–7.
7. Price CG, Suki WN. Newer modifications of peritoneal dialysis. Am J Nephrol 1981; pp 97–104.
8. Stephen RL. Reciprocating peritoneal dialysis with a subcutaneous peritoneal catheter. Dial Transplant 1978; 7: 834–8.
9. Miller JH, Blumenkrantz MJ, Lewin AJ, Roberts M, Marantz LB, Vegagomez G, McArthur MJ. Optimizing low flow peritoneal dialysis. (Abstract) Trans Am Soc Artif Intern Organs 1981; p 50.
10. Twardowski ZJ, Prowant BF, Nolph KD, Khanna R, Schmidt LM, Satslowich RJ. Chronic nightly tidal peritoneal dialysis. Trans Am Soc Artif Intern Organs 1990; 36: M584–8.
11. Keshaviah P. Personal communication.
12. Diaz-Buxo JA, Kay DA, Holt KL. Safe, simple, inexpensive disconnecting device for CCPD. Kidney Int 1985; 27: 179.
13. Diaz-Buxo JA, Burgess WP, Farmer CD, Chandler JT, Walker PJ, Adcock A. Multiple tubing set (MTS™)-making CCPD safe, simple and cost effective. Perit Dial Bull 1987; 7: 522.
14. Shen FH, Sherrard DJ, Scollard D et al. Thirst, hyponatremia and excessive weight gain in maintenance peritoneal dialysis. Trans Am Soc Artif Intern Organs 1978; 24: 142–5.
15. Nolph KD, Sorkin ML, Moore H. Autoregulation

of sodium and potassium removal during continuous ambulatory peritoneal dialysis. Trans Am Soc Artif Intern Organs 1980; 26: 334–8.
16. Twardowski ZJ, Nolph KD, Khanna R, Gluck Z, Prowant BF, Ryan LP. Daily clearances with continuous ambulatory peritoneal dialysis and nightly peritoneal dialysis. Trans Am Soc Artif Intern Organs 1986; 32: 575–80.
17. Brandes J, Emerson P, Campbell D, Keshaviah P. The relationship between body size, fill volume and mass transfer area coefficient (MTAC) in PD. (Abstract) J Am Soc Nephrol 1992; 3: 407.
18. Schoenfeld P, Diaz-Buxo JA, Keen M, Gotch FA. The effect of body position (P), surface area (BSA), and intraperitoneal exchange volume (Vip) on the peritoneal transport constant (KoA). (Abstract) J Am Soc Nephrol 1993; 4: 416.
19. Twardowski Z, Nolph K, Khanna R, Prowant B, Frock J, Dobbie J, Serkes K, Kenley R, Witsoe D, Garber J. Eight hr tidal peritoneal dialysis (TPD) matches 24 hr CAPD and surpasses 8 hr nightly intermittent peritoneal dialysis (NIPD) clearances (C). (Abstract) Perit Dial Bull 1987; 7: S79.
20. Diaz-Buxo JA, Farmer CD, Chandler JT, Walker PJ, Burgess WP. CCPD – wet is better than dry. Perit Dial Bull 1987: S22.
21. Lameire NH, Vanholder R, Veyt D, Lambert MC, Ringoir S. A longitudinal, five year survey of urea kinetic parameters in CAPD patients. Kidney Int 1992; 42: 426–32.
22. Diaz-Buxo JA. Is CAPD adequate long-term therapy for ESRD? A critical assessment. J Am Soc Nephrol 1992; 3: 1039–48.
23. Blumenkrantz MJ, Gordon A, Roberts M, Lewin AJ, Pecker EA, Moran JK, Coburn JW, Maxwell MH. Applications of the Redy® sorbent system to hemodialysis and peritoneal dialysis. Artif Organs 1979; 3: 230–6.
24. Twardowski ZJ, Nolph KD, Khanna R, Prowant BF, Frock JT Dobbie JW, Kenley RS, Serkes KD, Witsoe DA, Garber JW. Tidal peritoneal dialysis. In: Avran MM, Giordano C (eds), Ambulatory Peritoneal Dialysis. Plenum Publishing Corporation, New York 1990; pp 145–9.
25. Shah J, Lane D, Shrivastava D, Berlyne GM, Barth RH. Isovolemic tidal technique does not increase clearances in intermittent peritoneal dialysis (IPD). (Abstract) J Am Soc Nephrol 1992; 3: 419.
26. Gotloib L, Mines M, Garmizo L, Varka I. Hemodynamic effects of increasing intra-abdominal pressure in peritoneal dialysis. Perit Dial Bull 1981; 1: 41–3.
27. Twardowski ZJ, Prowant BF, Nolph KD, Martinez AJ, Lampton LM. High volume, low frequency continuous ambulatory peritoneal dialysis. Kidney Int 1983; 23: 64–70.
28. Diaz-Buxo JA. CCPD is even better than CAPD. Kidney Int 1985; 28: S26–8.
29. Curatola G, Zoccahi C, Cruccitti S, Siclani F, Maggionre Q. Effect of posture on peritoneal clearance. Perit Dial Int 1988; 8: 58–9.
30. Fukudome Y, Ozawa K, Shoji T, Tamura T, Nakanishi T, Kijima Y, Sasaoka T. How is the portal vein flow in CAPD? Evaluation of postural change by colour flow-doppler ultrasound (CFDU). (Abstract) Perit Dial Int 1992: S4.
31. Otero A, Esteban J, Canovas L. Does posture modify solute transport in CAPD? (Correspondence) Perit Dial Int 1992; 12: 399–400.
32. US Renal Data System, USRDS 1991 Annual Data Report, The National Institutes of Health, National Institute of Diabetes and Digestive and Kidney Diseases, Bethesda, MD, August 1991.
33. Diaz-Buxo JA. Patient selection and dialysis prescription in peritoneal dialysis. In: La Greca G, Olivares J, Feriani M, Passlick-Deetjen J (eds), CAPD – A Decade of Experience. Contrib Nephrol Karger, Basel 1991; 89: 224–30.
34. Diaz-Buxo JA. Current status of continuous cyclic peritoneal dialysis (CCPD). (Editorial) Perit Dial Int 1989; 9: 9–14.
35. Chormann ML, Staccone M, Edd P, Andrus CH, Ornt DB. Experience with automated peritoneal dialysis (APD) in a pediatric population. In: Khanna R, Nolph K, Prowant B, Twardowski Z, Oreopoulos D (eds), Advances in Continuous Ambulatory Peritoneal Dialysis. University of Toronto Press, Toronto 1987; 3: 66–72.
36. Diaz-Buxo JA. The place for automated peritoneal dialysis. In: Khanna R, Nolph K, Prowant B, Twardowski Z, Oreopoulos D (eds), Advances in Peritoneal Dialysis. University of Toronto Press, Toronto 1992; 8: 98–101.
37. Fine RN. Choosing a dialysis therapy for children with endstage renal disease. Am J Kidney Dis 1984; 4: 249–52.
38. Viglino G, Grasso PG, Mariano F, Cavalli PL. Need of a partner on home peritoneal dialysis (HPD): incidence and an alternative choice. In: Khanna R, Nolph K, Prowant B, Twardowski Z, Oreopoulos D (eds), Advances in Peritoneal Dialysis. University of Toronto Press, Toronto 1989; 5: 67–71.
39. Nolph KD, Cutler SJ, Steinberg SM, Novak JW. Special studies from the NHI USA CAPD Registry. Perit Dial Bull 1986; 6: 28–34.
40. Diaz-Buxo JA. Reverse osmosis machines and cyclers for peritoneal dialysis. In: Nissenson AR, Fine RN (eds), Dialysis Therapy, 2nd Edition, Hanley and Belfus, Philadelphia 1992; pp 55–60.
41. King LK, Kingswood JC, Sharpstone P. Comparison of the efficacy cost and complication rate of APD and CAPD as long-term outpatient treatments for renal failure. In: Khanna R, Nolph K, Prowant B, Twardowski Z, Oreopoulos D (eds), Advances in Peritoneal Dialysis. University of Toronto Press, Toronto 1992; 8: 123–6.
42. Teehan BP, Schleifer CR, Sigler MH, Gilgor GS. A quantitative approach to the CAPD prescription. Perit Dial Bull 1985; 5: 152–6.
43. Lysaght MJ, Pollock CA, Hallet MD, Ibels LS, Farrell PC. The relevance of urea kinetic modeling to CAPD. Trans Am Soc Artif Intern Organs 1989; 35: 784–90.
44. Lindsay RM, Spanner E. A hypothesis: the protein catabolic rate is dependent upon the type and

amount of treatment in dialyzed uremic patients. Am J Kidney Dis 1989; 13: 382–9.
45. Ku K, Anderson R, Schoenfeld P. Kinetic modeling of urea in peritoneal dialysis. Dial Transplant 1983; 12: 374–81.
46. Acchiardo SR, Kraus AP, Kaufman PA et al. Evaluation of CAPD prescription. In: Khanna R, Nolph KD, Prowant BF et al. (eds), Advances in Peritoneal Dialysis. University of Toronto Press, Toronto 1991; 7: 117–9.
47. Bergström J, Alvestrand A, Lindholm B, Tranaeus A. Relationship between KT/V and protein catabolic rate is different in continuous peritoneal dialysis and haemodialysis patients. (Abstract) J Am Soc Nephrol 1991; 2: 358.
48. Gotch F. The application of urea kinetic modeling to CAPD. In: La Greca G, Ronco C, Feriani M et al. (eds), Peritoneal Dialysis. Wichtig Editore, Milano 1991; pp 47–51.
49. Teehan BP, Schleifer CR, Brown JM, Sigler MH, Raimondo J. Urea kinetic analysis and clinical outcome in CAPD: a five year longitudinal study. In: Khanna R, Nolph KD, Prowant BF et al. (eds), Advances in Peritoneal Dialysis. University of Toronto Press, Toronto 1990; 6: 181–5.
50. Nolph KD, Moore HL, Twardowski ZJ, Khanna R, Prowant B, Meyer M, Ponferrada L. Cross-sectional assessment of weekly urea and creatinine clearances in patients on continuous ambulatory peritoneal dialysis. ASAIO J 1992; 38: M139–42.
51. Gotch FA. Adequacy of peritoneal dialysis. Am J Kidney Dis 1993; 21: 96–8.
52. Keshaviah PR, Nolph KD, Van Stone JC. The peak concentrations hypothesis: A urea kinetic approach to comparing the adequacy of continuous ambulatory peritoneal dialysis (CAPD) and hemodialysis. Perit Dial Int 1989; 9: 257–60.
53. Keshaviah P. Quantitative approaches to prescribing peritoneal dialysis. In: La Greca G, Ronco C, Feriani M et al. (eds), Peritoneal Dialysis. Wichtig Editore, Milano 1991; pp 53–60.
54. Teehan BP, Schleifer CR, Brown JM, Sigler MH, Raimondo J. Urea kinetic analysis and clinical outcome in CAPD: a five year longitudinal study. In: Khanna R, Nolph KD, Prowant BF et al. (eds), Advances in Peritoneal Dialysis. University of Toronto Press, Toronto 1990; 6: 181–5.
55. Keshaviah P. Adequacy of CAPD: a quantitative approach. Kidney Int 1992; 42: S160–4.
56. Keshaviah P. Urea kinetic and middle molecule approaches to assessing the adequacy of hemodialysis and CAPD. Kidney Int 1993; 43: S28–38.
57. Diaz-Buxo JA. Continuous ambulatory and continuous cycling peritoneal dialysis: In: La Greca G, Chiaramonte S, Fabris A, Feriani M, Ronco C (eds), Peritoneal Dialysis. Wichtig Editore, Milano 1985; pp 257–64.
58. Diaz-Buxo JA. Continuous cyclic peritoneal dialysis (CCPD). In: Franz HE (ed), Blood Purification, 3rd edition. Georg Thieme Verlag, Stuttgart 1985; pp 458–63.
59. Moncrief JW, Popovich RP, Nolph KD, Rubin J, Robson M, Nicholas D, deVaberga GA, Oreopoulos DG. Clinical experience with continuous ambulatory peritoneal dialysis. ASAIO J 1979; 2: 114–8.
60. Lamperi S, Icardi A, Carozzi S et al. Effect on CAPD on renal anemia. Intl J Nephrol Urol Androl 1981; 1: 43–52.
61. De Paepe MBJ, Schelstraete KHG, Ringoir SM Lameiri NH. Influence of continuous ambulatory peritoneal dialysis on the anemia of end-stage renal disease. Kidney Int 1983; 23: 474–8.
62. Lamperi S, Corozzi S, Icardi A. In vitro and in vivo studies of erythropoiesis during continuous ambulatory peritoneal dialysis. Perit Dial Bull 1983; 3: 94–6.
63. Lindblad AS, Novak JW, Nolph KD, Stablein DM, Cutler SJ, Steinberg SM, Vena DA. Hematocrit values in the CAPD/CCPD population. In: Final Report of the National CAPD Registry of the National Institute of Health 1988; pp 6–13 to 6–20.
64. Nissenson AR. National cooperation rHu erythropoietin study in patients with chronic renal failure: a phase IV multicenter study. Report of National Cooperative rHu Erythropoietin Study Group. Am J Kidney Dis 1991; 18 (4 suppl 1): 24–33.
65. Rahman R, Heaton A, Goodship THJ et al. Renal osteodystrophy in patients on continuous ambulatory peritoneal dialysis: a five year study. Perit Dial Bull 1987; 7: 20–5.
66. Delmez JA, Fallon MD, Bergfeld MA, Gearing BK, Dougan CS, Teitelbaum SL. Continuous ambulatory peritoneal dialysis and bone. Kidney Int 1986; 30: 379–84.
67. Vincenti F, Hattner R, Amend WJ Jr et al. Decreased secondary hyperparathyroidism in diabetic patients receiving hemodialysis. J Am Med Assoc 1981; 245: 930–3.
68. Grodstein GP, Blumenkrantz MJ, Kopple JD, Moran JK, Coburn JU. Glucose absorption during continuous ambulatory peritoneal dialysis. Kidney Int 1981; 19: 564–7.
69. Blumenkrantz MJ, Gahl GM, Kopple JD. Protein losses during peritoneal dialysis. Kidney Int 1981; 19: 593–602.
70. Leichter HE. The optimal CCPD regimen for children. Perspect Perit Dial 1987; 5: 5–8.
71. Katirtzoglou A, Oreopoulos DG, Husdan H et al. Reappraisal of protein losses in patients undergoing continuous ambulatory peritoneal dialysis. Nephron 1980; 26: 230–3.
72. Moncrief JW, Pyle WK, Simon P et al. Hypertriglyceridemia, diabetes mellitus and insulin administration in patients undergoing CAPD. In: Moncrief JW, Popovich RP (eds), CAPD Update, Proc 2nd Intl Symp, Mason, NY 1981; pp 143–65.
73. Beardsworth SF, Goldsmith HJ, Stanbridge BR. Intraperitoneal insulin cannot correct hyperlipidemia of CAPD. Perit Dial Bull 1983; 3: 126–7.
74. Diaz-Buxo JA. Does CCPD lower the peritonitis rate? Contrib Nephrol 1987; 57: 191–6.
75. Diaz-Buxo JA, Walker PJ, Chandler JT, Burgess WP, Farmer CD. Experience with intermittent peri-

toneal dialysis and continuous cyclic peritoneal dialysis. Am J Kidney Dis 1984; 4: 242–8.
76. Cavoretto L, Jackson F. A decrease in peritonitis with CCPD: one unit's experience. Nephrol Nurse 1983; 5: 33–7.
77. Lindblad AS, Novak JW, Nolph KD, Stablein DM, Cutler SJ, Steinberg SM, Vena DA. Complications of treatment. In: Final Report of the National CAPD Registry of the National Institutes of Health 1988; pp 4-1 to 4-13.
78. Rottembourg J, Brouard R, Issad B, Allouache M, Nguyen J, Montassine MC, Kirstein E, Jacobs C. Prevention of peritonitis during continuous ambulatory peritoneal dialysis. Value of disconnectable systems. Presse Med 1988; 17: 1349–53.
79. Holley JL, Bernardini J, Piraino B. Continuous cycling peritoneal dialysis is associated with lower rates of catheter infections than continuous ambulatory peritoneal dialysis. Am J Kidney Dis 1990; 16; 133–6.
80. de Fijter CW, Oe PL, Nauta JJ, van der Meulen J, ter Wee PM, Snoek FJ, Conker AJ. A prospective randomized study comparing the peritonitis incidence of CAPD and Y-connector (CAPD-Y) with continuous cyclic peritoneal dialysis (CCPD). In: Khanna R, Nolph K, Prowant B, Twardowski Z, Oreopoulos D (eds), Advances in Peritoneal Dialysis. University of Toronto Press, Toronto 1991; 7: 186–9.
81. Brem AS, Toscano AM. Continuous cycling peritoneal dialysis for children: an alternative to hemodialysis treatment. Pediatrics 1984; 74: 254–8.
82. Southwest Pediatric Nephrology Study Group. Continuous ambulatory and continuous cyclic peritoneal dialysis in children. Kidney Int 1985; 27: 558–64.
83. Fine RN, Salusky CB. CAPD/CCPD in children: four year's experience. Kidney Int 1986; 30: S7–10.
84. Verrina E, Edefonti A, Bassi S, Perfumo F, Zachello G, Andreetta B, Caringella D, Lavoratti G, Picca M, Rinaldi S et al. Peritonitis in children undergoing chronic peritoneal dialysis (CPD): data from the Italian Registry of Pediatric CPD. In: Khanna R, Nolph K, Prowant B, Twardowski Z, Oreopoulos D (eds), Advances in Peritoneal Dialysis. University of Toronto Press, Toronto 1992; 8: 419–22.
85. Levy MM, Balfe JW, Geary DF, Fryer-Keene SP, Bannatyne RM et al. Factors predisposing and contributing to peritonitis during chronic peritoneal dialysis in children: a 10 year experience. Perit Dial Int 1990; 10: 263–9.
86. Bazzato G, Landini S, Coli U, Lucatello S, Francasso A, Moracchiello M. A new technique of continuous ambulatory peritoneal dialysis (CAPD): double-bag system for freedom to the patient and significant reduction of peritonitis. Clin Nephrol 1980; 13: 251–4.
87. Maiorca R, Cancarini GC, Broccoli R et al. Prospective controlled trial of a Y-connector and disinfectant to prevent peritonitis in continuous ambulatory peritoneal dialysis. Lancet 1983; 2: 642–4.
88. Suki WN, Walshe JJ, Ashebrook DW, Gentile DE, Tucker CT, Ash SR, Ahmad S. Multicenter evaluation of a bagless CAPD system. Trans Am Soc Artif Intern Organs 1986; 32: 572–4.
89. Diaz-Buxo JA, Walsh JJ, Flanigan M. Multicenter experience with Y-set CAPD system (Freedom Set). Perit Dial Bull 1987: S23.
90. Verger C, Faller B, Ryckelynck JPH, Cam G, Pierre D. Comparison between the efficacy of CAPD Y-lines without "in-line" disinfectant and standard systems: a multicenter prospective controlled trial. Perit Dial Bull 1987; 7: S82.
91. Verger C, Luzar MA. In vitro study of CAPD Y-line system. In: Khanna R, Nolph K, Prowant B, Twardowski Z, Oreopoulos D (eds), Advances in Peritoneal Dialysis. University of Toronto Press, Toronto 1986; pp 160–4.
92. de Fijter CW, Verbrugh HA, Oe LP, Peters ED, van der Meulen J, Donker AJ, Verhoef J. Peritoneal defense in continuous ambulatory versus continuous cyclic peritoneal dialysis. Kidney Int 1992; 42: 947–50.
93. Vlaanderen K, de Fijter CW, Bos HJ, van der Meulen J, Beelen RH, Oe PL, Verbrugh HA. The effect of dwell time on peritoneal phagocytic defense of chronic peritoneal dialysis patients. In: Khanna R, Nolph K, Prowant B, Twardowski Z, Oreopoulos D (eds), Advances in Peritoneal Dialysis. University of Toronto Press, Toronto 1989; 5: 151–3.
94. de Fijter CW, Verbrugh HA, Peters ED, Oe PL, van der Meulen J, Donker AJ, Verhoef J. Another reason to restrict the use of a hypertonic glucose-bases peritoneal dialysis fluid: its impact on peritoneal macrophage function in vivo. In: Khanna R, Nolph K, Prowant B, Twardowski Z, Oreopoulos D (eds), Advances in Peritoneal Dialysis. University of Toronto Press, Toronto 1991; 7: 150–3.
95. Piraino B, Bernardini J, Holley JL, Perlmutter JA. Increased risk of staphylococcus epidermidis peritonitis in patients on dialysate containing 1.25 mmol/L calcium. Am J Kidney Dis 1992; 19: 371–4.
96. Burkart JM, Jordan JR, Durnell TA, Case LD. Comparison of exit-site infections in disconnect versus nondisconnect systems for peritoneal dialysis. Perit Dial Int 1992; 12: 317–20.
97. Diaz-Buxo JA, Geissinger WT. Single cuff versus double cuff Tenckhoff catheter. Perit Dial Bull 1984; 4: S100–2.
98. Chan MK, Baillod RA, Tanner A et al. Abdominal hernias in patients receiving continuous ambulatory peritoneal dialysis. Brit Med J 1981; 283: 826.
99. Digenis GE, Khanna R, Oreopoulos DG. Abdominal hernias in patients undergoing continuous ambulatory peritoneal dialysis. Perit Dial Bull 1982; 2: 115–7.
100. Jorkasky D, Goldfarb S. Abdominal wall hernia complicating chronic ambulatory peritoneal dialysis. Am J Nephrol 1982; 2: 323–4.

101. Rubin J, Raju S, Teal N et al. Abdominal hernia in patients undergoing continuous ambulatory peritoneal dialysis. Arch Int Med 1982; 142: 1453–5.
102. Tucker CT, Cunningham JT, Nichols AM et al. Cannulography with peritoneal air contrast study. Contemp Dial 1982; 3: 9–13.
103. US Renal Data System, USRDS 1991 Annual Data Report, The National Institutes of Health, National Institute of Diabetes and Digestive and Kidney Diseases, Bethesda, MD, August 1991.
104. Port FK, Held PJ, Nolph KD, Turenne MN, Wolfe RA. Risk of peritonitis and technique failure by CAPD connection technique: a national study. Kidney Int 1992; 42: 967–74.
105. National CAPD Registry of the National Institute of Health, Bethesda, Maryland, 1987.
106. Diaz-Buxo JA. Continuous cyclic peritoneal dialysis. In: Nolph KD (ed), Peritoneal Dialysis, 3rd edition. Martinus Nijhoff, Boston 1988; pp 169–83.
107. Suki WN, Muniz E, Nishioka J. Drop-out in patients undergoing continuous cycled peritoneal dialysis. In: Khanna R, Nolph KD, Prowant B, Twardowski ZJ, Oreopoulos DG (eds), Advances in Peritoneal Dialysis. University of Toronto Press, Toronto 1987; pp 183–5.
108. Diaz-Buxo JA, Walker PJ, Chandler JT, Burgess WP, Farmer CD. Experience with intermittent peritoneal dialysis and continuous cyclic peritoneal dialysis. Am J Kidney Dis 1984; 4: 242–8.
109. Aujla NS, Piraino B, Sorkin MI. An intraperitoneal insulin regimen for diabetics on continuous cyclic peritoneal dialysis. ASAIO Trans 1990; 36: 119–21.
110. Posen GA, Luiscello J. Continuous equilibration peritoneal dialysis in the treatment of acute renal failure. Perit Dial Bull 1980; 1: 6.
111. Katirtzoglou A, Kontesis P, Myopoulou-Synvoulidis D, Digenis GE, Synvoulidis A, Komminos Z. Continuous equilibration peritoneal dialysis (CEPD) in hypercatabolic renal failure. Perit Dial Bull 1983; 3: 178–80.
112. Gaillou PJ, Will EJ, Davison AM, Giles GR. CAPD – a risk factor in renal transplantation? Br J Surg 1984; 71: 878–80.
113. Gelfand M, Kois J, Quillan B et al. CAPD yields inferior transplant results compared to hemodialysis (HD). Perit Dial Bull 1984; 4: S26.
114. Giacchino F, Alloatti S, Quarello F et al. The influence of peritoneal dialysis on cellular immunity. Perit Dial Bull 1982; 2: 165–8.
115. Giangrande A, Cantu P, Limido A, de Francisco D, Malacrida V. Continuous ambulatory peritoneal dialysis and cellular immunity. Proc EDTA 1982; 19: 372–7.
116. Walker JF, Oreopoulos DG, Uldal PR et al. The effect of pretransplant blood transfusion on graft outcome in patients on peritoneal dialysis prior to renal transplantation. Trans Proc 1982; 17: 687–9.
117. Cardella CJ. Renal transplantation in patients on peritoneal dialysis. Perit Dial Bull 1982; 2: 165–8.
118. Gokal R, Ramos JM, Veitch P et al. Renal transplantation in patients on continuous ambulatory peritoneal dialysis. Proc EDTA 1981; 18: 222–7.
119. Stefanidis C, Balfe JW, Arbus GS et al. Renal transplantation in children treated with continuous ambulatory peritoneal dialysis. Perit Dial Bull 1983; 1: 5–8.
120. Leichter HE, Salusky IB, Fine RN. Renal transplantation in patients on CAPD and CCPD – special focus in pediatrics. Perspect in Perit Dial 1986; 4: 12–5.
121. Wood C, Thomson NM, Scott DF et al. Results of renal transplantation in patients on CAPD. Perit Dial Bull 1984; 4: S72.
122. Diaz-Buxo JA, Walker PJ, Burgess WP et al. The influence of peritoneal dialysis on the outcome of transplantation. Int J Artif Organs 1986; 9: 359–62.
123. Hutchison A, Turner K, Gokal R. Effect of longterm therapy with 1.25 mmol/l calcium dialysis fluid on the incidence of peritonitis in CAPD. Perit Dial Int 1992; 12: 321–3.

14 Adequacy of peritoneal dialysis

PRAKASH KESHAVIAH

1. Introduction 419
2. Clinical approach to adequacy 420
3. Quantitating the therapy prescription: small solute indices 421
   3.1. The peritoneal equilibration test 421
   3.2. Dialytic solute clearance 421
   3.3. Residual solute clearance 421
   3.4. Normalized weekly clearances 422
   3.5. Dialysis index 423
   3.6. Creatinine efficacy number (EN) 423
4. Middle and large molecular weight toxins 423
5. Automated PD and adequacy 429
6. The relationship between peritoneal volume and peritoneal surface area 430
7. Review of clinical studies of peritoneal dialysis adequacy 432
   7.1. Multicenter studies, studies involving large patient populations and risk factor analyses 433
   7.2. Longitudinal studies relating clinical outcome to dialysis prescription 434
   7.3. Cross-sectional and short term studies of dialysis dose and clinical outcomes 436
   7.4. $(KT/V)_{urea}$ and weekly creatinine clearance 437
   7.5. Residual renal function, KT/V and PCR 437
8. Concluding remarks 438
References 440

1. Introduction

The subject of adequacy of peritoneal dialysis has attracted considerable attention only recently. It is interesting to note that this subject has not been explicitly addressed in either of the two major textbooks devoted to peritoneal dialysis – *Continuous Ambulatory Peritoneal Dialysis* edited by Gokal [1] or *Peritoneal Dialysis* edited by Nolph [2]. This is possibly because peritonitis and catheter problems such as exit site and tunnel infections have been the major areas of focus, these being the predominant reasons for switching patients from peritoneal dialysis to hemodialysis. With the advent of disconnect systems like the Y-system and twin bag [3, 4], there is the expectation of significant reductions in the incidence of peritonitis with a consequent favorable impact on therapy survival. In the past, the combined impact of transplantation, peritonitis, and catheter problems resulted in a 3 year technique survival of less than 35% [5, 6]. Now, it is not unreasonable to expect that a significant number of patients on peritoneal dialysis will be able to remain on peritoneal dialysis for durations exceeding 3 years. This expectation has some important implications – firstly, the magnitude of residual renal function will decline in 3 years to levels too low to provide a major contribution to the total dose of therapy [7, 8]; secondly, the consequences of an inadequate therapy prescription will now become evident and reflected in the morbidity and mortality statistics of the peritoneal population because of the cumulative effects of prolonged exposure. The few longitudinal studies that have been published to date [9, 10 11] attest to this. In the past, transplantation, peritonitis, and catheter problems have masked the problem of inadequate dialysis. This may no longer be the case in the future. Therefore, it is timely that the issue of adequacy of peritoneal dialysis has become a subject of considerable importance and concern with a spate of recent publications [9, 10, 11, 12, 13, 14, 15, 16, 17, 18] concerning the definition of dialysis adequacy, its quantification, and the need to establish criteria for individualizing the therapy prescription.

Inadequate dialysis is easier to define and recognize than adequate dialysis. Defining inadequate dialysis is the first step, and allows the establishment of a minimum acceptable dose of dialysis that is compatible with short-term well-being and the absence of overt symptoms of uremia. It is harder to establish the optimum dose of dialysis which must, of necessity, include favorable long-term outcomes such as survival, rehabilitation and quality of life. There is now sufficient data in the literature to establish the minimum acceptable dose of dialysis for CAPD. Few patients have remained on peritoneal dialysis long enough to document long-term clinical outcomes and test the effect of therapy prescription on these long-term outcomes. Long-term outcomes may also often be inextricably intertwined with other parameters such as the primary cause of renal failure, patient demographics, and comorbid conditions. Sophisticated analyses such as the Cox Proportional Hazards Model [19] need to be applied to large multicenter study populations followed for long periods of time before the influence of primary disease, demographics, comorbid conditions, dose of therapy, and patient nutrition on long-term outcomes is quantifiable separately, in order to arrive at an optimum therapy prescription. While it is hoped that large studies such as the CAN-USA Multicenter Study [20] will, in the future, shed light on the optimum dose of dialysis, at the present, we must content ourselves with establishing the minimum acceptable therapy prescription and ensuring that this information is rapidly and widely disseminated amongst clinical practitioners prescribing peritoneal dialysis. The subject of dialysis adequacy has been of concern to researchers in the area of hemodialysis for over two decades. There is a lot more information available regarding the adequacy of hemodialysis because of the large number of patients on this modality, the high therapy survival associated with it, and long-term follow-up of such populations. It will, therefore, be useful to consider how the data on hemodialysis adequacy is relevant to peritoneal dialysis and whether similar quantitative approaches apply to both dialysis modalities.

2. Clinical approach to adequacy

The most commonly used and obvious approach to assessing dialysis adequacy is to prescribe the dose of dialysis based on patient symptoms. One example of the clinical approach is summarized in Table 1. Another example is the scale of adequacy that is symptom-based as shown in Fig. 1. At one extreme is the ultimate and irreversible symptom – death. At the other extreme, the patient is free of all uremic symptoms, eating well, and active. This approach to dialysis is a trial and error, subjective, reactive approach that, in a sense, treats the patient like a guinea pig. The symptoms manifested by the patient are titrated against the amount of therapy prescribed, and the approach requires a well-trained, observant clinician and frequent observations. An objective, quantitative approach to therapy that is pro-active rather than reactive has obvious advantages. While such an approach cannot be divorced

Table 1. Clinical approach to assessing dialysis adequacy (Twardowski & Nolph [25]).

No clinical signs of uremia (insomnia, weakness, nausea, dysgeusia, etc).
Hct > 25% (without anabolic steroids/EPO)
Stable nerve conduction velocities
Controlled blood pressures

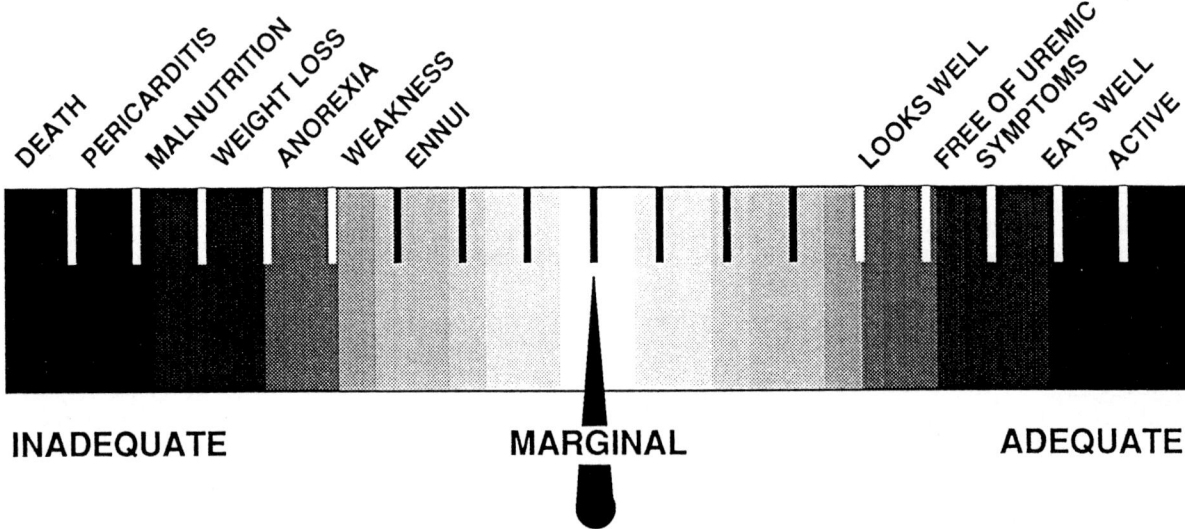

Figure 1. An adequacy scale calibrated by clinical symptoms (modified from P. Lundin, M.D. (personal communication)).

from careful clinical observation of the patient, it can reduce the amount of guess work and trial and error involved, thus sparing the patient some of the ordeal of uremic symptoms.

The quantitative approach also allows the dose of dialysis to be individualized to the needs of the patient unlike the commonly used approach of prescribing a standard regimen of dialysis that does not take into consideration patient size, residual renal function, nutrition, and disease-specific requirements. During the first few years on peritoneal dialysis, there are significant increases in body weight and significant decreases in residual renal function [11] both of which require an increase in the dose of dialytic therapy. The quantitative approach allows such adjustments to be made reliably without resorting to trial and error.

3. Quantitating the therapy prescription: small solute indices

3.1. The peritoneal equilibration test

The peritoneal equilibration test (PET) was introduced by Twardowski [21] as an easy and convenient method for characterizing the transport characteristics of the peritoneal membrane. This test uses a standardized approach to study the rates of equilibration of small solutes like creatinine and glucose using the dialysate to plasma ratio (D/P) at 2 and 4 hours. Based on data from a study population of 101 patients and the 4 hour D/P ratio, Twardowski has classified peritoneal permeability into 4 categories, low, low average, high average, and high. This scheme of categorization also allows the clinician to decide which mode of peritoneal dialysis (CAPD, NIPD, CCPD, etc.) is most suitable for a given patient.

There has been some confusion regarding the relationship between the PET and therapy adequacy requirements. To use the analogy of hemodialysis, the PET measures the mass transfer-area characteristics of the biological dialyzer whereas the operating conditions of blood and dialysate flow rates and treatment time decide the adequacy of the hemodialysis therapy prescription. In peritoneal dialysis, the blood flow and mass transfer-area coefficients are given, but the volume of dialysis fluid used per exchange, the number of exchanges, and the treatment time determine the dose of peritoneal dialysis. (In research settings, the blood flow and mass transfer-area coefficients can be pharmacologically manipulated).

3.2. Dialytic solute clearance

Solute clearance (K) during a peritoneal dialysis exchange is defined thus:

$$K = (V_d/T) \cdot (D/P)$$

where V_d is the volume of dialysate drained at the end of the exchange, T is the duration of the exchange, and D/P is the dialysate to plasma ratio for that exchange.

From the equation above, we get $KT = V_d \cdot (D/P)$ i.e., the clearance-time product is equal to the volume of dialysate drained times the D/P ratio. For CAPD, the KT product for a 24 hour period is calculated by pooling the drained volumes of all the exchanges during the 24 hour period, measuring the dialysate and plasma solute concentrations and multiplying the total drained volume by the D/P ratio of the pooled dialysate. Note that the D/P ratio used in this calculation applies to the 24 hour pooled volume and not the 4 hour D/P ratio for the PET test. For a patient on NIPD, the total drained volume of all nightly exchanges is pooled, the D/P ratio measured, and a similar KT calculation performed. As the plasma solute concentration may change over the period of NIPD, an average of pre and post dialysis plasma concentrations must be used. While the correct average to use is the log mean average, the change in plasma concentration is not as large as in hemodialysis, and the arithmetic average is a reasonable approximation for the log mean concentration. The weekly KT is obtained by multiplying the per session KT by the number of sessions per week (7 for CAPD, NIPD, and CCPD and 3 for thrice weekly IPD).

3.3. Residual solute clearance

Rottembourg [7, 22], Cancarini [23], and Lysaght [8] have documented that residual renal clearance is better preserved in peritoneal dialysis patients compared to patients on hemodialysis. In hemodialysis, the contribution of residual clearance to total solute clearance is not significant for small solutes but may be significant for middle molecular weight and larger solutes. However, in peritoneal dialysis, even for small solutes, the residual renal contribution is significant. A residual GFR of 1 ml/min is equivalent to a weekly clearance of 10 L, which, for a small solute like creatinine, represents 20–25% of the total weekly clearance.

The relationship between residual urea and creatinine clearance is shown in Fig. 2. The residual creatinine clearance is 1.7 times the residual urea clearance because creatinine is secreted in the tubules, whereas urea undergoes some tubular reabsorption. The residual clearance, therefore, overestimates the GFR and the residual urea clearance underestimates the GFR. It was shown by Milutinovic et al. [24] almost 2 decades ago, that in patients with ESRD, the average of the residual urea and creatinine clearances is a good approximation for the GFR.

In considering the contribution of residual renal function to the weekly creatinine clearance, it may, therefore, be more appropriate to use the average of the residual urea and creatinine clearances rather than the residual creatinine clearance. However, in calculating the weekly urea clearance, using the residual urea clearance alone, rather then the average of residual urea and creatinine clearances, provides a more conservative approach.

3.4. Normalized weekly clearances

In order to individualize the dose of dialysis to patient size to make meaningful comparisons across patients of varying size, it is necessary to normalize the weekly solute clearance by some parameter reflecting patient size. Traditionally, acute body weight, ideal body weight, and body surface area are some of the measures of body size used for such normalization. In the case of the weekly creatinine clearance, Twardowski [25] has recommended normalizing the weekly creatinine clearance to body surface area and standardizing the clearance to a body surface area of $1.73 M^2$. In the case of the weekly urea clearance, the volume of body water in which urea is distributed has been traditionally used for normalization. The advantage of this approach to normalizing the urea clearance is that it results in the parameter KT/V which governs the kinetics of urea removal during hemodialysis, being the exponent of the rate of decay of urea concentration. Body surface area and the volume of body water are strongly correlated, this correlation being the basis of the Hume & Weyers nomogram [26] for determining total body water.

The weekly creatinine clearance normalized to $1.73 M^2$ of body surface area and KT/V are, therefore, both indices of small solute clearance with slightly different normalization schemes to account for body size. As we will see later, these two indices are highly correlated and there is internal consistency in the clinically recommended ranges for these therapy prescription indices.

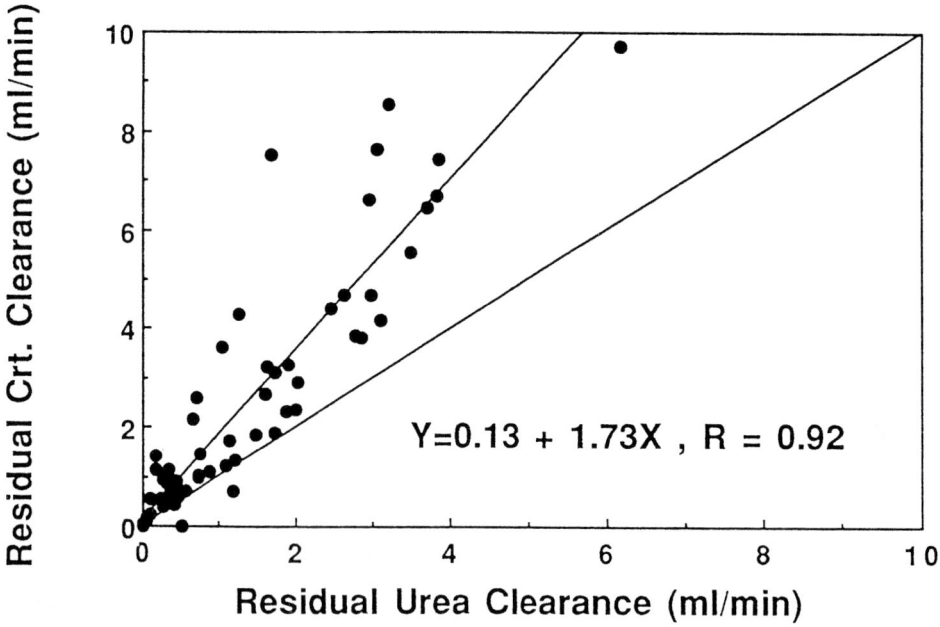

Figure 2. Relationship between residual urea and residual creatinine clearances. The slope is greater than unity because creatinine is secreted in the tubules, whereas urea is reabsorbed in the tubules. An average of residual urea and creatinine clearances is a good estimate of GFR.

3.5. Dialysis index

The dialysis index was introduced by Teehan in 1985 [27] as an index of CAPD therapy prescription based on the information gleaned from the urea kinetic studies of hemodialysis adequacy. This index is based on the targeting of a desirable steady state BUN level of 70 mg/dl in a patient with a dietary protein intake of 1.2 gm/kg/day. Based on the urea kinetic model, the drained dialysate volume (*DV*) required to achieve this target is calculated thus:

$$DV = 0.23 \, IBW - (2.7 + 1.44 \, K_r)$$

where IBW is the ideal body weight (kg) and K_r the residual renal urea nitrogen clearance (ml/min). The constants in this formula arise from assuming protein and amino acid nitrogen losses of 1900 mg, other miscellaneous nitrogen losses of 31 mg/kg, and total equilibration between plasma and dialysate urea nitrogen. The dialysis index is the ratio of the actual drained volume to the desired volume based on the above calculation. Values less than 1 connote underdialysis.

The dialysis index is highly correlated to the KT/V urea index [13, 17]. This is not surprising, since they are both based on the single pool urea kinetic model. This dialysis index was proposed by Teehan on the basis of the urea kinetic model but was not clinically tested in a prospective study as being a valid index of dialysis adequacy. However, Teehan has subsequently tested the validity of this index in a retrospective analysis of longitudinal clinical observations in 51 CAPD patients [17], showing a high correlation between the dialysis index and KT/V.

The dialysis index is based on a target BUN of 70 mg/dl in a patient consuming 1.2 gm of protein per kg of body weight per day. Several studies in stable CAPD patients who appear to be adequately dialyzed suggest that few CAPD patients achieve such a high intake of protein, the actual protein intake averaging 0.9 to 1.0 gm/kg/day [12, 16, 17]. The dialysis index can be reformulated on the basis of this level of protein intake. However, as the KT/V and the dialysis index are so highly correlated, and as the KT/V index has gained increasing acceptance in hemodialysis, the KT/V index is preferred to the dialysis index.

3.6. Creatinine efficacy number (EN)

Brandes introduced this index of CAPD adequacy in 1990 [28] with subsequent clinical validation in 1992 [15]. The EN is based on creatinine kinetics as inferred from the standardized 4 hour PET.

$$EN \, (L/gm \, of \, creatinine/day) = (D/P)_{crt} \cdot V/ACP_{PD}$$

where the $(D/P)_{crt}$ is the 4 hour dialysate to plasma ratio of creatinine from the 4 hour PET, V is the prescribed volume exchanged per day (L/day), and ACP_{PD}, the adjusted creatinine production is the sum of the creatinine appearance over 24 hours and the amount of creatinine cleared by the extra-renal route.

$$ACP_{PD}(gm/24 \, hr) = [(D_{crt} \cdot V_d \cdot 6) + (0.4 \cdot S_{crt} \cdot BW_t)].$$

The 24 hour creatinine appearance rate is estimated from the 4 hour dialysate concentration (D_{crt}, mg/L) and the drained volume per exchange V_d(dl), assuming 6 exchanges of 4 hour duration. The extra-renal clearance according to the data of Mitch and Walser [29] depends on the serum creatinine (S_{crt}, mg/dl) and body weight (B.wt, kg). Based on a short-term study of CAPD adequacy in 18 patients followed for 12 months, Brandes indicates that EN values of the order of 7 are associated with good clinical outcomes, levels around 5 with intermediate outcome, and values around 3.5 with poor clinical outcome. The classification of clinical outcome was based on a composite outcome scale that included clinical symptoms like insomnia, nausea, weakness, hospitalization, death, biochemical indices (BUN, albumin, nPCR), and therapy failure.

4. Middle and large molecular weight toxins

All of the quantitative indices that we have considered above are based on the small molecular weight toxins, urea and creatinine. Middle molecules were invoked by Babb and Scribner [30, 31, 32] as hypothetical toxins in the molecular weight range of 1000–2000 daltons that were poorly removed by the thick cellulosic hemodialysis membranes that were widely used in the mid-seventies. Babb and Scribner hypothesized that uremic lesions like peripheral neuropathy, anemia, and lipid abnormalities that stable hemodialysis patients continued to manifest must be a consequence of the retention of middle molecular weight uremic toxins that were not cleared by cellulosic membranes. On the basis of this reasoning, they developed the square meter-hour hypothesis and the middle molecule index. The square meter-hour hypothesis is based on the concept of optimizing the product of membrane surface area (square meters) and the duration of dialysis (hours) in order to achieve adequate removal of the so called middle molecules. The surface area-time product needed to be adjusted so as to achieve a middle molecule index of 1 or greater. The middle molecule index was based on the surrogate middle molecule vitamin B_{12} whose molecular weight is 1355 daltons. Vitamin B_{12} was used as an exogenous marker to characterize the permeability and clearance characteristics of various dialyzers. Scribner had made the empirical observation that patients with a residual renal function of 3 ml/min (30 liters/week) or greater did not have peripheral neuropathy, which in those days, was the classic hallmark of inadequate dialysis. Reasoning that residual renal function was capable of clearing toxic middle molecules, this target of 30 liters of middle molecule clearance per week was established. The middle molecule index is the ratio of actual weekly clearance of middle molecules to the desired clearance of 30 liters/week (normalized to a normal body surface area of 1.73 M^2).

It is interesting to note that Scribner, in making the empirical observation of the absence of peripheral neuropathy in patients with a residual renal function of 3 ml/min, also observed that peripheral neuropathy was not common in patients on peritoneal dialysis, suggesting that the peritoneal membrane like residual renal function, was capable of clearing middle molecules. Boen who had collaborated with Scribner in some of the earliest studies of peritoneal dialysis quantification [33, 34] also noted that patients on peritoneal dialysis appeared to be of 'comparable good health' relative to patients on hemodialysis despite much lower small solute clearances. This was also consistent with the middle molecule paradigm.

Babb [35] set out to quantitate the comparative permeability of the peritoneal membrane and cellulosic hemodialysis membranes using a wide spectrum of solute markers from urea (60 daltons) to inulin (5200 daltons). This data is summarized in Table 2. The mass transfer area coefficients for the peritoneal membrane are much lower than those of cellulosic membranes for urea and creatinine but are of the same order of magnitude for molecules like inulin. This comparison of mass transfer-area coefficients needs critical examination. The comparison was based on 1.0 M^2 of surface area for hemodialysis membranes compared to a nominal surface area of 1.7 M^2 for the peritoneal membrane. Also, the data for inulin was derived by infusing inulin intraperitoneally and measuring its disappearance rate from the peritoneal cavity. The disappearance of inulin from the peritoneal cavity is the combined effect of two transport mechanisms – diffusion and lymphatic drainage [36, 37]. As the contribution of lymphatic drainage, though significant, was not recognized by Babb, the peritoneal mass transfer-area coefficient for inulin was overestimated, because all of the transport was ascribed to diffusive transport. Measurements by Struijk [36] based on intravenous infusion of inulin and appearance of inulin in the peritoneal cavity indicate much smaller mass transfer-area coefficients for inulin (1.8 vs 4.7). Struijk's data is the average of measurements in 9 patients, whereas the data of Babb was derived from a single patient.

The cellulosic membranes used for hemodialysis in the seventies were 3 times as thick as those currently in use (20–25 μm vs 6–8 μm today). Also high flux cellulosic membranes like the cellulose triacetate (CT) membrane are available today. Table 3 is a more realistic comparison of the permeability characteristics of peritoneal and hemodialysis membranes, based on a nominal surface area of 1.7 M^2 for both peritoneal and hemodialysis membranes. These data are compiled from several sources [36, 37, 38] and do account for the lymphatic contribution to transport. On the basis of this comparison, one sees that even for a large molecule like inulin, the peritoneal mass transfer-area coefficient is lower than that of an 8 μ Cuprophan membrane and is much lower than that of a high flux membrane.

Table 2. Comparison of mass transfer area coefficients of peritoneal and hemodialysis mebranes (modified from Reference [18]).

Solute	Mol. Wt. (daltons)	Mass transfer area coefficients (ml/min)	
		Peritoneal membrane (~1.7 M^2)	Cuprophane (1.0 M^2)
Urea	60	24	133
Creatinine	113	11	90
Vitamin B_{12}	1355	5.4	18
Inulin	5200	4.7	5

However, for a larger molecule like Beta-2 microglobulin, the peritoneal membrane is intermediate between conventional Cuprophan and high flux membranes.

Even the comparison of Table 3 is not a suitable comparison of the solute removal capabilities of peritoneal and hemodialysis membranes. This is because time has not been factored in. CAPD, for instance, is performed 24 hours per day, 7 days per week. On the other hand, hemodialysis is conventionally performed 3–5 hours per session, 3 sessions weekly. As suggested by the square meter-hour hypothesis, time plays a significant role in the transport of middle and large molecules. A more realistic comparison of weekly solute clearances of peritoneal and hemodialysis membranes is made in Table 4. This table indicates that for small solutes, peritoneal dialysis is less efficient than even standard hemodialysis. However, for middle and large molecules, peritoneal dialysis is intermediate between standard and high flux dialysis. Though not shown in Table 4, peritoneal dialysis is comparable to high efficiency dialysis in the removal of middle molecules like VB_{12} and is more efficient than high efficiency dialysis in the removal of larger solutes like Beta-2 microglobulin.

It is matter of common clinical experience that when CAPD patients manifest uremic symptoms suggestive of underdialysis, these symptoms are alleviated by an increase in the number of exchanges or an increase in the volume of each exchange. If the number of exchanges is increased, what impact does this change have on small, middle, and large molecular weight clearances? We set up a mathematical model of peritoneal transport based on well established principles to study the effect of increasing the number of exchanges on solute clearance over a wide molecular weight spectrum [14]. The results of the modeling are shown in Figure 3. It is clear from this figure that clearance of middle and large molecular weight solutes are not appreciably affected by increasing the number of exchanges from 2 exchanges to 5 exchanges per day, whereas there is almost a doubling of small solute clearances with increase in the number of exchanges. These results fit with intuition and the model is required only to quantify the magnitude of the ensuing changes. With middle and large molecular weight solutes, because of slow transport across the peritoneal membrane, rapid equilibration between dialysate and blood does not occur, so that at the end of the normal exchange duration (4–6 hours) there is still a large concentration gradient between blood and dialysate. With 2 exchanges/day, each exchange lasts 12 hours and as the concentration gradient for large solutes is not rapidly dissipated as with small solutes, diffusive transport continues to occur over the long duration. Increasing the number of exchanges reduces the duration of each exchange but does not appreciably increase clearance because of the slow transport of middle and large molecules. With a small solute like urea, almost complete equilibration between blood and dialysate occurs in 4–6 hours and no further transport occurs unless the gradient is reestablished by draining the equilibrated dialysate and replenishing the peritoneal cavity with a fresh volume of dialysate. Increasing the number of exchanges and reducing the time per exchange therefore has a significant effect on small solute clearances.

If small solute clearances alone are appreciably increased with increasing the number of exchanges, and if, as common clinical experience indicates, there is alleviation of the symptoms of under-

Table 3. Mass transfer area coefficient comparison of peritoneal, conventional hemodialysis, and high flux hemodialysis membranes for 1.7 M^2 of membrane surface area (modified from Reference [18]).

Solute	Mass transfer area coefficient (ml/min)		
	Peritoneal	Cuprophane (8 μ)	Cellulose triacetate
Urea	20	692	818
Creatinine	12	404	583
Vitamin B12	3.5	6.8	248
Inulin	1.8	35	125
Beta-2-Microglobulin	0.8	0	70

Table 4. Comparison of weekly clearances (liters/week) with CAPD, conventional hemodialysis, and high flux hemodialysis (modified from Reference [18]).

Solute	Peritoneal	Cuprophane*	Cellulose triacetate**
Urea	64	119	139
Creatinine	57	96	126
Vitamin B12	37	27	86
Inulin	17	14	51
Beta-2-Microglobulin	18	0	38

* Cuprophane: CF1511 (Baxter Healthcare Corporation) Qb/Bd = 200/500 ml/min, 12 hr/week
** Cellulose triacetate: CT190 (Baxter Healthcare Corporation) Qb/Bd = 200/500 ml/min, 12 hr/week

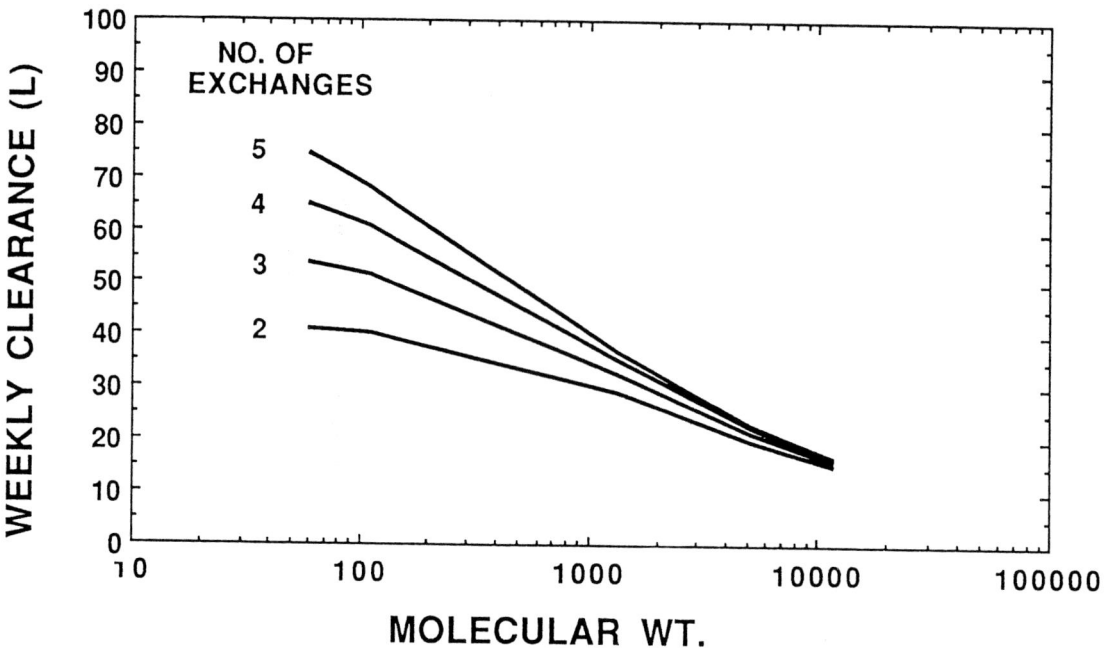

Figure 3. Influence of the number of CAPD exchanges on weekly solute clearances over a wide range of molecular weights derived from a mathematical model of peritoneal transport. Small solute clearances are appreciably influenced by the number of exchanges whereas middle and large molecular clearances are not significantly altered. (Reprinted by permission of Blackwell Scientific Publications, Inc, Reference [14]).

dialysis, it stands to reason that the commonly observed symptoms of underdialysis are related to inadequate removal of small solutes. This fits with our knowledge of dialysis adequacy in the hemodialysis setting where the value of the KT/V urea index in determining the adequacy of the therapy prescription has been clearly established.

Having thus established the importance of adequate small solute clearances even in the peritoneal dialysis setting, let us go back and look at the weekly clearances of small solutes by peritoneal dialysis compared to hemodialysis in Table 4. It is clear from this table that the weekly clearances of urea achieved with the standard CAPD regimen of 4 daily 2 liter exchanges is only of the order of 54% of that achieved with conventional hemodialysis with cellulosic membranes. The lower small solute clearances of CAPD relative to hemodialysis are also reflected in a KT/V calculation. This calculation for an average size patient on the standard CAPD regimen and with no residual renal function is detailed in Table 5. The daily KT/V = 0.214 and multiplying by 7, the weekly KT/V = 1.498. To compare with hemodialysis, we divide the weekly KT/V by 3 as hemodialysis is traditionally performed thrice weekly. The equivalent KT/V for comparison to hemodialysis is 0.50 or approximately half the minimum KT/V established for hemodialysis based on the Gotch analysis [39] of the data from the National Cooperative Dialysis Study [40].

In the hemodialysis setting, a KT/V of 0.5 is lower than the KT/V achieved in Groups II and IV of the National Cooperative Dialysis Study. These groups had an extremely high morbidity, and failure rates as high as 40–70% within a few months of being randomized to this level of KT/V. The failure rate in Group IV, the short time, low KT/V group, was so high as to pose ethical concerns about the continuation of this study group. Patients in this group were removed from the study, and it is

Table 5. KT/V calculation for the standard CAPD regimen.

KT (liters)	= Drained volume (liters) × $(D/P)_{24hr}$ Ratio (volume instilled + ultrafiltrate)		
	= 9.5 × 0.9		
	= 8.55 liters		
V (liters)	= Volume of body water estimated from sex, age, height, & weight		
	= 40 liters		
therefore	$(KT/V)_{day}$	= 8.55/40	= 0.214
	$(KT/V)_{week}$	= 0.21 × 7	= 1.498
	$(KT/V)_{HD\ equivalent}$	= 1.47/3	= 0.50

noteworthy that even after removal from the study, these patients continued to have a high incidence of mortality as a carry-over phenomenon related to the inadequate study prescription. The overt symptoms, hospitalization rates, medical problems, withdrawal from study, and high mortality left little doubt about the inadequacy of therapy prescription (KT/V ~0.5–0.6) in Groups II and IV.

At the same low level of KT/V with the standard CAPD regimen, it is clear that these drastic clinical outcomes are not commonly observed. In fact, the literature clearly indicates that clinical outcomes in CAPD are, in general, comparable to those observed in hemodialysis relative to survival [41, 42] and morbidity as reflected in non-peritonitis related hospitalizations [43, 44]. CAPD outcomes are in no way comparable to those of Groups II and IV of the NCDS. In fact according to the Best Demonstrated Practices database maintained by the Baxter Healthcare Corporation [45], only 10% of the patients withdrawn from CAPD to other modalities are withdrawn for reasons of inadequate dialysis. This percentage may, to some extent, be an underestimation of the true incidence of inadequate dialysis in CAPD as there were additional medical withdrawals that, upon closer scrutiny, may fall into the inadequate dialysis category. However, some of the withdrawals classified as inadequate dialysis are related to inadequate ultrafiltration secondary to peritoneal membrane changes rather than inadequate solute removal. It should also be borne in mind that much of this data was gathered before the widespread acceptance of disconnect systems. As a consequence, peritonitis often intervened as a reason for therapy failure before residual renal function declined to insignificant levels. As peritonitis becomes a less frequent cause for therapy failure, patients will stay on CAPD for longer durations of time with loss of residual function and need for greater attention to the dialytic therapy prescription. Despite all these caveats, it is clear that a paradox exists in comparing CAPD and hemodialysis outcomes using KT/V as a basis of comparison. This paradox has been addressed by the peak concentration hypothesis [46]. According to this hypothesis, a direct comparison between CAPD and hemodialysis on the basis of KT/V is untenable because CAPD is a continuous therapy whereas hemodialysis is an intermittent therapy. Being an intermittent therapy, hemodialysis is associated with peaks and troughs of small solute concentrations. If the same weekly KT/V is prescribed for both therapies, the time averaged small solute concentrations will be the same in both therapies. With CAPD, the actual and time-averaged concentrations are not different because of its continuous nature. However, with hemodialysis, despite the same time-averaged concentration, for about half the duration of the week, small solute concentrations will be higher than with CAPD, and for the rest of the week, the concentrations will be lower with CAPD (Fig. 4). The hypothesis postulates that if toxicity is correlated to peak rather than time-averaged concentrations, then hemodialysis will be associated with a higher toxicity than CAPD at the same KT/V, and hence, same time-averaged concentrations. Or put another way, in order to reduce the peak hemodialysis concentration to the CAPD level, a higher KT/V is required for hemodialysis. An approximate formula for matching peak hemodialysis concentrations to steady state CAPD concentrations is given below from the paper by Nolph, Keshaviah, and Popovich [47].

$$C_{HD}/C_{CAPD} = (KT/V)_{CAPD}/(1 - \exp(-KT/V)_{HD})$$

where C_{HD} is the pre-dialysis hemodialysis concentration, C_{CAPD}, the steady state CAPD concentration, and $(KT/V)_{CAPD}$ is the thrice weekly equivalent KT/V for comparison to $(KT/V)_{HD}$. A more accurate matching of the two therapies based on the variable volume single pool urea kinetic model is shown in Fig. 5. The approximate matching formula is also plotted in Fig. 5. According to this figure, which is based on matching the peak hemodialysis BUN concentration to the steady state CAPD concentration, a per hemodialysis session KT/V of 0.9 is equivalent to a weekly CAPD KT/V of 1.7. As 0.9 is the minimum acceptable KT/V based on Gotch's analysis of the NCDS data, according to the peak concentration hypothesis, a weekly KT/V of 1.7 is the minimum acceptable therapy prescription for CAPD. It is becoming apparent in the hemodialysis setting that higher values of KT/V (> 0.8) are associated with improved survival outcomes. Many clinicians are targeting KT/V values of 1.2 and higher for more optimal outcomes. Translating this to the CAPD setting based on the peak concentration hypothesis, weekly KT/V values of 1.9 or greater may be required for optimal outcomes. At the other end of the spectrum, the dismal results of Groups II and IV of the NCDS were at KT/V levels between 0.5 and 0.6. Corresponding levels for CAPD based on the peak concentration hypothesis would be a weekly KT/V of around 1.2. Extrapolating from the hemodialysis experience in

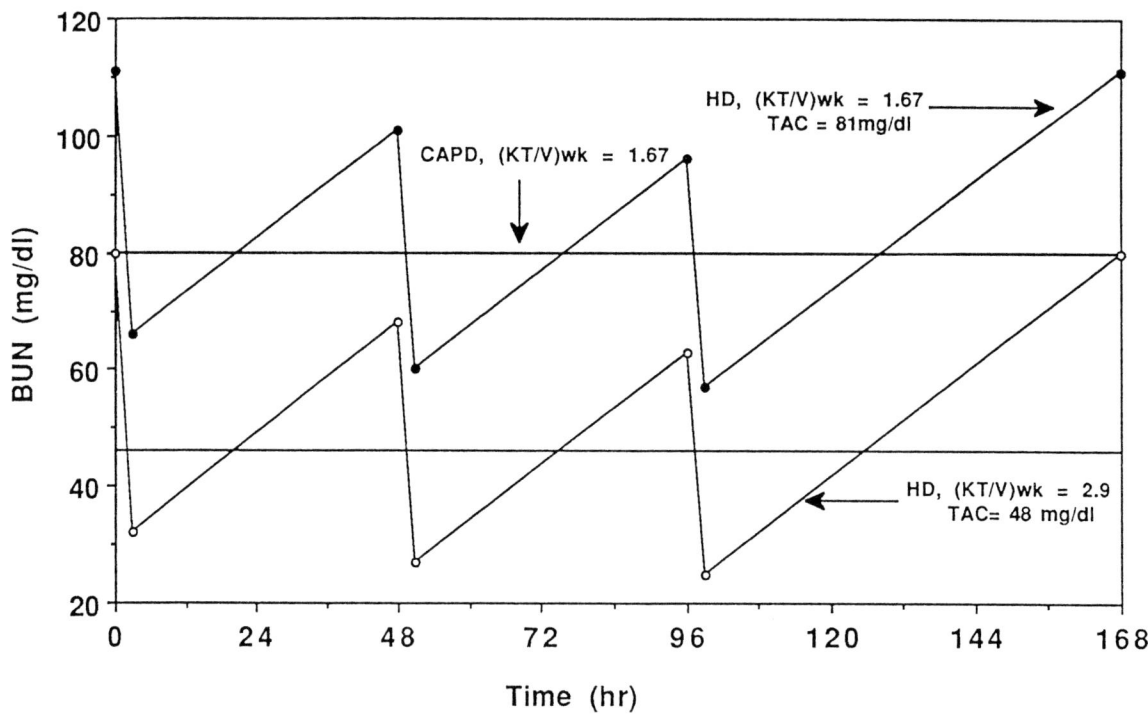

Figure 4. BUN profile for hemodialysis (thrice weekly) and CAPD over the duration of the week. The TACurea for hemodialysis is the same as the steady state CAPD BUN for the same KT/V (KT/V = 1.67). Matching of peak BUN for hemodialysis with steady state BUN for CAPD requires a higher KT/V for hemodialysis (KT/V = 2.9 vs 1.67).

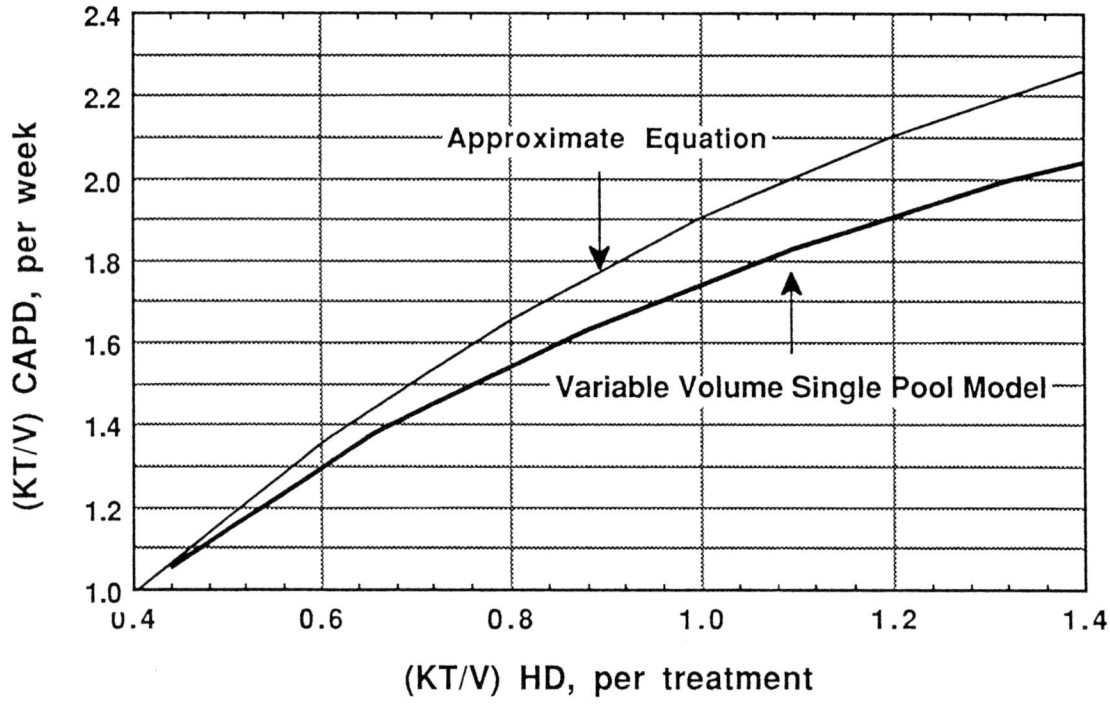

Figure 5. Scaling weekly KT/V for CAPD to the per session KT/V for hemodialysis based on the peak concentration hypothesis, peak BUN for hemodialysis being matched to the steady state BUN for CAPD. The approximate matching equation from reference [47] and the more rigorous matching using a variable value single pool urea kinetic model are both shown on this plot.

conjunction with the peak concentration hypothesis, therefore, yields a weekly KT/V scale for CAPD that is illustrated in Fig. 6. While a direct validation of the peak concentration hypothesis is not easy, an indirect validation of this hypothesis is possible by examining if these predictions of inadequate, minimum, and optimum weekly KT/V ranges fit with clinical observations. We will consider the few available clinical studies of PD adequacy in a succeeding section.

5. Automated PD and adequacy

According to the glossary of Twardowski [48], there are many possible combinations of day time and night time PD therapies. In the early days of peritoneal dialysis before the advent of CAPD, peritoneal dialysis was typically used in center, thrice weekly for periods as long as 12–14 hours per session. It was a matter of common clinical experience that patients did not thrive on this therapy modality. Let us quantitate the magnitude of therapy that these patients were receiving. Machines that prepare fluid on site using R.O. water and concentrate were used with pumped inflow rates of 500 ml/min and gravity outflow. Typically, 2 liter exchanges were used with inflow, dwell, and outflow durations of 4, 40, and 16 minutes respectively. Each exchange, therefore, lasted 1 hour with a total of 12–14 exchanges (24–28 liters of fluid exchanged). In order to estimate the clearance achieved with this mode of therapy, we need to determine typical D/P ratios for a half hour dwell based on the peritoneal equilibration test. For an average permeability patient, according to the data of Twardowski [21], D/P ratios for urea and creatinine for a dwell period of 40' are of the order of 0.4 and 0.25 respectively. Using the clearance equation described earlier, we arrive at urea and creatinine clearances of 13.3 and 8.3 ml/min respectively based on 28 liters of fluid exchanged over a total duration of 14 hours. The clearance-time product (KT) values for urea and creatinine are 11.2 and 7 liters respectively. Assuming an average body size (70 kg body weight, 1.73 M^2 body surface area and body water = 58% of body weight), we arrive at KT/V of 0.28 per treatment (3 treatments per week) and a weekly creatinine clearance of 21 liters per week. These are clearly inadequate therapy prescription indices if we use a minimum acceptable KT/V of 0.8 per treatment for thrice weekly therapy or a weekly creatinine clearance of 40–50 liters per week 1.73 M^2 of body surface area. Let us consider a more aggressive therapy schedule that some centers had adopted of 2 exchanges per hour for a total volume of 56 liters and D/P ratios of 0.30 and 0.20 respectively for urea and creatinine. The KT product with this schedule is 14 liters for urea and

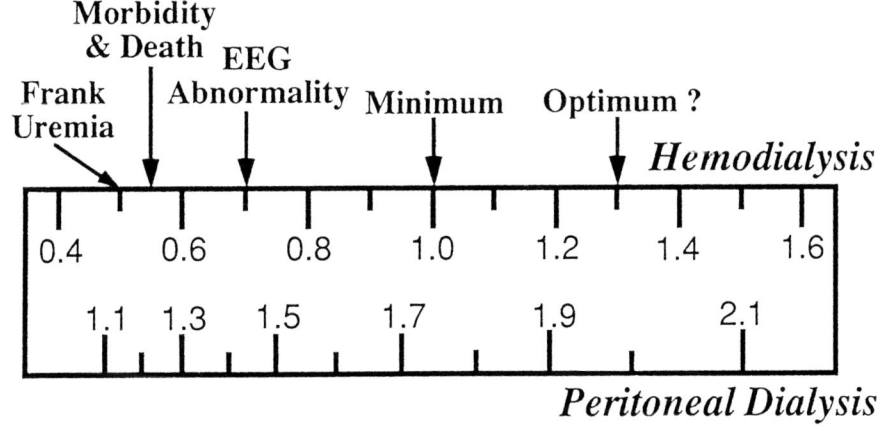

Figure 6. Composite KT/V scale for hemodialysis based on studies in the literature with a corresponding CAPD scale based on the peak concentration hypothesis scaling factor. (Reprinted by permission of Blackwell Scientific Publications, Inc, Reference [14]).

8.4 liters for creatinine. The KT/V for urea is 0.34 and the weekly creatinine clearance is 25.2 liters. Even these indices represent grossly inadequate therapy. It is, therefore, not surprising that patients did poorly on this mode of therapy and that peritoneal dialysis fell into disrepute until the introduction of CAPD.

The modes of automated peritoneal dialysis currently in vogue are continuous cycling peritoneal dialysis (CCPD) and nightly intermittent peritoneal dialysis (NIPD). CCPD may be considered to be a combination of NIPD and a day time exchange ('wet day'). We will first consider typical therapy indices with NIPD. This therapy mode is usually performed 7 nights a week with a duration of 10 hours and 5 exchanges per night with a total fluid usage of 10 liters. Inflow and outflow are usually by gravity with inflow times of around 10 minutes and outflow times of 16–20 minutes. For a total exchange time of 2 hours, the dwell phase is about 90 minutes. D/P ratios for this duration are of the order of 0.6 for urea and 0.4 for creatinine. We, therefore, get KT products of 6 liters for urea and 4 liters for creatinine or weekly values of 42 liters and 28 liters respectively. The weekly KT/V is of the order of 1.03 for urea and the weekly creatinine clearance is 28 liters. In the absence of residual renal function, these indices connote inadequate dialysis. If we consider the day time exchange with total equilibration (D/P = 1) for urea and a D/P of 0.8 for creatinine, the additional KT products for the day time exchange ('wet day') on a weekly basis are 14 liters for urea and 11.2 liters for creatinine for a total weekly KT/V of 1.4 and a weekly creatinine clearance of 39.2 liters. These are on the threshold of being minimum acceptable therapy indices. We can use the CAPD scale of adequacy with CCPD because of the continuous nature of CCPD. However, for NIPD with 'dry days', one has to change the scaling factor, as NIPD is an intermittent therapy. Using the approximate equation from the paper by Nolph et al. [47] we calculate that for a 10 liters per day, 7 days per week therapy, the weekly KT/V should be of the order of 2.0 for the minimum acceptable prescription corresponding to a weekly KT/V of 1.7 for CAPD. In the patient with average permeability and no residual renal function, the 10 liters per day NIPD regimen does not come close to being acceptable therapy. Surveys conducted by Baxter Healthcare Corporation [49] suggest that the average usage of fluid for NIPD has decreased from 11–12 liters per day in the late Eighties to between 9–10 liters per day in the early Nineties. Unless these patients have significant residual renal function, there is risk of underdialysis relative to small solute clearances. It is, therefore, recommended that the usage of fluid be increased in anuric patients on NIPD or that CCPD be considered as an alternative to boost weekly clearances.

6. The relationship between peritoneal volume and peritoneal surface area

An exchange volume of 2 liters has become the standard of practice on the basis of empiricism. Few systematic studies have been performed aimed at optimizing exchange volume relative to body size. Recently we studied [50] the influence of peritoneal volume on the mass transfer-area coefficient and hence on the peritoneal surface area. To study these relationships, we performed 120 minute peritoneal equilibration tests in a group of 10 patients with a range of peritoneal exchange volumes from 0.5 to 3.0 liters. The order in which different peritoneal volumes were studied was randomized and the rate of transport of 3 solutes – urea, creatinine, and glucose, were quantitated for these equilibration studies. At each peritoneal exchange volume, the mass transfer-area coefficient for the 3 solutes was calculated and average data for the group studied are shown in Fig. 7. The mass transfer-area coefficients were then normalized to the mass transfer-area coefficient at a 2 liter exchange volume, and the normalized values for the 3 solutes were found to collapse onto the same trend line as shown in Fig. 8. This, therefore, leads us to conclude that this trend line represents the surface area vs volume relationship because by normalizing the mass transfer-area coefficient K_oA at each volume to that at 2 liters, the K_o gets canceled leaving the A vs volume relationship. This conclusion is further strengthened by the fact that all 3 solutes – urea, creatinine, and glucose, fall on the same trend line through this normalization process. As Fig. 8 indicates, the area A increases almost linearly with volume V between 1 and 2 L and begins to plateau thereafter with only a 10% increase in A between V of 2 and 3 L. So the empirical choice of an exchange volume of 2 L in the average patient is validated by this analysis. However, if we plot the optimum volume at which surface area is maximized as a function of body surface area, we arrive at the relationship in Fig. 9. This figure suggests

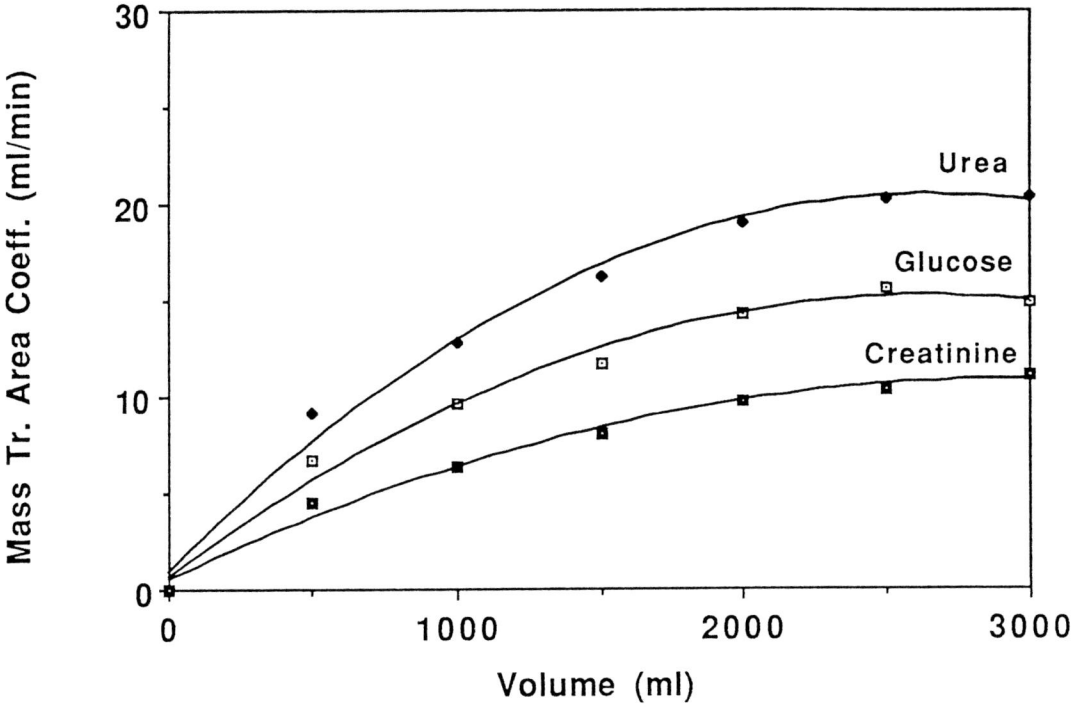

Figure 7. The influence of peritoneal volume on the mass transfer area coefficients (MTAC) for urea, creatinine, and glucose. A significant almost linear increase in the MTAC is seen when volume is increased from 0.5–2 liters, but between 2 and 3 liters, the increase is relatively small.

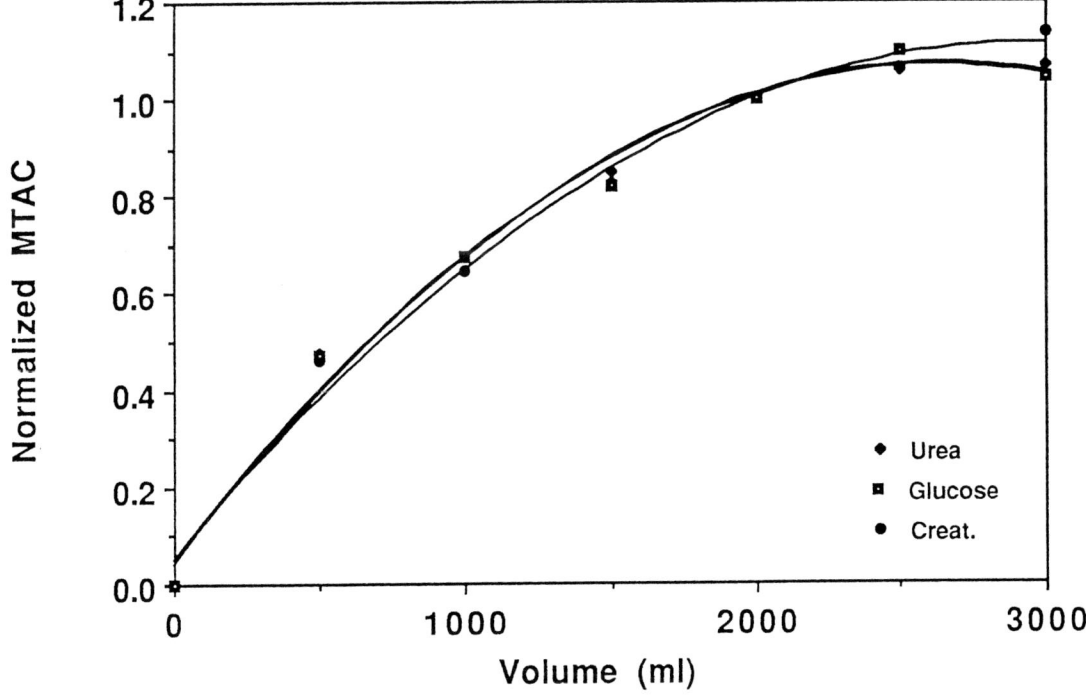

Figure 8. Influence of peritoneal volume on the normalized MTAC, normalization being done using the MTAC at 2 liters instilled volume. The collapse of the data for the 3 solutes onto the same trend line strongly indicates that the trend line represents peritoneal surface area vs peritoneal volume.

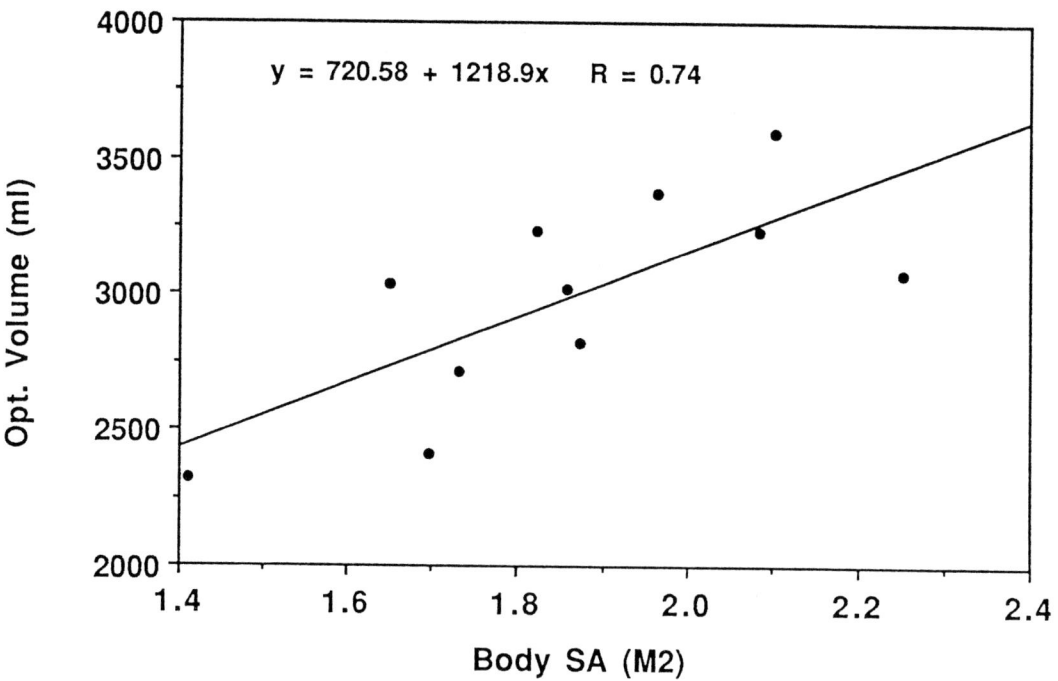

Figure 9. The optimum volume (peak MTAC) increases with increasing body surface area. The therapy prescription for larger patients can be optimized by using larger instilled volumes.

that for larger patients, one should choose larger exchange volumes in order to maximize surface area A, and hence K_oA, resulting in improved solute transport and an improved therapeutic efficiency. This approach to improving therapeutic efficiency has not been widely exploited and even large patients continue to be treated with an exchange volume of only 2 liters. The importance of using larger exchange volumes in larger patients can be appreciated better when one realizes that indices like KT/V and weekly creatinine clearance/$1.73 M^2$ are all normalized to patient size so that it is harder to achieve the desired targets in larger patients. This optimization approach is analogous to choosing a larger surface area dialyzer (hence higher K_oA) for larger patients in order to improve the clearance K and hence KT/V. The larger exchange volume provides for a higher K_oA and hence higher K in order to achieve the desired KT/V.

7. Review of clinical studies of peritoneal dialysis adequacy

The clinical studies in the current literature on peritoneal dialysis adequacy may be classified into 3 categories. First there are the large patient population studies, usually multicenter, with statistical analyses of risk factors using models like the Cox proportional hazards model. Unfortunately, most of these studies do not include in their analyses, the dose of prescribed therapy, but instead focus on risk factors such as patient demographics and comorbid conditions. The second category includes longitudinal studies with follow-up durations of the order of 2–5 years involving much smaller numbers of patients. There are currently only a handful of such studies and they all suffer from the lack of a prospective design, most being retrospective analyses. The last category, possibly the most numerous and detailed relative to quantitative indices of adequacy, are single center, cross-sectional studies or short term longitudinal studies that attempt to correlate clinical outcomes with dose of prescribed therapy.

None of these three types of studies can appropriately address the issue of what constitutes adequate dialysis. An ideal study would be a longitudinal, multicenter, prospective cohort study with randomized assignment of patients to two distinct levels of therapy dose with a period of follow-up that is long enough for a significant decline of residual renal function and allows the cumulative effects of underdialysis to become manifest. Recently, a multicenter, longitudinal, prospective cohort study has begun that will have a follow-up period of approximately 3 years [20].

However, this study does not randomize patients to two distinct levels of therapy but will instead rely on statistical techniques to determine the effect of therapy dose on clinical outcomes such as mortality and morbidity, the number of patients enrolled being large enough for statistical validity. With CAPD, there are logistical problems with trying to assign patients randomly to two distinct levels of therapy that have a separation wide enough to provide statistically meaningful conclusions. Residual renal function provides a significant contribution to total therapy dose. As residual function declines, the dialytic prescription has to be increased to provide the same total prescribed dose. At the higher dose level, this could be a very difficult problem especially in patients with large body weights. The volume per exchange, the number of exchanges, and the dextrose concentration are the only variables that can be manipulated, and in order to fulfill the desired prescription in a large patient who becomes anuric, the volume per exchange and the number of exchanges may increase to a point where patient compliance and patient drop out from the study can endanger the continuation of the study. On the other hand, in a small patient with significant residual function, it may be difficult to achieve the lower therapy dose without significantly curtailing the number of daily exchanges. In this case, the therapy dose relative to urea or creatinine may be met, but fluid removal, electrolyte balance, and acid-base balance may be adversely affected. In addition to logistical issues and issues related to patient life style and compliance there are ethical issues concerning the level of the lower prescribed dose for providing a distinct separation between the two doses of therapy. In the National Cooperative Dialysis Study of hemodialysis, Group IV, the short time, high BUN (low KT/V) group had to be discontinued mid-study for ethical reasons. When the study was designed, practitioners of dialysis knew less about the lower limits of therapy dose. Group IV patients experienced significant morbidity and medical withdrawals resulting in a premature discontinuation of this study group. Further, patients in this group continued to suffer the cumulative ill effects of inadequate dialysis even twelve months later, manifested as a high mortality rate post study. With current knowledge of the lower limits of therapy, ethical concerns will prevent the lower weekly KT/V level in a randomized, prospective study from being any lower than 1.4–1.6. The higher weekly KT/V dose will therefore have to be of the order of 1.9–2.1 for a distinct separation. It may be well nigh impossible to achieve a KT/V of 2.1 in a large patient with little or no residual renal function. With CAPD, one has far fewer choices in manipulating therapy dose than one has with hemodialysis.

7.1. Multicenter studies, studies involving large patient populations and risk factor analyses

Gokal et al. [43] in England reported in 1987, the results of a prospective 7 center study of 610 new CAPD patients and 329 new hemodialysis patients who started dialysis between 1983 and 1985. The Kaplan-Meier patient survival estimates at 2 years were 74% for hemodialysis and 62% for CAPD. Technique survival was 91% for hemodialysis and 61% for CAPD. The Cox proportional hazards regression analysis identified cerebrovascular/cardiovascular disease, age over 60 years, and diabetes mellitus as important predictors of survival in CAPD patients. The only significant risk factor in the hemodialysis group was age over 60 years. There were no predictive risk factors for permanent change from CAPD to hemodialysis. About 51% of the transfers from CAPD to hemodialysis were due to peritonitis and tunnel infections. Inadequate dialysis listed as loss of ultrafiltration, loss of peritoneal cavity, and loss of biochemical control accounted for 16% of the transfers from CAPD to hemodialysis. The average number of hospital days per patient year was 14.8 for CAPD and 12.4 for hemodialysis with more days for peritonitis and catheter problems (5.7 days per patient year) in the CAPD group than for vascular access problems (3.1 days per patient year) in the hemodialysis group. Therapy prescription was not quantitated or used as a predictive risk factor in the analysis of survival.

Burton and Walls [51] also published in 1987 a study of risk factors in a group of 389 patients accepted for renal replacement therapy in Leicester between July 1974 and July 1985, analyzed retrospectively with respect to a wide range of pretreatment variables (6 scaled variables and 115 binary variables) using the Cox proportional hazards model to adjust for selection bias. There were 106 CAPD patients, 150 patients on hemodialysis, and 133 transplant patients in the study. The total number of deaths in the study were 22 on CAPD, 60 on hemodialysis, and 14 in the transplant group. Nine independent variables were identified as having a significant influence on survival. Of these, the five adverse factors were older age, amyloidosis, ischemic heart disease, convulsions, and acute presentation. The four beneficial factors were male sex, parenthood, pyelonephritis, and residence near the hospital. For the study population as a whole, the 5 year survival was 70% and the 10 year survival was 50%. A bias-adjusted analysis of the relative risk of death provided values of 1.00 for CAPD, 1.30 for hemodialysis, and 1.09 for transplantation. The authors concluded that after correction for selection bias, all three principal forms of renal replacement therapy seemed equally effective at preserving life. They also sharply refuted the suggestions that CAPD was inferior in its ability to preserve life. It is interesting to note that neither diabetes nor left ventricular failure showed up as adverse factors in their analysis. As with the Gokal study, no attempt was made in this study to quantitate the dose of therapy and use therapy dose as a prognosticating risk factor.

In 1986, Nissenson et al. [52] reported on 775 CAPD patients in 42 centers in the Southwestern US between 1979 and 1983. Most of these patients (82%) were not new to dialysis but transfers from another modality. Patient survival was predicted by age and diabetes. Technique survival was beneficially influenced by age < 20 years. The majority of the technique failures (56%) were related to infection.

Nolph et al. [53] analyzed the data of the National CAPD Register in 1987 and found that the combination of diabetes and age (> 60 years and < 20 years) was predictive of peritonitis, hospitalizations, and death. These outcomes were more likely in black patients and those with prior exposure to dialysis therapy.

Maiorca et al. [54] reported in 1991 the results of a multicenter (6 center) Italian study involving 450 CAPD patients and a comparison group of 378 hemodialysis patients. They found, using the Cox proportional hazards model, that the primary risk factors influencing survival were age, cardiovascular disease, diabetes, malignancy, and multisystem disease. After adjusting for significant risk factors, there were no differences in survival between CAPD and hemodialysis. Also, when peritonitis was eliminated as a cause for technique failure, technique failure was similar in CAPD and hemodialysis.

Pollock et al. [55] in Australia reviewed the records of 134 patients on CAPD at the Royal North Shore Hospital in New South Wales between 1980 and 1988. Of the 134 patients on CAPD, 39 had been transferred from hemodialysis and 21 had failed renal transplantation. Using univariate analysis, older age and diabetes were adverse risk factors for patient survival. There were no risk factors associated with technique failure. The serum albumin was lower in those who died compared to those remaining alive as well as in those frequently hospitalized compared to those with infrequent hospitalizations.

As stated earlier, in none of these large patient populations studies of patient survival, morbidity and technique failure is there quantification of dialysis dose and inclusion of dialysis dose as a predictor of clinical outcome.

7.2. Longitudinal studies relating clinical outcome to dialysis prescription

The longest longitudinal study relating clinical outcome to dialysis dose is that of Lameire et al. [11] who retrospectively analyzed data in 16 CAPD patients selected because they had been on uninterrupted CAPD at a constant dialytic dose for at least 5 years. During the same time period a total of 126 patients had started CAPD at the University Hospital of Gent. In the study cohort, the mean age at initiation of CAPD therapy was 56 years. All but one patient had a CAPD prescription of 2 L × 4 exchanges per day. The one exception used 3 L × 4 exchanges per day. Patients were seen as outpatients every 2–3 months and brought in with them a 24 hour collection of spent dialysate and urine. In the retrospective analysis, correlations were sought between the KT/V urea index and a number of clinical and biochemical parameters. The clinical outcomes include hospital days per year, peritonitis rate, and nerve conductive velocities in the lateral peroneal nerve. In 12 of the 16 patients, the protein catabolic rate (PCR) was calculated between 24 and 48 months of treatment. The weekly total KT/V index (dialytic and residual renal) declined over time from an initial value of 2.78 ± 0.18 to 1.65 ± 0.15 at 5 years. This decline was related to two significant changes – a gradual decline in residual renal function and an increase in body weight over time. The residual renal contribution to KT/V declined from 27% initially to 8% at 4 years and 0% at 5 years. The dry body weight increased from 58 ± 2.8 kg at the start of therapy to 71 ± 3.3 kg at 5 years, most of the increase being in the first 18–24 months of being on CAPD. The PCR at 24 months was 0.98 ± 0.05 gm/kg/day, decreasing slightly to 0.87 ± 0.05 gm/kg/day at 48 months. There was a significant positive correlation ($r = 0.56$, $p < 0.001$) between PCR and KT/V. No significant correlations were found between KT/V and a number of hematological and biochemical parameters such as hemoglobin, hematocrit, plasma albumin, or PTH. However, there was a significant positive correlation ($r = 0.29$, $p < 0.05$) between individual KT/V indices and individual nerve conductive velocities over 5 years. In an arbitrary grouping of 5 patients with a weekly KT/V < 2.4 and 9 patients with a weekly KT/V > 2.4, it was seen that the low KT/V group has a significant fall in nerve conduction velocities over the 5 years whereas the high KT/V group maintained stable nerve conduction velocities. These differences were highly significant over the time period of 36–60 months. A significant negative correlation was noted between KT/V and the hospital days per year ($r = -0.46$, $p < 0.001$). The incidence of peritonitis was once every 53 months in patients with a weekly KT/V > 2.4 compared to once every 14 patient months in the patients with weekly KT/V < 2.4. It should be noted that KT/V values quoted above were based on a value of V assumed to be 60% of ideal body weight in males and 55% of ideal weight in females. Ideal body weight was defined as weight in the absence of signs or symptoms of either volume depletion or hypervolemia. The high values of KT/V noted in this study are probably a consequence of low body weights as well as significant initial residual renal function.

Teehan et al. [17] presented in 1990 the results of a retrospective study of 56 patients followed over a 5 year period with quarterly assessments of parameters such as KT/V and nPCR (normalized PCR). Clinical outcomes included survival, hospital days per year, and transfusion requirements. The predictors of clinical outcomes considered were age, serum albumin, KT/V, duration on CAPD, and comorbid factors such as diabetes, coronary artery disease and hypertension. Both univariate and multivariate analyses were used. A death discriminant analysis which accurately classified 80% of the deaths indicated that the predictors of death were a low serum albumin, older age, longer duration on CAPD and low KT/V. A low serum albumin was the most significant predictor of death and the factors influencing a low serum albumin were low KT/V, low BUN, and a short duration on CAPD. Hospitalizations were correlated with a low serum albumin and a longer duration on CAPD. Transfusion requirements were correlated with a low KT/V, low hematocrit, and a low nPCR. In summary, the study of Teehan indicates that CAPD outcome is related to patient variables such as age and duration on CAPD, nutritional state (serum albumin and nPCR) and therapy prescription (KT/V).

Teehan et al. have extended their retrospective analysis to include 91 patients followed over a period of approximately 8 years [10]. They have included Kaplan-Meier survival analysis and the Cox proportional hazards model in their extended study. In this extended study, they still find that survival is predicted by lower age, higher KT/V, and higher serum albumin. Kaplan-Meier survival curves predict a half life of > 48 months with a serum albumin > 3.5 gm/dl, compared to 25 months at a serum albumin < 3.5 gm/dl ($p < 0.006$). Also mortality was more than 2.5 times higher at weekly KT/V $\leq$ 1.7 compared to higher values of KT/V. However, this difference was apparent only after 12–24 months of exposure to these levels of KT/V, unlike the survival curves at low and high serum albumin where a significant difference was apparent fairly early in the follow-up period (~6 months).

The results of Blake et al. [16] contradict those of Lameire and Teehan. Blake et al. studied 76 CAPD patients over a period of 3 years with a mean follow-up of 20 months. They were unable to detect differences in deaths or hospitalizations between one subgroup with a high KT/V and high nPCR compared to another subgroup with a low KT/V and low nPCR. KT/V and nPCR were correlated to each other ($r = 0.6$). Of 13 total deaths, there were 2 deaths in the high KT/V and nPCR group and 2 deaths in the low KT/V and nPCR group. There were 8.8 hospital days per 6 months in the high KT/V and nPCR subgroups compared to 10.7 days per 6 months in the low KT/V and nPCR subgroup. In analyzing hospitalization, all causes of hospitalizations including peritonitis were considered. As peritonitis is often technique related, the inclusion of these hospitalizations clouds the interpretation of the data. Blake noted that nPCR was directly correlated with urea and inversely correlated with creatinine. Also there were inverse correlations between KT/V and serum creatinine, urea, potassium and phosphate, and a direct correlation with serum bicarbonate.

Comparing the Blake and Teehan studies, some important differences emerge. In the Blake study, KT/V was estimated rather than measured, a D/P of 1.0 being assumed for all patients and V being based on a fixed percentage of body weight. The median study duration was only 12 months in the

Blake study compared to 24 months in the Teehan study. As the survival curve of Teehan suggests, a follow-up duration of 2 years or more may be required to detect cumulative effects of low KT/V on survival. In both the Blake and Teehan studies, the number of patients studied is relatively small to draw statistically significant conclusions regarding dose of dialysis and survival. No attempt was made to adjust for age, diabetes, prior history of cardiovascular disease, etc. in the survival analysis and the number of deaths were too small for meaningful analysis. As the large multicenter studies quoted above indicate, age, diabetes, prior exposure to CAPD, cerebrovascular and cardiovascular disease are all significant risk factors and should not be ignored in an analysis of survival. Finally, in the Blake study, the dialytic KT/V was adjusted periodically on clinical grounds and the residual renal KT/V declined significantly over time. No attempt was therefore made to keep the dose of therapy fixed and it is difficult to draw meaningful conclusions with a moving target for dose of therapy.

In a subsequent analysis of this data [56], Blake et al. did find an excess mortality in patients with a weekly KT/V less than 1.5 or a weekly creatinine clearance less than 48 L/week per 1.73 M^2 of body surface area. These lower limits are of the same order of magnitude as the predictions of the peak concentration hypothesis and are consistent with Teehan's studies.

7.3. Cross-sectional and short term studies of dialysis dose and clinical outcomes

One of the first studies to explore the validity of urea kinetic indices for quantitating CAPD adequacy was by Keshaviah et al. in 1990 [12]. This study was a cross-sectional study in 19 stable CAPD patients with a clinical assessment score that included 12 parameters, 8 of which were based on symptoms such as insomnia, weakness and nausea, and scored 1, 2, or 3 (frequent, occasional, no problem, respectively) and 4 objective parameters, namely serum albumin, hematocrit, creatinine, and lean body mass. They showed that the relationships between serum urea nitrogen, KT/V, and PCR were compatible with the predictions of the urea kinetic model (Fig. 10). PCR and dietary protein intake were well correlated and there was also a high degree of positive correlation between PCR and KT/V. In 74% of the patients, the clinical assessment of adequacy was in agreement with the KT/V domains of adequacy established by the peak concentration hypothesis. In a subsequent update

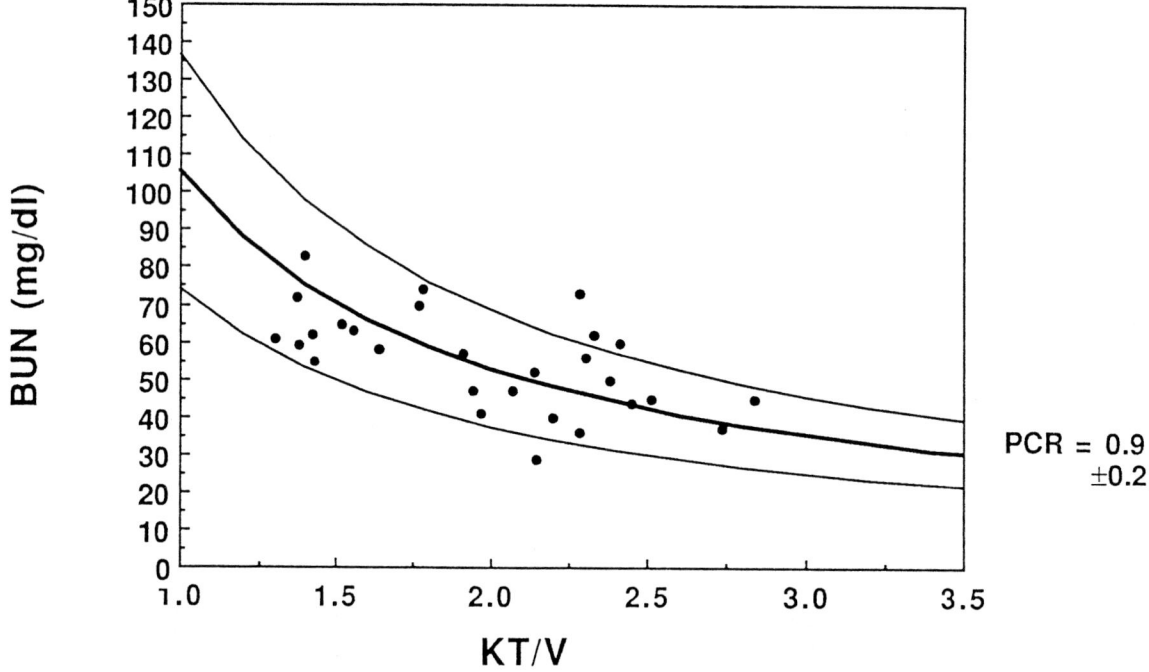

Figure 10. The relationship between BUN, KT/V, and PCR. The plotted points are clinical measurements for a PCR range of 0.9 ± 0.2 and the solid lines are derived from the single pool urea kinetic model for the same range of PCR. (Reprinted by permission of Blackwell Scientific Publications, Inc, Reference [14]).

with 28 CAPD patients, Keshaviah et al. [57] showed a positive correlation between the clinical assessment score and KT/V ($r = 0.33$, $p = 0.06$).

Brandes et al. [15, 28] performed a cross-sectional study of 18 CAPD patients using a weighted clinical outcome score that included symptoms, hospitalizations, transfer to hemodialysis, and deaths. Three quantitative indices of therapy prescription were used, the KT/V urea index, the weekly creatinine clearance, and the creatinine efficacy number that has been defined earlier in this chapter. This number is the ratio of KT creatinine to the adjusted creatinine production. Based on the weighted clinical score, patients were divided into good ($N = 6$), intermediate ($N = 4$), and poor ($N = 8$) outcome subgroups with mean KT/V values of 2.3 ± 0.2, 1.8 ± 0.2, and 1.5 ± 0.1 respectively. There was a significant difference in the KT/V between the good and poor outcome groups but not between good and intermediate and the intermediate and poor outcome groups. The weekly creatinine clearance per 1.73 M^2 was 71 ± 8 L/week in the good group and 44 ± 3 and 35 ± 1 L/week in the intermediate and poor outcome groups. The creatinine efficacy number for the 3 groups was 7.4 ± 0.8, 4.9 ± 0.4, and 3.0 ± 0.2 respectively. With both weekly creatinine clearance and the creatinine efficacy number, there were statistically significant differences between good and intermediate as well as between the good and poor outcome groups. Brandes concluded that KT/V and the creatinine indices were all able to predict clinical outcome but that the two creatinine indices were more sensitive indicators than KT/V.

Recently, Gotch [58, 59] has developed a domain map for CAPD correlating BUN, nPCR, and KT/V analogous to the hemodialysis domain map [39]. In a multicenter study sample of 132 CAPD patients from 15 facilities, Gotch et al. [60] measured a mean weekly KT/V of 1.96 with a range from 0.7 to 3.5. The residual renal contribution to KT/V was of the order of 25%. Mean nPCR was 0.8 gm/kg/day and significantly correlated to KT/V ($r = 0.61$, $p < 0.001$). In 80% of the patients, the standard therapy regimen of 2 L × 4 exchanges/day was prescribed without regard to patient size or residual renal function. Assuming a match between the steady state CAPD BUN and the pre-dialysis BUN for hemodialysis (peak concentration hypothesis), they derived the equivalent hemodialysis KT/V in this patient group using an empirical relationship. They found that 65% of the patients had a hemodialysis equivalent KT/V of < 1.0, the mean being 1.07. Some patients had a hemodialysis equivalent KT/V as low as 0.5. Using the HCFA clinical consensus criterion of a weekly CAPD KT/V = 1.5, however, more than 90% of the patients were judged to be adequately dialyzed. Based on this finding, Gotch et al. have suggested the need for a prospective, randomized study comparing clinical outcomes at two distinct weekly KT/V levels of 1.4 and 2.1 in order to better define adequate CAPD therapy.

7.4. $(KT/V)_{urea}$ and weekly creatinine clearance

According to the peak concentration hypothesis, weekly KT/V values of the order of 1.2 connote significant underdialysis and minimum acceptable levels are on the order of 1.7. For optimal outcomes, KT/V values of 2.0 or higher may be required. The clinical studies of Keshaviah, Brandes, Teehan, Blake, and Lameire lend credence to these predictions. A minimum weekly creatinine clearance of 40–50 liters/1.73 M^2 has been recommended based on clinical observations and experience [25]. According to the data of Blake, weekly creatinine clearances < 48 liters/1.73 M^2 are associated with a higher morbidity. Brandes found an intermediate clinical outcome at a creatinine clearance of 44 liter/week and a poor outcome at 35 liter/week. Keshaviah et al. [14] correlated KT/V to weekly creatinine clearances in 50 CAPD patients with 71 observations (Fig. 11). Dialytic and residual renal contributions were included for both indices, the residual renal clearance used in the creatinine clearance being the average of the residual urea and creatinine clearances to better estimate GFR. There is a higher degree of correlation between the indices ($r = 0.71$), and there is internal consistency in ranges of KT/V and weekly creatinine clearance. A weekly creatinine clearance of 40–50 liters/week corresponds to a KT/V range of 1.3 to 1.7, a range that is consistent with clinical outcomes and the predictions of the peak concentration hypothesis.

7.5. Residual renal function, KT/V and PCR

As seen in the study of Lameire [11], residual renal function provides a significant contribution to the total dose of therapy when CAPD is first initiated but declines significantly thereafter. The residual renal contribution was 28% at initiation, declining to 8% at 4 years, and 0% at 5 years. Blake et al.

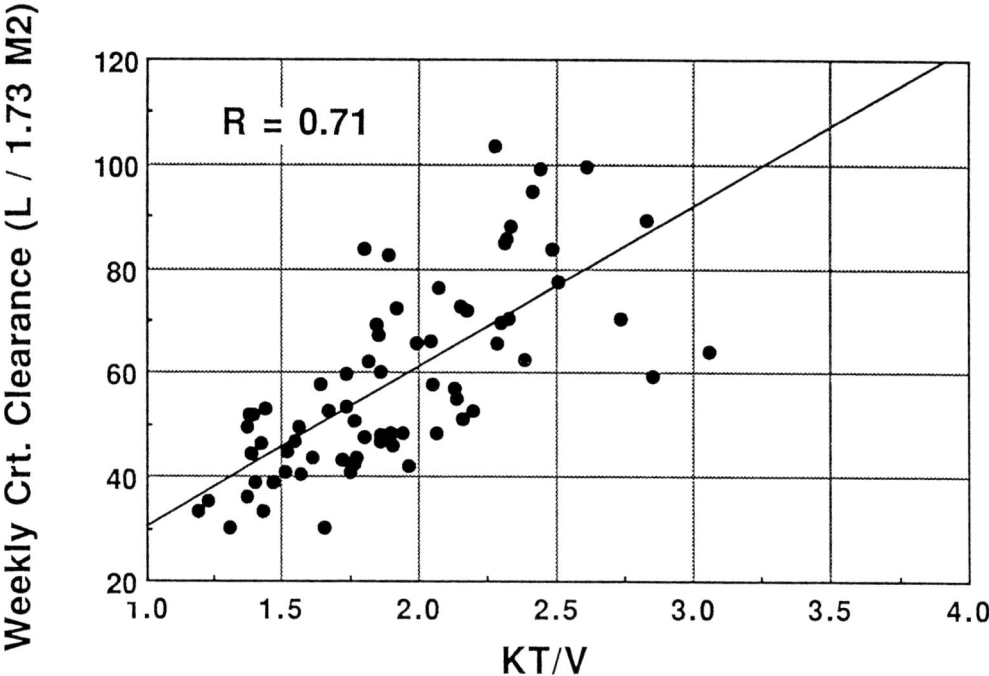

Figure 11. Weekly creatinine clearance and $(KT/V)_{urea}$ are highly correlated and the empirically derived minimum acceptable weekly creatinine clearance is consistent with the KT/V adequacy domain predicted by the peak concentration hypothesis. (Reprinted by permission of Blackwell Scientific Publications, Inc, Reference [14]).

[16] also noted a significant decline in total KT/V related to a decline in residual renal function.

With significant reductions in the incidence of peritonitis consequent to the use of disconnect schemes, it is anticipated that therapy survival will improve substantially with patients staying on CAPD for longer durations of time than in the past. Many CAPD patients will therefore be faced with the declining contribution of residual renal function and a need to increase dialytic prescription to compensate for the loss of the residual renal contribution. This may require increased instilled volumes per exchange as well as increased number of exchanges. Unless this is done, significant underdialysis may ensue.

We have made 21 sequential sets of measurements in 16 stable CAPD patients to study the influence of declining residual renal function on therapy adequacy [61, 14]. No adjustments were made to dialytic prescription as long as the weekly total KT/V was above 1.7. As shown in Fig. 12, there was a high degree of correlation between the change in residual renal function and delta KT/V. Also there was a strong correlation (Fig. 13) between delta KT/V and delta PCR suggesting that dietary intake was reduced with a reduced KT/V consequential to a decline of residual renal function.

This finding is consistent with the hypothesis of Lindsay *et al.* [62, 63] linking nutrition with dialysis adequacy. Retention of small molecular weight toxins may therefore be associated with decreased dietary intake and consequent malnutrition. As it is well recognized that malnutrition is associated with significant morbidity, these data emphasize the need to monitor residual renal function periodically and to adjust the total dose of therapy to compensate for the declining renal contribution.

8. Concluding remarks

The longitudinal and cross-sectional studies available in the literature suggest that attention must be paid to small solute clearances in order to avoid morbidity and mortality associated with inadequate dialysis. Weekly creatinine clearances of the order of 50 liters/week and weekly KT/V of around 1.7 are current recommendations for a minimum acceptable therapy prescription. For a more optimum prescription, higher values for these indices may be required.

Middle molecule and large molecule clearances are not sensitive to changes in the number of daily exchanges, and the weekly clearances of the middle and large molecular weight solutes are higher than

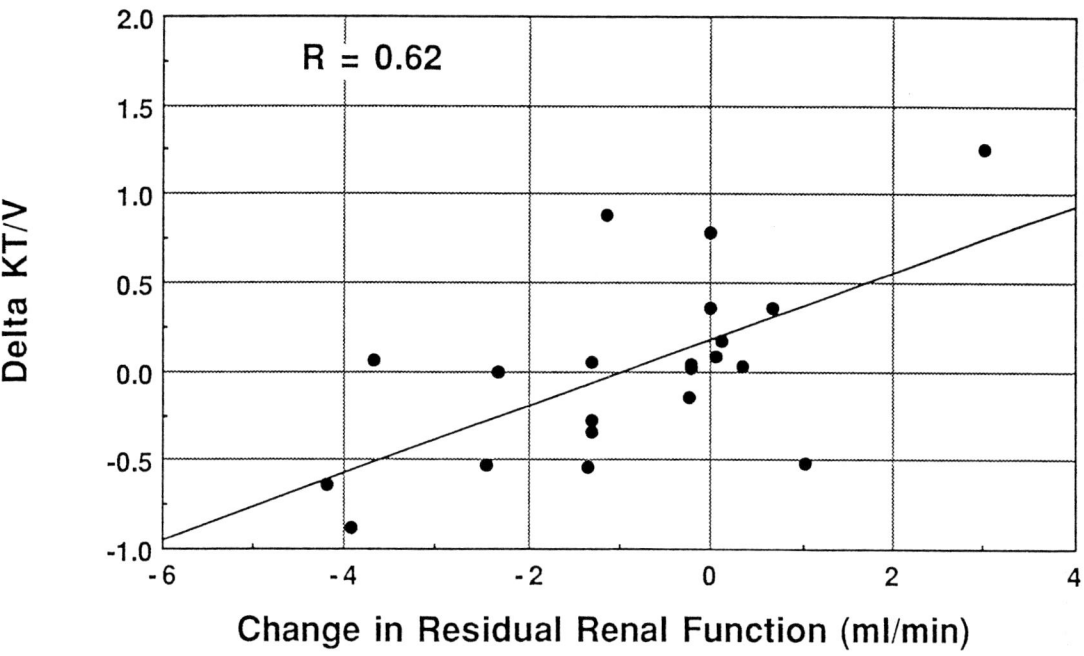

Figure 12. Decreasing residual renal function results in a significant decrease in KT/V. Data from 21 sequential measurements in 16 CAPD patients. (Reprinted by permission of Blackwell Scientific Publications, Inc, Reference [14]).

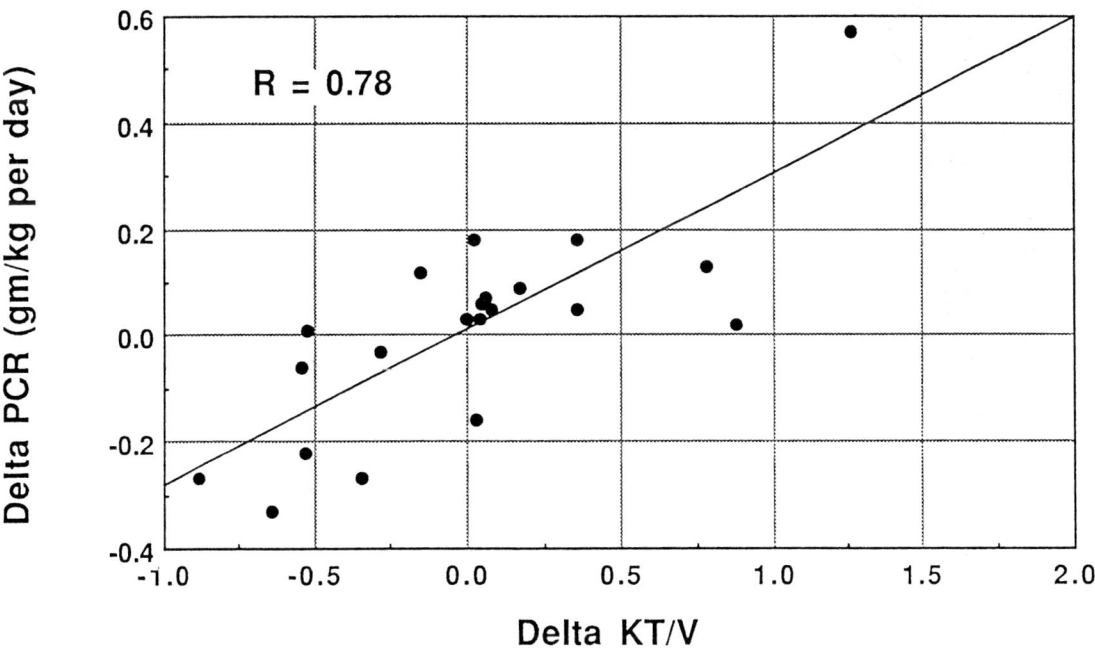

Figure 13. The change in KT/V consequent to declining residual renal function is highly correlated to the change in PCR. (Reprinted by permission of Blackwell Scientific Publications, Inc, Reference [14]).

those of standard hemodialysis but less than those currently achievable with high flux hemodialysis.

The importance of residual renal function cannot be emphasized enough. This significant contribution to total therapy dose must be monitored regularly, and the dialytic prescription adjusted to achieve the total desired dose of therapy.

There are associative relationships between KT/V and PCR and the data suggest that malnutrition may ensue if an adequate dose of dialysis is not prescribed. The significance of serum albumin as a risk factor in both hemodialysis and CAPD settings underscore the need to pay attention to nutrition, PCR being a convenient parameter to track changes in nutritional state.

The need for prospective, longitudinal studies with large numbers of patients and a long follow-up period to detect the cumulative effects of dialytic therapy prescription and the influence of declining renal function is still unmet. In the next few years, more longitudinal studies relating therapy prescription to clinical outcomes are expected and our understanding of adequacy of peritoneal dialysis will hopefully increase.

References

1. Continuous Ambulatory Peritoneal Dialysis, Gokal R (ed), Churchill-Livingston, New York 1986.
2. Peritoneal Dialysis, Nolph KD (ed), Kluwer Academic Publishers, Dordrecht, Boston, London, third Edition 1988.
3. Maiorca R, Cancarini GC, Camerini C. Is CAPD competitive with hemodialysis for long-term treatment of uremic patients? Neph Dial Transplant 1989: 244–53.
4. Canadian CAPD Clinical Trials Group. Peritonitis in CAPD: a multicenter randomized clinical trial comparing the Y-connector disinfectant system to standard systems. Perit Dial Int 1989; 9: 159–63.
5. Nolph KD. Clinical results with peritoneal dialysis and hemodialysis-registry experiences. In: Twardowski ZJ, Nolph KD, Khanna R, Stein J (eds), Contemporary Issues in Nephrology: Peritoneal Dialysis. Churchill-Livingston, New York 1990: 127–44.
6. Disney APS. Twelfth Report of the Australia and New Zealand Combined Dialysis and Transplant Registry. Woodville, Queen Elizabeth Hospital, South Australia 1989.
7. Rottembourg J, Issad B, Gallego JL. Evolution of residual renal function in patients undergoing maintenance hemodialysis or continuous ambulatory peritoneal dialysis. Proc Eur Dial Transplant Assoc 1982; 19: 397–401.
8. Lysaght M, Vonesh E, Ibels L. Decline of residual renal function in hemodialysis and CAPD patients: a risk adjusted growth function analysis. Neph Dial Transplant 1989: p 499.
9. Teehan B, Schleifer C, Brown J. Urea kinetic modeling is an appropriate assessment of adequacy. Sem Dial 1992; 5(3): 189–92.
10. Teehan B, Schleifer B, Brown J, McDonald B. Factors predicting clinical outcome in CAPD patients. (Abstract) Am Soc Artif Int Organs 1993; 22: 112.
11. Lameire NH, Vanholder R, Veyt D. A longitudinal, five year survey of urea kinetic parameters in CAPD patients. Kidney Int 1992; 42: 426–32.
12. Keshaviah P, Nolph KD, Prowant B. Defining adequacy of CAPD with urea kinetics. Adv Perit Dial 1990; 6: 173–7.
13. Keshaviah P. Quantitative approaches to prescribing peritoneal dialysis. In: Peritoneal Dialysis: Proceedings Fourth International Course on Peritoneal Dialysis. Wichtig Editore, Milano 1991; pp 83–60.
14. Keshaviah P. Adequacy of CAPD: a quantitative approach. Kidney Int 1992; 42 (Suppl 38): S160–4.
15. Brandes JC, Piering WF, Beres JA. Clinical outcome of continuous ambulatory peritoneal dialysis by urea and creatinine kinetics. J Am Soc Nephrol 1992; 2: 1430–5.
16. Blake P, Sombolos K, Abraham G. Lack of correlation between urea kinetic indices and clinical outcomes in CAPD patients. Kidney Int 1991; 39: 700–6.
17. Teehan B, Schleifer C, Brown J. Urea kinetic analysis and clinical outcome on CAPD. A five-year longitudinal study. Adv Perit Dial 1990; 6: 181–5.
18. Keshaviah P. Urea kinetic and middle molecule approaches to assessing the adequacy of hemodialysis and CAPD. Kidney Int 1993: 43 (suppl 40): S28–38.
19. Cox DR. Regression models and life tables. JR Statis Soc 1972; B34: 197–220.
20. Churchill DN, Taylor W, Members of the CANUSA Peritoneal Study Group. Canada–USA (CANUSA) multicenter study of peritoneal dialysis adequacy; description of the study population and preliminary results. In: Khanna R, Nolph K, Prowant B, Twardowski Z, Oreopoulos D (eds), Advances in Peritoneal Dialysis 1992. Peritoneal Publications Inc 1992; 8: 88–92.
21. Twardowski ZJ. Clinical value of standardized equilibrium tests in CAPD patients. Blood Purif 1989; 7: 95–108.
22. Rottembourg J, Issad B, Poignet JL. Residual renal function and control of blood glucose levels in insulin dependent diabetic patients treated by CAPD. In: Keen H, Legrain M (eds), Prevention and Treatment of Diabetic Nephropathy. Boston: Lancaster MPT Press 1983; pp 339–59.
23. Cancarini GC, Brunori G, Camerini C, Brasa S, Manili L, Maiorca R. Renal function recovery and maintenance of residual diuresis in CAPD and hemodialysis. Perit Dial Bull 1986; 6: 77–9.
24. Milutinovic J, Cutler RE, Hoover P, Meijsen B, Scribner BH. Measurement of residual glomerular

filtration rate in the patient receiving repetitive hemodialysis. Kidney Int 1975; 8: 185–90.
25. Twardowski Z, Nolph K. Peritoneal dialysis: how much is enough? Sem Dial 1988; 1(2): 75–6.
26. Hume R, Weyers E. Relationship between total body water and surface area in normal and obese subjects. Clin Path 1971; 24: 234–8.
27. Teehan B, Schleifer C, Sigler M, Gilgore G. A quantitative approach to the CAPD prescription. Perit Dial Bull 1985; 5: 152–6.
28. Brandes J, Piering W, Beres J. A method to assess efficacy of CAPD: preliminary results. Adv Perit Dial 1990; 6: 192–6.
29. Mitch WE, Walser M. A proposed mechanisms for reduced creatinine excretion in severe chronic renal failure. Nephron 1978; 21: 248–54.
30. Babb A, Popovich R, Christopher T, Scribner B. The genesis of the square meter-hour hypothesis. Trans Am Soc Artif Int Organs 1971; 17: 81–91.
31. Scribner BH, Babb AL. Evidence for toxins of "middle" molecular weight. Kidney Int 1975; 7(Suppl 2): S349–51.
32. Scribner BH, Baccay PD, Holar EM. The current status of research on middle molecules. Workshop on dialysis and transplantation. Am Soc Artif Int Organs 1972; 1: 76–9.
33. Boen ST. Kinetics of peritoneal dialysis. Medicine 1981; 40: 243–87.
34. Boen S. Long-term peritoneal dialysis and a peritoneal dialysis index. Dial & Transplant 1978; 7: 377–8.
35. Babb AL, Johansen PJ, Strand MJ, Tenckhoff H, Scribner BH. Bidirectional permeability of the human peritoneum to middle molecule. Proc Eur Dial Transplant Assoc 1973; 10: 247–57.
36. Struijk D, Krediet R, Koomen G, Boeschoten E, Reijden H, Arisz L. Indirect measures of lymphatic absorption with inulin in continuous ambulatory peritoneal dialysis (CAPD) patients. Perit Dial Int 1990; 10: 141–5.
37. Hallett M, Lysaght M, Farrell P. The role of lymphatic drainage in peritoneal mass transfer. Artif Organs 1989; 13(1): 28–34.
38. Mistry C, O'Donoghue D, Nelson S, Gokal R, Ballardie F. Kinetic and clinical studies of Beta-2 microglobulin in continuous ambulatory peritoneal dialysis: influence of renal and enhanced peritoneal clearances using glucose polymer. Neph Dial Transplant 1990; 5(7): 513–9.
39. Gotch F, Sargent J. A mechanistic analysis of the National Cooperative Dialysis Study (NCDS). Kidney Int 1985; 28: 526–34.
40. Lowrie E, Laird N, Parker T. Sargent J. Effect of the hemodialysis prescription on patient morbidity. N Eng J Med 1981; 305(20): 1176–81.
41. Maiorca R, Vonesh E, Cancarini GC. A six-year comparison of patient and technique survivals in CAPD and HD. Kidney Int 1988; 34: 518–24.
42. Wolfe RA, Port FK, Hawthorn VM. A comparison of survival among dialytic therapies of choice: in-center hemodialysis versus continuous ambulatory dialysis at home. Am J Kidney Dis 1990; 15: 433–40.
43. Gokal R, King J, Bogel S. Outcome of patients on continuous ambulatory peritoneal dialysis and hemodialysis: four year analysis of a prospective multicenter study. Lancet 1987: 1105–8.
44. Maiorca R, Cancarini GC, Brunori G, Camerini C, Manili L. Morbidity and mortality of CAPD and hemodialysis. Kidney Int 1993; 43 (suppl 40): S4–15.
45. Holden A, Gaumer G. Best demonstrated practices program promoting CAPD patient retention in the United States. Advances in CAPD, Proc 7th Annual CAPD Conf, Kansas City, MO 1987; 3: 186–91.
46. Keshaviah P, Nolph K. The peak concentration hypothesis: a urea kinetic approach to comparing the adequacy of continuous ambulatory peritoneal dialysis (CAPD) and hemodialysis. Perit Dial Int 1989; 9: 257–60.
47. Nolph KD, Keshaviah P, Popovich R. Problem in comparison of clearances prescription in hemodialysis and continuous ambulatory peritoneal dialysis. Perit Dial Int 1991; 11: 298–300.
48. Twardowski ZJ. Peritoneal Dialysis Glossary III. Perit Dial Int 1990; 10: 173–5.
49. Westman J. Personal communication, Unpublished Baxter Survey, 1992.
50. Brandes J, Emerson P, Campbell D, Keshaviah P. The relationship between body size, fill volume and mass transfer coefficient (MTAC) in PD. (Abstract) J Am Soc Neph September 1992; 3(3): 407.
51. Burton PR, Walls J. Selection-adjusted comparison of life expectancy of patients on continuous ambulatory peritoneal dialysis, hemodialysis, and renal transplantation. Lancet 1987; 1: 1115–9.
52. Nissenson AR, Gentile DE, Soderblom RE, Oliver DF, Brax C. Morbidity and mortality of continuous ambulatory peritoneal dialysis. Regional experience and long-term prospects. Am J Kidney Dis 1986; 7: 229–34.
53. Nolph KD, Cutler SJ, Steinberg SM, Novak JW, Hirschman GH. Factors associated with morbidity and mortality among patients on CAPD. Trans Am Soc Artif Int Organs 1987; 33: 57–65.
54. Maiorca R, Vonesh EF, Cavalli PL, DeVecchi A, Giangrande A, La Greca G, Scarpioni LL, Bragantini L, Cancarini GC, Cantaluppi A, Castinovo C, Castiglioni A, Poisetti PG, Viglino G. A multicenter, selection adjusted comparison of patient and technique survivals on CAPD and hemodialysis. Perit Dial Int 1991; 11: 118–27.
55. Pollock CA, Ibels LS, Caterson RJ, Mahony JF, Waugh DA, Cocksedge B. Continuous ambulatory peritoneal dialysis; eight years experience at a single center. Medicine (Baltimore) 1989; 68: 293–308.
56. Blake P, Balaskas E, Blake R, Oreopoulos D. Urea kinetics has limited relevance in assessing adequacy of dialysis in CAPD. Adv Perit Dial 1992; 8: 65–70.
57. Keshaviah P. Quantitative approach to prescribing peritoneal dialysis. In: La Greca G, Ronco C, Feriani M, Chiaramonte S, Conz P (eds), Peritoneal Dialysis: Proceedings of the Fourth International Course on Peritoneal Dialysis, Vicenza, Italy. Wichtig Editore, Milano 1991: 53–60.
58. Gotch FA. Application of urea kinetic modeling to

adequacy of CAPD therapy. Adv Perit Dial 1990; 6: 178–80.
59. Gotch FA. The application of urea kinetic modeling in CAPD. In: La Greca G, Ronco C, Feriani M, Chiaramonte S, Conz P (eds), Peritoneal Dialysis: Proceedings of the Fourth International Course on Peritoneal Dialysis, Vicenza, Italy. Wichtig Editore, Milano 1991: 47–51.
60. Gotch FA, Gentile DE, Schoenfeld PV. CAPD in current clinical practice. Adv Perit Dial 1993; 9: (in press).
61. Keshaviah P, Nolph K, Moore H, Prowant B. The influence of declining residual renal function on therapy adequacy: a longitudinal study. (Abstract) Am Soc Artif Int Organs 1992 Abstracts 1992; p 110.
62. Lindsay R, Spanner E. A hypothesis: the protein catabolic rate is dependent upon the type and amount of dialyzed uremic patients. Am J Kidney Dis 1989; 8(5): 382–9.
63. Lindsay RM, Spanner E, Heidenheim RP, LeFebree JM, Hodsman A, Baird J, Allison MEM. Which comes first, KT/V or PCR – chicken or egg? Kidney Int October 1992; 42 (suppl 38).

15 Nutritional requirements of peritoneal dialysis patients

BENGT LINDHOLM AND JONAS BERGSTRÖM

1. Introduction 443
   1.1. Intermittent peritoneal dialysis 444
   1.2. Continuous ambulatory peritoneal dialysis (CAPD) 444
2. Protein-energy malnutrition in peritoneal dialysis patients 445
   2.1. Causes of protein energy malnutrition in uremia 445
   2.2. Signs of protein-energy malnutrition 445
   2.3. Prevalence of protein-energy malnutrition 446
3. Protein intake, malnutrition and clinical outcome 447
4. Protein and energy requirements in peritoneal dialysis patients 448
5. Protein catabolic factors in peritoneal dialysis patients 449
   5.1. Low energy intake 449
   5.2. Metabolic acidosis 450
   5.3. Loss of metabolizing renal tissue 451
   5.4. Recurrent peritonitis and other infections 451
   5.5. Dialysis procedure as stimuli of net protein catabolism in HD vs CAPD 451
   5.6. Loss of glucose in HD vs glucose absorption in CAPD 452
   5.7. Loss of amino acids 452
   5.8. Protein losses in CAPD 452
   5.9. Biocompatibility and protein catabolism in HD vs CAPD 452
6. Dialysis dose, anorexia and nutritional intake 453
   6.1. Prevention and treatment of malnutrition in CAPD 455
7. Amino acid-based dialysis fluids 456
8. Glucose and insulin metabolism 457
   8.1. Glucose absorption and glucose intolerance in CAPD 457
9. Disturbances in lipid metabolism 458
   9.1. Hyperlipidemic effect of CAPD 459
   9.2. Hypertriglyceridemia in CAPD 459
   9.3. Hypercholesterolemia in CAPD 460
   9.4. Transitory changes of serum lipoprotein levels during CAPD 460
   9.5. Increased plasma lipoprotein (a) in CAPD 460
10. Carnitine depletion 460
11. Mineral metabolism and nutrition 461
    11.1. Calcium and phosporous 461
    11.2. Potassium and magnesium 461
12. Anemia and erythropoietin 461
13. Vitamins and trace elements 462
    13.1. Water-soluble vitamins 462
    13.2. Fat-soluble vitamins 462
    13.3. Trace elements 463
14. Recommended nutritional intakes and treatment of malnutrition 463
    14.1. Protein and energy intakes 463
    14.2. Minerals, vitamins and trace elements 464
15. Summary 465
Acknowledgements 466
References 466

1. Introduction

Patients with chronic renal failure display a variety of metabolic and nutritional abnormalities and a large proportion of the patients demonstrate signs of protein-energy malnutrition. This may be a consequence of multiple factors including disturbances in protein and energy metabolism, hormonal derangements, infections and other superimposed illnesses, and poor food intake because of anorexia, nausea and vomiting, caused by uremic toxicity. With maintenance dialysis therapy some of these factors, but far from all, can be partly or fully corrected. On the other hand, metabolic and nutritional problems may be caused by the method of dialysis [1-3].

When evaluating the nutritional effects of dialysis therapies it should be kept in mind that the patient starting dialysis is often suffering from malnutrition and wasting. During the period prior to the institution of dialysis therapy the patients are often treated with low protein diets and a variety of drugs that may worsen anorexia. In addition, underlying disease, such as diabetes mellitus, rheumatoid arthritis and vasculitis, and medical complications such as infections, pericarditis, congestive heart failure, and complications of therapy, in particular corticosteroid therapy, may result in the patient initiating dialysis being in an already severely debilitated state.

Once dialysis therapy begins, accompanied by reduction of uremic symptoms and liberalisation of the diet, some patients may show improved nutritional status. However, many of the indicators of malnutrition that are present at the onset of therapy remain abnormal and some aspects of malnutrition may become even more severe. One example of this is that renal replacement therapy such as hemodialysis and peritoneal dialysis may induce catabolism and increase protein requirements above the baseline of non-dialyzed uremic patients.

1.1. Intermittent peritoneal dialysis

The long-term experiences mainly in the 1960s' and 1970s' with maintenance intermittent peritoneal dialysis for the definitive management of patients with end-stage renal failure generally were not favourable in terms of nutritional aspects (Table 1). Although capable of transiently improving uremic symptoms, intermittent peritoneal dialysis is frequently associated with progressive tissue wasting and malnutrition. Dialysate protein, amino acid and trace mineral losses are substantial and the combination of insufficient dialysis and inadequate nutrient intake are major factors contributing to the frequently observed development of malnutrition and wasting.

1.2. Continuous ambulatory peritoneal dialysis (CAPD)

Following the preliminary experiences with CAPD in the late 1970s', several favourable effects were reported (Table 2). The patients starting on CAPD appeared to thrive, their body weight and hematocrit increased and the control of serum biochemistries, acid base equilibrium, and fluid balance was reported to be comparable to, or better, than in patients undergoing other forms of dialysis therapy. These effects, which suggested an anabolic state, were attributed to the continuous dialytic process and to an effective removal of uremic middle molecules.

Table 1. Nutritional problems with intermittent peritoneal dialysis.

1. Anorexia due to insufficient dialysis, especially of small solutes.
2. Substantial dialysate protein and amino acid losses.
3. Physical inactivation (bedridden during long dialysis sessions).
4. High incidence of peritonitis.
5. Hyperglycemia.

However, CAPD can potentially involve several catabolic factors, such as loss of appetite, insufficient removal of small solutes, dialysate loss of proteins (5 to 15 g/24 hr) and amino acids (2 to 4 g/24 hr), and recurrent peritonitis [1]. In addition, the continuous supply of glucose (100 to 200 g/24 hr) and lactate from the dialysate represents a sizable and perhaps undesirable energy load that may induce or accentuate hyperglycemia, hyperinsulinemia, hypertriglyceridemia, and other metabolic abnormalities (Table 3). These factors, superimposed on the already deranged metabolism and nutritional state of patients with chronic renal failure, may have serious consequences in the form of aggravated malnutrition, susceptibility to infection, anemia, cardiovascular dysfunction, progressive neuropathy, hyperlipidemia, failure of rehabilitation, and increased morbidity and mortality.

This chapter will focus on nutritional requirements of the adult non-diabetic patient undergoing continuous ambulatory peritoneal dialysis (CAPD). After describing the syndrome of malnutrition in patients with chronic renal failure and a comparative analysis with the situation in patients undergoing hemodialysis (HD) as a general background, we describe specific nutritional problems in CAPD patients. We also review the current experience of using amino acids instead of glucose as osmotic agent in the dialysis fluid to improve metabolic and nutritional abnormalities in peritoneal dialysis

Table 2. Nutritional advantages with CAPD.

1. Stable metabolite levels due to continuous dialysis
2. Prevention of hyperkalemia and other electrolyte disorders
3. Improved control of metabolic acidosis
4. Effective removal of middle molecules
5. Continuous energy supply
6. Net protein catabolism due to blood-membrane contact (such as in HD) is avoided
7. Better preservation of residual renal function

Table 3. Potential nutritional problems with CAPD.

1. Anorexia (due to insufficient dialysis, glucose absorption, abdominal filling)
2. Loss of protein (5–15 g/d) and amino acids (2–4 g/d)
3. Catabolic effects of peritonitis
4. Hyperglycemia and hyperinsulinemia
5. Hyperlipidemia and dyslipoproteinemia
6. Obesitas

2. Protein-energy malnutrition in peritoneal dialysis patients

Several reports have documented that protein-energy malnutrition and wasting are frequently present in nondialyzed as well as in patients undergoing maintenance dialysis therapy even in those patients who appear to be normal and who have had a successful clinical course.

2.1. Causes of protein-energy malnutrition in uremia

A variety of causes (Table 4) contribute to impaired nutritional status in uremic patients [1–3]. The most important are: 1) Abnormal protein and amino acid metabolism secondary to the influence of uremia per se, loss of renal tissue, and proteinuria. 2) Poor food intake because of anorexia, nausea and vomiting, caused by uremic toxicity. 3) Intercurrent illnesses such as infections, hyperparathyroidism, pericarditis and congestive heart failure, resulting in increased metabolic stress and sometimes profound hypercatabolism. 4) Decreased biological activity of anabolic hormones such as insulin and somatomedins and increased circulating levels of catabolic hormones such as glucagon and parathyroid hormone. 5) Dialytic losses of amino acids, water-soluble vitamins and other essential small molecular solutes. 6) Protein losses into the dialysate (in peritoneal dialysis). 7) Catabolic effects of the dialytic procedure (in hemodialysis). 8) Frequent blood sampling. 9) Low physical activity. 10) Abnormal cell energy metabolism, carbohydrate intolerance, and impaired lipid metabolism, contributing to negative energy balance.

2.2. Signs of protein-energy malnutrition

In order to diagnose malnutrition in dialysis patients, it is important to appropriately assess the nutritional status [1–3]. Validation of nutritional status may be based on clinical evaluation, diet history, anthropometric measurements and various biophysical and biochemical methods (Table 5).

Signs of malnutrition in dialysis patients are reduced muscle mass assessed by anthropometric methods, low concentration of albumin, transferrin, and other liver-derived proteins, low alkali-soluble protein in muscle in relation to dry fat-free weight and DNA, abnormal plasma amino acid and intracellular amino acid profiles, similar to those found in untreated uremia, indicating that dialysis does not reverse these abnormalities (Table 6).

Table 4. Causes of protein-energy malnutrition and wasting in uremic patients.

1. Increased net protein catabolism (uremic toxicity)
2. Anorexia, nausea, vomiting (uremic toxicity)
3. Intercurrent illnesses such as infections resulting in hypercatabolism
4. Decreased biological activity of anabolic hormones (insulin, somatomedins)
5. Increased circulating levels of catabolic hormones (glucagon, PTH)
6. Impaired cell energy metabolism and negative energy balance
7. Urinary protein loss
8. Frequent blood drawing
9. Dialytic losses of amino acids and vitamins (HD, PD)
10. Blood-membrane contact as stimuli of catabolism (HD)
11. Dialysate protein loss (PD)

Table 5. Methods to assess nutritional status.

Clinical evaluation with physical examination
  Muscle wasting?
  Loss of subcutaneous fat?
  Edema?
  Subjective global assessment
Evaluation of nutritional intake
  Dietary history and dietary records
  Urea appearance
Anthropometric methods
  Body weight, body mass index, weight loss
  Skinfold thickness (triceps and other sites)
  Mid arm muscle circumference
  Muscle strength (handgrip)
  Bioelectrical impedance
  Total body H_2O, total body K, total body N
  Dual Energy X-ray Absorptiometry (DEXA)
Biochemical methods
  Total (renal plus dialysate) creatinine and urea clearances and calculation of urea appearance
  Plasma proteins (albumin, prealbumin, transferrin, IGF-1)
  Other plasma and blood chemistries (Hb, urea, creatinine, lipids, amino acids)
  Muscle protein, RNA, DNA, amino acids
Immunological methods
  Total lymphocyte count
  Acute phase protein complement C_3
  Delayed hypersensitivity, skin test

2.3. Prevalence of protein-energy malnutrition

Malnutrition is frequently present in patients treated with maintenance dialysis therapy. In various studies of HD patients [4–7], a low percent ideal body weight or low body mass index was found in 10–30%, a low triceps skinfold thickness in 20–60%, and low arm muscle circumference in 0–44%. Low serum albumin was observed in 13–70% and low transferrin in 30–60% of HD patients. Muscle alkali-soluble protein (ASP) to DNA ratio was found to be on average reduced to 67% of normal, indicating cellular protein depletion [4], but a normal ASP/DNA ratio in HD patients has also been reported [9].

The anthropometric data may suggest that energy malnutrition is more prevalent than protein malnutrition in HD patients. However, results of a recent study using total body N determination by neutron activation analysis indicate that anthropometric measurements may underestimate the degree of protein malnutrition in HD patients [10].

There is also a high prevalence of protein energy malnutrition in CAPD patients, with 18–56% of CAPD patients showing anthropometric and biochemical evidence of malnutrition [1]. Some data provide evidence of an increased net anabolism during the first year of CAPD with weight gain and improvement in anthropometric parameters and a rise in plasma proteins [11–13]. However, prospective studies of total body protein show a gradual deterioration in nutritional status, indicating that the body protein mass decreases, especially in male patients, with large protein stores at the beginning of treatment [11, 14, 15].

The most extensive evaluation of nutritional status in CAPD patients included 224 patients from six centers in Europe and North-America [16]. A total of 224 patients, 132 males and 92 females, ranging in age from 14 to 87 years, were selected. All patients had been maintained on CAPD for more than 3 months and had remained free from peritonitis for at least 1 month before the study. A total of 113 patients from altogether 337 patients of the total CAPD population at the six centres were excluded due to non-medical reasons such as non-compliance and duration of treatment less than 3 months, transfer to hemodialysis, transplantation and hospitalization. Thus, 224/237 patients (66%) were included in the study. The patients had a mean (±SD) age of 53 ± 15 years and had been maintained on CAPD 32 ± 27 months. Their residual renal function was 1.3 ± 2.0 ml/min.

A "subjective nutritional assessment" was made, using 21 variables derived from history and clinical examination, or anthropometry and biochemistry. Eighteen patients (8%) were severely malnourished, 73 (32.6%) were mildly to moderately malnourished, and 133 (59.4%) did not show evidence for malnutrition.

There was a higher incidence of mild to moderate malnutrition in diabetics that in non-diabetics. A statistical analysis identified 12 variables, seven objective and five subjective, that correlated with subjective nutritional assessment. Actual intercenter differences for the incidence of malnutrition were related to patient age, nutritional status at the commencement of continuous ambulatory peritoneal dialysis (CAPD), the length of time of CAPD, and residual renal function.

Variables that were most frequently correlated with subjective nutritional assessment and with one another included plasma albumin, mid-arm muscle circumference (MAMC), weight loss, and the clinical judgement of muscle wasting and loss of subcutaneous fat. Loss of residual renal function correlated with muscle wasting and months on CAPD. In women there was a trend for more anorexia, greater weight loss from muscle wasting and a larger decrease in albumin, whereas in men there was a more gradual decrease in nutritional status.

Variables that did *not* correlate with other estimates of nutritional status included: peritonitis rate, patient age, serum transferrin, dialysate protein loss, and serum cholesterol and triglycerides.

Patients with severe malnutrition (8%) had minimal or no residual renal function and were either older or had been on CAPD longer than other patients.

From this study [16] one may conclude that progression of malnutrition may occur in CAPD

Table 6. Evidence of malnutrition in uremic patients.

1. Subjective global assessment of nutritional status indicates a high prevalence of malnutrition.
2. Body weight (% relative body weight, % pre-uremic body weight) is low
3. Skinfold thickness (triceps and other sites) is low
4. Midarm muscle circumference (MAMC) is low
5. Visceral proteins (serum total protein, albumin, transferrin, immunoglobins, C_3, C_4) are low
6. Essential amino acids (plasma, muscle) are low
7. Non-essential amino acids (plasma, muscle) are high
8. Muscle intracellular alkali-soluble protein (ASP): DNA is low

patients due to the synergistic effects of loss of residual renal function, anorexia and inadequate dietary intake. In some patients, especially patients with minimal or no residual renal function, more efficient dialysis may be required before nitrogen depletion can be reversed by either dietary supplementation or alternative therapies.

Marckmann [8], who studied 32 patients on HD and 16 patients on CAPD, found an equally high prevalence of malnutrition in both groups (54% and 52%, respectively). In a multicenter study, comparing 609 HD and 138 CAPD patients, Nelson et al. [17] noted no difference in nutritional status between the two groups. However, Maiorca et al. [18] reported that CAPD patients, unlike HD patients, failed to correct the slight hypoalbuminemia present at the beginning of treatment.

Non-dialyzed chronic renal failure patients have several abnormalities in plasma and muscle free amino acid patterns with among others low concentrations of several of the essential amino acids, suggesting the presence of protein malnutrition [19]. Some of these abnormalities are corrected in maintenance dialysis patients whereas other abnormalities are not restored to normal [20, 21]. The concentration of plasma amino acids are generally lower in CAPD patients than in HD patients, whereas more intracellular amino acid abnormalities are present in HD than in CAPD patients [2].

In conclusion, the prevalence of protein energy malnutrition is high both in HD and CAPD patients. No conclusions can be drawn from the data available in the literature as to which method is superior, regarding adequacy of nutrition, especially since the patient populations in the various studies differed with regard to age, incidence of complicating diseases, socioeconomic conditions, time on dialysis, dialysis dose and dietary recommendations.

3. Protein intake, malnutrition and clinical outcome

It is generally accepted that suboptimal nutritional status is associated with increased morbidity and may impair rehabilitation and the quality of life. Cutaneous energy and other immune alterations strikingly similar to those observed in malnutrition, which have been documented both in HD and CAPD patients [22, 23], suggest that protein-energy malnutrition may entail the risk of infection and septicemia.

Several studies suggest that low protein intake and malnutrition are important risk factors for morbidity and mortality in HD patients [5, 7, 8, 24–27]. In the National Cooperative Dialysis Study it was observed that a PCR of < 0.8 g/kg body weight (BW)/day was associated with treatment failure [27]. Among 120 HD patients, Acchiardo et al. [26] found that a subgroup with a mean protein intake of 0.63 g/kg/day (estimated from the urea appearance rate) had a mortality rate of 14% per year, while groups of patients with higher intakes, 0.93, 1.02, and 1.29 g/kg/day, had mortality rates of only 4%, 3%, and 0%, respectively. The number of hospitalizations per year was also much higher in the group of patients having the lowest intake of protein, with higher frequencies of heart disease, pericarditis, infections, and gastrointestinal manifestations than in the other patient groups.

More recently, Lowrie and Lew [5] reported that there was a strong association between a low serum albumin concentrations and mortality in a population of more than 12,000 HD patients. The annual risk of death was seven times higher in patients with an albumin level below 30 g per l, than in those with an albumin level above 40 g per l, and no less than 14 times higher when adjusted for other risk factors that influence mortality by using logistic regression analysis. The risk of death was inversely related to the predialysis serum creatinine level, which is a marker of the size of the muscle mass. Patients with the lowest BUN levels also ran a considerably increased risk of death suggesting that a low protein intake is also a risk factor. An association between low BUN values and an increased mortality rate has also been observed in other studies [24, 25].

In CAPD patients there is also some evidence that malnutrition is an important risk factor. Teehan et al. [28] retrospectively analyzed the clinical outcome in 51 CAPD patients, followed longitudinally for five years, and found a strong association between low serum albumin and increased mortality and number of hospitalisation. It was also observed that a low protein intake (low PCR) was associated with increased number of hospital admissions, and that low BUN, reflecting a low protein intake, was a risk factor for low serum albumin. However, in another retrospective study by Blake et al. [29] concerning 76 new patients on CAPD, followed over an average of 20 months, there was no association between PCR and clinical outcome, although some of these patients had protein intakes clearly below the recommended intake. Obviously prospective studies in larger patient groups are required to enable an evaluation of to what extent malnutrition is a risk factor for a poor outcome in CAPD patients. It is conceivable that malnutrition is equally important as a risk factor in HD and CAPD.

It should be kept in mind that the relationship between malnutrition and increased morbidity and mortality is not necessarily a cause-effect one. In addition to renal failure, a large proportion of maintenance dialysis patients have complicating diseases, such as severe cardiovascular disease, diabetic vascular complications, gastrointestinal and liver diseases, and other systemic diseases with an unfavorable prognosis. Such sick patients may become anorectic and malnourished and malnutrition may be a marker of illness, but not the direct cause of death.

Among the causes of death in patients with end-stage renal failure on renal replacement therapy, cardiovascular diseases predominate, followed by septicemia and infection, whereas according to the EDTA Registry, cachexia is a rare cause of death (3% in patients aged 15–64 years and 9% in older patients [30]. In the U.S. Renal Data System Annual Report, cachexia and malnutrition are not listed among the causes of death [31]. However, malnutrition may have contributed to the high death rate, due to infection, and it may have been partly the reason why some of the patients were taken off dialysis or died from unknown causes.

4. Protein and energy requirements in peritoneal dialysis patients

To maintain a satisfactory nutritional status the intake of protein and energy must be sufficient to meet the requirements. A low intake of protein is especially detrimental in case the protein requirements are increased, which seems to be the case in patients on renal replacement therapy.

The average minimum protein requirements in normal adult subjects are about 0.5–0.6 g/kg body weight/day and the safe requirement, i.e. the protein intake on which practically all individuals are in nitrogen equilibrium or in positive nitrogen balance, is about 0.75 g/kg body weight/day [32]. The protein requirements are critically dependent on the energy intake so that with a low intake the requirements of protein are increased above those needed when the energy intake is adequate or high. Non-dialyzed uremic patients may be in nitrogen balance on 0.5-0.6 g/kg day of high-quality protein, or less, if the diet is supplemented with essential amino acids or their keto analoques.

Results of nitrogen balance studies in patients on HD twice a week suggested that approximately 0.75 g/kg BW/day of high biological value protein is necessary to maintain nitrogen equilibrium [33] or a slightly positive nitrogen balance [34]. However, according to more recent long-term studies, this amount of protein may not be adequate. Signs of malnutrition have been observed in many apparently well-rehabilitated patients on maintenance HD, who had a daily protein intake of about 1 g/kg BW/day [35]. On the basis of clinical results with protein and energy supplements to the diet, it was suggested that 1.2 g of protein, primarily of high biological value, and an energy intake of 35 kcal/kg BW/day should be prescribed for HD patients [35].

Protein catabolic rate (PCR), estimated from the urea appearance rate, reflects the protein intake in metabolically stable patients [36]. In the National Cooperative Dialysis Study, a PCR > 1.0 was associated with a low morbidity, provided that the blood urea concentration was adequately controlled [37–39]. Gotch and Sargent [38] performed a "mechanistic" analysis of the NCDS data resulting in a nomogram which is now widely accepted for assessing the adequacy of dialysis. This nomogram expresses the relationship between the mid-week BUN, PCR and Kt/V with a region labeled adequate, within which the patient data should fit if the patient is adequately treated. According to this nomogram, the lower limit for an adequate PCR is 0.8 g/kg BW/day.

Protein requirements in CAPD patients also appear to be increased, compared to normal individuals. The results of nitrogen balance studies, in a group of CAPD patients, using two levels of protein intake, 0.98 and 1.44 g protein/kg body weight/day, suggest that the protein requirements for CAPD patients are considerably higher than those for normal individuals [40]. On the basis of these results a protein intake of ≥ 1.2 g/kg BW/day was recommended for patients treated with CAPD to ensure nitrogen equilibrium or a positive nitrogen balance. It should be noted however that it is the experience of our group and others in general, that the protein intake in most CAPD patients is considerably lower than the generally recommended intake of 1.2 g/kg body weight/day, and that the high intake recommended is rarely obtained.

Lysaght et al. [42] observed that the estimated protein intake (urea kinetics) was about 18% lower in CAPD compared to HD patients (0.91 and 1.13/kg BW/day, respectively). Retrospective observations by our group also demonstrate that the protein intake in CAPD patients is generally lower than in HD patients. In spite of this, CAPD patients do not seem to fare worse than HD patients from the nutritional point of view, raising the question whether the protein requirements, though increased in comparison to those of normal individuals, are lower than those of HD patients.

It is therefore of interest to note that in another study, in which nitrogen balance was measured in CAPD patients receiving a diet that closely corresponded to their spontaneous daily intake of protein and energy, some of the patients were in neutral or positive nitrogen balance with a protein intake as low as 0.70 g/kg BW/day [41]. In this study a strong correlation between nitrogen balance and dietary protein intake was noted after 3.4 ± 1.2 months on CAPD (Fig. 1). A strong correlation between nitrogen balance and energy intake was noted both during the initial period of CAPD as well as after 12.1 ± 2.6 months (Fig. 1).

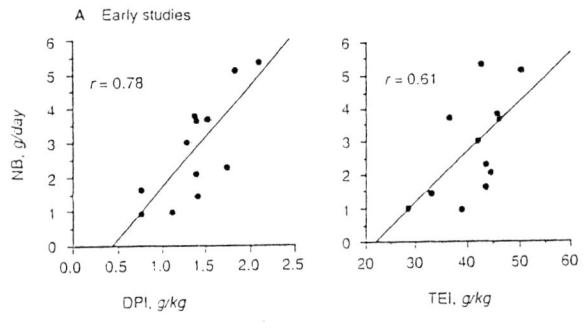

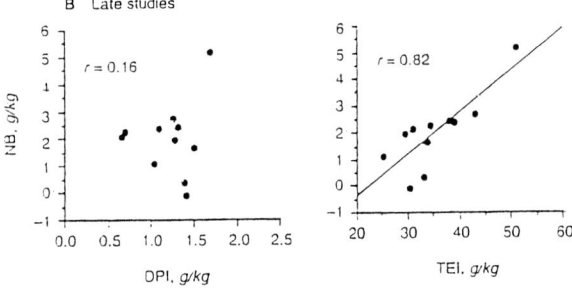

Figure 1. Relationships between nitrogen balance (NB) not corrected for "Unmeasured" nitrogen losses and dietary protein intake (DPI) and total energy intake (TEI) during early (3.4 ± 1.2 months on CAPD) and late 12.1 ± 2.6 months on CAPD studies in altogether 23 NB studies in 12 CAPD patients. (Reproduced with permission from reference [41]).

The energy requirements depend on the level of physical activity, an intake of 35–40 kcal/kg BW/day being recommended for individuals not performing heavy physical exercise [32]. There is no evidence that the energy requirements of maintenance dialysis patients are usually different from those of normal subjects. Monteon *et al.* [43] measured energy expenditure in normal subjects, non-dialyzed patients with chronic renal failure and maintenance HD patients and found no difference among the three groups with the subjects sitting, exercising or in the post-prandial state. This finding suggests that during a given physical activity the energy expenditure of chronic HD patients does not differ from that in normal subjects. Nor is there any evidence that the energy requirements in patients on CAPD differ from normal (see also section 5.1 in this chapter).

5. Protein catabolic factors in peritoneal dialysis patients

The observation that HD and CAPD patients seem to have a diminished utilization of ingested protein and increased protein requirements, compared to normal individuals indicates that metabolic factors, not fully corrected for by dialysis treatment, as well as the treatment *per se*, may enhance net protein catabolism and impair the utilization of dietary protein (Table 7). Many patients on renal replacement therapy are physically inactive for various reasons such as fatigue, anemia, skeleto-muscular disease, and psychological factors. Physical inactivity may result in muscle-wasting and a negative nitrogen balance [44].

In maintenance HD patients, investigated by ^{13}C leucine kinetics, the protein breakdown was the same as that in controls, but the protein oxidation rate was higher and net the protein synthesis was lower, which was thought to contribute to muscle-wasting [45]. In contrast, kinetic leucine studies in CAPD patients showed that the protein turnover and the rate of protein oxidation were lower than in controls and that the balance between synthesis and breakdown was higher before the start of dialysis and after three months on CAPD suggesting protein anabolism [46].

5.1. Low energy intake

Metabolic studies indicate that the utilization of protein is greatly dependent on the energy intake, so that a low energy intake reduces utilization, whereas a high energy intake has a protein-saving effect [47]. Slomowitz et al. [48] demonstrated that this also applies to HD patients. In six patients on a constant protein intake, averaging 1.13 g/kg desirable BW/day, the nitrogen balance, adjusted for unmeasured losses, was negative when the energy intake was 25 kcal/kg BW/day, but neutral or positive when the energy intake was 35 or 45 kcal/kg/day. In CAPD patients also, the nitrogen balance is strongly correlated to the total energy intake [41]. Glucose is absorbed from the dialysate, averaging 8 kcal/kg BW/day and varying between 5–20 kcal/kg BW/day, which should be advantageous regarding the utilization of protein. However, despite glucose uptake, many CAPD patients have a total energy intake below 35 kcal/kg BW/day [1, 41, 49, 50]. Considering that many patients on maintenance dialysis ingest less than 35 kcal/kg BW/day, energy deficiency may be an important factor contributing to poor utilization of dietary protein [41].

5.2. Metabolic acidosis

It has become increasingly evident that metabolic acidosis is an important stimulus for net protein catabolism. In non-dialyzed chronic uremic patients the correction of metabolic acidosis improves the nitrogen balance [51]. A study of leucine kinetics in normal subjects during acute acidosis and alkalosis showed that total body protein breakdown as well as apparent leucine oxidation increase more during acidosis than during alkalosis [52]. In the aforementioned studies of leucine kinetics in HD patients [45], demonstrating an increased protein oxidation and reduced protein synthesis, the patients were acidotic with a plasma bicarbonate pre-dialysis averaging 18 mmol/l, suggesting that acidosis might have been a factor of importance. In rats with chronic renal failure, acidosis, rather than uremia *per se*, appears to enhance protein catabolism [53]. This effect seems to be mediated by the stimulation of skeletal muscle branched-chain keto acid decarboxylation, which increases the catabolism of the branched-chain amino acids (valine, leucine and isoleucine), which are mainly metabolized in muscle tissue [54]. It was recently reported that metabolic acidosis also elicits the transcription of genes for proteolytic enzymes in muscle [55]. Our group has recently reported that the intracellular valine concentration in the muscle of patients treated with maintenance HD is low [20]. The concentration showed a correlation with the pre-dialysis blood standard bicarbonate level which varied between 18 and 24 mmol/l, suggesting that even slight and intermittent acidosis may have stimulated the catabolism of valine in muscle, resulting in a valine depletion that may be a limiting factor for protein synthesis. In contrast, CAPD patients in whom plasma standard bicarbonate levels are more normal have well-maintained muscle intracellular pools of valine and other essential amino acids [21].

In our experience, acidosis is common in HD patients, despite the use of bicarbonate as the buffer in the dialysis fluid. In a group of 129 HD patients, we observed that 41% of the HD patients had pre-dialysis plasma bicarbonate concentrations ≤ 21 mmol/l and 17% ≤ 19 mmol/l [2]. In 44 CAPD patients, most of whom were not taking oral sodium

Table 7. Catabolic effects of the dialytic proedure.

	CAPD	HD
Loss of amino acids	2–4 g/d (14–28 g/week)	9–13 g/dialysis (27–39 g/week)
Loss of glucose	(uptake)	~25 g/dialysis (glucose-free dialysate)
Loss of protein	5–15 g/d (higher with peritonitis)	0
Inflammatory stimuli	Low-grade inflammation? (particles, chemicals)	Blood-membrane contact
	Cytokine release due to – Peritonitis	Cytokine release due to – Complement activation – Endotoxins – Acetate

bicarbonate, the steady state plasma bicarbonate concentration was in general less abnormal than in the HD patients predialysis [2]. We therefore speculate whether the intermittent acidosis in HD patients with a nadir concentration of plasma bicarbonate before each dialysis may act as a stimulus for protein catabolism, which is less prominent or absent in the CAPD patients, who are either only slightly acidotic or have a normal steady state plasma concentration.

It should be pointed out that acidosis is today the only identified uremic "toxic" factor, which induces catabolism and impairs nitrogen utilization. Full correction of acidosis is consequently an obvious goal for treatment both in HD and CAPD patients. This goal is more easily obtained in CAPD patients.

5.3. Loss of metabolizing renal tissue

The normal kidneys actively take part in the metabolism of amino acids where, among other processes, phenylalanine hydroxylation to tyrosine [56, 57] and glycine conversion to serine take place [58]. In patients with chronic renal failure the concentration of free tyrosine is low and the phenylalanine/tyrosine ratio is increased in plasma and muscle, serine in plasma is low and glycine increased [30, 31]. We observed that HD patients exhibit a more severe serine depletion with significantly reduced intracellular levels in muscle than do controls, non-dialyzed chronic uremic patients and CAPD patients [20]. One possible explanation is that the non-dialyzed patients and CAPD patients still had some functioning renal tissue left, by means of which serine conversion could take place.

5.4. Recurrent peritonitis and other infections

Uremia leads to disturbances in the immune response, with cutaneous anergy and impaired granulocyte function, thus increasing the susceptibility to infections. A severe infection is an important stimulus for protein catabolism. HD patients are especially at risk for developing sepsis from infections in arteriovenous fistulas, grafts and indwelling venous catheters.

Recurrent peritonitis is one of the most serious complications of CAPD and may result in markedly negative introgen balance [49]. Adverse effects of recurrent peritonitis on nutritional status were demonstrated by Rubin *et al.* [59, 60], who observed that changes in total body potassium correlated negatively with the number of episodes of peritonitis per month and that patients with a high incidence of peritonitis had a lower arm muscle circumference and lower plasma protein than did patients with a lower incidence of peritonitis. Peritonitis is associated with increased losses of protein in the dialysate (vide infra). In addition the inflammatory response may be a strong catabolic stimulus superimposed on the enhanced protein losses.

5.5. Dialysis procedure as stimuli of net protein catabolism in HD vs CAPD

The dialytic procedure *per se* may induce net catabolism of protein (Table 7). The mechanisms differ in several ways in HD and CAPD patients (see sections 5.6–5.9 in this chapter). Borah *et al.* [36] observed in five HD patients on low and high protein intakes, respectively, that the nitrogen balance (corrected for changes in total body urea) was negative on the dialysis days, but less negative (with a protein intake of 0.5 g/kg BW/day) or positive (with a protein intake of 1.4 g/kg BW/day) on the days between the dialysis. Farrell, Ward and co-workers [61, 62] reported that the urea appearance rate is 30% higher during the HD procedure than in the interdialytic period. These results suggest that the HD procedure is a strong intermittent stimulus for net protein catabolism. An increase in the urea appearance rate or a decrease in nitrogen balance may be due to reduced protein synthesis [63, 64], enhanced breakdown of protein or a combination of both. With regard to the catabolic effect of the HD procedure the data suggest that both processes are involved.

Lim *et al.* [64] studied leucine and alpha-ketoisocaproate kinetics by use of stable isotopes before, during and after cuprophane HD with acetate. They concluded that HD is a catabolic event, characterized not by enhanced protein degradation but by reduction in protein synthesis. However, there is also evidence that proteolysis is enhanced as a result of blood membrane interaction. The mechanism by which HD elicits a reduction in protein synthesis remains unknown, but one may speculate whether amino acid depletion induced by the dialysis procedure might somehow trigger this effect. As discussed below the catabolic effect of the dialysis procedure *per se* is much weaker in CAPD, except for the losses of protein into the dialysate.

5.6. Loss of glucose in HD vs glucose absorption in CAPD

When a glucose-free dialysis fluid is used for HD about 28 g of glucose is removed during 4 h of HD, whereas the addition of glucose (11 mmol/l) to the dialysis fluid results in a gain of about 23 g of glucose by the patient [65]. To avoid symptomatic hypoglycemia, glucose removed from the extracellular fluid by dialysis must be replaced by ingested carbohydrate, by breakdown of liver glycogen or by gluconeogenesis from amino acids; the latter should result in an enhanced protein breakdown and urea synthesis. Observations by Wathen et al. [65] showing that pyruvate decreased during glucose-free dialysis, but was unchanged during glucose dialysis, indicate that gluconeogenesis may be stimulated by glucose-free dialysis. However, Ward et al. [61], and Farrell and Hone [62] have reported that the urea appearance rate is stimulated to a similar extent by dialysis, whether glucose is present in the dialysis fluid or not.

In contrast, CAPD patients are provided with glucose continuously by the peritoneal route, which is potentially beneficial by providing an additional energy supply. However, glucose uptake may also have negative metabolic effects, such as hyperglycemia, hyperinsulinemia, hyperlipidemia and obesity [1].

5.7. Loss of amino acids

During HD the average loss of free amino acids in the dialysis fluid has been reported to be 5–8 g/dialysis, of which about one third are essential amino acids [66–68]. Moreover, 4–5 g of peptide-bound amino acids are lost per dialysis [66]; thus, the total losses of amino acids are about 10–13 g/dialysis.

The losses of free amino acids into the dialysate during CAPD are of the same magnitude (per week) or smaller than with HD (Table 7). The reported average dialysate losses of free amino acids during CAPD vary between 1.2 and 3.4 g/24 h in different studies. About 30% of the amino acids lost into the dialysate are essential amino acids. Obviously, the losses of amino acids *per se* by dialysis are too small to fully account for the increased protein requirements in maintenance dialysis patients.

5.8. Protein losses in CAPD

Substantial loss of protein into the dialysate is a major drawback with peritoneal dialysis which is not present in HD (Table 7). In CAPD the reported average loss of protein into the dialysate varies between 5 and 15 g in different studies with large interindividual differences. Thus, dialysate protein loss may vary between 20 and 140 g/week in different patients.

In CAPD patients with mild peritonitis the dialysate protein losses increased by 50–100% to an average of 15.1 ± 3.6g/day [69], and remained elevated for several weeks [11, 70].

It should be noted that protein losses indirectly may contribute to various nutritional and metabolic disturbances in patients on CAPD: for example, hypercholesterolemia, altered amino acid metabolism, and metabolic bone disease due to losses of vitamin D binding protein.

5.9. Biocompatibility and protein catabolism in HD vs CAPD

A major difference between CAPD and HD (Table 7) is that the HD procedure may give rise to an inflammatory reaction, the intensity of which depends on the membrane material that is used [71–76]. IL-1 and TNF may act in concert and induce *inter alia* lysosomal catabolism of muscle protein [77], an effect which is mediated by the release of prostaglandin E2 [78]. More recently it has been observed that IL-1, TNF and endotoxin may induce net catabolism of muscle protein by stimulating branched-chain keto acid dehydrogenase, which leads to an enhanced oxidation of branched-chain amino acids [79].

Blood membrane contact during sham-HD in normal individuals may elicit an enhanced release of amino acids from the leg tissue (mainly skeletal muscle), corresponding to an enhanced protein breakdown of 15–20 g [80, 81]. By giving indomethacin before and during the procedure this catabolic response was abolished, a finding which suggests that the catabolic effect is mediated by prostaglandins. With a more biocompatible membrane there was no increase in amino acid release [80, 81]. These studies demonstrate that *in vivo* blood membrane interaction in a dialyzer without dialysate stimulates net protein catabolism, especially when the membrane has a low biocompatibility.

Sham-HD with cuprophane, but not with more biocompatible membranes, elicited an increased release from the leg musculature and an elevation in the plasma concentration of 3-methylhistidine

[81]. This amino acid is formed post-translationally by the irreversible methylation of histidine in actinomyosin proteins and cannot be reutilized after being released during protein degradation [82]. The increase in leg efflux and elevated arterial concentration of 3-methylhistidine following HD therefore indicates that increased protein breakdown plays an important part in the net catabolic process induced by blood-membrane contact.

Apparently the peritoneal dialysis procedure is not such a strong catabolic stimulus as HD, provided that the patient is free from peritonitis. However, there is a possibility that in CAPD the dialytic procedure *per se* elicits a low-grade inflammatory response, induced by substances other than live bacteria, thereby stimulating protein catabolism. These substances could be microbial products (endotoxins), acetate, plastics, silicon, glucose, or other products from the system which elute into the peritoneal cavity.

6. Dialysis dose, anorexia and nutritional intake

Even though low protein and energy intakes are known to be harmful in dialysis patients, it may be difficult to fulfill the nutritional requirements, since some seem to loose their appetite, and thus reduce their protein intake spontaneously. This may in part be due to a gradual loss of residual renal function and failure to increase the dialysis dose accordingly, resulting in underdialysis and thus anorexia (Table 8).

Nutritional surveys indicate that the mean intake

Table 8. Causes of anorexia in maintenance dialysis patients.

General factors
Uremic toxicity (underdialysis, especially in patients with minimal GFR!)
Unpalatable or inadequate diets
Gastropathy (diabetic patients)
Inflammation, infection, sepsis
Medications
Psychosocial and socioeconomic factors
    Loneliness
    Depression
    Ignorance
    Poverty
    Alcohol and drug abuse

Effects of the HD procedure	*Effects of the PD procedure*
Cardiovascular instability	Abdominal discomfort
Nausea, vomiting	Glucose absorption
Post-dialysis fatigue	Peritonitis

of protein in HD patients is less than 1 g/kg BW/day in a large proportion of maintenance HD patients [4, 6, 8]. Jacob *et al.* [6] noted in 61 HD patients that 45% had a protein intake less than 1 g/kg BW/day. The energy intake is also low in groups of HD patients, with a mean intake of 26–29 kcal/kg BW/day [6, 8, 83], i.e. much less than the 35 kcal/kg BW/day generally recommended. This is in keeping with observations that a high proportion of HD patients show signs of energy depletion.

Nutritional problems may occur in CAPD patients due to a decreased intake of both protein and total energy with time on CAPD. After one year in CAPD the average dietary protein intake is reported to fall to about 1.0 g/kg/day and the average total energy intake to about 30 kcal/kg/day [49].

A large proportion of CAPD patients thus ingest considerably lower amounts of protein than the recommended intake of 1.2 g/kg BW/day [4, 41, 42, 49]. Lysaght *et al.* [42] observed that the estimated protein intake in some CAPD patients was as low as 0.4–0.5 g/kg BW/day.

The energy intake in CAPD patients has been reported to be low in spite of the additional supply of energy as glucose by the peritoneal route [49, 50]. There is also a decrease of protein and energy intake with time which is paralleled by a fall in nitrogen balance [14, 41, 48]. The reduced nutritional intake with time during CAPD seems to be caused by anorexia with a reduced nutritional intake as a consequence, probably because CAPD patients become underdialyzed as the total solute clearance falls, due to a decrease in residual renal function.

Some factors which may contribute to a low intake of protein and energy are listed in Table 8. Anorexia may be due to unpalatable or inadequate diets, gastropathy (in diabetic patients with autonomic neuropathy), medications, psychosocial and socioeconomic factors such as loneliness, depression, ignorance and poverty, especially in elderly patients, and those with alcohol and drug problems. Nausea and vomiting may lead to a reduction in food intake. In CAPD patients abdominal distension may lead to feelings of fullness and discomfort and the glucose uptake may suppress appetite. However, by far the most important anorectic factor, common to both HD and CAPD patients, is persistent uremia due to underdialysis.

An adaptive decrease in protein intake in HD patients dialyzed for a short time and with low efficacy was observed in the National Cooperative Dialysis Study [83]. More recently, Lindsay and

Spanner [85] reported a correlation between the dose of dialysis (Kt/V$_{urea}$) and the protein catabolic rate (PCR), which in metabolically stable patients, reflects the protein intake. They increased the dose of dialysis (Kt/V) in individual patients and observed that the protein intake (PCR) increased spontaneously. The relationship between Kt/V and PCR seemed to vary with the type of membrane, so that with a more permeable and biocompatible membrane PCR increased more for the same increase in Kt/V than with cuprophane [85].

There is also evidence that the daily dose of dialysis is of critical importance for the intake of protein in CAPD patients, based on recent reports demonstrating a correlation between Kt/V for urea and protein intake, as assessed from the urea appearance rate [42, 84, 85]. In addition, we observed a correlation between Kt/V for urea and dietary protein intake as assessed from diaries kept concerning diets and recall interviews by a dietitian [41]. (Fig. 2).

In general, CAPD patients have a lower weekly dialytic clearance of urea than do HD patients. The dietary protein intake has been reported to decrease in patients after switching from HD to CAPD, and to increase in patients after switching from CAPD to HD [86]. This suggests that a less efficient removal of critical uremic toxins in CAPD may have suppressed appetite. However, a positive factor in favor of CAPD as compared to HD, is that the residual renal function seems to be better preserved in CAPD patients than in HD patients after starting dialysis [87].

We performed a retrospective analysis of Kt/V and PCR in a group of 115 unselected HD patients and a group of 29 patients on continuous peritoneal dialysis and found that the relationship between Kt/V and PCR in the CAPD patients differed from that in the HD patients, most of whom were treated with cellulosic membrane [88]. At the same low Kt/V levels the protein intake (PCR) in the CAPD patients was higher than in the HD patients and the protein intake increased more for the same increase in Kt/V in the CAPD than in the HD patients.

An attractive hypothesis for explaining the different relationships between Kt/V and PCR in CAPD patients and HD patients might be that the anorectic factor(s) are molecules of larger size than urea, which are relatively more efficiently dialyzed by the peritoneal route than by the cellulosic membranes in the artificial kidney. This hypothesis is supported by the challenging observation by Lindsay and Spanner mentioned earlier [85], indicating that with a permeable membrane protein intake increases proportionally more with the same increase in Kt/V$_{urea}$ than with cellulosic membranes. The peak concentration hypothesis, recently presented by Keshaviah *et al.* affords an alternative explanation, namely that the periodic peak concentrations of urea and other toxins in HD patients, is more important than the time average concentration [89]. Accordingly, a higher KT/V$_{urea}$ is required in intermittent HD patients than in CAPD patients for dialysis to be adequate. Today there is no proof that any of these hypothesis are more true than the other.

From the results of previous studies one may conclude that: 1) KT/V for urea is easy to calculate in CAPD patients, 2) the weekly Kt/V in CAPD patients is often about 40% less than in HD patients, 3) despite low Kt/V CAPD patients seem to fare not worse than HD patients with much higher Kt/V, 4) a prospective study similar to the NCDS study has so far not been established, 5) the appropriate interpretation and clinical meaning of Kt/V in CAPD is thus unclear, 6) the apparent "Kt/V paradox" in CAPD patients (see above) has not yet been resolved although some possible explanations have been provided such as the "peak concentration hypothesis", feed-back mechanisms between clearance, serum urea concentration, appetite and protein intake, and improved maintenance of residual renal function in CAPD. In addition, the catabolic effects of HD and the unphysiology of intermittent HD,

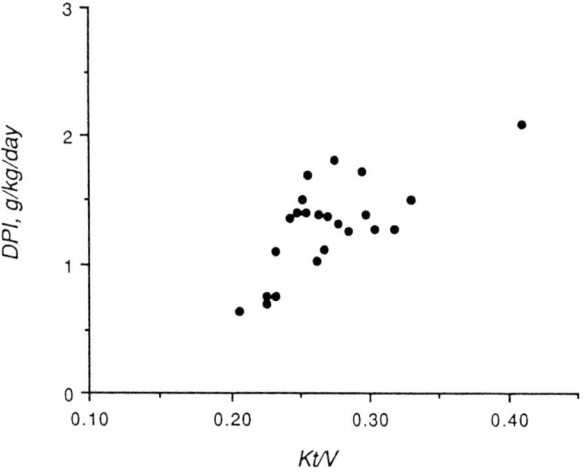

Figure 2. Relationship between daily Kt/V for urea and dietary protein intake (DPI) at the time of 23 nitrogen balance studies in 12 CAPD patients. DPI was assessed from diaries kept concerning diets and recall interviews by a dietitian. Kt/V for urea and DPI were correlated; r = 0.45. P = 0.032. (Reproduced with permission from reference [41]).

improved middle molecule removal in CAPD, the anabolic effects of the continuous intraperitoneal glucose supply in CAPD patients and last, but not least, the stable metabolite levels and improved control of acidosis in CAPD are all factors which may explain why CAPD patients seem to tolerate a lower Kt/V than HD patients.

6.1. Prevention and treatment of malnutrition in CAPD

The previous discussion has underlined that the incidence of malnutrition is high in maintenance dialysis patients, irrespectively whether they are treated with HD or CAPD, and is strongly associated with increased morbidity and mortality. Contributing factors are increased protein requirements and low supply of energy and protein in relation to the needs. CAPD patients generally have a lower protein intake than HD patients, but there is indirect evidence that CAPD patients may have lower average protein requirements than HD patients. In HD the dialytic procedure is a strong intermittent stimulus of net catabolism, which is not present in CAPD patients. On the other hand, the protein losses by the dialysate in CAPD patients are unparalleled in the HD patients. Peritonitis when present, is a strong catabolic stimulus in CAPD patients. Anorexia with low protein and energy intake results from a variety of factors of which underdialysis with insufficient control of uremic toxicity seems to be a major one. The relationship between the dose of dialysis expressed as Kt/V for urea and the protein intake (assessed from urea appearance) is more favourable in CAPD patients than in HD patients, suggesting that control of potential uremic toxins which cause anorexia is better in CAPD patients than in HD patients, at the same dose of dialysis, evaluated from the efficacy of urea removal. Underdialyzed CAPD patients may enter a vicious circle of low protein and energy intake, and enhanced protein catabolism, leading to progressive malnutrition and muscle wasting and a fatal outcome. To break this vicious circle the intensity of dialysis should be increased, acidosis corrected and measures should be taken to increase the supply of energy and protein.

Since malnutrition may entail increased risk of morbidity and mortality in maintenance dialysis patients, measures should be taken to minimize or eliminate factors that result in inadequate nutritional intake (see Table 8) aiming at a protein intake of ≥ 1.2g/ kg BW/day and an energy intake of ≥ 35 kcal/kg BW/day.

Patients undergoing CAPD require relatively few restrictions concerning their dietary intakes of water, salt and other nutrients. In fact, this is one of the main advantages with CAPD as compared to intermittent dialysis. However, a major problem is that many CAPD patients have insufficient nutritional intakes. Individualized dietary prescriptions are therefore necessary. *Ad libitum* diets should be discouraged. Recommended nutritional intakes in patients undergoing CAPD are given in Table 9.

Underdialysis, when present or suspected, should be corrected by increasing the dose of dialysis, in

Table 9. Recommended nutritional intakes for patients treated by CAPD.

Protein	≥1.2 g/kg (approximately 50% of high biologic value)
Energy (including glucose absorption)	≥35 kcal/kg/d
Fat	35% (high content of unsaturated lipids)
Water and sodium	As tolerated by fluid balance
Potassium	40–80 mmol
Calcium	1000 mg (supplements may be required)
Phosphorous	8–17 mg/kg (phosphate binder is often needed)
Magnesium	200–300 mg
Iron	10–15 mg (supplements may be required)
Zinc	15 mg (supplements may be required)
Vitamins (recommended supplementation, mg/d)	
Pyridoxine (B_6)	10
Ascorbic acid	100
Thiamine (B_1)	2.0 (not routinely)
Folic acid	1.0 (not routinely)
Other water soluble vitamins	Daily allowances as for healthy subjects
Vitamins A and K	None
Vitamin D	See text

CAPD patients by increasing the number of daily exchanges and/or the exchange volumes. CAPD patients who remain underdialyzed in spite of these measures may have to be switched over to HD, which is less limited regarding weekly dialysis dose. Metabolic acidosis should be corrected by oral medication with sodium bicarbonate or other alkaline salts, or by increasing the base concentration in the dialysis fluid. If severe malnutrition develops despite dialysis being adequate and measures having been taken to eliminate various anorectic and catabolic factors, enteral or parenteral nutritional supplementation with energy and amino acids may be warranted [90, 91]. Intradialytic parenteral nutrition, i.e. intravenous supply of amino acids, glucose and lipids during the HD sessions, has become increasingly popular in recent years for treatment of malnourished HD patients [7, 92–95] and favourable effects on nutritional status have been recorded in some of these studies [7, 92, 93]. However, the long-term impact on rehabilitation and survival remains open. Parenteral nutrition has been used successfully in infected HD and CAPD patients [93, 96]. In CAPD patients amino acids have been used instead of glucose as osmotic agents with the dual purpose of acting as a glucose-free osmotic agent and for nutritional support to correct protein malnutrition and amino acid abnormalities [97–116]. Although promising results have been recorded, suggesting a future role of AA solutions in malnourished CAPD patients, the experiences are still limited and untowards effects such as nausea, increase in BUN and enhanced metabolic acidosis have been observed (see below).

7. Amino acid based dialysis fluids

To overcome problems with malnutrition and insufficient dietary protein intake in CAPD patients the use of amino acids (AA) instead of glucose as osmotic agent has been proposed by Oreopoulos *et al.* [98]. The growing insight and concern that CAPD is associated with protein malnutrition and various adverse effects of glucose absorption from the dialysate has stimulated the industry and several investigators to develop and test different AA solutions for CAPD [98–106].

The effect of a daily use of Travasol-based AA solutions have been tested in several studies. Oren *et al.* [104] evaluated the daily use of 1% AA solution over 4 weeks in 6 CAPD patients which resulted in slightly improved nutritional status, increased total body nitrogen, increased serum transferrin, minor changes in plasma AA, increased BUN (+59%) and lowered standard bicarbonate levels (24 to 19 mmol/l).

Schilling *et al.* [105] evaluated the effects of 1% or 2% Travasol based AA solutions over 5–6 months in 3 patients and found rather discouraging results with anorexia in two patients using the 2% AA solution. Schilling *et al.* [106] also reported on the use of a 1% Travasol based AA solution (two exchanges per day) over 1–4 weeks in 12 CAPD patients with peritonitis. The results were discouraging. There was no improvement of nitrogen balance, plasma AA pattern or nutritional status. BUN increased by +50% and 9 out of twelve patients lost their appetite.

In a more recent study Dombros *et al.* [107] evaluated the use of a 1% Travasol based AA solution over 6 months in 5 CAPD patients and found: no improvement of nutritional status, total body nitrogen tended to decrease, there was no change in plasma AA, and BUN increased by +27%.

However the AA composition in the Travasol based solutions (with large amounts of non-essential amino acids) is not tailored to meet the need of uremic patients. Furthermore, they contain an inadequate amount of buffer. Therefore they are not able to normalize the amino acid abnormalities in uremia. Furthermore, they contribute to acidosis. These disadvantages are well recognized by the authors [104–107]. Also, the energy intake of the patients in these four studies was too low; the intraperitoneal supply of AA was therefore probably used as a source of energy.

The importance of combined energy and AA supply was evaluated by Okamura *et al.* [108], who studied the use of a combined of 0.7% AA plus 1.5% glucose solution over 4 weeks in 5 CAPD patients. The AA solution contained essential amino acids. This study resulted in increased plasma concentrations of the essential amino acids, increased plasma transferrin and increased BUN (+20%).

Pedersen *et al.* [109] evaluated the use of a 1% AA solution (two exchanges per day) over 3 months in 6 CAPD patients. The AA solution contained essential as well as non-essential AA. This study resulted in improved plasma AA pattern with increased plasma concentrations of branched-chain AA, increased serum triglycerides and increased serum urea (+30%).

In 1985 a new 1% AA solution based on Renamin (Baxter/Travenol) became available. This AA solution contained amino acids in proportions which takes the amino acid abnormalities in uremic patients into account [19]. Thus, it contained mainly essential AA. The content of lactate was 35 mmol/l.

Young et al. [110] found that the use of a 1% Renamin based AA solution over 12 weeks in 8 CAPD patients resulted in: no change in fasting plasma AA levels, increased plasma transferrin, decreased plasma cholesterol and apolipoprotein B, decreased standard bicarbonat (−13%) and increased serum urea levels (+36%). As part of the same study Dibble et al. [111] reported on decreased 6–8 hour profiles of total cholesterol, LDL cholesterol and apolipoprotein B.

Bruno et al. [112] reported on the use of the 1% Renamin based AA solution over 6 months in 6 CAPD patients and found: improved estimated nitrogen balance (−1.3 g nitrogen/day to +3.1 g nitrogen/day), improved plasma AA profiles (all essential AA except leucine increased), decreased standard bicarbonate (−17%) and increased plasma urea (+29%).

Arfeen et al. [113] evaluated the effect of the same solution (two exchanges per day) over 8 weeks in 7 CAPD patients and found: improved plasma AA 24 hour profiles (especially increased concentrations of branched-chain amino acids), improved plasma albumin, metabolic acidosis (standard bicarbonate −31%) and increased plasma urea (+63%).

These studies show that 1) the improvement of the composition of AA in Renamin-based vs Travasol-based solutions was beneficial, 2) the amount of lactate should be further increased to prevent acidosis, 3) patients included should have signs of protein malnutrition combined with low dietary protein intake to benefit from intraperitoneal supply of AA and 4) energy intake should be sufficient to prevent utilization of AA as an energy source.

For this purpose a new improved 1.1% AA solution has been developed, containing an increased amount of essential AA and an increased amount of lactate (40 mmol/l). The increased concentration of AA (to 1.1%) was needed to provide the same osmotic effect as the 1.36% standard glucose based solution. The 1.1% AA solution has been tested in an international multicenter study in CAPD patients with signs of protein malnutrition [114]. The effect of the AA solution on nitrogen balance was evaluated in patients on a fixed diet containing 0.8 g protein and 25–30 kcal/kg/day. After a control period of 15 days on standard glucose based solutions, the patients were given AA solutions (one or two exchanges per day) to obtain a target protein intake of 1.1–1.3 g/kg/day during the treatment period of 20 days. The results [114] suggest that this AA solution is effective in improving nutritional status of malnourished CAPD patients who have a low protein intake (mean pretrial protein intake of 0.8 g/kg/day). Mean nitrogen balance in the patients increased significantly during the treatment period. Statistically significant increases were also observed in serum transferrin and midarm muscle circumference [114].

These results suggest a promising future role of AA solutions in malnourished CAPD patients. However, increased BUN levels and an increased tendency towards acidosis remain as problems. Furthermore, the cost of commercially available AA solutions will certainly be higher than standard glucose solutions. Nevertheless, the possibility to use AA solutions in malnourished patients should be of value for the role of CAPD treatment in chronic renal failure.

8. Glucose and insulin metabolism

Uremic patients have disturbances in glucose and insulin metabolism with glucose intolerance, hyperinsulinemia, and reduced peripheral sensitivity to insulin [117]. Impaired response to a glucose load in uremic patients seems in part to be due to hyperparathyroidism, since PTH has been shown to produce an inhibiting effect on insulin secretion by the pancreatic beta cells and lack of $1,25 (OH)_2 D_3$ seems also to play a role. In chronic uremic patients the peripheral sensitivity to insulin almost normalized 10 weeks after the start of HD and also improved after treatment with a low-protein diet, suggesting that an accumulation of some dialyzable toxic product from protein metabolism is responsible for the deranged glucose tolerance [117]. A factor from uremic serum, that has a molecular weight between 1000 and 2000 daltons and contains a protein component, has been described which inhibits glucose metabolism in vitro [118]. The underlying disturbances in glucose and insulin metabolism are however only slightly modified by treatment with CAPD despite the efficient removal of middle molecules (see below).

8.1. Glucose absorption and glucose intolerance in CAPD

The alterations in carbohydrate metabolism in uremia are of particular importance in peritoneal dialysis in view of the impact of glucose absorption from the dialysate. The normal pancreatic response to overcome the peripheral insulin resistance in uremia is to further increase the secretion of insulin; however, if the insulin response is inadequate glucose intolerance may become overtly impaired. A potential hazard with peritoneal dialysis is therefore that the intraperitoneal glucose load might exhaust the secretory capacity of the pancreatic beta-cells.

The effects of CAPD on glucose tolerance and serum immunoreactive insulin and glucagon responses to oral glucose were studied in 13 patients undergoing their first year of therapy [119]. Before the start of CAPD, about 50% of the patients displayed decreased glucose tolerance characterized by: an increased peak glucose concentration and a delayed return of blood glucose towards the fasting level; normal fasting blood glucose (< 6.7 mmol/l); and either normal or high serum immunoreactive insulin and glucagon levels. These alterations represent typical findings in uremic patients.

The follow-up studies after 3 and 12 months treatment with CAPD showed no significant changes of any of these variables. The blood glucose concentration over time curves during the tests were in fact almost inseparable. Thus, the treatment with CAPD for one year appeared to have no effect on glucose tolerance and insulin secretory response. Also, there was no statistically significant relationship between the peritoneal glucose supply and any of the variables expressing glucose tolerance (fasting blood glucose, blood glucose during tests, and total and incremental areas under the glucose curve).

These data therefore seem to refute the hypothesis that the continuous glucose load during CAPD results in further impairment of glucose tolerance by exhausting insulin secretion capacity.

It should be noted that the oral glucose tolerance tests in our studies were performed after a 10–14 h interruption of dialysis. In patients performing regular CAPD the presence of glucose intolerance together with the hyperglycemic stress of the continuous absorption of glucose may result in manifest diabetes mellitus.

Although exchanges with isotonic dialysate have only a marginal effect on blood glucose and insulin levels, there is a constant tendency in CAPD patients towards hyperglycemia along with hyperinsulinemia. This tendency is reflected by increased plasma C-peptide levels as well as by an increased ratio between C-peptide and insulin in CAPD patients compared with HD patients, indicating that CAPD patients have continuously increased production of proinsulin [120].

Since sustained hyperinsulinemia may possibly increase atherogenesis, the elevated circulating insulin levels – rather than the relatively small de novo incidence of insulin-dependent diabetes mellitus – constitute a potential risk factor for the majority of the patients during long-term treatment with CAPD. In addition, hyperglycemia in CAPD may lead to formation of both abnormal circulating proteins and abnormal – and potentially atherogenic – structural proteins in the capillary basement membrane. Possible effects of glucose absorption in CAPD are summarized in Table 10.

9. Disturbances in lipid metabolism

Chronic renal failure is associated with deranged lipid metabolism, resulting in typical serum lipoprotein abnormalities and an increased prevalence of hypertriglyceridemia. The "uremic dyslipoproteinemia" shares several similarities with both the type III and type IV hyperlipoproteinemia [121].

The plasma lipid and lipoprotein abnormalities of uremia consists of the following: triglyceride enrichment mainly in very low density lipoprotein (VLDL), high VLDL cholesterol and intermediate density lipoprotein (IDL) cholesterol, reduced high-density lipoprotein (HDL) cholesterol, increased ratio of LDL to HDL cholesterol, impaired catabolism of lipoproteins, a variety of apolipoprotein

Table 10. Glucose absorption in CAPD.

Benefits
Continuous energy supply resulting in improved energy balance
Hyperinsulinemia may promote anabolism
Continuous glucose supply may prevent hypoglycemia
Continuous dialysis with potassium free solutions with glucose contributes to improved control of hyperkalemia

Disadvantages
Hyperglycemia results in formation of abnormal glycosylated proteins
Hyperinsulinemia may promote atherogenesis
Hyperglycemic stress may result in exhaustion of pancreatic betacells
Hyperlipidemia due to continuous glucose supply and hyperinsulinemia
Obesity
Anorexia
Amino acid alterations
Toxic effects on peritoneum

abnormalities and an increased concentration of lipoprotein (a) [121–123]. An improved control of uremia by dialysis does not result in correction of these abnormalities [121–123]. Longitudinal studies in HD patients demonstrate that plasma lipids, apolipoproteins and risk ratios remain unchanged over time [124]. A reduction of total cholesterol with time has been observed which is thought to be a sign of inadequate nutrition [125].

Patients on renal replacement therapy have a high prevalence of arteriosclerotic cardiovascular disease. The lipid abnormalities in dialysis patients with high plasma levels of triglycerides and lipoprotein (a) and low HDL cholesterol are recognized risk factors for arteriosclerosis. However, lipid changes are poor predictors of cardiovascular disease in dialysis patients and the role of the lipid abnormalities in the development of arteriosclerosis in dialysis patients has not been determined.

Studies have documented the efficacy of low-cholesterol, low-saturated-fat isocaloric diets in patients with renal failure. Typically, levels of triglyceride, LDL, and LDL cholesterol decrease, and HDL and HDL cholesterol/total cholesterol ratio increase. The cost of such diets, their acceptability, and their long-term benefits remain to be defined [122]. Diets rich in omega-polyunsaturated fatty acids produce a modulating effect on serum lipids in HD patients showing a decrease in VLDL triglycerides and an increase in HDL-cholesterol, suggesting that such diets could be of value for ameliorating the lipid abnormalities [126]. Interestingly, low total cholesterol in plasma has been shown to be associated with increased mortality in a cohort of more than 13,000 HD patients, presumably because hypocholesterolemia reflects malnutrition in general which is a risk factor for increased morbidity and mortality [5].

9.1. Hyperlipidemic effect of CAPD

A hyperlipidemic effect of CAPD was demonstrated in several studies after introduction of CAPD, and it became apparent that hypertriglyceridemia and serum lipoprotein abnormalities were accentuated within the first months of the treatment [49].

In a study from our group, the effects of CAPD on serum lipids and lipoproteins over the initial year of therapy were studied in 23 patients who were investigated before the start of CAPD, and again after 3 months (17 patients) and 13 months on CAPD [121].

The patients showed a significant and persistent increase of the VLDL-fraction and a smaller, and transitory, increase in LDL-CHOL. These changes resulted in a significant increase of both serum CHOL and serum TG during the first months of the treatment, and the rise in serum CHOL remained statistically significant also after one year on CAPD. VLDL-TG, VLDL, CHOL, and serum TG, and the changes of these variables over the study period, correlated with the amount of glucose supplied intraperitoneally in the dialysis fluid [121]. The results of this study indicate that the continuous peritoneal absorption of glucose (100–200 g/24 hr) during CAPD contributes to potentially atherogenic changes in serum lipids and lipoproteins. However, these changes were, in part, transitory, indicating an adaptation to the peritoneal glucose load in CAPD.

Other studies have demonstrated a hyperlipidemic effect on CAPD [49, 127]; however, the results differ considerably between different reports due to large interindividual variations, varying energy intakes and fluctuations of serum lipids over time in the individual patient [49]. Nevertheless, the results may be summarised as follows. At the start of CAPD, many patients show hypertriglyceriderma, while most have normal serum cholesterol levels. During the first year of CAPD both serum triglycerides and serum cholesterol levels usually increase, at least during the initial months of the treatment. These changes are due to concurrently increased lipid concentration in the VLDL and LDL fractions, whereas the changes in HDL usually are less marked. These changes are more marked in patients already hyperlipidemic at the start of CAPD.

9.2. Hypertriglyceridemia in CAPD

The prevalence of hypertriglyceridemia in patients undergoing long-term treatment with CAPD is reported to be 60–80% [49, 121]. Although many patients on CAPD may develop very high triglyceride concentrations the changes of this variable often fail to reach statistical significance due to large interindividual differences.

Differences in circulating lipid levels between patients, and within individual patients over time, may be due to varying energy intake of the patients. Many centres recommend their patients a restricted use of hypertonic PD fluid, as well as decreased dietary energy intake. These interventions seem to effectively reduce the development of hypertriglyceridemia.

9.3. Hypercholesterolemia in CAPD

The initial hyperlipidemic effect of CAPD involves all three lipoprotein fractions. About 15–30% of the patients develop hypercholesterolemia de novo during their first year on CAPD [49, 121]. The rise in serum cholesterol levels are due to increased levels of both VLDL cholesterol and LDL cholesterol. In addition, an increased HDL cholesterol level has also been observed [128].

Many patients are treated with low protein diets containing 20–40 g of protein/day before the start on CAPD. During CAPD, their dietary protein intake increases to, on the average, about 80 g/day. Since both the quantity and the quality of protein intake are reported to affect serum cholesterol levels it is possible that changes in dietary protein intake may contribute to the observed hypercholesterolemia in the CAPD patients.

This is supported by the finding of a positive correlation between serum albumin and VLDL cholesterol levels, suggesting and interrelationship between protein and lipid status [121]. On the other hand, it has been suggested that protein losses into the dialysate during the CAPD may induce a hypercholesterolemia similar to that observed in the nephrotic syndrome [129]. This suggestion is supported by observations of a significant correlation between serum cholesterol levels and dialysate protein losses in children undergoing CAPD [130]. However, Breckenridge et al. found little indication that loss of apolipoproteins, or lipoproteins, into the dialysate could account for any changes in plasma lipoproteins during CAPD [128].

9.4. Transitory changes of serum lipoprotein levels during CAPD

Changes in serum lipid concentrations during CAPD are transitory, except in a small group of patients who show steadily increasing concentrations especially of the VLDL fraction. Peak levels of serum cholesterol and triglycerides are usually reached within 3–12 months, with a subsequent fall during the following months to pretreatment levels as noted previously [121, 127].

Thus, the uremic dyslipoproteinemia remains essentially unchanged after 1 yr of CAPD compared to the pretreatment status, with the exception of a small group of patients in whom serum triglyceride levels increase significantly. In fact, serum lipid levels after one year on CAPD are approximately the same in HD and CAPD patients; CAPD patients may even show better (less reduced) HDL cholesterol levels than HD patients [116, 131].

The finding that the hyperlipidemic effect of CAPD is transitory in many patients may indicate a metabolic adaptation to the glucose load during CAPD but it may also be due to changes in energy intake over time [121].

9.5. Increased plasma lipoprotein (a) levels in CAPD

Increased plasma Lp (a) levels is a strong independent risk factor for coronary heart disease, similar to and synergistic with increased LDL cholesterol levels [132]. Hitherto only a few clinical conditions have been found to significantly affect plasma Lp (a) concentrations [132]. In patients with chronic renal failure Lp (a) levels have been reported to be markedly increased in CAPD patients [133–138] with only one exception [139], whereas increased [134, 135, 138–142] as well as normal [133] levels have been reported in HD patients. In most comparative studies, Lp (a) levels seem to be higher in CAPD compared to HD patients. In transplanted patients Lp (a) levels have been reported to be normal or only slightly elevated [138, 142, 143], and furthermore, high plasma levels of apo (a) in terminal renal failure patients have been reported to fall after renal transplantation [143].

The mechanisms behind the increased Lp (a) levels in CAPD patients are however largely unknown, but the difference in Lp (a) levels observed in several studies between CAPD and HD patients suggest that the choice of dialysis procedure might be of importance. Our group has recently observed that the increased Lp (a) levels in CAPD patients correlate to parameters related to the peritoneal transport rate of beta-2-microglobulin and albumin, suggesting that the increased Lp (a) levels may in part be due to the protein losses in CAPD [144].

10. Carnitine depletion

L-carnitine (L-3-hydroxy-4-N-trimethylaminobutyrate) is an amino acid which transfers long-chain fatty acids from the cytoplasm through the inner mitochondrial membrane, the myocardial and skeletal muscle exhibiting the highest concentrations of this compound. A deficiency of L-carnitine may lead to impaired oxidation of long-chain fatty acids, inefficient energy production and derangements of intermediary metabolism.

The data in the literature disagree as to whether CAPD patients develop carnitine depletion; low as well as normal plasma and muscle concentrations of carnitine and carnitine esters have been reported [145, 146]. In a recent review it was concluded that only a minor part of HD patients seem to exhibit severe carnitine deficiency [147]. Several positive clinical affects of L-carnitine administration to HD patients have been reported, including increased well-being and muscle strength, improved nutritional status and reduction of cardiac arrhythmias and angina, suggesting that carnitine depletion may be a pathogenic factor in skeletal muscle weakness and uremic heart disease [147]. Reports of the effects of L-carnitine supplementation on blood lipids and lipoproteins are inconsistent.

The role, if any, of L-carnitine supplementation in CAPD remains to be elucidated. Patients eating well will probably have well-maintained carnitine stores due to an adequate intake of both carnitine and the carnitine precursors, lysine and methionine, in the food. However, CAPD patients with a poor nutritional intake may be at risk of developing a carnitine deficiency.

11. Mineral metabolism and nutrition

11.1. Calcium and phosphorous

Uremia is associated with accumulation of phosphorous, mainly in the form of phosphate, and reduced intestinal absorption of calcium caused by vitamin D deficiency and resistance to the actions of vitamin D. The goal of management is the achievement of normal serum calcium and phosphate levels, reduction of secondary hyperparathyreoidism, and restoration of normal vitamin D activity. This is discussed elsewhere in this book.

It has been recognized for many years that patients with primary hyperparathyroidism may show evidence of weight loss, weakness, and muscle atrophy. Whether this is caused by a specific effect of parathyroid hormone (PTH) on protein synthesis or breakdown, or is indirectly mediated by its generalized effects in causing fatigue, anorexia, neuropsychiatric disturbances, myopathy, and bone disease is an open question [148].

Secondary hyperparathyroidism is a common complication in chronic renal failure patients. In some cases with severe hyperparathyroidism the nutritional status may improve markedly after parathyroidectomy. However, the role of hyperparathyroidism as a protein catabolic factor in such patients has not been determined.

Both calcium and phosphorous balances were greater with a higher protein diet (1.44 g/kg/day) vs a lower protein diet (0.98 g/kg/day) in the study by Blumenkrantz et al. [40]. Calcium balance was always neutral or positive when dietary intake was equal to 720 mg/day or greater. Calcium uptake, or loss, from dialysate was rather small compared with the calcium intake from the diet. These observations concerning mineral metabolism in CAPD show that adult patients undergoing CAPD may go into positive mineral balance, especially with high protein diets [116].

11.2. Potassium and magnesium

In the study by Blumenkrantz et al. [40] potassium balance was neutral with a protein diet of 0.98 g/kg/day and significantly positive with a diet containing 1.44 g/kg/day. Potassium balance was positive when potassium intake was 67 mmol/day or greater. Dialysate losses accounted for approximately 70% of potassium output and about 30% was from feces.

In the same study, dietary magnesium intake and balance were greater with the higher protein diet and magnesium balance was significantly positive with both diets (see above) [40]. Patients using dialysis fluids containing 0.75 mmol/l have only small losses of magnesium into the dialysate.

12. Anemia and erythropoietin

Renal anemia is usually present in the most dialysis patients and may be severe, especially in anephric patients and in patients who are inadequately dialyzed. Anemia leads to fatigue, diminishing exercise capacity, and physical inactivity, which may contribute to muscle wasting, and malnutrition. A correction of anemia with recombinant human erthropoietin (rHu-EPO) is reported to improve nutritional status to a moderate degree in HD patients [9], which is presumably a secondary effect of anemia correction on general well-being, appetite and physical work capacity rather than a specific effect of rH-EPO. Although anemia is often less severe in CAPD patients than in HD patients, correction of anemia with rHu-EPO in CAPD patients may contribute to improved nutritional status.

13. Vitamins and trace elements

The metabolism, concentrations and requirements of trace elements and vitamins in chronic renal failure patients, HD patients and CAPD patients have recently been extensively reviewed [149]. Inadequate dietary intake, altered metabolism in uremia, and vitamin loss into dialysate may lead to vitamin deficiencies, in particular deficiencies of water-soluble vitamins [116, 149]. In addition, trace element metabolism is frequently altered in chronic renal failure patients [116, 149].

13.1. Water-soluble vitamins

The serum levels of pyridoxine (B_6), thiamine (B_1), folic acid and ascorbic acid have been reported to be low in various studies of dialysis patients [149]. Vitamin B_6 coenzymes play a vital role in every aspect of amino acid utilization. Vitamin B_6 deficiency impairs the synthesis, interconversion, catabolism and cellular uptake of amino acids; the need for vitamin B_6 is particularly critical if amino acid intake is limited [150]. Changes in fasting plasma amino acid and serum high-density lipoprotein levels after correction of the biochemical deficiency of vitamin B_6 in dialysis patients indicates its role in the pathogenesis of the abnormal amino acid and lipid metabolism [151]. There are data suggesting that the daily requirement of pyridoxine is higher in dialysis patients than in normal subjects and that such patients should be supplemented with a minimum of 10 mg/day [150]. Supplementation of the diet and vitamin C has also been recommended. However, high intake of vitamin C may aggravate hyperoxalemia in dialysis patients.

Blumberg et al. [152] studied vitamin status in 10 CAPD patients who were on an unrestricted diet and not receiving vitamin supplements. The fat-soluble vitamin A and E showed increased plasma levels, while vitamin B_1, vitamin B_6, folic acid, and vitamin C levels were low or borderline low due to losses into the dialysate and inadequate dietary intake of these vitamins. Vitamin B_2 and B_{12} were normal, Blumberg et al. suggested that CAPD patients should receive 30–40 mg of vitamin B_1, 10–15 mg of vitamin B_6, 0.5–1 mg of folic acid and 100–200 mg of vitamin C.

Henderson et al. [153] studied 9 patients who were investigated before starting CAPD, after 6 months of CAPD with oral water-soluble vitamin supplementation, and after a further 6 months without vitamin supplementation. they observed normal plasma levels of vitamins A and E. Vitamin C levels were increased before the commencement of CAPD and did not change after 6 months of dialysis with supplementation of 100 mg of vitamin C. After a further 6 month period without supplementation, levels fell significantly. Vitamin B_1 and B_2 levels were normal during the study period, but vitamin B_6 levels decreased significantly after 6 months of CAPD without any supplementation. Vitamin B_{12} status and serum and red-cell folate levels were either normal or increased. Henderson et al. suggested that CAPD patients should receive vitamin C and B_6, but probably not folic acid [153].

Boeschoten et al. [154] investigated vitamin status and dialysate losses of vitamins in 31 patients who had been maintained on CAPD for 0.5 to 36 months. The patients did not receive vitamins supplements for at least 4 weeks before sampling. In 24 h dialysates only losses of vitamin C and folic acid exceeded their excretions in the urine of healthy subjects. Deficiencies of vitamin B_6 – which could not be explained by increased loss via dialysates – were found in 58% of the patients, vitamin C was deficient in 50%, and folic acid in 17% of the patients. The authors concluded that CAPD patients should be given vitamin B_6, vitamin C, folic acid and probably also thiamine (vitamin B_1) [154].

13.2. Fat-soluble vitamins

Vitamin A tends to accumulate in CAPD patients as well as in other patients with renal failure and may have potentially harmful effects. Administration of vitamin A supplements should therefore be avoided. Vitamin D and its active forms should not be prescribed as a routine but should be given on the basis of an evaluation of the calcium-phosphate status and bone metabolic status and taking the risks of hyperphosphatermia and hypercalcermia into consideration.

Vitamin E acts as a scavenger for oxygen – free radicals to function as an antioxidant. Blood levels of vitamin E have been found to be normal or high in most studies in uremic patients [149]. Selenium is also involved in the scavenger system that protects against free oxygen radicals. Selenium deficiency has been reported in CAPD patients [155]. Deficiency of vitamin K has not been reported in renal failure patients.

13.3. Trace elements

Uremic patients have altered blood and tissue concentrations of many trace elements [116, 149]. High levels have been attributed to impaired renal elimination or contamination of dialysis fluid and low levels of trace elements may occur due to inadequate dietary intake or loss of protein bound trace elements into the peritoneal dialysate. The single most important abnormality is the consistent finding of accumulation of aluminum in uremic patients; this problem is discussed elsewhere in this book.

Several groups have found decreased levels of zinc in serum, leucocytes and muscle of CAPD patients [149]. Zinc deficiency has been reported to be associated with hypogeusia, anorexia, hyperprolactinemia and impotence which have been alleviated by zinc administration. However, these results have not been generally confirmed and the role of zinc deficiency and requirements for extra supply of zinc in the diet of CAPD patients remains at present controversial [116, 149].

Thomson et al. [155] investigated trace element status in 31 patients who were on CAPD for at least 3 months. The predominant abnormalities were a marked reduction in red cell concentrations of zinc and copper; however, the clinical significance, if any, of these alterations could not be established. Whole blood chromium concentrations were increased to twice normal in the CAPD patients [155]. Wallaeys et al. [156] observed major deviations from normality for bromine (low), chromium (high) and cobalt (high serum concentrations) in CAPD patients.

The clinical significance of these alterations have not been established as yet. However, supplementation with zinc has been suggested in patients with hypogeusia, anorexia and muscle weakness.

14. Recommended nutritional intakes and treatment of malnutrition

14.1. Protein and energy

To ensure a safe supply of protein it is recommended that CAPD patients should have a protein intake of at least 1.2 g/kg BW/day of which a large part should preferably be of high biological value – i.e., have a high content of essential amino acids (usually animal proteins from milk, eggs and meat). Some patients probably require less than this to maintain nitrogen equilibrium [41]; however, it is difficult to identify such patients by simple methods. Other patients may benefit by eating as much as 1.4–2.1 g protein/kg/day, especially during the initial months of the treatment [41]. Estimation of protein intake by the use of urea kinetic modeling may help to identify patients with a suboptimal protein intake; repeated values below 1.0 g/kg BW/day should arouse the suspicion that the protein intake is too low and the patient should be advised to increase the intake of dietary protein. Those who are initially malnourished or later develop signs of protein-energy malnutrition may require higher amounts of protein (and energy) for repleting the protein and energy stores.

A regular follow-up of estimated protein intake assessed by urea kinetics is strongly advisable. In CAPD patients, this is very simple but requires the condition of steady-state as regards nitrogen balance. In patients with even slight variations in body weight or serum urea level which could suggest net protein catabolism or anabolism the estimation of protein intake based on urea kinetic modelling should be interpreted with great caution [41, 157]. Formulas for calculations of the estimated protein intake in CAPD patients based on urea appearance are provided in [41].

In these formulas [41] we used data from 34 nitrogen balance studies (23 studies from our own investigation [41], and 11 studies from the investigation by Blumenkrantz et al. [40]) to calculate regression equations describing the relationship between total nitrogen appearance (TNA) and non-protein nitrogen appearance (NPNA), respectively, and urea nitrogen appearance (UNA). Equations were derived by which the *protein equivalent* of TNA (PNA), i.e. 6.25 TNA, and the *protein equivalent* of NPNA (PNPNA), i.e. 6.25 NPNA, may be *calculated directly from UNA* which is directly measured (in 24 h collection of drained dialysate plus urine). In stable CAPD patients who are not strongly catabolic or anabolic, PNA may be used to estimate dietary protein intake (DPI) and PNPNA may be used to estimate the net protein intake (NPI) (DPI – total protein losses (PL)). The following equations can be used for estimating PNPNA from UNA:

PNPNA (g/day) =
13 + 7.31 UNA (g/day) (Eq. 3A [41])

or, using urea appearance (UA) instead of UNA:

PNPNA (g/day) =
13 + 0.261 (mmol/day) (Eq. 3B [41])

In adult stable CAPD patients estimated PNPNA reflects NPI, i.e., DPI – PL. To estimate DPI from these two equations above, the 24 h PL (in dialysate plus urine) should be determined and added to PNPNA.

Equations based on the relationship between UNA and TNA can be used for estimating PNA from UNA and UA, respectively:

PNA (g/day) =
19 + 7.62 × UNA (g/day)   (Eq. 4A [41])

and

PNA (g/day) =
19 + 0.272 UA (mmol/day)   (Eq. 4B [41])

Estimations of DPI from PNA according to equations 4A and 4B are valid only in the absence of excessive PL.

The addition of oral essential amino acids to the diet may increase the total intake and the biological value of ingested protein and may improve the nutritional status. Special amino acid formulas have been developed with a modified amino acid composition (high valine, addition of tyrosine and serine) designed to compensate for amino acid deficiencies present in uremia [158].

As pointed out previously, energy depletion may be at least as common as protein depletion in CAPD patients. An energy intake of ≥ 35 kcal (145 kJoule)/kg BW/day is generally recommended, higher intakes being necessary if the patient is energy-depleted or is regularly doing physical exercise. It is recommended that 35% of the energy should be given as fat, a substantial part of which should be unsaturated. Obese patients, on the other hand, may be recommended restrictions in the use of hypertonic dialysis fluid and a low energy intake for body weight reduction which may have salutary effects regarding glucose tolerance and lipid abnormalities. If the dietary energy supply is considered insufficient, liquid or powder mixtures of glucose polymers may be used as supplement.

For a more complete supplementation of both protein and energy several liquid formulas containing large amounts of protein of high biological value, lipids and carbohydrates and having a low content of phosphate, potassium and sodium in a small amount of fluid are available, which are suitable for the supplementary nutrition of dialysis parents. Patients may drink such supplements; they may prefer to sip small amounts with meals or slowly during the day.

If severe malnutrition develops in CAPD patients despite adequate dialysis and measures to eliminate anorectic and catabolic factors, enteral or parenteral nutritional supplementation with energy and amino acids may be necessary. Severely malnourished patients may have to be hospitalized temporarily for such treatment. Enteral nutrition through a thin nasogastric tube is less expensive than parenteral nutrition and does not carry the risk of catheter sepsis and is therefore preferable whenever possible.

In patients who need parenteral nutrition with amino acids, a mixture of essential and non-essential amino acids seems better than a solution with only essential amino acids. Special amino acid solutions designed to compensate for the specific disturbances in amino acid metabolism of renal failure patients have been designed and used successfully [92, 95]. Tyrosine which may be indispensable for patients with renal failure has a low water solubility and can therefore only be provided in small amounts as free amino acid in solutions for parenteral nutrition. However, dipeptides of tyrosine which have a higher water solubility are effectively utilized in uremic patients [159] and glycyl-tyrosine has been used to increase the tyrosine content of an amino acid solution for parenteral nutrition of dialysis patients [92]. Energy should be provided simultaneously as hypertonic glucose or a mixture of glucose and lipid emulsion.

Recombinant human growth hormone administration enhances the growth velocity of children undergoing CAPD [160] and may reduce urea generation and improve the efficiency of dietary protein utilization in stable adult HD patients [161]. Growth hormone may turn out to be a useful adjunctive therapy to diminish body protein catabolism in CAPD patients in the future.

14.2. Minerals, vitamins and trace elements

Sodium and water can be removed easily with CAPD and most patients can therefore be allowed a liberal intake of salt and water. This is a major advantage with CAPD compared with HD. Some patients may even require a high dietary intake of salt to prevent hypotension. A high dietary intake of sodium (6–8 g/day) and water (1500–300 ml/day) may enable the patient to use more hypertonic exchanges. This results in increased dialysate outflow volumes, increased dialysate clearances of small molecules, and increased energy intake in the form of glucose absorption. However, this treatment may be undesirable in obese patients or in patients with marked hypertriglyceridemia. It should be noted that extensive use of hypertonic solutions may result in hypernatremia [162, 163].

In some CAPD patients a lower sodium intake may be required to prevent excessive weight gain, extracellular fluid overload edema, hypertension, and cardiac congestion. However, most patients find a low-salt diet tasteless and unpalatable. Although a dietician may advise the patient how to compose individual menus that are palatable in spite of salt restriction one often has to allow patients a higher salt intake to increase the palatability in order to ensure an adequate intake of energy and protein.

The minimum requirements for potassium and magnesium are probably met by any diet that meets energy and protein requirements. Note that hypokalemia may indicate a poor nutritional intake whereas hyperkalemia is often due to excessive intake of fruits or vegetables. However, elimination of fruit and vegetables from the diet introduces problems of diet palatability and potential vitamin deficiencies. It is therefore preferable to administer potassium-binding ion exchange resins to CAPD patients with hyperkalemia. Potassium restriction is thus rarely necessary in CAPD patients. This is a major advantage with CAPD vs HD.

The recommended intake of calcium in CAPD patients is about 0.8–1.0 g/day; however, a low concentration of calcium in the dialysis fluid may allow a higher intake (see Chapter 18). This intake is fulfilled provided that the intake of protein and energy from natural foodstuffs is adequate, especially since the majority of CAPD patients are in addition treated with calcium carbonate or calcium acetate as phosphate binder. The need of oral calcium supplements is probably lower in CAPD patients than in HD patients. However, oral calcium supplementation e.g. in the form of calcium carbonate may reduce not only intestinal phosphate absorption but it may also correct mild acidosis. Therefore oral calcium supplementation is recommended for CAPD patients as tolerated by serum calcium. The requirement of phosphorous is probably met by any diet that meets energy and protein requirements. Hypophosphatemia may suggest insufficient intakes of protein and energy. A relatively low intake of phosphate (0.6–1.0 g of elementary phosphorous) is however recommended since the dialytic treatment *per se* may be insufficient to remove the excess phosphate. Hyperphosphatemia may be due to excessive intakes of milk or cheese, resulting also in hypercalcemia, and some dietary restrictions may be necessary. In general however, restrictions of dietary phosphorous intake may be difficult to combine with a sufficient dietary protein intake.

The advent of rH-EPO for correction of renal anemia, necessitates an increased supply of iron to non-overloaded patients as the hemoglobin mass increases. The increasing use of rH-EPO in CAPD patients requires assessment of iron stores because iron depletion will impair the response to rH-EPO and rH-EPO can cause iron deficiency. The increased iron requirements should be met if possible by oral substitution with iron [149].

It is questionable whether CAPD patients who have an adequate nutritional intake need additional vitamins. Whether vitamin supplements need to be prescribed in CAPD patients depends on the dietary intake, concurrent medication and nutritional status. There is no or little evidence that supplements of cobolamine, biotin, niacin, pantothenic acid, vitamin A or vitamin E are required [149]. However, it is generally recommended that CAPD patients take water-soluble vitamins, since some of these vitamins are lost in the dialytic procedure and since deficiencies of vitamins, especially low pyridoxine (vitamin B_6) levels, have been recorded in groups of patients. Depletion of vitamin C, vitamin B_1, vitamin B_2 vitamin B_6 and folic acid may occur during CAPD and the patients may benefit from supplementation with these vitamins. However, the need of supplemental folic acid, thiamine (vitamin B_1, riboflavin (vitamin B_2) appears to be low.

Polyvitamin preparations containing vitamin A should be avoided because of the possibility of vitamin A toxicity. No supplemental vitamin B_{12}, vitamin K or E is recommended. Supplementation with 10 mg pyridoxine as well as supplements of ascorbic acid 100 mg/day are usually recommended. In patients with a poor nutritional intake supplementation with folic acid 1 mg/day and thiamine (vitamin B_1) 2 mg/day can be considered (see Table 9). Multivitamin tablets containing these water-soluble vitamins (but not fat-soluble vitamins) may be given routinely as a safety precaution to all CAPD patients.

15. Summary

A large proportion of peritoneal dialysis patients demonstrate signs of protein-energy malnutrition due to disturbances in protein and energy metabolism, hormonal derangements, infections and other superimposed illnesses, and poor food intake because of anorexia, nausea and vomiting, caused by uremic toxicity, in particular in underdialyzed patients. These factors may have serious consequences in the form of failure of rehabilitation, and increased morbidity and mortality.

The most extensive evaluation of nutritional status in CAPD patients included 224 patients from six centers in Europe and North-America. In this study, a subjective nutritional assessment based on 21 variables derived from biochemical measurements, history and clinical examinations, showed that 41% of the patients had mild (33%) or severe (8%) malnutrition. The variables that were most correlated with the subjective nutritional assessment score and with another included: albumin, midarm muscle circumference (MAMC), signs of muscle wasting, loss of subcutaneous fat, and history of anorexia. Malnutrition was more common in females than in males and in diabetics vs non-diabetics. Patients with severe malnutrition had minimal or no residual renal function and were either older or had been on CAPD longer than other patients.

The safe protein requirement in CAPD patients appears to be increased to about twice that of normal individuals. Thus, about 1.2 g protein/kg/day may be required to obtain a positive nitrogen balance in CAPD patients; however, some patients are in neutral balance with as low protein intake as 0.7g/kg/day. The nitrogen balance is strongly dependent on the energy intake which often is lower than 35 kcal/kg/day in CAPD patients.

CAPD patients generally have a lower protein intake than HD patients, but may have lower average protein requirements than HD patients. In HD the dialytic procedure is a strong intermittent stimulus of net catabolism. On the other hand, the protein losses by the dialysate in CAPD patients are unparalleled in the HD patients. Peritonitis, when present, is a strong catabolic stimulus. Anorexia with low protein and energy intake results from a variety of factors of which underdialysis with insufficient control of uremic toxicity seems to be a major one. The daily dose of dialysis is of critical importance for the intake of protein in dialysis patients.

The relationship between the dose of dialysis expressed as Kt/V for urea and the protein intake (assessed from urea appearance) is more favourable in CAPD than in HD patients, suggesting that control of potential uremic toxins which cause anorexia is better in CAPD patients than in HD patients, at the same Kt/V dose of dialysis.

Underdialyzed CAPD patients may enter a vicious circle of low protein and energy intake and enhanced protein catabolism, leading to progressive malnutrition and muscle wasting and a fatal outcome. To break this vicious circle the intensity of dialysis should be increased, acidosis corrected and measures should be taken to increase the supply of energy and protein.

Amino acid based dialysis fluids may provide new opportunities to improve the nutritional status in malnourished CAPD patients; however increased serum urea levels and a tendency towards acidosis are still problems.

Ackowledgements

The present study was supported by grants from the Swedish Medical Research Council (Project No. 1002) and Baxter Healthcare Corporation. The authors wish to thank Ann Hellström and Katarina Dagfjord for excellent secretarial assistance.

References

1. Lindholm B, Bergström J. Nutritional aspects on peritoneal dialysis. Kidney Int 1993; 42 (Suppl 38): 165–71.
2. Bergström J, Lindholm B. Nutrition and adequacy of dialysis. How do hemodialysis and CAPD compare? Kidney Int 1993; 43 (Suppl 40): 39–50.
3. Bergström J. Protein catabolic factors in patients on renal replacement therapy. In-depth Review. Blood Purific 1985; 3: 215–36.
4. Guarnieri G, Toigo G, Situlin R, Faccini L, Coli U, Lannini S, Bazzato G, Dardi F, Campanacci L. Muscle biopsy studies in chronically uremic patients: evidence for malnutrition. Kidney Int 1983; 24 (Suppl 16): 187–93.
5. Lowrie EG, Lew NL. Death risk in hemodialysis patients: the predictive value of commonly measured variables and an evaluation of death rate differences between facilities. Am J Kidney Dis 1990; 15: 458–82.
6. Jacob V, Le Carpentier JE, Salzano S, Naylor V, Wild G, Brown CB, El Nahas AM. IGF-I, a marker of undernutrition in hemodialysis patients. Am J Clin Nutr 1990; 52: 39–44.
7. Bilbrey GL, Cohen TL. Identification and treatment of protein calorie malnutrition in chronic hemodialysis patients. Dial Transplant 1989; 18: 669–77.
8. Marckmann P. Nutritional status and mortality of patients in regular dialysis therapy. J Intern Med 1989; 226: 429–32.
9. Bárány P, Pettersson E, Ahlberg M, Hultman E, Bergström J. Nutritional assessment in anemic hemodialysis patients treated with recombinant human erythropoietin. Clin Nephrol 1991; 35: 270–9.
10. Rayner HC, Sroud DB, Salamon KM, Strauss BJG,

Thomson NM, Atkins RC, Wahlqvist ML. Anthropometry underestimates body protein depletion in hemodialysis patients. Nephron 1991; 59: 33–40.
11. Williams P, Kay R, Harrison J, Mcneil K, Petit J, Kellman B, Mendez M, Klein M, Ogilvie R, Khanna R, Carmichael D, Oreopoulos DG. Nutritional and anthropometric assessment of patients on CAPD over one year: Contrasting changes in total body nitrogen and potassium. Perit Dial Bull 1981; 1: 82–7.
12. Nolph KD, Sorkin MN, Rubin J, Arfania D, Prowant BF, Fruto L, Kennedy D. Continuous ambulatory peritoneal dialysis. Three-year experience at one center. Ann Intern Med 1980; 92: 609–13.
13. Kurtz SB, Wong VH, Anderson CF, Vogel JP, McCarthy JT, Mitchell JC. Continuous ambulatory peritoneal dialysis. Three years' experience at the Mayo Clinic. Mayo Clin Proc 1983; 58: 633–9.
14. Heide B, Pierratos A, Khanna R, Petit J, Ogilvie R, Harrison J, McNeil K, Siccion Z, Oreopoulos DG. Nutritional status of patients undergoing continuous ambulatory peritoneal dialysis (CAPD). Perit Dial Bull 1983; 3: 138–41.
15. Schilling H, Wu G, Petit J, Harrison J, Mcneil M, Siccion Z, Oreopoulos DG. Nutritional status of patients on long-term CAPD. Perit Dial Bull 1985; 5: 12–8.
16. Young GA, Kopple JD, Lindholm B, Vonesh EF, de Vecchi A, Scalamogna A, Castelnova C, Oreopoulos DG, Anderson GH, Bergström J, Dichiro J, Gentile D, Nissenson A, Sakhrani L, Brownjohn AM, Nolph KD, Prowant BF, Algrim CE, Martis L, Serkes KD. Nutritional assessment of continuous ambulatory peritoneal dialysis patients: An international study. Am J Kidney Dis 1991; 27: 462–71.
17. Nelson EE, Hong CD, Pesce AL, Peterson DW, Singh S, Pollak VE. Anthropometric norms for the dialysis population. Am J Kidney Dis 1990; 16: 32–7.
18. Maiorca R, Cancarini GC, Camerini C, Brunori G, Manili L, Movilli E, Feller P, Mombelloni S. Is CAPD competitive with haemodialysis for long-term treatment of uraemic patients? Nephrol Dial Transplant 1989; 4: 244–53.
19. Alvestrand A, Fürst P, Bergström J. Plasma and muscle free amino acids in uremia: influence of nutrition with amino acids. Clin Nephrol 1982; 18: 297–305.
20. Bergström J, Alvestrand A, Fürst P. Plasma and muscle free amino acids in maintenance hemodialysis patients without protein malnutrition. Kidney Int 1990; 38: 108–14.
21. Lindholm B, Alverstrand A, Fürst P, Bergström J. Plasma and muscle free amino acids during continuous ambulatory peritoneal dialysis. Kidney Int 1989; 35: 1219–26.
22. Bansal VK, Popli S, Pickering J, Ing TS, Vertuno LL, Hano JE. Protein-calorie malnutrition and cutaneous anergy in hemodialysis maintained patients. Am J Clin Nutr 1980; 33: 1608–11.
23. Young GA, Young JB, Young SM, Hobson SM, Hildreth B, Brownjohn AM, Parsons FM. Nutrition and delayed hypersensitivity during continuous ambulatory peritoneal dialysis in relation to peritonitis. Nephron 1986; 43: 177–86.
24. Degoulet P, Legrain M, Reach I, Aime F, Devries C, Rojas P, Jacobs C. Mortality risk factors in patients treated by chronic hemodialysis. Nephron 1982; 31: 103–10.
25. Shapiro JI, Argy WP, Rakowski TA, Chester A, Siemsen AS, Schreiner GE. The unsuitability of BUN as a criterion for prescription dialysis. Trans Am Soc Artif Intern Organs 1983; 29: 129–34.
26. Acchiardo SR, Moore LW, Latour PA. Malnutrition as the main factor in morbidity and mortality of hemodialysis patients. Kidney Int 1983; 24 (Suppl 16): 199–203.
27. Hartier HR. Review of significant findings from the National Cooperative Dialysis Study and recommendations. Kidney Int 1983; 23 (Suppl 13): 107–12.
28. Teehan BP, Schleifer CR, Brown JM, Sigler MH, Raimondo J. Urea kinetic analysis and clinical outcome on CAPD. A five year longitudinal study. Adv Perit Dial 1991; 6: 181–5.
29. Blake PG, Sombolos K, Abraham G, Weissgarten J, Pemberton R, Lian Chu G, Oreopoulos DG. Lack of correlation between urea kinetic indices and clinical outcomes in CAPD patients. Kidney Int 1991; 39: 700–6.
30. European Dialysis and Transplant Association-European Renal Association, EDTA/ERA Registry Report, Demography of Dialysis and Transplantation in Europe, 1984. Nephrol Dial Transplant 1986; 1: 1–8.
31. Excerpts from United States Renal Data System, 1991 Annual Data Report, V. Survival probabilities and causes of death. Am J Kidney Dis 1991; 18 (suppl 2): 49–60.
32. Fao/Who. Energy and protein requirements. Report of a joint Fao/Who ad hoc Expert Committee. Tech Rep Ser No 522, Geneva, World Health Organization, 1973.
33. Ginn He, Frost A, Lacy WW. Nitrogen balance in hemodialysis patients. Am J Clin Nutr 1968; 21: 385–93.
34. Kopple JD, Shinaberger JH, Coburn JW, Sorensen MK, Rubini ME. Optimal dietary protein treatment during chronic hemodialysis. Trans Am Soc Artif Organs 1969; 15: 302–8.
35. Kluthe R, Lüttgen FM, Capetianu T, Heinze V, Katz N, Südhoff A. Protein requirements in maintenance hemodialysis. Am J Clin Nutr 1978; 31: 1812–20.
36. Borah MF, Schoenfeld PY, Gotch FA, Sargent JA, Wolfson M, Humphreys MH. Nitrogen balance during intermittent dialysis therapy of uremia. Kidney Int 1978; 14: 491–500.
37. Laird NM, Berkey CS, Lowrie EG. Modeling success or failure of dialysis therapy: The National Coorperative Dialysis Study. Kidney Int 1983; 23 (Suppl 13): 101–6.
38. Gotch FA, Sargent JA. A mechanistic analysis of

the National Cooperative Dialysis Study. Kidney Int 1985; 28: 526–34.
39. Parker TF, Reed RB, Lowrie EG. Description of the participating centers and the patient population in the National Cooperative Dialysis Study. Kidney Int 1983; 23 (Suppl 13): 37–41.
40. Blumenkrantz MJ, Kopple JD, Moran JK, Coburn JW. Metabolic balance studies and dietary protein requirements in patients undergoing continuous ambulatory peritoneal dialysis. Kidney Int 1982; 21: 849–61.
41. Bergström J, Fürst P, Alvestrand A, Lindholm B. Protein and energy intake, nitrogen balance and nitrogen losses in patients treated with continuous ambulatory peritoneal dialysis. Kidney Int 1993; 44: 1048–57.
42. Lysaght MJ, Pollock CA, Hallet MD, Ibels LS, Farrell PC. The relevance of urea kinetic modeling to CAPD. Trans Am Soc Artif Intern Organs 1989; 35: 784–90.
43. Monteon FJ, Laidlaw SA, Shaib JK, Kopple JD. Energy expenditure in patients with chronic renal failure. Kidney Int 1986; 30: 741–7.
44. Schoenheyder F, Heilskov NSC, Olsen K. Isotopic studies on the mechanism of negative nitrogen balance produced by immobilization. Scand J Clin Bal Invest 1954; 6: 178–88.
45. Berkelhammer CH, Baker JP, Leither LA, Uldall PR, Whittall R, Slater A, Wolman SL. Whole-body protein turnover in adult hemodialysis patients as measured by ^{13}C-leucine. Am J Clin Nutr 1987; 46: 778–83.
46. Goodship THJ, Lloyd S, Clague MB, Bartlett K, Ward MK, Wilkinson R. Whole body leucine turnover and nutritional status in continuous ambulatory peritoneal dialysis. Clin Sci 1987; 73: 463–9.
47. Kishi K, Miytani K, Inoue G. Requirement and utilization of egg protein by Japanese young men with marginal intakes of energy. J Nutr 1978; 198: 658–69.
48. Slomowitz LA, Monteon FJ, Grosvenor M, Laidlaw SA, Kopple JD. Effect of energy intake on nutritional status in maintenance hemodialysis patients. Kidney Int 1989; 35: 704–11.
49. Lindholm B, Bergström J. Nutritional management of patients undergoing peritoneal dialysis in Peritoneal Dialysis, edited by Nolph KD, Boston Kluwer Academic Publishers 1989; pp 230–60.
50. Von Baeyer H, Gahl GM, Riedinger H, Borowzak R, Averdunk R, Schurig R, Kessel M. Adaptation to CAPD patients to the continuous peritoneal energy uptake. Kidney Int 1983; 23: 29–34.
51. Papadoyannakis NJ, Stefanidis CJ, Mcgeown M. The effect of the correction of metabolic acidosis on nitrogen and potassium balance of patients with chronic renal failure. Am J Clin Nur 1984; 40: 623–7.
52. Straumann E, Keller U, Küry D, Bloesch D, Thélin A, Arnaud MJ, Stauffacher W. Effect of acute acidosis and alkalosis on leucine kinetics in man. Clin Physiol 1992; 12: 39–51.
53. Hara Y, May RC, Kelly RC, Mitch WE. Acidosis, not azotemia, stimulates branched-chain, amino acid catabolism in uremic rats. Kidney Int 1987; 32: 808–14.
54. May RC, Hara Y, Kelly RA, Block KP, Buse M, Mitch WE. Branched-chain amino acid metabolism in rat muscle: Abnormal regulation in acidosis. Am J Physiol 1987; 252: 712–8.
55. Greiber S, Mitch WE. Mechanisms for protein catabolism in uremia: metabolic acidosis and activation of proteolytic pathways. Miner Electrolyte Metab 1992; 18: 233–6.
56. Tizianello A, Deferrari G, Garibotto G, Gurreri G, Robaudo C. Renal metabolism of amino acids and ammonia in subjects with normal renal function and in patients with chronic renal insufficiency. J Clin Invests 1980; 65: 1162–73.
57. Fukuda S, Kopple JD. Uptake and release of amino acids by the kidney of dogs made chronically uremic with uranyl nitrate. Min Electr Metab 1980; 3: 248–60.
58. Pitts RF, Macleod MB. Synthesis of serine by the dog kidney in vivo. Am J Physiol 1972; 222: 394–8.
59. Rubin J, Flynn MA, Nolph KD. Total body potassium – a guide to nutritional health in patients undergoing continuous ambulatory peritoneal dialysis. Am J Clin Nutr 1981; 34: 94–8.
60. Rubin J, Kirchner K, Barnes T, Teal N, Ray R, Bower JD. Evaluation of continuous ambulatory peritoneal dialysis. Am J Kidney Dis 1983; 3: 199–204.
61. Ward RA, Shirlow MJ, Hayes JM, Chapman GV, Farrell PC. Protein catabolism during hemodialysis. Am J Clin Nutr 1979; 32: 243–2449.
62. Farrell PC, Hone PW. Dialysis-induced catabolism. Am J Clin Nutr 1980; 33: 1417–22.
63. Löfberg E, Wernerman J, Noree LO, Decken A, Vinnars E. Ribosome and free amino acid content in muscle during hemodialysis. Kidney Int 1991; 39: 984–9.
64. Lim VS, Bier DM, Flanigan M, Symreng T. The effect of hemodialysis on protein metabolism. J Am Soc Nephrol 1990; 1: 366.
65. Wathen RL, Keshaviah P, Hommeyer P, Cadwell K, Comty CM. The metabolic effects of hemodialysis with and without glucose in the dialysate. Am J Clin Nutr 1978; 31: 1870–5.
66. Kopple JD, Swendseid ME, Shinaberger JH, Umezawa CY. The free and bound amino acids removed by hemodialysis. Trans Am Soc Artif Intern Organs 1973; 19: 309–13.
67. Wolfson M, Jones MR, Kopple JD. Amino acid losses during hemodialysis with infusion of amino acids and glucose. Kidney Int 1982; 21: 500–6.
68. Tepper T, Hem GK, van der Klip HG, Donker AJM. Loss of amino acids during hemodialysis: effect of oral essential amino acid supplementation. Nephron 1981; 29: 25–9.
69. Bannister DK, Acchiardo SR, Moore LW, Kraus AP. Nutritional effects of peritonitis in continuous ambulatory peritoneal dialysis (CAPD) patients. J Am Diet Ass 1987; 87: 53–6.
70. Verger C, Larpent L, Dumontet M. Prognostic value of peritoneal equilibration curves (EC) in

71. Cheung AK. Biocompatibility of hemodialysis membranes. J Am Soc Nephrol 1990; 1: 150–61.
72. Betz M, Haensch GM, Rauterberg EW, Bommer J, Ritz E. Cuprammonium membranes stimulates interleukin-1 release and arachidonic acid metabolism in monocytes in the absence of complement. Kidney Int 1988; 34: 67–73.
73. Haefener-Cavaillon N, Cavaillon MJ, Laude M, Kazatchkine MD. C3a/C3adesArg induces production and release of interleukin-1 (IL-1) by cultured human monocytes. J Immunol 1987; 139: 794–9.
74. Lonnemann G, Bingel M, Floege J, Koch KM, Shaldon S, Dinarello CA. Detection of endotoxin-like interleukin-1-inducing activity during in vitro dialysis. Kidney Int 1988; 33: 29–35.
75. Evans RC, Holmes CJ. In vitro study of the transfer of cytokine-inducing substances across selected high-flux hemodialysis membranes. Blood Purif 1991; 9: 92–101.
76. Bingel M, Lonnemann G, Koch KM, Dinarello CA, Shaldon S. Enhancement of in-vitro human interleukin-1 production by sodium acetate. Lancet 1987; 1: 14–6.
77. Flores EA, Bistrian BR, Pomposelli JJ, Dinarello CA, Blackburn GL, Istfan NW. Infusion of tumor necrosis factor. Cachectin promotes muscle catabolism in the rat. J Clin Invest 1989; 83: 1614–22.
78. Baracos V, Rodeman HP, Dinarello CA, Goldberg AL. Stimulation of muscle protein degradation and prostaglandin E2 release by leukocytic pyrogen (interleukin-1). N Engl J Med 1983; 308: 553–8.
79. Nawabi MD, Block KP, Chakrabarti MC, Buse MG. Administration of endotoxin, tumor necrosis, or Interleukin-1 to rats activates skeletal muscle branched-chain alpah-keto acid dehydrogenase. J Clin Invest 1990; 85: 256–63.
80. Gutierrez A, Alvestrand A, Wahren J, Bergström J. Effect of in vivo contact between blood and dialysis membranes on protein catabolism in humans. Kidney Int 1990; 38: 487–94.
81. Gutierrez A, Bergström J, Alvestrand A. Protein catabolism in sham hemodialysis: The effect of different membranes. Clin Nephrol 1992, 38: 20–9.
82. Young VR, Munro HN. Methylhistidine and muscle protein turnover: an overview. Fed Proc 1978; 37: 2291–300.
83. Schoenfeld PY, Henry RR, Laird NM, Roxe DM. Assessment of nutritional status of the National Cooperative Study population. Kidney Int 1983; 23 (Suppl 13): 80–8.
84. Oreopoulos DG, Marliss E, Anderson GH, Oren A, Dombros N, Williams P, Khanna R, Rodella H, Brandes L. Nutritional aspects of CAPD and the potential use of amino acid containing dialysis solutions. Perit Dial Bull 1983; 3: 10–5.
85. Lindsay RM, Spanner E. A hypothesis: The protein catabolic rate is dependent upon the type and amount of treatment in dialyzed uremic patients. Am J Kidney Dis 1989; 13: 382–9.
86. Farrell PC, Randerson DH. Comparison of CAPD with HD and IPD. In: Gahl GM, Kessel M, Nolph KD (eds), Advances in Peritoneal Dialysis. Excerpta Medica, Amsterdam 1981; pp. 131–7.
87. Lysaght MJ, Vonesh EF, Gotch F, Ibels L, Keen M, Lindholm B, Nolph KD, Pollock CA, Prowant B, Farrell PC. The influence of dialysis treatment modality on the decline of remaining renal function. Trans Am Soc Artif Intern Organs 1991; 37: 598–604.
88. Bergström J, Alvestrand A, Lindholm B, Tranæus A. Relationship between Kt/V and protein catabolic rate (PCR) is different in continuous peritoneal dialysis (CPD) and haemodialysis (HD) patients. J Am Soc Nephrol 1991; 2: 358.
89. Keshaviah PR, Nolph KD, van Stone JC. The peak concentration hypothesis: A urea kinetic approach to comparing the adequacy of continuous ambulatory peritoneal dialysis (CAPD) and hemodialysis. Perit Dial Int 1989; 9: 257–60.
90. Bergström J, Alvestrand A. Therapy with branched-chain amino acids and keto acids in chronic uremia. In: Adibi SA, Fekl W, Langenbeck U, Schaunder P (eds), Branched-chain amino and keto acids in health and disease. Basel S. Karger, 1984; pp 391–422.
91. Bergström J. Nutritional requirements of hemodialysis patients. In: Mitch WE, Klahr S (eds), Nutrition and the kidney. Little, Brown and Company, Boston 1993; pp 263–89.
92. Cano N, Labastile-Coeyrehourq J, Lacombe P, Stroumza P, Di Costanzo-Dufetel J, Durbec JP, Coudray-Lucas C, Cynober L. Perdialytic parenteral nutrition with lipids and amino acids in malnourished hemodialysis patients. Am J Clin Nutr 1990; 52: 726–30.
93. Vehe KL, Brown RO, Moore LW, Acchiardo SR, Luther RW. The efficacy of nutrition support in infected patients with chronic renal failure. Pharmacotherapy 1991; 11: 303–7.
94. Snyder S, Bergen C, Sigler MH, Teehan BP. Intradialytic parenteral nutrition in chronic hemodialysis patients. ASAIO Trans 1991; 37: M373–5.
95. Toigo G, Situlin R, Tamaro G, del Bianco A, Giuliani V, Dardi F, Vianello S, Toffoletto P, Faccini L, Guarnieri G. Effect of intravenous supplementation of a new essential amino acid formulation in hemodialysis patients. Kidney Int 1989; 27: 278–81.
96. Rubin J. Nutritional support during peritoneal dialysis-related peritonitis. Am J Kidney Dis 1990; 15: 551–5.
97. Lindholm B, Bergström J. Amino acids in CAPD solutions: lights and shadows. In: La Greca G, Ronco C, Feriani M, Chiaramonte S, conz P (eds), Peritoneal dialysis.Wichtig Editore, P. Milano 1991; pp 139–43.
98. Oreopoulos DG, Grassweller P, Katirtzoglow A et al.: Amino acids as an osmotic agent (instead of glucose) in continuous ambulatory peritoneal

dialysis. In: Legrain M (ed), Continuous ambulatory peritoneal dialysis. Excerpta Medica: Amsterdam, 1980; 335–40.
99. Williams P, Marliss EB, Anderson GH et al. Amino acid absorption following intraperitoneal administration in CAPD patients. Perit Dial Bull 1982; 2: 124–30.
100. Goodship THJ, Lloyd S, McKenzie PW et al. Short term studies on the use of amino acids as an osmotic agent in continuous ambulatory peritoneal dialysis. Clinical Science 1987; 73: 471–8.
101. Lindholm B, Werynski A, Bergström J. Peritoneal dialysis with amino acid solutions: fluid and solute transport kinetics. Artificial Organs 1988; 12: 2–10.
102. Young GA, Dibble JB, Taylor AE, Kendall S, Brownjohn AM. Effects of amino acid based CAPD fluid on protein and amino acid losses during a 5 month study (abstract). Fifth Int Congr on Nutrition and Metabolism in Renal Disease. Strasbourg, France, 1988.
103. Steinhauser HB, Lubrich-Birker I, Kluthe R, Hörl WH, Schollmeyer P. Amino acid dialysate stimulates peritoneal prostaglandin E2 generation in humans, in Advances in Continuous Ambulatory Peritoneal Dialysis. In: Khanna R et al. (eds), Peritoneal Dialysis Bulletin. Inc: Toronto 1988; 21–6.
104. Oren A, Wu G, Anderson GH et al. Effective use of amino acid dialysate over four weeks in CAPD patients. Perit Dial Bull 1983; 3: 66–73.
105. Schilling H, Wu G, Petit J, Mitwalli A, Anderson HG, Ogilvie R, Oreopoulos DG. Effects of prolonged CAPD with amino acid-containing solutions in three patients, in Advances in Continuous Ambulatory Peritoneal Dialysis. In: Khanna R et al. (eds), Peritoneal Dialysis Bulletin. Inc: Toronto, 1985; 49–55.
106. Schilling H, Wu G, Petit J, Mittwalli A, Anderson HB, Ogilvie R, Oreopoulos DG. Use of amino acid containing solutions in continuous ambulatory peritoneal dialysis patients after peritonitis: results of a prospective controlled trial. Proc EDTA-ERCA 1985; 22: 421–5.
107. Dombros NV, Prutis K, Tong M et al. Six-month overnight intraperitoneal amino-acid infusion in continuous ambulatory peritoneal dialysis (CAPD) patients – no effect on nutritional status. Perit Dial Int 1990; 10: 79–84.
108. Okamura K, Yamauchi J, Nakahamma H, Ohmura N, Okada M, Shirai D, Kitaoka T. The effects of adding essential amino acids to the dialysis solution of continuous ambulatory peritoneal dialysis patients, in Machine Free Dialysis for Patient Convenience: The Fourth ISAO Official Satellite Symposium on CAPD, edited by Maekawa M et al., ISAO Press: Cleveland, 1984; 103–7.
109. Pedersen FB, Dragsholt C, Frifelt JJ, Trostman AF, Ekelund S, Paaby P. Alternate use of amino acid and glucose solutions in CAPD. Perit Dial Bull 1985; 5: 215–8.
110. Young GA, Dibble JB, Hobson SM, Tompkins L, Gibson J, Turney JH, Brownjohn AM. The use of an amino-acid-based CAPD fluid over 12 weeks. Nephrol Dial Transplant 1989; 4: 285–92.
111. Dibble JB, Young GA, Hobson SM, Brownjohn AM. Amino-acid-based continuous ambulatory peritoneal dialysis (CAPD) fluid over twelve weeks: effects on carbonhydrate and lipid metabolism. Perit Dial Bull 1990; 10: 71–7.
112. Bruno M, Bagnis C, Marangella M, Roocra L, Cantaluppi A, Linari F. CAPD with an amino acid dialysis solution: a long-term cross-over study. Kidney Int 1990; 35: 1189–94.
113. Arfeen S, Goodship THJ, Kirkwood A, Ward MK. The nutritional/metabolic and effects of 8 weeks of continuous ambulatory peritoneal dialysis with a 1% amino acid solution. Clin Nephrol 1990; 33: 192–9.
114. Jones MR, Martis L, Algrim CE, Bernard D, Swartz R, Messana J, Bergström J, Lindholm B, Lim V, Serkes KD, Vonesh E, Kopple JD. Amino acid solutions for CAPD: rationale and clinical experience. Miner Electrolyte Metab 1992; 18: 309–15.
115. Lindholm B, Park MS, Bergström J. Supplemented dialysis: Amino acid-based solutions in peritoneal dialysis, in Evolution in Dialysis Adequacy. In: Bonomini V (ed), Contrib. Nephrol. Basel, Karger 1992; 103: 168–82.
116. Kopple JD, Hirschberg R. Nutrition and peritoneal dialysis, in Nutrition and the Kidney, edited by Mitch WE, Klahr S, Boston, Little, Brown and Co, 1993; pp 290–313.
117. Mak RHK, De Fronzo RA. Glucose and insulin metabolism in uremia. Nephron 1992; 61: 377–82.
118. McCaleb ML, Izzo MS, Lockwood DH. Characterization and partial purification of a factor from uremic human serum that indices insulin resistance. J Clin Invest 1985; 75: 391–6.
119. Lindholm B, Karlander SG. Glucose tolerance in patients undergoing continuous peritoneal dialysis. Acta Med Scand 1986; 220: 447–83.
120. Wideröe TE, Smeby LC, Myking OL. Plasma concentrations and transperitoneal transport of native insulin and C-peptide in patients on continuous ambulatory peritoneal dialysis. Kidney Int 1984; 25: 82–7.
121. Lindholm B, Norbeck HE. Serum lipids and lipoproteins during continuous ambulatory peritoneal dialysis. Acta Med Scand 1986; 220: 143–51.
122. Appel G. Lipid abnormalities in renal disease. Kidney Int 1991; 39: 169–83.
123. Attman PO, Alaupovic P. Lipid abnormalities in chronic renal insufficiency. Kidney Int 1991; 39 (Suppl 31): 16–23.
124. Burrell D, Antignani A, Fein PA, Goldwasser P, Mittman N, Avram MM. Longitudial survey of apolipoproteins and atherogenic risk in hemodialysis and continuous ambulatory peritoneal dialysis patients. ASAIO Trans 1990; 36: 331–5.
125. Lapuz M, Avram MM, Lustig A, Goldwasser P, Antignant A, Fein PA, Mittman N. Fall of cholesterol with time on dialysis: impact on atherogenicity. ASAIO Trans 1989; 35: 258–60.

126. Bilo HJG, van der Heide H, Gans Rob, Donker AJM. Omega-3 polyunsaturated fatty acids in chronic renal insufficiency. Nephron 1991; 57: 385–93.
127. Ramos JM, Heaton A, McGurk JG, Wark MK, Kerr DNS. Sequential changes in serum lipids and their subfractions in patients receiving continuous ambulatory peritoneal dialysis. Nephron 1983; 35: 20–3.
128. Breckenridge WC, Roncari DAK, Khanna R, Oreopoulos DG. The influence of continuous ambulatory peritoneal dialysis on plasma lipoproteins. Atherosclerosis 1982; 45: 249–58.
129. Gokal R, Ramos JM, McGurk JG, Ward MK, Kerr DNS. Hyperlipidemia in patients on continuous ambulatory peritoneal dialysis. In: Gahl GM, Kessel M, Nolph KD (eds), Advances in Peritoneal dialysis Amsterdam, Excerpta Medica 1981; pp 430–3.
130. Broyer M, Niaudet P, Champion G, Jean G, Chopin N, Czernichow P. Nutritional and metabolic studies in children on continuous ambulatory peritoneal dialysis. Kidney Int 1983; 24 (suppl 15): 106–10.
131. Chan MK, Baillod RA, Chuah P, Sweny P, Raftery MJ, Varghese Z, Moorhead JF. Three years' experience of continuous ambulatory peritoneal dialysis. Lancet 1981; 1: 1409–12.
132. Scanu AM. Lipoprotein (a), a genetic risk factor for premature coronary heart disease. JAMA 1992; 267: 3326–9.
133. Haffner SM, Gruber KK, Aldrete G, Morales PA, Stern MP, Tuttle KR. Increased lipoprotein (a) concentrations in chronic renal failure. J Am Soc Nephrol 1992; 3: 1156–62.
134. Shoji T, Nishizawa Y, Nishitani H, Yamakawa M, Norii H. High serum lipoprotein (a) concentrations in uremic patients treated with continuous ambulatory peritoneal dialysis. Clin Nephrol 1992; 38: 271–6.
135. Webb AT, Reavely DA, O'Donnell M, O'Connor B, Seed M, Brown EA. Lipoprotein (a) in patients on maintenance haemodialysis and continuous ambulatory peritoneal dialysis. Nephrol Dial Transplant 1993; 8: 609–13.
136. Anwar N, Bhatnagar D, Short CD, Mackness MI, Durrington PN, Prais H, Gokal R. Serum lipoprotein (a) concentrations in patients undergoing continuous ambulatory peritoneal dialysis. Nephrol Dial Transplant 1993; 8: 71–4.
137. Thillet J, Faucher C, Issad B, Allouace M, Chapman J, Jacobs C. Lipoprotein (a) in patients treated by continuous ambulatory peritoneal dialysis. Am J Kidney Dis 1993; 22: 226–32.
138. Barbagallo CM, Averna MR, Sparacino V, Galione A, Caputo F, Scafidi V, Amato S, Mancino C, Defalù AB, Notarbartolo A. Lipoprotein (a) levels in end-stage renal failure and renal transplantation. Nephron 1993; 64: 560–4.
139. Kandoussi A, Cachera C, Paginez D, Dracon M, Fruchart JC, Tacquet A. Plasma level of lipoprotein Lp (a) is high i predialysis or hemodialysis, but not in CAPD. Kidney Int 1992; 42: 424–5.
140. Parra HJ, Mezdour H, Cachera C, Dracon M, Tacquet A, Fruchart JC. Lp (a) lipoprotein in patients with chronic renal failure treated by hemodialysis. Clin Chem 1987; 33: 721.
141. Cressman MD, Heyka RJ, Paganini EP, O'Neil J, Skibinski CI, Hoff HF. Lipoprotein (a) is an independent risk factor for cardiovascular disease in hemodialysis patients. Circulation 1992; 86: 475–82.
142. Heimann P, Josephson MA, Fellner SK, Thistlethwaite Jr JR, Stuart FP, Dasgupta A. Elevated Lipoprotein (a) levels in renal transplantation and hemodialysis patients. Am J Nephrol 1991; 11: 470–4.
143. Black IW, Vilcken DEL. Decrease in apolipoprotein (a) after renal transplantation: Implications for lipoprotein (a) metabolism. Clin Chem 1992; 38: 353–7.
144. Heimbürger O, Stenvinkel P, Berglund L, Tranæus A, Lindholm B. Lipoprotein (a) correlates with peritoneal albumin clearance in CAPD (abstract). 14th Annual Conference on Peritoneal Dialysis 1994. Perit Dial Int 1994; 14 (Suppl 1): S97.
145. Moorthy AV, Rosenblum M, Rajaram R, Shug AL. A comparison of plasma and muscle carnitine levels in patients on peritoneal or hemodialysis for chronic renal failure. Am J Nephrol 1983; 3: 205–8.
146. Amair P, Gregordiadis A, Rodela H, Ogilvie R, Khanna R, Brandes L, Roncari DAK, Oreopoulos DG. Serum carnitine in patients on continuous ambulatory peritoneal dialysis (CAPD). Perit Dial Bull 1982; 2: 11–2.
147. Wanner C, Hörl WH. Carnitine abnormalities in patients with renal insufficiency. Nephron 1988; 50: 89–102.
148. Kopple JD, Cianciaruso B, Massry SG. Does parathyreoid hormone cause protein wasting? Contr Nephrol 1980; 20: 138–48.
149. Gilmour ER, Hartley GH, Goodship THJ. Trace elements and vitamins in renal disease, in Nutrition and the Kidney, edited by Mitch WE, Klahr S, Boston, Little, Brown and Co, 1993; pp 114–31.
150. Kopple JD, Mercurio K, Blumenkrantz MJ, Jones MR, Tallos J, Roberts C, Card B, Saltzman R, Casciato DA, Swendseid ME. Daily requirement for pyridoxine supplements in chronic renal failure. Kidney Int 1981; 19: 694–704.
151. Kleiner MJ, Tate SS, Sullivan JF, Charmi J. Vitamin B6 deficiency in maintenance dialysis patients: metabolic effects of repletion. Am J Clin Nutr 1980; 33: 1612–9.
152. Blumberg A, Hanck A, Sander G. Vitamin nutrition nutrition in patients on continuous ambulatory peritoneal dialysis (CAPD). Clin Nephrol 1983; 20: 244–50.
153. Henderson IS, Leung ACT, Shenkin A. Vitamin status in continuous ambulatory peritoneal dialysis. Perti Dial Bull 1984; 4: 143–5.
154. Boeschoten EW, Schrijver J, Krediet RT, Arisz L. Deficiencies of vitamins in CAPD patients: the effect of supplementation. Nephrol Dial Transplant 1988; 2: 187–93.
155. Thomson MM, Stevens BJ, Humphrey TJ, Atkins

RC. Comparison of trace elements in peritoneal dialysis, hemodialysis and uremia. Kidney Int 1983; 23: 9–14.
156. Wallaeys B, Cornelis R, Mees L, Lameire N. Trace elements in serium, packed cells, and dialysate of CAPD patients. Kidney Int 1986; 30: 599–604.
157. Lindholm B, Heimbürger O, Ahlberg A, Werynski A, Waniewski J. Urea kinetic modelling (UKM) in peritoneal dialysis, in Urea Kinetic Modelling, edited by Lopot F, EDTNA-ERCA Series, Vol 4, Ruddervoorde, D. Verlinde 1990; pp 133–46.
158. Garibotto G, Deferrari G, Robaudo C, Saffioti S, Sala MR, Paoletti E, Tizianello A. Effects of a new amino acid supplement on blood AA pools in patients with chronic renal failure. Amino Acids 1991; 1: 319–29.
159. Druml W, Lochs H, Roth E, Hübl W, Balcke P, Lenz K. Utilization of tyrosine dipeptides and acetyltyrosine in normal and uremic humans. Am J Physiol 260 (Endocrinol Metab) 1991; 23: 280–5.
160. Fine RN. Growth in children undergoing CAPD/CCPD/APD. Perit Dial Int 1993; 13 (Suppl 2): S247–50.
161. Ziegler TR, Lazarus JM, Young LS, Hakim R, Wilmore DW. Effects of recombinant human growth hormone in adults receiving maintenance hemodialysis. J Am Soc Nephrol 1991; 2: 1130–5.
162. Heimbürger O, Waniewski J, Werynski A, Tranæus A, Lindholm B. Peritoneal transport characteristics in CAPD patients with permanent loss of ultrafiltration. Kidney Int 1990; 38: 495–506.
163. Heimbürger O, Waniewski J, Werynski A, Lindholm B. A quantitative description of solute and fluid transport during peritoneal dialysis. Kidney Int 1992; 41: 1320–32.

16 Peritonitis

WILLIAM F. KEANE AND STEPHEN I. VAS

1. Introduction — 473
2. Pathogenesis of peritonitis — 474
   2.1. Portals of entry — 475
      2.1.1. Intraluminal infections — 476
      2.1.2. Periluminal infections — 476
      2.1.3. Transmural (intestinal) infections — 476
      2.1.4. Haematogenous infections — 476
      2.1.5. Other endogenous infections — 477
      2.1.6. Environmental infections — 477
      2.1.7. Biofilm — 477
   2.2. Inflammatory response — 477
      2.2.1. Inflammatory mediators — 477
      2.2.2. Fibrin, fibronectin — 477
      2.2.3. Cellular response — 477
3. Defense mechanisms of the peritoneum — 478
   3.1. Humoral factors — 478
   3.2. Cellular factors — 478
4. Microbiological diagnosis of peritonitis — 479
   4.1. Specimen — 479
   4.2. Gram stain — 479
   4.3. Culture procedure — 479
   4.4. Antibiotic sensitivities — 480
   4.5. Cell count — 480
5. Presenting signs and symptoms of peritonitis — 480
6. Clinical course of peritonitis — 480
   6.1. Incubation period — 480
   6.2. Length of symptoms — 480
   6.3. Exit site and tunnel infections — 480
   6.4. Relapse, recurrence or reinfection — 481
7. Causative organisms of peritonitis — 481
   7.1. Viruses — 481
   7.2. Protozoa, parasites — 482
   7.3. Bacteria — 482
      7.3.1. Gram positive organisms — 482
      7.3.2. Gram negative organisms — 483
      7.3.3. Anaerobic organisms — 483
      7.3.4. Mycobacteria — 483
   7.4. Fungi — 484
   7.5. Cryptogenic — 484
      7.5.1. "Sterile" or aseptic peritonitis — 484
      7.5.2. Eosinophilic peritonitis — 484
      7.5.3. Neutrophilic peritonitis — 484
      7.5.4. Bloody fluid — 485
8. Treatment of peritonitis — 485
   8.1. General considerations — 485
   8.2. Antibiotics — 485
   8.3. Length of treatment — 489
   8.4. Side effects — 489
   8.5. Peritoneal lavage — 489
   8.6. The role of heparin — 489
   8.7. Treatment protocols — 489
   8.8. Treatment of exit site and tunnel infections — 489
   8.9. Catheter removal — 490
9. Complications of peritonitis — 490
   9.1. Intestinal perforation and diverticulitis — 490
   9.2. Adhesions, sclerosing peritonitis — 490
   9.3. Mortality — 490
10. Differential diagnostic problems — 490
    10.1. Constipation — 491
    10.2. Appendicitis — 491
    10.3. Pancreatitis — 491
    10.4. Cholecystitis — 491
    10.5. Perforated ulcer — 491
    10.6. Malignancy — 491
11. Prevention of peritonitis — 491
    11.1. Sterile connections — 491
       11.1.1. U.V. box and sterile weld — 491
       11.1.2. O-Z connection — 491
       11.1.3. Disconnect systems — 491
       11.1.4. Millipore filter — 492
       11.1.5. Auxiliary devices for the handicapped — 492
    11.2. Antibiotic prophylaxis — 492
    11.3. Patient selection — 492
    11.4. New catheters — 492
    11.5. Alternate dialysis solutions — 492
12. Evaluation of peritonitis rate — 492
13. Future considerations — 493
Reference — 493

1. Introduction

The frequent occurrence of peritonitis – one of the major complications of peritoneal dialysis – has hindered the development and acceptance of this technique.

In the mid-1940's, Seligman [1], Fine [2] and Frank [3] reported a method of continuous peritoneal lavage, but the high incidence of infection and technical difficulties, as well as the introduction of the artificial kidney, discouraged its supporters. In 1951, Grollman [4] drew attention again to the value of peritoneal dialysis in the treatment of acute renal failure when he introduced intermittent peritoneal lavage. Later, Doolan [5] confirmed its safety and effectiveness in human subjects. Another major advance, the introduction of the nylon catheter which allowed safe access to the peritoneal cavity [6, 7], made possible intermittent peritoneal dialysis with infection rates of 5.2 to 7.5 episodes of peritonitis per patient year of dialysis [8, 9].

In 1964 Palmer and associates [10] began to provide longterm intermittent peritoneal dialysis employing an indwelling silicone rubber irrigating catheter device which Tenckhoff [11] later modified to its present form. This technique reduced infection rates to 0.23 to 1.2 episodes of peritonitis per patient year [12–18].

In 1976 Popovich and colleagues [19] described the technique of continuous ambulatory peritoneal dialysis (CAPD) for the treatment of chronic renal failure. The incidence of peritonitis with this method, employing bottled dialysate, was 4.6 episodes of peritonitis per patient year [20]. This technique was subsequently modified and replaced the bottled dialysate with a plastic dialysate bag [21]. This arrangement was more convenient for the patients and substantially reduced the number of manipulations of the catheter and therefore the infection rate. Subsequently, many workers using this technique have reported rates of peritonitis varying from 1.2 to 6.3 episodes per patient year [20–26]. As noted above, these high rates of infection have been the major criticism of the procedure [27–30], but with increasing control of peritonitis, CAPD could become the dialysis of choice for many patients with endstage renal disease.

Changes in the connecting technique of the transfer sets (titanium connector), and use of long-life tubing – less frequent tubing changes – further reduced the peritonitis risk.

The major change came with reports [273, 257] from Italy on the use of the so-called Y set. The use of this method reduced peritonitis to 1/24–1/36 month. Successively, a multicenter trial in Canada confirmed the results [258].

The "flush-before-fill" or the "disconnect" method, as these systems came to be known, have become widely accepted in their many variations, making it possible for the average unit to report one episode of peritonitis every two years though many units report even better results [236].

Connection devices were also introduced (UV flash, Sterile Connection Device [128, 129]), which helped in lowering chances of contamination for the manually or visually handicapped.

In a recent study [179] it was found that about 40% of US patients are on some form of disconnect system. The time to first peritonitis of patients on Y sets was 20.6 months compared to the standard (spike) connection where the time to first peritonitis was 11.4 months.

Intermittent peritoneal dialysis has a lower rate of peritonitis. It is not unusual to observe peritonitis rates of one every 3 to 5 years. The reason for this difference is not quite clear. It is tempting to speculate that the shorter time patients are on peritoneal dialysis means fewer connections and smaller volumes of fluid used, and that this has something to do with this decreased rates. This argument is fallacious. If one compares certain parameters of intermittent peritoneal dialysis with continuous ambulatory peritoneal dialysis it becomes obvious that the number of connections made during intermittent peritoneal dialysis is larger, the total volume of fluid used is more, and therefore none of these factors may be important in the development of peritonitis. The only factor which is different in the two populations is that intermittent peritoneal dialysis patients do not have dialysis fluid in the abdominal cavity for the major part of their program (usually 2 days off, 12 to 18 hours on). It is speculative but plausible that peritoneal defense mechanisms are operating better when the peritoneum does not contain large volumes of fluid (see discussion on defense mechanisms below).

CCPD or continuous cycling peritoneal dialysis and APD (automated peritoneal dialysis) have reported peritonitis rates between CAPD and IPD [32]. These modalities of treatment are becoming increasingly popular.

2. Pathogenesis of peritonitis

Initially, those who had to deal with peritonitis episodes in peritoneal dialysis patients conceived peritonitis as similar to the experience with surgical peritonitis [33]. While this was a reasonable approach, it soon became clear that peritonitis developing in dialysis patients has considerable differences from that of surgical peritonitis.

While small amounts of contamination do not usually cause surgical peritonitis, as evidenced by the large number of laparotomies which heal without any evidence of clinical peritonitis, minor contaminations in the peritoneal dialysis patient will lead to peritonitis. Similarly, surgical peritonitis develops mainly when the abdominal cavity has a major soil, usually by fecal content, and therefore removal of the contaminating material is essential. In peritoneal dialysis such large amounts of contaminants are rare. Finally, in surgical peritonitis about 30% of the patients will show bacteraemia as part of the disease [33], while in peritonitis of peritoneal dialysis patients positive blood cultures are the rare exception rather than a frequent event, and when positive blood cultures are observed they are usually the harbinger of a haematogenous source of peritoneal infection [70]. Finally, the distribution of organisms isolated from CAPD peritonitis shows predominantly gram positive organisms (Table 1).

This distribution changed somewhat due to the introduction of methods reducing the so-called intraluminal infections and therefore reducing the contribution of gram positive skin organisms with a slight proportionate increase of gram negative organisms.

Therefore, peritonitis in CAPD patients has now been accepted as a special disease entity whose management requires a different approach.

More similar to peritonitis in PD patients is the disease called spontaneous bacterial peritonitis [34-39] which is occasionally seen in patients suffering from cirrhosis of the liver with ascites. It is believed that the lack of reticuloendothelial function of the liver is the primary reason why these patients develop spontaneous peritonitis. These patients also have large volumes of fluid in their abdominal cavity which may also explain some of the similarities.

2.1. Portals of entry

Microbial environment and host are living in a symbiotic relationship. The occasional penetrations of infectious organisms into an intact host are met with defense and usually the small number of invaders is destroyed [40]. The outcome, therefore, is dependent on the delicate balance of the number of invaders vs. defense. Bacterial penetration is probably a frequent event (it is known, for example, that minor exertions like brushing of teeth or bowel movements will lead to transient shortlasting bacteremias in many normal individuals) and will only rarely lead to major infections.

We do not know how frequently infectious events occur in peritoneal dialysis patients. It is conceivable that these events are more frequent than the episodes of peritonitis [184, 185]. Since the conditions which lead to peritonitis are not known, all portals of entry have to be considered seriously, and to reduce peritonitis all of them have to be managed with great care.

Surveillance cultures from abdominal skin site, and nostrils, hands of peritoneal dialysis patients before they enter a dialysis program have been done in our unit. The results of such surveillance are shown in Table 2.

These are the areas from which incidental contaminations of peritoneal dialysis patients can occur. In fact, if one compares the Staphylococcus aureus phagetype or the Staphylococcus epidermidis biotype isolated from the peritoneal fluid of these patients during peritonitis episodes with the skin biotype, as shown in Table 3, it is obvious that the patients are at high risk from their own flora rather than from acquiring infections from the environment or other people. This observation has been confirmed by others [234].

It is therefore possible to generate a listing (Table 4) which estimate the probable route of entry from

Table 1. Distribution of organisms isolated from peritonitis episodes.

Coagulase negative staphylococci	30–40%
Staphylococcus aureus	20%
Streptococcus sp	10–15%
Neisseria sp	1–2%
Diphtheroid sp	1–2%
E. Coli	5–10%
Pseudomonas sp	5–10%
Enterococcus	3–6%
Klebsiella sp	1–3%
Proteus sp	3–6%
Acinetobacter sp	2–5%
Anaerobic organisms	2–5%
Fungi	2–10%
Other (mycobacteria, etc)	2–5%
Culture negative	0–30%

Table 2. Surveillance cultures of 47 CAD patients.

Organism	Hand	Abdomen	Nostril	Total
CN Staph	66 (76%)	56 (69%)	59 (63%)	181 (69%)
S aureus	3 (3%)	4 (5%)	7 (7%)	13 (5%)
Gram negative	3 (3%)	4 (5%)	8 (9%)	15 (6%)
Dipht, yeast etc	15 (7%)	18 (22%)	20 (21%)	53 (20%)

Table 3. Correlation of isolates of skin and peritonitis of CAPD patients.

Organism	Same type	Different type
S epidermidis (biotype)	45 (94%)	–
S epidermidis (plasmid)	3 (50%)	3 (50%)
S aureus (phagetype)	19 (86%)	3 (14%)

the type of organisms isolated. For example, it is assumed that 2/3 of S. epidermidis infections occur through the intraluminal route while only 1/2 of S. aureus infections occur through the same route. Such a listing is helpful (and by experience close to accurate) in understanding the role of various portals of entry.

2.1.1. Intraluminal infections

Intraluminal infections occur when bacteria enter the internal pathway of peritoneal dialysis tubing through the internal surface or through cracks in the tubing. The commercial dialysis fluids are prepared with great care and they can be considered sterile. There have been no episodes ascribed to peritoneal dialysis from commercial sources in the last few years [41]. Additions through the port to the peritoneal dialysis bag have to be made with sterile precautions and fresh vials of drugs should be used for each addition.

Intraluminal infections may occur more frequently than believed, but do not result in peritonitis. In a study done by us [184], it was shown that if one cultures routinely clear bags from patients not showing signs of peritonitis a certain number will grow organisms. These organisms usually are Propionobacteria though occasionally other organisms are grown. All these cultures require prolonged growth (usually 8–12 days) indicating that their number is very small. The patients do not require treatment. This observation emphasizes the experience that routine surveillance cultures of bags from patients not showing symptoms are unnecessary and misleading [185].

Most of the intraluminal infections develop after accidental touch contamination of the connector site or disconnections of the dialysis tubing.

Table 4. Routes of infections in CAPD patients.

Route	Organism	%
Transluminal	S epidermidis	
	Acinetobacter	30–40
Periluminal	S epidermidis	
	S aureus	
	Pseudomonas	20–30
	Yeast	
Transmural	Enteric gram negative	
	Anaerobes	25–30
Hematogenous	Streptococcus	
	M tuberculosis	5–10
Ascending	Yeast	
	Lactobacillus	2–5

2.1.2. Periluminal infections

The Silastic catheter never forms a completely sealed junction with the skin or subcutaneous tissues [42]. While the purpose of the cuffs (single or double) was to reduce the penetration of bacteria around the catheter, it does not always achieve its goal. Therefore, bacterial penetration around the catheter is a possibility. However, casual penetration of bacteria around the catheter is probably not a factor, in the absence of an exit site or a tunnel infection. Studies in our unit have shown that, while originally the exit site was kept under occlusive dressings, the removal of such occlusive dressing (in fact, permitting the patient to shower daily without covering the exit site) does not lead to increased incidence of peritonitis. It is therefore probable that an infectious process has to establish itself in the tissues of the exit site or the subcutaneous tunnel to produce a peritoneal infection. Bacteria may enter from these subcutaneous infections occasionally leading to clinical symptoms. Detailed studies on exit sites raised many important possibilities on the development of exit site infections but were not conclusive [260].

2.1.3. Transmural (intestinal) infections

The isolation of intestinal organisms from peritoneal dialysis fluid, especially if they belong to more than one group of bacteria or anaerobic organisms, is indicative of a fecal leak [182]. There is some evidence that bacteria may migrate through intact intestinal wall [43] and, rarely, ischemic bowel disease may lead to more frequent penetration [36]. It is more likely that the source of intestinal leak is pre-existing diverticulosis in these patients. It is known that diverticulosis increases with age and that there is an increased incidence of diverticulosis in polycystic kidney disease patients. A study done by us showed that diverticulosis was a major source of faecal peritonitis [44].

2.1.4. Haematogenous infections

It has been shown that haematogenous spread is a frequent cause of spontaneous bacterial peritonitis of cirrhotics [34, 35] We have observed that Streptococcus viridans peritonitis developed in patients who had acute upper respiratory infections. Some of these patients preceded the development of peritonitis with positive blood cultures from which the same organism, usually Streptococcus viridans, was isolated. It is also probable that tuberculous peritonitis develops through this route [45].

2.1.5. Other endogenous infections

Rarely, other sources can be implicated in the development of peritonitis. We [46] and others [47, 48, 69] have observed women who had a vaginal leak of peritoneal dialysis fluid. Some of these developed Candida peritonitis. Tubal ligation was indicated in some of these patients after which the vaginal leak disappeared and there was no recurrence of peritonitis. The intrauterine contraceptive device [183] was also recognized as a possible source of infection. Women on CAPD therefore should be advised of contraceptive practices, especially in view of the fact that rifampin, a frequently used antibiotic in treatment of peritonitis, interferes with oral contraceptive pills.

2.1.6. Environmental infections

Peritonitis from which Xanthomonas maltophilia, Acinetobacter [49] or other environmental bacteria are isolated, are occasionally observed. It is possible that these infections develop by contact with water [50] (showering, swimming pool) entering through the exit site. In peritoneal dialysis patients, episodes of infections with atypical Mycobacteria [51, 52] have been described where the source was ascribed to tap water entering the peritoneal cavity.

2.1.7. Biofilm

The formation of a biofilm is a property of certain organisms and surfaces [188]. Biofilm on peritoneal catheters has been described [154]. The biofilm appears to be present on catheter surfaces regardless of the peritonitis history of the patient [187]. The role of the biofilm in initiating peritonitis is questioned [189]. It appears that the presence of biofilm on the catheters does not necessarily lead to peritonitis and an added injury (decrease in defense mechanisms, chemical injury, etc.) is needed. Further studies on the formation and role of biofilms are needed to answer this question. The presence of the biofilm is also stimulating research for better non-adhesive catheter material.

2.2. Inflammatory response

The normal homeostasis of the peritoneal cavity is disrupted if bacteria or chemical stimuli enter the peritoneal cavity.

2.2.1. Inflammatory mediators

Bacteria combining with normal opsonins present in the peritoneal cavity in the presence of complement will result in the release of chemotactic factors which will stimulate the outflow of polymorphonuclear cells thus increasing the cell number present in the peritoneal cavity and shifting it from a predominantly mononuclear cell population [143] to a polymorphonuclear cell population [33]. Other inflammatory mediators like histamine and serotonin will be released [53], which results in vasodilatation leading to an increase in protein outflow. Some of the mediators will produce the typical peritoneal pain.

2.2.2. Fibrin, fibronectin

The normal peritoneal cavity fluid contains fibrinogen and fibrinolysin [54] which breaks down the fibrin formed and maintains the shiny slippery surface of the peritoneum. During inflammation, the fibrinolysis is affected and while an increased amount of fibrinogen enters the peritoneal cavity, the resulting fibrin will not be broken down rapidly enough because of the lack of fibrinolysis. The result is the formation of fibrin filaments and fibrin clot.

Myhre-Jensen [55] and Porter [56] have shown that the fibrinolytic activity of the mesothelial surface of the peritoneum resides in the mesothelial cells. The presence of fibrinolytic activities suggests that fibrinolysis may assist in removing fibrin deposits from these surfaces. However, it has been demonstrated that certain stimuli such as cutting abrasion and ischemia are associated with local depression of peritoneal fibrinolysis activity [57–59]. Also, Hau et al. [60] were able to decrease fibrinolytic activity by inducing bacterial peritonitis. Thus it appears that the depression of fibrinolytic activity of the peritoneum is an important mechanism in the development of fibrin formation and probably in intraperitoneal adhesions.

Fibronectin, a normal constituent of biological fluids, has been studied in CAPD patients [180, 181]. While its concentration increases in peritoneal fluid of CAPD patients during peritonitis, it has no predictive value for susceptibility to peritonitis.

2.2.3. Cellular response

The normal peritoneal cell population is primarily mononuclear cells, probably macrophages of blood origin and some mesothelial cells from the peritoneal lining [202, 205]. On inflammation, rapid migration of polymorphonuclear cells occurs [143, 196]. The rapidity of this migration is truly amazing. It may take only a few hours for a completely clear peritoneal fluid to turn cloudy. The estimation of the peritoneal cell population is a useful adjunct during diagnosis of peritonitis [143]. The cellular response also follows the improvement of peritonitis during therapy and is a useful sign to follow. Occasionally, eosinophilic cells enter the peritoneal cavity (see below 7.3.2).

Abscess formation is an infrequent complication of peritoneal dialysis related peritonitis. Onderdonk et al. [84] demonstrated that intra-abdominal abscess formation appeared to be related to the presence of both anaerobes and gram negative aerobic bacteria. Since isolation of anaerobes is a rare occurrence in peritonitis in peritoneal dialysis patients, abscess formation in peritonitis due to faecal flora should also be suspected. Staphylococcus aureus is an organism that may be associated with abscess formation due to its effect on fibrin around the organisms [144].

3. Defense mechanisms of the peritoneum [247, 248]

The peritoneal membrane lines the interior of the abdominal wall (parietal peritoneum) and the abdominal viscera (visceral peritoneum) forming a potential space of the peritoneal cavity. The peritoneal membrane consists of a surface layer of mesothelial cells which lie on a basement membrane with deeper layers of capillaries and lymphatics. Transport through the peritoneal membrane moves from the capillaries through the basement membrane through intercellular junctions. Small particles may have two methods for transport; moving through cellular junctions or through pinocytosis by mesothelial cells [148, 149]. The principal route for movement of small particles from the peritoneum is via the lymphatics, primarily through the lymphatics below the diaphragmatic surface [150]. The exact mechanism of this movement is not clear although Courtice and Simmonds [151] have postulated that openings exist between the peritoneal cavity and the diaphragmatic lymphatics. During peritonitis the primary flow is towards the peritoneal cavity. This may explain the extremely low rate of bacteraemia in peritoneal dialysis patients during peritonitis. In secondary surgical peritonitis the rate of bacteraemia is 30% [152]. In cirrhotic patients with spontaneous peritonitis the rate of bacteraemia is between 39 to 76% (34, 35, 61). The rate of bacteraemia in patients on intermittent peritoneal dialysis was originally reported as high as 15% [8]. However, most studies have not observed bacteraemia to exceed 1–2%. We have not observed a single positive blood culture in several hundred episodes of bacterial peritonitis in CAPD patients except as noted above where the bacteraemia preceded peritonitis. The defense mechanism of the peritoneum is probably the single most important factor in the removal of small amounts of microorganisms from the peritoneal cavity.

3.1. Humoral factors

Immunoglobulins and complement are present in normal peritoneal fluid. The normal level of these components is not established. Presumably they would reflect serum concentrations. Most patients on CAPD have demonstrated near normal serum levels of immunoglobulins [62]. However, peritoneal concentrations appear diluted largely due to the volume of dialysis fluid that is instilled in the peritoneal cavity [63, 207, 208]. The relative lack of opsonin has been postulated to be a factor in the repeated episodes of peritonitis of so-called high risk patients [198, 199, 208, 209]. The lack of ability to produce adequate amounts of interleukin-1 and the release of large amounts of prostaglandin E2 by the macrophages of certain patients has also been postulated as contributing to the development of recurrent peritonitis [197].

3.2. Cellular factors

The normal self-clearing mechanism of the peritoneum is primarily dependent on mesothelial cells and mononuclear cells. During inflammation a large number of active phagocytic polymorphonuclear cells enter the peritoneal cavity participating in the removal of bacteria. Whether these cells have a reduced bactericidal capacity is subject to controversy [201, 203, 204, 206]. During peritoneal dialysis, fluid with a low pH and high osmolality is instilled into the peritoneal cavity. Both of these factors temporarily decrease the efficiency of phagocytic cells [64, 193–195]. Although urea, creatinine and other low molecular weight substances enter the peritoneal cavity during peritoneal dialysis they are not deleterious to phagocytosis in the concentrations present in the peritoneal dialysis fluid. Similarly, heparin, which is added to reduce fibrin formation, does not appear to inhibit phagocytosis.

The relative ratio of bacteria to cell is also important in the efficiency of phagocytosis. The large volume present in the peritoneal cavity during peritoneal dialysis dilutes this ratio and the chance of phagocytosis is diminished.

The role of the eosinophils in peritoneal dialysis fluid is not established. While some phagocytosis is performed by eosinophilic cells, they probably represent reaction to inflammatory agents rather than a primary defense mechanism.

The role of lymphocyte mediators in peritoneal defenses is also not clear. While it is known that end stage renal failure inhibits cellular immune functions, the role of such inhibition is not established in peritonitis [65, 66]. Patients with renal failure are considered more susceptible to infections [72]. Although, considering the exposure these patients are subjected to, other explanations for their increased rate of infections could be just as important. Whether altered production of mediators or inhibitors of cellular immunity contribute to increased infections has been continuously debated [197].

The release of free radicals during the phagocytic process is a double-edged sword. These highly potent radicals, though necessary for bactericidal action, may participate in damage to the peritoneum [265].

4. Microbiological diagnosis of peritonitis

4.1. Specimen

Several studies have dealt in the recent past with the conditions necessary for improved diagnosis in CAPD peritonitis [155–159]. In order to establish accurate microbiological diagnosis of peritonitis, the following points are important:

a) Cultures should be taken as early as possible from suspected cases of peritonitis; the first cloudy bag is the best specimen. A delay of several hours from the time of collection to the time of culture does not seem to decrease the accuracy of bacteriological diagnosis [68].
b) Large volumes should be concentrated for improving recovery rate.
c) Washing of the specimens with sterile saline or using antibiotic removing resin may be necessary in patients already receiving antibiotic therapy.
d) Identification and sensitivity testing should be done as soon as possible to achieve rational antibiotic therapy [67].

4.2. Gram stain

Gram stain from the sediment of the peritoneal dialysis bag establishes the presence of microorganisms only in about 20 to 30% of the cases. This is not a sufficiently sensitive test to permit rational therapy. While gram stains are customarily done, presumptive therapy of most of these patients will have to be initiated. Gram stains may be helpful for the diagnosis of fungal peritonitis.

4.3. Culture procedure

The microbiological culturing [241] of peritoneal dialysis samples is of utmost importance to establish the proper etiological agent and the appropriate antibiotic therapy. In addition, the type of organism indicates the possible source of infection. Culture methods have been reviewed recently [159]. Initially, peritoneal dialysis fluid was handled in the laboratories as any other specimen, culturing small amounts of fluid [157, 158]. Culturing of large amounts of fluid improves the accuracy of diagnosis [73, 22]. Most methods presently employed incorporate a concentration method [156], filtration or centrifugation. The removal of possible antibiotics present in the specimen may further improve the isolation rate. [155].

Centrifugation of 50 ml of suspected peritoneal drainage fluid at 3000 G for 15 minutes followed by resuspension of the sediment in 3–5 ml of sterile saline and inoculation of this material into a standard blood culture medium is usually adequate for primary isolation of the causative organisms. The use of anaerobic blood culture media for inoculation is optional; some laboratories find the use advantageous.

The speed with which bacteriological diagnosis can be established is important [70]. The concentration method increases not only the proper identification but also reduces the length of time necessary for bacteriological cultures. The majority of cultures will become positive after the first 24 hours and in over 75% of cases diagnosis can be established in less than 3 days.

Several reports have suggested the use of the Limulus lysate test for the diagnosis of Gram negative peritonitis [160, 161, 162]. The test, based on sensitive demonstration of endotoxin, appeared to correlate with the Gram negative peritonitis cases making the routine initial use of aminoglycosides unnecessary and thereby reducing potential toxicity. The test did not make inroads into clinical practice.

4.4. Antibiotic sensitivities

Antibiotic sensitivities of the isolated organisms are established by normal laboratory procedures against the primary and secondary antibiotics used in the treatment of peritonitis. It is important to be informed of local antibiotic sensitivity patterns of organisms since this varies from hospital to hospital. Such knowledge of local sensitivity patterns is useful in establishing the initial antibiotic treatment until sensitivity results become available.

4.5. Cell count

Cell counts are routinely obtained from the first dialysis fluid and at regular intervals thereafter to follow the efficiency of therapy [143]. Centrifugal (Cytospin) smears for differential cell counts help in judging the clinical course of peritonitis. Normal white cell count in the peritoneal dialysis fluid is considered 0–100 cells per cubic millimeter. Above 100 white blood cells per cubic millimeter, the peritoneal dialysis fluid becomes visibly cloudy. In an emergency a so-called "cloudy fluid" is enough for strong suspicion of peritonitis.

5. Presenting signs and symptoms of peritonitis

The literature contains only general reference to presenting signs and symptoms of patients presenting with peritonitis [16]. These manifestations include mild abdominal pain, low grade temperature, and usually mild abdominal tenderness. Conn [35] described clinical features of patients with spontaneous peritonitis. Fever was present in these patients in 81%, abdominal pain in 78% and physical signs of peritonitis in 65%. In 103 episodes of peritonitis of CAPD patients fever of > 37.5° was present in 53%, abdominal pain was present in 79%, 70% showed abdominal tenderness and 50% rebound pain. 31% experienced nausea and 7% complained of diarrhea. All but 1 patient had cloudy fluid before admission.

A practical definition [73] of peritonitis requires the presence of two of the following criteria in any combination:

a) Presence of organisms on Gram stain or subsequent culture of PD fluid
b) Cloudy fluid (cell count > 100 cells with > 50% polymorphonuclear cells)
c) Symptoms of peritoneal inflammation

This working definition is reliable.

Besides the above mentioned presenting signs and symptoms patients sometimes present with profound hypotension and shock. This presentation is usually a sign of either Staphylococcus aureus peritonitis [70] or faecal peritonitis.

Many of the patients will have only very mild symptoms and do not require hospitalization.

6. Clinical course of peritonitis

6.1. Incubation period

The incubation period of peritonitis in peritoneal dialysis is not well known. It is estimated from touch contamination incidents that the incubation period usually is 24 to 48 hours. Occasionally, incubation periods may be as short as 6 to 12 hours. The appearance of the symptoms may be very rapid [70] and develop during one peritoneal dialysis period. The incubation period of endogenous infections is not known but probably is much shorter than exogenous infections.

6.2. Length of symptoms

In most cases of peritonitis the symptoms decrease rapidly after initiation of therapy and disappear within 2 to 3 days. During this period the cell counts decrease and bacterial cultures become negative. In the majority of the cases positive peritoneal cultures are present only for 3 to 4 days [70]. Any prolongation of symptoms is indicative of a complicated course or a possible organism which does not respond well to antibiotics used and requires further investigation.

6.3. Exit site and tunnel infections

Exit site and tunnel infections are rarely presenting problems. Usually they are discovered on routine investigation of the exit site or the patient complaining of some purulent discharge. The exit site is inflamed with a serous or purulent discharge and occasionally painful infiltrate can be seen. Tunnel infections are much more difficult to diagnose if they are present without exit site infections. Recently, radioactive scanning [142] has been recommended as a diagnostic procedure. Ultrasonography for fluid collections in the tunnel may be also useful. Exit site and tunnel infections may be present for prolonged periods without leading to peritonitis but they are always a potential danger for the development of the disease [74].

6.4. Relapse, recurrence or reinfection

Those concepts are not well defined in the peritoneal dialysis population. Relapse is the reappearance of symptoms, the appearance of positive cultures after cultures have become negative or an increase of polymorphonuclear cells in the peritoneal dialysis fluid after they have declined. It indicates either inadequate treatment or possibly the opening of an abscess cavity which was previously inaccessible to treatment.

Recurrence is the term used of reappearance of symptoms of infection after the therapy has been stopped but within a four week period. It indicates probably either inadequate therapy or the presence of an endogenous focus like exit site or tunnel infection from which seeding occurred.

Reinfection is a new peritonitis episode beyond the four week period either with the same organism or a different organism. If reinfection happens with the same organism as before an internal focus should be suspected.

7. Causative organisms of peritonitis

The overwhelming majority of peritonitis episodes are caused by bacteria (Table 5). While a small number (4 to 8%) of peritonitis episodes are caused by fungi, most commonly Candida species, a few episodes are caused by Torulopsis or filamentous fungi (Dermatophyton, Mucor, Penicillium, Fusarium, etc.) as shown in Table 6 [75, 81].

7.1. Viruses

The role of viruses in peritoneal dialysis patients is not certain. One report [210] has claimed viral peritonitis, a culture negative peritonitis with concomitant rise in Enterovirus serum titer. Certainly if viral peritonitis was a more common event, evidence would have surfaced by now.

More interesting is the observation that viral infections predispose to peritonitis [211]. While this is a coincidental observation it deserves further study.

Dialysis of a patient infected with a virus is occasionally necessary when the patient develops renal failure. This does not present a problem generally [270].

The dialysis of Hepatitis B surface antigen positive patients presented problems in dialysis

Table 5. Bacteria isolated from peritonitis of CAPD patients.

Acinetobacter sp	Micrococcus mucilaginous
Actinomyces israeli	Mycobacterium chelonei
Aeromonas hydrophylia	Mycobacterium fortuitum
Alcaligenes fecalis	Mycobacterium tuberculosis
Bacillus cereus	Neisseria
Bacteroides fragilis	Neisseria gonorrhoeae
Bordetella bronchiseptica	Pasteurella multiocida
Campylobacter fetus	Propionobacteria
Campylobacter jejuni	Proteus sp
Citrobacter sp	Pseudomonas aeruginosa
Corynebacteria	Pseudomonas cepacia
Corynebacterium aquaticum	Pseudomonas maltophilia
Clostridium difficile	Pseudomonas stutzeri
Clostridium perfringens	Serratia sp
E. coli	Staphylococcus aureus
Enterobacter agglomerans	Staphylococcus epidermidis
Enterococcus	Stomatococcus mucilaginous
Gardnerella vaginalis	Streptococcus faecalis
CDC Group IV c-2	Streptococcus pneumoniae
CDC Group Ve-1	Streptococcus pyogenes
CDC Group Ve-2	Streptococcus viridans
Klebsiella sp	Vibrio alginolyticus
Listeria monocytogenes	

While an attempt has been made to make the listing comprehensive it may not be complete. From [174]. Sp = species.

Table 6. Yeast, fungi, algae isolated from peritonitis of CAPD patients.

Yeasts	Filamentous fungi
Candida albicans	Alternaria alternans
Candida guillermondii	Aspergillus fumigatus
Candida krusei	Aspergillus flavus
Candida parapsilopsis	Curvularia lunata
Candida tropicalis	Drechslera spicifera
Coccidioidomyces immitis	Dermatophyton
Pityrosporum ovale	Exophiala jenselmei
Pityrosporum pachydermatis	Fusarium moniliforme
Cryptococcus neoformans	Fusarium oxysporum
Rhodotorula rubra	Fusarium verticilloides
Torulopsis glabrata	Lecythophora mutabilis
	Mucor
	Penicillium sp
	Trichisporon cutaneum
	Trichoderma viride
	Trichoderma koningii
Algae	
Prothotheca wickerhamii	

While an attempt has been made to make the listing comprehensive it may not be complete. From [174]. Sp = species.

units which had experience in the haemodialysis of HBsAg positive patients. The precautions developed for haemodialysis were not suitable for PD. Special precautions became especially important with the demonstration [212, 213] of surface antigen in the dialysis fluid.

Small outbreaks of infections have been reported from PD units [214]. Adequate precautions (universal precautions or body substance precautions) have been developed in most units to cover this risk [215]. Both patients and staff are recommended to be vaccinated against hepatitis B with resulting decrease of contact risk to patients or staff.

More important is the recent controversy of nonA nonB hepatitis and AIDS in dialysis centers [163–168]. This controversy relates to several problems:

a) AIDS is presently an incurable, fatal disease.
b) Dialysis patients may have a higher incidence of AIDS or nonA nonB hepatitis due to previous multiple transfusions.
c) Previous outbreaks of hepatitis B in haemodialysis units sensitized staff to risks. Incidence of AIDS antibodies in dialysis patients is not adequately established. While there have been limited studies no national or international figures are available [166, 167]. A relatively high percentage of false positive tests have been reported.

The incidence of renal failure appears to be slightly increased in AIDS patients. Some of these patients may require dialysis [168].

The precautions necessary to dialyse AIDS patients is not difficult. Precautions already in place to prevent the spread of hepatitis B are adequate [171, 172].

A special problem is the recent observation that patients who have AIDS antibodies or are Hepatitis B antigen carriers may have a higher incidence of transplant rejection [170, 173]. Since most dialysis patients are transplant candidates, this may result in the elimination of some patients from the transplant lists.

Routine serological screening of dialysis patients or staff is not justified at present.

7.2. Protozoa, parasites

No protozoan or parasitic causes of peritonitis have been described.

7.3. Bacteria

7.3.1. Gram positive organisms

Coagulase Negative Staphylococcus (CN-S)
Staphylococcus epidermidis is the most common coagulase negative staphylococcus isolated from CAPD peritonitis although other biotypes [76, 177] have been identified (Table 7). It is generally a benign form of peritonitis. Its origin is from the skin by the transluminal route or from an exit site infection periluminally. It responds well to appropriate antibiotic treatment and usually it is symptomless within 2 to 3 days. This is a form of peritonitis most suitable for home treatment with oral antibiotics. Staphylococcus epidermidis proper is the leading cause of peritonitis in these patients. The role of slime formation of this group of organisms in the attachment to the catheter and its potential role of relapse deserves further study [77, 154, 175, 176].

S. Aureus
Staphylococcus aureus peritonitis [224] is a much more serious inflection. Patients who develop this infection can be hypotensive, or in septic shock. Frequently they complain of extensive abdominal pain. Patients with Staphylococcus aureus peritonitis with symptoms of toxic shock syndrome have also been reported [70, 78]. While the infection presents with severe symptoms, it usually responds well to antibiotic treatment. Typically the clinical improvement is much slower than with Staphylococcus epidermidis infections. We have found it useful to treat these patients with a combination of a penicillin type antibiotic (penicillin or cloxacillin depending on the sensitivity of the organisms) and rifampin which shows synergy against this organism [70]. The infection subsides slower and sometimes residual abscesses are found

Table 7. Biotypes of coagulase negative Staphylococci isolated from CAPD peritonitis.

Biotype	Vas %	Gruer et al. [175] %
S. epidermidis	77	79
S. warneri	7	5
S. haemolyticus	6	5
S. hominis	4	5
S. capitis	2	0
S. simulans	2	5
S. saprophyticus	1	0
S. xilosus	1	0
No of strains	91	43

[144]. Exit site and tunnel infections frequently recur and catheter removal may be necessary.

Alpha-Haemolytic Streptococci Streptococcus viridans, probably the most commonly isolated organism from this group of organisms in CAPD peritonitis is a milder form though patients often complain of severe pain. The infection usually responds promptly to penicillin type antibiotics. Several types of alpha-haemolytic streptococci (Table 8) may be participating in these infections [79]. We assume that this infection is caused by haematogenous spread as well as direct intraluminal infection from the oral flora. While it is possible that this infection is preceded by upper respiratory infections, antibiotic prophylaxis for this purpose has not been investigated.

Enterococcus Enterococcus, while belonging to the Gram-positive cocci, clearly is a fecal organism and indicates transmural infection. Peritonitis caused by this organism has no distinguishing features from Gram-negative peritonitis (see below) and warrants further investigation for intestinal leak. It generally is sensitive to vancomycin though recently vancomycin resistant strains have been reported.

Diphtheroids, Propionobacteria Diphtheroids, or the anaerobic variety Propionobacteria, are skin organisms indicating intraluminal infections. They may be clinically insignificant contaminants [184]. Although some are quite resistant to antibiotics, most of them respond quite readily to a variety of antibiotics [80].

7.3.2. Gram negative organisms

Enterobacteria Gram negative enterobacteria are an indication of fecal contamination of the peritoneal cavity. While a small number of Gram negative organisms may colonize the skin (Table 2) it is more likely that peritonitis with these organisms indicates direct faecal contamination. If more than a single gram negative organism is isolated from the peritoneal fluid, it is a strong indication of perforation. They usually respond well to appropriate treatment with aminoglycosides or cephalosporins.

Pseudomonas Pseudomonas infections [223] are usually more difficult to treat, are frequently accompanied or preceded by exit site infections, and may cause multiple abscesses in the patient [82]. Patients with this infection are frequently septic. Besides S. aureus, this infection is the most frequent cause of catheter removal. Treatment with aminoglycoside and an anti-pseudomonas antibiotic (see below) should be started.

Acinetobacter Acinetobacter [49], while it has no distinguishing features, may suggest an environmental contamination usually from water. It readily responds to appropriate antibiotic treatment.

Miscellaneous organisms Single episodes of peritonitis caused by various organisms (Hemophilus, Neisseria, Campylobacter etc.) have been described (Table 5) suggesting that most organisms have the potential to cause infections if inoculated into the peritoneal cavity of CAPD patients in large enough numbers.

7.3.3. Anaerobic organisms

Clostridium, Bacteroides When Clostridium and/or Bacteroides species are isolated from peritoneal fluids they are indicative of fecal contamination (see below). Some centers question the importance of doing anaerobic cultures on peritoneal fluids [83]. While they are only present in a small number of infections, our experience with infections containing anaerobic organisms is that they are very severe infections usually requiring laparotomy and there is a high propensity for abscess formation [84]. Aggressive surgical management is necessary [85–87] and therefore we consider it important to culture peritoneal fluids for these organisms.

7.3.4. Mycobacteria

M. Tuberculosis Mycobacterium tuberculosis occurs in patients with a high prevalence of tuberculosis. It most likely infects the peritoneum by haematogenous spread. It occurs in patients who have had a previous infection with this organism which was inadequately treated. It should be con-

Table 8. Biotypes of alpha hemolytic streptococci isolated from CAPD peritonitis.

Biotype	Number
Strep sanguinis II	12
Strep bovis (var)	2
Strep anguinosus (constellatus)	1
Strep MG (intermedius)	1
Strep mitis	1

sidered in high risk groups (88). If the cell counts are elevated and consistently showing predominance of mononuclear cells and cultures are repeatedly negative mycobacterial peritonitis should be considered in the high risk group [89, 90]. The treatment of the disease requires long term anti-tuberculous chemotherapy and the removal of the catheter. Peritoneal biopsy through direct laparotomy or laparoscopy may be indicated [91, 92].

A tuberculin test in diagnosing this disease is of no great value since skin reactivity to tuberculin is an unreliable response in patients with end-stage renal failure. One should consider anti-tuberculous prophylactic chemotherapy of patients who have a positive tuberculin test [93] in view of the fact that many of the patients who are on peritoneal dialysis will later enter a transplant program and therefore be at high risk for reactivation of tuberculosis.

Other Mycobacterium Peritoneal infections with Mycobacterium chelonei have been observed in intermittent peritoneal dialysis units. It has been suggested that these infections are a result of water contaminants [51, 52]. M. fortuitum infection has also been observed [233].

7.4. Fungi

Yeasts Yeasts are the most common organisms causing fungal peritonitis in peritoneal dialysis patients [75, 81, 94, 95, 218–221). They probably enter the peritoneal cavity intraluminally or periluminally though in a few cases vaginal infection was considered the source.

Yeast infections of the peritoneal cavity are difficult to treat with antifungal antibiotics [75, 95, 216–221]. These organisms are resistant to normal mechanisms like phagocytic killing [200, 225]. 5 fluorocytosin, an antifungal agent often used in the treatment of Candida cystitis, is not suitable for treatment alone since resistance emerges against it fairly rapidly. Amphotericin B cannot be administered intraperitoneally because it is irritating and painful. Treatment with amphotericin, miconazole, ketoconazole – with or without 5 fluorocytosin – while described in a few cases, is erratic, therefore catheter removal has to be considered early in these patients [75, 95–98, 216–221). After catheter removal the symptoms subside rapidly. If the patient cannot be considered for catheter removal and antibiotic therapy has to be attempted, placing the patient on intermittent peritoneal dialysis may be helpful.

Filamentous fungi Filamentous fungi rarely contaminate the catheter and cause peritoneal infections [75, 81, 95, 99, 221]. Since most filamentous fungi are resistant to antifungal antibiotics early catheter removal may be necessary.

The resistance of fungal peritonitis may be related to the ease with which these organisms colonise the surface of silastic catheters and form an antibiotic resistant biofilm. This may be the reason why catheter removal is frequently required to eliminate the infection [153].

7.5. Cryptogenic

7.5.1. "Sterile" or aseptic peritonitis

This condition is usually due to inappropriate culture procedures or specimens taken while the patient was on antibiotics. The incidence of sterile peritonitis varies among units from 2 to 20% [70, 100] depending on the methods used in the laboratory.

7.5.2. Eosinophilic peritonitis

This is usually observed early after catheter implantation [101, 120]. It may or may not be associated with peripheral eosinophilia. It usually is not associated with isolation of bacteria. Usually these patients do not have pain or fever, only cloudy fluid. The condition subsides in a couple of days without further complications and therapy. It is assumed to be associated with chemical stimuli leached from the catheter or the equipment for peritoneal dialysis [102]. Eosinophilia in the peritoneal fluid may be observed with use of antibiotics or other drugs in patients who are hypersensitive to these drugs.

7.5.3. Neutrophilic peritonitis

Diarrhoea Neutrophilia in the peritoneal fluid has been observed during diarrhoeal illness of patients without having any bacteria isolated from the peritoneal fluid.

Endotoxin Endotoxin entering the peritoneal cavity may be also associated with an increase of neutrophils in the peritoneal fluid [145].

Chemical peritonitis Aseptic chemical peritonitis was described in the beginning of the peritoneal dialysis experience [145]. Recently several episodes were reported [191] of cloudy fluids immediately after intraperitoneal administration of vancomycin. Such chemical peritonitis is rare considering the frequent application of i.p. vancomycin in the treatment of peritonitis.

7.5.4. *Bloody fluid*

Menstruation, ovulation During menstruation or ovulation, some patients will observe bloody peritoneal dialysis fluid. While initially this may be of concern it has no consequences and usually resolves after a few exchanges.

Intraperitoneal bleeding Intraperitoneal bleeding, especially in patients who are treated with anticoagulants, is of concern. If patients are on intraperitoneal heparin it should be suspended for a few days while in patients on coumadine immediate assessment of the coagulation status is warranted. If the intraperitoneal bleeding is profuse, surgical intervention may be considered.

8. Treatment of peritonitis

Treatment of peritonitis has to be initiated in the absence of appropriate diagnostic information and therefore certain arbitrary decisions have to be taken on the appropriateness of the antibiotic treatment based on the considerations discussed above on causative organisms.

8.1. General considerations

The usual method for dosing antibiotics during peritonitis used the "steady state" principle. This meant that appropriate antibiotics in appropriate concentration were placed in the dialysis fluid in each exchange [239, 240]. This approach equilibrated the antibiotic in the body at a certain level usually equivalent to the dialysate concentration.

An alternate approach for the use of antibiotics is to administer them in an intermittent fashion. For vancomycin administration of 1–2 gr/bag in dialysis fluid for one 6 hour dwell time once a week is appropriate. This dosage provides adequate levels for the length of required treatment [252–254].

For aminoglycosides the principle of intermittent therapy is based on two experimental observations. The first is the fact that the bactericidal action of aminoglycosides is proportionate to its concentration. This does not apply to penicillin or cephalosporin type antibiotics. The second observation is the so-called "post-antibiotic" effect [242–246]. This means that after the application of appropriate concentration of aminoglycoside the majority of susceptible bacteria are killed while the remaining ones have an increased susceptibility to the antibiotic.

On the basis of the above, a once a day aminoglycoside therapy for a localized infection like CAPD peritonitis becomes feasible. This approach, besides being cheaper and easier to use has also been shown to reduce toxic side effects [261, 262]. Although limited experiences with intermittent dosing for peritonitis have been reported, its success in other closed space infections suggests a useful role in the treatment of peritonitis.

8.2. Antibiotics

The antibiotics selected for initial treatment should be effective against the most frequent organisms observed in peritonitis. The antibiotic sensitivity pattern of the organisms isolated from peritonitis episodes does not differ from the sensitivity organisms prevalent in the hospital. It is important to know and develop an approach jointly with the infectious disease specialist in each hospital since certain differences in the sensitivity against antibiotics of various organisms can be observed depending on the hospital.

Recommended antibiotic dosages as modified for peritoneal use are listed in Table 9.

Since no reliable microbiological information is usually available at the start of treatment the first choice of antibiotics should cover the most frequent organisms causing these infections. Therefore it should give coverage against most gram positive organisms as well as gram negative organisms. Most centers use as initial choice for gram positive coverage vancomycin though cephalothin or cephazolin in appropriate concentrations is still widely used. These antibiotics provide good cover against Staphylococcus epidermidis, some Staphylococcus aureus and a certain number of gram negatives. If one wants to cover the more threatening intestinal organisms the addition of an aminoglycoside is justified. If the patient is hypersensitive against cephalosporins the use of vancomycin in conjunction with an aminoglycoside is the first choice. Also, in areas where methicillin resistance of staphylococci is prevalent vancomycin is a proper initial choice. After the organisms have been identified and an antibiotic sensitivity is available adjustments should be made to the therapy.

Penetration of antibiotics from the peritoneal cavity to serum is good and rapid [103, 104, 253, 256]. It is therefore not necessary in most cases to

Table 9. Pharmacokinetics of antibiotics in CAPD patients and proposed regimens for the treatment of CAPD peritonitis.

	Half-life (H)				Dose (per 70 kg adult)[a] Maintenance dose	
	Normal	ESRD	CAPD	Initial dose (mg/2-L bag)	Intermittent mg/2-L bag per dosing interval	Continuous (mg/2-L bag)
Aminoglycosides						
Amikacin	1.6	39	40	500	120/d	12–24
Gentamicin	2.2	53	32	70–140	40/d	8–16
Netilmicin	2.1	42	18	70–140	40/d	8–16
Tobramycin	2.5	58	36	70–140	40/d	8–16
Cephalosporins						
First generation						
Cefazolin	2.2	28	30	500–1000	1000/d	250–500
Cefonicid	4.0	68	50	250	ND	50
Cephalothin	0.2	3.7	ND	1000	ND	200
Cephradine	0.9	12	ND	500	ND	250
Cephalexin	0.8	19	9	1000 PO	500/QID PO	NA
Second generation						
Cefamandole	1.0	10	8.0	1000	1000/d	500
Cefmenoxime	1.3	11.3	6.0	2000	1000/d	100
Cefoxitin	0.8	20	15	1000	ND	200
Cefuroxime	1.3	18	15	1000	400/d IV/PO	150–400
Third generation						
Cefixime	3.2	11.5	15	400 PO	400/d PO	NA
Cefoperazone	1.8	2.3	2.2	2000	ND	400–1000
Cefotaxime	0.9	2.5	2.4	2000	2000/d	500
Cefsulodin	1.8	11	11	1000	500/d	50
Ceftazidime	1.8	26	13	1000	1000/d	250
Ceftizoxime	1.6	28	11	1000	1000/d	250
Ceftriaxone	8.0	15	12	1000	1000/d	250–500
Moxalactam	2.2	20	16	1000	1000/d	350
Penicillins						
Azlocillin	0.9	5.1	ND	500	ND	500
Mezlocillin	1.0	4.3	ND	3000 IV	3000/BID IV	500
Piperacillin	1.2	3.9	2.4	4000 IV	4000/BID IV	500
Ticarcillin	1.2	15	ND	1000–2000	2000/BID	250
Quinolones						
Ciprofloxacin	4.0	8.0	11	500 PO	500/TID PO	50
Fleroxacin	13	27	27	800 PO	400/d PO	NA
Ofloxacin	7.0	30	25	400 PO	200/d PO	NA
Vancomycin and others						
Vancomycin	6.9	161	92	1000–2000	1–2000/7 d	30–50
Teicoplanin	50	260	260	400	400/BID	40[b]
Aztreonam	2.0	7.0	9.3	1000	1000/d	500
Clindamycin	2.8	2.8	ND	300	ND	300
Erythromycin	2.1	4.0	ND	ND	500/QID PO	150
Metronidazole	7.9	7.7	11	500 PO/IV	500/TID PO/IV	ND
Minocycline	15.5	20	ND	NA	100/BID PO	NA
Rifampin	4.0	8.0	ND	600 PO	600/d PO	NA
Antifungal agents						
Amphotericin B	360	360	ND	NA	20–30/d IV	2–8
Flucytosine	4.2	115	ND	2000–3000 PO	1000/d PO	NA
Fluconazole	22	125	72	NA	150 mg q 2d	ND
Ketoconazole	2.0	1.8	2.4	400 PO	200–800/d PO	NA
Miconazole	24	25	ND	200	ND	100–200

Table 9. *(Continued)*

	Half-life (H)				Dose (per 70 kg adult)[a] Maintenance dose	
	Normal	ESRD	CAPD	Initial dose (mg/2-L bag)	Intermittent mg/2-L bag per dosing interval	Continuous (mg/2-L bag)
Combinations						
Amphicillin	1.3	15	9.5	1000–2000	1000/BID	100
Sulbactam	1.0	19	9.7	1000–2000	1000/BID	100
Imipenem	0.9	3.0	6.4	1000	500/BID	200
Cilistatin	0.8	15	19	5000–1000	500/BID	100–200
Sulfamethoxazole	10	13	14	1600 PO	1600/1–2 d PO	400
Trimethoprim	14	33	34	320 PO	320/1–2 d PO	80

[a] The route of administration is intraperitoneal unless otherwise specified. The pharmacokinetic data and proposed dosage regimens presented here are based on published literature reviewed through April 1992.
There is no evidence that mixing different antibiotics in dialysis fluid (except for aminoglycosides and penicillins) is deleterious for the drugs or patients. Do not use the same syringe to mix antibiotics.
[b] This is in each bag × 7 days, then in 2 bags/day × 7 days, and then in 1 bag/day × 7 days.
ESRD = creatinine clearance < 10 mL/min, patient not in dialysis; NA = not applicable; ND = no data; IV = intravenous; PO = oral; d = once a day; BID = twice a day; TID = three times a day; QID = four times a day.

give an intravenous loading dose since peritoneal administration of antibiotics will achieve high enough concentrations in the serum in a few hours.

Recently an expert committee [178] reviewed the earlier therapeutic recommendations.

A simplified schedule (from 178) is shown below (Table 10).

The addition of more than one antibiotic or other therapeutic agent to the dialysis fluid has been studied. Commonly used antibiotics do not interact deleteriously in peritoneal dialysis fluid, neither

Table 10. Treatment of CAPD peritonitis.

General rules in treatment of CAPD peritonitis
All treatment should be guided by antibiotic sensitivity of causative organism.
If no clinical improvement or decrease in cell count of dialysis fluid in 3–4 days repeat culture.
If after 5 days cultures are consistently positive consider catheter removal especially in the presence of exit site infection with same organism.
Length of treatment for Gram positive peritonitis is 14 days (3 doses of Vancomycin), Gram negative peritonitis is 21 days, Pseudomonas/Xanthomonas peritonitis 28 days.
Fungal peritonitis can be attempted to be treated. If no improvement in clinical course, cell count or cultures, catheter should be removed.

Initial treatment

Vancomycin		2 gr I.P. if BW > 40 kg
		1 gr I.P. if BW < 40 kg
	and	
Ceftazidime		Loading dose 500 mg/L I.P.
		Maintenance 125 mg/L I.P.
	or	
Aminoglycoside[1,2]		Loading dose 1.7 mg/kg bw I.P.
		Maintenance 8 mg/L
	or	
Aminoglycoside		20 mg/l in one exchange/day
	and	
Heparin		1000 μ/l each exchange while fluid is cloudy

[1] Aminoglycoside includes Netilmycin < Tobramycin < Gentamicin in increasing order of toxicity.
[2] For Amikacin dose multiply aminoglycoside dose by 3, e.g., Aminoglycoside 8 mg/L = Amikacin 24 mg/L.

Table 10. *(Continued).*

Culture: No growth in 2–3 days	Culture: Gram positive	Culture: Gram negative
Continue vancomycin For 2 more doses Every 7 days 2 gr I.P. if BW > 40 kg 1 gr I.P. if BW < 40 kg Stop aminoglycoside	Continue vancomycin For 2 more doses Every 7 days 2 gr I.P. if BW > 40 kg 1 gr I.P. if BW < 40 kg Stop aminoglycoside	Continue Ceftazidime 125 mg/L each exchange or Aminoglycoside 8 mg/L each exchange for 7 days then 6 mg/L each exchange or Aminoglycoside 20 mg/L one exchange/day
Oral therapy depending on antibiotic Sensitivity	Culture: Staph aureus	Fecal peritonitis
Ciprofloxacin 750 mg B.I.D. or Ofloxacin 300 mg/day or Septra 1 ds tabl B.I.D. or Cephalexin 250 mg T.I.D. plus Rifampin 300 mg B.I.D. P.O.	Continue vancomycin for 2 more doses Every 7 days 2 gr I.P. if BW > 40 kg 1 gr I.P. if BW < 40 kg add Rifampin 300 mg B.I.D. P.O. Stop aminoglycoside	As in gram negative peritonitis add Metronidazole 500 mg/8 hours P.O. or I.V. or Rectal Suppository Consider surgery
Fungal peritonitis	Patient sensitive to vancomycin	Pseudomonas/xanthomonas peritonitis
Fluconazole 150 mg I.P. in one bag Every 2nd day and Flucytosine Loading dose 2000 mg P.O. Maintenance 1000 mg P.O./day or Amphotericin B 25 mg/day I.V. and Flucytosine As above	Clindamycin 150 mg/L in each exchange	Aminoglycoside 8 mg/L each exchange for 7 days then 6 mg/L each exchange for 21 days or Aminoglycoside 20 mg/L one exchange/day for 21 days add Anti-pseudomonas antibiotic for 28 days see below

Antibiotics with anti-pseudomonas/anti-xanthomonas (*) activity

Antibiotic	Dosage
Ceftazidime	125 mg/L I.P. each exchange
Piperacillin	4 gr every 12 hours I.V.
Ciprofloxacine	750 mg B.I.D. P.O.
Aztreonam	Load 500 mg/L maint: 250 mg/L I.P.
Imipenem	Load 500 mg/L maint: 100 mg/L I.P.
Sulfamethoxazole/Trimethoprim (*)	Load 1600/320 mg I.P. Maint: 200/40 mg I.P.
Minocyclin (*)	100 mg B.I.D. P.O.

do other additions like heparin and insulin [105–109].

8.3. Length of treatment

No clinical trials have established the optimal length of therapy for peritonitis. Antibiotics for 7 days after the last positive culture has been obtained are frequently used as the endpoint. Since antibiotic elimination will be slow after cessation of treatment this adds additional days of effective therapy; therefore the length of treatment is probably 14–21 days. Some causative organisms require longer therapy (see Recommendations Table 10). If no clinical improvement and decrease in cell counts is evident after 4–5 days repeat cultures are necessary and change in antibiotics or catheter removal should be considered.

8.4. Side effects

Hypersensitivity reactions against antibiotics have been observed in peritoneal dialysis patients. If antibiotics are used intraperitoneally in these patients eosinophilia in the peritoneal fluid may be observed. Skin rash may appear in patients with antibiotic hypersensitivity during peritoneal application.

Recently chemical peritonitis after use of a preparation of vancomycin has been reported [191, 250, 251].

Aminoglycosides are known to have renal, vestibular and ototoxic effects [261, 262]. All attempts should be made to preserve residual renal functions since the loss of such functions may necessitate one extra peritoneal dialysis cycle per day [110]. In the concentrations recommended evidence of nephrotoxicity has not been reported. Ototoxicity has been observed in patients where gentamicin was used [261]. Tobramycin [262], netilmicin or amikacin are believed to have less ototoxicity or vestibular toxicity. Vestibular or ototoxicity is rare except in patients who accidentally overdose themselves severalfold with intraperitoneal antibiotics.

The use of rifampin occasionally results in elevation of liver enzymes or nausea, necessitating the discontinuation of the drug. 600 mg of rifampin per day in divided doses has less toxic effect. Rifampin interferes with the effect of oral contraceptives and therefore patients should be advised against the use of oral contraceptives.

Peritoneal dialysis patients on antibiotics may develop pseudomembranous enterocolitis [111, 274]. Therapy for this complication is the same as in non-renal cases.

8.5. Peritoneal lavage

Peritoneal lavage has been instituted in the treatment of dialysis related peritonitis based on experience with this treatment in the surgical field [112]. The reason for peritoneal lavage in surgical peritonitis is to remove detritus and faecal contamination from the peritoneal cavity.

It has been shown that in CAPD patients the effect of lavage may reduce peritoneal defenses and remove necessary phagocytic cells [64]. Peritoneal lavage with added iodine has been advocated [113] but the use of such treatment has not been clinically substantiated [114]. There is evidence to suggest peritoneal antibiotic treatment using 1–2 brief lavages is clinically efficacious and less costly [115–118, 146].

8.6. The role of heparin

Heparin addition to the peritoneal dialysis fluid during peritonitis is important. Since the inflammatory process will result in the diapedesis of large amounts of fibrinogen into the peritoneal fluid, the inhibition to fibrin formation is helpful. In addition, it appears that heparin will reduce subsequent adhesion of the peritoneal membrane, therefore reducing postinfectious complications [147].

8.7. Treatment protocols

Development of standard treatment protocols for CAPD peritonitis is useful for efficient treatment of patients especially in the emergency room where experience with this condition is limited. Appropriate microbiological diagnosis will not be available for 24 to 72 hours and until that time arbitrary antibiotic combinations have to be used to cover the most likely pathogens [178, 179].

8.8. Treatment of exit site and tunnel infections

Catheter related infections are a major problem of peritoneal dialysis [226]. The 1987 report of the National CAPD Registry of NIH showed that about 31% of the patients developed exit site infections within the first year and probably about 1/2 of these patients required catheter replacement during this period [31]. The tunnel infection rate was reported to be 0.17 per year for males and 0.23 per year for females. Diabetic females had a rate 0.35/y and diabetic males 0.20/y [235].

Their treatment is not very successful and often requires removal of the catheter [237]. Most commonly exit sites are infected with Staphylococcus epidermidis or Staphylococcus aureus though Pseudomonas or Proteus infections can be observed. The exit site is erythematous, elevated, with drainage of pus or serous fluid but it is not generally painful. For tunnel infections [238] sometimes an abscess can be palpated under the skin along the canula tract. Ultrasonography for establishing fluid collection in the tunnel can be useful.

A culture swab should be obtained from the depth of the exit site, without touching adjoining skin. Alginate swabs used to take urethral specimens are most suitable because of their size. Since the organisms present in tunnel and exit site infections are the same as skin organisms care has to be exercised to avoid contamination with skin organisms.

Treatment of exit site infections can be attempted with local disinfectant or oral antibiotics. The use of antibiotic ointment should be discouraged since its effectiveness is questionable and may lead to the emergence of resistant organisms. In addition, the ointment forms a crust over the exit site making cleaning difficult.

With daily cleaning and local care with hydrogen peroxide, exit site infections sometimes can be cured.

Recent recommendations for exit site care have been published [178, 186, 271]. If the outer cuff (double-cuffed catheters) appears in the exit site or is extruded, catheter shaving [74, 119] can be attempted, though with no great success in reducing the incidence of exit site infections [190].

8.9. Catheter removal

The most common cause for catheter removal is a persistently infected exit site or tunnel [121]. Replacement can be done on these patients usually one to two weeks after catheter removal usually into a different site.

If peritonitis is not responding to adequate therapy, a catheter replacement should be considered. If the catheter has to be removed because of frequent recurrence of peritonitis with the same organism or other infectious causes, the catheter usually can be replaced after three weeks of termination of successful treatment of peritonitis.

Replacement of catheters at the same time as removal [222] has been reported. However this approach should be used cautiously and probably not in patients with fungal, pseudomonas, mycobacterial or fecal infections.

9. Complications of peritonitis

9.1. Intestinal perforation and diverticulitis

A small prospective study [44] has shown diverticulosis to be a risk factor for development of faecal peritonitis. Aggressive treatment, including laparotomy and sometimes surgical resection will be necessary. Surgery resulting in a colostomy will delay the reinstitution of peritoneal dialysis.

9.2. Adhesions, sclerosing peritonitis

As a consequence of peritonitis, fibrous adhesions may develop between the peritoneal membranes [140, 141]. This is especially frequent as a consequence of Staphylococcus aureus or faecal peritonitis.

Lysis of adhesions on implantation of the peritoneal catheter may be attempted by blunt dissection but this procedure increases the risk of producing microperforations with resulting peritonitis. Sclerosing peritonitis [122–124] in which thick fibrinous exudate develops making the exchange of fluid and solutes impossible has been described [264]. It is not clear whether this is due to repeated injuries to the peritoneum like frequent peritonitis or due to some chemical injury.

9.3. Mortality

It is difficult to establish the accurate mortality due to peritonitis. One report puts the mortality at 2 to 3% [125, 126, 249]. While this is certainly high it is not surprising since the patients with peritonitis suffer from an ultimately fatal disease. Many of the causes of death during peritonitis are not directly attributable to the infection but may be related to the patients frequent comorbidity.

10. Differential diagnostic problems

Various diseases may mimic peritonitis or may be the initiating event which leads to peritonitis but without treatment of the underlying problem the peritonitis will not improve. In general, the early involvement of a surgeon in the evaluation of the patient with atypical peritonitis is advisable [228].

10.1. Constipation

Constipation may lead to diffuse abdominal pain mimicking peritonitis but will not lead to cloudy fluid or positive cultures. In the absence of the latter, treatment with antibiotics should not be initiated. Careful history for bowel habits and a radiographic examination without contrast material should be done for appropriate diagnosis. Constipation should be treated with mild laxatives, enema or if necessary, disimpaction.

10.2. Appendicitis

Appendicitis in a patient on peritoneal dialysis may mimic peritonitis producing a cloudy fluid with an elevated polymorphonuclear cell count due to inflammation of the bowel wall extending to the serosa [227]. Unfortunately the early diagnosis is difficult and patients are treated for peritonitis delaying accurate diagnosis. It is important to diagnose appendicitis in a peritoneal dialysis patient early since the delay of treatment may lead to perforation and resulting faecal peritonitis.

10.3. Pancreatitis

Acute pancreatitis or an infected pseudocyst may lead to symptoms suggestive of peritonitis such as pain, fever, and cloudy fluid. Elevated serum amylase level is an early indication of such infection. Sometimes amylase may be measured in the peritoneal dialysis fluid though this test is not reliable.

10.4. Cholecystitis

Cholecystitis may also mimic peritonitis in dialysis patients. Early ultrasound demonstrating the presence of stones may be a diagnostic clue. Sometimes cholecystitis may lead to perforation of the gallbladder resulting in true peritonitis. A positive blood culture with a gram negative organism may be suggestive of cholecystitis or cholangitis.

10.5. Perforated ulcer

Perforation of a gastric or duodenal ulcer may also lead to peritonitis. Usually the organisms cultured from such peritonitis are gram positive, most commonly alpha haemolytic streptococci. Occasionally fungal peritonitis can be the result of a perforated gastric ulcer. Surgical management of this complication is essential [228].

10.6. Malignancy

Rarely, asymptomatic cloudy fluid may be observed in malignancies with widespread metastases. Cytologic examination of the dialysis fluid is usually diagnostic.

11. Prevention of peritonitis

11.1. Sterile connections

Obviously the most sensible approach to peritonitis is the prevention of infectious events which may lead to the development of the disease. The observance of strict sterile conditions during connections and disconnections, the use of disinfectants on all areas exposed to possible contaminations, the wearing of appropriate face masks, scrubbing and gloves, etc. is essential. The single most important prophylactic approach for prevention of peritonitis is the development of appropriate procedural protocols and the careful training of patients [127].

11.1.1. *U.V. box and sterile weld*
An ultraviolet device producing sterile connections (UV System Travenol [230, 231]) and a sterile weld device (Sterile Connection Device SCD DuPont [232]) have been reported to reduce infections. While these devices show benefits, especially in high risk populations, their expense limits their widespread use.

11.1.2. *O-Z connection*
For patients who have had repeated peritonitis episodes and are at high risk for developing others a special connection has been designed. This connection maintains the spike between dialysis in a disinfectant and makes a connection in the presence of this disinfectant (Betadine). Reduction of peritonitis episodes in high risk patients has been reported [127].

11.1.3. *Disconnect systems*
The widespread use of disconnect systems (flush-before-fill, Y set with or without disinfectant) has certainly reduced the incidence of peritonitis [259]. The ultimate in disconnect systems, the so-called

double bag or twin bag system, where both fill bag and drainage bag are integral units and are disconnected after each exchange, have been recently introduced [266]. These systems have reduced mainly the incidence of gram positive bacterial peritonitis without any appreciable effect on gram negative peritonitis. As a result the relative frequency of gram negative peritonitis has increased.

11.1.4. *Millipore filter*

To prevent intraluminal infections a bacterial retaining device close to the peritoneal surface would be useful. To solve this problem a bacteriological filter (Peridex, Millipore Corporation) has been developed which fits into the tubing set used for peritoneal dialysis and which incorporates a bypass valve to facilitate drainage of the fluid. Although some reduction in peritonitis from use of such device has been reported [130], it is no longer used routinely.

11.1.5. *Auxiliary devices for the handicapped*

Several auxiliary devices have been developed for use of patients handicapped in movement or vision. The development of such devices was essential to facilitate self care in these patients.

11.2. Antibiotic prophylaxis

Previous clinical studies have examined the use of prophylactic antibiotics in patients on intermittent peritoneal dialysis [131–133]. It is difficult to draw conclusions from these studies because of the small number of events and the otherwise low incidence of peritonitis in these patients. One double blind prospective study [134] failed to show that the use of oral cephalexin twice daily prevented peritonitis. Another prospective study using oral Septra for prophylaxis was also unsuccessful [192].

No prospective studies have demonstrated that prophylactic antibiotics used at the time of catheter insertion result in a decrease in catheter related infections or peritonitis. However based on other, surgical, experience their use has been considered acceptable.

11.3. Patient selection

It is difficult to predict which patients are going to have frequent peritonitis episodes. Analysis of patient populations and peritonitis rates do not yield significant differences for prediction [135]. It is quite obvious that the compliant patients who have reasonable intellectual capabilities to absorb training and have good family support are doing better on peritoneal dialysis and have lower peritonitis rates. There are very few absolute contraindications to peritoneal dialysis at present and it is hoped that future analysis of peritonitis episodes in large populations of peritoneal dialysis patients may result in some understanding of risk factors that might predict peritonitis [272]. Assessment of humoral or cellular defense of the peritoneal cavity has not proven sufficiently sensitive to identify high risk patients.

Caution should be exercised in considering the following patients for CAPD:

a) Patients with extensive skin disease (pemphigus, eczema)
b) Patients with colostomy
c) Patients who are blind and have no helper
d) Patients with extensive intraabdominal adhesions

11.4. New catheters

The present peritoneal dialysis catheters whether they are single cuffed or double cuffed models do not show significant differences in peritonitis rates [179]. It is hoped that new catheters will be developed and the implant will form a complete integrated seal with the skin, thereby reducing exit site infections and the periluminal penetration of organisms.

An expert committee recently has made recommendations on peritoneal catheter implantation and the use of various catheters [186].

11.5. Alternate dialysis solutions

Presently used dialysis solutions are not ideal since they allegedly decrease defense mechanisms against infections [64]. Research for solutions containing alternate buffering agents continues [267, 268].

12. Evaluation of peritonitis rate

Initially, the ratio of peritonitis episodes over exposure months was used as an index of peritonitis frequency. While this ratio is a useful initial evaluation, it is not capable of expressing the true differences in peritonitis rates. This lies in the fact that patients enter and leave peritoneal dialysis programs at different times, and are in a program for different lengths of time. The combined experience is different for each period or group and therefore they are not readily suitable for statistical maneuvers.

Statistical approaches [136–139] based on an actuarial analysis have been developed. These methods define the time elapsed till the first peritonitis episode of a patient expressing the probability at different times for the development of peritonitis in a population of peritoneal dialysis patients. These show that the probability of developing the first episode of peritonitis is approximately 45% in the first 6 months while approximately 25% of the patients develop exit site infections during this period. Using such a statistical approach it has been found that there are no significant differences in peritonitis rates in the two sexes. The age related incidence is not significantly different though it appears to be less in the older age groups, and certain diseases (for example, diabetes) do not represent significantly increased risk factors.

Another statistical approach to evaluate peritonitis rates is based on the negative binomial probability model and appears to approach peritonitis morbidity rates more closely.

The selection of the appropriate model [263] is of importance to most accurately predict peritonitis rates.

13. Future considerations

It appears from experience acquired in the last few years that we have reached a relative plateau in the frequency of peritonitis. A peritonitis rate of one every two patient years may be acceptable. New developments in catheter technology and improved connections may lead to reduction in exit site and tunnel infections, which are a major problem at present. It may be that development in these areas will lead to the next major impact on peritonitis rates. Better understanding of patient selection and training programs, improved diagnostic and therapeutic methods in the management of peritonitis, and the possibility of some sort of immune prophylaxis are developments eagerly awaited [269].

References

1. Seligman AM, Frank HA, Fine J. Treatment of experimental uremia by means of peritoneal irrigation. J Clin Invest 1946; 25: 211–9.
2. Fine J, Frank HA, Seligman AM. The treatment of acute renal failure by peritoneal irrigation. Ann Surg 1946; 124: 857–78.
3. Frank HA, Seligman AM, Fine J. Further experiences with peritoneal irrigation for acute renal failure. Ann Surg 1948; 128: 561–608.
4. Grollman A, Turner LB, McLean JA. Intermittent peritoneal lavage in nephrectomized dogs and its application to the human being. Arch Intern Med 1951; 87: 379–90.
5. Doolan PD, Murphy WP, Wiggins RA, Carter NW, Cooper WC, Watten RH, Alpen EL. An evaluation of intermittent peritoneal lavage. Am J Med 1959; 26: 831–44.
6. Weston RE, Roberts M. Clinical use of stylet-catheter for peritoneal dialysis. Arch Intern Med 1965; 115: 659–62.
7. Maxwell MH, Rockney RE, Kleeman CR, Twiss MR. Peritoneal dialysis I. Technique and applications. JAMA 1929; 170: 917–24.
8. Cohen SL, Percival A. Prolonged peritoneal dialysis in patients awaiting renal transplantation. Br Med J 1968; 1: 409–13.
9. Leigh DA. Peritoneal infections in patients on long-term peritoneal dialysis before and after human cadaveric renal transplantation. J Clin Pathol 1969; 22: 539–44.
10. Palmer RA, Quinton WE, Gray JE. Prolonged peritoneal dialysis for chronic renal failure. Lancet 1964; 1: 700–2.
11. Tenckhoff H, Schecter H. A bacteriologically safe peritoneal access device. Trans Am Soc Artif Intern Organs 1968; 14: 181–7.
12. Tenckhoff H, Curtis FK. Experience with maintenance peritoneal dialysis in the home. Trans Am Soc Artif Intern Organs 1970; 16: 90–5.
13. Brewer TE, Caldwell FT, Patterson RM, Flanigan WJ. Indwelling peritoneal (Tenckhoff) dialysis catheter. Experience with 24 patients. JAMA 1972; 219: 1011–5.
14. Lankisch PG, Tonnis HJ, Fernandez-Redo E, Girndt J, Kramer P, Quellhorst E, Scheller F. Use of Tenckhoff catheter for peritoneal dialysis in terminal renal failure. Br Med J 1973. 4: 712–3.
15. Palmer RA. Peritoneal dialysis by indwelling catheter for chronic renal failure 1963–1968. Can Med Assoc J 1971; 105: 376–80.
16. Rae A, Pendray M. Advantages of peritoneal dialysis in chronic renal failure. JAMA 1973, 225: 937–41.
17. Devine H, Oreopoulos DG, Izatt S, Mathews R, deVeber GA. The permanent Tenckhoff catheter for chronic peritoneal dialysis. Can Med Assoc J 1975; 113: 219–21.
18. Petrie JJB, Jones EOP, Hartley LCJ, Olife KP, Clunie CJA. The use of an indwelling peritoneal catheter in the treatment of chronic renal failure. Med J Aust 1976; 2: 119–22.
19. Popovich RP, Moncrief JW, Decherd JB, Bomar JB, Pyle WK. The definition of a novel portable/wearable equilibrium peritoneal dialysis technique (abstract). Abstr Am Soc Artif Intern Organs 1976; 5: 64–8.
20. Popovich RP, Moncrief JW, Nolph KD, Ghods AJ, Twardowski ZJ, Pyle WK. Continuous ambulatory peritoneal dialysis. Ann Intern Med 1978; 88: 449–56.

21. Oreopoulos DG, Robson M, Izatt S, Clayton S, deVeber GA. A simple and safe technique for continuous ambulatory peritoneal dialysis (CAPD). Trans Am Soc Artif Intern Organs 1978; 24: 484–7.
22. Rubin J, Rodgers WA, Taylor HM, Everett ED, Prowant BF, Fruto LU, Nolph KD. Peritonitis during continuous ambulatory dialysis. Ann Intern Med 1980; 92: 7–13.
23. Oreopoulos DG. Continuous ambulatory peritoneal dialysis in Canada. Can Med Assoc J 1979; 120: 16–9.
24. Oreopoulos DG, Clayton S, Dombros N, Zellerman G, Katirtzoglou A. Experience with continuous ambulatory peritoneal dialysis (CAPD). Trans Am Soc Artif Intern Organs 25: 95–7.
25. Fenton SSA, Cattran DC, Ahlen AF, Rutledge P, Ampil M, Dadson J, Locking H, Smith D, Wilson DR. Initial experiences with continuous ambulatory peritoneal dialysis. Artif Organs 1979; 3: 206–9.
26. Oreopoulos DG, Khanna R, McCready W, Katirtzoglou A, Vas S. Continuous ambulatory peritoneal dialysis in Canada. Dial Transpl 1980; 9: 224–6.
27. Blagg CR, Scribner BH. Long-term dialysis; current problems and future prospects. Am J Med 1980; 68: 633–5.
28. Peritoneal dialysis in chronic renal failure (editorial). Lancet 1978; 2: 303.
29. Moncrief JW. Continuous ambulatory peritoneal dialysis. Dial Transpl 1979; 8: 1077–8.
30. Home peritoneal dialysis for end-stage renal disease. Med Lett Drugs Ther 21: 69–70.
31. National CAPD Registry of the NIH (1987). Characteristics of participants and selected outcome measures for the period January 1, 1981 through August 31 1986.
32. Diaz-Buxo JA, Walker PJ, Farmes CD, Chandler JT, Holt KL. Continuous cyclic peritoneal dialysis – The Nalle Clinic experience. In: Price JDE (ed), Peritoneal Dialysis. The State of the Art. Communication Media for Education, Princeton, NY 1983; pp 23–5.
33. Hau T, Ahrenholz DH, Simmons RL Secondary bacterial peritonitis: The biologic basis of treatment. In: Current problems in Surgery. Vol 16 No. 10 Year Book Medical Publ Inc Chicago 1979.
34. Correia JP, Conn HO. Spontaneous bacterial peritonitis in cirrhosis: endemic or epidemic? Med Clin North Am 1975; 59: 963–81.
35. Conn HO, Fessel JM. Spontaneous bacterial peritonitis in cirrhosis: variations on a theme. Medicine (Balt) 1971; 50: 161–97.
36. Bar-Meir S, Conn HO. Spontaneous bacterial peritonitis induced by intraarterial vasopressin therapy. Gastroenterology 1976; 70: 418–21.
37. Conn HO. Bacterial peritonitis: spontaneous or paracentric? (editorial). Gastroenterology 1979; 77: 1145–6.
38. Targan SR, Chow AW, Guze LB. Role of anaerobic bacteria in spontaneous peritonitis of cirrhosis. Report of two cases and review of the literature. Am J Med 1977; 62: 397–403.
39. Stephen CG, Meadows JG, Kerkering TM, Markowitz SW, Nisman RM. Spontaneous peritonitis due to Hemophilus influenzae in an adult. Gastroeinterology 1979; 77: 1088–90.
40. Hau T, Hoffman R, Simmons RL. Mechanisms of the adjuvant effect of hemoglobin in experimental peritonitis. I. In vivo inhibition of peritoneal leukocytosis. Surgery 1978; 83: 223–9.
41. Stewart WK, Anderson DC, Wilson MI. Hazard of peritoneal dialysis: contaminated fluid. Br Med J 1967; 1: 606–7.
42. Helfrick GB, Pechau BW, Alijani MR, Barnard WF, Rakowski TA, Winchester JF. Reduction of catheter complications with lateral placement. Perit Dial Bull 1983; 4 (suppl 3): 2–4.
43. Schweinburg FB, Seligman AM, Fine J. Transmural migration of intestinal bacteria. A study based on the use of radioactive Escherichia coli. N Engl J Med 1950; 242: 747–51.
44. Wu G, Khanna R, Vas S, Oreopoulos DG. Is extensive diverticulosis of the colon a contraindication to CAPD. Perit Dial Bull 1983; 3: 180–3.
45. Singh MM, Bhargawa AN, Jain KB. Tuberculous peritonitis: An evaluation of pathogenic mechanisms, diagnostic procedures and therapeutic measures. New Eng J Med 1969; 281: 1091–4.
46. Khanna R, Oreopoulos DG, Vas SI, McCready W, Dombros N. Fungal peritonitis in patients undergoing chronic intermittent or continuous peritoneal dialysis. Proc EDTA 1980; 17: 291–6.
47. Coward RA, Gokal R, Mallick NP. Recurrent peritonitis associated with vaginal leak. Perit Dial Bull 1983; 3: 164–5.
48. Dias-Buxo JA, Burgess P, Walker PJ. Peritoneovaginal fistula-unusual complication of peritoneal dialysis. Perit Dial Bull 1983; 3: 142–3.
49. Abrutyn E, Goodhart GL, Roos K, Anderson R, Buxton A. Acinetobacter calcoaceticus outbreak associated with peritoneal dialysis. Am J Epidemiol 107: 328–35.
50. Mader JT, Reinarz JA. Peritonitis during peritoneal dialysis. the role of the preheating water bath. J Chron Dis 1978; 31: 635–64.
51. Baud JD, Ward J, Fraser DW, Peteroon NJ, Silcox VA, Good RC, Ostroy PR, Kennedy J. Peritonitis due to a mycobacterium chelonei like organism associated with intermittent chronic peritoneal dialysis. J Inf Dis 1982; 145: 9–17.
52. Poisson M, Beromicide V, Falardeau C, Vega C, Morisset R. Mycobacterium chelonei peritonitis in a patient undergoing continuous ambulatory peritoneal dialysis (CAPD). Perit Dial Bull 1983; 3: 86–8.
53. Majno G, Palade GE. Studies on inflammation. I. The effect of histamine and serotonin on vascular permeability: an electron microscopic study. J Biophys Cytol 1961; 11: 571–600.
54. Ellis H. The cause and prevention of post-operative intraperitoneal adhesions. Surg Gynecol Obstet 1971; 133: 497–511.
55. Myhre-Jensen O, Larsen SB, Astrup T. Fibrinolytic activity in serosal and synovial membrane. Arch Pathol 1969; 88: 623–57.

56. Porter JM, McGregor FH, Mullen DC, Silver D. Fibrinolytic activity of mesothelial surfaces. Surg Forum 1969; 20: 80–2.
57. Ellis H. The aetiology of post-operative abdominal adhesions. An experimental study. Br J Surg 1962; 50: 10–6.
58. Buckman RF, Woods M, Sargent L, Gervin AS. A unifying pathogenetic mechanism in the etiology of intraperitoneal adhesions. J Surg Res 1976; 20: 1–5.
59. Gervain AS, Puckett CL, Silver D. Serosal hypofibrinolysis. A cause of post-operative adhesions. Am J Surg 1973; 125: 80–8.
60. Hau T, Payne WD, Simmons RL. Fibrinolytic activity of the peritoneum during experimental peritonitis. Surg Gynecol Obstet 1979; 148: 415–8.
61. Weinstein MP, Iannini PB, Stratton CW, Eickhoff TL. Spontaneous bacterial peritonitis. A review of 28 cases with emphasis on improved survival and factors influencing prognosis. Am J Med 1978; 64: 592–8.
62. Gilmour J, Tymiansky R, Pierratos A, Vas S, Klein M, Khanna R, Digenis D, Cuff S, Oreopoulos DG. Changes in some inflammatory proteins during peritonitis in CApd patients. Perit Dial Bull 1983; 3: 201–4.
63. Verbough HA, Keane WF, Hoidal JR, Freiberg MR, Elliott GR, Peterson PK. Peritoneal macrophages and opsonins: Antibacterial defense in patients undergoing chronic peritoneal dialysis. J Inf Dis 1983; 147: 1018–29.
64. Duwe A, Vas SI, Weatherhead JWS. Effect of composition of peritoneal dialysis fluid on chemiluminescence, phagocytosis and bactericidal activity in vitro. Infec Immun 1981; 33: 130–5.
65. Collart F, Tielemaus C, Schandene L, Dupont E, Wybrau Y, Dratwe M. CAPD and cellular immunity: No different than hemodialysis patients. Perit Dial Bull 1983; 3: 163–4.
66. Giaccino F, Alloatti S, Guarello F, Coppo R, Pellerey M, Piccoli G. The influence of peritoneal dialysis on cellular immunity. Perit Dial Bull 1982; 2: 165–8.
67. Vas SI, Low DE, Layne S, Khanna R, Dombros N. Microbiological diagnostic approach to peritonitis in CAPD patients (1981). In: Atkins RC et al. (ed), peritoneal Dialysis. Churchill Livingstone, Edinburgh 1981; pp 269–71.
68. Vas SI. Peritoneal fluid cultures remain positive for days. Perit Dial Bull 1982; 2: 144.
69. Swartz RD, Campbell DA, Stone D, Dickinson C. Recurrent polymicrobial peritonitis from a gynecological source as a complication of CAPD. Perit Dial Bull 1983; 3: 32–3.
70. Vas SI. Microbiologic aspects of chronic ambulatory peritoneal dialysis. Kidney International 1983; 23: 83–92.
71. Dobbelstein H. Immune system in uremia. Nephron 1976; 17: 409–14.
72. Montgomery YZ, Kalmanson GR, Guze LB. Renal failure and infection. Medicine 1968; 47: 1–32.
73. Vas SI. Peritonitis during CAPD. A mixed bag. Perit Dial Bull 1981; 1: 47–9.
74. Nichols WK, Nolph KD. A technique for managing exit site and cuff infection in Tenckhoff catheters. Perit Dial Bull 1983; 3 (suppl): S4–5.
75. Khanna R, McNeely DJ, Oreopoulos DG, Vas SI, McCready W. Treating fungal infections: fungal peritonitis in CAPD. Br Med J 1980; 280: 1147–8.
76. Kloos WE, Schleifer HK. Simplified scheme for the routine identification of human staphylococcus species. J Clin Microbio 1975; 1: 82–8.
77. Peter G, Locci R, Pulverer G. Adherence and growth of coagulase negative staphylococci on surfaces of intravenous catheters. J Infect Dis 1982; 146: 479–82.
78. Gregory MC, Duffy DP. Toxic shock following staphylococcal peritonitis. Clin Nephrol 1983; 20: 101–4.
79. Facklam RR. Physiological differentiation of viridans streptococci. J Clin Microbiol 1977; 5: 184–201.
80. Pierard D, Lauwers S, Monton MC, Sennesael J, Verbeelen D. Group JK Corynebacterium peritonitis in a patient undergoing continuyous ambulatory peritoneal dialysis. J Clin Microbiol 1983; 18: 1011–4.
81. Arfania D, Everett ED, Nolph K, Rubin J. Uncommon causes of peritonitis in patients undergoing peritoneal dialysis. Arch Int Med 1981; 141: 61–64.
82. Kolmos HJ, Anderson KEH. Peritonitis with Pseudomonas aeruginosa in hospitalized patients treated with peritoneal dialysis. Scand J Infect Dis 1979; 11: 207–10.
83. Matthews P. Primary anaerobic peritonitis. Br Med J 1979; 2: 903–4.
84. Onderdonk AB, Bartlett JG, Louie T, Sullivan-Seigler N, Gorbach SL Microbial synergy in experimental intra-abdominal abscess. Infect Immun 13: 22–6.
85. Simkin EP, Wright FK. Perforating injuries of the bowel complicating peritoneal catheter insertion. Lancet 1968; 1: 64–6.
86. Rubin J, Oreopoulos DG, Lio TT, Mathews R, deVeber GA. Management of peritonitis and bowel perforation during chronic peritoneal dialysis. Nephron 1976; 220–5.
87. Wu G. Review of peritonitis episodes that caused interruption of CAPD. Perit Dial Bull 1983; 3 (suppl): S11–3.
88. Sasaki S, Aliba T, Suenaga M, Tornura S, Yoobiyama N, Nakagawa S, Shoji T, Sasavka T, Takenchi J. Ten years survey of dialysis associated tuberculosis. Nephron 1979; 24: 141–5.
89. O'Connor J, MacCormick M. Tuberculous peritonitis in patients on CAPD: The importance of lymphocytosis in the peritoneal fluid. Perit Dial Bull 1: 106.
90. Morford DW. High index of suspicion for tuberculous peritonitis in CAPD patients. Perit Dial Bull 1982; 2: 189–90.
91. Dineen P, Hornan WP, Grafe WP. Tuberculous peritonitis: 43 years experience in diagnosis and treatment. Am Surg 1976; 184: 712–7.

92. Wolfe JHN, Behn AR, Jackson BT. Tuberculous peritonitis and role of diagnostic laparoscopy. Lancet 1978: Lancet 1: 852–853.
93. Vas SI Editorial comment. Perit Dial Bull 1982; 2: 190.
94. Bayer AS, Blumenkrantz MY, Montgomerie JZ, Galpin JE, Coburn JW, Gruze LB. Candida peritonitis. Am J Med 1976; 61: 832–40.
95. Kerr CM, Perfect JR, Craven PC, Jorgensen JH, Drutz DJ, Shelburne JD, Gallis HA, Gutman RA. Fungal peritonitis in patients on continuous ambulatory peritoneal dialysis. Ann Int Med 1983; 99: 334–7.
96. Holdsworth SR, Atkins RC, Scott DF, Jackson R. Management of Candida peritonitis by prolonged peritoneal lavage containing 5-fluorocytosine. Clin Nephrol 1975; 4: 157–9.
97. Lempert KD, Jones JM. Flucytosine – miconazole treatment of Candida peritonitis: Its use during continuous ambulatory peritoneal dialysis. Arch Int Med 1982; 142: 577–8.
98. Chapman JR, Warnoch DW. Ketoconazole and fungal CAPD peritonitis. Lancet II: 1983; 510–1.
99. Pearson JG, McKinney TD, Stone WJ. Penicillium peritonitis in a CAPD patient. Perit Dial Bull 1983; 3: 20–1.
100. NIH CAPD Patient Registry Report. 1987; Characteristics of participants and selected outcome measures for the period January 1 1981 through August 31 1986.
101. Steiner R. Clinical observations on the phathogenesis of peritoneal dialysate eosinophilia. Perit Dial Bull 1982; 2: 118–9.
102. Verger C, Berry JP, Galle P, Pavergue A, Hoang C, LeCharpentier Y. Foreign material inclusions in the peritoneum of CAPD patients: a study with X-ray microanalysis. Perit Dial Bull 1982; 2: 138–9.
103. Williams P, Khanna R, Simipson H, Vas SI. Tobramycin blood levels of CAPD patients during peritonitis. Perit Dial Bull 1982; 2: 48.
104. Manuel MA, Paton TW, Cornish WR. Drugs and peritoneal dialysis. Perit Dial Bull 1983; 3: 117–25.
105. Sewell DL, Golper TA. Stability of antimicrobial agents in peritoneal dialysate. Antimicrob Agents Chemother 21: 528–9.
106. Sewell DL, Golper TA, Brown SD, Nelson E, Knower M, Kimbrough RC. Stability of single and combination antimicrobial agents in various peritoneal dialysates in the presence of insulin and heparin. Am J Kidney Dis 1983; 3: 209–12.
107. Rubin J, Jumphries J, Smith G, Bower J. Antibiotic activity in peritoneal dialysate. Am J Kidney Dis 1983; 3: 205–8.
108. Bunke CM, Aronoff GR, Luft C. Pharmacokinetics of common antibiotics used in continuous ambulatory peritoneal dialysis. Amer J Kidney Dis 1983; 3: 114–7.
109. Vas SI. Letter. Perit Dial Bull 1981; 1: 67.
110. Gokal R, Vas SI. Risk of tobramycin use in CAPD patients with peritonitis. Perit Dial Bull 1982: 2: 139–41.
111. Silva J, Fekety R. Clostridia and antimicrobial enterocolitis. Am Rev Med 1981; 32: 327–33.
112. Antibiotic lavage for peritonitis. Editorial (1979) Brit Med Jour Sept 22, 1979; pp 691–2.
113. Stephen RL. Kablitz C, Kitahara M, Welson JA, Duffin DP, Kolff WJ. Peritoneal dialysis: peritonitis: saline iodine flush. Dial Transpl 1979; 8: 584–95.
114. Nolph KD. In: Continuous Ambulatory Peritoneal Dialysis, ed. by Legrain M. Excerpta Medica, New York, 1980; p 272.
115. Digenis GE, Khana R, Pierratos A, Vas S. Morbidity and mortality after treatment of peritonitis with prolonged exchanges and intraperitoneal antibiotics. Perit Dial Bull 1982; 2: 45–6.
116. Cantaluppi A, Scalamogna A, Guerra L, Graziani G, Ponticelli C. Treatment of peritonitis in patients on CAPD. Perit Dial Bull 1982; 2: 142.
117. DeGroc F, Rottembourg J, Jacq D, Jaslier V, N'Guyen J, Legrain M. Les peritonites au cours de la dialyse peritoneal continue ambulatoire. Traitment par lavage ou non? Etude prospective. Nephrologie (SWZ) 1983; 4: 24–7.
118. De Tremont JF, Khissi H, Thomas D, Tolain M, Lawrence G, Coevoet B, Fournier A, Orfica J. Traitment des peritonites ou dialyse peritoneal. Comparison entre lavage continue avec machine et lavage intermittent par quatre sac/jour de DPCA. Pathol Biol (Paris) 1983; 31: 544–7.
119. Helfrich GB, Winchester JF. Shaving of external cuff or peritoneal catheter. Perit Dial Bull 1982; 2: 183.
120. Digenis GE, Khanna R, Pantalony D. Eosinophilia after implantation of the peritoneal catheter. Perit Dial Bull 1982; 2: 98–9.
121. Vas SI. Indications for removal of peritoneal catheter. Perit Dial Bull 1981; 1: 145–6.
122. Gandhi VC, Humayun HM, Ing TS, Daugirdas JT, Jablokow VR, Iwantsuki S, Geis WP, Hano JE. Sclerotic thickening of the peritoneal membrane in maintenance peritoneal dialysis patients Arch Int Med 1980; 140: 1201–3.
123. Schmidt RW, Blumenkrantz M. Peritoneal sclerosis. A sword of Democles for peritoneal dialysis. Arch Int Med 141: 1265–7.
124. Sclerosing Peritonitis, Letters to the editor (1983) Lancet July 9 August 13, September 3, September 24, November 5, 1983.
125. Fenton SSA. Peritonitis related deaths among CAPD patients. Perit Dial Bull 1983; 3 (suppl 3): S9–11.
126. Wu G. Cardiovascular deaths among CAPD patients. Perit Dial Bull 1983; 3 (suppl 3): S23–6.
127. Oreopoulos D, Vas S, Khanna R. Prevention of peritonitis during continuous ambulatory peritoneal dialysis. Perit Dial Bull 1983; 3 (suppl 3): S18–20.
128. Hamilton RW, Disher BA, Dillingham GA, Nicholas AF. The sterile weld a new method for connection in continuous ambulatory peritoneal dialysis. Perit Dial Bull 1983; 2 (suppl 4): S8–10.
129. Buonchristiani U, Cozzari M, Quintiliani G, Carobi C. Abatement of exogenous peritonitis using the Perugia CAPD system. Dial Transplant 1983; 12: 14–25.

130. Ash SR, Hoswell R, Heefer EM, Bloch R. Effect of the Peridex filter on peritonitis rates in a CAPD population. Perit Dial Bull 1983; 3: 89–93.
131. Eremin J, Marshall VC. The place of prophylactic antibiotic in peritoneal dialysis. Aust Ann Med 1969; 18: 264–6.
132. Sharma BK, Smith EC, Rodriguez H, Pillay UKG, Gandhi VC, Dunea G. Trial of oral neomycin during peritoneal dialysis. Am J Med Sei 1971; 262: 175–8.
133. Axelrod J, Meyers BR, Hirschman SZ, Stein R. Prophylaxis with cephalothin in peritoneal dialysis. Arch Intern 1973; 132: 368–71.
134. Low DE, Vas SI, Oreopoulos DG, Manuel RA, Saiphoo CS, Finer C, Dombros N. Randomized Clinical trial of prophylactic cephalexin in CAPD. Lancet 1980; 2: 753–4.
135. Corey PN, Steele C. Risk factors associated with time to first infection and time to failure on CAPD. Perit Dial Bull 1983; 3 (suppl 3): S14–7.
136. D'Apice AJF, Atkins RC. Analysis of peritoneal dialysis data. Peritoneal Dialysis Edited: Atkins RC, Thomas NM, Farrell PC, Churchill Livingstone, Edinburge, pp 440–4.
137. Randerson DH, Farrell PC. Analysis of peritonitis data in CAPD 2nd Int. Symposium in Peritoneal Dialysis, Berlin, 1981; p 52.
138. Corey P. An approach to the statistical analysis of peritonitis data from patients on CAPD. Perit Dial Bull 1981; Suppl Vol 1 No 6: S29–32.
139. Pierratos A, Amair P, Corey P, Vas SI, Khanna R, Oreopoulos DG. Statistical analysis of the incidence of peritonitis in continuous ambulatory peritoneal dialysis. Perit Dial Bull 1982; 2: 32–6.
140. Ryan GB, Grobety J, Majno G. Post-operative peritoneal adhesions. A study of the mechanisms. Am J Pathol 65: 1971; 117: 117–38.
141. Mion CM, Boen ST, Scribner P. Analysis of factors responsible for the formation of adhesions during chronic peritoneal dialysis. Am J Med Sci 1965; 250: 675–9.
142. Steiner RW, Kipper S, Savoia MC, Witztum KF. Identification of peritoneal dialysis catheter tunnel infection by scanning with Indium-111 labelled leukocytes. Ann Int Med 1983; 99: 44–5.
143. Williams P, Pantalony D, Vas SI, Khanna R, Oreopoulos DG. The value of dialysate cell count in the diagnosis of peritonitis in patients on continuous ambulatory peritoneal dialysis. Perit Dial Bull 1981; 1: 59–62.
144. Kapral FA, Godwin JR, Dye ES. Formation of intraperitoneal abscesses by Staphylococcus aureus. Infec Immun 1980; 30: 204–11.
145. Karanicolas S, Oreopoulos DG, Frath Sh, Shiminer A, Manning RF Sepp H, de Veber GA, Darby T. Epidemic of aseptic peritonitis caused by endotoxin during chronic peritoneal dialysis. N Engl J Med 1972; 296: 1336–7.
146. Williams P, Khanna R, Vas S, Layne S, Pantalony D, Oreopoulos DG. Treatment of peritonitis in patients on CAPD: To lavage or not. Perit Dial Bull 1980; 1: 14–7.
147. O'Leary JP, Malik FS, Donahoe RR, Johnston AD. The effects of a minidose of heparin on peritonitis in rats. Surg Gynecol Obstet 1979; 148: 571–5.
148. Cotran RS, Karnowsky MJ. Ultrastructural Studies on the permeability of the mesothelium to horse radish peroxidase. J Cell Biol 1968; 37: 123–37.
149. MacCallum WG. On the mechanism of absorption of granular materials from the peritoneum. Bull Johns Hopkins Hosp 1903; 14: 105–10.
150. Casley-Smith JR. An electron microscopical study of the passage of ions through the endothelium of lymphatic and blood capillaries, and through the mesothelium. Quart J Exp Physiol 1967; 52: 105–13.
151. Courtice FC, Simmonds WJ. Physiological significance of lymph drainage of the serous cavities and lungs. Physiol Rev 1954; 34: 419–49.
152. Lorber B, Swenson RM, The bacteriology of intra-abdominal infections. Surg Clin North Am 1975; 55: 1349–54.
153. McNeely D, Vas SI, Dombros N, Oreopoulos DG. Fusarium peritonitis: an uncommon complication. Perit Dial Bull 1981; 1: 94–6.
154. Marrie TJ, Noble MA, Costerton JW. Examination of the morphology of bacteria adhering to peritoneal dialysis catheters by scanning and transmission electron microscopy. Jour Clin Microbiol 1983; 18: 1388–98.
155. Vas, SI and Low L. Microbiological diagnosis of peritonitis in patients on continuous ambulatory peritonel dailysis. J Clin Microb 1985; 21: 522–3.
156. Rubin SJ. Continuous ambulatory peritoneal dialysis: Dialysate fluid cultures. Clin Microbiol Newsl 1984; 6: 3–5.
157. Fenton P. Laboratory diagnosis in patients undergoing continuous ambulatory peritoneal dialysis. J Clin Path 1982; 35: 1181–4.
158. Knight KR, Rolak A, Crump J Maskell R. Laboratory diagnosis and oral treatment of CAPD patients. Lancet 1982; 2: 1301–4.
159. Buggy BP. Culture methods for continuous ambulatory peritoneal dialysis associated peritonitis. Clin Microb Newsletter 1986; 8: 12–4.
160. Smalley DL, Baddour LM, Kraus AP. Rapid detection of Gram-negative bacterial peritonitis by the Limulus amoebocyte lysate assay. J Clin Microbiol 1986; 24: 882–3.
161. Clayman MD, Raymond A, Colen D, Moffit C, Wolf C, Neilson E. The Limulus amebocyte lysate assay. Arch Int Med 1987; 147: 337–40.
162. Oreopoulos DG, Vas SI. Peritonitis in continous ambulatory peritoneal dialysis: Making therapeutic decisions easier. Arch Int Med 1987; 147: 818–9.
163. Heering PJ, Bach D, Henzler P, Grabensee B, Dialysis and HIV infection. Nephron 1987; 47: 158–159.
164. Berlyne GM, Rubin J, Adler AJ. Dialysis in AIDS patients. Nephron 1987; 44: 265–6.
165. Robles R, Lopox-Gomez Jm, Muino A, Valderrabano F. Dialysis in AIDS Patients: A new problem. Nephron 1987; 44: 375–6.
166. DeRossi A, Vertoli U, Romagnoli G, Bertoli M,

Dalla Grassa O, Chieco-Bianchi L, LAV/HTLV–III and HTLV–I antibodies in hemodialysis patients. Nephron 1987; 44: 377–8.
167. Morrison AJ, Freer CV, Poole CL, JOHNSTON DO, Westervelt F, Normansell DE, Wenzel RP. Prevalence of human lymphotropic virus type III antibodies among patients in dialysis programs at a university hospital. Ann Int Med 1986; 104: 805–7.
168. Humphreys MH, Scoenfield PY, Aids and renal disease. The Kidney 1987; 20: 7–12.
169. Rubin RH, Jenkins RL, Shaw BW, Shaffer D, Pearl RH, Erb S, Monaco AP, VanThiel DH. The aquired immunodeficiency syndrome and transplantation. Transplantation 1987; 44: 1–4.
170. Olivera DBG, Winearls CG, Cohen J, Ind PW, Williams G. Severe immunosuppression in a renal transplant recipient with HTLV–III antibodies. Transplantation 1986; 41: 260–2.
171. Favero MS. Recommended precautions for patients undergoing hemodialysis who have AIDS or non-A non-B hepatitis. Infection Control 1985; 6: 301–5.
172. Recommendations for providing dialysis treatment to patients infected with human T-Lymphotropic virus type III/lymphadenopathy-associated virus. MMWE 1986; 35: 376–83.
173. Harnett JD, Zeldis JB, Parfrey PS, Kennedy M, Sircar R, Steinmann TI, Guttmann RD. Hepatitis B disease in dialysis and transplant patients. Transplantation 1987; 44: 369–76.
174. Vas SI. Peritonitis of peritoneal dialysis patients: Pathogenesis and treatment. Medical Microbiology Vol 5: ed: Easmon CSF and Jeljaszewicz J. Academic Press London 1986; pp 21–63.
175. Gruer LD, Bartlett R, Aycliffe AJ. Species identification and antibiotic sensitivity of coagulase negative staphylococci from CAPD peritonitis. J Antimic Chemother 1984; 13: 577–83.
176. Baddour LM, Smalley DL, Kraus AP, Lamoreaux WJ, Christensen GD. Comparison of microbiologic characteristics of pathogenic and saprophytic coagulase negative staphylococci from patients on continuous ambulatory peritoneal dialysis. Diagn Microbiol Infect Dis 1986; 5: 197–205.
177. Horsman GB, Macmillan L, Amatnieks Y, Rifkin O, Vas SI. Plasmid profile and slime analysis of coagulase negative staphylococci from CAPD patients with peritonitis. Perit Dial Bull 1986; 6: 195–8.
178. Keane WF, Everett ED, Golper TA, Gokal R, Halstenson C, Kawaguchi Y, Riella M, Vas SI, Verbrugh HA. Peritoneal dialysis related peritonitis treatment recommendations: 1993 Update. The Ad Hoc advisory committee on peritonitis management. Perit Dial Intern 1993; 13: 14–28.
179. VI. Catheter related factors and peritonitis risk in CAPD patients. USRDS 1992 Annual Report. Am J Kidney Dis 20 (suppl. 2): 48–54.
180. Goldstein CS, Garrik RE, Polin RA, Gerdes JS, Kolski GB, Neilson EG, Douglas SD. Fibronectin and complement secration by monocytes and peritoneal macrophages in vitro from patients undergoing continuous ambulatory peritoneal dialysis. J Leucocyte Biol 1986; 39: 457–64.
181. Khan RH, Klein M, Vas S. Fibronectin in the normal peritoneal fluids of patients on chronic ambulatory peritoneal dialysis and during peritonitis. Perit Dial Bull 1987; 7: 69–73.
182. Holley J, Seibert D, Moss A. Peritonitis following colonoscopy and polypectomy: A need for prophylaxis? Perit Dial Bull 1987; 7: 105.
183. Stuck A, Seiler A, Frey FJ. Peritonitis due to an intrauterine contraceptive device in a patient on CAPD. Perit Dial Bull 1986; 7: 158–9.
184. Sombolos K, Vas S, Rifkin O, Ayomamitis A, McNamee P, Oreopoulos DG. Propionibacteria isolates and asymptomatic infections of the peritoneal effluent in CAPD patients. Nephrol Dial Transplant 1986; 1: 175–8.
185. Williams PS, Hendy MS, Ackrill P. Routine daily surveillance cultures in the management of CAPD patients. Peri Dial Bull 1987; 7: 183–6.
186. Gokal R, Ash S, Helfrich GB, Holme C, Joffe Pe, Nichols K, Oreopoulos DG, Riella M, Slingeneyer A, Twardowski ZJ, Vas SI. Peritoneal catheters and exit site practices: Toward optimum peritoneal access. Perit Dial Intern 1993; 13: 29–39.
187. Dasgupta MK, Bettcher KB, Ulan RA, Burns V, Lam K, Dossetor JB, Costerton JW. Relationship of adherent bacterial biofilms to peritonitis in chronic ambulatory peritoneal dialysis. Perit Dial Bull 1987; 7: 168–73.
188. Holmes CJ, Evans R. Biofilm and foreign body infection – The significance to CAPD associated peritonitis. Perit Dial Bull 1986; 6: 168–77.
189. Verger C, Chesneau AM, Thibault M, Bataille N. Biofilm on Tenckhoff catheters: A negligible source of contamination. Perit Dial Bull 1987; 6: 174–8.
190. Piraino B, Bernardini J, Peitzman A, Sorkin M. Failure of peritoneal cuff shaving to eradicate infection. Perit Dial Bull 1987; 7: 179–82.
191. Piraino B, Bernardini J, Johnston J, Sorkin M. Chemical peritonitis due to intraperitoneal vancomycin (Vancoled). Peri Dial Bull 1987; 7: 156–9.
192. Churchill DN, Oreopoulos DG, Taylor DW, Vas SI, Manuel MA, Wu G. Peritonitis in CAPD patients- A randomized clinical trial of trimethoprim-sulfamethoxazole prophylaxis. Abstr. 20th Ann Meeting of the American Societ of Nephrology, 1987; p 97A.
193. Harvey DM, Sheppard KJ, Morgan AG, Fletcher J. Effect of dialysate fluids on phagocytosis and killing by normal neutrophils. J Clin Microbiol 1987; 25: 1424–7.
194. McGregor SJ, Brock JH, Briggs JD, Junor BJ. Bactericidal activity of peritoneal macrophages from continuous ambulatory peritoneal dialysis patients. Nephrol Dial Transplant 1987; 2: 104–8.
195. Alobaidi HM, Coles GA, Davies M, Lloyd D. Host defence in continuous ambulatory peritoneal dialysis: the effect of dialysate on phagocyte function. Nephrol Dial Transplant 1986; 1: 16–21.
196. Lewis SL, Van Epps DE. Neutrophil and monocyte

alterations in chronic dialysis patients. Am J Kidney Dis 1987; 9: 381–395.
197. Lamperi S, Carozzi S. Suppressor resident peritoneal macrophages and peritonitis incidence in continuous ambulatory peritoneal dialysis. Nephron 1986; 44: 219–25.
198. Clark LA, Easmon CS. Opsonic activity of intravenous immunoglobulin preparations against Staphylococcus epidermidis. J Clin Pathol 1986; 39: 856–60.
199. Clark LA, Easmon CS. Opsonic requirements of Staphylococcus epidermidis. J Med Microbiol 1986; 22: 1–7.
200. Peterson PK, Lee D, Suh HJ, Devalon M, Nelson RD, Keane WF. Intracellular survival of Candida albicans in peritoneal macrophages from chronic peritoneal dialysis patients. Am J Kidney Dis 1986; 7: 146–52.
201. Peterson PK, Gaziano E, Suh HJ, Devalon M, Peterson L, Keane WF, Antimicrobial activities of dialysate-elicited and resident human peritoneal macrophages. Infect Immun 49: 212–8.
202. Goldstein CS, Bomalaski JS, Zurier RB, Neilson EG, Douglas SD. Analysis of peritoneal macrophages in continuous ambulatory peritoneal dialysis patients. Kidney Int 26: 733–40.
203. Wierusz-Wysocka B, Wysocki H, Michta G, Wykretowicz A, Czarnecki R, Baczyk K,. Phagocytosis and neutrophil bactericidal capacity in patients with uremia. Folia Haematol 1984; 111: 589–94.
204. Huttunen K, Lampainen E, Silvennoinen-Kassinen S, Tiilikainen A. The neutrophil function of uremic patients treated by hemodialysis or CAPD. Scand J Urol Nephrol 1984; 18: 167–72.
205. Maddox Y, Foegh M, Zeligs B, Zmudka M, Bellanti J, Ramwell P. A routine source of human peritoneal macrophages. Scand J Immunol 1984; 19: 23–9.
206. Cichocki T, Hanicki Z, SuLowicz W, Smolenski O, Kopec J, Zembala M. Output of peritoneal cells into peritoneal dialysate. Cytochemical and functional studies. Nephron 1983; 35: 175–82.
207. Rubin J, Lin LM, Lewis R, Cruse J, Bower JD. Host defense mechanisms in continuous ambulatory peritoneal dialysis. Clin Nephrol 1983; 20: 140–4.
208. Verbrugh HA, Keane WF, Hoidal JR, Freiberg MR, Elliott GR, Peterson PK. Peritoneal macrophages and opsonins: antibacterial defense in patients undergoing chronic peritoneal dialysis. J Infect Dis 1983; 147: 1018–29.
209. Lamperi S, Carozzi S. Defective opsonic activity of peritoneal effluent during continuous ambulatury peritoneal dialysis (CAPD): Importance and prevention. Perit Dial Bull 1986; 6: 87–92.
210. Struijk RG, van Ketel RJ, Krediet RT, Boeschoten EW, Arisz L. Viral peritonitis in a continuous ambulatory peritoneal dialysis patient. Nephron 1986; 44: 384.
211. Goodship THJ, Heaton A, Rodger RSC. Ward MK, Wilkinson R, Kerr DNS. Factors affecting development of peritonitis in continuous ambulatory peritoneal dialysis. Br Med J 1984; 289: 1485–6.
212. Goodman W, Gallagher N, Sherrard DJ. Peritoneal dialysis fluid as a source of hepatitis antigen. Nephron 1981; 29: 107–9.
213. Salo RJ, Salo AA, Fahlberg WJ, Ellzey JT. Hepatitis B surface antigen (HB(s)Ag) in peritoneal fluid of HB(s) Ag carriers undergoing peritoneal dialysis. J Med Virol 1980; 6: 29–35.
214. Spector D. Hepatitis B Miniepidemic in a peritoneal dialysis unit. Arch Int Med 1977; 137: 1030–1.
215. Vas SI, Oreopoulos DG. Handle with care: Hepatitis B antigen carriers in peritoneal dialysis units. Nephron 1981; 29:105–6.
216. Eisenberg ES, Leviton I, Soeiro R. Fungal peritonitis in patients receiving peritoneal dialysis: Experience with 11 patients and review of the literature. Rev Inf Dis 1986; 8: 309–21.
217. Oh SH, Conley SB, Rose GM, Rosenblum M, Kohl S, Pickering LK. Fungal peritonitis in children undergoing peritoneal dialysis. Pediatr Inf Dis 1985; 4: 62–6.
218. Vargamezis V, Papadopoulou ZL, Liamos H, Belechri AM, Natscheh T, Vergoulas G, Antoniadou R, Kilintzis V, Papadimitriou M. Management of fungal peritonitis doring continuous ambulatory peritoneal dialysis (CAPD). Perit Dial Bull 1986; 6: 17–20.
219. Cecchin E DeMarchi S, Panarello G, Tesio F. Chemotherapy and/or removal of the peritoneal catheter in the management of fungal peritonitis complicating CAPD? Nephron 1985; 40: 251–2.
220. Tapson JS, Mansy H, Freeman R, Wilkinson R. The high morbidity of CAPD fungal peritonitis-Description of 10 cases and review of treatment strategies. Quart J Med 1986; 61: 1047–53.
221. Kravitz SP, Berry PL. Successful treatment of Aspergillus peritonitis in a child undergoing continuous cycling peritoneal dialysis. Arch Int Med 1986; 146: 2061–2.
222. Paterson AD, Bishop MC, Morgan AG, Burden RP. Removal and replacement of Tenckhoff catheter at a single operation: Successful treatment of resistant peritonitis in continuous ambulatory peritoneal dialysis. Lancet 1986; 2: 1245–7.
223. Craddock CF, Edwards R, Finch RG. Pseudomonas peritonitis in continuous ambulatory peritoneal dialysis: laboratory predictors of treatment failure. J Hosp Infec 10: 179–86.
224. West TE, Walshe JJ, Krol CP, Amsterdam D. Staphylococcal peritonitis in continuous peritoneal dialysis. J Clin Microbiol 1986; 23: 809–12.
225. Peterson PK, Lee D, Suh HJ, Devalon M, Nelson RD, Keane WF. Intracellular survival of Candida albicans in peritoneal macrophages from chronic peritoneal dialysis patients. Am J Kidney Dis 1986; 7: 146–52.
226. Piraino B, Bernardini J, Sorkin M, The influence of peritoneal catheter exit site infections on peritonitis, tunnel infections and catheter loss in patients on continuous ambulatory peritoneal dialysis. Am J Kidney Dis 1986; 8: 435–40.

227. Beasley SW, Meech PR, Neale TJ, Hatfield PJ, Morrison RB. Continuous ambulatory peritoneal dialysis and acute appendicitis. NZ Med J 1986; 99: 145–6.
228. Spence PA, Mathews RE, Khanna R, Oreopoulos DG. Indications for operation when peritonitis ocurs in patients on chronic ambulatory peritoneal dialysis. Surg Gynecol Obstet 1985; 161: 450–2.
229. Lempert KD, Kolb JA, Swartz RD, Campese V, Golper TA, Winchester JF, Bolph KD, Husserl FE, Zimmerman SW, Kurtz SB. A multicenter trial to evaluate the use of the CAPD "O" set. ASAIO Trans 1986; 32: 557–9.
230. Holmes CJ, Miyake C, Kubey W. In vitro evaluation of an ultraviolet germicidal connection system for CAPD. Perit Dial Bull 1984; 3: 215–8.
231. Nolph KD. Randomized multicenter clinical trial to evaluate the effects of an ultraviolet germicidal system on peritonitis rates in continuous ambulatory peritoneal dialysis. Perit Dial Bull 1985; 19–24.
232. Hamilton RW, Disher BA, Dillingham SA, Nicholas AF. The sterile weld: A new method for connections in continuous ambulatory peritoneal dialysis. Perit Dial Bull 1983; 3 (suppl. 4): 8–10.
233. LaRocco MT, Mortensen JE, Robinson A. Mycobacterium fortuitum peritonitis in a patient undergoing chronic peritoneal dialysis. Diagn Microbiol Infect Dis 1986; 4: 161–4.
234. Eisenberg ES, Ambalu M, Szylagi G, Aning V, Soeiro R. Colonization of skin and development of peritonitis due to coagulase negative staphylococci in patients undergoing peritoneal dialysis. J Inf Dis 1987; 156: 478–82.
235. VI. Catheter related factors and peritonitis risk in CAPD patients. USRDS 1992 Annual Report. Am J Kidney Dis 20 (suppl. 2): 48–54.
236. Port FK, Held PJ, Nolph kd, Truenne MN, Wolfe RA. Risk of peritonitis and technique failure by CAPD connectin technique: A national study. Kidney Int 1992; 42: 967–74.
237. Scalamogna A, Castelnovo c, DeVecchi A, Ponticelli C. Exit-site and tunnel infections in continuous ambulatory peritoneal dialysis patients. Am J Kidney Dis 1992; 18: 674–7.
238. Holley JL, Bernardini J, Pirano B. Risk factors for tunnel infections in continous peritoneal dialysis. Am J Kidney Dis 1992; 18: 344–52.
239. Peterson PK, Matzke GR, Keane WF. Current concepts in the management of peritonitis in continuous ambulatory peritoneal dialysis patients. Rev Infec Dis: 9: 604–12.
240. Millikin SP, Matzke GR, Keane WF. Antimicrobial treatment of peritonitis associated with continuous ambulatory peritoneal dialysis. Perit Dial Int 1991; 11: 252–60.
241. Von Graevenitz A, Amsterdam D. Microbiological aspects of peritonitis associated with continuous ambulatory peritoneal dialysis. Clin Microbiol Rev 1992; 5: 26–48.
242. Gilbert DB. Once – daily aminoglycoside therapy. Antimicrob Agents Chemother 1991; 35: 399–405.
243. Nordstrom L, Lerner SA. Single daily dose therapy with aminoglycosides. J Hosp Inf 1991; 18 (suppl A): 117–29.
244. Levison ME. New dosing regimens for aminoglycoside antibiotics. Ann Int Med 1992; 117: 693–4.
245. Parker, SE, Davey PG. Once daily aminoglycoside dosing. Lancet 1993; 341: 346–7.
246. Odenholt-Tornquist I, Lowdin E, Cars O. Postantibiotic sub-MIC Effects of Vancomycin, Roxithromycin, Sparfloxin and Amikacin. Antimicrob Chemother 1992; 36: 1852–8.
247. Lewis S, Holmes C. Host defense mechanisms in the peritoneal cavity of continuous ambulatory peritoneal dialysis patients. Part 1 Perit Dial Int 1992; 11: 14–21.
248. Holmes C, Lewis S. Host defense mechanisms in the peritoneal cavity of continuous ambulatory peritoneal dialysis patients. Part 2 Perit Dial Int 1992; 11: 112–7.
249. Digenis G, Abraham G, Savin E, Blake P, Dombros N., Sombolos K, Vas S, Matthews R, Oreopoulos DG. Peritonitis related deaths in continuous ambulatory peritoneal dialysis (CAPD) patients. Perit Dial Int 1990; 10: 45–7.
250. Johnson CA. Intraperitoneal vancomycin administration. Perit Dial Int 1991; 11: 9–11.
251. Freiman JP, Graham DJ, Reed TG, McGoodwin EB. Chemical Peritonitis following the intraperitoneal administration of vancomycin. Perit Dial Int 1992; 12: 57–60.
252. Magera BE, Arroyo JC, Rosansky SJ, Postic B. Vancomycin pharmacokinetics in patients with peritonitis on peritoneal dialysis. Antimicrob Agents Dhemother 1983; 23: 710–4.
253. Harford AM, Sica DA, Tartaglione T, Polk RE, Dalton HP, Poynor W. Vancomycin pharmacokinetics in continouous ambulatory peritoneal dialysis patients with peritonitis. Nephron 1986; 43: 217–22.
254. Bastani B. Freer K, Read D, Bailey S, Sherman RA, Davis M, Engels D. Treatment of gram positive peritonitis with two intraperitoneal doses of vancomycin in continuous ambulatory peritoneal dialysis patients. Nephron 1987: 45: 283–5.
255. Boyce NW, Wood C., Thomson NM, Kerr P, Atkins RC. Intraperitoneal (IP) vancomycin therapy for CAPD peritonitis- a prospective randomized comparison of intermittent v continuous therapy. Am J Kidney Dis 1988; 12: 304–6.
256. Brown J, Altman P, Cunningham of J Chaw E, Marsk F. Pharmacokinetics of once daily intraperitoneal aztreonam and vancomycin in the treatment of CAPD peritonitis. J Antimicr Chemother 1990; 25: 141–7.
257. Fellin G, Gentile MG, Manna GM et al. Peritonitis prevention: Y connector and sodium hypochlorite. Three years' experience. Report of the Italian study group. In: Khanna R. Nolph KD, Prowant B, Twardowski ZJ, Oreopoulos DG (eds), Advances in Peritoneal Dialysis. Perit Dial Int Inc. Toronto 1987; 3: 114–8.
258. Canadian CAPD Clinical Trials Group. Peritonitis in continuous ambulatory peritoneal dialysis

258. (CAPD): A multi-center randomized clinical trial comparing the Y connector disinfectant system to standard systems. Perit Dial Int 1989; 9: 159–63.
259. Viglino G, Cancarini G, Catizone L, Cocchi R, de Vecchi A, Lupo A, Salomone M, Segoloni GP, Giangrande A. The impact of peritonitis on CAPD results. In: Khanna R, Nolph DK 1992; Prowant B, Twardowski ZJ, Oreopoulos DG (eds), Advances in Peritonal Dialysis Perit Dial Int Inc, Toronto 1992; 8: 270–5.
260. Twardowski ZJ, Dobbie JW, Moore HL, Nichols WK, De Spain JD, Anderson PC, Khanna R, Nolph KD, Loy TS. Morphology of peritoneal dialysis catheter tunnel. I, Macroscopy and light microscopy. Perit Dial Int 1991; 11: 237–51.
261. Chong TK, Piraino B, Bernardini J. Vestibular toxicity due to gentamicin in peritoneal dialysis patients. Perit Dial Int 1991; 11: 152–5.
262. Nikolaidis P, Vas S, Lawson V, Kennedy-Vosu L, Bernard A, Abraham G, Izatt S, Khanna S, Bargman JM, Oreopoulos DG. Is intraperitoneal tobramycin ototoxic in CAPD patients? Perit Dial Int 1991; 11: 156–61.
263. Vonesh EF. Which statistical method to use when analyzing the incidence of peritoneal dialysis related inmfections. Perit Dial Int 1991; 11: 301–4.
264. Dobbie JW. Pathogenesis of peritoneal fibrosing syndromes (sclerosing peritonitis) in peritoneal dialysis. Perit Dial Int 1992; 12: 14–27.
265. Breborowicz A. Free radicals in peritoneal dialysis: agents of damage. Perit Dial Int 1992; 12: 194–8.
266. Dasgupta MK, Fox S, Gagnon D, Bettcher K, Ulan RA. Significant reduction of peritonitis rate by the use of twin-bag system in a Canadian regional CAPD program. In: Khanna R, Nolph KD, Prowant B, Twardowski ZJ, Oreopoulos DG (eds), Advances in Peritoneal Dialysis. Perit Dial Int Inc, Toronto 1992; 8: 223–6.
267. Hutchison A, Gokal R. Peritoneal dialysis fluids for the future: Do we have the solution? Dialysis Transplant. 1992; 12: 199–203.
268. Ing TS, Zhou XJ, Yu AW, Vazir ND. Lactate-containing versus bicarbonate-containing peritoneal dialysis solutions. Perit Dial Int 1992; 12: 276–7.
269. Oreopoulos DG. Peritoneal dialysis research for the 1990's. Perit Dial Int 1992; 12: 278–80.
270. Vas SI. Primary and secondary role of viruses in chronic renal failure. Kidney Intrnational 1991; 40 (suppl 35): 2–4.
271. Prowant BF, Warady BA, Nolph KD. Peritoneal dialysis exit site care: Results of an international survey. Perit Dial Int 1993; 13: 149–54.
272. Korbet SM, Vonesh EF, Firanek CA. A retrospective assessment of risk factors for peritonitis among an urban CAPD population. Perit Dial Int 1993; 13: 126–31.
273. Maiorca R, Cantalupppi A, Cancarini GC, Scalamogna A, Broccoli R, Graziani G, Brasa S, Ponticelli C (1989) Prospective controlled trial of a Y-connector and disinfectant to prevent peritonitis in continuous ambulatory peritoneal dialysis (CAPD). Lancet 1983; 2: 642–4.
274. Gokal R, Ramos M, Francis D et al. Peritonitis in CAPD. Lancet 1982; 2: 1388–91.

17 Host defence and effects of solutions on peritoneal cells

GERALD A. COLES, SHARON L. LEWIS AND JOHN D. WILLIAMS

1.	Introduction	503	2.6.	Humoral defences	511
2.	Peritoneal cavity in CAPD patients	504	2.7.	Effect of dialysate on host defence	513
	2.1. WBC yields and differentials	504	2.8.	Catheter and biofilm	515
	2.2. Monocytes/Macrophages (cellular defences)	504	3.	Peritoneal cavity in CAPD patients during non infectious contamination	516
	2.2.1. Peripheral monocyte function	505	4.	Peritoneal cavity in CAPD patients during infectious contamination	517
	2.2.2. Peritoneal macrophage function	505		4.1. Inflammatory response	517
	2.2.3. Macrophage function as related to incidence of peritonitis	505		4.2 Cell-cell interaction and the mediator network in the peritoneal cavity	517
	2.3. Neutrophils	507		4.2.1. Peritoneal macrophages	518
	2.4. Lymphocytes	508		4.2.2. Peritoneal mesothelial cells	518
	2.4.1. Peripheral lymphocyte function	508		4.3. Humoral defences	519
	2.4.2. Peritoneal lymphocyte function	508	5.	Conclusions and clinical significance	521
	2.4.3. Relationship of peritonitis and lymphocyte function	509	References		522
	2.5. Mesothelial cells	510			

1. Introduction

It is general experience that some patients receiving long-term peritoneal dialysis suffer from repeated episodes of peritonitis while others remain relatively free of this complication. It has been suggested that differences in the ability of individual subjects to resist infection, i.e., their host defence, are at least partly responsible for this clinical observation. This hypothesis was strengthened by the report by Verbrugh *et al.* on the potential efficacy of peritoneal macrophages and opsonins in the antibacterial defence of such patients [1]. In this chapter we review the available evidence on the various components of host defences of peritoneal dialysis patients including the effect of the dialysate.

Any discussion on host defence must first consider the general medical state of the patients which may affect resistance to infection independently of the presence of uraemia or the use of dialysis. Certain specific diseases may directly impair host defence. It is generally held that subjects with diabetes are more liable to infection than normals. Evidence has been presented that diabetic CAPD patients have a higher nasal carriage of *S. aureus* and thus be more liable to exit site infection and possible subsequent peritonitis with this organism [2]. Individuals suffering from myeloma or other blood dyscrasias may well have immune alterations limiting host defence.

Immunosuppressive therapy for conditions such as systemic lupus erythematosus is well known to be associated with morbidity from infection. Finally as AIDS progresses, repeated and persistent infections occur due to unusual organisms, again because of immunosuppression induced by the disease.

Malnutrition is well known to be associated with an increased risk of infection. Since varying degrees of protein-calorie depletion are common in CAPD patients (see Chapter 15) the question as to whether these could contribute to the risk of peritonitis has been raised. Two studies have found an association between a low serum albumin and subsequent peritonitis [3, 4]. This has not, however, been confirmed by other centres [5]. The discrepancy may be in part explained by the fact that infection tends to occur mainly in the severely malnourished non-uraemic subject whereas mild to moderate degrees of malnutrition are seen in CAPD patients.

One further factor that may affect host defence is age. There is evidence that elderly individuals have a decreased immune response and consequent increased chances of infection such as tuberculosis. This immunodeficiency is at least in part aggravated by nutritional deficiencies [6]. Thus, since many

CAPD subjects have an age greater then 65 years, it is likely that they will be, as a group, more susceptible to infection irrespective of any influence of the uraemic state or the dialysis treatment.

2. Peritoneal cavity in CAPD patients

2.1. WBC yields and differentials

Studies of the normal human peritoneal cavity have primarily been done on women undergoing laparoscopy for diagnostic evaluation of infertility or for tubal ligation. Normally the peritoneal cavity contains less than 50 ml of fluid with cell yields ranging from 7 to 12 million in 3–15 ml of this fluid. Differentials of WBC in this fluid consist of about 90% macrophages, 5–10% lymphocytes, and less than 5% polymorphonuclear neutrophils (PMN) [7–10].

In peritoneal dialysis patients without peritonitis the WBC recovery from 1 to 3 liters of peritoneal dialysate effluent ranges from less than 1 million to 45 million cells [1, 7–15]. This represents about a 100 to 1000 fold decrease in the concentration of WBC within the peritoneal cavity of peritoneal dialysis patients as compared to "normal" controls. With increasing time on CAPD there is a decrease in WBC yields [9, 14]. However, there are no correlations between WBC yields and susceptibility to infection [9, 14]. When peritoneal dialysis patients with high and low incidences of peritonitis are compared, there are no significant differences between total WBC yields [15].

Peritoneal WBC differentials from uninfected peritoneal dialysis patients are diverse, ranging from 20–95% macrophages, 2–84% lymphocytes, and 0–27% neutrophils [1, 7–15]. The reasons for this wide diversity remain unknown and are not related to age, sex, frequency of peritonitis, or underlying renal disease [12, 15]. It has been shown in longitudinal studies that although there is a great deal of intrapatient variability in WBC differentials over time, interpatient variability is remarkable low [15, 16].

In general, data related to WBC yields and differentials of peritoneal dialysate effluents seem to indicate that these factors are not important in the prevention or in predicting the incidence of peritonitis in peritoneal dialysis patients.

2.2. Monocytes/Macrophages (cellular defenses)

The predominant cell type isolated from the effluent of CAPD patients is the macrophage (PMØ). Macrophages can be classified into resident and exudative inflammatory cells. The macrophages found in dialysate are exudative (inflammatory) macrophages having recently arrived from circulating blood in response to various stimuli within the peritoneal cavity. Both resident and exudative macrophages originate from monocytes in circulation.

There does not seem to be any conclusive data that certain subtypes of monocytes are destined for any particular tissue to become resident macrophages. It seems that monocytes leave the circulation randomly, and once in a given tissue, transform into a specific type of resident macrophage in response to tissue-specific stimuli. Once in tissues, monocytes/macrophages do not re-enter the circulation [17].

In the normal, unstimulated peritoneal cavity, 90% of PMØ are resident cells (as measured by peroxidase staining of the rough endoplasmic reticulum and nuclear envelope). In contrast, in CAPD patients exudative macrophages (peroxidase staining only in lysosomal granules) and peroxidase-negative PMØ are found [12]. Exudative macrophages lose the peroxidase-containing lysosomes very quickly and transform into peroxidase-negative macrophages.

The data related to peroxidase staining of macrophages suggest that PMØ from CAPD patients are stimulated or activated macrophages rather than resident peritoneal macrophages. Furthermore, it has been shown that dialysis fluid is an inducer of exudative PMØ [18]. The data related to peroxidase staining patterns of macrophages suggest that a permanent state of chronic activation exists in the peritoneal cavity of CAPD patients.

During CAPD it has been estimated that $3-4 \times 10^7$ PMØ are lost each day in dialysate effluent [7]. Because there is only about a two-fold reserve of monocytes in bone marrow, it has been postulated that this continual removal of PMØ (which have influxed from circulating blood) may stimulate the release of immature monocytes into circulation. Support for this postulate arises from a study by Bos *et al.* who have shown a decreased level of maturation of PMØ as compared to normal peritoneal macrophages [19]. In addition, Moughal *et* al. have shown that there are immature monocytes in the circulation of CAPD patients as determined by transferrin-receptor positive cells [20].

The functions of monocytes/macrophages include 1) recognition and phagocytosis of foreign material and 2) participation in the immune response. Figure 1 depicts the steps involved in effective phagocytosis and intracellular killing of microorganisms by monocytes/macrophages and PMN.

2.2.1. *Peripheral monocyte function*
There have been few studies that have investigated peripheral monocyte function of CAPD patients. It has been shown that peripheral monocytes have a decreased ability to bind C5a (a complement-derived chemotactic factor) as has also been found in hemodialysis patients [21]. It is possible that chronic complement activation may be occurring in the peritoneal cavity with sufficient C5a produced to cross the peritoneal membrane and block C5a receptors in the peripheral blood.

Oxidative metabolic functions of peripheral monocytes vary depending on the stimulus. When phorbol myristate acetate (PMA) is used as a stimulus, no differences can be detected in the production of H_2O_2 or O_2^- as compared to control cells. However, when C5a or fMLP (a synthetic chemotactic factor similar to bacterial-derived chemotactic factor) were used as stimulants, there was a decrease (as compared to controls) in the generation of H_2O_2 or O_2^- from monocytes of CAPD patients [22].

In general, these data suggest that alterations in chemotactic-mediated signal transduction exist that could affect 1) mobilization of cells to the site of injury or infection and 2) generation of reactive oxygen products needed for intracellular killing of microorganisms.

2.2.2. *Peritoneal macrophage function*
Studies on peritoneal macrophages have used *in vitro* assays to determine phagocytosis, bactericidal killing, and oxidative metabolic responses (Table 1). How the results of these *in vitro* studies relate to the *in vivo* situation is not really known.

Results of studies investigating phagocytosis of microorganisms *in vitro* indicate that PMØ from CAPD patients can function as effectively a normal PMN or PMØ [1, 8, 9, 23]. However, Brando *et al.* found that the phagocytic function of PMØ from CAPD patients was decreased as compared to peripheral monocytes [24].

Studies investigating bactericidal ability of PMØ have provided conflicting results. Goldstein *et al.* [7] and Verbrugh *et al.* [1] found normal bactericidal capacity while McGregor *et al.* [9] reported decreased capacity compared to normal PMØ.

The evaluation of oxidative metabolism of PMØ has also yielded varied results. When patients' PMØ were compared to normal peripheral PMN or peritoneal PMN from patients with peritonitis, they had a decreased oxidative metabolic response [1, 25]. However, when PMØ were compared to the patients' peripheral monocytes or normal PMØ, they had an enhanced oxidative metabolic response [8, 26, 27] suggesting that dialysate-elicited PMØ not only are functionally intact but are probably activated or stimulated cells.

Cell surface receptors and antigens on patients' PMØ have been characterized and compared to the patients' peripheral monocytes [28]. When PMØ were compared to the peripheral monocytes, they had increased binding of C5a, enhanced expression of Fc receptors (which binds IgG), and increased expression of Ia (HLA-DR) and CD14 antigens. CD14, commonly used to identify monocytes/macrophages in blood and tissues, is thought to be a growth factor receptor [29]. These results suggest that patients' PMØ are activated cells with increased expression of receptors and antigens important in host defence mechanisms.

The results of studies on PMØ from CAPD patients do not lead to a clearcut model of antibacterial capabilities of these cells. Different results may be due, in part, to using differing cell types for comparative studies (Table 1). In general, it seems that PMØ from most CAPD patients, when studied in dialysate-free media, have intact phagocytic and bactericidal capacities.

2.2.3. *Macrophage function as related to incidence of peritonitis*
Many studies have attempted to characterize PD patients into distinct groups as related to incidence of peritonitis and tried to identify what could be possible predictive factors or correlating variables with peritonitis.

Studies which have shown there is no difference between high peritonitis incidence (HPI) and low peritonitis incidence (LPI) patients have investigated phagocytosis and killing of *S. epidermidis* [9], phagocytosis of *S. epidermidis* and *E. coli* [30], and C2 secretion from cultured macrophages [31]. A variety of receptors (i.e., C5a, fMLP, Fc, complement receptors CR1 and CR3) on PMØ from HPI

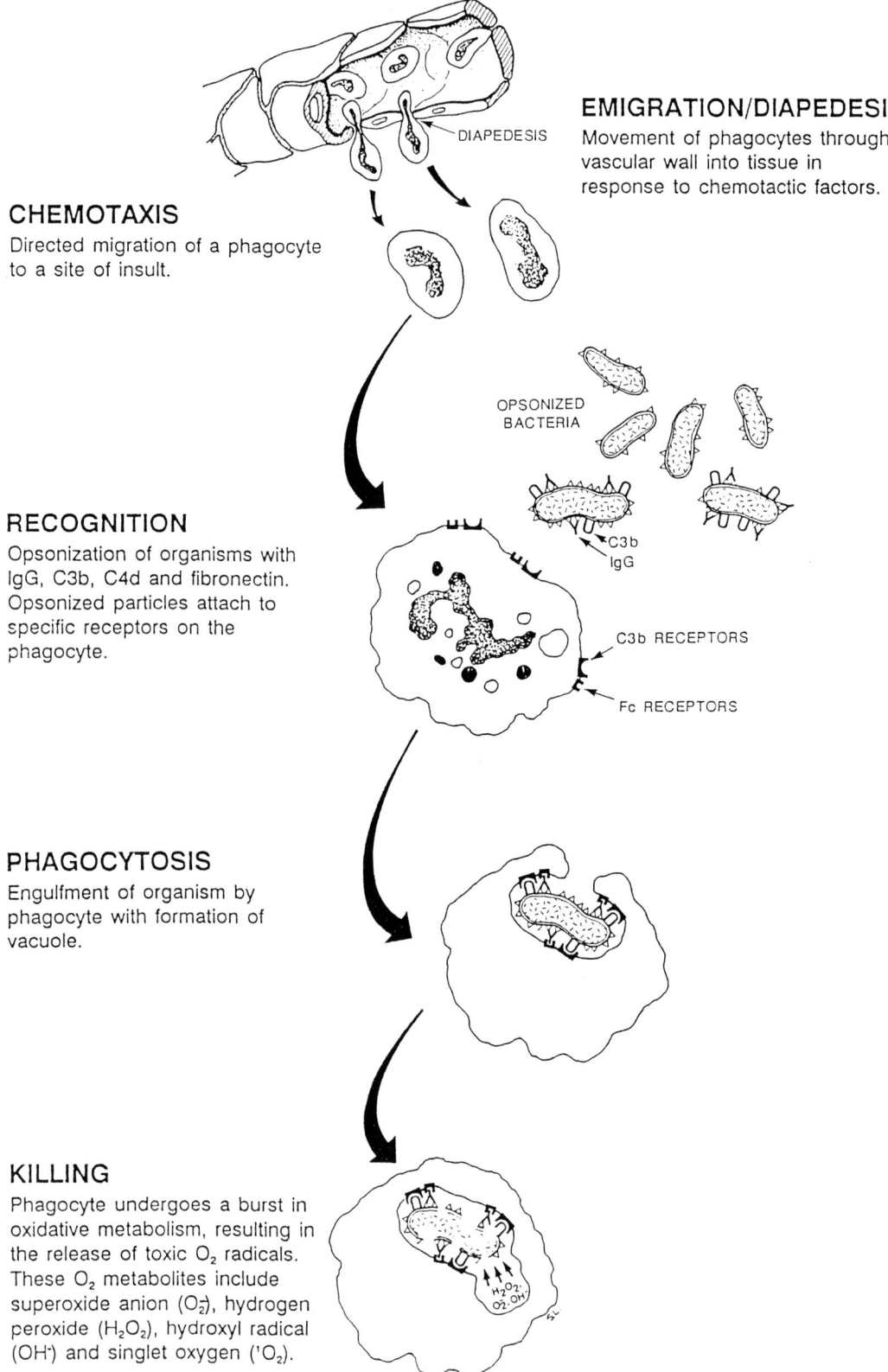

Figure 1. Representation of events involved in phagocytosis and killing of bacteria by phagocytic WBC. (Used with permission – Lewis S and Holmes C. Host defense mechanisms in the peritoneal cavity of CAPD patients. Peritoneal Dial Int 1991; 11: 14–21).

and LPI patients were analyzed on patients who were followed longitudinally for six months [15]. The results indicated that although there was a trend toward increased expression of these receptors in HPI patients, there were no significant differences between the two patient groups.

In contrast, Lamperi and Carozzi [32, 33] have identified many variables where differences were found between PMØ from patients with HPI as compared to those with LPI. These include decreased IL-1 secretion, increased PGE_2 release, decreased bactericidal activity and H_2O_2 production, and decreased IgG Fc receptors. Results of studies of other investigators that have found differences when HPI patients were compared to LPI patients, have found that PMØ from HPI patients have decreased fibronectin secretion [31], decreased expression of RFD1, a marker of maturation status [34], and decreased chemiluminescent response [34]. In addition, Bos et al. found that the total number of phagocytosing macrophages and the phagocytic capacity of PMØ were enhanced in HPI patients [19].

Reasons for discrepancies in the results of these studies are obscure. However, it should be noted that these studies have been cross-sectional in design and thus, cause and effect remain unknown.

Because the causes of peritonitis are multifactorial, it is highly unlikely one will find any significant correlation between peritonitis rates and a single parameter assessing host defence mechanisms. It is more likely that there is a continuum of peritonitis rates and risk factors rather than distinct groups of patients with high or low risks of peritonitis. Tranaeus et al. state that although there are differences in the occurrence rate of peritonitis among patients, the difficulties in identifying individual high risk factors can be explained by a random distribution of risk factors among patients [35].

2.3. Neutrophils

Because of the low numbers of cells normally found in dialysate, it is difficult to study peritoneal neutrophils. In CAPD patients 0–27% of peritoneal WBC are neutrophils as compared to less than 5% in normal subjects. Peritonitis is accompanied by a marked increase (as much as 100 fold) in cellularity usually due to an increase in PMN. (PMN response to microbial invasion in the peritoneal cavity is discussed later in this chapter).

Studies of peripheral PMN from CAPD patients have shown that these cells have decreased ability to bind C5a relative to normal controls [21] and decreased chemotactic and oxidative metabolic responses to the chemotactic factors C5a and fMLP [22].

Table 1. Peritoneal macrophage function in CAPD patients.

Parameter measured	Finding	Comparative cells	Reference
1. Phagocytic capacity	Normal	Normal peritoneal macrophages	8, 9, 23
	Normal	Normal PMN	1
	↓	CAPD peripheral monocytes	24
2. Bactericidal ability	Normal	Normal PMN	1
	Normal	Normal blood monocytes & peritoneal macrophages	7
	↓	Normal peritoneal macrophages	9
3. Oxidative metabolism			
– H_2O_2 generation	Normal	Normal peritoneal macrophages	7
– Chemiluminescence	↓	Normal peripheral or peritoneal PMN	1, 25
	↑	Normal peritoneal macrophages	8
	↑	CAPD peripheral monocytes	26
4. Maturation level	↓	Normal peritoneal macrophages	19
	↑	CAPD peripheral monocytes	26
5. Receptors			
– C5a	↑	Normal and CAPD peripheral monocytes	27
– Complement receptors CR1 & CR3	Normal	Normal and CAPD peripheral monocytes	27
– Fc receptors	↑	Normal and CAPD peripheral monocytes	27
	↑	CAPD peripheral monocytes	26

Adapted from Lewis SL and Holmes CJ. Host defense mechanisms in the peritoneal cavity of CAPD patients. Peritoneal Dial Int 1991; 11: 14–21.

Harvey et al. investigated phagocytosis and killing capability of circulating PMN from CAPD patients with and without peritonitis, and peritoneal PMN function from patients with peritonitis [36]. They found that peripheral PMN from uninfected patients showed reduced phagocytosis of both *Candida guilliermondii* and *S. epidermidis* due to an intrinsic defect in the neutrophils and also to an opsonic defect of CAPD serum. In contrast, both peripheral and peritoneal PMN from infected patients were found to phagocytose normally when tested in the presence of normal serum. Furthermore, in this study there was decreased bacterial killing by both peritoneal and peripheral PMN for *S. epidermidis* but not *Candida guilliermondii*. This defect indicates that *S. epidermidis* may be sequestered intracellularly during peritonitis, protected from antibiotics, and act as a nidus of infection.

The significance of PMN to peritoneal host defence is their ability to mobilize from the circulation to the peritoneum and phagocytose and kill invading microorganisms. It is unknown if PMN alterations in chemotactic, phagocytic, or killing responses have a major contributing role in overall peritoneal host defence mechanisms.

2.4. Lymphocytes

Lymphocytes consist primarily of T cells (thymus-dependent cells) and B cells (bursa-equivalent or thymus-independent) cells. T cells comprise 70–80% of circulating lymphocytes and are primarily responsible for immunity to intracellular viruses, tumor cells, and fungi. B cells account for about 10–20% of circulating lymphocytes. When B cells are sensitized to a specific antigen, they differentiate into plasma cells, which in turn produce immunoglobulins (antibodies).

T lymphocytes can be classified into T cytotoxic, T helper, and T suppressor cells. T cytotoxic cells are involved in attacking the cell membrane of foreign antigens and releasing cytolytic substances that destroy the antigen. T helper and T suppressor cells serve as immunoregulatory cells, facilitating antibody production by B cells and the cytotoxic activity of T lymphocytes, either positively (T helper) or negatively (T suppressor).

2.4.1. Peripheral lymphocyte function
Similar to HD patients, peripheral lymphopenia is characteristic in many CAPD patients [37, 38]. A 12 month longitudinal study has shown there are no significant changes over time in the peripheral WBC count or lymphocyte percentages for CAPD patients [39]. Although there are only a few reports of peripheral lymphocyte studies in CAPD patients (Table 2), in general these studies indicate there are no differences in the percentages of peripheral blood T and B cells as compared to normal controls [38, 39, 40]. Furthermore, no significant changes in these lymphocyte subsets have been observed over the first 6–12 months of CAPD therapy [39, 40].

CAPD patients have significantly higher percentages of peripheral natural killer (NK) cells and activated T cells than normal controls [39, 41]. When T helper (CD4) cells are divided into helper-inducer (CD4$^+$/CD29$^+$) cells and suppressor-inducer (CD4$^+$/CD45RA$^+$) cells, CAPD patients have significantly more CD4$^+$/CD29$^+$ and fewer CD4$^+$/CD45RA$^+$ cells [39]. Similar lymphocyte subset distributions are found in patients with various autoimmune diseases (e.g., multiple sclerosis, diabetes mellitus, systemic lupus erythematosus) [42, 43, 44]. The significance of these findings in the patients' peripheral lymphocytes suggests an activated and proinflammatory environment.

2.4.2. Peritoneal lymphocyte function
There have been several studies that have investigated peritoneal lymphocytes from CAPD patients [45–49]. In the peritoneum of normal controls about 5–10% of the WBC are lymphocytes [7–10].

Table 2. Characteristics and functions of peripheral and peritoneal lymphocytes from CAPD patients.

Parameter measured	Peripheral lymphocytes [Ref]*	Peritoneal lymphocytes [Ref]**
T Cells (%)	Normal [40, 45, 54, 97]	Normal [47] ↓ [39, 46]
T helper cells (%)	Normal [39]	↓ [39, 49]
T suppressor cells (%)	Normal [39]	↑ [39, 49, 50]
CD4/CD8 ratio	Normal [40, 45, 92]	Normal [39, 45, 48]
B cells (%)	Normal [54, 97]	Normal [47] ↑ [39, 46]
NK cells (%)	↑ [39]	↑ [39, 49]
Activated T cells (%)	↑ [39, 48, 49]	↑ [39, 46, 48, 49]
Interleukin-2 production	↓ [37, 53]	↓ [53]

*As compared to normal controls
** As compared to CAPD patients' peripheral lymphocytes
Adapted from Lewis SL, Kutvirt SG, Cooper CL, Bonner PN, Holmes CJ. Characteristics of peripheral and peritoneal lymphocytes from CAPD patients. Peritoneal Dial Int 1993; 13 (Suppl 2).

Reported peritoneal lymphocyte percentages in CAPD patients range from 2–84% with mean ranges of 20–30% [1, 7–15]. The reasons for this considerable variability among patients are unknown. In general, with continued CAPD therapy there is a slight trend for lymphocyte percentages in the dialysate to increase [14, 46], mainly from the beginning to the one month time period [39]. Although there is a great deal of interpatient variability, after the first month of CAPD and during peritonitis-free periods, an individual's percentage of peritoneal lymphocytes remains relatively stable [39, 50]. Following the resolution of peritonitis, there is an increase in lymphocyte percentages and by one to two months the patients' WBC count and cell pattern distribution gradually returns to their baseline values [39, 50]. There are no differences in the percentage of lymphocytes between HPI patients compared to LPI patients [15, 51].

When the percentages of T and B cells in the peripheral blood are compared to the peritoneal lymphocytes, there are decreased peritoneal T cells and increased peritoneal B cells [39, 46, 50]. In addition, there are decreased peritoneal T helper cells and increased peritoneal T suppressor cells [39, 49]. Although the percentage of peritoneal T and B cells differs somewhat from patient to patient, the percentages remain relatively similar over time for individual patients [39, 46]. In spite of increased peritoneal B cells, Davies et al. found that in vitro these B cells failed to produce a significant amount of any immunoglobulin when stimulated with pokeweed mitogen [52].

A consistent finding in studies of lymphocytes isolated from dialysate has been the presence of a high percentage of activated T lymphocytes as compared to peripheral lymphocytes [39, 46, 48, 49]. These activated T cells include both T suppressor and T helper cells [39, 49]. The presence of activated lymphocytes in the peritoneal cavity suggests that some degree of local activation is continuously present in the peritoneum of patients even in the absence of clinical evidence of infection. In addition, these lymphocytes can be further activated (as indicated by cell surface phenotypic markers) following exposure in vivo to an infectious agent [39]. The effects of activated peritoneal T cells on other cells of the immune system or on the peritoneal membrane are not known. It is likely that this activation is nonspecific as Davies et al. could find no evidence of lymphocyte proliferation within the peritoneum [46]. Although the peritoneal lymphocytes are activated, they are functionally impaired. In current ongoing studies we have shown significantly impaired IL-2 production by peritoneal lymphocytes [53].

When peripheral and peritoneal lymphocyte phenotypes were analyzed over the first 12 months of CAPD, there were no significant changes in the immunophenotypes of these cells [39]. This indicates that although lymphocyte activation is occurring, the characteristics of the lymphocyte populations are stable over time.

Whether lymphocytes are fulfilling a specific role in the peritoneal cavity or are just part of the generalized inflammatory process is open to speculation. Although there is evidence of activation, lymphocyte proliferation does not seem to be occurring in the peritoneal cavity. This may imply that the activation is nonspecific. To some extent changes in peritoneal lymphocytes reflect increased cytokine production by activated macrophages. Subsequently activated lymphocytes produce cytokines that can regulate other aspects of the immune and inflammatory responses. Thus, peritoneal lymphocytes are actively involved in the various aspects of host defence in the peritoneal cavity.

2.4.3. Relationship of peritonitis and lymphocyte function

The possibility that the frequency of peritonitis is related to the state of the immune system is speculative. Largely unanswered is the question of which may come first: depressed immune responses or frequent episodes of peritonitis.

Giacchino et al. have reported a slightly higher percentage of peritoneal suppressor T cells and a decreased percentage of B cells expressing surface IgA in a HPI group indicating that in these patients there may be an alteration in peritoneal lymphocytes [54]. Lamperi and Carozzi have also found that stimulated peritoneal lymphocytes from a HPI group showed a decreased ability to produce gamma-interferon as compared to a LPI group [33, 55]. Davis et al. found that the expression of HLA-DR antigen on lymphocytes from HPI patients was significantly less than in patients with medium or low incidences of peritonitis [46]. Although Young et al. found a relationship between peritonitis episodes and hypoalbuminemia, they found no association between peritonitis episodes and peripheral cell-mediated immunity as measured by delayed hypersensitivity skin testing [4].

Our studies have shown that after the onset of peritonitis, there was an increase in the percentage of peritoneal activated T cells and suppressor T cells [39]. However, there were no changes in peripheral lymphocyte phenotypes when patients developed peritonitis. This is an interesting finding as it may indicate that peritonitis is a localized infection as has been validated by such clinical observations as lack of positive blood cultures when patients develop peritonitis.

2.5. Mesothelial cells

Any consideration of cellular defences relating to the peritoneal cavity must clearly take into account the role played by the limiting membrane of the cavity, the peritoneal membrane. It acts as a barrier between the peritoneal cavity and the systemic circulation, all inflammatory cells that enter the cavity must traverse this barrier, and lastly the intrinsic cells of the barrier may themselves contribute significantly to the process of host defence and inflammation within the cavity.

The peritoneal membrane is a translucent semi-permeable membrane that consists of a monolayer of mesothelial cells resting on a basal lamina. Below this lamina is a discontinuous band of elastic fibrils and interwoven bundles of collagen fibrils embedded in a connective tissue stroma of glycoproteins and proteoglycans. Embedded in this stroma are fibroblasts, mast cells, blood capillaries and lymphatics [56, 57].

The mesothelial cells themselves are squamous epithelial cells of mesodermal origin. The nature of cell to cell apposition in the surface mesothelial cell layer is unclear. Both desmosomes and tight junctions have been located near to the luminal surface. Tight junctions are the most commonly found but gap junctions and cell process junctions have been described. Intracellularly, in the perinuclear areas of the cytoplasm, there is a well developed Golgi and an abundance of endoplasmic reticulum and mitochondria. Taken together these findings indicate that they are cells of potential secretory capacity. Electron microscopic examination has revealed the presence of lamellar bodies within mouse peritoneal mesothelium [58]. These resemble the lamellar bodies of type II pneumocytes and are thought to contain a lipid-laden material rich in phosphatidylcholine [59, 60] which may contribute to lubrication of the peritoneal surface. More recently studies with cultured mesothelial cells have established their capacity to synthesize a variety of proteoglycans [61]. These include not only molecules intended for structural purposes (basement membranes) but also charged cell surface molecules and molecules secreted into the peritoneal cavity including hyaluronic acid [62].

Their serosal surface has a well defined microvillus border [56] which is thought by some to result in an increased surface area to facilitate absorption [63] and by others to reduce the friction between apposing viscera [64]. The use of cationic markers such as cationised ferritin and ruthenium red [65, 66] have clearly demonstrated that the surface of the mesothelial cells and its villi are coated in a glycocalyx which confers negative charge to the peritoneal membrane. Such a finding has given rise not only to the hypothesis that the membrane may act as a selective barrier to the passage of molecules but also influence the ability of bacteria to bind and to colonise the peritoneal cavity.

The factors governing the initiation of an infection within the peritoneal cavity are numerous but of necessity must include the ability of an inoculum of organisms to adhere to an intraperitoneal surface and to establish colonies [67]. Bacterial-cell interaction and adherence is the result of either specific receptor ligand binding or the result of a non-specific physicochemical interaction [68, 69]. Whilst there are both anionic and cationic sites on the surfaces of bacteria, the presence of anionic polysaccharides in surface glycoproteins and structural carbohydrates usually results in a net negative charge. Thus the effect of a negatively charged peritoneal membrane will be to discourage bacterial adherence and to limit colonisation. Conversely any damage to the ability of the mesothelium to maintain its anionic barrier [70], the presence of cationic binding proteins, or the variation of bacterial charge by an increase in cationic surface structures may facilitate bacterial colonisation.

The *in vitro* binding of staphylococci to mesothelial cells has recently been examined [71]. It was clearly demonstrated that *S. aureus* but not *S. epidermidis* adhered well to mesothelial cell monolayers and that this binding was facilitated by the bacterial cell wall components lipoteichoic acid, and protein A. Lipoteichoic acid has also been demonstrated to be of importance in *Staphylococcus saprophyticus* adherence and this appears to be a direct interaction between the lipid moiety of the molecule with a cell surface binding residue [72]. The greater binding of *S. aureus* is also of clinical significance since it may partly explain its greater virulence in CAPD infection.

In addition to the role of colonisation in establishing infection, there is also morphological evidence that phagocytosis occurs at the surface of the membrane during peritonitis. Early studies by Verger and colleagues [73] demonstrated in a rat model that during episodes of peritonitis there were significant changes to the peritoneum. There were areas of denudation with loss of mesothelial cells. Bacteria were seen adherent to mesothelial cells, which themselves appeared to have lost their close apposition to each other. Leukocytes were observed in these gaps between mesothelial cells and phagocytosis appeared to be taking place on the mesothelial surface.

The direct effect of bacteria on mesothelial cells has received little attention. There is limited evidence to suggest that mesothelial cells may ingest bacteria and that these may survive intracellularly [74]. Short term cultures of mesothelial cell monolayers with a number of clinical isolates of *S. epidermidis* confirmed cell viability but demonstrated a significant inhibition of prostaglandin synthesis by the mesothelial cells [75]. After 18 h of incubation there was up to 90% inhibition of prostacylin and 60% inhibition of prostaglandin E_2. Whether a longer exposure will result in cell death and whether other metabolic functions of the cells are similarly inhibited remains to be examined.

In contrast there is evidence that prostaglandin levels increase during peritonitis [76, 77] and that the mesothelial cell is an important source of arachidonic acid metabolites within the peritoneal cavity [75, 78, 79].

Thus it appears that during infection although those cells of the peritoneal membrane directly affected by bacterial colonisation may be down-regulated, other unaffected areas have the potential for mediator synthesis.

The ability of the mesothelial cell to act as a source of cytokines has recently been investigated. Cultured human mesothelial cells contain mRNA for and secrete significant quantities of interleukins 6 and 8 [80, 81]. In addition the group of Rapoport and colleagues have demonstrated that human peritoneal mesothelial cells (HPMC) synthesize both interleukins 1α and β [82].

2.6. Humoral defences

The normal peritoneal fluid contains protein presumed to derive from the plasma of peritoneal capillaries. Concentrations. of IgG and C3 appear to be similar in this fluid to those in normal serum [83]. The exact role of the proteins of normal peritoneal fluid in host defence is still uncertain. That they may be of importance is suggested by studies of non-uraemic ascites. Patients with cirrhotic ascites tend to have a lower protein concentration, particularly of complement, in their fluid compared to non-cirrhotic causes and the values correlate with a reduced opsonic activity for gram negative organisms [83]. Furthermore, spontaneous bacterial peritonitis is much more likely to occur in subjects with relatively low levels of complement or total protein in their ascites irrespective of the cause [84, 85]. It is known that complement, especially C3 is essential for opsonisation of gram negative bacteria and thus it is assumed that a relative deficiency of this opsonin in the peritoneal cavity of such patients contributes to the development of clinical infection.

The humoral immune response in uraemic individuals and in particular those receiving CAPD has been reported as being both normal and impaired. In general CAPD patients have normal serum levels of immunoglobulins and complement components despite continuing losses in the dialysis effluent [86]. In adults, however, raised concentrations of IgG_3 have been reported [87]. In contrast children have been noted to have depressed values of serum IgG_2 [88]. During treatment with CAPD, systemic concentrations of immunoglobulins and complement remain stable [89] though C3 levels have been reported to correlate negatively with time on CAPD [90]. Whether this latter observation is significant is uncertain since in the same study serum concentrations of C3 did not change during a subsequent year's observation [90].

The response to immunisation of CAPD patients appears variable. A lower percentage of subjects develop protective levels of antibody after hepatitis B vaccination compared to normal controls [87, 91]. There is a tendency to an impaired humoral response following exposure to pneumococcal polysaccharide or tetanus toxoid [87, 89]. Antibody formation after influenza immunisation has been reported to be both normal [92] and depressed [93]. Interestingly one report has suggested that the response to hepatitis B immunisation is inversely correlated with the number of previous blood transfusions [94].

The mechanisms underlying any impairment in humoral immunity in uraemia are still unclear. Elevated plasma levels of complement fragment Ba have been reported [95]. This factor is known to suppress B lymphocyte function *in vitro*. Furthermore, the concentrations in plasma were higher in a group of uraemic subjects who failed to respond to hepatitis B vaccination compared to those who had an effective response [95]. There is also evidence that in experimental chronic renal failure raised levels of PTH contribute to impaired humoral immunity [96]. Unfortunately, there is no information on the relation of PTH levels to antibody formation in human studies.

In vitro studies suggest that B cells from uraemic patients have reduced proliferation when stimulated with *Staphylococcus aureus* and impaired immunoglobulin production both spontaneously and when exposed to *Staphylococcus aureus* or pokeweek mitogen [97]. However, when exposed to a polyclonal B cell activator, immunoglobulin secretion by both normal and uraemic lymphocytes is augmented. This suggests that the intrinsic ability to make antibody is retained but output is suppressed by abnormal T cell function.

Interest in humoral immune factors in the peritoneal cavity of PD patients was generated by the observation that the dialysis effluent contained opsonins. Opsonins are soluble factors which bind to particles, particularly microorganisms, rendering them much more susceptible to ingestion by phagocytes [98]. The opsonic activity of overnight dwell fluid approximates 1% of that in normal serum when tested against gram positive organisms [99]. It appears to be both heat-stable and heat-labile suggesting that both immunoglobulin and complement are involved [1]. Studies using chelation by EGTA or Mg-EDTA implicate both the classical and alternative pathways of complement activation [100].

Concentrations of IgG after an overnight dwell are on average about 0.1 g/l or slightly less [23, 99, 100, 101]. These is, however, little or no correlation with serum values in individual patients. IgG levels slowly rise with increasing dwell time. During the first few months of CAPD treatment concentrations tend to decline and then remain stable [14, 102] though there is a considerable variation in values when an individual patient is repeatedly tested [89, 103, 104].

Complement levels, particularly C3, also fluctuate in a similar manner. Analysis of effluent has shown evidence of C3 activation *in vivo*, though the results bear no relation to episodes of peritonitis [105].

Several studies have suggested that levels of opsonic activity or IgG in dialysate are lower in patients with a high incidence of peritonitis in particular due to *S. epidermidis* [23, 99, 100]. This suggests that subjects with low levels of opsonins represent a high risk group. Figure 2 shows the overnight dialysate IgG concentrations from 48 CAPD patients who were then subsequently followed for 6 months. There is a continuum of results over a nearly 10-fold range. As can be seen most individuals who developed *S. epidermidis* infection during the follow up period had relatively low levels of IgG in their dialysate. It is possible to calculate a discriminant value for separating the concentrations into high and low risk groups.

Similar results were obtained when measures of opsonic activity or C3 levels were assessed [100]. However, it is important to realise that more than half the patients classified into a high risk group did not develop this complication. Thus analysis of effluent for opsonins cannot predict peritonitis for an individual.

Not all studies have been able to confirm these findings [106, 107]. There are a number of possible reasons. In some cases retrospective analyses alone have been undertaken and will have included the period immediately after starting PD when dialysate IgG levels are highest. In addition, the variation in an individual patient's results could easily lead to misclassification. A further compounding problem is the fact that an individual dialysate will have marked variations in its opsonic acitivity for different strains of *S. epidermidis* [108–110]. Those

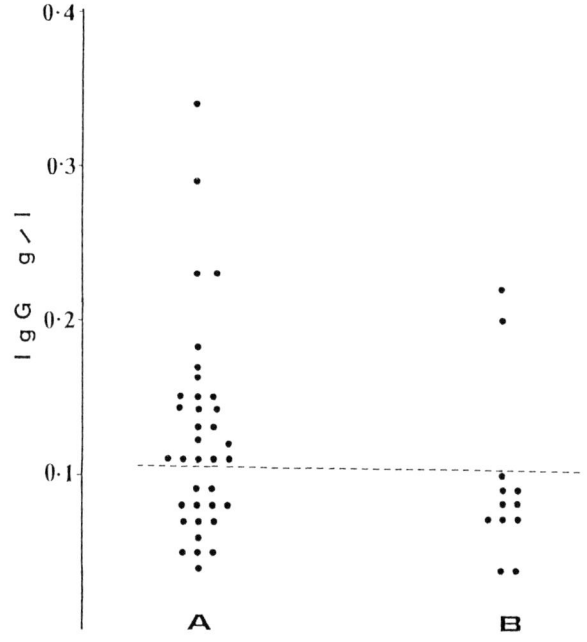

Figure 2. The IgG levels in overnight dialysate obtained from 48 CAPD patients who subsequently continued this treatment for at least 6 months. The results in the right hand column (B) are from these who developed *S. epidermidis* peritonitis during follow up. The results on the left (A) are from those who did not experience this infection. The horizontal line represents the calculated cut off point between "high" and "low" values. Adapted from Coles *et al.* [100]. (Reproduced with permission).

studies suggesting that patients can be assigned to high and low risk groups has each used only one isolate of this organism. Finally the introduction of flush before fill systems has considerably reduced the incidence of coagulase negative staphylococcal infection making it much more difficult to show the influences of any opsonin.

If there are patients with an increased risk of peritonitis it should clearly be of value to know as soon as possible after starting PD. Two studies have looked at levels of both IgG and specific anti-staphylococcal antibodies in dialysate at the beginning of treatment but neither was able to classify subjects into high and low risk groups [102, 104].

Opsonic activity for gram-negative organisms in PD effluent is considerably lower than for gram-positive bacteria [23, 99]. This has been related to the very low concentrations of complement components since these are essential as opsonins for gram-negative bacilli. This may explain the apparent clinical severity of peritonitis caused by this group of organisms. However, it is interesting that one patient with a complete absence of serum C3 underwent CAPD for 6 months with no peritonitis [111].

Fibronectin can act as an opsonin for gram-positive organisms and is found in low concentrations in the dialysate. Goldstein *et al.* [32] reported that the concentration of fibronectin was significantly lower in the dialysate of patients with a high incidence of peritonitis compared to those with a low rate. They furthermore suggested that peritoneal macrophages from the former group had a lower *in vitro* rate of fibronectin secretion. In contrast Khan *et al.* [112] and Davies *et al.* [113] were unable to relate the dialysate concentration to peritonitis rate. Part of the discrepancy may be methodological since fibronectin can be unstable if care is not taken when samples are thawed for the assay. Furthermore, as with other opsonically active proteins there is a considerable variation in dialysate concentrations from individual patients.

Fibrinogen can be found in peritoneal effluent and may polymerise to fibrin being visible macroscopically, particularly during episodes of peritonitis. The addition of *S. aureus* to used dialysate also induces fibrin formation which traps most of the bacteria. It is known that organisms sequestered in fibrin are not susceptible to phagocytosis but the addition of urokinase enhances the opsonic activity of PD effluent for *S. aureus* [114]. This suggests that intraperitoneal fibrinogen through its ability to transform to fibrin may have an adverse effect on host defence.

2.7. Effect of dialysate on host defence

The fresh dialysate which enters the peritoneal cavity has a major influence on the patient's ability to resist infection. The immediate effect is to dilute all aspects of host defence found in the cavity. The number of macrophages present in CAPD fluid are similar to those in the normal abdomen. However, the dilution by 2 litres reduces these phagocytes to concentrations of the order of 10^4 to 10^5/ml. Most studies of macrophage function *in vitro* have used concentrations of 10^6/ml with an excess of bacteria. The *in vitro* growth of gram positive organisms in CAPD effluent is only inhibited when more than 5×10^5/ml phagocytes are present [115]. In addition, rats given *E. coli* intraperitoneally have a higher mortality if the volume of injection but not the number of bacteria is increased [116]. During peritonitis it is unusual to find bacterial counts much above 10^2/ml. Thus, the chances of phagocytes and microorganisms interacting in the dialysate are remote. These considerations have led to the suggestion that any bacterial-phagocyte interaction must take place on a surface such as the mesothelium or possibly the catheter. Each exchange removes macrophages from the body. Thus the effect of dialysis is to facilitate the constant recruitment of new, possibly immature, cells into the peritoneum. In addition to the cells, the fluid also markedly dilutes humoral factors especially the opsonins. At the end of an overnight dwell, IgG concentrations in the effluent are approximately 1% those of serum [23, 99–101]. Values are considerably lower when fresh dialysate is instilled. Thus, for a large part of each cycle there may be insufficient amounts of antibody or complement present to act as effective opsonins.

In addition to its dilutional effect, dialysate is directly toxic to phagocytes, both macrophages and polymorphonuclear neutrophils, as well as mesothelial cells. Duwe *et al.* were the first to report that fresh dialysate inhibited peripheral blood leucocyte function [117]. Several studies have confirmed this finding and also shown that peritoneal macrophages are affected [7, 118–120]. A number of cell functions are inhibited. With increasing incubation there is loss of cell viability, neutrophils being more susceptible than macrophages [118]. There is also a severe depression of phagocytic capacity even after only 15 minutes exposure when most cells are still viable [118]. Neutrophils obtained from the peritoneal cavity of CAPD patients are similarly affected [119]. The fluid also suppresses oxygen uptake by both types of phagocyte as well as their chemiluminescent response and in particular superoxide generation [25, 120, 121]. As little as 5 minutes incubation in dialysate is sufficient to decrease superoxide production [122]. Neutrophils show morphological changes after exposure to unused dialysate [123].

Other aspects of phagocyte function are also affected. Stimulated release of the leukotrienes LTB_4 and combined $LTC_4/LTD_4/LTE_4$ from both peripheral blood and peritoneal neutrophils is suppressed [124]. Lipopolysaccharide-induced production of $TNF\alpha$ from peripheral blood mononuclear cells is similarly depressed [125]. The main effects of fresh dialysate on phagocytes are shown in Table 3.

Other studies have shown toxicity of fresh dialysate to uraemic mouse peritoneal cells [126], fibroblasts [127] and most importantly human mesothelial cells in culture [128, 129]. Fluids from different manufacturers were tested and all caused more than 50% release of ^{51}Cr from mesothelium after 18 hours incubation. There was, however, considerable variation in cytotoxicity induced by the different fluids with only 4 hours exposure [128].

Fresh dialysate can also interfere with humoral aspects of host defence. Using *E. coli* as the test organism, complement-mediated opsonisation and lysis by neutrophils are inhibited [130]. Both classical and alternative pathways of complement activation are affected. Unused fluid also depresses C3 deposition on *S. epidermidis* [131].

A number of investigators have attempted to delineate the factors in commercial dialysate responsible for altered phagocyte function. Possible toxic constituents include the low pH, usually about 5.2, lactate, osmolality, glucose itself and any compounds produced by the heat sterilisation process. Several studies have noted that raising the pH of dialysate to 6.5 or higher prevents impairment of many of the cell functions [25, 118, 119, 121, 131]. Exposure of phagocytes to fluids of pH 5.2 which do not contain lactate, however, does not have such a deleterious effect. It appears, therefore, that the combination of low pH and lactate are responsible.

Respiratory burst activation as judged by chemiluminescence or superoxide generation is affected by this combination probably by inducing a rapid intracellular acidosis [132, 133]. It is known that NADPH oxidase, a major component of the neutrophil respiratory burst mechanism, is inhibited at low pH. Non-lactate containing fluids such as phosphate buffered saline at low pH do induce intracellular acidosis but at a much slower rate.

Other aspects of phagocyte function such as LTB_4 release appear not to be affected by pH and lactate [133]. However, phagocytosis and LTB_4 release are inhibited by increased osmolality [134]. In contrast, cytotoxicity of neutrophils is caused by higher concentrations of D-glucose (2.7% or greater) independently of osmolality. L-glucose and D-mannitol which have identical molecular weights did not affect cell death suggesting a specific effect of D-glucose. Stimulated release of $TNF\alpha$ and IL-6 from mononuclear cells is depressed at higher osmolality but also by high concentrations of monosaccharides and not specifically glucose. In contrast respiratory burst activation is not affected by glucose concentrations or osmolality [62].

Finally it has been postulated that the heat sterilisation process may induce the formation of toxic compounds from glucose. Wieslander et al. found that heat sterilised fluid inhibited fibroblast growth *in vitro* whereas filter sterilised dialysate had no effect [127]. The nature of the toxic substance(s) produced by the high temperature remains uncertain.

The full clinical significance of the deleterious effects of unused dialysate on cells *in vitro* remains uncertain. *In vivo* the pH of peritoneal fluid rises to approximately 7 within 30 minutes of installation of a new bag [118]. Lactate concentrations also fall quickly. In contrast, over a 4 hour period, dialysate with an initial dextrose concentration of 3.86% will still be hyperosmolar. Short dwell time fluids inhibit the chemiluminescent response and phagocytic capacity of phagocytes whereas effluents obtained after periods of 8 hours or more *in vivo* do not affect these cellular functions [13, 25, 118]. Four hour dwell dialysate does not impair neutrophil function as judged by the nitroblue tetrazoline test [135]. Peritoneal macrophages obtained after a 1.5 hour period *in vivo* show diminished phagocytosis compared to those isolated from 15 hour effluent [13].

Table 3. Effects of unused dialysate on phagocyte function.

PMN	PMØ
Cytotoxicity	Cytotoxicity
Decreased respiratory burst	Decreased respiratory burst
Decreased phagocytosis	Decreased phagocytosis
Decreased LTB_4 release	Decreased $TNF\alpha$ production

Thus the effect of pH and lactate may be transient or not significant, though the fact that as little as 5 minutes of exposure affected superoxide production is cause for concern [122]. It is more likely that impaired phagocytosis could occur for a considerable part of the usual CAPD dwell times particularly if a hyperosmolar fluid is being used. In confirmation of this suggestion it has recently been shown that PMØ obtained from patients exposed to a dialysate of pH 7 *in vivo* for 30 minutes are significantly better able to phagocytose and kill as compared to cells affected by a fluid of pH 5 for the same length of time [136]. In addition it has also been found that mononuclear cell cytokine release remains impaired for at least 4 hours of the CAPD dwell [137]. This may be due to the accumulation of inhibitors.

The mechanism by which unused dialysate causes toxicity to mesothelial cells is still uncertain. Glucose at high concentrations (30 mM or greater) will inhibit cell proliferation [138]. Glycine at the same concentrations has a similar effect but mannitol and glycerol are less toxic. The role of pH and lactate remain unclear. During severe peritonitis denudation of mesothelial cells can occur and in this situation hypertonic fluids may impair regeneration of the mesothelium. Unfortunately, in the clinical situation there is often a reduction in ultrafiltration necessitating the use of increased concentrations of glucose.

Though there is no doubt that unused dialysate can seriously impair a variety of host defences *in vitro* there is one positive factor namely that the same fluid inhibits bacterial growth. Several investigators have found that *S. epidermidis* will not grow in fresh fluid and in fact there is a slow decline in bacterial numbers with time, effectively due to starvation [129, 139–141]. In contrast *Ps. aeruginosa* can survive and may even increase in numbers to a limited extent [129].

2.8. Catheter and biofilm

The peritoneal dialysis catheter may be detrimental to host defence. It is clearly a potential port of entry for certain pathogens. In experimental animals the implantation of a Tenckhoff catheter is followed by the progressive colonisation both externally and internally of the cannula by bacteria forming a biofilm [142]. Using CAPD in these animals accelerates the spread of the organisms. In humans *S. epidermidis* can certainly reach the peritoneal cavity via the catheter lumen, being flushed through after touch contamination. *S. aureus* can enter the same way but can also spread down the catheter in a periluminal manner particularly if the exit site is colonised.

If infection becomes established, the cannula will, as with any foreign body, make it more difficult to eradicate the microorganisms. Whether this is solely due to the colonisation of the catheter by a biofilm is as yet unclear. In uraemic mice *S. epidermidis* is cleared rapidly from the peritoneum, even if a catheter is present, as long as the bacteria are injected directly into the peritoneal cavity [143]. In contrast, if the organisms are administered through the lumen of the cannula then the latter remains heavily colonised. In normal rabbits intraperitoneally injected *Pseudomonas aeruginosa* is cleared rapidly [144]. However, in the presence of silicone discs in the peritoneal cavity, the same dose of organisms is associated with peritonitis and a biofilm forms rapidly on the foreign material.

When any foreign material is left in the body, it rapidly becomes coated with protein. On occasions microorganisms may also adhere to the device forming a biofilm [145]. Electron microscopy shows that the bacteria are embedded in a matrix which consists particularly of saccharides often called a glycocalyx. The matrix appears to be secreted by the organisms. There is evidence that these microbes are resistant to host defence. They are not so easily ingested by phagocytes [146, 147] and reduce binding of C3b [148]. Furthermore, bacteria embedded in a biofilm are more resistant to antimicrobial agents in the usual concentrations employed during peritoneal dialysis [149].

Biofilms have been found on peritoneal catheters. Most studies have suggested a prevalence of 80 to 100% [150–152]. However, Verger *et al.* found biofilm on only 2 of 12 examined cannula [153]. The discrepancy is as yet not fully explained but in the latter report the patients were all using a flush before fill system. It is still not clear whether the biofilm acts as a source of infection in recurrent peritonitis. One study noted that biofilm was found in all catheters removed whether for repeated peritonitis or because the patient had had a successful renal transplant [152].

It has been suggested that dissemination of bacteria from the biofilms occurs within the peritoneal cavity and that on some occasions this will be sufficient to overcome host defence and clinical peritonitis will result. On the other hand, the ubiquitous nature of biofilm may mean it has no relevance to recurrence or relapse. The study of

Zappacosta and Perras which reported that treatment was effective in 99% of cases of so-called uncomplicated peritonitis without catheter removal implies that the biofilm does not have a major role in relapse [154].

3. Peritoneal cavity in CAPD patients during noninfectious contamination

Microbial invasion of the peritoneal cavity in CAPD occurs via a variety of portals of entry with the most common being intraluminal (via internal pathway of PD catheter) and periluminal (penetration through skin at catheter exit site). The incubation period for exogenous contamination is not really known, although clinical experience indicates that signs and symptoms often occur within 24 to 48 hours after "touch" contamination. Occasionally appearance of symptoms may be very rapid (i.e., less than 6 to 12 hours). The incubation period for endogenous contamination is not known but is probably shorter than exogenous contamination.

Microbial contamination of the peritoneal cavity may occur in some patients without the development of "clinical" peritonitis [155]. Bacteria have been isolated from as many as 25% of tested dialysate effluents taken from CAPD patients without clinical manifestations of peritonitis [156–159]. The fate of bacteria invading the peritoneal cavity depends on multiple factors. The pathogenesis of peritonitis will depend on the balance between host defence mechanisms and the pathogenicity of the contaminating microorganism. Pathogenicity of the organism is determined by its virulence and dose. Relatively avirulent *Staphylococcus epidermidis* and *Propionibacteria* have frequently been isolated from asymptomatic patients. In contrast, organisms such as *Staphylococcus aureus* that are more virulent are only found in the context of symptomatic peritonitis [156]. Consequently, it can be hypothesized that healthy peritoneal host defence mechanisms can effectively eradicate a small inoculum of bacteria, especially if they are avirulent in nature but may be ineffective against virulent pathogens. Examination of peritoneal cells from patients without clinical evidence of peritonitis will reveal occasional macrophages laden with intracellular bacteria [160]. This observation supports the concept of a first line of macrophage defence.

In experimental animals there is good evidence that bacteria inoculated into the peritoneal cavity are partly cleared via lymphatics in the diaphragm [161]. Ligation of the thoracic duct leads to significantly higher numbers of organisms remaining in the peritoneum. Thus the lymphatics together with resident macrophages appear to provide the first line of host defence [162]. There is no direct evidence that the same mechanism occurs in human subjects but the frequent occurrence of bacteraemia during peritonitis in non dialysis patients suggests that lymphatic removal leading to entry into the circulation of bacteria must occur.

It is still unclear if the same is true of CAPD subjects. The rarity with which bacteraemia occurs during PD associated peritonitis suggests that the lymphatics may not be important. The contrast may, however, be due to the different natural history of the infections. In non uraemic patients, infections are usually gram negative as compared to gram positive in the CAPD subject. Furthermore, it is likely that the inoculum size is much greater in conditions such as bowel perforation than with touch contamination induced *S. epidermidis* peritonitis. Thus in the latter condition bacteria may pass up the lymphatics but in sufficiently small numbers that they can be effectively removed by lymph nodes before reaching the circulation. Lymphatic flow is considered further in Chapter 5.

Peritoneal drainage of dialysate in CAPD itself may be of benefit in eradicating contaminating microorganisms. Glancey et al. have shown that the actual drainage of dialysate effluent from CAPD patients removes bacteria from the peritoneal cavity [163]. In their study the effectiveness of bacterial clearance was related to the volume of peritoneal fluid remaining after drainage. A residual volume of less than 800 ml (normal ~400 ml) prevented survival of *S. epidermidis* whereas a residual volume of less than 200 ml was needed to eliminate *S. aureus*. Thus, physical removal of bacteria may be another contributing method to prevent microbial contamination from progressing to peritonitis.

When peritonitis-free CAPD patients were followed for six months, cyclic changes in the percentage and absolute number of PMN and an occasional increase in activated complement components in the peritoneal effluents were found in some of these patients [15, 105]. This finding may reflect occasional microbial contamination of the peritoneum resulting in a localized "infection" with an influx of neutrophils that can eradicate the microorganisms.

4. Peritoneal cavity in CAPD patients during infectious contamination

4.1. Inflammatory response

In order for contamination to progress to peritonitis, first lines of host defence have to be overwhelmed. As previously mentioned, the macrophage is classically considered the primary component of first line defence. However, the concentration of PMØ in dialysate may not be sufficient to eradicate bacteria, especially if contamination results in a large inoculum. The concentration of macrophages in effluent is only 10^4 cells/ml or 10 cells/µL. Verbrugh et al. have shown that in vitro a minimum of 5×10^5 cells/ml is required to achieve bacteriostasis for coagulase-negative Staphylococci and 5×10^6 cells/ml for Staphylococci aureus [115]. Given the low cell concentration in dialysate, there is a low probability of "collisions" between fluid phase phagocytes and bacteria in such a dilute phagocyte mixture. In contrast to the uninfected state, during clinical peritonitis the concentration of macrophages and neutrophils increase to $0.5–12 \times 10^6$ cells/ml and the chances of phagocytosis increase significantly. In addition to insufficient phagocytes, the unphysiological nature of peritoneal dialysis fluid with its low pH and high osmolality may interfere with WBC function [164].

Although speculative, it is possible that surface adherent macrophages may be more effective than fluid-suspended macrophages in host defense. However, scanning electron micrographs do not indicate any surface adherent macrophages [56]. Submesothelial macrophages have been found on biopsy specimens taken from patients both at the time of their first PD catheter insertion and following periods on CAPD therapy [165]. Although these cells may be resident cells or responding to chemotactic stimuli, their function is unknown.

When contamination of the peritoneal cavity goes unchecked, a dynamic process is set in motion resulting in clinical peritonitis. Following microbial-induced injury, a variety of chemotactic factors are released (Table 4). Interaction of the WBC and chemotactic factor via receptors on the WBC causes the cell to emigrate out of circulation and into the area of injury. The role of chemotactic factors is to ensure an accumulation of WBC in the injured site.

Neutrophils from peripheral blood arrive at the site of injury with a usual maximum response by 12–24 hours. These WBC have a short life span (24 to 48 hours) in tissues. Within hours following the microbial insult there is a dramatic increase in peritoneal WBC with PMN being the predominant influxing cell. The speed of migration is amazing as it takes only a few hours for completely clear peritoneal fluid to turn turbid. Peritoneal fluid turbidity becomes evident visually when greater than 100 WBC/µL are present and is usually obvious by the time there are 200–300 WBC/µL. In the peritoneal cavity PMN will phagocytose and kill the invading organisms. However, during peritonitis they may also release elastase, a potent proteolytic enzyme, as judged by raised levels of elastase-α 1 anti-proteinase complex in the dialysate [166]. In some instances free elastase may be found in the effluent and this could contribute to mesothelial damage [167].

Before a phagocyte can ingest bacteria, recognition must occur. Opsonization of an antigenic surface involves C3b (from complement activation) and IgG antibody (Fig. 1). Once coated with the opsonin, the microorganism can then be recognized by binding to specific receptors for C3b or the Fc fragment of IgG present on the cell surface of neutrophils and monocytes. Compared with blood, uninfected peritoneal dialysate effluent has about 1% of IgG and C3 levels as compared to serum [99, 107]. During episodes of peritonitis these levels increase secondary to the augmented permeability of the peritoneal membrane.

4.2. Cell-cell interaction and the mediator network in the peritoneal cavity

It has been well recognised for some time that the cell which likely triggers the peritoneal inflammatory response is the peritoneal macrophage [7]. The initial interaction of bacteria and phagocyte results in not only the phagocytosis of the organism and its killing but also the release of an array of mediators

Table 4. Chemotactic factors.

Bacteria-derived chemotactic factors
Complement-derived chemotactic factors (C5a)
Lipid-derived chemotactic factors (LTB$_4$)
Coagulation-related chemotactic factors (e.g., kallikrein)
Mesothelial-cell produced IL-8
Interleukin-1 (from macrophages)
Dialysate solution
Peritoneal cell-derived chemotactic factor
Endotoxin (lipopolysaccharide)

designed to amplify the response. This process includes a direct recruitment system for other phagocytes, the interaction of the peritoneal macrophage with the mesothelial cell and the subsequent release of both pro- and anti-inflammatory molecules by this latter cell.

4.2.1. Peritoneal macrophages

These cells form the first line of defence against invading microorganisms and their secretion of mediators forms the initial reaction of the host to infection. Interestingly those macrophages isolated from the peritoneal cavity of CAPD peritonitis appear already to be in an elicited state [168] and have an increased capacity to generate interleukin-1β when compared to resident macrophages. The direct recruitment of neutrophils into the peritoneal cavity may be mediated following the secretion of leukotriene B_4 and interleukin-8 from PMØ [169–171].

Among the earliest studies highlighting the release of mediators during infection was the observation that vasoactive prostanoid synthesis was significantly induced [76]. Both PGE_2 and prostacyclin are recovered in significant quantities from the peritoneal cavity during the earliest stages of infection [76, 77]. The source of prostaglandin synthesis in the peritoneal cavity, however, is not known. Studies by Fieren and coworkers demonstrated that PMØ isolated from the peritoneal cavity of patients during episodes of peritonitis demonstrate a marked decrease in cyclooxygenase metabolites [172]. This finding was confirmed by in vitro studies [169] which demonstrated down regulation of cyclooxygenase enzyme synthesis in PMØ exposed to *S. epidermidis*. Interestingly in the same series of studies lipoxygenase product synthesis (LTB_4 and LTC_4) was increased by the interaction of *S. epidermidis* with PMØ. More recently cytokine synthesis has been examined following bacteria-PMØ interaction [173]. These experiments demonstrated that unstimulated PMØ released measurable quantities of interleukin-1 (IL-1α and IL-1β), interleukin-6 (IL-6), interleukin-8 (IL-8) and tumor necrosis factor α (TNFα). Following stimulation with *S. epidermidis* these levels were all increased significantly.

These data indicate that the interaction of PMØ with invading pathogens results in the modulation of mediator synthesis with the inhibition of cyclooxygenase products but an increase in chemotactic molecules as well as both pro- and anti-inflammatory cytokines.

4.2.2. Peritoneal mesothelial cells

As noted previously the permeability of the peritoneal membrane correlates directly with intraperitoneal prostaglandin levels [76, 77]. It is unlikely, however, that the source of cyclooxygenase products is the peritoneal macrophage. Indeed more recent studies have indicated that the peritoneal mesothelial cells may contribute significantly to the cylooxygenase products of the peritoneal cavity [78, 79, 173–175].

Similarly the secretion of cytokines by mesothelial cells is comprehensive. These cells contain mRNA and secrete significant quantities of biologically active IL-6 and IL-8 following stimulation with macrophage conditioned medium. In addition these same cells also secrete interleukin-1α and β [82]. The significance of the findings can be appreciated when one considers that the total number of mesothelial cells by the peritoneal cavity is approximately 10^8 whereas the maximum number of PMØ in the resting peritoneal cavity is 10^7.

The mesothelial cells are also likely to contribute to the trafficking of leukocytes into the peritoneal cavity. In their morphological studies Verger & colleagues [73] demonstrated the apparent movement of leukocytes into the peritoneal cavity between mesothelial cells. The secretion of the neutrophil chemoattractant, IL-8 and monocyte chemotactic protein by mesothelial cells is established [81, 176]. In addition recent studies have demonstrated that mesothelial cells can synthesize and express the adhesion molecules intercellular adhesion molecule 1 (ICAM-1) and vascular cell adhesion molecule 1 (VCAM-1) [176].

These data indicate that mesothelial cells may play a central role in the recruitment of leukocytes to the sites of infection as well as contributing to the upregulation of the inflammatory response. In addition they have shown that the host defence response is a network of interactions between PMØ, mesothelial cells and PMN.

IL-1 and TNF released by PMØ in response to bacterial stimulation cause a significant generation of PGE_2, 6-keto-$PGF_{1\alpha}$, IL-6 and IL-8 by mesothelial cells. When combined there is an additive rise in prostaglandins and IL-6 and a synergistic release of IL-8 synthesis by the mesothelial cells. These findings complement the data from experimental animals when a combined injection of IL-1 and TNF into the peritoneal cavity results in a significant increase in neutrophil infiltration [177]. During clinical peritonitis levels of IL-6 in the dialysate increase markedly, probably due to increased production by both PMØ and more importantly the mesothelial cells. At the same time serum concentrations of this cytokine are also raised [178].

Thus to summarise the sequence of events involved in the inflammatory response to bacterial invasion of the peritoneal cavity probably involves the following. There is an initial interaction of the PMØ and the organism probably on the mesothelial surface. This leads to increased LTB_4 release which acts as a chemotactic agent for PMN. In addition various cytokines such as IL-1, TNF, IL-6 and IL-8 are also secreted (Fig. 3). The IL-1 and TNF will stimulate the mesothelial cells and IL-8 will also attract PMN.

The mesothelial cells respond by synthesizing PGE_2 and prostacyclin. These will increase capillary permeability allowing more opsonins such as IgG and complement to pass from the blood into the peritoneum (Fig. 4). PGE_2 in the peritoneal cavity could also act as a negative feedback on the PMØ which prevents excessive cytokine release. The mesothelium also makes IL-6 which systemically will activate the acute phase response, a non specific protective mechanism against infection. In the peritoneum IL-6 down regulates the PMØ again helping to control the extent of the inflammatory response. The IL-8 will also help to recruit PMN (Fig. 4). Migration of these cells is enhanced by increased mesothelial expression of integrins such as ICAM-1 (Fig. 5). Finally both types of phagocyte aided by opsonins will ingest and kill the bacteria.

4.3. Humoral defences

During peritonitis there is a rapid increase in the appearance of plasma proteins in the peritoneal cavity. This includes immunoglobulins and complement components which will significantly improve the opsonic capacity of the dialysate. How much these humoral factors contribute to the clearing of infection is as yet uncertain. During the early stage of peritonitis there is a marked increase in concentrations of the vasodilatory prostaglandins PGE_2 and PGI_2 in the effluent which correlate with the total protein levels [77]. This suggests that these prostanoids, by augmenting peritoneal capillary permeability allow plasma proteins to more rapidly diffuse into the peritoneum.

Though the increased concentration of proteins will locally improve defence mechanisms, if continued for more than a few days the increased loss

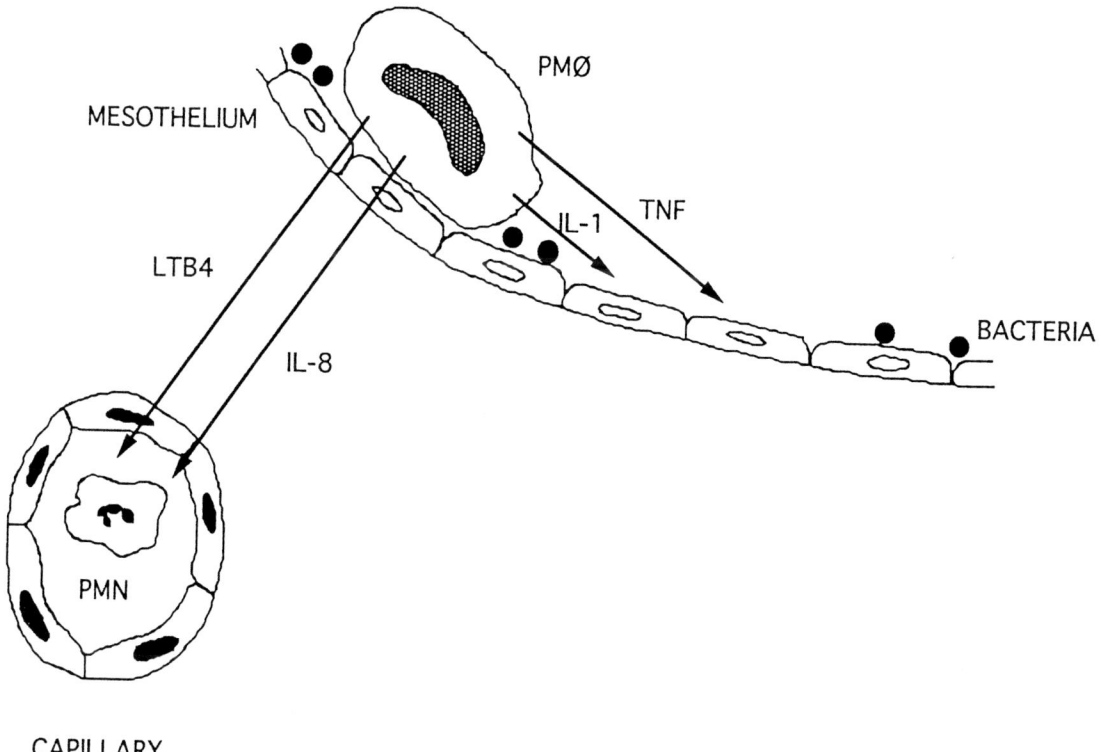

Figure 3. The effect of bacteria on PMØ. There is a stimulated release of LTB_4, IL-1, TNF and IL-8.

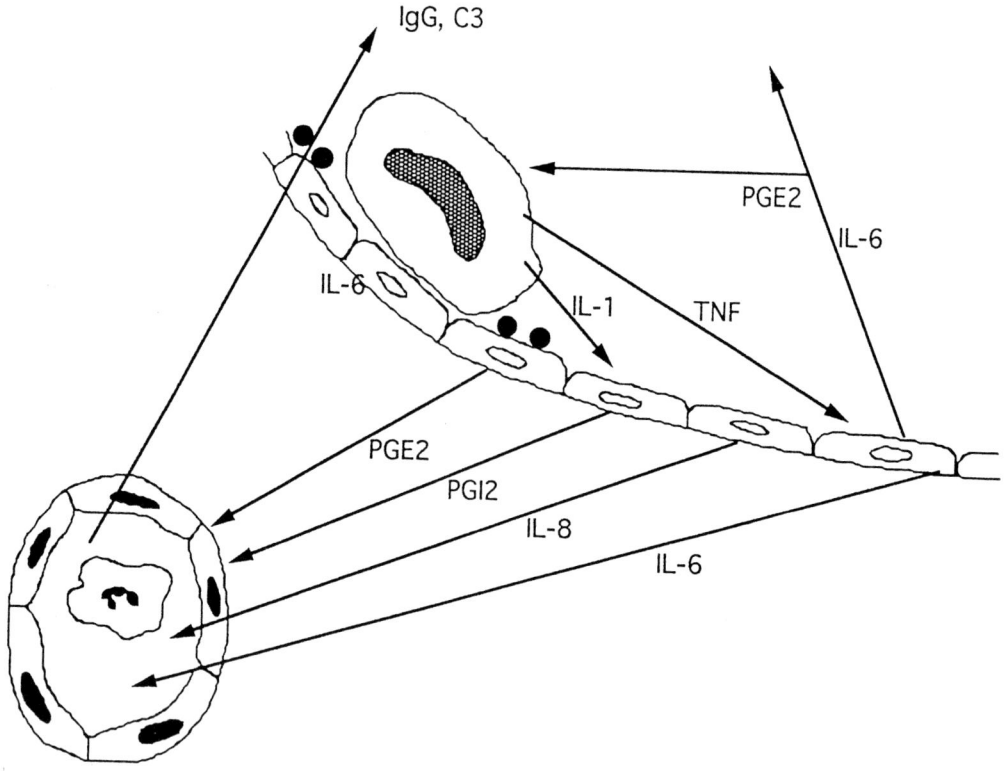

Figure 4. The effect of stimulated PMØ on the mesothelium. The latter release PGE_2, PGI_2, IL-6 and IL-8 in response to PMØ IL-1 and TNF.

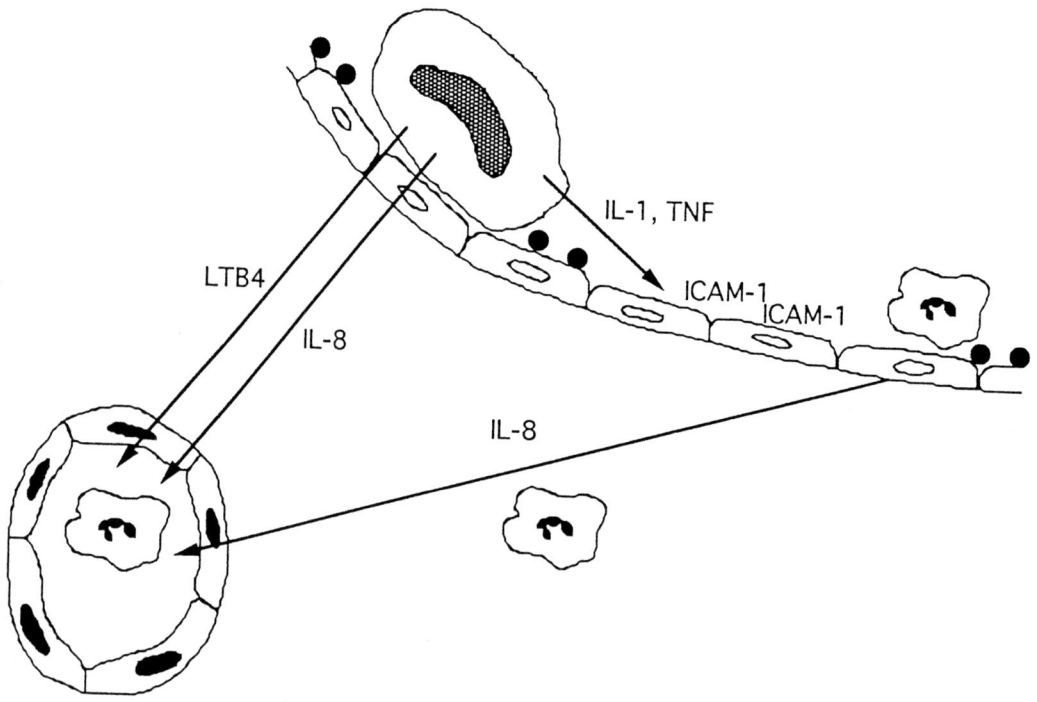

Figure 5. The recruitment of PMN into the peritoneal cavity. Chemotactic factors such as IL-8 and LTB_4 attract the PMN. IL-1 and TNF enhance integrin expression facilitating the passage of PMN which subsequently participate in phagocytosis and intracellular killing.

will have an adverse effect on host nutrition (see Chapter 15) which in turn could decrease resistance to infection.

5. Conclusions and clinical significance

It can be seen from the information presented in this chapter that host defence in the peritoneum of PD patients is a complex scenario involving humoral and cellular responses as well as exogenous factors such as the catheter and the dialysate. The relative importance of each component probably varies from individual to individual.

Since peritonitis remains an important cause of morbidity in PD subjects as well as a reason for transfer to haemodialysis, it is not surprising that clinicians have looked for possible means of augmenting host defence and thereby hopefully improving outcome. Various suggestions have been made and these will now be discussed.

Logically if peritonitis is to be avoided, then the best way is to prevent bacterial entry. In general organisms arrive in the peritoneal cavity via the catheter or from the bowel. In line filters have been proposed as a means of stopping bacterial entry. However, there is evidence that organisms can survive on the filter exposing the patient to endotoxins. Sometimes microbes will actually grow through the filter. Furthermore they may not reduce the incidence of peritonitis [179]. For these reasons these filters have largely been abandoned.

In contrast, flush before fill systems with or without an antiseptic agent have been proven to be effective in preventing peritonitis in controlled trials and are now in widespread use [180].

Prevention of migration of organisms from the bowel is not currently possible.

There is evidence that nasal carriage of *S. aureus* is associated with an increased risk of exit site infections [2]. Furthermore, episodes of *S. aureus* peritonitis only occurred in patients with this organism in the nares. Thus, logically, eradication of nasal carriage might lead to a reduction in infections due to *S. aureus*. This has been proven to occur in haemodialysis subjects [181]. At the time of writing a large multi-centre, randomly allocated prospective trial of nasal mupirocin is underway to determine if there is also a benefit for PD patients.

One possible measure that would improve cellular defence would be to make the dialysate more biocompatible. *In vitro* studies have shown that by adjusting the pH, phagocyte function is improved [25, 119, 120, 131]. This occurs irrespective of the method used to increase pH since both a bicarbonate based fluid and one containing histidine (a dibasic amino acid) are better than current commercial dialysate [129, 182]. The osmolar effects on phagocytosis might be abolished by using an isoosmolar fluid which still induces ultrafiltration (see Chapter 6). Though short term trials of bicarbonate dialysate have been undertaken there is no data as yet on whether this fluid will be associated with a decreased incidence of peritonitis. An alternative approach is to treat an episode of peritonitis completely by stopping PD for a period of some days while continuing antibiotics [183]. If necessary, the patient is given temporary haemodialysis. The potential benefits of this approach are that phagocytes and opsonins are not washed out and diluted by the dialysate. In addition it avoids the possibility that the fluid will have a detrimental effect on phagocyte function *in vivo*. In effect the peritoneal cavity is allowed to respond as in a non-dialysed subject except for the presence of the catheter. Though there are theoretical advantages in interupting dialysis, there are as yet no controlled trials to prove this regime is more effective than standard methods of treating peritonitis in PD patients. As noted earlier it is unclear if there are abnormalities in peritoneal macrophage function independent of the effect of the dialysate. There are certainly no controlled trials proving that treatment of supposed defects in peritoneal macrophage or PMN function will reduce the incidence or severity of peritonitis.

Since the level of opsonins in the peritoneal cavity during PD are critically low, it might seem reasonable to add IgG or complement to the dialysate. *In vitro* IgG will markedly improve opsonic activity of peritoneal effluent [110, 184]. It has been suggested that regular addition of IgG to the bags will decrease the incidence of peritonitis [23]. To date, however, there are no controlled trials to prove the efficacy of this treatment. It was originally suggested that the levels of immunoglobulin remained elevated in the effluent for many days after a 24 hour dose. Others have been unable to confirm this finding and report an immediate washout after the treatment ceases [185]. The discrepancy has not yet been explained.

An alternative approach would be to increase levels of specific antibody in the peritoneal cavity by immunization. A booster dose of tetanus toxoid is followed by a marked increase in concentrations of antitoxin in the PD effluent [89]. Administration of a staphylococcal vaccine also induces a rise in specific anti-staphylococcal antibody in the peritoneal cavity [186]. An uncontrolled study suggested that vaccination was accompanied by a decrease in infection rate [187] but a subsequent controlled trial has shown no benefit [186]. Thus at present there is no evidence that increasing antibody levels in dialysate either endogenously or exogenously will reduce the rate of peritonitis.

Increasing the concentration of complement in the peritoneal fluid might help in the elimination of gram negative infections. To date no studies have been published using this approach and there is no suitable preparation for human use.

In view of the known influence of nutrition on immunity then it is important to keep patients as fit as possible and treat any protein-calorie depletion. This is considered further in Chapter 15. It should be pointed out, however, that no prospective study has shown that improving the nutrition of PD subjects reduces the peritonitis rates.

As discussed earlier the biofilm may contribute to clinical infection. Various antiseptic agents can eradicate a biofilm *in vitro* but these are not suitable for routine human use. One unconfirmed report suggested that use of a flush before fill system considerably reduced biofilm formation [153]. Antibiotics such as rifampicin are effect against the encased bacteria [188] but at present long term prophylactic use is not recommended.

As outlined in section 2.6, *in vitro* urokinase enhances the opsonic activity of dialysis effluent for *S. aureus*. Several studies have suggested a beneficial effect of a fibrinolytic agent in relapsing peritonitis [189–191]. In contrast, Williams *et al.* found that catheter replacement was more effective than urokinase [192]. Thus, to-date, though fibrinolytics are of proven value in the management of a blocked catheter their use in enhancing host defence remains questionable.

In summary no measure currently available is of proven benefit in augmenting host defence and thus reducing the incidence of peritonitis in PD subjects. It is hoped that as knowledge of the mechanisms involved in host defence of CAPD patients continues to grow there will eventually be some benefit to our patients.

References

1. Verbrugh HA, Keane WE, Hoidal JR, Freiberg MR, Elliott GR, Peterson PK. Peritoneal macrophages and opsonins: Antibacterial defense in patients undergoing chronic peritoneal dialysis. J Infect Dis 1983; 147: 1018–29.
2. Luzar MA, Coles GA, Faller B et al. Staphylococcus aureus nasal carriage and infection in patients on continuous ambulatory peritoneal dialysis. New Eng J Med 1990; 322: 505–9.
3. Corey PN, Steels C. Risk factors associated with time to first infection and time to failure on CAPD. Perit Dial Bull 1983; S14–7.
4. Young GA, Young JB, Young SM et al. Nutrition and delayed hypersensitivity during continuous ambulatory peritoneal dialysis in relation to peritonitis. Nephron 1986; 43: 177–86.
5. Spiegel DM, Anderson M, Campbell U et al. Serum albumin: a marker for morbidity in peritoneal dialysis patients. Am J Kid Dis 1993; 21: 26–30.
6. Chandra RK. Nutritional regulation of immunity and risk of infection in old age. Immunol 1989; 67: 141–7.
7. Goldstein CS, Bomalaski JS, Zurier RB, Nelson EG, Douglas SD. Analysis of peritoneal macrophages in continuous ambulatory peritoneal dialysis patients. Kidney Int 1984; 26: 733–40.
8. Peterson PK, Gaziano E, Suh HJ, Devalon M, Peterson L, Keane WF. Antimicrobial activities of dialysate-elicited and resident human peritoneal macrophages. Infect Immun 1985; 49: 212–8.
9. McGregor SJ, Brock JH, Briggs JD, Junor BJR. Bactericidal activity of peritoneal macrophages from CAPD patients. Nephrol Dial Transplant 1987; 2: 104–8.
10. Ganguly R, Milutinovich J, Lazzell V, Waldman RH. Studies of human peritoneal cells: A normal saline lavage technique for isolation and characterization of cells from peritoneal dialysis patients. J Reticuloendothelial Soc 1987; 27: 303–10.
11. Cichocki T, Hanicki Z, Suowicz W, Smolenski O, Kopec J, Zembala M. Output of peritoneal cells into peritoneal dialysate. Nephron 1983; 35: 175–82.
12. Bos HJ, van Bronswijk H, Helmerhorst TJM, Oe PL, Hoefsmit ECM, Beelen RHJ. Distinct subpopulations of elicited human macrophages in peritoneal dialysis patients and women undergoing laparoscopy: A study of peroxidatic activity. J Leukocyte Biol 1988; 43: 172–78.
13. Bos HJ, Vlaanderen K, Van der Meulen J, de Veld JC, Oe PL, Beelen RHJ. Peritoneal macrophages in short dwell time effluent show diminished phagocytosis. Perit Dial Int 1988; 8: 199–202.
14. McGregor SJ, Brock JH, Briggs JD, Junor BJR. Longitudinal study of peritoneal defence mechanisms in patients on continuous ambulatory peritoneal dialysis (CAPD). Perit Dial Int 1989; 9: 115–9.
15. Holmes CJ, Lewis SL, Kubey WY. Comparison of peritoneal white blood cell parameters from CAPD patients with a high or low incidence of peritonitis. Am J Kidney Dis 1990; 15: 258–64.
16. Dez de Castro MF, Selgas R, Bajo MA et al. A study of cellular populations in the nocturnal effluent (NPE) on CAPD: It relationship with peri-

toneal antecedents and functions. Perit Dial Int 1993; 13 (suppl 1): 532.
17. Van Furth R, Raeburn JA, van Zwet TL. Characteristics of human mononuclear phagocytes. Blood 1979; 54: 485–500.
18. Bos HJ, Meyer F, de Veld JC. Peritoneal fluid induces change of mononuclear phagocyte proportions. Kidney Int 1989; 36: 20–6.
19. Bos HJ, Struijk DG, Tuk CW et al. Characterization of peritoneal cells from continuous ambulatory peritoneal dialysis (CAPD) patients: An immunological and functional study. J Leukocyte Biol 1989; 46: 313.
20. Moughal NA, McGregor SJ, Brock JH, Briggs JD, Junor BJR. Expression of transferrin receptors by monocytes and peritoneal macrophages from renal failure patients treated by CAPD. Eur J Clin Invest 1991; 21: 592–6.
21. Lewis SL, Van Epps DE, Chenoweth DE. C5a receptor modulation on neutrophils and monocytes from chronic hemodialysis and peritoneal dialysis patients. Clin Nephrol 1986; 26: 37–44.
22. Lewis SL, Van Epps DE, Chenoweth DE. Alterations in chemotactic factor-induced responses of neutrophils and monocytes from chronic dialysis patients. Clin Nephrol 1988; 30: 63–72.
23. Lamperi S, Carozzi S. Defective opsonic activity of peritoneal effluent during CAPD: Importance and prevention. Perit Dial Bull 1986; 6; 87–92.
24. Brando B, Galato R, Seveso M et al. Flow cytometric study of immunocompetent cell phenotypes and phagocytosis in CAPD effluent. Trans Am Soc Artif Inter Organs 1988; 34: 441–4.
25. Topley N, Alobaidi HM, Davies M, Coles GA, Williams JD, Lloyd D. The effect of dialysate on peritoneal phagocyte oxidative metabolism. Kidney Int 1988; 34: 404–11.
26. Lewis SL, Holmes CJ. Host defence mechanisms in the peritoneal cavity of CAPD patients. Perit Dial Int 1991; 11: 14–21.
27. Lewis SL, Norris PJ. Monocyte/macrophage function in continuous ambulatory peritoneal dialysis patients. Contrib Nephrol 1990; 85: 1–9.
28. Lewis SL, Norris PJ, Holmes CJ. Phenotypic characterization of monocytes and macrophages from CAPD patients. Trans Am Soc Artif Intern Organs 1990; 36: M575–7.
29. Goyert SM, Ferrero E, Rettig WJ, Yenamandra AK, Obata F, LeBeau MM. The CD14 monocyte differentiation antigen maps to a region encoding growth factors and receptors. Science 1988; 239: 497–50.
30. Lamperi S, Carozzi S, Nasini MG. Peritoneal membrane defense in CAPD. Contrib Nephrol 1987; 57: 69–78.
31. Goldstein CS, Garrick RE, Polin RA et al. Fibronectin and complement secretion by monocytes and peritoneal macrophages in vitro from patients undergoing CAPD. J Leukocyte Biol 1986; 39: 457–64.
32. Lamperi S, Carozzi S. Suppressor resident macrophages and peritonitis incidence in CAPD. Nephron 1986; 44: 219–25.
33. Lamperi S, Carozzi S. Interferon-gamma as an in vitro enhancing factor of peritoneal macrophage defectivity of bacterial activity during continuous ambulatory peritoneal dialysis (CAPD). Am J Kidney Dis 1988; 11: 225–30.
34. Davies SJ, Ogg CS, Cameron JS. Peritoneal macrophage markers and phagocytic function in patients on CAPD. Nephrol Dial Transplant 1988; 3: 837–45.
35. Tranaeus A, Heimburger O, Lindholm B. Peritonitis during CAPD: Risk Factors, Clinical severity, and pathogenic aspects. Perit Dial Int 1988; 8: 253–63.
36. Harvey DM, Shepard KJ, Morgan AG. Neutrophil function in patients on CAPD. Br J Haematol 1988; 68: 273–8.
37. Lin CY, Huang TP. Serial cell-mediated immunological changes in terminal uremic patients on CAPD therapy. Am J Nephrol 1988; 8: 355–62.
38. Giacchino F, Peyretti F, Piccoli G. Association between lymphocyte antigens B8, DR 3, and response to peritonitis in patients undergoing continuous ambulatory peritoneal dialysis. Nephron 1985; 40: 496–7.
39. Lewis SL, Bonner PN, Cooper CL, Holmes CJ. Prospective comparison of blood and peritoneal lymphocytes from CAPD patients. J Clin Lab Immunol 1992; 37: 3–19.
40. Singh S, Hurtubise P, Michael G, Pesce A, Pollak V. Preliminary observations on the laboratory markers of cell-mediated immunity in patients transferring from hemodialysis to CAPD. Contrib Nephrol 1983; 36: 73–81.
41. Shohat B, Boner G, Waller A, Rosenfeld JB. Cell-mediated immunity in uremic patients prior to and after 6 months' treatment with continuous ambulatory peritoneal dialysis. Israel J Med Sci 1986; 22: 551–5.
42. Macor S, Porrini AM. Giampietro A et al. Multiple sclerosis: an immune system activation disease. Acta Neurol (Napoli) 1991; 13: 590–6.
43. Al Kassab AS, Raziuddin S. Immune activation and T cell subset abnormalities in circulation of patients with recently diagnosed type I diabetes mellitus. Clin Exp Immunol 1990: 81: 267–71.
44. Morimoto C, Steinberg AD, Letvin NL et al. A defective immunoregulatory T cell subset in systemic lupus erythematosus patients demonstrated with anti-2H4 antibody. J Clin Invest 1987: 79: 762–70.
45. Giacchino F, Pozzato M, Formica M, Piccoli G. Improved cell-mediated immunity in CAPD patients as compared to those on hemodialysis. Perit Dial Bull 1984; 4: 209–12.
46. Davis SJ, Suassuna J, Ogg CS, Cameron JS. Activation of immunocompetent cells in the peritoneum of patients treated with CAPD. Kidney Int 1989; 36: 661–8.
47. Chandrasekaran B, Schultz EF, Debari VA et al. Surface marker characterization of peritoneal dialysis patients' intraperitoneal leukocytes by monoclonal antibodies. In Maher JF, Winchester

JP, eds. Frontiers in Peritoneal Dialysis. New York: Field, Rich, and Assoc, 1986: 583–5.
48. Valle MT, Degl'innocenti ML, Giordano P et al. Analysis of cellular populations in peritoneal effluents of children on CAPD. Clin Nephrol 1989; 32: 235–8.
49. Brando B, Galato R, Seveso M et al. Flow cytometric study of immunocompetent cell phenotypes and phagocytosis in CAPD effluent. Trans Am Soc Artif Inter Organs 1988; 34: 441–4.
50. Galato R, Seveso M, Brando B et al. Flow cytometric characterization of immunoincompetent cells of peritoneal effluent [abstract]. Nephrol Dial Transplant 1987; 2: 453.
51. Betjes MGH, Bos HJ, Kredict RT, Arisz L. The mesothelial cells in CAPD effluent and their relationship to peritonitis incidence. Perit Dial Int 1991; 11: 22–6.
52. Davis SJ. Peritoneal lymphocyte populations in CAPD patients. Contrib Nephrol 1990; 85: 16–23.
53. Lewis SL, Kutvirt SG, Holmes CJ. Interleukin-2 production by peritoneal and peripheral lymphocytes from CAPD patients [Abstract]. Perit Dial Int 1992; 12 (suppl 1): 137.
54. Giacchino F, Pozzato M, Formica M et al. Lymphocyte subsets assayed by numerical tests in CAPD. Int J Artif Organs 1984; 7: 81–4.
55. Lamperi S, Carozzi S. Immunological defenses in CAPD. Blood Purif 1987; 7: 126–43.
56. Dobbie JW, Azki MA. The ultrastructure of the parietal peritoneum in normal and uremic man and in patients on CAPD. In: Maher JF, Winchester JF (eds), Frontiers in Peritoneal Dialysis. Field, Rich, and Associates, Inc, New York 1985; pp 3–10.
57. Digenis GE. Anatomy of the peritoneal membrane. Perit Dial Bull 1984; 4: 63–9.
58. Lloyd JK, Dobbie JW, Hauck WN, Manning KA. Localisation of surfactant phospholipids in the peritoneal mesothelium. In: Bailey GW (ed), Proceedings of the 46th annual meeting of the Electron Microscopy Society of America. San Francisco: Press Inc, 1988.
59. Dobbie JW, Pavlina T, Lloyd J, Johnson RC. Phosphatidylcholine synthesis by peritoneal mesothelium: its implications for peritoneal dialysis. Am J Kid Dis 1988; 12: 31–6.
60. Beavis J, Jarwood JL, Coles GA, Williams JD. Intraperitoneal phosphatidylcholine levels in patients on CAPD do not correlate with adequacy of ultrafiltration. J Am Soc Nephrol 1993; 3: 1954–60.
61. Davies M, Stylianou E, Yung S, Thomas GJ, Coles GA, Williams JD. Proteoglycans of CAPD-dialysate fluid and metabolism. In: Coles GA, Davies M, Williams JD (eds). Contrib Nephrol 1990; 85: 134–41.
62. Davies M, Yung S, Coles GA. The possible significance of hyaluronan in the peritoneal cavity of CAPD patients. J Am Soc Nephrol 1992; 3: 408 (abstract).
63. Odon DL. Observations of the rat mesothelium with electron and phase microscopies. Am J Anat 1954; 95: 433–65.
64. Andrews PM, Porter KR. The ultrastructural morphology and possible functional significance of mesothelial microvilli. Anat Rec 1973; 177: 409–26.
65. Leak LV. Distribution of cell surface changes on mesothelium and lymphatic endothelium. Microvasc Res 1986; 31: 18–30.
66. Gotloib L, Shostack A, Jaichenko J. Ruthenium-red-stained anionic charges of rat and mice mesothelial cells and basal lamina: The peritoneum is a negatively charged dialyzing membrane. Nephron 1988; 48: 65–70.
67. Christiensen GD, Simpson WA, Beachey EH. Microbial adherence in infection. In: Mandell GL, Douglas RG Jr, Bennett JE (eds), Principles and practice of infectious diseases. 2nd ed. John Wiley and Sons, New York 1983; pp 6–23.
68. Steadman R, Topley N, Knowlden JM, Mackenzie RK, WIlliams JD. The assessment of relative surface hydrophobicity as a factor involved in the activation of human polymorphonuclear leukocytes by uropathogenic strains of E. coli. Biochim Biophys Acta 1989; 1013: 21–9.
69. Steadman R, Knowlden JM, Lichodziejewska M, Williams JD. The influence of net surface charge on the interaction of uropathogenic Escherichia coli with human neutrophils. Biochim Biophys Acta 1990; 1053: 37–42.
70. Gotloib L, Shustak A, Jaichenko J. Loss of mesothelial electronegative fixed charges during murine septic peritonitis. Nephron 1989; 51: 77–83.
71. Haagen IA, Heezius HC, Verkooyen RP, Verhoef J, Verbrugh HA. Adherence of peritonitis-causing Staphylococci to human peritoneal mesothelial cell monolayers. J Infect Dis 1990; 161: 266–73.
72. Teti G, Chiofalo MS, Tamasello F, Fava C, Mastroeni P. Mediation of Staphylococcus saprophyticus adherence to uroepithelial cells by lipoteichoic acid. Infect Immun 1987; 55: 839–42.
73. Verger C, Luger A, Moore HL, Nolph KD. Acute changes in peritoneal morphology and transport properties with infectious peritonitis and mechanical injury. Kidney Int 1983; 23: 823–31.
74. Muijsken MA, de Fijter CHW, Heezius ECJ et al. Intracellular survival of Staphylococci in both peritoneal macrophages and mesothelial cells as a possible cause of relapsing peritonitis. J Am Soc Nephrol 1991; 2: 366.
75. Stylianous E, Mackenzie RK, Davies M, Coles GA, Williams JD. The interaction of organism, phagocyte and mesothelial cell. Contrib Nephrol 1989; 85: 30–8.
76. Steinhauer HB, Günter B, Schollmeyer P. Stimulation of peritoneal synthesis of vasoactive prostaglandins during peritonitis in patients on continuous ambulatory peritoneal dialysis. Eur J Clin Invest 1985; 15: 1–5.
77. Steinhauer HB, Schollmeyer P. Prostaglandin mediated loss of proteins during peritonitis in continuous ambulatory peritoneal dialysis. Kidney Int 1986; 29: 584–590.
78. Coene M-C, Solheid C, Claeys M, Herman AG.

Prostaglandin production by cultured mesothelial cells. Arch Int Pharmacodyn 1981; 249: 316–318.
79. Coene MC, van Hove C, Claeys M, Herman AG. Arachidonic acid metabolism by cultured mesothelial cells. Biochim Biophys Acta 1982; 710: 437–45.
80. Topley N, Jörres A, Luttmann W et al. Human peritoneal mesothelial cells (HPMC) synthesize interleukin-6: induction by interleukin-1β and tumor necrosis factor α. Kidney Int 1993; 43: 226–33.
81. Topley N, Brown Z, Jörres A et al. Human peritoneal mesothelial cells synthesize IL-8; synergistic induction by interleukin-1β and tumor necrosis factor α. Am J Pathol 1993; 142: 1–11.
82. Rapoport J, Douvdevani A, Conforti A, Zlotnik M, Chaimowitz C. Peritoneal mesothelial cells synthesize IL-1. J Am Soc Nephrol 1992: 3: 416 (abstract).
83. Simberkoff MS, Moldover NH, Weiss G. Bactericidal and opsonic activity of cirrhotic ascites and non-ascitic peritoneal fluid. J Lab Clin Med 1978: 91: 831–9.
84. Runyon BA. Low protein concentration ascitic fluid is predisposed to spontaneous bacterial peritonitis. Gastroenterology 1986; 91: 1343–6.
85. Such J, Guarner G, Enriquez J, Rodriguez JL, Seres I, Vilandell F. Low C3 cirrhotic ascites predisposes to spontaneous bacterial peritonitis. Journal of Hepatology 1988; 6: 80–4.
86. Chan MK, Baillod RA, Varghese Z, Sweny P, Moorhead JF. Immunoglobulins and complement components (C3, C4) in CAPD and hemodialysis patients. Dial Transplant 1983; 12: 777–8.
87. Beaman M, Michael J, Maclennan ICM, Adu D. T-cell independent and T-cell dependent antibody responses in patients with chronic renal failure. Nephrol Dial Transplant 1989; 4: 216–21.
88. Schroder CH, Bakkeren JA, Weemaes CM, Monnens LA. IgG2 deficiency in young children treated with continuous ambulatory peritoneal dialysis. Perit Dial Int 1989; 9: 216–5.
89. Coles GA, Knight PA, Dharmasena AD. The secondary immune response of CAPD patients. Adv Perit Dial 1988; 4: 153–6.
90. Young GA, Taylor A, Kendall S, Brownjohn AM. Longitudinal study of proteins in plasma and dialysate during continuous ambulatory peritoneal dialysis (CAPD). Perit Dial Int 1990; 10: 257–61.
91. Balart LA, Husserl FE. The immunogenicity of hepatitis B vaccine (Heptavax-B) in chronic ambulatory peritoneal dialysis (CAPD) patients. Perit Dial Bull 1987; 7: 261.
92. Verslius DJ, Beyer WEP, Masurel N et al. Intact humoral immune response in patients on CAPD. Nephron 1988; 49: 16–9.
93. Saga T, Niki H, Niikura M et al. Influenza antibody titers after vaccination of chronic renal failure patients; before and during hemodialysis, or on continuous ambulatory peritoneal dialysis. Tokai J Exp Clin Med 1990; 15: 245–51.
94. Reddy PV, Zielezny M, Cunningham E, Walshe JJ. Efficacy of hepatitis B vaccine (Heptavax B). Perit Dial Bull 1987; 7 (suppl.): 62.
95. Opperman M, Kurts C, Zierz R, Quentin E, Weber MH, Gotze O. Elevated plasma levels of the immunosuppressive complement fragment Ba in renal failure. Kidney Int 1991: 40: 939–47.
96. Gaciong Z, Alexiewicz JM, Massry SM. Impaired in vivo antibody production in CRF rats: role of secondary hyperparathyroidism. Kidney Int 1991; 40: 862–7.
97. DeGiannis D, Mowat AM, Galloway E et al. In vitro analysis of B lymphocyte function in uraemia. Clin Exp Immunol 1987; 70: 463–70.
98. Winkelstein JA. Opsonins: their function, identity and clinical significance. Journal of Pediatrics 1973; 82: 747–53.
99. Keane WF Comty CM, Verbrugh HA et al. Opsonic deficiency of peritoneal dialysis effluent in CAPD. Kidney Int 1984; 25: 539–43.
100. Coles GA, Alobaidi H, Topley N, Davies M. Opsonic activity of dialysis effluent predicts those at risk of Staphylococus epidermidis peritonitis. Nephrol Dial Transplant 1987; 2: 359–65.
101. McGregor S, Brock J, Briggs J, Junor B. Relationship of IgG, C3, and transferrin with opsonising and bacteriostatic activity of peritoneal fluid from CAPD patients and the incidence of peritonitis. Nephrol Dial Transplant 1987; 2: 551–6.
102. Coles GA, Minors SJ, Horton JK, Fifield R, Davies M. Can the risk of peritonitis be predicted for new continuous ambulatory peritoneal dialysis (CAPD) patients? Perit Dial Int 1989; 9: 69–72.
103. Holmes C, Lewis S. Host defense mechanisms in the peritoneal cavity of continuous ambulatory peritoneal dialysis patients. 2. Humoral defenses. Perit Dial Int 1991; 11: 112–7.
104. Nielsen H, Espersen F, Kharazmi A et al. Specific opsonic activity for staphylococci in peritoneal dialysis effluent during continuous ambulatory peritoneal dialysis. Am J Kid Dis 1992; 20: 372–5.
105. Holmes CJ, Lewis SL, Evans RC et al. Periodic elevation of complement activation products in peritoneal dialysis effluent. ASAIO Trans 1989; 35: 587–9.
106. De Vecchi A, Castelnovo C, Failla N, Scalamonga A. Clinical significance of peritoneal dialysate IgG levels in CAPD patients. Adv Perit Dial 1990; 6: 98–101.
107. De Vecchi AF, Kopple JD, Young GA et al. Plasma and dialysate immunoglobulin G in continuous ambulatory peritoneal dialysis patients: A multicenter study. Am J Nephrol 1990; 10: 451–6.
108. Clark LA, Easmon CSF. Opsonic requirements of Staphylococcus epidermidis. J Med Microbiol 1986; 22: 1–7.
109. van Bronswijk H, Verbrugh HA, Heezius HCJM et al. Heterogeneity in opsonic requirements of Staphylococcus epidermidis: relative importance of surface hydrophobicity, capsules and slime. Immunol 1989; 67: 81–6.
110. Bennett-Jones DN, Yewdall VM, Gillespie CM,

Ogg CS, Cameron JS. Strain difference in the opsonization of Staphylococcus epidermidis. Perit Dial Int 1989; 9: 334–9.
111. Cozma G, Aburumeih S, Malik-Cozma MC, Johny KV. CAPD in a patient with complete absence of C3. Clin Nephrol 1987; 27: 269.
112. Khan RH, Klein M, Vas S. Fibronectin in the normal peritoneal fluids of patients on chronic ambulatory peritoneal dialysis (CAPD) and during peritonitis. Perit Dial Bull 1987; 7: 69–73.
113. Davies SJ, Animashun A, Taylor AE, Young GA, Turney JH. Fibronectin and fibrinogen in the plasma and dialysate of patients on CAPD. Perit Dial Bull 1987; 7: 233–6.
114. Davies SJ, Yewdall VM, Ogg CS, Cameron JS. Peritoneal defence mechanisms and Staphylococcus aureus in patients treated with continuous ambulatory peritoneal dialysis (CAPD). Perit Dial Int 1990; 10: 135–40.
115. Verbrugh HA, Keane WF, Conroy WE et al. Bacterial growth and killing in CAPD fluids. J Clin Microbiology 1984; 20: 199–203.
116. Dunn DL, Barke RA, Ahrenholz DH, Humphrey EW, Simmons RL. The adjuvant effect of peritoneal fluid in experimental peritonitis. Ann Surg 1984; 20: 199–203.
117. Duwe AK, Vas SI, Weatherhead JW. Effects of the composition of peritoneal dialysis fluid on chemiluminescence, phagocytosis and bactericidal activity in vitro. Infect Immun 1981; 33: 130–5.
118. Alobaidi HM, Coles GA, Davies M, Lloyd D. Host defence in continuous ambulatory peritoneal dialysis: The effect of the dialysate on phagocyte function. Nephrol Dial Transplant 1986; 1: 16–21.
119. Van Bronswijk H, Verbrugh HA, Heezius HC, Van der Meulen, J, Oe PL, Verhoef J. Dialysis fluids and local host resistance in patients on continuous ambulatory peritoneal dialysis. Eur J Clin Microbiol Inf Dis 1988; 7: 368–73.
120. Harvey DM, Sheppard KJ, Morgan AG, Fletcher J. Effect of dialysate fluids on phagocytosis and killing by normal neutrophils. J Clin Microbiol 1987; 25: 1424–7.
121. Ing BL, Gupta DK, Nawab ZM, Zhou FQ, Rahman MA, Daugirdas JT. Suppression of neutrophil superoxide production by conventional peritoneal dialysis solution. Int J Artif Organs 1988; 11: 351–4.
122. Yu A, Zhow F, Song R, Nawab Z, Rahman M, Ing T. Peritoneal dialysis solution pH and lactate in the inhibition of neutrophilic superoxide formation. J Am Soc Nephrol 1990; 2: 393.
123. Yu AW, Vedere AR, Agrawall A et al. Morphologic changes in human neutrophils after exposure to peritoneal dialysis solution (PDS). J Am Soc Nephrol 1991; 2: 370.
124. Jörres A, Jörres D, Topley N, Gahl GM, Mahiout A. Leukotriene release from peripheral and peritoneal leukocytes following exposure to peritoneal dialysis solutions. Nephrol Dial Transplant 1991; 6: 495–501.
125. Jörres A, Jörres D, Gahl GM et al. Leukotriene B4 and tumor necrosis factor release from leukocytes: Effect of peritoneal dialysate. Nephron 1991; 58: 276–82.
126. Gallimore B, Gagnon RF, Stevenson MM. Cytotoxicity of commercial peritoneal dialysis solutions towards peritoneal cells of chronically uremic mice. Nephron 1986; 43: 283–9.
127. Wieslander AP, Nordin MK, Kjellstrand PTT, Boberg UC. Toxicity of peritoneal dialysis fluids on cultured fibroblasts, L-929. Kidney Int 1991; 40: 77–9.
128. Van Broswijk H, Verbrugh H, Bos H et al. Cytotoxic effects of commercial continuous ambulatory peritoneal dialysis (CAPD) fluids and of bacterial exoproducts on human mesothelial cells in vitro. Perit Dial Int 1989; 9; 197–202.
129. Topley N, Mackenzie R, Petersen MM et al. In vitro testing of a potentially biocompatible continuous ambulatory peritoneal dialysis fluid. Nephrol Dial Transplant 1991; 6: 574–81.
130. Verburgh H, Verkooyen R, Verhoef J. Oe PL, van der Meulen J. Defective complement-mediated opsonization and lysis of bacteria in commercial peritoneal dialysis solutions. In: Maher JF, Winchester JF (eds), Frontiers in Peritoneal Dialysis. New York: Field and Rich, 1986; pp 559–64.
131. Gordon DL, Rice JL. Avery VM. Surface phagocytosis and host defence in the peritoneal cavity during continuous ambulatory peritoneal dialysis. Eur J Clin Microbiol Inf Dis 1990; 9: 191–7.
132. Yu AW, Zhou XJ, Nawab ZM, Gahndi VC, Ing TS, Vaziri ND. Neutrophilic intracellular acidosis induced by conventional, lactate-containing peritoneal dialysis solutions. Int J Artif Organs 1992; 15: 661–5.
133. Liberek T, Topley N, Jörres A et al. Peritoneal dialysis fluid inhibition of neutrophil (PMN) respiratory burst activation is related to the lowering of intracellular pH $[pH]_i$, Nephron 1993; 65: 260–5.
134. Liberek T, Topley N, Jörres A, Coles GA, Gahl GM, Williams JD. Peritoneal dialysis fluid inhibition of phagocyte function: effects of osmolality and glucose concentration. J Am Soc Nephrol 1993; 3: 1508–15.
135. Rubin J, Lin LM, Lewis R, Cruse J, Bowen JD. Host defense mechanisms in continuous ambulatory peritoneal dialysis. Clin Nephrol 1983; 20: 140–4.
136. de Fijter CWH, Verbrugh HA, Peters EDJ et al. In vivo exposure to the currently available peritoneal dialysis fluids decreases the function of peritoneal macrophages in CAPD. Clin Nephrol 1993; 39: 75–80.
137. Jörres A, Topley N, Steenweg L, Müller C, Köttgen E, Gahl GM. Inhibition of cytokine synthesis by peritoneal dialysate persists throughout the CAPD cycle. Am J Nephrol 1992; 12: 80–5.
138. Breborowicz A, Rodela H, Oreopoulos DG. Toxicity of osmotic solutes on human mesothelial cells in vitro. Kidney Int 1992; 41: 1280–5.
139. Flournoy DJ, Perryman FA, Qadri SMH. Growth of bacterial clinical isolates in continuous ambu-

latory peritoneal dialysis fluid. Perit Dial Bull 1983; 3: 144–5.
140. Sketh NK, Bartell CA, Roth DA. In vitro study of bacterial growth in continuous ambulatory peritoneal dialysis fluids. J. Clin Microbiol 1986; 23: 1096–8.
141. Macdonald WA, Watts J, Bowmen MI. Factors affecting Staphylococcus epidermidis growth in peritoneal dialysis solutions. J. Clin Microbiol 1986; 24: 104–7.
142. Read RR, Eberwein P, Dasgupta MK et al. Peritonitis in peritoneal dialysis: Bacterial colonization by biofilm spread along the catheter surface. Kidney Int 1989; 35: 614–21.
143. Gallimore B, Gagnon RF, Richards GK. Role of an intraperitoneal catheter implant in the pathogenesis of experimental Staphylococus epidermidis peritoneal infection in renal failure mice. Am J Nephrol 1988; 36: 406–13.
144. Ward KH, Olson ME, Lam K, Costerton JW. Mechanism of persistent infection associated with peritoneal implants. J Med Microbiol 1992; 36: 406–13.
145. Holmes CJ, Evans R. Biofilm and foreign body infection – the significance to CAPD-associated peritonitis. Perit Dial Bull 1986; 6: 168–77.
146. Schwarzmann S, Boring JR. Antiphagocytic effects of slime from a mucoid strain of Pseudomonas aeruginosa. Infect Immun 1971; 3: 762–7.
147. Laharrague PF, Corberand JX, Fillola G, Gleizes BJ, Fontanilles AM, Gyrard E. In vitro effect of the slime of Pseudomonas aeruginosa on the function of human polymorphonuclear neutrophils. Infect Immun 1984; 44: 760–2.
148. Verbrugh HA, van Dijk WC, van Erne ME, Peters R, Peterson PK, Verhoef J. Quantitation of the third component of human complement attached to the surface of opsonized bacteria: opsonin deficient sera and phagocytosis-resistant strains. Infect Immun 1979; 26: 808–12.
149. Evans RC, Holmes CJ. Effect of vancomycin hydrochloride on Staphylococcus epidermidis biofilm associated with silicone elastomer. Antimicrobial Agents and Chemotherapy 1987; 31: 889–94.
150. Marine TJ, Bobel MA, Costerton JW. Examination of the morphology of bacteria adhering to peritoneal dialysis catheters by scanning and transmission electron microscopy. J Clin Microscopy 1983; 18: 1388–98.
151. Reed WP, Light PD, Newman KA. Biofilm on Tenckhoff catheters: A possible source for peritonitis. In: Maher JF, Winchester JF (eds), Frontiers in Peritoneal Dialysis. Field and Rich, New York 1986; pp 176–80.
152. Dasgupta MK, Bettehen KB, Ulan RA et al. Relationship of adherent bacterial biofilms to peritonitis in chronic ambulatory dialysis. Perit Dial Bull 1987; 7: 168–73.
153. Verger C, Chesneau AM, Thibault M, Bataille N. Biofilm on Tenckhoff catheters: a negligble source of contamination. Perit Dial Bull 1987; 7: 174–8.
154. Zappacosta AR, Perras ST. Role of catheter removal in therapy of bacterial peritonitis of continous ambulatory dialysis. Trans Am Soc Artif Intern Organs 1989; 35: 40–5.
155. Fijen JQ, Struijk DG, Krediet RT et al. Dialysate leukocytosis in CAPD patients without clinical infection. Netherlands J Med 1988; 33: 270–80.
156. Sombolos K, Vas S, Rifkin O et al. Propionibacteria isolates and asymptomatic infections of the peritoneal effluent in CAPD patients. Nephrol Dial Transplant 1986; 1: 175–8.
157. Van Bronswijk H. Microbial invasion and peritoneal defence in CAPD patients. Doctoral thesis submitted to Free University of Amsterdam, 1988.
158. Rubin J, Rogers WA, Taylor HM et al. Peritonitis during continuous ambulatory dialysis. Ann Intern Med 1980; 92: 7–13.
159. Riera G, Bushinsky D, Emmanuel DS. First exchange neutrophilia: an index of peritonitis during chronic intermittent peritoneal dialysis. Clin Nephrol 1985; 24: 5–9.
160. Peterson PK, Keane WF. Infections in chronic peritoneal dialysis patients. In: Remington JS, Swartz MN (eds), Current Clinical Topics in Infectious Diseases. McGraw-Hill, New York 1985; 6: 239–60.
161. Dunn DL, Barke RA, Knight NB et al. Role of resident macrophages, peripheral neutrophils, and translymphatic absorption in bacterial clearance from the peritoneal cavity. Infect Immun 1985; 49: 257–64.
162. Dunn DL, Barke RA, Ewald DC, Simmons RL. Macrophages and translymphatic absorption represent the first line of host defence of the peritoneal avity. Arch Surg 1987; 122: 105–10.
163. Glancey GR, Cameron JS, Ogg CS. Peritoneal drainage: an important element in host defense against Staphylococcal peritonitis in patients on CAPD. Nephrol Dial Transplant 1992; 7: 627–31.
164. Van Bronswijk H, Verbrugh HA, Heezius EZ et al. Host defence in CAPD treatment: The effect of the dialysate on cell function. Contrib Nephrol 1990; 85: 67–72.
165. Suassuna J, Neves F, Glancey G et al. Activation markers on leucocytes within the peritoneum of CAPD patients. Abstracts Vth Cong. Int Soc Perit Dial. Kyoto 1990: 43.
166. Mariano F, Tetta C, Montrucchio G, Cavalli PL, Camussi G. Role of α-1-proteinase inhibitor in restraining peritoneal inflammation in CAPD patients. Kidney Int 1992; 42: 735–42.
167. Donovan KL, Pacholok S, Humes JL, Coles GA, Williams JD. Intraperitoneal free elastase in CAPD peritonitis. Kidney Int 1993; 44: 87–90.
168. Fieren MWJA, van den Bemd GJCM, Bonta IL. Endotoxin-stimulated peritoneal macrophages obtained from continuous ambulatory peritoneal dialysis patients show increased capacity to release interleukin-1β in vitro during peritonitis. Eur J Clin Invest 1990; 20: 453–7.
169. Mackenzie RK, Coles GA, Williams JD. Eicosanoid synthesis in human peritoneal macrophages stimulated with S. epidermidis. Kidney Int 1990; 37: 1316–24.

170. Rankin JA, Sylvester I, Smith S, Yoshimura T, Leonard EJ. Macrophages cultured in vitro release leukotriene B_4 and neutrophil attractant/activation protein (interleukin-8) sequentially in response to stimulation with lipopolysaccharide and zymosan. J Clin Invest 1990; 86: 1556–64.
171. Mackenzie RK, Coles GA, Williams JD. The response of human peritoneal macrophages to stimulation with bacteria isolated from episodes of continuous ambulatory pertioneal dialysis-related peritonitis. J Infect Dis 1991; 163: 837–42.
172. Fieren MWJA, Adolfs MJP, Bonta IL. Alterations in sensitivity and secretion of prostaglandins of human macrophages during CAPD related peritonitis. Contrib Nephrol 1987; 57: 55–62.
173. Topley N, Jörres A, Petersen MM et al. Human peritoneal mesothelial cell prostaglandin (PG) metabolism: induction by cytokines and peritoneal macrophage conditioned medium. J Amer Soc Nephrol 1991; 2: 432.
174. Bult H, Coene M-C, Rampart M, Herman AG. Complement derived factors and prostacyclin formation by isolated rabbit peritoneum and cultured mesothelial cells. Agents Actions 194: 14: 237–47.
175. Satoh K, Prescott SM. Culture of mesothelial cells from bovine pericardium and characterisation of their arachidonate metabolism. Biochim Biophys Acta 1987; 930: 283–96.
176. Jonjic N, Peri G, Bernasconi S et al. Expression of adhesion molecules and chemotactic cytokines in cultured human mesothelial cells. J. Exp Med 1992; 176: 1165–74.
177. Sayers TJ, Wiltrout TA, Bull CA, Denn AC, Pilaro AM, Lokesh B. Effects of cytokines on polymorphonuclear neutrophil infiltration in the mouse: prostaglandin- and leukotriene-independent induction of infiltration by IL-1 and tumor necrosis factor. J Immunol 1988; 141: 1670–77.
178. Nakahama H, Tanaka Y, Shirai D et al. Plasma interleukin-6 levels in continuous ambulatory peritoneal dialysis and hemodialysis patients. Nephron 1992; 61: 132–4.
179. Tranaeus A, Heimburger O, Lindholm B. Peritonitis in continuous ambulatory peritoneal dialysis (CAPD): diagnostic findings, therapeutic outcome and complications. Perit Dial Int 1989; 9: 179–90.
180. Canadian CAPD Clinical Trials Group. Peritonitis in continuous ambulatory peritoneal dialysis (CAPD): a multi-center randomized clinical trial comparing the Y connector disinfectant system to standard systems. Perit Dial Int 1989; 9: 159–63.
181. Boelaert JR, De Smedt RA, De Baere YA, Godard CA, Matthys EG, Schurgers ML, Daneels RF, Gordts BZ, Van Landuyt HW. The influence of calcium mupirocin ointment on the incidence of Staphylococcus aureus infections in haemodialysis patients. Nephrol Dial Transplant 1989; 4: 278–81.
182. Manahan FJ, Ing BL, Chan JC et al. Effects of bicarbonate-containing versus lactate-containing peritoneal dialysis solutions on superoxide production by human neutrophils. Artif Organs 1989; 13: 495–7.
183. Kant KS, Goetz D, Marzkuff C, Motz D. Relapsing peritonitis in continuous ambulatory peritoneal dialysis (CAPD): treatment by interuption of CAPD and prolonged antibiotic therapy. Perit Dial Int 1988; 8: 155–7.
184. Keane WF, Peterson WK. Host defense mechanisms of the peritoneal cavity and continuous ambulatory peritoneal dialysis. Perit Dial Bull 1984; 4: 122–7.
185. Glancey GR, Cameron JS, Ogg CS, de Fijter CWH, van der Meulen J. The washout kinetics of intraperitoneal IgG in CAPD patients. Nephrol Dial Transplant 1990; 5: 78.
186. Poole-Warren LA, Hallett MD, Hone PW, Burden SH, Farrell PC. Vaccination for prevention of CAPD-associated staphylococcal infection: results of a prospective multicentre clinical trial. Clin Nephrol 1991; 35: 198–206.
187. Scatizzi A, Strippoli P. Prophylaxis against Staphylococcus aureus peritonitis in continuous ambulatory peritoneal dialysis. Proceedings of the EDTA 1985; 22: 392–6.
188. Obst G, Gagnon RF, Harris A, Prentis J, Richards GK. The activity of rifampicin and analogs against Staphylococcus epidermidis biofilms in a CAPD environment model. Am J Nephrol 1989; 9: 414–20.
198. Block RA, Taylor B, Frederich G. Intraperitoneal infusion of streptokinase in the treatment of recurrent peritonitis. Perit Dial Bull 1983; 3: 162–3.
190. Norris KC, Shinaberger JH, Reyes GD, Kraut JA. The use of intra catheter instillation of streptokinase in the treatment of recurrent bacterial peritonitis in continuous ambulatory peritoneal diaysis. Am J Kid Dis 1987; 10: 62–5.
191. Pickering SJ, Fleming SJ, Bowley JA et al. Urokinase: a treatment for relapsing peritonitis due to coagulase-negative staphylococci. Nephrol Dial Transplant 1989; 4: 62–5.
192. Williams AJ, Boletis I, Johnsson BF et al. Tenckhoff catheter replacement or intraperitoneal urokinase: a randomized trial in the management of recurrent continuous ambulatory peritoneal (CAPD) peritonitis. Perit Dial Int 1989; 9: 65–7.

18 Calcium, phosphate and renal osteodystrophy

ALASTAIR J. HUTCHISON AND RAM GOKAL

1. Introduction 529
2. Classification of renal osteodystrophy 530
   2.1. High turnover bone diseases 530
   2.2. Low turnover bone diseases 530
3. Pathogenesis of renal osteodystrophy 531
   3.1. Parathyroid hormone and calcium metabolism 532
   3.2. Vitamin D metabolism 533
   3.3. Phosphate metabolism 534
   3.4. Magnesium metabolism 535
   3.5. Aluminium and osteodystrophy 535
   3.6. Acid-base balance 535
   3.7. Calcitonin 535
4. Clinical and radiological features of renal osteodystrophy 536
   4.1. Extraskeletal manifestations 536
   4.2. Skeletal manifestations 536
   4.3. Radiological features 536
5. Renal osteodystrophy and CAPD 537
   5.1. Calcium and phosphorus balance in CAPD 537
       5.1.1. Gastrointestinal absorption 537
       5.1.2. The role of calcium salts in renal osteodystrophy 538
       5.1.3. Peritoneal flux and reduced calcium dialysis fluid 539
   5.2. Serum magnesium in CAPD 540
   5.3. Acid-base balance and 40 mmol/L lactate PD fluid 540
   5.4. Parathyroid hormone in CAPD 541
   5.5. Vitamin D in CAPD 541
   5.6. The role of calcitriol therapy in CAPD 542
       5.6.1. Oral pulse calcitriol therapy 542
       5.6.2. Calcitriol analogues 542
   5.7. Renal osteodystrophy in diabetic patients 543
   5.8. The idiopathic adynamic bone lesion in CAPD 543
6. Recommendations for management of osteodystrophy in CAPD 544
   6.1. Biochemical monitoring 545
   6.2. Radiological monitoring 546
   6.3. Transiliac bone biopsy 546
7. Summary 547
References 547

1. Introduction

The first association between uraemia and bone disease was made by Lucas and reported in The Lancet of 1883 [1]. However it was not until nearly forty years later that the major clinical and radiological manifestations of the skeletal changes were accurately defined [2, 3]. In 1943 the histopathology of osteitis fibrosa and osteomalacia was described [4] and, in the same year, the term 'renal osteodystrophy' was coined by Liu and Chu [5]. Subsequently the abnormalities of bone mass that occur in osteopaenia and osteosclerosis were also described [6]. Following the research of Stanbury and Lumb [7, 8], there began a period of rapid advance in the understanding of the processes behind altered divalent ion metabolism, and the abnormalities of parathyroid hormone and vitamin D_3 production that are seen in end-stage renal disease. Despite these advances, and the introduction of vitamin D_3 replacement therapy, osteodystrophy remains a common complication of end-stage renal failure, and continues to pose diagnostic and therapeutic dilemmas for clinical nephrologists. It has become apparent that the spectrum of bone lesions seen in dialysis patients is changing with hyperparathyroid disease becoming less common [9, 10], and furthermore, a different pattern of bone lesions is found in CAPD and haemodialysis patients [9–11]. In a histological study of 259 chronic dialysis patients in Canada the commonest bone lesion was found to be hyperparathyroid disease (50%) in haemodialysis patients, and adynamic bone (61%) in peritoneal dialysis patients [10]. In contrast, Malluche and Monier-Faugere (Kentucky, USA) reported that in a retrospective survey of 602 patients from 1982 to 1991 the mixed lesion was the commonest diagnosis [9], regardless of mode of dialysis (56% in CAPD and 49% in haemodialysis). The difference between these reports is noteworthy in itself, since both are large and reliable studies, but from centres many hundreds of miles apart. Whilst differing diagnostic criteria may account for some of the difference, it emphasizes the fact that in dialysis patients, histomorphometric data represent the result of pathological processes, treatment regimes and environmental effects that have been on-going for years.

2. Classification of renal osteodystrophy

In this chapter the term *renal osteodystrophy* is used to include all its skeletal manifestations such as osteitis fibrosa, osteomalacia, mixed lesions, the adynamic bone lesion, osteoporosis, osteosclerosis, and in children, retardation of growth. A variety of extra-skeletal problems is associated with this syndrome including myopathy, vascular and visceral calcification, and peripheral ischaemic necrosis.

Since the introduction of the undecalcified bone biopsy, significant advances have been made in the understanding of the histological changes underlying all forms of renal osteodystrophy. Renal bone disease has its origins early in the course of renal failure [12, 13], so that by the time GFR has fallen to 50% of normal, at least 50% of the patients exhibit abnormal bone histology [14, 15]. In a study of 16 patients with creatinine clearances between 20 and 59 mls/min, Baker *et al.* found all of them to have abnormal bone histology [16].

The classification of renal osteodystrophy is simplified by the recognition that there are essentially two groups of diseases:

2.1. High turnover bone diseases

Osteitis fibrosa cystica – the characteristic findings include a marked increase in bone resorption, osteoblastic and osteoclastic activity, and endosteal fibrosis (Fig. 1). In particular, the number of osteoclasts is markedly increased, and they may be larger than normal with multiple nuclei. There may be a great increase in surface resorption with dissecting cavities where the osteoclasts have tunnelled through the trabecular bone. This results in deposition of fibrous tissue in the marrow spaces (peritrabecular fibrosis), and the formation of so-called 'woven bone', new bone matrix which is not lamellar but disorganised in structure. Although the bone may show increased osteoid, the use of tetracycline labelling prior to biopsy demonstrates that mineralisation proceeds relatively normally. Skeletal mass may diminish as the rate of resorption exceeds that of formation.

The term "*osteitis*" implies inflammation of bone, which is not present, so that is it preferable to refer to this lesion as "*severe*" or "*predominant hyperparathyroid bone disease*" [9].

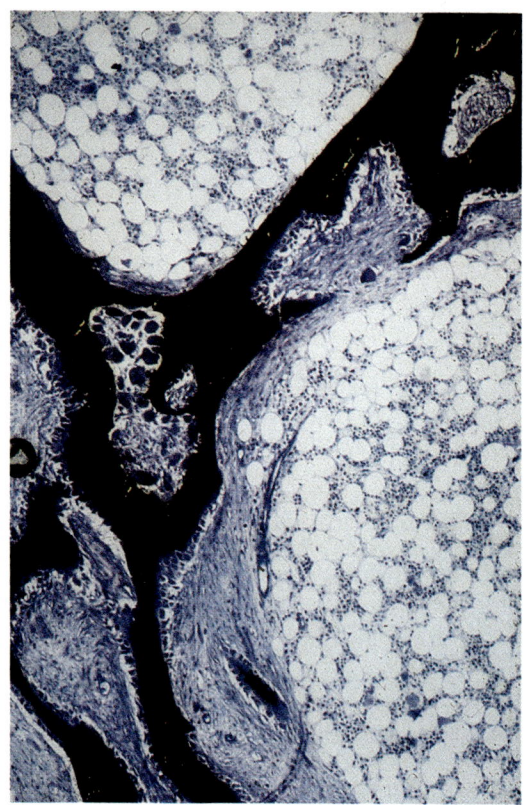

Figure 1. Bone histology in severe hyperparathyroid disease. Numerous large, multinucleate osteoclasts can be seen tunnelling into mineralized trabecular bone. Osteoblasts are also numerous, and peritrabecular fibrous tissue has been deposited in the marrow cavity (toluidine blue stain, × 100).

Mild hyperparathyroidism – here elevated parathyroid hormone levels increase bone turnover but peritrabecular fibrosis is minimal or absent.

2.2. Low turnover bone diseases

Osteomalacia – defective mineralization of bone, due to deficiency of 1,25-dihydroxyvitamin D_3, results in a relative increase in the amount of osteoid or unmineralized bone matrix (Fig. 2). Osteitis fibrosa can also increase osteoid mass, simply as a result of increased bone turnover, but bone biopsy with dual tetracycline labelling will reliably distinguish these diseases. Aluminium accumulation can also lead to an osteomalacic-type osteodystrophy even in the presence of adequate 1,25-dihydroxyvitamin D_3 levels [17]. In bone, the site of aluminium deposition is at the interface between mineralized bone and unmineralized osteoid. Here it appears to reduce osteoblast numbers and delay the process of mineralization, as

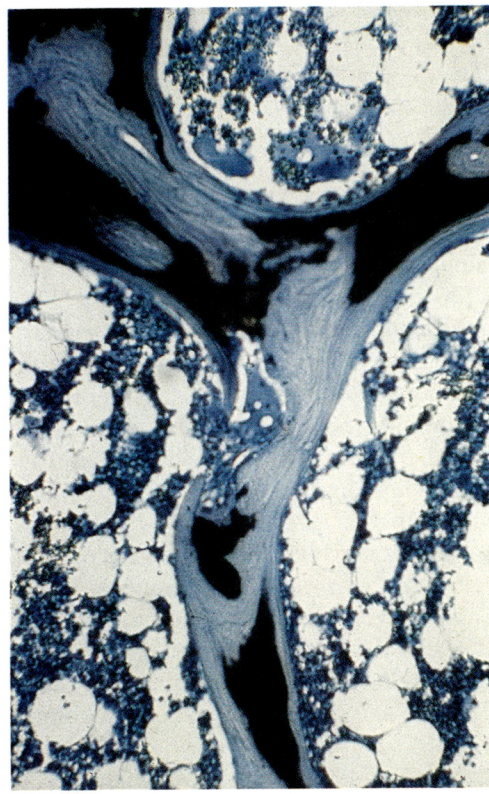

Figure 2. Bone histology in osteomalacia (not aluminium-related). Broad lamellar osteoid seams surround the calcified trabecular bone. In some areas the failure of mineralization has resulted in "islands" of calcified bone so that the mechanical strength of the trabeculum is greatly reduced (toluidine blue stain, × 100).

demonstrated by diminished uptake of tetracycline into trabecular bone [18]. Studies have established an inverse relationship between bone aluminium accumulation and the rate of bone formation [19] and, even in cell-free laboratory studies, aluminium has been shown to reduce both the formation and growth of hydroxyapatite crystals [20].

Adynamic bone lesion (Fig. 3) – previously thought to be a result of aluminium accumulation in bone, this entity has now been shown also to occur in the absence of stainable bone aluminium and is characterised by an abnormally low bone formation rate, a defect of bone mineralization, normal or decreased osteoid thickness, decreased osteoblastic surfaces, and normal or decreased osteoclastic surfaces [15, 21]. This appearance is also referred to as *aplastic*, a term usually reserved for structures that are congenitally absent, whereas *adynamic* more accurately conveys the inactivity of bone cells in this lesion. Little is known about its aetiology, and even less about its natural history,

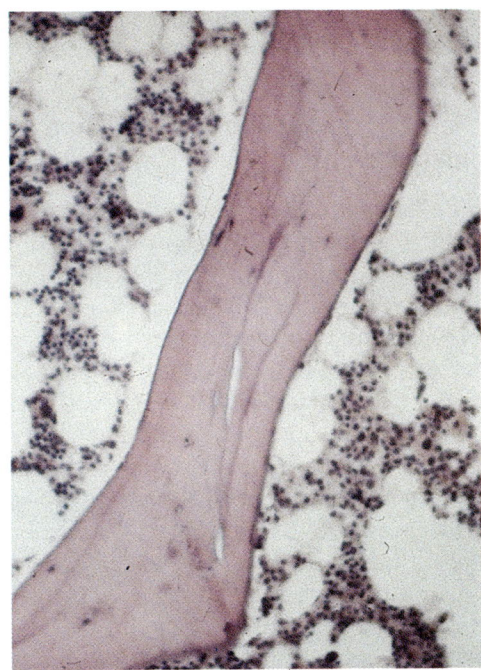

Figure 3. Bone histology in the adynamic lesion. Osteoid seams are very thin or almost absent. Numbers of osteoclasts and osteoblasts are greatly reduced and unrepaired microfractures can be seen within the mineralized bone (H & E stain, × 100).

although there is some evidence to suggest that it is commoner in patients with diabetes [10, 22], elderly dialysis patients [23], and those on CAPD [9, 10].

Mixed bone disease – hyperparathyroidism and defective mineralization can often coexist in chronic renal failure with variable bone volume and rates of bone turnover.

3. Pathogenesis of renal osteodystrophy

Renal osteodystrophy is recognised to be a common complication of end-stage renal failure and is believed to have its origins early in the onset of renal impairment [24]. The mechanism of its development is both multifactorial and controversial, but since normal kidneys maintain calcium, phosphorus, magnesium and bicarbonate balance, synthesize 1,25- and 24,25-dihydroxyvitamin D_3, act as a major target organ and excretory organ for parathyroid hormone, and also excrete aluminium, it is self-evident that renal failure will have numerous profound effects on mineral metabolism. These various factors all interact to a greater or lesser extent, but for simplicity are considered separately in the following sections.

3.1. Parathyroid hormone and calcium metabolism

Bone is continually being remodelled, and in health a balance is maintained between synthesis of bone matrix(osteoid formation), its mineralization, and subsequent resorption. This balance is governed by the relative activity of osteoblasts, osteoclasts and osteocytes. Increased secretion of parathyroid hormone (PTH) increases both the activity and numbers of these bone cells, causing an overall increase in bone turnover. Excessive production may result in deposition of fibrous tissue in the marrow spaces (osteitis fibrosa), endosteal fibrosis, and the formation of so-called 'woven bone', new bone matrix which is not lamellar but disorganised in structure. Skeletal mass may diminish as the rate of resorption exceeds that of formation, and recent results from the European Dialysis and Transplant Association Registry [25] show that in patients dialysed for up to 15 years, parathyroidectomy is still required in up to 40%. Similarly there is increasing evidence to suggest that, in the uraemic patient, low/normal levels of PTH may result in excessively low bone cell activity and overall bone turnover with or without the presence of aluminium [9, 10, 21, 23, 26–28].

PTH is a single-chain protein of 84 amino acids, the sequence of which was established by Keutmann *et al.* in 1978 [29]. It is synthesized in the parathyroid chief cell via two precursors, pre-pro-PTH and pro-PTH (115 and 90 amino acids respectively). PTH secretion occurs approximately 20 minutes after synthesis of the original pre-pro-PTH [30].

Significant elevations of serum parathyroid hormone have been reported in patients with only moderately abnormal glomerular filtration rates of 60–80 ml/min [16, 31, 32]. The secretion of PTH is controlled by many factors, but in renal impairment the most important stimulus is thought to be reduction in the level of serum-ionised calcium (Fig. 4). Factors which contribute to hypocalcaemia and elevation of serum PTH are phosphate retention, defective vitamin D metabolism, skeletal resistance to the calcaemic action of PTH, elevation of the 'set point' at which serum calcium suppresses PTH release and impaired degradation of circulating PTH [32].

Secretion of PTH is primarily controlled by the concentration of ionised calcium in the extracellular space so that hypocalcaemia stimulates, and hypercalcaemia suppresses PTH release [33]. This

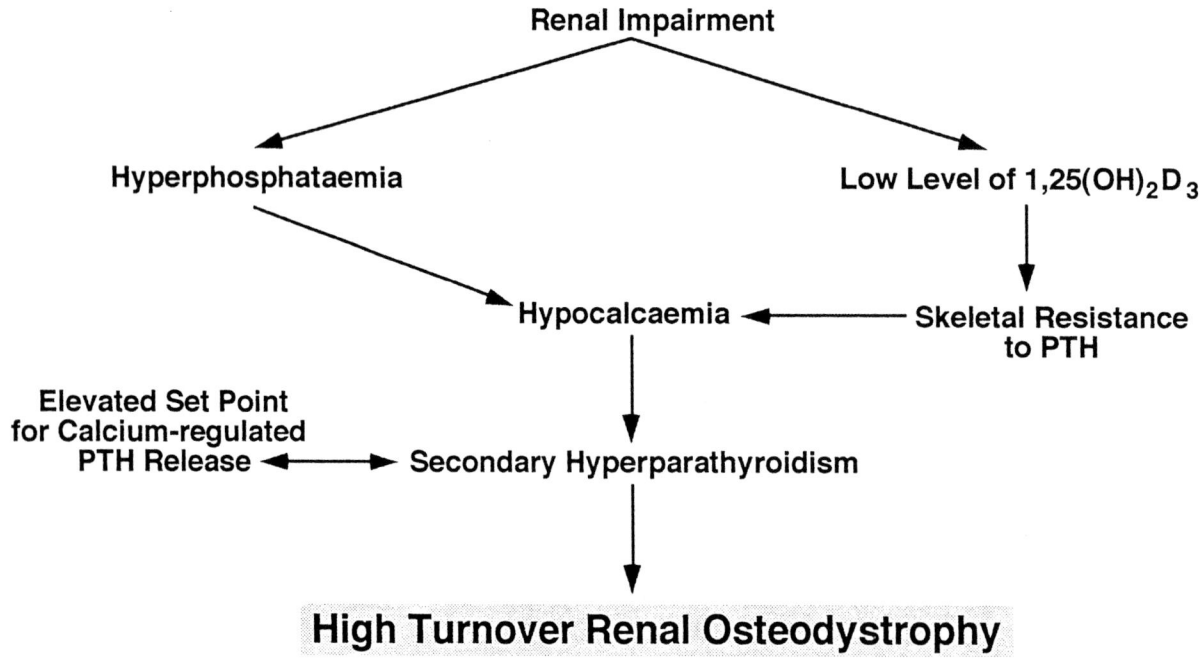

Figure 4. Factors contributing to the production of excess parathyroid hormone in dialysis patients.

relationship between PTH and serum calcium can be represented as a sigmoidal curve, with a basal rate of secretion persisting even during hypercalcaemia [34]. In normal individuals the basal PTH level is approximately 25% of the maximally stimulated PTH level and is positioned in the initial part of the steep ascent of the sigmoidal curve. Therefore, a small decrease in serum calcium produces a large increase in serum PTH secretion. Felsenfeld observed that for the same ionised calcium level, serum PTH was higher during the induction of hypocalcaemia than during the recovery from hypocalcaemia [35]. Conversely, the PTH level was greater when hypercalcaemia was induced from the nadir of hypocalcaemia than when hypercalcaemia was induced from basal serum calcium. Furthermore the set point of calcium was greater during the induction of hypocalcaemia than during the recovery from hypocalcaemia. This differential response of PTH to the direction of change of serum calcium is known as "hysteresis" and there is evidence that the PTH-calcium curves may differ in different forms of renal osteodystrophy or after a specific form of therapy such as desferrioxamine or calcitriol [35–37].

As well as suppressing PTH secretion, hypercalcaemia is also known to decrease parathyroid cell cyclic adenosine monophosphate (cAMP) but it is not clear whether this is the means by which PTH is controlled or whether it is a secondary phenomenon [38].

Hyperplastic parathyroid glands are less sensitive to ionised calcium levels than are normal glands, suggesting that one cause of elevated PTH in chronic renal failure may be a shift in the 'set point' for calcium-regulated PTH secretion, in addition to the increase in parathyroid mass. The set point is defined as a calcium ion concentration necessary to suppress the secretion of PTH by 50%. Furthermore the degree of responsiveness across the calcium-sensitive range is altered so that hyperparathyroidism is a product of the increase in tissue mass (because the non-suppressible, basal secretion is increased) and the lack of suppression by calcium in the normocalcaemic range. Thus normal concentrations of ionised calcium may not be sufficient to suppress hyperplastic parathyroid glands and serum levels have to be increased to the upper limits of normal to control the release of PTH in patients with secondary hyperparathyroidism [34]. However, there is evidence that once the parathyroid gland size exceeds a certain limit, the non-suppressible basal secretion alone becomes sufficient to increase serum parathyroid hormone to hyperparathyroid levels [39]. When this occurs parathyroidectomy is required.

Firm evidence now exists that parathyroid cells possess specific nuclear receptors for 1,25-dihydroxyvitamin D_3 [39, 40]. When given intravenously to a group of 20 haemodialysis patients calcitriol produced a marked suppression (70.1 ± 3.2%) of PTH levels without a significant change in serum calcium, confirming that it is an important regulator of PTH secretion at least in states of calcitriol depletion [41]. Substantial degradation of calcitriol occurs in the intestine so that oral vitamin D increases intestinal calcium absorption but the delivery of calcitriol to peripheral target organs is limited [42]. This could explain the much greater effect of intravenous compared to oral calcitriol. PTH secretion is also affected by ionised magnesium; however only severe hypomagnesaemia seems to have any clinical relevance in that it has been shown to inhibit PTH secretion [43].

In addition to the abnormalities of secretion that occur in chronic renal failure, the process of degradation is incomplete. Normally, intact PTH is degraded by the liver and kidneys, resulting in the production of amino (N)- and carboxy (C)-terminal fragments. The fragments are further metabolized by the kidney so that in the absence of renal function they accumulate. C-terminal fragments are detectable up to two weeks after parathyroidectomy in chronic renal failure, yet decrease by 80% within 24 hours of a successful renal transplant. Various portions of the PTH molecule may be measured by radioimmunoassay but it has been shown that the results of sandwich assays specific to the whole, or intact, 1–84 PTH molecule correlate best with the biological effects of PTH on bone in chronic renal failure [44].

3.2. Vitamin D metabolism

The similarity between the bone disease caused by simple vitamin D deficiency and that which occurs in chronic renal failure has been recognised for many years, both at clinical [1] and histological levels [4]. It was also known that renal failure was associated with impaired intestinal absorption of calcium [5]. In renal failure both the bone lesions and the defect in calcium absorption were shown to be correctable by oral calciferol, but the amount required to have an effect is much larger than in simple deficiency states. The disease is 'vitamin D resistant'. Vitamin D_3 (calciferol) circulates in the blood bound to vitamin D-binding protein, after having been synthesized in the skin or absorbed from the diet. In the liver it is metabolized by the enzyme vitamin-D-25-hydroxylase to form 25-hydroxyvitamin D (calcidiol; 25-OH–D). In most patients with chronic renal failure 25-OH–D levels are normal if they eat a balanced diet and their skin is not completely covered from the sun.

In the kidney 25-OH–D is further metabolized by a mitochondrial cytochrome P-450 oxidase, 25-OH–D-1 alpha-hydroxylase, to form 1,25-dihydroxyvitamin D_3 (calcitriol), the biologically active form of vitamin D. The exact location of the 1 alpha-hydroxylase enzyme in human kidney is unknown. In 1973, Mawer *et al.* showed that calcitriol could not be detected in the serum of patients with chronic renal failure, after injection of radioactive cholecalciferol, and suggested that it was the inability to form this metabolite that was the cause of the vitamin D resistance [45]. This is now known to be the case, and is a result of reduced renal 1 alpha-hydroxylase activity caused by loss of renal mass, hyperphosphataemia and possibly by uraemic toxins [46]. In addition to renal production of 1,25-OH–D_3 humans can, in certain pathological states produce it extrarenally. In sarcoidosis cultured alveolar macrophages and lymph node homogenates can convert 25-OH–D to 1,25-OH–D_3 and a similar process probably accounts for the hypercalcaemia and hypercalciuria sometimes seen in other granulomatous diseases such as tuberculosis, silicosis, berylliosis and fungal diseases. In CAPD patients who have had one or more episodes of peritonitis cultured peritoneal macrophages are also able to convert 25-OH–D_3 to 1,25-OH–D_3 [47].

Once synthesized in the kidney, 1,25-OH–D_3 is transported by vitamin D-binding protein to its target cells. It enters the cell by a mechanism that is poorly understood and is then transported to the nucleus. Here it interacts with its nuclear receptor, phosphorylating it to bring about interaction with chromatin and transcription of specific genes. In the small intestine this results in expression of the gene coding for calbindin, the calcium binding protein. The activity of other proteins is also affected, with the net result that calcium and phosphate absorption from the intestine is stimulated. The effect of 1,25-OH–D_3 on bone is to increase removal of calcium. A small decrease in serum ionised calcium stimulates PTH production which in turn stimulates the kidney to produce 1,25-OH–D_3. 1,25-OH–D_3 in conjunction with PTH increases osteoclastic activity and release of calcium, returning the ionised calcium level to normal.

1,25-OH–D_3 has been conclusively shown to suppress PTH secretion in dialysis patients when administered orally or intravenously [41, 48–54]. It undoubtedly also has important immunoregulatory functions and is able to decrease the rate of proliferation of certain tumour cells, such as the HL-60 (human promyelocytic) cell, and even transform them into mature macrophages. 1,25-OH–D_3 can also inhibit the proliferation of cultured human keratinocytes, an ability which has important clinical implications in that it has been shown to dramatically improve psoriasis in seventy five per cent of a group of patients given up to 2 µg per day [55]. It has recently been suggested that vitamin D deficiency may be an important factor in the pathogenesis of hypertension and insulin resistance in end-stage renal failure [56].

3.3. Phosphate metabolism

In the past, overactivity of the parathyroid glands in renal failure was explained by the trade-off hypothesis of Bricker [57]. He postulated that as renal failure progresses there is a tendency for serum phosphate levels to rise and ionised calcium levels to fall resulting in a compensatory rise in PTH. The increase in PTH reduces tubular reabsorption of phosphate in the remaining nephrons and increases serum calcium. Thus serum values of phosphate and calcium may be kept within, or near, the normal range at the expense of rising PTH levels and its resultant effects on the skeleton. However, more recent work has cast doubt on this with the observations that hyperparathyroidism can develop even in the presence of a high serum calcium [58], and that hyperphosphataemia stimulates PTH secretion independent of serum calcium concentration [59, 60]. However, increased phosphate excretion results in decreased activity of 25-OH–D-1 alpha-hydroxylase, and consequently decreased production of 1,25-dihydroxyvitamin D_3 [55]. This in turn stimulates increased synthesis and secretion of PTH in an attempt to stimulate renal production of 1,25-dihydroxyvitamin D_3. As renal failure progresses the compensatory effect of PTH on 1,25-dihydroxyvitamin D_3 deficiency is overcome and an absolute deficiency develops [15]. This further stimulates PTH levels and decreases gastro-intestinal calcium absorption [61]. With further progression of renal failure, to a glomerular filtration rate of around 10 ml/min, phosphate excretion can no longer be increased and hyperphosphataemia occurs, exacerbating the hypocalcaemia. At this stage hypocalcaemia further stimulates PTH secretion, although doubt remains as to its role in the earlier stages of renal failure. In addition hyperphosphataemia can lead to extraskeletal calcification in soft tissues and, more worryingly, in blood vessels.

3.4. Magnesium metabolism

Although magnesium metabolism is affected by decreasing renal function, the clinical relevance of this is unknown. In normal subjects magnesium is absorbed from the small intestine and excreted in the urine, so that elevated serum levels are seen in renal failure [62, 63]. In vitro, magnesium is an inhibitor of crystallisation and may increase bone levels of pyrophosphate – another inhibitor of mineralization [64]. In uraemia, bone magnesium is correlated with serum magnesium, and serum pyrophosphate is increased [65]. Hence it is theoretically possible that elevated serum magnesium could play a role in the development of osteomalacia, but there is no evidence in the literature that this is the case.

Moderate hypomagnesaemia can contribute to elevation of serum PTH [66], whereas severe hypomagnesaemia has been shown to inhibit PTH secretion [43].

3.5. Aluminium and osteodystrophy

In 1978 Ward *et al.* made the association between aluminium and bone disease in dialysis patients [17]. Since then the importance attached to reducing exposure to aluminium has gradually increased but the use of aluminium hydroxide as a phosphate binder is still quite widespread.

A normal human daily intake of aluminium ranges from 2 to 20 mg but gastrointestinal uptake is estimated to be only 0.5 to 1% of this. The normal urinary aluminium excretion varies between 20–50 μg per day but was shown to increase to 200–400 μg per day when normal individuals were given aluminium hydroxide in amounts commonly given to dialysis patients [67]. In end stage renal failure the loss of urinary excretion plus exposure to aluminium in dialysate solutions, phosphate binders, and volume replacement fluids can result in the total body content rising by a factor of up to 20. Serum levels are a poor guide to total body load, since it is strongly protein bound and largely deposited in tissues such as bone, liver and spleen.

Aluminium accumulates at the interface between mineralized bone and unmineralized osteoid, where it delays the process of mineralization. Aluminium also accumulates in parathyroid glands and suppresses their secretion of PTH. In patients with aluminium-related bone disease and renal failure, PTH levels are commonly lower than would be expected and may be suppressed to normal levels, giving some degree of protection from hyperparathyroid bone disease [68], but possibly resulting in development of the adynamic bone lesion [44].

It is to be hoped that aluminium-related bone disease will gradually disappear as more physicians change to calcium-based phosphate binders, and exposure from other sources is sought out and reduced to minimal levels.

3.6. Acid-base balance

The role of acidosis in the pathogenesis of renal osteodystrophy is unclear. However, acidosis is involved in both calcium balance and PTH release. Acidotic azotaemic patients show increased losses of urinary and faecal calcium which can be reduced by alkali treatment, resulting in restoration of a neutral calcium balance [69]. In a study of 54 uraemic patients, infusion of sodium bicarbonate produced a rise in arterialyzed capillary blood pH and a proportional fall of around 20% in serum PTH [70]. No significant change in serum ionized calcium was observed during the study. The clinical significance of these findings remains to be elucidated but it seems likely that, as with changes in magnesium metabolism, the effects are of much less importance than those associated with PTH and Vitamin D.

3.7. Calcitonin

Calcitonin is a 32-amino acid single chain peptide, and the major stimulus for its secretion is hypercalcaemia. Circulating calcitonin has a short half-life (around 10 minutes) and depends on renal function for degradation and excretion, so that high circulating levels are found in patients with renal failure [71]. Its role in normal human subjects is debated, since neither the absence of this hormone (as in completely thyroidectomized patients) nor its thousandfold excess (as in patients with thyroid medullary carcinoma) is generally associated with any abnormality of calcium homeostasis or skeletal integrity [72]. However, there is around 40% structural homology between PTH and calcitonin receptors, the latter being found in bone, kidney, central nervous system, testis, placenta and on some tumour cells.

4. Clinical and radiological features of renal osteodystrophy

Clinical features of the altered mineral and skeletal metabolism that occurs in renal failure may be considered under two broad headings, extraskeletal and skeletal manifestations (Table 1).

4.1. Extraskeletal manifestations

Extraskeletal manifestations are mainly a result of deposition of calcium in soft tissues. Hyperphosphataemia can cause an increase in the calcium × phosphate product to a point where its solubility product is exceeded and precipitation can occur in many sites. It has been suggested that calcium deposition in the skin may contribute to the pruritus that in severe cases can be quite disabling for dialysis patients, preventing sleep and resulting in widespread excoriations with skin sepsis. Calcification in the conjunctiva is another common problem leading to the intensely painful 'red-eye', with flecks of calcium often clearly visible on examination.

Perhaps the most important extraskeletal manifestation is calcification of the vascular tree which frequently becomes visible on plain X-rays. The abdominal aorta, femoral and digital arteries are often clearly outlined on films taken for skeletal survey, but the same process is undoubtedly occurring in the cerebral and coronary vasculature, resulting in considerable morbidity and mortality in dialysis and transplant patients [23]. In severe cases, vascular calcification in the iliac and femoral vessels may render a patient untransplantable because anastomosis of the vessels becomes impossible. Furthermore the risk of per-operative myocardial infarction is greatly increased, and heart failure, controlled by strict attention to fluid balance while on dialysis, may be unmasked by renal transplantation.

4.2. Skeletal manifestations

Skeletal signs and symptoms of renal osteodystrophy include bone pain, bone tenderness, spontaneous fractures, retardation of growth and joint disease. With the exception of adolescents with tubulo-interstitial pathology, symptoms are unusual in patients with end-stage renal disease, unless the decline in renal function has been particularly slow. However, those with tubulo-interstitial disease and adolescent patients are more prone to overt bone disease. The prevalence of symptoms among dialysis patients varies greatly from unit to unit which may reflect differences in reporting or true differences due to a dialysis-induced cause such as aluminium intake [73, 74].

Both osteomalacia and osteitis fibrosa may be associated with bone pain, tenderness and proximal muscle weakness. In addition lower back and lower limb pain contribute to the reduced exercise ability that is common in dialysis patients. This in turn worsens muscle weakness and loss of skeletal mass.

Periosteal new bone growth and osteosclerosis are usually asymptomatic but may often be seen on skeletal radiography.

4.3. Radiological features

Although regular radiological assessment, using plain radiographs, is the most frequently used

Table 1. Clinical and radiological features of renal osteodystrophy.

Clinical manifestations:

Skeletal	Extraskeletal
Bone tenderness	Renal "red-eye"
Bone pain	Pruritus
Joint pains	Myopathy
Spontaneous fracture	Tumoural calcification
Growth retardation	Peripheral ischaemic necrosis

Radiological manifestations:

Hyperparathyroidism
Erosion of tips of terminal phalanges, radial aspects of middle phalanges, distal ends of clavicals
"Pepper-pot" skull
Thinning of cortex in tubular bones
Osteopaenic vertebral bodies with sclerotic upper and lower surfaces, results in "rugger jersey spine" appearance
Visceral/vascular calcification

Osteomalacia
Looser's zones (most often in public bones or femur), otherwise no specific features in milder cases

Adynamic lesion
No specific features, but associated with increased risk of vascular calcification

method of monitoring renal osteodystrophy it is undoubtedly insensitive and only reliably detects advanced cases. Malluche and Faugere state that information obtained from skeletal X-rays is limited and often misleading, and that most radiologic signs considered to be pathognomonic of severe osteitis fibrosa can be found in any of the three histological types of renal osteodystrophy [15].

The earliest radiological feature of hyperparathyroidism is subperiosteal erosion occurring at the tufts of the terminal phalanges, the radial aspect of the middle phalanges and the distal ends of the clavicals. In a study of 30 end stage renal failure patients, performed immediately prior to commencing dialysis, erosion of the terminal phalanges was seen in five of the eight patients ,who had severe hyperparathyroid disease on bone biopsy [75]. However, plain radiographs did not identify patients with mild hyperparathyroid disease, and the majority of patients were judged to have essentially normal skeletal surveys. These findings are in agreement with those of Owen et al., who compared plain skeletal radiology with bone histology in 82 patients with renal failure, and found no correlation between radiological and histological indices [76]. We would therefore agree with the previously quoted statements of Malluche and Faugere [15], and question the need for the traditional annual skeletal survey which provides a significant dose of ionizing radiation.

Apart from a generalised increase in radiolucency, radiological signs are uncommon in osteomalacia. However, Looser's zones may sometimes be seen and are characteristic of this condition.

In recent years, other radiological techniques have been developed for examining bone in a more quantitative fashion, including skeletal scintigraphy, measurement of bone density and mineral content by single or dual photon densitometry, plus single and dual energy quantitative computed tomography (QCT) scan [77, 78]. These techniques are discussed later in the chapter.

5. Renal osteodystrophy and CAPD

The introduction of CAPD in the 1970's has provided new opportunities for the investigation and management of renal osteodystrophy. However, reports of its control and development in CAPD remain confusing with some showing improvement [73, 79, 80] and others showing deterioration [81–3].

The different pattern of bone lesions seen in CAPD and haemodialysis is now well described [9–11, 84]. There are several differences between the dialysis modalities which may affect mineral metabolism [11]. CAPD is associated with far greater losses of middle and large molecular weight protein fractions, thereby removing more transferrin-bound aluminium, as well as 25-hydroxyvitamin D_3. With CAPD, weekly phosphate removal is greater than haemodialysis, and it provides a steady state biochemical profile unlike the "sawtooth" pattern of haemodialysis. Furthermore, the high calcium concentration in standard peritoneal dialysis fluids may have a significantly suppressive effect on PTH levels, contributing to the higher incidence of low-turnover bone disease seen in CAPD. In contrast, a haemodialysis patient will experience episodes of relative hypocalcaemia two or three times each week and this may well stimulate PTH production.

5.1. Calcium and phosphorus balance in CAPD

In end-stage renal disease serum phosphate levels begin to rise and ionised calcium levels begin to fall once the GFR is less than 20 mls/min. These abnormalities can be at least partially corrected by the administration of oral calcium carbonate. However, ionised calcium levels may still below (0.9–1.1 mmol/L) when patients start CAPD even though total serum calcium levels are normal [85]. Serum levels usually rise once CAPD has begun, since the majority of dialysis fluids currently in use have a calcium concentration of 1.75 mmols/litre. Gastrointestinal absorption and peritoneal flux of calcium during dialysis are the two major determinants of overall calcium mass-balance in peritoneal dialysis patients.

5.1.1. Gastrointestinal absorption
The gastrointestinal absorption of calcium has been studied by several groups and is known to be dependent on many factors including the degree of uraemia, serum phosphate level, PTH level, 1,25-dihydroxyvitamin D_3 level and total calcium intake. In uraemic subjects Recker and Saville [86] found that calcium absorption ranged from 5 to 59%, whilst Clarkson and colleagues [87] and Ramirez et al. [88] reported figures of 8 and 28% respectively. In a study of CAPD patients in our own unit calcium absorption rate was subnormal in 18 of 19 subjects, although significant variation existed between patients. Percentage absorption ranged

from 3.2 to 23.9%, results not dissimilar to those in uraemics [89]. Blumenkrantz examined absorption of dietary calcium in CAPD patients over the range 500 to 2500 mg/day [90] and suggested that it can be represented by the empirical relationship $Y = 0.42X - 277$ (where Y = amount absorbed, X = intake in mg/day). Therefore if the daily intake is around 730 mg/day, approximately 30 mg of calcium is absorbed by the patient.

If calcium salts are to be used as first line therapy for hyperphosphataemia then oral intake and gastrointestinal absorption will be necessarily high. Once a patient is established on dialysis, control of hyperphosphataemia is very important, not only to minimise further stimulation of PTH secretion, but also to keep the calcium × phosphate product within the normal range. Failure to do this can result in rapid progression of vascular and soft tissue calcification. The CAPD patient's high protein diet (recommended minimum protein intake 1.2 g/kg/day) provides an obligatory phosphate intake of up to 1200 mg daily [90, 91]. Although peritoneal dialysis controls the hyperphosphataemia of end stage renal disease more effectively than does haemodialysis [83, 92, 93] it removes only 310–320 mg/day [90, 94] – rather less than one third of the amount required to bring phosphate levels into the normal range. Therefore if a neutral phosphate balance is to be achieved, the gastrointestinal elimination of phosphorus needs to be around 700 mg/day [95]. Since 40 to 80% of dietary phosphorus is absorbed by patients with renal failure [93] the fraction of phosphate absorbed must be reduced, and hence gastrointestinal elimination increased, by oral phosphate-binding agents.

5.1.2. *The role of calcium salts in renal osteodystrophy*

Available phosphate binders, suitable for clinical use, include aluminium hydroxide and carbonate, calcium carbonate, acetate and citrate, magnesium carbonate, keto-analogues of amino acids, and finally polyuronic acids (Table 2). Each of these binders has advantages and disadvantages, but only three are in widespread use – aluminium hydroxide, calcium carbonate and calcium acetate. Calcium carbonate is probably the most commonly used phosphate binder in CAPD patients, where maintenance of optimal serum calcium and phosphate levels is central to the treatment of hyperparathyroidism.

When CAPD was first introduced aluminium gels were the standard phosphate binders, and a high calcium concentration in the dialysis fluid (1.75 mmol/L–3.5mEq/L) was therefore beneficial, rapidly bringing serum calcium levels into the normal range. Now that the dangers of aluminium accumulation have become apparent [68, 96], aluminium containing phosphate binders have been replaced by calcium salts as first line therapy for hyperphosphataemia in most renal units. Unfortunately calcium salts frequently result in hypercalcaemia when given in sufficiently large oral doses to control serum phosphate [97–99], so that aluminium containing phosphate binders continue to be used. It has been suggested that when used in low doses, with careful monitoring of serum aluminium, these binders are safe [15]. However, although only about 1% of the oral dose of aluminium is absorbed [100], even on modest doses this represents between 5 and 10 mg of elemental aluminium daily. Since CAPD removes only 40–50 µg daily [101] it is evident that tissue accumulation is inevitable and significant. If aluminium salts are to be completely avoided, then the hypercalcaemia associated with calcium salts must be prevented. Reduction of dialysis fluid calcium concentration is one means of achieving this end and has been studied in haemodialysis [102, 103] and peritoneal dialysis patients [104–110].

Maintenance of a high/normal serum ionised calcium and control of hyperphosphataemia can be beneficially employed to suppress PTH production, even in patients not taking vitamin D_3 supplements. This is obviously desirable in patients with significantly elevated PTH levels, but in patients with normal, or only mildly elevated levels, it is not necessarily so. Many of these patients will have the adynamic bone lesion, and a small rise in PTH levels may be beneficial. One method of achieving this would be to allow the serum ionised calcium to fall below the "set point" for calcium-mediated PTH release, but at the same time one would want to maintain strict control of serum phosphate.

Table 2. Available compounds for use as phosphate binders in dialysis patients.

Calcium-based	Others
Calcium carbonate	Aluminium carbonate
Calcium acetate	Magnesium carbonate
Calcium citrate	Aluminium hydroxide
Calcium gluconate	Magnesium hydroxide
Calcium alginate	Polyuronic acids
Calcium-ketovalin	

This is not easy when the calcium supplement and phosphate binder are one and the same tablet, but such manoeuvres are undoubtedly facilitated by the availability of reduced calcium dialysis fluids. In this way, hypercalcaemic over-suppression of PTH can be minimised, whilst still allowing the ingestion of sufficiently large doses of calcium carbonate to enable good control of serum phosphate.

Control of serum phosphate is not only important in terms of its effect on PTH, but also for prevention, and sometimes treatment, of extraskeletal calcification. This potentially lethal aspect of renal osteodystrophy is a particular hazard in patients who have persistent hypercalcaemia and hyperphosphataemia. It is traditional to prescribe aluminium-containing binders for such patients on the grounds that the aluminium absorbed is likely to be less harmful than allowing the process of vascular calcification to continue unchecked. Utilization of reduced calcium dialysis fluid offers a better alternative for a least 50% of patients, with the other 50% achieving a reduction in aluminium intake although no change in the calcium × phosphate product (see below).

5.1.3. *Peritoneal flux and reduced calcium dialysis fluid*

During an exchange of 2 litres of 1.36% glucose solution there is a net influx of calcium to the patient, although the amount varies from one study to the next (84 ± 18 mg/day [90]; 300 mg/day [111]). The transfer of calcium is also influenced by ultrafiltration rate and volume [112] so that a 1.36% glucose solution results in a 10 mg calcium uptake by the patient but the greater ultrafiltration from a 3.86% solution leads to a loss of 20 mg. This gives a net daily absorption of 10mg if one hypertonic bag is used per day [112]. In another study, Kwong et al. [113] found an uptake of 29 mg per 1.36% exchange and a loss of 6 mg per 3.86% exchange suggesting a larger net gain of around 80 mg daily. However, a lower PD fluid calcium concentration of 1.5 mmols/litre causes the balance to become negative with a loss of 50 ± 36 mg/day [74]. These findings suggest that patients using dialysis solutions containing 1.75 mmol/L of calcium are in a significantly positive calcium balance even before considering the additional gut absorption from oral calcium carbonate and vitamin D therapy.

The theoretical work by Martis et al. [95] formed the basis for the commercial production of a peritoneal dialysis fluid with a calcium concentration of 1.25 mmol/L, in an attempt to decrease the incidence of hypercalcaemia in CAPD patients taking oral calcium salt phosphate binders. Clinical studies have now confirmed this theoretical work [109, 114]. Although dialysis fluids with other concentrations of calcium can be obtained (0, 0.60, 1.00, 1.45 mmol/)), 1.25 mmol/L would appear to be the logical choice for a new standard CAPD fluid because it is so close to normal serum ionised calcium levels. This results in a homeostatic effect, with calcium being lost into the peritoneum when serum levels are above 1.25 mmol/L, but being absorbed from the peritoneum during times of relative hypocalcaemia. All other proposed calcium concentrations are outside the normal range of serum ionised calcium and therefore cannot exert this homeostatic effect.

Convective effects of ultrafiltration increase the removal of calcium from the peritoneum so that patients using one or more 3.86% glucose exchanges per day will have a significantly greater negative peritoneal calcium balance than patients using only 1.36% exchanges. Whilst in theory this could result in some degree of hypocalcaemia, in practise it rarely occurs as calcium absorption from oral phosphate binders is usually sufficient to compensate.

A two year prospective biochemical, radiological and histological study of 1.25 mmol/L calcium PD fluid showed it to be safe in compliant, well monitored patients [115]. It allowed administration of larger doses of calcium carbonate and achievement of good control of serum phosphate and calcium × phosphate product. Parathyroid hormone levels were suppressed in the majority of patients, and bone histology and density did not deteriorate. By utilising this more physiological dialysis fluid, aluminium containing phosphate binders may be completely avoided in most CAPD patients.

In a smaller study of 1.25 mmol/L calcium dialysis solution, 11 CAPD patients were selected on the basis of persistent hypercalcaemia and uncontrolled hyperphosphataemia [106]. After three months these patients were changed from standard 1.75 mmol/ calcium, to 1.25 mmol/L calcium solution and followed for a further 6 months. Overall mean calcium × phosphate product changed little, however in a subgroup of six patients it fell significantly, while in the other five it tended to rise. The group's mean serum aluminium fell significantly and although geometric mean iPTH rose slightly (but non-significantly) there was an association between phosphate control and iPTH at

6 months. In the subgroup of patients whose calcium × phosphate product fell, there was a much smaller rise in iPTH than in the others (57.3 to 73.2 vs 52.8 to 167.1 pg/ml). This suggests that in those patients using standard solutions, with apparently poor calcium and phosphate control, around 50% of them may, by changing to 1.25 mmol/L calcium solution, achieve a normal calcium × phosphate product whilst still avoiding aluminium salts. In this group of patients a lower calcium solution (0.75–1.00 mmol/L) may well prove appropriate.

Cunningham et al. [110] have used a similar low calcium dialysis fluid to enable the use of calcium carbonate plus alfacalcidol in a group of CAPD patients. In 17 CAPD patients taking oral calcium carbonate, reductions in dialysis fluid calcium concentration to 1.45 mmol/L or 1.00 mmol/L enabled most of the patients to also take oral alfacalcidol. Parathyroid hormone, serum aluminium and alkaline phosphatase levels were all decreased during the 11 months of the study, with the authors concluding that a dialysate calcium concentration of 1.75 mmol/L is too high for the majority of calcium carbonate treated patients, and that substantial reductions of the dialysate calcium concentration are required. Other workers have used 1.0 mmol/L calcium fluid in hypercalcaemic CAPD patients, again with similar results [28, 116]. Utilization of solutions with calcium concentrations of 1.00 mmol/L and below put the patient into a permanent negative calcium balance, so that very close attention must be given to PTH levels and compliance with oral calcium and vitamin D therapy.

5.2. Serum magnesium in CAPD

Magnesium levels are consistently elevated in CAPD patients managed with standard dialysate containing 0.75 mmol/L of magnesium [85, 111]. No toxicity has been reported at these levels and indeed hypermagnesaemia may have a suppressive effect on PTH release and retard the development of arterial calcification in CAPD patients [117]. Hypermagnesaemia may therefore be beneficial, but it has also been shown that normalization of serum magnesium is associated with an improvement in bone histology in haemodialysis patients [118]. Reducing the magnesium content to 0.25 mmol/L normalises serum magnesium levels in CAPD patients [92, 114]. Parsons et al. [119, 120] have described the use of a low calcium/zero magnesium CAPD fluid with a combination of calcium carbonate and magnesium carbonate in liquid form as the phosphate binder. Using this approach, mean serum phosphate levels of 1.4 to 1.5 mmol/L were obtained without causing hypermagnesaemia, although hypomagnesaemia was seen in 2 of 32 patients. Zero magnesium fluids have also been studied by Shah et al. [121], and offer the advantage of permitting larger doses of magnesium salt phosphate binders, but there are two disadvantages. Firstly patients may experience gastrointestinal upset, since magnesium salts have a laxative effect [122], and secondly monitoring of compliance and serum magnesium levels becomes obligatory, as hypomagnesaemia has been associated with cardiac rhythm disturbances [123–125] and electrocardiographic abnormalities [126].

5.3. Acid-base balance and 40 mmol/L lactate PD fluid

There is considerable evidence that as renal mechanisms for acid excretion fail, bone mineral stores become an important source of buffer [127, 128]. Acetazolamide produces a metabolic acidosis in normal subjects by inhibiting carbonic anhydrase in the proximal tubular epithelium, resulting in a bicarbonate diuresis. In virtually anuric haemodialysis patients it might therefore be expected to have little effect, but in fact produces a severe metabolic acidosis [129], suggesting that it is interfering with extra-renal buffering. Carbonic anhydrase is present in osteoclasts [130], and may be activated by PTH to promote bone resorption by release of H^+ ions [131]. The availability of bone buffers and bicarbonate would therefore depend on the activity of PTH and could be inhibited by acetazolamide. It can be seen therefore that during a time of prolonged metabolic acidosis, such as exists in many CAPD patients using PD fluid with only 35 mmol/L lactate [132], buffering by bone would be linked to bone resorption and increased PTH levels.

The use of PD fluid containing 40 mmol/L lactate corrects the mild acidosis experienced by most CAPD patients using the lower lactate concentration that is common in most European countries. Optimal correction of acidosis has been shown to change the progression of osteodystrophy in haemodialysis patients by Lefebvre et al. who, over 18 months prospectively studied two groups of patients dialysed against either standard dialysis fluid (32–24 mmol/L), or against fluid supplemented with 7–15 mmol/L of bicarbonate to achieve a pre-dialysis plasma bicarbonate of 24 mmol/L.

The supplemented group had a decreased rate of progression of secondary hyperparathyroidism in patients with high bone turnover, and stimulated bone turnover in those with low bone formation rates [133].

5.4. Parathyroid hormone in CAPD

Although the prevalence of symptomatic bone disease has decreased in recent years, the 1989 EDTA Registry report showed that around 40% of all patients dialysed for up to 15 years still required parathyroidectomy [25]. This partly reflects the poor understanding of the pathogenesis of secondary hyperparathyroidism that existed in the 1970's and 80's, and partly the difficulty of monitoring vitamin D and PTH levels.

In the last five years considerable progress has been made with the introduction of sensitive and specific assays for calcium-regulating hormones [44, 134]. This has resulted in new concepts for prophylaxis and treatment of renal osteodystrophy which hopefully will further improve long-term results.

CAPD has been shown to clear significant amounts of PTH from the serum. Using a C-terminal assay Delmez et al. [112] found a clearance rate of 1.5 ml/min or 13.6 ± 3.2% of the estimated total extracellular iPTH. Despite this, there is no clear-cut consensus on the effect of CAPD on PTH levels although the weight of evidence is in favour of a steady decline with time [73, 79, 135–137]. However, other reports show no change [112], an increase in the levels [81, 138] or a variable response [82]. The reason for these differences lies in the widely varying practices between centres with regard to the use of calcium carbonate, aluminium hydroxide, vitamin D_3 treatment and also the different radioimmunoassays used for measurement of iPTH and its fragments.

Until recently, CAPD tended to be seen as a prescription in itself, with a standard set of guidelines that were suitable for every patient. As a result, the majority were treated with four 2 litre exchanges, a phosphate binder, vitamin supplements and a small oral dose of 1,25-dihydroxyvitamin D_3. PTH levels were rarely measured, and the dosage of calcitriol was only changed if hypercalcaemia occurred or evidence of osteitis fibrosa appeared on plain radiology of the hands.

Maintenance of a high serum ionised calcium (1.2–1.3 mmol/L) and strict control of serum phosphate, from the time of first starting dialysis, has been shown to decrease PTH levels in CAPD patients without the addition of Vitamin D_3 therapy [107, 115] but Hercz et al. [10, 28] has shown that such suppression can result in a hitherto infrequently recognised form of renal osteodystrophy, the non aluminium-related, or "idiopathic", adynamic bone disease. Hence the question now is not only "what is the best way to suppress PTH", but also "can PTH be over suppressed?".

5.5. Vitamin D in CAPD

Vitamin D metabolism is well known to be abnormal in uraemia, with very low levels of 1,25-dihydroxyvitamin D_3 [45]. However there are additional factors affecting Vitamin D levels relating to the CAPD itself. Levels of 1,25-dihydroxyvitamin D_3 are known to be very low, and sometimes undetectable, at the start of CAPD [75, 137]. 25-hydroxyvitamin D_3 levels are usually within the normal range at start of CAPD but begin to decline thereafter [73, 94]. This is not unexpected since peritoneal dialysis effluent contains significant amounts of vitamin D binding protein, an alpha$_2$-globulin of molecular weight 59,000 Daltons, which binds all three vitamin D metabolites (1,25-dihydroxyvitamin D_3, 25-hydroxyvitamin D_3 and 24,25-hydroxyvitamin D_3). Losses of 1,25-dihydroxyvitamin D_3 and 24,25-dihydroxyvitamin D_3 have been shown to average approximately 6–8% of the plasma pool per day [139]. Thus, CAPD patients probably require 2–3 times the maintenance doses used in haemodialysis patients if it is thought necessary to bring serum levels of 1,25-dihydroxyvitamin D_3 into the normal range, These doses frequently produce the problem of hypercalcaemia.

In England a seasonal variation in 25-hydroxyvitamin D_3 levels was found by Cassidy et al. [140] and in sunnier climates, patients may be able to maintain 25-hydroxyvitamin D_3 levels within the normal range throughout the year. Whether 24,25-dihydroxyvitamin D_3 plays an important role in bone mineralization remains to be proved, but Dunstan et al. [141] have shown that the combination of 1,25-dihydroxyvitamin D_3 and 24,25-dihydroxyvitamin D_3 given orally did not appear to confer any additional benefit compared with 1,25-dihydroxyvitamin D_3 alone. This result is challenged by the work of Chaimovitz and colleagues who suggest that 24,25-dihydroxyvitamin D_3 plays a role in the regulation of PTH levels [142], and when given in conjunction with 1,25-dihydroxyvitamin D_3 suppressed osteoclastic parameters without causing hypercalcaemia.

5.6. The role of calcitriol therapy in CAPD

In CAPD patients with serum PTH levels of greater than 400 pg/ml there is increasing evidence that the best way to administer oral vitamin D_3 is in once or twice weekly pulses to reduce the incidence of hypercalcaemia [54, 143], a technique now being adopted in many centres. The idea of pulse therapy was initially investigated in haemodialysis patients, where thrice weekly intravenous pulses of 1,25-$(OH)_2D_3$ were administered at the end of a haemodialysis session [41]. This regime resulted in marked suppression of iPTH levels with a mean decrement of around 70%, although Slatopolsky surmised that this was largely as a result of the rise in serum ionized calcium that occurred during the study. Furthermore, this study also demonstrated that when equal doses of intravenous or oral calcitriol were given, the serum concentration of calcitriol was six to eight times higher with the IV preparation, resulting in a greater delivery to non-intestinal target tissues and allowing greater expression of its biological effect on the parathyroid glands. However, even this degree of suppression was insufficient to restore iPTH to satisfactory levels, because of the large non-suppressible basal secretion rate of hypertrophied glands. Interestingly, it has also been shown that administering calcitriol at night reduces both the incidence and severity of hypercalcaemia in haemodialysis patients [144]!

Korkor demonstrated that the parathyroid glands from patients with chronic renal failure contained only one third as many calcitriol receptors as are found in parathyroid adenomas [145], and in animal studies it is known that uraemia results in a two- to fourfold decrease in receptor numbers as compared to normal values [146, 147]. Thus it is likely that reduced receptor numbers in the parathyroid glands of uraemic patients render them less responsive to the inhibitory effects of calcitriol, so that suppression requires high peak serum levels.

Since the initial work of Slatopolsky several other workers have confirmed that both pulse intravenous 1,25-dihydroxyvitamin D_3 and alpha-calcidol are effective in reducing serum PTH levels in haemodialysis patients [48, 50, 53, 148–50], although all found difficulty in distinguishing direct effects on parathyroid secretion from indirect effects mediated by raising serum calcium. It is however, clear that 1,25-dihydroxyvitamin D_3 does have a direct suppressive effect on parathyroid cells by influencing transcription of the parathyroid gene [40, 151]. Delmez et al. demonstrated that calcitriol could also be given intraperitoneally in CAPD patients where again it produced a rise in serum ionised calcium levels and a significant fall in serum PTH [80].

5.6.1. Oral pulse calcitriol therapy

The discovery that intermittent dosage of 1,25-dihydroxyvitamin D_3 was very effective in suppressing PTH levels led to a Japanese group trying oral pulse therapy in haemodialysis patients. 19 patients received 4.0 μg of oral calcitriol twice weekly after dialysis which resulted in a fall of more than 45% in PTH levels after six months of treatment, despite a small fall in serum ionised calcium [51]. Similar results were then reported by Martin et al. in CAPD patients, using an initial twice weekly oral dose of 5 μg of calcitriol [54]. Once again the decrease in PTH levels was not associated with any rise in serum calcium, and this mode of administration would appear to be the most appropriate to CAPD patients.

5.6.2. Calcitriol analogues

The discovery of a non-calcaemic calcitriol analogue, 22-oxa-calcitriol, may alter therapeutic strategies once again in the near future, although no studies of its use in humans have yet been reported. In rats with normal renal function 22-oxa-calcitriol has been shown to have very little calcaemic activity [152], yet it suppresses PTH mRNA levels equally as effectively as 1,25-$(OH)_2D_3$ [153]. A similar effect is reported in 7/8 nephrectomized rats [40], and in dogs with over 12 months of renal failure administration of a single intravenous dose of 5 μg of 22-oxa-calcitriol decreased PTH by 80% over 24 hours without any change in serum calcium or phosphate levels [153]. However, Drueke and co-workers found similar degrees of hypercalcaemia in rats with chronic renal failure treated with either 1,25-$(OH)_2D_3$ or 22-oxa-calcitriol [154], so clearly further studies are required. Other analogues, such as 2β-3-hydroxypropoxy calcitriol, CB 966 and KH 1060 are under investigation as immunosuppressive agents, as well as for their effects on divalent ion metabolism.

5.7. Renal osteodystrophy in diabetic patients

A number of reports over the last 12 years have suggested that insulin dependent diabetes mellitus is associated with lower serum levels of PTH [84, 155, 156], and decreased responsiveness to acute hypocalcaemia [157]. Therefore it has been suggested that diabetic patients may be more prone to low turnover bone disease, and relatively protected from severe hyperparathyroidism. However, until recently it has been difficult to separate the effects of diabetes from those of aluminium accumulation, but Pei et al. [84] have now shown that diabetes mellitus is an important risk factor for both aluminium related bone disease and, the non-aluminium related, idiopathic adynamic bone lesion. These authors also noted that diabetes appears to enhance the risk of developing aluminium bone disease, possibly by increasing gastrointestinal absorption and bone surface accumulation of aluminium. This finding adds further impetus to the drive to eliminate use of aluminium-based phosphate binders wherever possible.

5.8. The idiopathic adynamic bone lesion in CAPD (Fig. 3)

The spectrum of bone disease has changed over the last 10 years with the emergence of the adynamic bone lesion, now present in over 20% of dialysis patients [9, 10, 21, 23], and the welcome decline in the usage of aluminium containing phosphate binders. The association of adynamic bone with low PTH levels has resulted in a reassessment of attempts to suppress serum PTH to "normal" levels in both pre-dialysis and dialysis patients [21, 158] and acknowledgement that blanket prescription of continuous low dose oral calcitriol therapy for all dialysis patients is unwise [159].

This lesion occurs more commonly in patients aged over 50 years at start of dialysis (Table 3), in those with a longer duration of pre-dialysis renal failure [23], and in diabetic patients [84]. In a longitudinal histological study of bone disease in CAPD [115], five of eight patients who completed a full two years of follow-up were found to have developed the adynamic lesion (Fig. 5). None of the patients reported symptoms attributable to the

Table 3. Associations of the idiopathic adynamic bone lesion.

Clinical
Age > 50 years
Diabetes mellitus
Commoner in CAPD than haemodialysis patients

Biochemical
Low/normal parathyroid hormone
High/normal ionised calcium
Low/normal bone alkaline phosphatase and other markers of bone turnover

Radiological
Increased incidence of vascular calcification

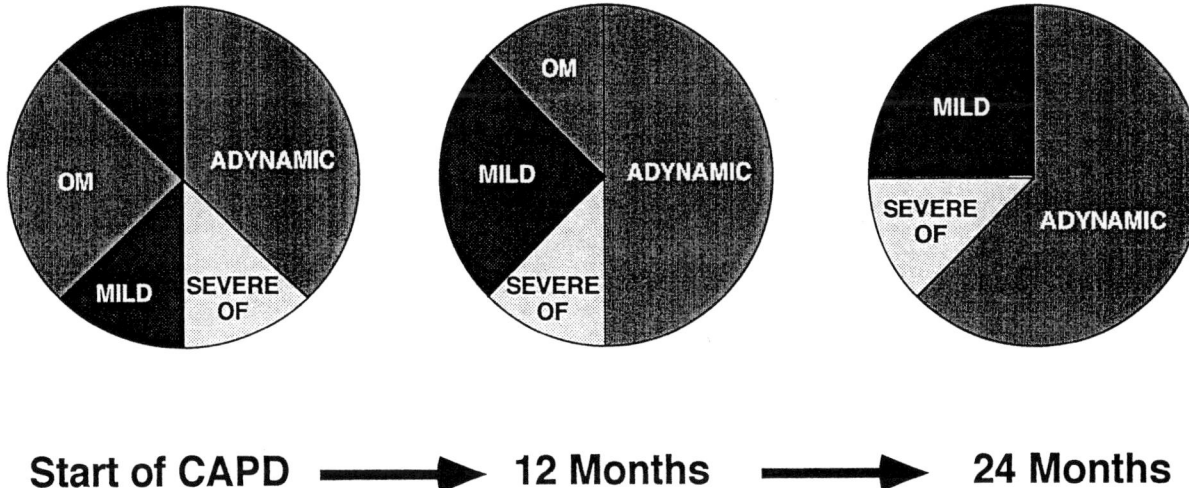

Figure 5. Changes in bone histology in eight patients over 24 months of continuous ambulatory peritoneal dialysis.

lesion, and it has no characteristic radiological findings. Bone mineral density did not to decline over the two years, but even longer follow-up may be required for signs and symptoms to appear. It is associated with normal, or suppressed levels of parathyroid hormone [9, 10, 44, 75], and high or high/normal levels of ionized calcium. Sherrard et al. noted that the adynamic bone lesion was the commonest histological diagnosis in their study of 267 dialysis patients [10], and that it occurred more frequently in PD (61%) than in haemodialysis patients (36%). They suggest that this may be due to the more sustained and higher calcium levels associated with PD which may result in more effective suppression of PTH than the intermittent calcium load of haemodialysis.

In a 10 year retrospective study of 1,803 patients on chronic maintenance dialysis Malluche and Faugere report a gradual increase in the incidence of the adynamic bone lesion, so that in 1991 it affected 20% of patients. The primary factors associated with the occurrence of this lesion were found to be aluminium accumulation, increased age, diabetes mellitus, and possibly CAPD. In addition these authors noted a tendency towards hypercalcaemia, and accumulation of microfractures which they suggest might ultimately lead to clinical bone fracture.

In our own patients we have found an association between adynamic bone and the presence of significant vascular calcification, which may be related to the higher serum calcium levels found in patients with this lesion. This is a worrying association since many of these patients will be hoping for renal transplantation which may become impossible when vascular calcification is severe. Furthermore it seems likely that adynamic bone would be significantly more prone to the osteoporotic effects of high dose steroid immunosuppression, as well as avascular necrosis of the femoral head. Under normal circumstances the skeleton provides a large buffering capacity for both serum calcium and phosphate. If the bone is adynamic, its buffering ability may be significantly reduced, and serum levels are therefore much more easily influenced by dietary intake or absorption from the dialysis fluid. Under these conditions there is a greater likelihood of the calcium × phosphate product being exceeded, and the process of metastatic calcification beginning. If this is the case then it would be very important to allow PTH levels to rise slightly and stimulate bone turnover, whilst maintaining strict control of serum phosphate. In this way one would also hope to induce resorption of vascular calcium deposits.

It is evident that the use of calcitriol, a powerful modulator of calcium and PTH, should be tailored to the individual patient's clinical situation, not merely prescribed in an unthinking fashion as a "vitamin supplement". Tailoring of any therapy requires the clinician to gather certain data in order to determine appropriate management. In this case one needs to examine the patient's serum calcium, phosphate and parathyroid hormone levels, in conjunction with bone histology data in certain cases. On the basis of these findings one can plan individual treatment along the lines of the clinical algorithm shown in Fig. 6.

6. Recommedndations for management of osteodystrophy in CAPD

Techniques for monitoring renal osteodystrophy in CAPD patients are still evolving. In the past different units have approached the problem in widely differing ways, with some only monitoring serum calcium, phosphate and alkaline phosphatase plus annual skeletal surveys, and others performing much more detailed (and expensive) investigations, sometimes including bone biopsy. If we consider the available techniques under three broad headings – biochemical, radiological and histological – certain recommendations can be made, given the present state of understanding (Table 4).

Table 4. Recommendations for the management of renal osteodystrophy in adult CAPD patients (see also Fig. 6).

1) Restrict dietary phosphate, as far as possible within the confines of a 1.2 g/kg/day protein diet.
2) Use 1.25 mmol/L (2.5 mEq/L) calcium dialysis fluid to minimize hypercalcaemia. Individual patients may require higher or lower concentrations depending on serum ionized calcium (or total corrected calcium) and phosphate levels.
3) Calcium carbonate/acetate given twice daily with main meals. Dose titrated to serum calcium and phosphate levels. Educate patients to distribute dose according to phosphate intake.
4) Measure serum parathyroid hormone every three months (see Fig. 6) and use pulse oral vitamin D3 therapy if necessary. Replace 25-hydroxyvitamin D3 if serum levels are low.
5) Measure serum magnesium and aluminium every six months, unless patients is taking oral aluminium (then measure every three months).

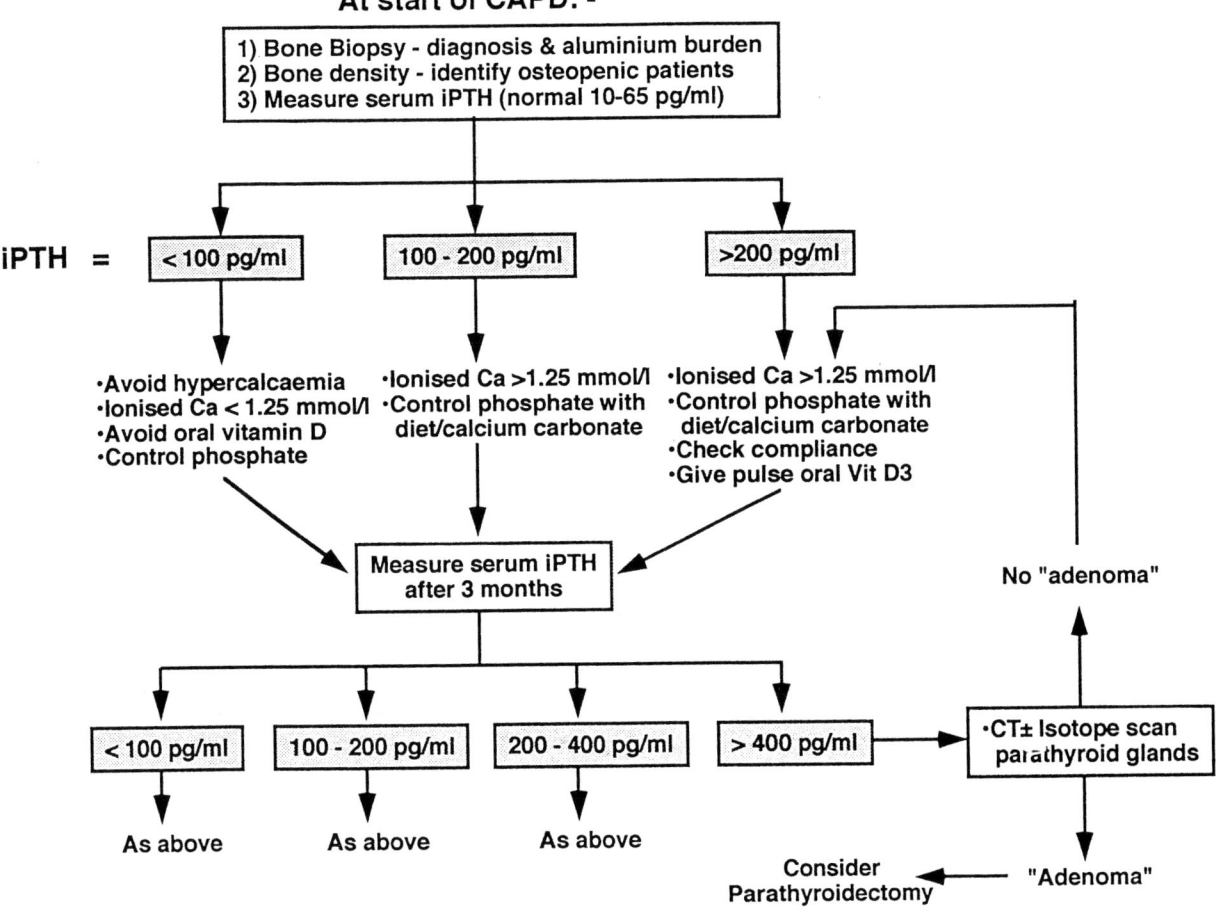

Figure 6. Clinical algorithm for the monitoring and management of renal osteodystrophy in CAPD patients.

6.1. Biochemical monitoring

In dialysis patients, changes in serum calcium and phosphate do not reflect disease processes within the skeleton as they may do in patients with normal renal function. They are primarily influenced by the patient's diet and oral intake of phosphate binders plus the amount of dialysis they are receiving. A rise in serum alkaline phosphatase is more indicative of increased bone turnover, but is only seen in advanced hyperparathyroidism. A rising level is generally associated with histologically severe osteitis fibrosa. The bone isoenzyme of alkaline phosphatase is a more sensitive indicator and low levels are associated with a greater likelihood of adynamic bone histology [23]. However, regular estimation of intact molecule PTH remains the most useful biochemical investigation. More recently measurement of serum osteocalcin has become possible, providing a marker of osteoblast activity, but the very short half-life of the molecule means that unless the serum is spun and frozen within 20 minutes any subsequent assay is likely to be invalid. For this reason it seems unlikely to be helpful in clinical practise, and in any case reports show a close correlation with intact PTH levels in dialysis patients [160]. Another marker of hyperparathyroid bone disease, tartrate resistant acid phosphatase (TRAP) has recently been reported to be sensitive indicator of high- and low-turnover bone states [161, 162]. This enzyme is produced by actively resorbing osteoclasts, and can be measured in serum by immunoassay or colorimetrically. Experience with this marker is limited at present.

The most widely available, and generally useful marker at present, is intact PTH, which should be measured every three or four months in all CAPD patients. Regular measurement of total alkaline phosphatase is unnecessary, although it will continue to be performed as part of the "liver screen"

6.2. Radiological monitoring

Routine, full skeletal surveys are unnecessary, and could be replaced by regular monitoring of serum PTH with plain X-rays of the hands plus a single lateral view of the lumbar spine [115, 163, 164]. This would greatly reduce the dose of radiation received by CAPD patients without detriment to patient care. In addition significant financial savings could be made. Some measurement of skeletal bone density should be made at the time of starting dialysis in all patients so that those with subnormal bone density can be identified and special efforts made to improve the situation. Whether this measurement is best performed by QCT, SPA, DPA or DEXA scan would depend on local facilities and expertise.

Skeletal scintigraphy may be performed using technetium labelled 99m-methylene diphosphonate, but correlation of scan results with bone histology is poor, although increased uptake has been demonstrated in severe hyperparathyroid bone disease [165–167].

Single photon absorptiometry (SPA): This is the most widely used method of quantifying bone mineral density in renal osteodystrophy. A highly collimated beam of photons is used with ^{125}I as a source. However, the single energy beam requires a constant thickness of soft tissue around the bone to produce reliable results, and it cannot distinguish between trabecular and cortical bone. Studies have found that mineral content tends to be lower than normal in patients with renal failure [75, 168–170], but it does not allow differentiation between different types of osteodystrophy.

Dual photon absorptiometry (DPA): DPA utilises an isotope with two energies (^{153}Gd), thereby overcoming the requirement of SPA for a constant thickness of soft tissue around the bone. It can therefore be used to measure bone mineral density in any skeletal site, but normal scan results have been seen in haemodialysis patients with histologically proven osteodystrophy [164].

Quantitative computed tomography (QCT): The principle of this technique is the same as for standard CT scanning, and a calibration phantom placed under the patient is used to relate bone mineral density to Hounsfield units. True bone density is measured in g/cm^3 and it is less affected by artefacts such as soft tissue calcification. However, it delivers a relatively high radiation dose.

In our own experience, bone density measurements are if anything, less helpful than plain radiographs, since there is no correlation with histological diagnosis. Although end stage renal failure patients were found to have reduced bone density, compared to age and sex matched normal values, the majority of patients had both QCT and SPA results within 2SD of normal. Piraino *et al.* used QCT to measure bone mineral density in a group of 31 patients who had been on dialysis (19 peritoneal dialysis, 10 haemodialysis) for a mean of 5.3 years [171]. It is now known that the type of dialysis influences bone histology [11] and therefore it may be misleading to consider peritoneal dialysis and haemodialysis patients together. However, as in our study, Piraino *et al.* found that serum PTH was a better indicator of the type of bone disease present than was QCT-determined bone density, and concluded that the usefulness of this technique in patients with renal failure is limited.

Dual-energy X-ray absorptiometry (DEXA): Less experience is available with the more recently developed DEXA scan. It has several theoretical advantages over the other techniques, including low radiation dose, greater precision and rapidity of scanning. Despite this, measurements can be distorted by several artefacts such as osteophytes, calcification of the aorta or other soft tissues, and previous vertebral collapse. In 25 dialysis patients, no correlation was found between QCT and DEXA measurements of vertebral bone mineral density [172].

Whilst single bone density measurements may be unhelpful, sequential studies might be more so, having initially established the hsitological diagnosis by biopsy. Decreasing bone density in a patient known to previously have osteitis fibrosa would suggest deterioration, especially if associated with a high iPTH.

6.3. Transiliac bone biopsy

Bone biopsy with tetracycline labelling is undoubtedly the only reliable method of diagnosing the type and severity of renal osteodystrophy. It is rarely performed in clinical practise because of patients' and doctors' perceptions of its painfulness and invasiveness. In our experience, it is no more painful than Jamshidi marrow biopsies which are routinely performed in many clinical situations if the blood film suggests it is necessary.

Local expertise permitting, CAPD patients ought to undergo a tetracycline labeled bone biopsy at the time of starting dialysis, to establish the exact histology of their bone plus the degree of aluminium accumulation. In many cases this could be performed under general anaesthetic by the surgeon as the Tenckhoff catheter is inserted. Thereafter, one can probably surmise what is happening to the histology on the basis of regular PTH measurements once the initial histology is known.

These recommendations can be formed into a clinical algorithm (Fig. 6). The implementation of this scheme depends firstly on maximal restriction of dietary phosphate, within the limitations of a diet providing 1.2 g protein/kg body weight per day, and secondly on the routine use of CAPD fluid with a calcium concentration of 1.25 mmol/L, magnesium of 0.25 mmol/L and lactate of 40 mmol/L. Calcium carbonate should be given in doses adequate to maintain serum phosphate below 1.8 mmol/L and aluminium containing binders should be avoided. Serum ionised calcium and iPTH should be measured every three months to provide a guide for treatment with oral calcitriol. If iPTH is less than 200pg/ml, vitamin D_3 is not required. If iPTH exceeds 200 pg/ml then attention should be paid to maintenance of a high/normal ionised calcium level and tighter dietary control of phosphate where possible. Calcitriol should be given as intermittent pulse doses [54], and iPTH remeasured after three months. If the level remains significantly elevated, or is rising, then appropriate scans should be ordered to search for a parathyroid adenoma with a view to possible parathyroidectomy (provided the patient does not have significant aluminium deposition).

Serum magnesium levels should be measured once every six months, especially in those patients whose dietary intake may be low, to check for hypomagnesaemia. Plasma aluminium levels should also be monitored every six months, even in patients not taking aluminium containing phosphate binders since there are other sources of this metal such as drugs and drinking water. It must be remembered that aluminium uptake can be significantly enhanced by citrate ingestion and oral vitamin D_3.

Utilisation of these guide-lines should enable good control of divalent ion metabolism, and prevention or amelioration of osteodystrophy in the majority of CAPD patients. Further advances will hinge on a greater understanding of the vitamin D/parathyroid axis in renal failure along with the development of safe, non-calcaemic analogues of vitamin D_3 plus more efficient phosphate binders, possibly based on substances other than aluminium or calcium.

7. Summary

Disorders of calcium, magnesium, phosphate, vitamin D_3, and parathyroid hormone can combine to produce a variety of skeletal and extraskeletal pathologies in CAPD patients. The recognition of the long-term toxicity of aluminium containing phosphate binders, and their withdrawal, is a significant step in the drive towards combating renal osteodystrophy. However, the replacement of aluminium by calcium containing phosphate binders has been primarily hampered by the occurrence of hypercalcaemia in many patients. This problem is further compounded by the increased gastrointestinal absorption brought about by oral vitamin D_3, and the probably unnecessary peritoneal absorption of calcium from PD fluid. An increasing range of dialysis solutions is becoming available, so that in the future, it will be possible to tailor peritoneal dialysis treatment to the needs of the individual patient.

The judicious use of a variety of biochemical and radiological investigations, plus bone histomorphometry where appropriate, can provide a rational basis for the monitoring and management of divalent ion metabolism and renal osteodystrophy in CAPD patients.

References

1. Lucas R. On a form of late rickets associated with albuminuria, rickets of adolescence. Lancet 1883; 1: 993–4.
2. Fletcher H. Case of infantilism with polyuria and chronic renal disease. Proceedings Royal Society Medicine, London 1911; pp 95–7.
3. Barber H. The bone deformities of renal dwarfism. Lancet 1920; 1: 18–20.
4. Follis R, Jackson D. Renal osteomalacia and osteitis fibrosa. Bulletin Johns Hopkins Hospital 1943; 72: 232–4.
5. Liu S, Chu H. Studies of calcium and phoshorus metabolism with special reference to pathogenesis and effects of dihydrotachysterol (A.T. 10) and iron. Medicine 1943; 22: 103–7.
6. Garner A, Ball J. Quantitative observations on mineralised and unmineralised bone in chronic renal azotaemia and intestinal malabsorption syndrome. Journal of Pathology and Bacteriology 1966; 91: 545–9.
7. Stanbury S, Lumb G. Metabolic studies of renal osteodystrophy. Medicine 1962; 41: 1–28.
8. Stanbury S, Lumb G. Parathyroid function in chronic renal failure: A statistical survey of the plasma biochemistry in azotaemic renal osteodystrophy. Quarterly Journal of Medicine 1966; 35: 1–12.

9. Malluche H, Monier-Faugere M. Risk of adynamic bone disease in dialyzed patients. Kidney International 1992; 42 (suppl 38): S62–7.
10. Sherrard D, Hercz G, Pei Y, Maloney N, Greenwood C, Manuel A, Saiphoo C, Fenton S, Segre G. The spectrum of bone disease in end-stage renal failure – An evolving disorder. Kidney International 1993; 43: 436–42.
11. Coburn J. Mineral metabolism and renal bone disease: Effects of CAPD versus hemodialysis. Kidney International 1993; 43 (suppl 40): S92–100.
12. Llach F, Massry S, Singer F, Yurokawa K, Kaye J, Coburn J. Skeletal resistance to endogenous parathyroid hormone in patients with early renal failure. A possible cause of secondary hyperparathyroidism. J Clin Endocrinol Metab 1975; 41: 339–45.
13. Avioli L. The renal osteodystrophies. In: Brenner B, FC R (ed), The Kidney. Saunders, WB, Philadelphia 1986; 1: 1542–80.
14. Malluche H, Ritz E, Kutschera J, Krause K, Werner E, Gati A, Seiffert U, Lange H. Calcium metabolism and impaired mineralization in various stages or renal insufficiency. In: Normal A, Scaeffer K, Grigoleit H, Herrath D, Ritz E (ed), Vitamin D and Problems Related to Uremic Bone Disease. Walter de Gruyter & Co, Berlin-New York 1975; pp 513–22.
15. Malluche H, Faugere M. Renal bone disease 1990: An unmet challenge for the nephrologist. Kidney International 1990; 38: 193–211.
16. Baker L, Abrams S, Roe C, Faugere M, Fanti P, Subayti Y, Malluche H. 1,25-dihydroxyvitamin D_3 administration in moderate renal failure: A prospective double-blind trial. Kidney International 1989; 35: 661–9.
17. Ward M, Feest T, Ellis H et al. Osteomalacic dialysis osteodystrophy: evidence for a waterbourne aetiological agent, probably aluminium. Lancet 1978; 1: 841–5.
18. Cournot-Witmer G, Plachot J, Borudeau A, Lieberherr M, Jorgetti V, Mendes V, Halpern S, Hemmerle J, Drueke T, Balsan S. Effect of aluminum on bone and cell localization. Kidney International 1986; 29 (suppl 18): S37–40.
19. Ott S, Maloney N, Coburn J, Alfrey A, Sherrard D. The prevalence of bone aluminum depostion in renal ostedystrophy and its relation to the response to calcitriol therapy. N Engl J Med 1982; 307: 709–14.
20. Posner A, Blumenthal N Boskey A. Model of aluminum-induced osteomalacia: Inhibition of apatite formation and growth. Kidney International 1986; 29 (suppl.18): S17–9.
21. Fournier A, Moriniere P, Cohen Solal M, Boudailliez B, Achard J, Marie A, Sebert J. Adynamic bone disease in uremia: May it be idiopathic? Is it an actual disease? Nephron 1991; 58: 1–12.
22. Cuevas X, Aubia J, Bosch J, Serrano S, Marinoso L, Ramirez-Orellano M, Rio M. Histomorphometric bone patterns of diabetic-uremic patients on dialysis are established in pre-dialysis stage already (abstract). Nephrology Dialysis Transplantation 1992; 7: 756.
23. Hutchison A, Whitehouse R, Boulton H, Adams J, Freemont A, Mawer E, Gokal R. Histological, radiological and biochemical features of the adynamic bone lesion in CAPD patients. Am J Nephrol 1994; 227: In press.
24. Coburn J. Renal Osteodystrophy. Kidney International 1980; 17: 677–93.
25. Fassbinder W, Brunner F, Brynger H, Ehrich J, Geerlings W, Raine A, Rizzoni G, Selwood N, Tufveson G, Wing A. Combined report on regular dialysis and transplantation in Europe, XX, 1989. Nephrology Dialysis Transplantation 1991; 6 (suppl 1): 5–35.
26. Dunstan C, Evans R, Hills E, Wong S, Alfrey A. Effect of aluminum and parathyroid hormone on osteoblasts and bone mineralization in chronic renal failure. Calcified Tissue International 1984; 36: 133–8.
27. Charhon S, Chavassieux P, Chapuy M, Boivin G, Meunier P. Low rate of bone formation with or without histologic appearance of osteomalacia in patients with aluminum intoxication. Journal of Laboratory and Clinical Medicine 1985; 106: 123–31.
28. Hercz G, Pei Y, Manuel A, Saiphoo C, Goodman W, Segre G, Sherrard D. Aplastic osteodystrophy without aluminum staining in dialysis patients (abstract). Kidney International 1990; 37: 449.
29. Keutmann H, Sauer M, Hendry G et al. Complete amino-acid sequence of human parathyroid hormone. Biochemistry 1978; 17: 5723–9.
30. Chu L, MacGregor R, Hamilton J et al. Conversion of proparathyroid hormone to parathyroid hormone: The use of amines as specific inhibitors. Endocrinology 1974; 95: 1431–8.
31. Arnaud C. Hyperparathyroidism and renal failure. Kidney International 1973; 4: 89–92.
32. Slatopolsky E, Martin K, Morrissey J, Hruska K. Parathyroid Hormone: Alterations in chronic renal failure. In: Robinson R (ed), Nephrology. Springer-Verlag, New York 1985; 1: 1292–304.
33. Sherwood L, Mayer G, Ramberg C et al. Regulation of parathyroid hormone secretion: Proportional control by calcium, lack of effect of phosphate. Endocrinology 1968; 83: 1043–51.
34. Slatopolsky E, Lopez-Hilker S, Dusso A et al. The interrelationship between Vitamin D and parathyroid hormone secretion in health and disease. In: Davison A (ed), Nephrology. Balliere Tindall, London 1988; 2: 1067–75.
35. Felsenfeld A, Ross D, Rodriguez M. Hysteresis of the parathyroid hormone response to hypocalcemia in haemodialysis patients with low turnover aluminum bone disease. Journal of the American Society of Nephrology 1991; 6: 1136–43.
36. Dunlay R, Rodriguez M, Felsenfeld A, Llach F. Direct inhibitory effect of calcitriol on parathyroid function (sigmoidal curve) in dialysis patients. Kidney International 1989; 36: 1093–8.
37. Cunningham J, Altmann P, Gleed J, Butter K,

Marsh F, O'Riordan J. Effect of direction and rate of change of calcium on parathyroid hormone secretion in uraemia. Nephrology Dialysis Transplantation 1989; 4: 339–44.
38. Brown E, Gardener D, Windeck R et al. Relationship of intracellular 3′,5′-adenosine monophosphate accumulation to parathyroid hormone release from dispersed bovine parathyroid cells. Endocrinology 1978; 103: 2323–33.
39. Kitaoka M, Fukagawa M, Tanaka Y, Ogata E, Kurokawa K. Parathyroid gland size is critical for long-term prognosis of calcitriol pulse therapy in chronic dialysis patients (abstract). Journal of the American Society of Nephrology 1991; 2: 637.
40. Fukagawa M, Kaname S, Igarashi T, Ogata E, Kurokawa K. Regulation of parathyroid hormone synthesis in chronic renal failure in rats. Kidney International 1991; 39: 874–81.
41. Slatopolsky E, Weerts C, Thielan J et al. Marked suppression of secondary hyperparathyroidism by intravenous administration of 1,25-dihydroxycholecalciferol in uremic patients. Journal of Clinical Investigation 1984; 74: 2136–43.
42. Salusky I, Goodman W, Norris K, Horst N, Fine R, Coburn J. Bioavailability of calcitriol after oral, intravenous, and intraperitoneal doses in dialysis paients. In: Norman A, Schaefer K, Griroleit H, Herrath D (eds), Vitamin D. Molecular, Cellular and Clinical Endocrinology. Walter de Gruyter & Co, Berlin 1988: 783–4.
43. Chase L, Slatopolsky E. Secretion and metabolic efficiency of parathyroid hormone in patients with severe hypomagnesemia. Journal of Endocrinology and Metabolism 1974; 38: 363–71.
44. Cohen Solal M, Sebert J, Boudailiez B, Marie A, Moriniere P, Gueris J, Bouillon R, Fournier A. Comparison of Intact, Midregion, and Carboxy Terminal Assays of Parathyroid Hormone for the Diagnosis of Bone Disease in Hemodialyzed Patients. Journal of Clinical Endocrinology and Metabolism 1991; 73(3): 516–24.
45. Mawer E, Taylor C, Backhouse J, Lumb G, Stanbury S. Failure of Formation of 1,25-dihydroxycholecalciferol in Chronic Renal Insufficiency. The Lancet 1973; 1: 626–8.
46. Rapoport J, Shany S, Chaimovitz C. Continuous Ambulatory Peritoneal Dialysis and Vitamin D. Nephron 1988; 48: 1–3.
47. Hayes M, O'Donoghue D, Ballardie F, Mawer E. Peritonitis induces the synthesis of 1-α-25, dihydroxyvitamin D_3 in macrophages from CAPD patients. FEBS 1987; 220: 307–10.
48. Lind L, Wengle B, Wide L, Wrege U, Ljunghall S. Suppression of serum parathyroid hormone levels by intravenous alphacalcidol in uremic patients on maintenance hemodialysis. Nephron 1988; 48: 296–9.
49. Andress D, Norris K, Coburn J, Saltopolsky E, Sherrard D. Intravenous cacitriol in the treatment of refractory osteitis fibrosa of chronic renal failure. New Engl J Med 1989; 321: 274–9.
50. Ljunghall S, Althoff P, Fellstrom B, Marjanovic B, Nisell J, Weiss L, Wide L. Effects on serum parathyroid hormone of intravenous treatment with alphacalcidol in patients on chronic hemodialysis. Nephron 1990; 55: 380–5.
51. Tsukamoto Y, Nomura M, Takahashi Y, Takagi Y, Yoshida A, Nagaoka T, Togashi K, Kikawada R, Marumo F. The "oral 1,25-dihydroxyvitamin D_3 pulse therapy" in hemodialysis patients with severe secondary hyperparathyroidism. Nephron 1991; 57: 23–8.
52. Gallieni M, Brancaccio D, Padovese P, Rolla D, Bedani P, Colantonio G, Bronzieri C, Bagni B, Tarolo G. Low-dose intravenous calcitriol treatment of secondary hyperparathyroidism in hemodialysis patients. Kidney International 1992; 42: 1191–8.
53. Moriniere P, Maurouard C, Boudailiez B, Westeel P, Achard J, Boitte F, EI Esper N, Compgnon M, Maurel G, Bouillon R, Pamphile R, Fournier A. Prevention of hyperparathyroidism in patients on maintenance dialysis by intravenous 1-alpha-hydroxyvitamin D_3 in association with $Mg(OG)_2$ as sole phosphate binder. Nephron 1992; 60: 154–63.
54. Martin K, Ballal H, Domoto D, Blalock S, Weindel M. Pulse oral calcitriol for the treatment of hyperparathyroidism in patients on continuous ambulatory peritoneal dialysis: Preliminary observations. American Journal of Kidney Diseases 1992; 19: 540–5.
55. Holick M. Vitamin D and the Kidney. Kidney International 1987; 32: 912–29.
56. Mak R, Wong J. The vitamin D.parathyroid hormone axis in the pathogenesis of hypertension and insulin resistance in uremia. Mineral and Electrolyte Metabolism 1992; 18: 156–9.
57. Bricker N. On the pathogenesis of the uremic state. An exposition of the "trade-off" hypothesis. N Engl J Med 1972; 286: 1093–9.
58. Faugere M-C, Friedler R, Fanti P, Malluche H. Lack of histologic signs of Vit D deficiency in early development of renal osteodystrophy. J Bone Miner Res 1988; 3 (supp 1): S95.
59. Lopez-Hilker S, Galceran T, Chan U-L, Rapp N, Martin K, Slatopolsky E. Hypocalcaemia may not be essential for the development of secondary hyperparathyroidism in chronic renal failure. J Clin Invest 1986; 78: 1097–102.
60. Ritz E, Matthias S, Seidel A, Reichel H, Szabo A, Horl W. Disturbed calcium metabolism in renal failure – Pathogenesis and therapeutic strategies. Kidney International 1992; 42 (suppl 38): S37–42.
61. Massry S, Tuma S, Dua S, Goldstein D. Reversal of skeletal resistance to parathyroid hormone in uremia by vitamin D metabolites. J Lab Clin Med 1979; 94: 152–7.
62. Brookfield R. The magnesium content of serum in renal insufficiency. Quarterly Journal of Medicine 1937; 6: 87–90.
63. Randall R, Cohen M, Spray C, Rossmeisl E. Hypermagnesaemia in renal failure. Annals of Internal Medicine 1964; 61: 73–88.
64. Moriniere P, Vinatier I, Westeel P, Cohen Solal M, Belbrik S, Abdulmassih Z, Hocine C, Marie A, Leflon P, Roche D, Fournier A. Magnesium

hydroxide as a complementary aluminium-free phosphate binder to moderate doses of oral calcium carbonate in uraemic patients on chronic haemodialysis: Lack of deleterious effect on bone mineralization. Nephrology Dialysis Transplantation 1988; 3: 651–6.
65. Alfrey A, Solomons C. Bone pyrophosphate in uremia and its association with extraosseous calcification. Journal of Clinical Investigation 1976; 57: 700–5.
66. MacIntyre I, Davidsson D. The production of secondary potassium depletion, sodium retention, nephrocalcinosis and hypercalcaemia by magnesium deficiency. Biochem J 1958; 70: 456–62.
67. Kaehny W, Hegg A, Alfrey A. Gastrointestinal absorption of aluminium from aluminium-containing antacids. New England Journal of Medicine 1977; 296: 1389–90.
68. de Broe M, D'Hasse P, Elseviers M, Clement J, Visser W, van de Vyver F. Aluminium and end-stage renal failure. In: Davidson A (ed), Nephrology: Proceedings of the Xth ICN. Balliere Tindall, Cambridge 1988; 2: 1086–116.
69. Litzow J, Lemann J, Lennon E. The effect of treatment of acidosis on calcium balance in patients with chronic azotemci renal disease. Journal of Clinical Investigation 1967; 46: 280–4.
70. Kuster S, Ritz E, Horl W. A role for metabolic acidosis in the genesis of renal secondary hyperparathyroidism (abstract). In: Eliahou H, Iaina A, Bar-Khayim Y (eds), Abstract Book, XIIth International Congress of Nephrology. Jerusalem, Israel 1993; p 467.
71. Lee J, Parthemore J, Deftos L. Immunochemical heterogeneity of calcitonin in renal failure. Journal of Clinical Endocrinology and Metabolism 1977; 45: 528–33.
72. Marcus R. Endocrine control of bone and mineral metabolism. In: Manolagas S, Olefsky M (eds), Metabolic Bone and Mineral Disorders. Churchill Livingstone, New York 1988; pp 21–2. (Olefsky J (ed), Contemporary Issues in Endocrinology & Metabolism; Vol 5).
73. Gokal R, Ramos J, Ellis H, Parkinson I, Sweetman V, Dewar J, Ward M, Kerr D. Histological renal osteodystrophy, and 25-hydroxycholecalciferol and aluminium levels in patients on CAPD. Kidney International 1983; 23: 15–21.
74. Calderaro V, Oreopoulos D, Meema H, Ogilvie R, Husdan H, Khanna R, Quinton C, Murray T, Carmichael D. The evolution of renal osteodystrophy in patients undergoing continuous ambulatory peritoneal dialysis. Proceedings of the EDTA 1980; pp 533–42.
75. Hutchison A, Whitehouse R, Boulton H, Adams J, Mawer E, Freemont A, Gokal R. Correlation of Bone Histology with Parathyroid Hormone, Vitamin D, and Radiology in End-Stage Renal Disease. Kidney International 1994; 44: 1071–7.
76. Owen J, Parnell A, Keir M, Ellis H, Wilkinson R, Ward M, Elliott R. Critical analysis of the use of skeletal surveys in patients with chronic renal failure. Clinical Radiology 1988; 39: 578–82.
77. Adams J, Chen S, Adams P, Isherwood I. Measurement of Trabecular Bone Mineral by Dual Energy Computed Tomography. Journal of Computer Assisted Tomography 1982; 6: 601–7.
78. Genant H, Block J, Steiger P, Glueer C, Ettinger B, Harris S. Appropriate Use of Bone Densitometry. Radiology 1989; 170: 817–22.
79. Rahman R, Heaton A, Goodship T, Rodger R, Tapson J, Sellars L, Ellis H, Wilkinson R, Ward M. Renal osteodystrophy in patients on CAPD: A five year study. Perit Dial Bull 1987; 7: 1–4.
80. Delmez J, Dougan C, Gearing B, Rothstein M, Windus D, Rapp N, Slatopolsky E. The effects of intrapertioneal calcitriol on calcium and parathyroid hormone. Kidney International 1987; 31: 795–9.
81. Digenis G, Khanna R, Pierratos A, Meema H, Rabinovich S, Petit J, Oreopoulos D. Renal osteodystrophy in patients managed on CAPD for more than three years. Peritoneal Dialysis Bulletin 1983; 3: 81–6.
82. Kurtz S. Clinical parameters of renal bone disease: A comparison of CAPD and haemodialysis. Dialysis and Transplantation 1985; 14: 30–6.
83. Bucciante G, Biachi M, Valenti G. Progress of renal osteodystrophy during CAPD. Clinical Nephrology 1984; 6: 279–83.
84. Pei Y, Hercz G, Greenwood C, Segre G, Manuel A, Saiphoo C, Fenton S, Sherrard D. Renal osteodystrophy in diabetic patients. Kidney International 1993; 44: 159–64.
85. Gokal R, Fryer R, McHugh M et al. Calcium and phosphate control in CAPD patients. In: Legrain M (ed). Excerpta Medica, Amsterdam 1980; pp 283–91.
86. Recker R, Saville P. Calcium absorption in renal failure: Its relationship to blood urea nitrogen, dietary calcium intake, time on dialysis, and other variables. Journal of Laboratory and Clinical Medicine 1971; 78: 380–8.
87. Clarkson E, Eastwood J, Koutsaimanis K et al. Net intestinal absorption of calcium in patients with chronic renal failure. Kidney International 1973; 3: 258–63.
88. Ramirez J, EmmettM, White M et al. The absorption of dietary phosphorus and calcium in haemodialysis patients. Kidney International 1986; 30: 753–9.
89. Hutchison A, Boulton H, Herman K, Prescott M, Gokal R. The use of oral stable strontium to provide an index of intestinal calcium absorption in Chronic Ambulatory Peritoneal Dialysis patients. Mineral and Electrolyte Metabolism 1992; 18: 160–5.
90. Blumenkrantz M, Kopple J, Moran J Coburn J. Metabolic balance studies and dietary protein requirements in patients undergoing CAPD. Kidney International 1982; 21: 849–61.
91. Lindholm B, Bergstrom J. Nutritional aspects of CAPD. In: Gokal R (ed), Continuous Ambulatory Peritoneal Dialysis. Churchill Livingstone, Edinburgh 1986; pp 228–55.
92. Nolph K, Prowant B, Serkes K et al. Multicenter

evaluation of a new peritoneal dialysis solution with a high lactate and a low magnesium concentration. Peritoneal Dialysis Bulletin 1983; 3: 63–6.
93. Hercz G, Coburn J. Prevention of phosphate retention and hyperphosphatemia in uremia. Kidney International 1987; 32 (suppl 22): S215–20.
94. Delmez J, Fallon M, Bergfeld M, Gearing B, Dougan C, Teitelbaum S. Continuous ambulatory peritoneal dialysis and bone. Kidney Int 1986; 30: 379–84.
95. Martis L, Serkes K, Nolph K. Calcium carbonate as a phosphate binder: Is there a need to adjust peritoneal calcium concentrations for patients using calcium carbonate? Peritoneal Dialysis International 1989; 9: 325–8.
96. Andreoli S, Briggs J, Junor B. Aluminium intoxication from aluminium-containing phosphate binders in children with azotemia not undergoing dialysis. New England Journal of Medicine 1984; 310: 1079–4.
97. Salusky I, Coburn J, Foley J, Nelson P, Fine R. Effects of oral calcium carbonate on control of serum phosphorus and changes in plasma aluminium levels after discontinuation of aluminium-containing gels in children receiving dialysis. Journal of Pediatrics 1986; 108: 767–70.
98. Slatopolsky E, Weerts C, Lopex-Hilker S, Norwood K, Zink M, Windus D, Delmez J. Calcium carbonate as a phosphate binder in patients with chronic renal failure undergoing dialysis. New England Journal of Medicine 1986; 315: 157–61.
99. Stein H, Yudis M, Sirota R. Calcium carbonate as a phosphate binder. New England Journal of Medicine 1987; 316: 109–10.
100. Ott S. Aluminum accumulation in individuals with normal renal function. American Journal of Kidney Diseases 1985; 4: 297–301.
101. Joffe P, Olsen F, Heaf J, Gammelgaard B, Podenphant J. Aluminium concentrations in serum, dialysate, urine and bone among patients undergoing continuous ambulatory peritoneal dialysis. Clinical Nephrology 1989; 32(3): 133–8.
102. Slatopolsky E, Weerts C, Norwood K, Giles K, Fryer P, Finch J, Windus D, Delmez J. Long-term effects of calcium carbonate and 2.5mEq/liter calcium dialysate on mineral metabolism. Kidney International 1989; 36: 897–903.
103. Van der Merwe W, Rodger R, Grant A, Logue F, Cowan R, Beastall G, Junor B, Briggs J. Low calcium dialysate and high-dose oral calcitriol in the treatment of secondary hyperparathyroidism in haemodialysis patients. Nephrology Dialysis and Transplantation 1990; 5: 874–7.
104. Gokal R, Hutchison A. Calcium, Phosphorus, Aluminium and Bone Disease in Continuous Ambulatory Peritoneal Dialysis Patients. In: Hatano M (ed), Nephrology. Spinger Verlag, Tokyo 1991; 2: 1602–9.
105. Hutchison A, Gokal R. Towards Tailored Dialysis Fluids in CAPD: The role of reduced calcium and magnesium dialysis fluids. Peritoneal Dialysis International 1992; 12: 199–203.
106. Hutchison A, Were A, Boulton H, Mawer E, Laing I, Gokal R. Control of hypercalcaemia, hyperphosphataemia and hyperaluminaemia in CAPD by reduction in dialysate calcium concentration (abstract). Nephrology Dialysis Transplantation 1992; 7: 1143.
107. Hutchison A, Freemont A, Boulton H, Gokal R. Low-calcium dialysis fluid and oral calcium carbonate in CAPD: A method of controlling hyperphosphataemia whilst minimizing aluminium exposure and hypercalcaemia. Nephrology Dialysis Transplantation 1992; 7: 1219–25.
108. Hutchison A, Gokal R. Improved Solutions for Peritoneal Dialysis: Physiological calcium solutions, osmotic agents and buffers. Kidney International 1992; 42 (suppl 38): S152–9.
109. Piraino B, Perlmutter J, Holley J, Johnston J, Bernardini J. The use of dialysate containing 2.5 mEq/L calcium in peritoneal dialysis patients. Peritoneal Dialysis International 1992; 12(1): 75–6.
110. Cunningham J, Beer J, Coldwell R, Noonan K, Sawyer N, Makin H. Dialysate Calcium Reduction in CAPD Patients Treated With Calcium Carbonate and Alfacalcidol. Nephrology Dialysis Transplantation 1992; 7(1): 63–8.
111. Parker A, Nolph K. Magnesium and calcium transfer during continuous ambulatory peritoneal dialysis. Transactions of the American Society of Artificial and Internal Organs 1980; 26: 194–6.
112. Delmez J, Slatopolsky E, Martin K, Gearing B, Herschel R. Minerals, vitamin D, and parathyroid hormone in continuous ambulatory peritoneal dialysis. Kidney International 1982; 21: 862–7.
113. Kwong M, Lee J, Chan M. Transperitoneal calcium and magnesium transfer during an eight hour dialysis. Peritoneal Dialysis Bulletin 1987; 7: 85–9.
114. Hutchison A, Merchant M, Boulton H, Hinchcliffe R, Gokal R. Calcium and Magnesium Mass Transfer in Peritoneal Dialysis Patients using 1.25 mmol/L Calcium, 0.25 mmol/L Magnesium Dialysis Fluid. Peritoneal Dialysis International 1993; 13: 219–23.
115. Hutchison A, Whitehouse R, Boulton H, Adams J, Freemont A, Mawer E, Gokal R. Reduction of Dialysis Fluid Calcium Concentration in CAPD: Long-term Effect on Renal Osteodystrophy, with special reference to the Adynamic Lesion. 1993; (in press).
116. Hamdy N, Brown C, Boletis J, Boyle G, Tindale W, Beneton M, Charlesworth D, Kanis J. Mineral Metabolism in CAPD. In: Coles G, Davies M, Williams J (eds), CAPD: Host Defence, Nutrition and Ultrafiltration. Karger, Basel 1990; pp 73–8. (Berlyne G, Giovannetti S (eds), Contributions to Nephrology; Vol 85).
117. Meema H, Oreopoulos D, Rapoport A. Serum magnesium level and arterial calcification in end-stage renal disease. Kidney International 1987; 32: 388–94.
118. Gonella M, Ballanti P, Della Rocca C, Calabrese G, Pratesi G, Vagelli G, Mazzotta A, Bonucci E. Improved bone morphology by normalizing serum magnesium in chronically hemodialyzed patients.

Mineral and Electrolyte Metabolism 1988; 14: 240–5.
119. Breuer J, Moniz C, Baldwin D, Parsons V. The effects of zero magnesium dialysate and magnesium supplements on ionized calcium concentration in patients on regular dialysis treatment. Nephrology Dialysis and Transplantation 1987; 2: 347–50.
120. Parsons V, Baldwin D, Moniz C, Marsden J, Ball E, Rifkin I. Successful control of hyperparathyroidism in patients on continuous ambulatory peritoneal dialysis using magnesium carbonate and calcium carbonate as phosphate binders. Nephron 1993; 63: 379–83.
121. Shah G, Winer R, Cutler R, Arieff A, Goodman W, Lacher J, Schoenfeld P, Coburn J, Horowitz A. Effects of a magnesium-free dialysate on magnesium metabolism during continuous ambulatory peritoneal dialysis. Americal Journal of Kidney Diseases 1987; 10(4): 268–75.
122. George C et al. Gastro-intestinal System. In: British National Formulary. The Bath Press, Bath 1991; p 46. (Prasad A (ed), Vol 21).
123. Dyckner T, Wester P. Relation between potassium and magnesium in cardiac arrhythmias. Acta Med Scand 1981; 647 (suppl): 163–9.
124. Whang R. Magnesium deficiency: Pathogenesis, prevalence, and clinical implications. American Journal of Medicine 1987; 82 (suppl 3A): 24–9.
125. Hollifield J. Magnesium depletion, diuretics, and arrhythmias. American Journal of Medicine 1987; 82 (suppl 3A): 30–7.
126. Seelig M. Electrocardiographic patterns of magnesium depletion appearing in alcoholic heart disease. Ann NY Acad Sci 1969; 162: 906–17.
127. Lemann J, Lennon E. Role of diet, gastrointestinal tract and bone in acid-base homeostasis. Kidney International 1972; 1: 275–9.
128. Kaye M, Frueh A, Silverman M. A study of vertebral bone powder from patients with chronic renal failure. J Clin Invest 1978; 49: 442–53.
129. De Marchi S, Cecchin E. Severe metabolic acidosis and disturbances of calcium metabolism induced by acetazolamide in patients on haemodialysis. Clinical Science 1990; 78: 295–302.
130. Maren T. Carbonic anhydrase. N Engl J Med 1985; 313: 179–81.
131. Waite L. Carbonic anhydrase inhibitors, parathyroid hormone and calcium metabolism. Endocrinology 1972; 91: 1160–5.
132. Nolph K, Sorkin M, Rubin J, Arfania D, Prowant B, Fruto L, Kennedy D. Continuous ambulatory peritoneal dialysis: Three-year experience at one center. Annals of Internal Medicine 1980; 92: 609–13.
133. Lefebvre A, de Vernejoul M, Gueris J, Goldfarb B, Graulet A, Morieux C. Optimal correction of acidosis changes progression of dialysis ostedystrophy. Kidney International 1989; 36: 1112–8.
134. Mawer E, Hann J, Berry J, Davies M. Vitamin D metabolism in patients intoxicated with ergocalciferol. Clinical Science 1985; 68: 135–41.
135. de Fremont J, Moriniere P, Roussel J. Control of hyperparathyroidism by CAPD. Kidney International 1982; 21: 122–6.
136. Teitelbaum S, Fallon M, Gearing G, Dougan C, Delmez J. The effects of CAPD on bone histomorphometry. Kidney International 1982; 21: 180–4.
137. Loschiavo C, Fabris A, Adami S, Tomelleri L, Valvo E, Oldrizzi L, Gammaro L, Rugui C, Maschio G. The effects of CAPD on renal osteodystrophy. Peritoneal Dialysis Bulletin 1985; 5: 53–5.
138. Nolph K, Ryan L, Prowant B, Twardowski Z. A cross sectional assessment of serum vitamin D and triglycerides in a CAPD population. Peritoneal Dialysis Bulletin 1984; 4: 232.
139. Aloni Y, Shany S, Chaimovitz C. Losses of 25-hydroxyvitamin D in peritoneal fluid: Possible mechangism for bone disease in uraemic patients treated with CAPD. Mineral and Electrolyte Metabolism 1983; 9: 82–6.
140. Cassidy M, Owen J, Ellis H, Dewar J, Robinson C, Wilinson R, Ward M, Kerr D. Renal osteodystrophy and metastatic calcification in long term CAPD. Quarterly Journal of Medicine 1983; 213: 29–48.
141. Dunstan C, Hills E, Norman A, Bishop J, Mayer E, Wong S, Eade Y, Johnson J, George C, Collett P, Kalowski S, Wyndham R, Lawrence J, Alfrey A, Evans R. Treatment of haemodialysis bone disease with 24,25-dihydroxyvitamin D_3 and 1,25-dihydroxyvitamin D_3 alone or in combination. Mineral and Electrolyte Metabolism 1985; 11: 358–68.
142. Burbea Z, Gibor Y, Ladkani D, Griffel R, Gery R, Rodoy Y, Zevin D, Chaimovitz C. Combined oral treatment with $24,25(OH)_2D_3$ & $1alpha(OH)D_3$ regulates PTH level in secondary HPT of hemodialysis patients. Nephrology Dialysis Transplantation 1992; 7: 755.
143. Gonzalez E, Bander S, Thieland B, Martin K. Comparison of intravenous and pulse oral calcitriol for suppression of PTH in patients on haemodialysis (abstract). Journal of the American Society of Nephrology 1991; 2: 636.
144. Schaefer K, Umlauf E, von Herrath D. Reduced risk of hypercalcaemia for hemodialysis patients by administering calcitriol at night. Am J Kidney Dis 1992; 19: 460–4.
145. Korkor A. Reduced binding of [^{3}H] 1,25-dihydroxyvitamin D_3 in the parathyroid glands of patients with renal failure. N Engl J Med 1987; 316: 1573–7.
146. Merke J, Hugel U, Zlotkowski A, Szabo A, Bommer J, Mall G, Ritz E. Diminished parathyroid $1,25-(OH)_2D_3$ receptors in experimental uremia. Kidney International 1987; 32: 350–3.
147. Brown A, Dusso A, Lopez-Hilker S, Lewis-Finch J, Grooms P, Slatopolsky E. $1,25-(OH)_2D_3$ receptors are decreased in parathyroid glands from chronically uremic dogs. Kidney International 1989; 35: 19–23.
148. Fockens P, Hillen P, van Boven W, van Buchem-Ramakers T, Juttman J. Treatment of secondary

hyperparathyroidism in haemodialysis patients by intravenous administration of vitamin D one-alpha derivatives. Calcif Tissue Int 1986; 39: A117.
149. Lind L, Lithell H, Wengle B, Wrege U, Ljunghall S. A pilot study of metabolic effects of intravenously given alpha-calcidol in patients with chronic renal failure. Scand J Urol Nephrol 1988; 22: 219–22.
150. Carmichael D, Hume B. Intermittent intravenous 1-alpha-hydroxycholecalciferol reduces intact plasma parathyroid hormone in patients with end stage renal failure on long-term hemodialysis. Kidney International 1989; 35: 149.
151. Russell J, Lettieri D, Sherwood L. Suppression by $1,25(OH)_2D_3$ of transcription of the parathyroid hormone gene. Endocrinology 1986; 119: 1864–6.
152. Brown A, Ritter C, Finch J, Morrissey J, Martin K, Murayama E, Nishii Y, Slatopolsky E. The non-calcaemic analogue of vitamin D, 22-oxacalcitriol, suppresses parathyroid hormone synthesis and secretion. Journal of Clinical Investigation 1989; 84: 728–32.
153. Brown A, Finch J, Lopez-Hilker S, Dusso A, Ritter C, Pernalette N, Slatopolsky E. New active analogues of vitamin D with low calcemic activity. Kidney International 1990; 38 (suppl. 29): S22–7.
154. Kubrusly M, Gagne E, Hanrotel C, Lacour B, Drueke T. Effect of calcitriol versus 22-oxa-calcitriol on intestinal calcium transport in rats with severe chronic renal failure. Nephrology Dialysis Transplantation 1992; 7: 761.
155. McNair P, Christensen M, Madsbad S, Christensen C, Transbol I. Hypoparathyroidism in diabetes mellitus. Acta Endocrinol 1981; 96: 81–6.
156. Andress D, Hercz G, Kopp J, Endres D, Norris K, Coburn J, Sherrard D. Bone histomorphometry of renal osteodystrophy in diabetic patients. Journal of Bone and Mineral Research 1987; 2: 525–31.
157. Heidbreder E, Gotz R, Schafferhans K, Heidland A. Diminished parathyroid gland responsiveness to hypocalcemia in diabetic patients with uremia. Nephron 1986; 42: 285–9.
158. Cohen Solal M, Sebert J, Boudalliez B, Westeel P, Moriniere P, Marie A, Agarabedian M, Fournier A. Non-aluminic adynamic bone disease in non-dialyzed uremic patients: A new type of osteopathy due to over treatment? Bone 1992; 13: 1–5.
159. Fournier A, Moriniere P, Ben Hamidi F, El Esjer N, Shenovda M, Ghazali A, Bouzeridj M, Achard J, Westeel P. Use of alkaline calcium salts as phosphate binder in uremic patients. Kidney International 1992; 42 (suppl 38): S50–61.
160. Mazzaferro S, Coen G, Ballanti P, Bondatti F, Bonucci E, Pasquali M, Sardella D, Tomei E, Taggi F. Osteocalcin, iPTH, alkaline phosphatase and hand X-ray scores as predictive indices of histomorphometric parameters in renal osteodystrophy. Nephron 1990; 56: 261–6.
161. Maruyama Y, Arai K, Yoshida K, Motomiya Y, Kaneko Y, Hirao Y, Okajima E. Study of tartrate resistant acid phosphatase in patients with chronic renal failure on maintenance hemdialysis. Nippon Jinzo Gakkai Shi 1991; 33: 297–402.
162. Stamatiades D, Stathakis C, Boletis J, Fragou I, Papastathi E, Kiriakides S, Kostakis A, Vosnides G. Serum Tartrate resistant acid phosphatase: A simple index for the evaluation of secondary hyperparathyroidism of patients on hemodialysis and CAPD. Peritoneal Dialysis International 1992; 12 (suppl 2): 82.
163. Mohini R, Dumler F, Rao D. Skeletal surveys in renal osteodystrophy. ASAIO Trans 1991; 37: 635–7.
164. DeVita M, Rasenas L, Bansal M, Gleim G, Zabetakis P, Gardenswartz M, Michellis M. Assessment of renal osteodystrophy in hemodialysis patients. Medicine 1992; 71: 284–90.
165. Olgaard K, Heerfordt J, Madsen S. Scintigraphic skeletal changes in uremic patients on regular hemodialysis. Nephron 1976; 17: 325–34.
166. Hodson E, Howman Giles R, Evans R, Bautovich G, Hills E, Sherbon K, Bach B, Horvath S, Tiller D. The diagnosis of renal osteodystrophy: a comparison of Technetium 99m-pyrophosphate bone scintigraphy with other techniques. Clinical Nephrology 1981; 16: 24–8.
167. Karsenty G, Vigneron N, Jogetti V, Fauchet M, Zingraff J, Drueke T, Cournot-Witmer G. Value of the 99mTc-methylene diphosphonate bone scan in renal osteodystrophy. Kidney International 1986; 29: 1058–65.
168. Heaf J, Nielsen L, Mogensen N. Use of bone mineral content determination in the evaluation of osteodystrophy among hemodialysis patients. Nephron 1983; 35: 103–7.
169. Rickers H, Christensen M, Rodbro P. Bone mineral content in patients on prolonged maintenance hemodialysis: a three-year follow-up study. Clinical Nephrology 1983; 20: 302–7.
170 Lindergard B, Johnell O, Nilsson B, Wiklund P. Studies of bone morphology, bone densitometry and laboratory data in patients on maintenance hemodialysis treatment. Nephron 1985; 39: 122–9.
171. Piraino B, Chen T, Cooperstein L, Segre G, Puschett J. Fractures and vertebral bone mineral density in patients with renal osteodystrophy. Clinical Nephrology 1988; 30: 57–62.
172. Funke M, Maurer J, Grabbe E, Scheler F. Comparitive studies with quantitative computed tomography and dual-energy X-ray absorptiometry on bone density in renal osteopathy. Rofo Fortschr Geb Rontgenstr Neuen Bildgeb Verfahr 1992; 157: 145–9.

19 Noninfectious complications of peritoneal dialysis

JOANNE M. BARGMAN

1. Introduction 555
2. Hernias 555
3. Genital edema 556
   3.1. Radiologic and isotopic diagnosis of hernias and genital edema 557
4. Hydrothorax 557
   4.1. Pathogenesis of hydrothorax 557
   4.2. Diagnosis of hydrothorax 558
   4.3. Treatment of hydrothorax 559
      4.3.1. Temporary hemodialysis (2 to 4 weeks) with subsequent return to CAPD 559
      4.3.2. Temporary hemodialysis with a return to a peritoneal dialysis regimen with lower IAP 559
      4.3.3. Obliteration of the pleural space ("Pleurodesis") 559
      4.3.4. Operative repair 559
5. Respiratory complications 560
   5.1. Changes in pulmonary function resulting from altered mechanics of breathing 560
   5.2. Substrate-induced changes in respiration 561
6. Acid base and electrolyte disorders 561
   6.1. Disorders of water metabolism 561
   6.2. Disorders of potassium metabolism 562
   6.3. Acid base balance 562
7. Cardiovoascular complications 563
8. Gastrointestinal complications of peritoneal dialysis 564
   8.1. Pancreatitis 564
   8.2. Hepatic complications 565
   8.3. Other gastrointestinal complications 565
9. Failure of ultrafiltration 566
10. Sclerosing encapsulating peritonitis 567
11. Calcifying peritonitis 569
12. Hemoperitoneum 570
13. Chyloperitoneum 572
14. Acquired cystic disease of the kidney 572
    14.1. Neoplastic transformation 573
    14.2. Other complications 573
15. Pruritus 573
16. Dialysis-associated amyloidosis 574
17. Tendonitis, tendon rupture and calcific periarthritis 575
18. Back pain 576
19. Oxalate metabolism and kidney stones 576
20. Immune function 577
21. Transplantation 578
22. Cancer 579
Acknowledgements 580
References 580

1. Introduction

The steady decrease in the incidence of bacterial peritonitis in patients on continuous ambulatory peritoneal dialysis (CAPD) has allowed us to focus on noninfectious complications of peritoneal dialysis. Many of the complications result from the increased intra-abdominal pressure caused by the instillation of litres of fluid into a cavity which usually holds much less. Other complications arise because of the long-term effect of peritoneal dialysate directly on the mesothelial cells with which it has almost continuous contact, and more indirectly from the long-term metabolic consequences of this solution on the body's physiochemistry. This chapter will address these and other complications of peritoneal dialysis.

2. Hernias

The presence of dialysis fluid in the peritoneal cavity leads to increased intra-abdominal pressure (IAP). Pressure within the abdomen rises in proportion to the volume of dialysate instilled [1, 2]. The supine patient generates the lowest IAP for a given volume of IP fluid. Coughing and straining in the sitting and upright positions results in the highest pressures. In addition, patients who are older and those who are more obese generate higher IAP for a given activity [2].

In accordance with Laplace's law, the tension on the abdominal wall increases with the instillation of dialysate, as a result of the rise in IAP and the larger radius of the abdomen. Increased abdominal pressure and abdominal wall tension lead to hernia formation in those with congenital or acquired defects in or around the abdomen. The areas of weakness are probably very important in the pathogenesis of hernias. Indeed, the IAP in patients with hernias is no different from the pressure measured in those without hernias [3]. A host of hernias has been described in peritoneal dialysis patients (Table 1). The most common hernia is incisional or through the catheter placement site [4, 5]; in other reports inguinal [6–9] or umbilical [10–12] hernias occur most frequently. Asymptomatic hernias are probably quite common and may not be detected until some complication such as bowel strangulation occurs. One review found that 11.5% of CAPD patients developed hernias during a five year follow-up. Patients with hernias tend to be older, female, multiparous, those who have experienced a higher frequency of post-operative leak at the time of catheter insertion [5] and those who have undergone a previous hernia repair [4].

Patients with polycystic kidney disease may be predisposed to hernia formation, either as a result of higher IAP caused by the lage kidneys, or as a manifestation of a generalized disorder of collagen [13]. The mean time for development of hernia is one year, and the risk increases by 20% for each year on CAPD [4].

A major potential area of weakness is the abdominal incision for the implantation of the dialysis catheter. When this incision is made in the midline there is a predilection for incisional hernia to develop because this is an anatomically weak area [14]. Change to a paramedian incision through the rectus muscle has resulted in less perioperative leak and hernia formation [15].

Another area of potential weakness for herniation is the processus vaginalis. After the migration of the testes in fetal life, the processus vaginalis normally undergoes obliteration. Frequently, this does not occur, and the increased abdominal pressure during CAPD may push bowel into the processus vaginalis resulting in an indirect inguinal hernia. Male pediatric patients may be predisposed to this complication, and if they develop a unilateral inguinal hernia, both sides should probably be repaired prophylactically [16].

Most hernias present as a painless swelling [5]. Bowel has been reported to herniate through the diaphragm at the foramen of Morgagni and present as a retrosternal air-fluid level [17]. The rare obturator hernia can present with increasing paresthesia and hyperesthesia in the thigh [18]. The most worrisome complications are incarceration and strangulation of bowel. This can occur through almost any kind of hernia, but especially a small one. It may present as a tender lump [19, 20], recurrent gram negative peritonitis, bowel obstruction or perforation [5, 21, 22]. Bowel incarceration or strangulation can mimic peritonitis [8, 20, 21] and this complication must be kept in mind, particularly if the site of herniation itself is not obvious.

Hernias warrant surgical repair. Although large ventral hernias carry little measurable risk of bowel incarceration [23] they are unsightly and prone to enlarge. The other types of hernias should be repaired because of the risk of bowel incarceration and strangulation. The patient can be maintained temporarily on low volume intermittent peritoneal dialysis postoperatively to allow time for wound healing. If hernias recur, other options include changing the patient to night-time cycler dialysis, where the patient dialyzes supine (and hence under lower IAP), or using lower volumes of dialysate but with more frequent exchanges.

3. Genital edema

Edema of the labia majora or scrotum and penis is a distressing complication of peritoneal dialysis. Early reports suggested that up to 10% of CAPD patients could experience genital edema [24–29] although more recent reports document a lower incidence of this complication [30, 31]. It appears that women have a much lower incidence of genital edema compared to men [30, 31]. This disparity may be the result of the processus vaginalis being patent more often in males; alternatively, labial swelling may not be as noticeable compared to swelling over the penis and scrotum.

Two mechanisms have been suggested to explain the edema [24]. Firstly, dialysate can track through the soft-tissue plane from the catheter insertion site, from a soft-tissue defect within a hernia, or from a peritoneo-fascial defect. In any of these cases,

Table 1. Hernias in patients on peritoneal dialysis.

Umbilical [4–6, 8–12]
Inguinal [4–10, 12]
Catheter Incision Site [4, 6, 9, 19, 21]
Ventral [6, 9, 12]
Catheter Exit Site
Epigastric [4, 5, 8]
Incisional [4–6, 8, 10, 15]
Cystocele [5]
Foramen of Morgagni [5, 17]
Richter's [20, 321]
Enterocele [5, 322]
Spigelian [323]
Obturator [18, 324]

genital edema can be associated with edema of the anterior abdominal wall [25]. Secondly, dialysis fluid can travel through a patent processus vaginalis to the labia or scrotum, where it may leak into the surrounding soft tissue. If bowel accompanies the dialysate through the processus vaginalis, there will be an associated inguinal hernia. In fact, the presence of scrotal edema may suggest a clinically occult indirect inguinal hernia [26].

The presence of abdominal wall edema suggests that the origin of the peritoneal leak is proximal to the inguinal region in one of the potential sites listed above. On clinical examination the patient should stand. Asymmetry of the abdomen may indicate dialysis leak into the abdominal wall. Moreover, when dialysate has dissected superficially, the abdominal wall can look paler than usual. The skin indentations made by the elastic waistband or underwear or by the catheter lying across the abdomen look deeper and more prominent than usual.

Treatment of genital edema includes bedrest, scrotal elevation, and the use of frequent low volume exchanges [24]. In the case of a leak, cessation of peritoneal dialysis for a week or two may allow a defect to seal on its own. Converting the patient to night-time cycling dialysis with an empty peritoneum during the day allows dialysate to dwell under conditions of relatively low presure and can allow closure of a leak without changing to hemodialysis. Many patients can eventually resume CAPD [25].

3.1. Radiologic and isotopic diagnosis of hernias and genital edema

Abdominal scintigraphy with Technetium 99m has proven successful in identifying and locating the site of abdominal leak or a patent processus vaginalis. Different radioligands have been used with the tracer, including DTPA, albumin colloid, and tin colloid. One to five millicuries are injected into one half to two litres of dialysate [24, 29, 32, 33]. It has been suggested that the patient sit up and lean forward to encourage the radiolabelled dialysate into the leaking sites [34]. Delayed images after ambulation may be necessary to detect the leak [35, 36]. In addition, multiple projections should be taken in order to separate an abdominal wall leak from the peritoneal dialysate directly posterior to it [35]. While the dose of isotope may seem hefty, much of the radiation is drained out of the body with the dialysate after the study. Therefore the net dose of radiation is only a fraction of that originally instilled in the peritoneal cavity [34].

Computerized tomographic (CT) scanning can be helpful in diagnosing leaks and the cause of genital edema. Different agents (iopamidol, diatrizoate) have been employed in various volumes of dialysis fluid. It makes sense to use the largest volume tolerable in conjunction with manoeuvres to raise the IAP in order to facilitate fluid egress from the peritoneal cavity [37]. Peritoneal instillation of radiocontrst dye with CT scanning detects more leaks and hernias compared to plain peritoneography without CT scanning [37, 38]. CT scanning can demonstrate collections of dialysate/dye in the anterior abdominal wall which can track inferiorly and collect in the scrotum. Alternatively, dye can be visualized in the processus vaginalis as a cord-like structure and subsequent cuts can follow this inferiorly to the genitalia. Within the scrotal sac it can often be discerned whether the contrast/dialysate forms a hydrocele, or whether the fluid has dissected through the tunica vaginalis into the scrotal wall itself.

4. Hydrothorax

Increased intra-abdominal pressure (IAP) can result in leak of dialysis fluid across the diaphragm and into the pleural space. The accumulation of dialysis fluid in the pleural cavity is called hydrothorax. It is not clear how often hydrothorax occurs in patients receiving peritoneal dialysis, but most studies estimate that the incidence is less than 5%, which would make it a less frequent consequence of raised IAP than abdominal hernias, for example [39–44]. However, it is possible that hydrothorax does occur more frequently, but does not come to medical attention if the patient is asymptomatic or minor complaints of shortness of breath are overlooked.

4.1. Pathogenesis of hydrothorax

A defect in the diaphragm must be present to allow flux of dialysis fluid from the peritoneal into the pleural cavity. Autopsy studies have revealed localized absence of muscle fibres in the hemidiaphragm [45, 46]. The missing muscle fibres are replaced with a disordered network of collagen. One or more defects in the tendinous part of the hemidiaphragm have been observed [45–48].

When hydrothorax has been investigated by surgery or pleuroscopy, "blisters" or "blebs" have sometimes been noted on the pleural surface of the diaphragm. Presumably these represent the areas of deficiency in the usual support structures of the diaphragm described at autopsy [48]. With the instillation of dialysis fluid into the peritoneal cavity, these blebs can be seen to swell, weep and even rupture, thus providing the pathway for the movement of dialysate into the pleural space.

In pediatric patients receiving peritoneal dialysis who develop hydrothorax, diaphragmatic eventration rather than hernia has been described at surgery [49].

It is likely that these defects in the musculotendinous part of the diaphragm are not rare occurrences, but, in a manner similar to patent processus vaginalis, come to medical attention only when there is fluid in the abdominal cavity under increased pressure. This explains why hydrothorax has been described in patients on peritoneal dialysis and in those with liver disease or with ovarian cancer and ascites.

The extent of the deficiency in the hemidiaphragm varies among patients. Those with a pre-existent clear connection between peritoneal and pleural space probably correspond to those patients who develop hydrothorax with their first-ever infusion of dialysis fluid. In contrast, there are patients who develop hydrothorax months to years after starting peritoneal dialysis. Presumably those patients have attenuated tissue separating pleural from peritoneal space, and it may take repeated exposure to raised IAP or an episode of peritonitis to remove the barrier between the two cavities.

4.2. Diagnosis of hydrothorax

Small pleural effusions can be asymptomatic and are detected by routine chest radiographs. Larger pleural effusions can lead to respiratory embarassment.

The shortness of breath which results from the pleural effusion can be mistaken for congestive heart failure. The patient may choose more hypertonic dialysis solutions in an effort to increase ultrafiltration. In the patient with hydrothorax, however, increased ultrafiltration will lead to even greater IAP with further flux of dialysate into the pleural space, worsening the symptoms. Therefore, a history of a patient complaining of dyspnea that appears to worsen with hypertonic dialysate should suggest the possibility of hydrothorax, particularly if effluent returns are less than normal. Physical examination is consistent with pleural effusion, with absent breath sounds and stony dullness to percussion in the lung base. Tension hydrothorax has rarely been reported [50].

Chest x-ray shows a pleural effusion which occurs on the right side in most patients. It is assumed that the defect in the diaphragm discussed in the previous section occurs more frequently on the right rather than left side, although the reason for this is obscure. Alternatively, the heart may cover any defects that might be present in the left hemidiaphragm.

Clearly other causes for pleural effusion should be ruled out, including local parenchymal lung disease, congestive heart failure or pleuritis. The scenario wherein a patient develops a large right-sided pleural effusion with the first few dialyses is strongly suggestive of hydrothorax. However, in a patient on CAPD for months who develops peritonitis, fluid overload and pleural effusion, making the correct diagnosis can be more difficult.

In the patient in whom the etiology of the pleural effusion is uncertain, a thoracentesis can be helpful in making the correct diagnosis. If the pleural fluid is composed of dialysate, the glucose concentration is very high (usually greater than 40 mmol/L), and the fluid has a low protein concentration consistent with a transudate. Some investigators have pointed out that the dextro-isomer of lactate is present in dialysis fluid but not in "endogenous" pleural effusions, and is another way of identifying dialysate in the pleural fluid [51]. However, most laboratories are not equipped to rapidly detect D-lactate, and certainly glucose concentration remains an easier and cheaper way to look for dialysis fluid.

It has been suggested that the dye methylene blue can be instilled in the peritoneal cavity before the pleural tap, and blue staining of the pleural fluid provides evidence of peritoneal-pleural communication. However, intraperitoneal methylene blue can lead to chemical peritonitis, and, furthermore, the blue staining may be so faint as to not be appreciated in the pleural fluid, leading to a false negative result.

Even when the diagnosis is certain, thoracentesis should also be used in patients who are short of breath from the hydrothorax. Evacuation of one or more liters of fluid should lead to significant improvement in the patients' respiratory status.

In the absence of thoracentesis, the presence of a peritoneal-pleural communication can be confirmed by isotopic scanning. In different studies, between 3–10 mCi of technetium-labelled macro-aggregated albumin or sulphur colloid has been instilled into the peritoneal cavity along with the usual volume of dialysis fluid. The patient should move around to ensure mixing of the radioisotope and dialysate and to raise the IAP. Subsequent scanning detects movement of the isotope above the hemidiaphragm. This usually is detectable in the first few minutes but sometimes late pictures (up to 6 hours) need to be taken. This method is convenient but not absolutely foolproof. Defects have been found in the diaphragm at surgery in patients in whom isotopic scanning was negative [52–55].

Other studies have reported the use of contrast peritoneography using diatrizoate and iopamidol, but experience with these non-isotopic methods is limited [56].

4.3. Treatment of hydrothorax

Thoracentesis is recommended for the immediate treatment of hydrothorax if respiratory compromise is present. Otherwise, simply discontinuing peritoneal dialysis often leads to rapid and dramatic resolution of the pleural effusion [43, 44, 57, 58]. In a small number of patients the effusion is very slow to resolve, suggesting that there may be a one-way or ball-valve type communication between peritoneal and pleural spaces. In this instance thoracentesis may be helpful to hasten the resolution of the pleural effusion.

Subsequent treatment depends on whether the patient is going to continue on peritoneal dialysis. The occurrence of hydrothorax occasionally is so distressing to the patient that he or she requests transfer to hemodialysis. In this case, the communication between peritoneal and pleural space should be of no consequence and nothing further needs to be done once the effusion has resolved.

If the patient is going to continue with peritoneal dialysis, there are a number of different options:

4.3.1. *Temporary hemodialysis (2 to 4 weeks) with subsequent return to CAPD*

Especially in the presence of peritonitis, there may be a transient loss of the integrity of the cell layers overlying a diaphragmatic defect. If peritoneal dialysis is temporarily discontinued and the mesothelium allowed to reconstitute itself over the defect, it is possible that the peritoneo-pleural communication may become re-sealed. It is less likely that this would be effective in those patients demonstrating pleural leak with the first dialysis, but even this phenomenon has been reported after a 2 month hiatus on hemodialysis. It has been suggested that the dialysate in the pleural space may act as a sclerosing agent and prevent subsequent leaks [59].

4.3.2. *Temporary hemodialysis with a return to a peritoneal dialysis regimen with lower IAP*

Patients who experience hydrothorax on CAPD are sometimes able to resume peritoneal dialysis by cycler. Even though the supine position might be thought of as conducive to the movement of fluid into the pleural cavity, it appears to be more than compensated by the reduction in IAP afforded by this posture [60]. The use of smaller dialysis volumes with more frequent exchanges is helpful in minimizing the increment in IAP.

4.3.3. *Obliteration of the pleural space ("Pleurodesis")*

Previous studies have reported the successful obliteration of the pleural cavity. In this instance the leaves of the pleura stick together and prevent the re-accumulation of pleural fluid.

There are different agents used to induce pleurodesis. Oxytetracycline (20 mg/kg) has been administered via a thoracostomy tube [44, 51, 57, 61]. It is important that the patient remain supine, up to 24 hours, and assume different positions, including head-down, to ensure exposure of the agent to all the pleural surfaces. The patient should also receive analgesia, as this procedure can be painful. Talc has also been reported as a successful agent for pleurodesis in a patient on peritoneal dialysis [62].

Obliteration of the pleural cavity has also been accomplished by the instillation of 40 ml of autologous blood. The patient should be maintained, if possible, on hemodialysis for a few weeks to allow the pleurodesis to take place. More than one instillation of blood may be necessary, but the benefit of the blood is that it appears to be a relatively painless procedure compared to the use of talc or tetracycline [63, 64]. There are reports from Japan of the use of OK-432, a hemolytic streptococcal preparation, and the use of *Nocardia rubra* cell wall skeleton to effect pleurodesis [44].

Finally, a combination of aprotinin-calcium-chloride-thrombin and "fibrin glue" instilled in the drained pleural cavity was reported to successfully prevent recurrent hydrothorax in a patient who had previously failed treatment with other agents [65].

4.3.4. *Operative repair*

At thoracotomy a communication between peritoneal and pleural space may be visualized. Sometimes the "blebs" or blisters are quickly recognized and these can be sutured and reinforced with Teflon felt patches [48]. It is recommended that two to three liters of dialysate be infused into the peritoneal cavity through the dialysis catheter. The diaphragm is inspected from the pleural side for seepage of dialysate through holes or blisters. It is important that the surgeon be patient as it may take time for the seepage to be recognized [66, 67].

In the case of eventration of the diaphragm, as reported in the pediatric literature, surgical repair can be effected by plication with nonabsorbable suture. These patients are able to return to peritoneal dialysis successfully [49].

In summary, hydrothorax is a well-described but relatively uncommon complication of peritoneal dialysis. Diagnosis is relatively simple once the possibility of peritoneal-pleural communication has been entertained. Thoracentesis may be necessary to confirm the diagnosis and is mandated by respiratory embarassment. If the patient is willing to continue with peritoneal dialysis, several treatment options are available.

5. Respiratory complications

The effect of CAPD on respiration can be divided into two. The first is related to the physical presence of dialysis fluid in the peritoneal cavity with subsequent increase in intra-abdominal pressure and alteration of the mechanics of breathing. The second effect results from the carbohydrate loading of dialysate glucose absorption, which can affect intermediary metabolism and change respiration in a substrate-driven manner.

5.1. Changes in pulmonary function resulting from altered mechanics of breathing

Early studies of peritoneal dialysis suggested that this procedure compromised respiratory function [68]. However, these and other studies were reported in acutely ill subjects, and many other factors could have affected the integrity of the lungs, pleura and respiratory muscles. Later studies of stable patients on chronic peritoneal dialysis demonstrated that two litres of dialysis fluid in the abdomen resulted in reduction of most lung volumes, including the functional residual capacity (FRC) [69-73]. These changes can persist [73] or normalize after only two weeks of CAPD [71].

It has been suggested that as the FRC decreases to less than the closing volume, small airways will collapse and cause ventilation-perfusion mismatch and arterial hypoxemia [74]. At the outset of dialysis, instillation of dialysate is associated with an average 5 mmHg fall in arterial pO2 in the sitting position and an average 8 mmHg decrease when the patient is supine. These changes are seen in association with a fall in FRC. When these patients are re-studied a few months later, there is no longer a decrement in arterial pO2, despite a similar fall in FRC. The authors have suggested that some long term adjustment takes place, such as redistribution of blood away from the more poorly ventilated lower segments of the lungs [72]. Other studies have not confirmed arterial hypoxemia in patients on peritoneal dialysis [69, 71, 75].

The changes in lung volumes have not been found to be any more severe in patients with chronic obstructive airways disease [71] and it has been advised that obstructive airways disease should not be regarded as a contraindication to the use of peritoneal dialysis [76]. It recently has been demonstrated by total body plethysmography that the presence of two liters of dialysis fluid has no effect on airways resistance [73]. Indeed, it is conceivable that the presence of dialysis fluid in the abdomen can facilitate pulmonary function. This change may be explainable by altered diaphragmatic contractility secondary to stretch of the diaphragm caused by the dialysate [70]; that is, with increased length of the muscle fibers, there is improved muscle function. Explained in another way, the presence of the intraperitoneal fluid increases the upward curvature of the diaphragm. The radius of the new curve is smaller. Laplace's law dictates that the diaphragm generates more pressure for a given amount of muscle tension when the radius is smaller. Therefore, the contractility of the diaphragm may increase in the presence of intraperitoneal fluid [77]. This effect is analogous to the benefit the patient with obstructive airways disease achieves by holding a pillow tightly against the abdomen. However, there is an upper limit to this relationship after which the diaphragm loses efficiency and compromise of ventilation occurs [77].

A recent study of pulmonary function in predialysis, peritoneal dialysis, hemodialysis and renal transplant patients showed that the diffusion factor for carbon monoxide, while reduced in all the groups, was significantly lower in the group of patients on CAPD, with a mean TLCO just under 70% of predicted value. The authors postulated that this surprising finding was most likely the result of subclinical pulmonary edema (potentiated by the low serum albumin in the CAPD group) or else the result of interstitial fibrosis caused by repeated episodes of pulmonary edema [78]. However, another intriguing possibility is that the raised intra-abdominal pressure leads to reflux, chronic aspiration and the consequent development of restrictive lung disease [79].

5.2. Substrate-induced changes in respiration

The nature and availability of energy substrate can alter intermediary metabolism and affect ventilation. This relationship has been described in patients undergoing total parenteral nutrition, where hypercaloric glucose and amino acid solutions produce significant increase in minute ventilation, carbon dioxide excretion and oxygen consumption [80]. A theoretical treatment of substrate absorption during CAPD predicts that the absorption of glucose, and, to a lesser extent, lactate, would drive intermediary metabolism and lead to the changes in respiration described above. The increase in metabolically-driven ventilation could prove dangerous to the patient with lung disease [80].

Studies in patients on CAPD confirm increased minute volume, oxygen consumption and carbon dioxide excretion compared to controls [81]. This suggests that the lactate and glucose absorbed are incorporated into the Krebs cycle. Moreover, because some of the glucose is metabolized in a manner that does not require oxygen but does produce carbon dioxide, the respiratory quotient increases. In the normal situation, however, the arterial pCO2 does not increase because the patient is stimulated to hyperventilate and "blow off" the extra carbon dioxide. In the patient who is too ill to hyperventilate, this may not be the case. Recently, Cohn and coworkers described a patient with systemic lupus erythematosus and renal and respiratory failure who developed acute respiratory acidosis each time a high-glucose dialysis solution was used. The acidosis would abate when the dialysis was changed to one with a lower concentration of glucose. The authors suggested that the carbohydrate loading led to lipogenesis, a process associated with a respiratory quotient (CO2 produced per O2 used) as great as 8. In the patient with compromised ventilatory status and respiratory muscle dysfunction, the extra carbon dioxide could not be exhaled quickly enough, and so hypercapnea ensued. The use of dialysis solutions with lower glucose concentration resulted in less net glucose absorption and hence less substrate-driven carbon dioxide production [82].

6. Acid base and electrolyte disorders

6.1. Disorders of water metabolism

In patients with endstage renal disease the serum sodium concentration will depend on the relative amount of salt and water being ingested and the amount of salt and water removed by dialysis. Sodium flux into the peritoneal cavity in the peritoneal dialysis patient is caused by diffusion and convection. Because sodium is sieved by the peritoneal membrane, the fluid entering the peritoneal cavity by osmotically-driven flow is hyponatremic, that is, more water than salt flows from plasma to peritoneal compartment [83]. In theory, this flux should leave the patient with a relative water deficit; the patient should become hypernatremic. However, hypertonicity is a powerful stimulant of ADH secretion which in turn stimulates thirst. The patient drinks water or some other hypotonic fluid until tonicity is restored. In fact, patients on CAPD may actually demonstrate plasma sodium concentrations slightly lower than normal. There are a number of reasons for the relative water excess, including increased water intake or low sodium concentration in the dialysis solution [84]. Infants undergoing peritoneal dialysis and fed normal infant formula may be prone to hyponatremia because sodium losses from ultrafiltration are greater than sodium gained from ingestion of formula. Moreover, the proprietary infant formulas have a high water to sodium ratio, leading to water accumulation and hyponatremia [85].

In a study of insulin-dependent diabetics with hyperglycemia, those on hemodialysis were able to nearly normalize the serum tonicity whereas peritoneal dialysis patients remained hypertonic owing to continued loss of water in excess of solute into the dialysate. In hyperglycemia, the increased extracellular glucose effects osmotic flux of water from the intracellular towards normal. The fall in serum sodium concentration resulting from this movement of water into the extracelluar compartment can be predicted. Patients on hemodialysis, however, demonstrate a greater fall in serum sodium concentration than do hyperglycemic patients not on dialysis. On the other hand, patients on peritoneal dialysis behave more like the nondialysis patients. One explanation is that the hemodialysis patient drinks water in response to increased plasma osmolality and, in the absence of ongoing osmotic diuresis, is able to lower plasma tonicity. In contrast, the patient on peritoneal dialysis undergoes continuous loss of water in excess of sodium (see above) and in this way mimics the effect of the osmotic diuresis seen in hyperglycemia with normal renal function. The excess loss of water can perpetuate the hyperosmolar state [86].

6.2. Disorders of potassium metabolism

Patients on hemodialysis who are noncompliant with dietary prescription may have problems with hyperkalemia on nondialysis days. On the other hand, in patients on CAPD, low serum potassium concentration can be the more prevalent problem. Hypokalemia is found in 10–36% of CAPD patients [87, 88]. Hypokalemia can be profound, as reported in a diabetic CAPD patient with vomiting and diarrhea [89]. Ongoing losses of potassium in the dialysate may contribute to hypokalemia in some patients. However, other factors such as cellular uptake and bowel losses play a role. Muscle biopsy studies show that muscle potassium content is increased in CAPD patients, presumably reflecting intracellular uptake [84].

It is recommended that the serum potassium concentration be maintained at greater than 3.0 mmol/L in the asymptomatic patient, and greater then 3.5 mmol/L in the patient on digoxin or with a history of cardiac arrhythmias [90]. Potassium supplementation should be monitored in dialysis patients because of the absence of renal reserve to excrete excess potassium. Potassium chloride can be added to the dialysate to diminish the concentration gradient for diffusion of potassium into the dialysis fluid. In the acute setting, up to 20 mmol/L of KCl can be added to the dialyate with a low incidence of side effects. This dose has been reported to increase the plasma potassium concentration by an average 0.44 mmol/L over 2–3 hours. However, the effect of this hyperkalemic solution on the peritoneal membrane is unknown and so this treatment should be used only in urgent settings [87].

Hyperkalemia is occasionally seen in acute PD and CAPD patients. It has been noted to occur after acute peritoneal dialysis [91, 92] and has been attributed to breakdown of glycogen with consequent release of potassium. Other factors which affect extrarenal potassium disposal, such as insulin deficiency, converting enzyme inhibitors and beta-blockers, should be considered.

6.3. Acid base balance

In health, the kidneys help to maintain acid base balance via excretion of acid and generation of new bicarbonate. As the kidneys fail, however, net acid excretion diminishes and metabolic acidosis develops. It is important, therefore, that any form of dialysis provide replenishment of buffer.

In the early years of peritoneal dialysis bicarbonate, the obvious choice, was employed as buffer. However, bicarbonate reacts with calcium chloride leading to precipitation of calcium carbonate. Therefore, other less reactive buffers had to be used, and experience has accumulated with lactate and acetate. Dialysate containing glucose must be kept at pH 5–6 to prevent caramelization. At equimolar concentration of acetate and lactate, acetate demonstrates higher titratable acidity. Therefore, when instilled into the peritoneal cavity, solutions containing acetate remain acidic longer than do lactate-based solutions [93]. The prolonged acidity of the solution may explain reports of abdominal pain and chemical peritonitis with the use of acetate-based dialysate [93, 94] (other long-term effects of acetate are discussed in the sections on sclerosing peritonitis and ultrafiltration failure). Serum lactate remains low in patients receiving lactate-containing dialysate. Patients receiving equimolar amounts of acetate-containing dialysate, on the other hand, demonstrate abnormally high levels of plasma acetate [95]. This finding suggests that less lactate is absorbed or it is more efficiently metabolized than acetate. The patients receiving lactate show normal serum bicarbonate levels [95, 96] suggesting that adequate amounts of lactate are being absorbed and converted to bicarbonate. The dialysate lactate is composed of both the easily metabolized L isomer and the slowly metabolized D isomer. Both isomers are absorbed from dialysate in equal amounts. The lack of accumulation of the D isomer in blood suggests that it is, indeed, metabolized to a significant extent [97], although previous investigations have suggested otherwise [98]. The fate of absorbed D-lactate is of concern because of reports of cerebral dysfunction in patients with high blood levels of this isomer [99]. During IPD, there is a net gain in body buffer of about 80 mmol, the result of lactate absorption surpassing bicarbonate loss from plasma to dialysate. High rates of ultrafiltration mitigate this effect via both increased loss of bicarbonate and diminished absorption of lactate. Presumably, this is on the basis of convective forces [97].

Ammonium chloride loading has demonstrated that patients on CAPD tolerate an acid load better than patients receiving hemodialysis. This tolerance does not seem to increase with time on CAPD [100].

Use of lactate does have its drawbacks. Its use in patients with lactic acidosis may worsen the metabolic derangement [101, 102]. In this setting, specially prepared bicarbonate-based solutions are recommended [103], or the use of a proportioning system similar to that used in bicarbonate-based hemodialysis [104]. Lactate may be an inappropriate buffer in patients with hepatic failure. In this setting, lactate may not be sufficiently converted to bicarbonate, leading to acidosis and lactate accumulation [92, 105].

Patients on peritoneal dialysis may develop metabolic or respiratory alkalosis. The metabolic alkalosis can result from contraction of the extracellular fluid volume, as reported in the treatment phase of hyperglycemia [106, 107] or with the frequent use of hypertonic dialysis solutions [108]. In patients with respiratory alkalosis, the normally functioning kidneys defend against alkalemia by excreting bicarbonate. The CAPD patient has no such mechanism. Furthermore, the constant infusion of buffer in the patient with respiratory alkalosis can lead to serious alkalemia [109].

Respiratory alkalosis may appear during the initial stages of dialysis. In the acidotic patient commencing dialysis, the infusion of buffer will correct the extracellular acidosis. However, because the bicarbonate anion crosses the blood-brain barrier relatively slowly, the cerebrospinal fluid bathing the respiratory centre will remain relatively acid. This cerebrospinal fluid acidosis will continue to stimulate respiratory drive and maintain hyperventilation in the face of now-normal extracellular fluid pH. Therefore, respiratory alkalosis will develop as a response to the hyperventilation [91, 110]. This phenomenon poses only a minor problem in peritoneal dialysis because the conversion of lactate to bicarbonate occurs slowly enough to allow cerebrospinal fluid equilibration with extracellular fluid.

7. Cardiovascular complications

The development of left ventricular hypertrophy (LVH) in nonuremic hypertensives confers a negative prognosis for cardiovascular morbidity and mortality [111]. This relationship appears to hold in the uremic population as well [112]. The pathogenesis of myocardial hypertrophy in uremic patients is varied and includes putative factors such as hypertension, chronic anemia, and extracellular fluid volume overload [113]. In addition, the uremic state is associated with intermyocardiocytic fibrosis, which further compromises ventricular compliance [114]. Echocardiographic studies have documented a decrease in left ventricular mass in the majority of CAPD patients in whom it was increased at the beginning of dialysis. These patients experienced near-normalization of the end-diastolic dimension, left ventricular fractional shortening, and ejection fraction [115]. These changes were thought to be the result of improved control of systemic blood pressure. However, not all studies have confirmed regression of LVH in patients on peritoneal dialysis. The discrepancy may be the result of different degrees of control of the extracellular fluid volume, different methodological approaches to the assessment of LVH, and the different pharmacologic approaches to the control of systemic hypertension [113].

The reduction in blood pressure can also have deleterious effects. Diabetic patients have been reported to experience exacerbation of peripheral vascular disease during CAPD. Risk factors for the worsening of peripheral perfusion include smoking, previous symptoms of peripheral vascular disease, and absent limb pulses. It has been suggested that the lowered blood pressure on CAPD compromises blood flow to the ischemic limbs [116].

Persistent hypocalcemia after parathyroidectomy has been implicated as a cause of congestive cardiomyopathy in CAPD patients. It was suggested that concomitant reduction in intracellular calcium compromised the force developed by the contractile elements of the heart. Cardiac function and dilatation improved in one patient with calcium repletion [117].

The elevated intra-abdominal pressure caused by the presence of dialysis fluid in the peritoneal cavity has the potential to affect cardiac function. In cirrhotic patients, drainage of ascitic fluid produces a fall in right and left atrial pressure with improvement in cardiac function [118]. There is no consensus on the influence of peritoneal dialysate on cardiac function. Studies have been unable to document a decrease in cardiac function with infusions of as much as three liters of dialysate [119], whereas others have reported up to a 20% decrease in cardiac index with two liters of intraperitoneal fluid [120, 121]. Perhaps what makes the most sense physiologically was a study that found that it was the subgroup of patients with LVH who showed echocardiographically-detectable changes in function with the infusion of large (3L or more) volumes of dialysate [122]. The reduction in LV systolic function was felt to be the result of reduction in preload, because a significant decrease in the LV internal diameter in diastole was found. It is predicted that the subgroup of patients with LVH are the patients in whom cardiac function is affected by preload reduction [113]. In other words, the patients with LVH and diminished LV compliance would be vulnerable to a decrease in LV preload resulting from decreased venous return [122]. However, decreased venous return could not explain the reduced cardiac output in all the patients. Some of these patients had no change in right heart pressure. In these patients, increased cardiac surface pressure from the bulging of the diaphragm into the thoracic cavity may have compromised cardiac function [122]. In this regard it is interesting to note that inferior attenuation on cardiac thallium-201 imaging has been noted in patients holding two liters of peritoneal dialysis fluid. The elevation of the diaphragm as a result of increased intra-abdominal pressure was thought to be the cause of the abnormal scan, as opposed to myocardial disease [123]. In summary, it appears that the presence of intraperitoneal dialysate usually does not exert a clinically significant effect on the cardiovascular system, although there is a potential for such an effect with the use of large (3L or more) volumes in patients with diminished cardiac compliance.

A discussion of coronary artery disease and the CAPD patient is beyond the scope of this chapter. However, ischemic heart disease and its complications remain a very significant cause of death in this population. Hypertension, unfavourable lipid profiles and glucose intolerance may all contribute to the development of or worsening of coronary artery disease in the patient on CAPD.

8. Gastrointestinal complications of peritoneal dialysis

8.1. Pancreatitis

The uremic milieu is associated with histological abnormalities in the pancreas. Postmortem studies have confirmed an increased incidence of pancreatic lesions in uremics compared to nonuremic controls [124]. In animal models of uremia, the pancreas shows hypertrophy and hyperplasia [125]. Pathological changes in the pancreas are prevalent in the majority of patients undergoing hemodialysis. Postmortem examination has revealed pancreatitis, pancreatic fibrosis, calcification and cystic changes [126]. Postmortem examinations in CAPD patients have revealed a similar prevalence of histological changes in the pancreas [127].

Patients on peritoneal dialysis may be at additional risk for the development of pancreatitis. Peritoneal dialysate can gain access to the lesser sac of the peritoneal cavity via the epiploic foramen. The posterior surface of the lesser sac is also the anterior surface of the pancreas. Therefore, any constituent of the dialysate has the potential to irritate the pancreas. Proposed irritants include the high glucose concentration of dialysis fluid, unidentified toxic byproducts of the dialysate, bags, or tubing [128], acidity of the dialysate [129] and, of course, infected dialysate as seen in peritonitis [129, 130]. Rechallenge with peritoneal dialysate after an episode of pancreatitis has resulted in a recurrent episode of pancreatitis [131]. In addition, there may be a predilection for pseudocyst formation [129].

Other risk factors for pancreatic inflammation in patients on CAPD include hypertriglyceridemia, which is prevalent in these patients. In addition, patients with aplastic bone disease (see Chapter 18) are prone to hypercalcemia when given calcium supplements and vitamin D, and the elevated serum calcium is another risk factor for acute pancreatitis [132].

Despite all the potential risk factors outlined above, it still remains controversial whether acute pancreatitis occurs more frequently in CAPD patients compared to those on hemodialysis. In a recent review of the literature, Gupta et al. concluded that, in fact, acute pancreatitis was not more common in CAPD patients, and that previous reports to the contrary were the result of reporting bias [133]. However, given the potential for contact between peritoneal dialysis fluid and the pancreas, and the frequency of at least transient episodes of hypercalcemia in CAPD patients, there remains a strong theoretical risk for a predisposition toward acute pancreatitis in this population compared to those on hemodialysis.

Diagnosis of acute pancreatitis may be difficult. It should be considered in cases of culture-negative peritonitis, especially if the abdominal pain fails to resolve or localizes in the epigastrium. Hiccoughs may be present [134]. The serum amylase will rise with pancreatitis. However, because patients with chronic renal failure can have elevated serum amylase levels, there is overlap between the elevated levels seen in patients with renal failure and pancreatitis and those with renal failure alone [129]. Serum amylase values greater than three times the upper limit of normal are suggestive of acute pancreatitis [135]. A review of the literature concerning pancreatitis in CAPD patients shows that the amylase level was elevated in eighteen of twenty-three patients. In the eighteen, the mean increase was 8.5 times the upper limit of normal [133]. In the other five patients, however, the serum amylase was normal. In summary, it seems that a markedly elevated serum amylase is strongly suggestive of acute pancreatitis, but normal levels do not rule out this diagnosis.

It has been reported that an increased amylase level in the dialysis effluent (greater than 100 U/L) indicates acute pancreatitis or other intra-abdominal pathology compared to the lower levels seen with dialysis-associated peritonitis [136]. However, this has not been confirmed in other centres [130, 133].

Ultrasound and CT scanning can demonstrate an engorged, edematous pancreas [128, 131], or pseudocyst formation. Unfortunately, these radiological studies are also frequently normal [128, 129]. The mortality is high, and part of the reason may be that time to diagnosis can be delayed on the assumption that the abdominal pain is the result of bacterial peritonitis.

8.2. Hepatic complications

The liver is at risk for abscess formation as a result of dialysis-associated peritonitis. This diagnosis should be considered in cases of persistent peritonitis. Ultrasound of the liver may be normal and exploratory laparotomy may be necessary [137]. Needle aspiration and drainage under CT guidance is a less invasive alternative.

In CAPD patients receiving intraperitoneal insulin, a unique hepatic lesion can develop. A layer of fat is deposited under the hepatic capsule exposed to the peritoneal cavity. The thickness of this fatty layer correlates with the degree of obesity, as well as the size of the dose of intraperitoneal insulin. It has been proposed that the insulin in the peritoneal dialysate causes increased concentration of this hormone at the capsule and at the level of the subcapsular hepatocytes. In the face of relative peripheral insulin deficiency, free fatty acids are delivered to the liver, where they are re-esterified in the presence of the high insulin levels under the hepatic capsule. Pathologically, there may be associated steatonecrosis, but liver function remains normal [138]. However, it is important that this complication be kept in mind. One of our CAPD patients on intraperitoneal insulin underwent CT scanning for abdominal pain and was reported to have metastatic carcinoma of the liver. However, the abnormality was distributed just under the liver capsule across the surface of the liver exposed to the dialysate. A needle biopsy confirmed that the lesion was not cancer, but the above-described subcapsular steatosis.

8.3. Other gastrointestinal complications

Many patients on CAPD complain of abdominal bloating and reflux. It has been assumed that the cause of these symptoms is the increased intra-abdominal pressure and volume. It might be expected that the increased abdominal pressure changes the pressure dynamics across the esophageal-gastric junction and leads to esophageal reflux or spasm. However, in a study using manometry to measure esophageal pressures and peristalsis, no increase in esophageal pressure or pressure at the lower esophageal sphincter was noted when 1.5L to 2.5L of dialysate was instilled in the peritoneal cavity [139].

The small bowel is vulnerable to catheter-related perforation. This complication results from pressure necrosis from the dialysis catheter. Small bowel perforation of this type has been reported not only in patients with an unused peritoneal dialysis catheter, but also in patients actively receiving CAPD [140].

There are rare reports of ischemic colitis and necrotizing enteritis as complications of peritoneal dialysis [141–143]. The likeliest cause is hypotension with consequent hypoperfusion of the bowel. However, the development of ischemic bowel in a normotensive 6-year old child on peritoneal dialysis with improvement upon transfer to hemodialysis suggests that peritoneal dialysis itself may play a role in the bowel ischemia [142]. Marked gastrointestinal bleeding from dilated submucosal vessels in the bowel have been reported in association with the use of hypertonic dextrose solutions. No such bleeding occurred when the patient changed to hemodialysis. It was suggested that peritoneal dialysis provoked mesenteric vasodilatation which promoted the gastrointestinal bleeding [144].

9. Failure of ultrafiltration

Early experience with acute peritoneal dialysis suggested that the peritoneal membrane could withstand the infusion of dialysate without serious side effects. With the advent of chronic peritoneal dialysis, however, it became apparent that the peritoneal membrane could fail. It was reported that subgroups of long-term CAPD patients needed increasing numbers of exchanges with hypertonic dialysate to maintain euvolemia [145].

In most of the descriptions of ultrafiltration failure the solute transport remained normal or was above normal (type I ultrafiltration failure). The inability to sustain an osmotic gradient across the peritoneal membrane because of rapid diffusion of glucose from the dialysate is the principal cause of this type of ultrafiltration failure. It is possible that increased lymphatic absorption also plays a role [146]. Less commonly, transport of solute is impaired as well as ultrafiltration. This generalized reduction in peritoneal transport (type II ultrafiltration failure) results from a reduction in the surface area available for transport. It can be seen in the patient with extensive adhesions or sclerosing encapsulating peritonitis [147].

There may be regional variation in this incidence and prevalence of ultrafiltration failure. Some centers in Europe have reported a high incidence of this problem [148-150] whereas it may not be as common in North America. An actuarial analysis by Slingeneyer suggested a risk rate for ultrafiltration failure of 10% in the first year and 30% by the second year of CAPD. The sex of the patient made no difference, nor did the frequency of peritonitis. Interestingly, younger patients had a higher incidence of ultrafiltration loss [148]. When patients were grouped with respect to their ability to ultrafilter large volumes, the low ultrafiltration group had been on CAPD almost as long as those able to ultrafilter large volumes. Not surprisingly, the patients with poor ultrafiltration demonstrated greater permeability to small solutes. Again, no difference in the incidence of peritonitis could be detected between the two groups [150]. These authors have recently extended their observations with different results. When patients who had been on CAPD for a mean of 5 years were matched to a cohort of patients who had just started CAPD, very different transport characteristics of the peritoneum became apparent. For example, almost twice the volume of fluid was ultrafiltered using hypertonic dialysate in the group of patients new to peritoneal dialysis compared to the long-term group. The mass transfer area coefficient for creatinine and glucose was higher in the long-term patients, although it was lower for large MW proteins typified by alpha-2-macroglobulin. The authors suggested that these findings could be reconciled by postulating an increased peritoneal surface area over time (leading to more rapid dissipation of the glucose gradient) along with the development of submesothelial fibrosis (leading to restriction in the transport of large proteins). In keeping with their earlier observations, the authors found no difference in peritoneal transport characteristics when the long-term patients were subgrouped according to the frequency of peritonitis [151].

A prospective study of patients on CAPD found that almost equal proportions of patients developed increased compared to decreased ultrafiltration over time. These differences were apparent within the first year of treatment. In fact, the patients who eventually showed reduction in ultrfiltration had higher peritoneal permeability to solutes at the outset [152]. However, as recently reviewed by Struijk [151], many studies have documented a general trend toward loss of ultrafiltration capacity over time with an incidence varying from 1.3 to 100%. Given the change in mesothelial structure with long-term peritoneal dialysis (see Chapter 2), this finding is not unexpected.

The role of acetate in the pathogenesis of ultrafiltration failure is suspect, but uncertain. Analysis of the incidence of ultrafiltration failure showed an association between this complication and the use of acetate as the buffer anion in the dialysis fluid [153, 154]. However, the link became more complex when it was noted that not only the buffer anion but also the specific manufacturer seemed to be associated with the development of ultrafiltration failure [155]. In summary, acetate must remain suspect in the ultrafiltration abnormalities reported from Europe, although this association is certainly not universal [156]. Other factors may play a role, including the underlying cause of renal failure, a previous severe or prolonged episode of peritonitis, or intercurrent abdominal surgery.

Treatment of ultrafiltration failure entails shortening dwell time to minimize dissipation of the glucose gradient. This can be done by shorter, more frequent exchanges, or by leaving the peritoneal cavity empty overnight. Rapid cycler dialysis can be substituted for CAPD in the form of night-time intermittent peritoneal dialysis, or NIPD. A six-month peritoneal "rest" was found to restore the capacity for ultrafiltration in a patient who previously became unable to ultrafilter [157]. Finally, there are reports that oral or intraperitoneal administration of phosphatidylcholine improves ultrafiltration in peritoneal dialysis patients with impaired water transport [158]. It has been suggested that contact of phosphatidylcholine with the mesothelial cells of the peritoneum causes them to become hydrophobic [157]. Alternatively, the phosphatidylcholine may interfere with lymphatic absorption of fluid, and in this way augment net ultrafiltration [159]. However, the reports are anecdotal, and there is likely bias in reporting only successful outcomes. On the other hand, the use of phosphatidylcholine seems relatively risk-free, particularly when given orally. There appears to be little harm in trying this treatment, especially if the alternative is a major disruption in the patient's treatment by changing the modality of dialysis.

10. Sclerosing encapsulating peritonitis

This unfortunate syndrome, consisting of progressive inanition, vomiting, intermittent bowel obstruction, and decreased peritoneal transport of water and solutes, has been reported mainly from Europe [141, 160-164], although sporadic cases have been found elsewhere. At surgery or postmortem examination, the small intestine is bound or encapsulated by a thick fibrous layer, rendering the peritoneal surface opaque. The fibrous layer resembles a 'thick shaggy membrane' [141], 'marble' [165], 'cocoon' or a 'fruit rind' which may or may not peel off the bowel relatively easily [166]. The bowel so exposed may appear normal [166]. A different form of sclerosing peritonitis has been described where the diffuse sclerosing process extends transmurally with incorporation of the inner circular muscular layer and myenteric plexus of the small bowel in the fibrosing process [167].

Patients with this syndrome do poorly, with at least 50% mortality [165], probably on the basis of severe malnutrition and recurrent bowel obstruction. Those whose symptoms lead to laparotomy have a mortality rate of close to 80% [165]. The diagnosis of bowel obstruction may be delayed because the fibrosing process does not allow the bowel to distend and display the typical radiologic findings [161].

Sclerosing encapsulating peritonitis (SEP) appears to be a distinct and devastating syndrome and the name should not be used interchangeably with 'peritoneal sclerosis'. The latter term should be reserved for the finding of non-encapsulating sclerosis and fibrous adhesions associated with ultrafiltration failure. This condition is seen in patients who have had prolonged peritoneal dialysis or recurrent episodes of peritonitis, but may be present at the initiation of dialysis (see section on ultrafiltration failure). Indeed, the lack of rigorous differentiation between these two entities may confuse any attempt to define etiological factors, particularly among different dialysis centers.

The cause of SEP is uncertain. There are numerous possibilities (see Table 2). The original reports came from centers where the dialysate buffer was primarily acetate rather than lactate [141, 164]. It has been suggested that acetate may be irritating to the peritoneal membrane and perhaps initiate the fibrosing process [141, 168]. Acetate-containing dialysate exposes mesothelium to concentrations of this buffer anion that are 350-450 times that normally found in the peritoneal cavity [169]. However, SEP has also been reported in patients dialyzing with lactate [170, 171], although in some cases the disease in question may be peritoneal sclerosis [170] or transmural bowel fibrosis [167].

Recurrent peritonitis or subclinical 'grumbling' peritonitis [172] has been suggested as a cause of this distressing syndrome, although clearly many patients have never had peritonitis (detectable clinically) or had a relatively low incidence of peritonitis [164]. Alternatively, it is possible that one severe episode of peritonitis may condition the peritoneal milieu for the development of this syndrome.

Shaldon and colleagues have postulated that the

Table 2. Postulated causes of sclerosing encapsulating peritonitis.

Acetate-containing dialysate [141, 164, 168]
Recurrent peritonitis [141, 161, 170]
Plastic particles [164, 325]
Formaldehyde [164]
Bacterial filter causing upstream multiplication of bacteria with pyrogen release into peritoneum stimulating interleukin-1 production [173]
Multiple abdominal surgeries [170]
Unrecognized subclinical peritonitis with fastidious bacteria or fungi [172]
IP contamination with chlorhexidine in alcohol sprayed on connector [171, 183]
Hypertonic acidic dialysate [164]
Catheter [164, 177, 326]
Beta blockers [160, 164, 168]
High interdialytic peritoneal content of fibrinogen [166]

use of a bacterial filter in the dialysis tubing may be linked to the high incidence of SEP. They suggested that bacteria trapped upstream of the filter secrete pyrogen which crosses the filter and enters the peritoneal cavity where it stimulates macrophages to secrete interleukin-1 [173]. This lymphokine stimulates fibroblast proliferation and so could accelerate the fibrosing process. Once again, however, only some patients with SEP have used bacterial filters.

As suggested by Dobbie, however, the large molecular weight of interleukin-1 would impede its transport through or around mesothelium to affect the more deeply situated fibroblasts. In addition, histologically, loss of the normal cellular constituents appears to be more important than fibroblast proliferation in the pathogenesis of peritoneal fibrosis and sclerosis [169]. Indeed, rather than fibroblast proliferation, it may be the loss of plasminogen activation from the damaged mesothelial cells that impairs normal fibrinolysis and allows fibrosis [169]. Markedly elevated levels of Type I and Type III procollagen propeptides have been found in the peritoneal fluid of a patient who subsequently developed peritoneal fibrosis [174].

A retrospective analysis in one dialysis unit demonstrated that all the patients who developed SEP were members of a subgroup who sprayed their connectors at each exchange with 0.5% chlorhexidine in 70% alcohol [171]. The authors studied the effect of this antiseptic over the short term in a rat model and demonstrated inflammation in submesothelial tissues. The incidence of SEP in this unit has diminished since changing the antiseptic protocol. On the other hand, a study in Y-set patients observed no difference in peritoneal transport characteristics in patients with or without accidental hypochlorite infusion, or in the same patient before and after this infusion [175]. However, in the first study the patients had regular exposure to the potential contaminant, chlorhexidine, as part of their connector care, whereas in the latter study there was a one-time exposure to the disinfectant. Therefore the studies are not comparable.

The presence of the dialysis catheter in the peritoneal cavity could promote an inflammatory or foreign-body response. In this regard, a similar encapsulating peritoneal sclerosis has been described in patients with ascites in whom LeVeen shunts have been implanted [176]. Given all the patients with implanted silastic catheters, the SEP-type response is very rare. In addition, it would not explain the predilection for European centers. It is interesting, however, that localized fibrosis and peritoneal pseudocyst formation may develop in relation to the peritoneal dialysis catheter. This phenomenon has also been observed in patients with a ventriculoperitoneal shunt [177].

Other factors include the use of beta blockers, which have been linked to peritoneal sclerosis [178, 179]. Finally, there are many potentially toxic factors related to the dialysis itself, including hypertonicity and acidity of the dialysate.

Taken in sum, there is no single factor which can be incriminated in the pathogenesis of SEP. It is likely that the etiology is multifactorial. Because of the association with the use of acetate in the dialysis solution most centers avoid its use.

The radiologic picture may be suggestive. Extensive plaque-like or eggshell calcification may be more indicative of the more benign calcifying peritonitis (see below). By ultrasound, changes that have been noted in SEP include increased small bowel peristalsis, tethering of the bowel to the posterior abdominal wall, echogenic strands and new membrane formation [180]. With CT scanning, the advanced picture is characteristic (see Fig. 1). In the early stages loculated ascites, adherent bowel loops, narrowing of the bowel lumen and thickening of the peritoneal membrane may be a marker of the subsequent development of SEP, although these changes may also represent those seen with peritoneal fibrosis [181].

Even though a causal relationship has never been established with certainly, most centers have abandoned the use of acetate as dialysis buffer because of its association with the sclerosing syndromes. Similarly, after the report of the potential relationship of chlorhexidine with development of SEP, use of this antiseptic declined rapidly. Indeed, as emphasized recently by Dobbie [169], the peritoneal mesothelium is sensitive to cytotoxic and even carcinogenic effects of a wide variety of substances. The use of any agent that might enter the peritoneum must be tempered with consideration of its long-term effects on this delicate membrane.

Surgical treatment of SEP is fraught with hazard and can lead to severe bleeding. In cases of life-threatening obstruction or necrosis of bowel, however, the surgeon may have no other choice but to operate. Postoperative mortality is high. It has been suggested that in cases of bowel resection primary anastomosis is best avoided. Instead, one suggestion is that the bowel be put to rest and the patient receive parenteral alimentation before anastomosis is attempted [182].

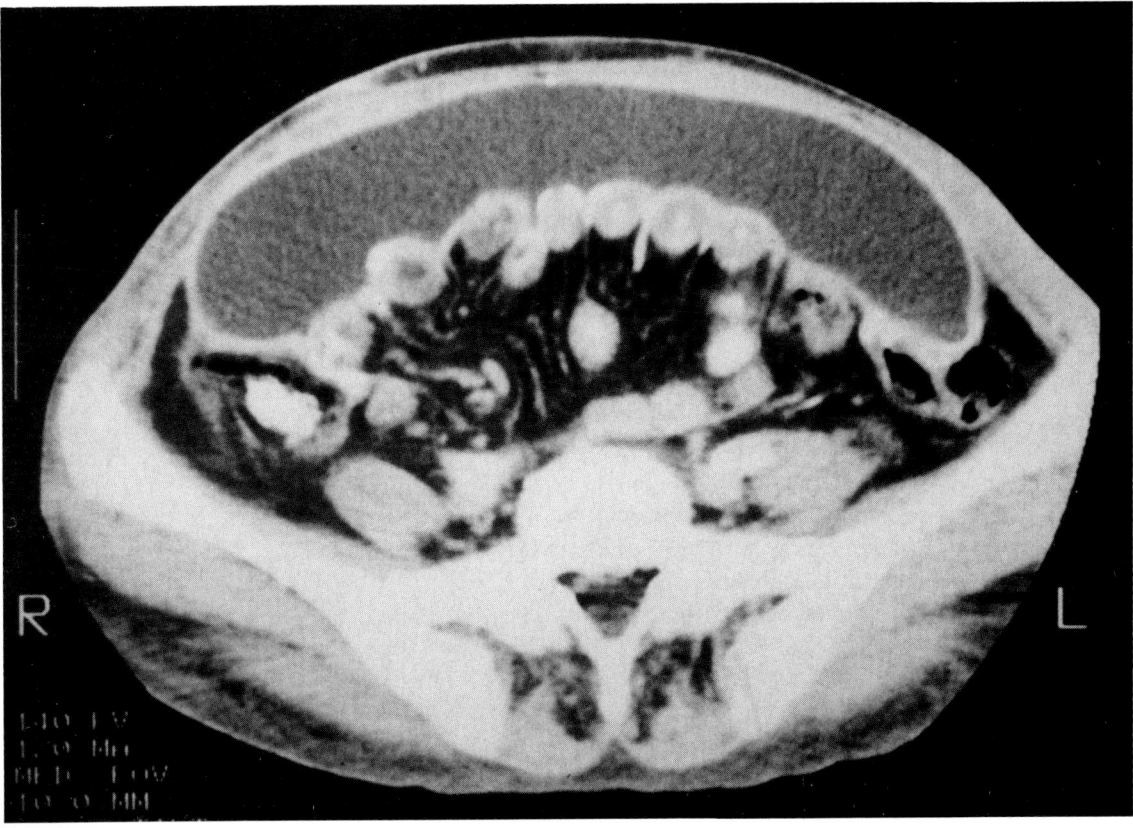

Figure 1. Computerized tomographic scan of the abdomen in a patient with sclerosing encapsulating peritonitis. Note the thickened, dense peritoneal membrane binding the bowel to the posterior aspect of the peritoneal cavity.

A very important but as yet unsolved management problem is whether the patient with early but definite SEP should be transferred to hemodialysis or deliberately maintained on peritoneal dialysis. The rationale for the latter decision is to keep bowel loops separate from one another "afloat" in dialysate so there is no opportunity for the bowel and peritoneal membrane to become matted down in the posterior peritoneum. Two of our patients with SEP appeared to develop their disease after they were transferred to hemodialysis. Others have noted that patients with chlorhexidine-associated SEP who were maintained on CAPD survived, whereas almost all of those transferred to hemodialysis died of progressive disease. The one patient who received a transplant, and presumably immunosuppression, died from intestinal obstruction (see below) [183]. Similarly, it has been noted that the onset of symptomatic SEP appeared soon after transfer to another treatment modality [184]. Therefore, while the first response would be to stop peritoneal dialysis, it is possible that the dry peritoneum can accelerate the encapsulating process.

If peritoneal transport is sufficient, a case could be made to continue peritoneal dialysis instead. However, there are too few cases documented to put forth firm recommendations.

A recent provocative report has suggested that the use of prednisone and azathioprine in patients with (mostly) chlorhexidine-associated SEP led to improved outcome with recovery of bowel function [185]. However, the report was observational and the number of patients small. If the effect is real, it is not clear whether the benefit derives from immunosuppression or the anti-inflammatory effect of the corticosteroid.

11. Calcifying peritonitis

Marichal *et al.* described 2 patients on CAPD who developed recurrent abdominal pain and incomplete bowel obstruction. Radiographs revealed multiple calcifications which had an eggshell pattern on the loops of the small bowel. One of the patients came to laparotomy, where the intestinal loops were found to be free, in contrast to the appearance in sclerosing encapsulating peritonitis. Pathologically the parietal peritoneum showed fibrous thickening and few cells. Also seen were bands of ossification and calcium deposits. The authors called this entity "progressive calcifying peritonitis". Other interesting aspects of these patients included that they dialyzed with acetate buffer, and one of the patients had hyperparathyroidism and recurrent hemoperitoneum. The patients had a benign course compared to that of sclerosing encapsulating peritonitis, and once peritoneal dialysis was discontinued bowel function improved [186].

The relatively benign outcome was substantiated by a report from Australia of a long-term CAPD patient with similar features, extensive plaque-like calcification on visceral and parietal peritoneum, and, again, hemoperitoneum. This patient had elevated levels of parathyroid hormone and increased calcium-phosphate product. After surgical excision of some of the plaques, the patient was able to return to peritoneal dialysis [187].

However, the optimistic outlook for calcifying peritonitis has been tempered by a recent report of a long-term CAPD patient who developed extensive peritoneal calcification but whose course was more typical of sclerosing encapsulating peritonitis. This patient had recurrent ileus which did not improve with transfer to hemodialysis. She ultimately sustained bowel infarction and died [188].

The etiology of calcifying peritonitis remains obscure. In the original report acetate was implicated as a cause [186] but subsecquent patients dialyzed with lactate buffer. As in the more sinister sclerosing encapsulating peritonitis, it is possible that the calcification is a reaction to multiple episodes of bacterial peritonitis. It has been suggested that hemoperitoneum could accelerate the calcification, because iron in the peritoneal cavity can serve as a nidus for precipitation of calcium [189] Not all the patients had hemoperitoneum, however.

Perhaps the likeliest cause is a disorder in the phosphate-calcium-parathyroid hormone axis. Some of the patients had markedly increased levels of PTH, and it is conceivable that the peritoneal calcification was a manifestation of calciphylaxis [190]. On the other hand, calcifying peritonitis has been reported in patients years after parathyroidectomy. In this setting it has been suggested that after parathyroidectomy the bone reverts to a low turnover state. Administration of calcium and vitamin D analogues results in extraosseous or metastatic calcification, one consequence of which is the peritoneal calcification [191].

Calcifying peritonitis has been reported so infrequently that it is difficult to provide any recommendations for management. Clearly it is advisable to avoid hypercalcemia or marked elevations of the calcium-phosphate product. It is possbile that the development of calcifying peritonitis may be an indication for parathyroidectomy if the level of hormone is markedly increased, particularly if there is uncontrolled hypercalcemia.

From the available reports it is not clear whether calcifying peritonitis is in itself an indication for transfer to hemodialysis, although the original report implied that bowel motility improved once peritoneal dialysis was stopped [186].

12. Hemoperitoneum

The presence of blood in the dialysis effluent can be distressing to the patient and a source of concern to the physician. As little as 2 mls of blood can render a litre of dialysis fluid noticeably blood-tinged [192].

Hemoperitoneum has a wide differential diagnosis, as listed in Table 3. A common and benign cause of blood in the peritoneal cavity is menstruation. In a recent review of hemoperitoneum, menstrual bleeding was the single most common cause, accounting for one third of the benign episodes [193]. The majority of regularly menstruating women on CAPD experience recurrent hemoperitoneum.

There are two mechanisms by which menstruation can lead to hemoperitoneum. If there is endometrial tissue in the peritoneal cavity, it will shed simultaneously with the intrauterine endometrium, and so bloody dialysate will occur simultaneously with menstrual flow. The alternative mechanism is that the shed uterine tissue and blood move out of both the uterine cervix and in retrograde fashion through the fallopian tubes into the peritoneal cavity. The peritoneal bleeding may start a few days prior to the appearance of blood per vagina [194]. It has been suggested that the timing of menstrual pain matches the appearance of peritoneal blood rather than vaginal menstrual flow so that the peritoneal blood may be an important cause of dysmenorrhea [194].

Women of reproductive age may also experience hemoperitoneum coincident with ovulation at midcycle [193, 195]. It is suggested that the source of blood is bleeding from the ovary with the rupture and release of the ovum. Other ovarian sources of bleeding include ruptured cysts which can bleed sufficiently to necessitate transfusion [196].

The episodes of hemoperitoneum associated with menstruation and ovulation are recognized by their periodicity and occurrence in women of reproductive age. While this cause of blood in the dialysate is considered benign, there are potential complications. The blood loss can exacerbate the anemia of chronic renal failure, and for this reason alone anovulant therapy may be indicated. A reported association between hemoperitoneum and staphylococcus epidermidis peritonitis suggests that the bloody dialysate may provide a rich growth medium for intraperitoneal bacteria. Moreover, the retrograde movement of blood from the uterine cavity through the fallopian tubes may passively carry bacteria into the peritoneum and lead to peritonitis [197, 198]. Other investigators, however, have been unable to document an increased frequency of peritonitis in relation to menstruation-generated hemoperitoneum [193].

In the patient who is not menstruating, hemoperitoneum must be carefully investigated. There are a number of surgical causes of blood in the peritoneal cavity, including cholecystitis [192], rupture of the spleen [199] and pancreatitis [193]. In these instances it should be apparent that the patient has a painful abdomen, and the localized tenderness in concert with the bloody effluent should mandate an urgent surgical consultation.

In the nondialysis patient there may be episodes of peritoneal bleeding that never come to medical attention because they are hidden from observation. The peritoneal dialysis patient, on the other hand, has a "window" into the peritoneal cavity and otherwise asymptomatic peritoneal bleeding is readily apparent. This explains the hemoperitoneum observed in patients with coagulation disorders [193, 200], polycystic kidney disease [201], post-colonoscopy [192, 193], leakage from a hematoma outside the peritoneal cavity [193, 202] and that seen after extracorporeal lithotripsy for kidney stones [203].

Recurrent hemoperitoneum may be a harbinger of disease of the peritoneal membrane itself. Bloody effluent has been described in patients with peritoneal calcification in association with hyperparathyroidism [187], in patients with radiation-induced peritoneal injury [204], and as the presenting abnormality in patients who develop sclerosing peritonitis [193, 205].

In patients with polycystic kidney disease, bleeding into a cyst can be associated with hematuria or hemoperitoneum [201]. Recently a patient with polycystic kidney disease on peritoneal dialysis was described with bloody effluent. In this case, however, the bleeding was painless, which is unusual if a kidney cyst had ruptured into the peritoneal cavity. Moreover, there was associated leukocytosis of the dialysis effluent. These unusual features lead to further investigations, which revealed that the patient had renal cell carcinoma [206]. Bloody dialysate has also been mentioned in association with adenocarcinoma of the colon [206], presumably from serosal spread of the tumour.

The patient with hemoperitoneum is at risk of the intraperitoneal blood coagulating in the catheter lumen. Therefore, it has been recommended to use intraperitoneal heparin 500–1000 U/L for as long as the dialysate still has visible blood or fibrin. In our experience the intraperitoneal heparin doesn't

Table 3. Causes of Hemoperitoneum.

Gynecologic
Menstruation [194, 195, 197]
Ovulation [195]
Bleeding ovarian cysts [193, 195, 196]

Neoplastic
Renal cell carcinoma [206]
Adenocarcinoma of colon [206]

Polycystic kidney disease [201]

Hematologic
Idiopthic thrombocytopenic purpura [193, 200]
Anticoagulant therapy [193]

Peritoneal membrane disease
Peritoneal calcification [187]
Radiation-induced peritoneal fibrosis [204]
Sclerosing peritonitis [193, 205]

Gastrointestinal
Acute cholecystitis [192]
Post-colonoscopy {192, 193]
Intraperitoneal connective tissue pouch [208]
Catheter-induced splenic rupture [199]
Pancreatitis [193]

Miscellaneous
Leakage from extraperitoneal hematoma [193, 202]
Tuberous sclerosis [209]
IgA nephritis [210]
Mixed connective tissue disease [211]
Extracorporeal lithotripsy [203]

worsen the bleeding nor lead to systemic anticoagulation. In some instances of hemoperitoneum the use of rapid exchanges with dialysate at room temperature leads to rapid resolution of the bleeding. It is postulated that the relatively cool dialysate induces peritoneal vasoconstriction and this leads to hemostasis [207].

13. Chyloperitoneum

The influx of triglyceride-rich chylomicrons into the peritoneal cavity is the result of interruption of the lymphatic drainage from the gut to the main lymphatic trunks. Compromise of the integrity of these lymphatic channels is most commonly the result of neoplasm, particularly lymphoma [212–214].

After a fatty meal, long-chain fatty acids are incorporated into chylomicrons, which enter the lymphatic circulation. Therefore chyloperitoneum is an intermittent event, occurring after the ingestion of fat and clearing sometime afterward. Because medium-chain triglycerides are not absorbed through the lymphatic channels, chylous complications have been treated by prescribing a diet in which fat is delivered in this form [215] thus obviating the need for lymphatic drainage of triglyceride.

In the patient not on peritoneal dialysis, chylous ascites is likely to present as increasing abdominal girth and peripheral edema [212]. For the patient on peritoneal dialysis, chyloperitoneum presents as milky-white effluent which can be mistaken for peritonitis.

Chyloperitoneum has been reported to be present at the time of insertion of the peritoneal catheter [216], or in the days to months after its insertion [217, 218]. The diagnosis is suggested by the white, milky appearance of the dialysate in conjunction with the absence of any indication of peritonitis. Lipoprotein electrophoresis showed lipid staining at the origin, characteristic of chylomicrons [216]. When the dialysate was separated into layers upon standing, the supernatant stained positively for fat with sudan black, and dissolved with ether [216, 217]. The triglyceride level of the dialysate was greater than the plasma triglyceride level, a characteristic of intestinal lymph [214].

The etiology of chyloperitoneum is obscure. In each case there must be communication between the peritoneal lymphatics and peritoneal cavity. The dialysis catheter or its trochar could sever a lymph vessel. Multiple previous episodes of peritonitis could result in peritoneal adhesions and lymphatic obstruction. In the non-dialysis patient bacterial peritonitis has been incriminated in the pathogenesis of chylous ascites and encapsulating peritonitis [219].

We recently puzzled over a CAPD patient who presented with recurrent episodes of cloudy peritoneal dialysate associated with low peritoneal cell counts and sterile bacteriologic cultures. Investigation revealed extensive retroperitoneal lymphoma and the episodes of cloudy dialysate likely represented chyloperitoneum. This phenomenon should be part of the differential diagnosis of "culture-negative" peritonitis.

14. Acquired cystic disease of the kidney

Acquired renal cystic disease (ARCD) is the term used to describe the progressive replacement of renal parenchyma by cysts in patients with chronic renal failure. This phenomenon was initially described in patients receiving chronic hemodialysis [220]. It had been suggested that a retained uremic toxin or one unique to hemodialysis stimulated cystic transformation in the endstage kidney [221]. However, in a manner similar to that seen with "hemodialysis-associated amyloid", it has become clear that ARCD is in no way unique to the subset of the population with chronic renal failure that receives hemodialysis. This complication has been reported in patients with renal failure who have never undergone dialysis and in patients on peritoneal dialysis who were never exposed to hemodialysis [222, 223]. These observations suggest that factor(s) in the uremic milieu are probably responsible for cystic transformation rather than something particular to the dialysis process itself.

At present there have been reports of ARCD in approximately 200 CAPD patients [224]. As in the hemodialysis literature, there is great variation reported for the prevalence of this condition. This variation is the result of the method used to diagnose ARCD i.e. postmortem examination of the kidneys versus ultrasound, the particular population being studied, and the criteria used for making the diagnosis. In a recent review by Ishikawa, the reported prevalence of this condition in CAPD patients varied from 3 to 100% with a mean prevalence of 41%. Methods of diagnosis included ultrasound, CT scanning, MRI and postmortem studies [224].

In comparing the prevalence of ARCD in hemodialysis and CAPD patients, a number of confounding factors need to be recognized. Cystic transformation has been reported to be more common in males than in females [225, 226]. Moreover, it has been associated with increasing age [225, 227] and with longer duration of dialysis [226, 228] (The latter factor likely explains why ARCD was described earlier in hemodialysis than in peritoneal dialysis patients, because there is a greater prevalence of long-term hemodialysis patients.) Therefore any comparison must take into account the patients' age and sex and duration of dialysis before the actual mode of dialysis can be implicated in facilitating cystic change. With these limitations in mind surveys of dialysis patients suggest that the prevalence of ARCD averages about 40–50% and is independent of the mode of dialysis [224, 225, 227].

14.1. Neoplastic transformation

In dialysis patients with ARCD, there is a small but significant risk of the development of renal malignancy. The prevalence of renal cancer will again vary depending on the method of detection. A recent review noted a prevalence of 1.3% for renal malignancy in a dialysis population with ARCD [229], which is a two-fold risk compared to renal failure patients without ARCD [230]. In CAPD patients, however, the incidence is 0.4%, or 2 out of 475 patients examined in one group analysis [224]. Overall, there are few reports of renal cell malignancy complicating ARCD in peritoneal dialysis patients, and two rare instances of metastatic disease. In one case the renal neoplasm was a poorly differentiated transitional cell carcinoma, and analgesic abuse could not be effectively ruled out as a causative factor [231]. In another instance, however, renal cell carcinoma was confirmed in a nephrectomy specimen with ARCD and subsequently hepatic metastases occurred [230].

The lower incidence of renal neoplasia in peritoneal dialysis patients with ARCD, when viewed in an optimistic light, might reflect the better-preserved immune function seen in these patients compared to those receiving hemodialysis (see below). In other words, tumour surveillance may be more effective as a result of improved immune function. Alternatively, peritoneal dialysis may provide some protection against exposure to potentially inflammatory or teratogenic agents which might occur with extracorporeal dialysis. On the other hand, it may simply be that the index of suspicion is lower in those managing patients on peritoneal dialysis consequent to the paucity of reports of renal neoplasms in this group [230–233].

Many reports of neoplastic transformation in dialysis patients with ARCD conclude by advising "regular" or annual surveillance by ultrasound. However, this approach must be tempered by consideration of the enormous cost involved to do this compared to the low incidence of renal cancer and even lower incidence of metastatic disease in the population of peritoneal dialysis patients. Perhaps, as suggested by Ishikawa [224], only those at high risk should be screened, that is, men on long-term CAPD with extensive cystic transformation of the kidneys.

14.2. Other complications

There have been reports of spontaneous hemorrhage into the cysts of PD patients with ARCD [233, 234]. This may occur less frequently than in hemodialysis because of the reduced need for systemic anticoagulation [224].

15. Pruritus

The sensation of itch commonly accompanies chronic uremia and is not necessarily ameliorated by dialysis therapy. To the dialysis patient, itch may range from a mild distraction to a burden sufficient to induce suicide.

Despite investigations along a number of different routes, the etiology of uremic pruritus remains obscure. Patients with chronic renal failure often have dry skin, or xerosis, and this condition contributes to itching in some [235].

Hyperparathyroidism and abnormalities in divalent iron metabolism have been implicated in uremic pruritus. It has been observed that itching will often dramatically improve in hyperparathyroid dialysis patients after removal of the parathyroid glands [236]. However, the correlation between parathyroid gland hypersecretion and pruritus is not tight; although studies have demonstrated that patients with itch overall have higher levels of parathyroid hormone, there is no correlation between the severity of pruritus and levels of the hormone [237]. Moreover, studies of skin mineral content in pruritic and non-pruritic dialysis patients have been conflicting [237].

The role of histamine is also not clear. It is recognized to cause itching in allergic skin reactions and has long been suspected to play a role in uremic pruritus. Mast cells, which release histamine, have been found in increased numbers in the skin of uremics [238, 239]. However, other studies could not confirm the increase in skin mast cells nor the relationship between plasma histamine levels and itch [240].

There are theoretical reasons why pruritus might be less prevalent and less severe in patients on CAPD compared to those on hemodialysis. Reactions with the extracorporeal circuit, including the sterilizers and plasticizers, are known to be immunogenic and can sometimes produce hypersensitivity reactions. If middle molecule retention is important in the pathogenesis of pruritus, it might be anticipated that the better clearance of these molecules by peritoneal dialysis may afford protection against pruritus [239]. Finally, improved divalent ion metabolism and control of hyperparathyroidism with CAPD (see Chapter 18) might also be expected to correlate with a reduced prevalence of pruritus. A study of severe pruritis in dialysis patients found a lower prevalence in CAPD compared to hemodialysis [241]. However, more recent surveys have been unable to document any difference in this complaint between the two dialysis modalities [240, 242]. Plasma histamine levels were not different among CAPD, hemodialysis or predialysis patients and there was no correlation between these levels and the extent of itch [240]. Perhaps the intervening appearance of high flux dialyzers and more careful management of calcium and phosphate have resulted in a more equal distribution of pruritic complaints among hemodialysis and peritoneal dialysis patients related to other, as yet unknown, factors.

Trying to study the treatment of pruritus is fraught with hazard. Meaurement is confounded by its subjective nature, the absence of animal models, and the lack of validated measurements. The effect of treatment is subject to bias on the part of investigator and patient [243]. It is likely that the placebo effect is significant.

Measures to relieve pruritus have included moisturizing agents for the skin, activated oral charcoal, cholestyramine, intravenous lidocaine, antihistaminics, the mast cell stabilizer ketotifen, and parathyroidectomy in these with evidence of hyperparathyroidism [244].

Many studies have reported relief of pruritus with ultraviolet phototherapy. The mechanism of this effect is unknown. A recent meta-analysis of published trials for uremic pruritus found that only ultraviolet B phototherapy fulfilled the criteria for clinically significant improvement. While noting that many of the studies were flawed, the authors concluded that this phototherapy was the treatment of choice in moderate to severe uremic pruritus. The effects of lidocaine, charcoal and nicergoline were statistically but not clinically significant, and the effect of the bile acid sequestrant cholestyramine was clinically insignificant [243].

16. Dialysis-associated amyloidosis

In the 1980s a new constellation of musculoskeletal disorders was described, including carpal tunnel syndrome, subchondral bone cysts, spondyloarthropathy and pathological fractures. These abnormalities could not be linked to hyperparathyroidism or aluminum intoxication [reviewed in 245]. The finding of amyloid deposits in the involved tissues led to the term "hemodialysis-associated amyloidosis". Subsequently, the amyloid was found to be composed of beta-2-microglobulin (B_2M) [246, 247].

This protein is a B cell product and is present on almost all cell membranes. It is measurable in plasma. These levels may be the result of production of the molecule by lymphocytes, or from normal cell turnover and release of membrane constituents. It is freely filtered at the glomerulus and absorbed and catabolized in the proximal tubule. With renal insufficiency, the filtration and catabolism of B_2M decreases and plasma levels increase.

Since the musculoskeletal syndrome was originally described exclusively in long term hemodialysis patients, many factors related to hemodialysis were postulated to play a role in the formation of B_2M amyloid. Firstly, B_2M levels were markedly elevated in long-term hemodialysis patients, especially in those patients using small pore membranes and those with negligible endogenous renal function. Secondly, the stimulation of the immune system by the repeated interface of blood with artificial membranes was postulated to lead to increased production of B_2M [245].

Serum levels of B_2M are also very high in patients receiving peritoneal dialysis, although not as high as levels in hemodialysis patients [248–250]. Explanations put forth to explain the discrepancy include better clearance of this middle molecule by the peritoneal than by the hemodialysis membrane [251], the lack of immune stimulation using the peritoneal membrane, and, in long-term patients, better preservation of endogenous renal function [252].

However, by the mid-1980's presumptive evidence of B_2M amyloidosis in CAPD patients began to emerge. The prevalence of carpal tunnel syndrome, subclinical median mononeuropathy, bone cysts, discitis and cervical spondyloarthropathy suggested that peritoneal dialysis patients were not protected from this articular complication [250, 253–256]. Subsequently B_2M amyloid was isolated from the tenosynovium of a long-term CAPD patient undergoing surgical release for a carpal tunnel syndrome [257]. Large interstitial B_2-M amyloid deposits were also isolated from the synovial tissue of the hip of a long-term CAPD patient undergoing prosthetic hip replacement [258]. Finally, postmortem studies in long-term peritoneal dialysis patients have confirmed the deposition of this type of amyloid in the intervertebral discs of the lumbosacral spine [259], the synovium of the scapulohumeral joint, hip and wrist [260] and the capsules of the shoulder joint and periarticular tissues [261].

A worrisome manifestation of B_2M amyloidosis is destructive cervical spondyloarthropathy. Again this complication had hitherto been documented only in long-term hemodialysis patients [262]. However, in our institution a patient who had received CAPD for 13 years developed this spondyloarthropathy, complicated by a compressive myelopathy. The cartilage removed at the time of fusion grafting was positive for amyloid composed of B_2-M (Fig. 2) [263].

In summary, levels of B_2M in patients on peritoneal dialysis are lower than those in patients receiving hemodialysis with conventional membranes. However, these levels are still much higher than those seen in controls. The relative paucity of reports of dialysis-associated amyloid in CAPD patients does not necessarily reflect a proportionately lower incidence of this arthropathy. There are fewer long-term peritoneal dialysis patients compared to hemodialysis patients. The level of suspicion for this complication may not be as high in those treating CAPD patients. In the coming years, as the proportion of long-term CAPD patients increases, we will likely witness a marked increase in the diagnosis of B_2M amyloidosis in this group.

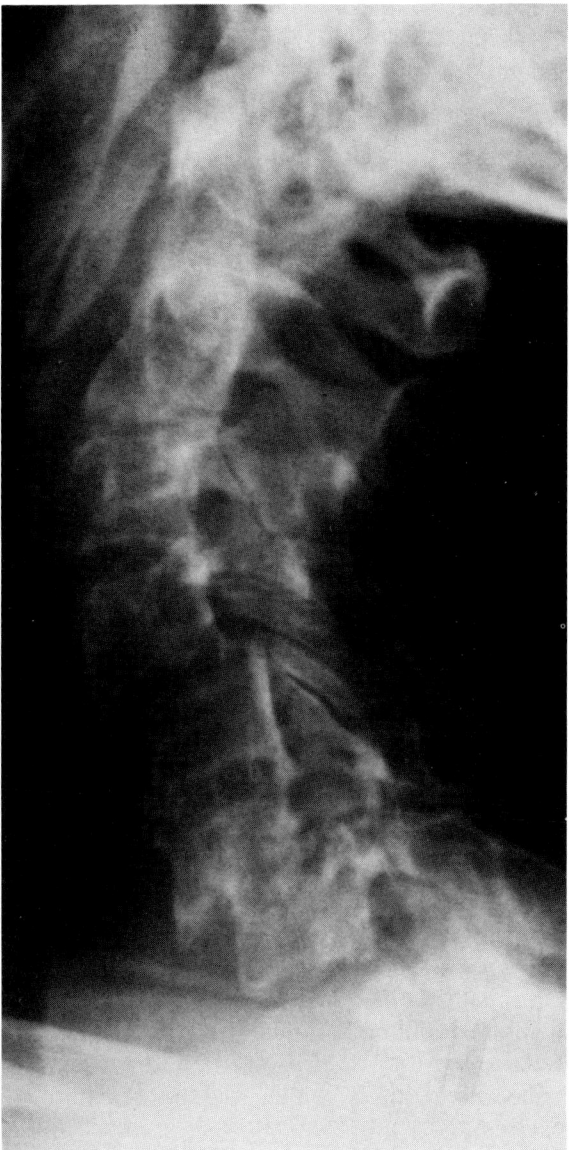

Figure 2. Radiograph of the cervical spine in a long-term CAPD patient who developed destructive spondyloarthropathy. Analysis of resected vertebral tissue revealed amyloid composed of B-2 microglobulin.

17. Tendonitis, tendon rupture and calcific periarthritis

Spontaneous tendon rupture can occur in dialysis patients and may be associated with hyperparathyroidism and osteodystrophy [264]. This complication has been described mainly in patients undergoing hemodialysis. However, we have seen a young patient on CAPD with rupture of the quadriceps femoris tendon. Bilateral rupture of the tendon of the long head of the biceps muscle has also been described [265] and was attributed to the strain of the spiking and hanging of the two-litre bag.

Lateral epicondylitis or "spike elbow" has also been described in CAPD [266]. This inflammation may be an overuse syndrome caused by the repetitive insertion of the spike with a twisting and pushing motion.

Calcific periarthritis has also been well described in patients on dialysis, although, again, it has been more frequently reported in patients on hemodialysis. Deposits of hydroxyapatite, calcium pyrophosphate dihydrate (CPPD) or calcium oxalate [267] can accumulate around the joints and led to acute attacks of synovitis or periarticular inflammation. This sydrome has been associated with an elevated calcium-phosphorus product and hyperparathyroidism. In CAPD patients there is no correlation between levels of PTH and periarticular calcification [268]. Similarly, there is no association between inflammatory arthritis or periarthritis and PTH-induced subperiosteal resorption in peritoneal dialysis patients. Furthermore, changing patients from intermittent to continuous peritoneal dialysis with improvement in the calcium-phosphorus product had no salutary effect on the arthritis or periarthritis [269]. These findings suggest that the calcific periarthritis may be related to factors other than parathyroid overactivity or increased calcium-phosphorus product. In a recent report a young lupus patient on CAPD with only modest elevation in the calcium-phosphorus product developed severe progressive calcific periarthritis resembling tumoral calcinosis which had to be surgically excised [270].

18. Back pain

The instillation of dialysis fluid into the peritoneal cavity can lead to alteration in spinal mechanics in the upright posture. In the patient with lax abdominal musculature, the abdomen protrudes under the weight and volume of dialysate, and this swings the centre of gravity anteriorly. The normal lumbar lordosis is inappropriately accentuated.

Many patients entering peritoneal dialysis programs are elderly, or have been deconditioned by years of illness and poor nutrition. Moreover, some patients have had treatment with corticosteroids or have undergone previous abdominal surgery. It is not surprising, therefore, that the abdominal musculature is often weak, leading to the alteration in spinal mechanics outlined above. In addition, the elderly uremic patient may be at risk for degenerative disc disease, spondylolysis, spondylolisthesis and osteoporosis. Therefore the combination of intraperitoneal fluid, poor abdominal muscle tone and intrinsic disease of the spinal column may culminate in back pain. This pain may be the result of paraspinal muscle spasm, posterior facet disease or sciatica [271].

Treatment includes simple back education, where the patient learns the appropriate way to stand, bend over, and so on, in a way to minimize strain on the back. Pelvic tilt exercises are simple and can be performed by patients on peritoneal dialysis [271].

In the patient complaining of persistent back pain, further evaluation is warranted. This includes vertebral radiographs to evaluate the bony structures. The opinion of a rheumatologist or physiatrist may be necessary. The dialysis regimen can be altered to use small volumes of dialysate in conjunction with more frequent exchanges to avoid underdialysis. Judicious use of skeletal muscle relaxants or anti-inflammatory agents may be necessary for short-term relief of symptoms. Dialysis in the supine position removes the lordotic stress to the lumbar vertebrae. Consideration should be given to dialysing the patient with persistent back pain in this position, employing night-time cycler peritoneal dialysis. The patient should have an empty peritoneal cavity or a minimal volume of dialysate during the daytime upright activities. With this regimen the adverse effect of intraperitoneal fluid on spinal mechanics is minimized and the patient may be able to successfully perform peritoneal dialysis.

19. Oxalate metabolism and kidney stones

Oxalate is freely filtered at the glomerulus and secreted in the proximal tubule. As renal function deteriorates, oxalate retention and hyperoxalemia supervene [272]. The retained oxalate is deposited as the poorly-soluble calcium salt in kidney, bone, hyaline and fibrocartilage, myocardium, lungs, central nervous system and blood vessels [reviewed in 264]. Chondrocalcinosis and pseudogout can be caused by calcium oxalate as well as calcium pyrophosphate dihydrate in patients with end stage renal disease [267].

In patients on CAPD, plasma levels of oxalate are three to five times higher than in controls [273] and are equivalent to predialysis levels in hemodialysis patients [274]. Because of its low molecular weight (90 daltons) it is rapidly cleared during hemodialysis and levels fall about 40%. On the other hand, CAPD clears about 300 µmol/day, which approximates the amount synthesized daily. Therefore, CAPD can maintain steady state plasma levels of oxalate, but at levels much higher than normal [274–276]. Previous studies of oxalate removal by peritoneal dialysis should be interpreted in the light of the recent finding of rising oxalate levels in the drained effluent, suggesting ongoing production of oxalate *ex vivo* in the dialysate [276]. Furthermore, ascorbic acid supplements cause a further increase in plasma oxalate levels. In a recent study, 100 mg of oral ascorbic acid resulted in nearly a 20% increase in plasma levels of oxalate [276].

In patients on CAPD taking vitamins, the benefit of vitamin C supplements should be weighed against the potential hazard of further elevating plasma oxalate values. These patients have normal plasma levels of ascorbic acid before receiving supplementation, so there may not be a need for vitamin C treatment. Concurrent treatment with 10 mg of vitamin B6 results in a 17% decrease in oxalate levels in patients already taking ascorbic acid, but these levels remain markedly elevated [276].

A significant number of patients on CAPD will pass kidney stones. In one survey [277], ten of 186 CAPD patients (5.4%) passed renal calculi after six to nine months on CAPD. Half of these stones were composed of calcium oxalate monohydrate and the rest were made of protein matrix alone or calcium apatite. Metabolic investigation of CAPD patients has demonstrated that, while the total excretion of calcium and oxalate is necessarily diminished, the concentration of oxalate is significantly elevated compared to normals and the ionic calcium concentration in the urine is lower than normal. However, the calcium oxalate activity product is in the 'labile' region and varies according to the urinary ionic calcium concentration. This dependence upon urinary calcium is differnt from normals, where the calcium oxalate activity product depends upon the concentration of both urinary oxalate and calcium. Therefore, although the urine ionic calcium concentration is low in renal failure, relative increases in this level will significantly influence the activity product and lead to crystallization. The administration of 1,25-dihydroxyvitamin D3 correlates with the urine ionic calcium concentration [277] and could be considered a risk factor for stone formation. With the move from aluminum-containing to calcium-containing phosphate binders, it will be interesting to see whether the incidence of calcium-containing stones increases in CAPD patients.

Interestingly, intraluminal lithiasis should be kept in mind as a rare cause of obstruction of the peritoneal dialysis catheter. A recent report demonstrated the impaction of a calcium-struvite calculus in the intraperitoneal tip of the catheter lumen. The authors suggested that a fibrin clot could have adhered to the catheter and served as a nidus for mineralization in this patient with an elevated calcium-phosphate product [278].

20. Immune function

It is difficult to arrive at any sound conclusion about the immunocompetence of patients on dialysis. It is even more difficult to compare immune function of patients on peritoneal dialysis with those receiving hemodialysis. As pointed out by Schollmeyer *et al.*, the experimental design and techniques used in different studies are not always comparable. The groups being compared may not be matched by age, sex, underlying disease, or length of time on dialysis [279]. Moreover, it is problematic to try to extrapolate from a single *in vitro* test a complex multifaceted *in vivo* immune response.

The abnormal immune response of uremia persists even in patients receiving what is considered to be adequate dialysis. It is possible that retained middle molecules may be responsible for the ongoing alteration in immune function. Since CAPD clears more of these molecules than does conventional hemodialysis, immune function may be more normal in patients on CAPD. On the other hand, about thirty to forty million peritoneal monocytes may be drained every day with the dialysate [280]. In addition, the same procedure may remove a significant amount of immunoglobulin [281]. Therefore, the CAPD patient could actually have compromised immune function as a result of these losses.

The uremic state is associated with T cell lymphopenia. However, upon starting CAPD the number of these cells normalize in the majority after a few months [282, 283] whereas a similar change is not seen in patients on hemodialysis or hemofiltration [282]. Not all studies have confirmed normalization of the number of T lymphocytes in CAPD patients [284, 285]. Peritoneal dialysis effluent inhibits E-rossette formation of normal lymphocytes. This inhibitory factor has a molecular weight of less than 500 daltons [283]. Since it is removed by peritoneal dialysis, the assumption is that immune function is improved by this procedure.

The ratio of 'helper/inducer' or CD4 T lymphocytes to 'suppressor/cytotoxic' or CD8 lymphocytes in CAPD patients is normal [283, 286] although a trend toward an increased ratio has been described, both as a result of higher CD4(+) lymphocytes [284] and lower CD8(+) lymphocytes [284, 287]. It is not clear to what extent therapy with 1,25-dihydroxyvitamin D3, which increases CD4:CD8 ratios, may have played in these results [288].

The in vitro proliferative response to the mitogens phytohemagglutinin and concanavalin A is less than [287] or the same as [289] that in nonuremic controls, and is better than the proliferative response in hemodialysis patients [287, 289]. Furthermore, while this response diminishes over time in patients on hemodialysis, they remain stable or improve on CAPD [284, 287]. The mixed lymphocyte response in CAPD patients is subnormal, but better than that seen in hemodialysis patients.

Other tests of T-cell function show that the delayed hypersensitivity response to intradermal antigens such as PPD or DNCB is better preserved in CAPD compared to hemodialysis [286]. Patients regain cutaneous reactivity over time on CAPD, but stay anergic on hemodialysis [282]. A xenogeneic graft-versus-host reaction improved over time in nondiabetic patients on CAPD [285].

The number of B lymphocytes are normal [282] or less than normal on CAPD [284]. Despite ongoing losses in the effluent, there is no parallel fall in serum immunoglobulin concentration in adults [282, 284]. However, children on peritoneal dialysis may be prone to hypogammaglobulinemia. In this population, daily loss of immunoglobulin into the effluent can be as high as 30% of the daily synthetic rate of IgG [290]. In addition, impaired synthesis of immunoglobulin may contribute to the low serum levels in these infants [291]. The hypogammaglobulinemia may render these infants susceptible to infection. Interestingly, all children in one study developed protective antibody responses to immunization [290] despite the low circulating immunoglobulin levels. Unlike hemodialysis patients, adults on CAPD also develop protective antibody responses to vaccination [292]. The level of circulating immune complexes, as measured by the C1q binding assay, is increased in CAPD patients when compared to controls, but less than the levels found in hemodialysis patients [293]. Uremics may be unable to eliminate antigens as well as nonuremics. The persisting antigens induce antibody formation with the subsequent development of immune complexes. The clinical significance of these complexes is unclear.

In summary, in vitro studies suggest that the patient on CAPD has more normal immune responses compared to patients on hemodialysis. The observation of flares of disease in patients with previously inactive systemic lupus erythematosus when starting CAPD or changing from hemodialysis to CAPD supports this asumption [294, 295]. On the other hand, a recent study found that there was no difference in disease activity or amount of medication used in lupus patients on CAPD versus hemodialysis, although low platelet counts and elevated levels of anti-double-stranded DNA were still found more frequently in the CAPD patients [296]. With the new generation of hemodialysis membranes, the greater clearance of middle molecules may result in better-preserved immune function, and results of in vitro testing and in vivo observations reported above may start to approach those seen in peritoneal dialysis patients and nonuremic controls.

21. Transplantation

As reviewed in this chapter and elsewhere [297, 298] the patient on CAPD may be more immunocompetent than the patient receiving hemodialysis. Theoretically, this more "normal" immune response may predispose the patient to rejection of a renal allograft.

Two early reports led to concern. A significant increase in the helper to suppressor T lymphocyte ratio in patients on long-term CAPD was associated with an increased incidence of graft rejection when compared to hemodialysis patients [299]. Similarly, a second study found decreased graft survival in patients previously receiving CAPD when compared to those on hemodialysis. This decreased survival was apparent as early as one month post-transplant. Again, the patients who had been on peritoneal dialysis had a higher ratio of circulating helper T lymphocytes and did not display the T-cell lymphopenia found in the hemodialysis patients [300]. Although the implication is that the increased ratio of circulating T lymphocytes is linked with graft rejection, it has not been demonstrated that the ratio of helper to suppressor T lymphocytes bears any consistent relationship to graft outcome [297]. Unlike hemodialysis patients, CAPD patients did not benefit from pre-transplant blood transfusions [300]. Indeed, a fall in panel reactive antibodies was noted in three children with their conversion from hemodialysis to peritoneal dialysis, which was attributed to a reduced need for blood transfusion during the latter treatment [301].

Since these two reports, many centers have compared patient and graft outcome in their peritoneal dialysis and hemodialysis patients. While there is some variation from center to center, there does not appear to be any consistent trend in the survival of either graft or patient between the two modalities of dialysis [302–313]. Many of the studies consisted of small numbers of peritoneal dialysis patients, which limits the power of statistical analysis and increases the chance of beta error. However, as pointed out in a recent review [298] even the studies involving large numbers of peritoneal dialysis patients have shown similar, if not identical, graft and patient survival. It is conceivable that the intense immunosuppressive therapy given to transplant patients negates any modest difference in innate immunocompetence between the two dialysis modalities.

The peritoneal dialysis patient may face extra risk of infection from the peritoneal cavity and catheter. Previous episodes of peritonitis could leave a nucleus of infection which could develop into overwhelming sepsis. The development of peritonitis could pose a life-threatening complication in patients receiving immunosuppressive drugs [302]. The incidence of peritonitis in the post-transplant period does appear to be significant, varying from 5 to 35% if the patient needs to resume peritoneal dialysis because of graft non-function [306, 309, 312]. Peritonitis is easily managed by antibiotics, lavage, and catheter removal if necessary [302, 304, 314] although in one patient it led to death from sepsis [307]. The simultaneous administration of cytotoxic agents does not hamper the response of bacterial peritonitis to antibiotic therapy.

Most centers electively remove the peritoneal dialysis catheter about two to three months post-transplant [303, 304, 306, 314, 315] although some remove it at the time of transplant and hemodialyze the patient as needed thereafter [316]. Because of the risk of bowel perforation, an unused catheter should be flushed regularly and removed no later than two to three months after successful transplantation. In patients with simultaneous transplant of kidney and pancreas, the catheter should be removed at surgery since the pancreas is placed intraperitoneally [298].

Post-transplant ascites has been reported in children [317] and adults [318] who were on CAPD before the transplant. In adults the ascites lasted up to 50 days, but ultimately resolved [318].

Finally, there is the risk of mechanical problems in the peritoneal dialysis patient undergoing transplant. The catheter exit site can be close to the transplant bed. (Initial implantation sites of peritoneal dialysis catheters should be chosen with this potential problem in mind.) If the peritoneum has not been disrupted during transplant surgery, peritoneal dialysis can be performed postoperatively if necessary. There have been reports of drainage of dialysate through the transplant incision [307, 309] and through the site of a transplant nephrectomy [308]. This complication is managed by temporarily stopping peritoneal dialysis and providing antibiotic coverage.

22. Cancer

As reviewed above, changes in immune function can be demonstrated in patients with chronic renal failure on dialysis. Since one important immune function is tumour surveillance, it is possible that impaired tumour surveillance exists in these patients and as such they are at increased risk for neoplasm. However, careful study of this risk is fraught with epidemiological hazard. Appropriate controls matched for age, sex, race and time are needed. Detection bias in a carefully followed dialysis population would mistakenly lead to the assumption of a higher cancer rate. For example, a recent survey of hemodialysis patients in Japan showed a higher incidence of cancer in patients dialyzing at university-affiliated hospitals rather than private hospitals. The authors suggested that closer follow-up and higher autopsy rates were responsible for this difference [319].

In a review of 328 CAPD patients at one institution, nine patients developed cancer after a mean duration of 21 months [320]. Three of these patients had received immunosuppressive drugs. If all nine patients are considered, there was a trend for a higher incidence of cancer in patients on CAPD, which was not statistically significant compared to the general population. If the three patients who received the immunosuppressive medications are excluded from the analysis, there was no difference in the incidence of cancer between the CAPD and matched general population. This negative finding could be a function of the relative small number of patients surveyed. On the other hand, it may reflect better immunocompetence in this population compared to patients on hemodialysis or with chronic renal failure not receiving dialysis.

Acknowledgements

The author thanks Maureen M. Kiely for excellent secretarial assistance.

References

1. Gotloib L, Mines M, Garmizo L, Varka I. Hemodynamic effects of increasing intra-abdominal pressure in peritoneal dialysis. Perit Dial Bull 1981; 1: 41–4.
2. Twardowski Z, Khanna R, Nolph K et al. Intraabdominal pressures during natural activities in patients treated with continuous ambulatory peritoneal dialysis. Nephron 1986; 44: 129–35.
3. Durand PY, Chanliau J, Gamberoni J, Hestin D, Kessler M. Routine measurement of hydrostatic intraperitoneal pressure. In Khanna R, Nolph KD, Prowant BF, Twardowski ZJ, Oreopoulos DG, eds. Advances in Peritoneal Dialysis. University of Toronto Press, Toronto 1992; 8: 108–12.
4. O'Connor J, Rigby R, Hardie I et al. Abdominal hernias complicating continuous ambulatory peritoneal dialysis. Am J Nephrol 1986; 6: 271–4.
5. Digenis G, Khanna R, Mathews R, Oreopoulos DG. Abdominal hernias in patients undergoing continuous ambulatory peritoneal dialysis. Perit Dial Bull 1982; 2: 115–7.
6. Rubin J, Raju S, Teal N, Hellems E, Bower J. Abdominal hernia in patients undergoing continuous ambulatory peritoneal dialysis. Arch Intern Med 1982; 142: 1453–5.
7. Kauffman H, Adams M. Indirect inguinal hernia in patients undergoing peritoneal dialysis. Surgery 1986; 99: 254–5.
8. Engeset J, Youngson G. Ambulatory peritoneal dialysis and hernial complications. Surg Clin North Am 1984; 64: 385–92.
9. Rocco M, Stone W. Abdominal hernias in chronic peritoneal dialysis patients: A review. Perit Dial Bull 1985; 5: 171–4.
10. Tzamaloukas A, Bevan M, Cox B et al. Clinical associations and effects of hernias in CAPD patients (Abstract). Perit Dial Bull 1986; 6 (suppl): S21.
11. Wise M, Manos, J, Gokal R. Small umbilical hernias in patients on CAPD (letter). Perit Dial Bull 1984; 4: 270–1.
12. Wetherington G, Leapman S, Robinson R, Filo RS. Abdominal wall and inguinal hernias in continuous ambulatory peritoneal dialysis patients. Am J Surg 1985; 150: 357–60.
13. Modi KB, Grant AC, Garret A, Rodger RSC. Indirect inguinal hernia in CAPD patients with polycystic kidney disease. In: Khanna R, Nolph KD, Prowant BF, Twardowski ZJ, Oreopoulos DG (eds), Advances in Peritoneal Dialysis. University of Toronto Press, Toronto 1989; 5: 84–6.
14. Apostolidis NS, Tzardis PJ, Manouras AJ, Kosenidou MD, Katirtzoglou AN. The incidence of postoperative hernia as related to the site of insertion of permanent peritoneal catheter. Am Surgeon 1988; 54: 318–9.
15. Spence P, Mathews R, Khanna R, Oreopoulos DG. Improved results with a paramedian technique for the insertion of peritoneal dialysis catheters. Surg Gynecol Obstet 1985; 161: 585–7.
16. Khoury AE, Charendoff J, Balfe JW, McLorie GA, Churchill BM. Hernias associated with CAPD in children. In: Khanna R, Nolph KD, Prowant BF, Twardowski ZJ, Oreopoulos DG (eds), Advances in Peritoneal Dialysis. University of Toronto Press, Toronto 1991; 7: 279–82.
17. Ramos, J, Burke D, Veitch P. Hernia of Morgagni in patients on continuous ambulatory peritoneal dialysis (letter). Lancet 1982; 1: 161–2.
18. Grossi C, Faiolo S, Tettamanzi F, Zani B, Mangano S, Scalia P. Obturator hernia, a rare complication in a CAPD patient: report of a case (Abstract). Perit Dial Int 1993; 13 (suppl 1): S11.
19. Griffin P, Coles G. Strangulated hernias through Tenckhoff cannula sites. Br Med J 1982; 284: 1837.
20. Power D, Edward N, Catto G, Muirhead N, MacLeod A, Engeset J. Richter's hernia: an unrecognised complication of chronic ambulatory peritoneal dialysis. Br Med J 1981; 283: 528.
21. Shohat J, Shapira Z, Shmueli D, Boner G. Intestinal incarceration in occult abdominal wall herniae in continuous ambulatory peritoneal dialysis. Isr J Med Sci 1985; 21: 985–7.
22. Steiner RW, Halasz NA. Abdominal catastrophes and other unusual events in continuous ambulatory peritoneal dialysis patients. Am J Kid Dis 1990; 15: 1–7.
23. Moffat F, Deitel M, Thompson D. Abdominal surgery in patients undergoing long-term peritoneal dialysis. Surgery 1982; 92: 598–604.
24. Kopecky R, Funk M, Kreitzer P. Localized genital edema in patients undergoing continuous ambulatory peritoneal dialysis. J Urol 1985; 134: 880–4.
25. Beaman M, Feehally J, Smith B, Walls J. Anterior abdominal wall leakage in CAPD patients: management by intermittent peritoneal dialysis (letter). Perit Dial Bull 1985; 5: 81–2.
26. Cooper JC, Nicholls AJ, Simms JM, Platts MM, Brown CB, Johnson AG. Genital oedema in patients treated by continuous ambulatory peritoneal dialysis: an unusual presentation of inguinal hernia. Br Med J 1983; 286: 1923–4.
27. Orfei R, Seybold K, Blumberg A. Genital edema in patients undergoing continuous ambulatory peritoneal dialysis (CAPD). Perit Dial Bull 1984; 4: 251–2.
28. Twardowski Z, Tully R, Nichols W, Sunderrajan

28. S. Computerized tomography CT in the diagnosis of subcutaneous leak sites during continuous ambulatory peritoneal dialysis (CAPD). Perit Dial Bull 1984; 4: 163–6.
29. Schurgers M, Boelaert J, Daneels R, Robbens E, Vandelanotte M. Open processus vaginalis. Perit Dial Bull 1983; 3: 30–1.
30. Tzamaloukas AH, Gibel LJ, Eisenberg B et al. Scrotal edema in patients on CAPD: Causes, differential diagnosis and management. Dial Transplant 1992; 21: 581–90.
31. Abraham G, Blake PG, Mathews RE, Bargman JM, Izatt S, Oreopoulos DG. Genital swelling as a surgical complication of continuous ambulatory peritoneal dialysis. Surg Gyn Obstet 1990; 170: 306–8.
32. Mandel P, Faegenburg D, Imbriano L. The use of technetium – 99m sulfur colloid in the detection of patent processus vaginalis in patients on continuous ambulatory peritoneal dialysis. Clin Nucl Med 1985; 10: 553–5.
33. Dubin L, Froelich J. Evaluation of scrotal edema in a patient on peritoneal dialysis. Clin Nucl Med 1985; 10: 173–4.
34. Johnson BF, Segasby CA, Holroyd AM, Brown CB, Cohen GL, Raftery AT. A method for demonstrating subclinical inguinal herniae in patients undergoing peritoneal dialysis: The isotope 'peritoneoscrotogram'. Nephrol Dial Transplant 1987; 2: 254–7.
35. Berman C, Velchik MG, Shusterman N, Alavi A. The clinical utility of the Tc – 99m SC intraperitoneal scan in CAPD patients. Clin Nuc Med 1989; 14: 405–9.
36. Sissons GRJ, Meecham Jones SM, Evans C, Richards AR. Scintigraphic detection of abdominal hernias associated with continuous ambulatory peritoneal dialysis. Br J Rad 1991; 53: 1158–61.
37. Twardowski ZJ, Tully RJ, Ersoy FF, Dedhia NM. Computerized tomography with and without intraperitoneal contrast for determination of intra-abdominal fluid distribution and diagnosis of complications in peritoneal dialysis patients. ASAIO Trans 1990; 36: 95–103.
38. Caimi F, Roveroe G, Phillipson M, Battaglia E. Contribution of peritoneography combined with computerized tomography, in the assessment of abdominal complications in patients undergoing continuous peritoneal dialysis. Radiologia Medica 1991; 81: 656–659.
39. Maher J, Schreiner G. Hazards and complications of dialysis. N Engl J Med 1965; 273: 370–7.
40. Edwards S, Unger A. Acute hydrothorax: a new complication of peritoneal dialysis. J Am Med Assoc 1967; 199: 189–91.
41. Bunchman T, Wood E, Lynch R. Hydrothorax as a complication of peritoneal dialysis. Perit Dial Bull 1987; 7: 237–9.
42. Scheldewaert R, Bogaerts Y, Pauwels R, Van DerStraeten M, Ringoir S, Lameire N. Management of a massive hydrothorax in a CAPD patient: A case report and a review of the literature. Perit Dial Bull 1982; 2: 69–72.
43. Abraham G, Shoker A, Blake P, Oreopoulos D. Massive hydrothorax in patients on peritoneal dialysis: a literature review. In: Khanna R, Nolph KD, Prowant BF, Twardowski ZJ, Oreopoulos DG (eds), Advances in Peritoneal Dialysis. University of Toronto Press, Toronto 4: pp
44. Nomoto Y, Suga T, Nakajima K et al. Acute hydrothorax in continuous ambulatory peritoneal dialysis – a collabortive study of 161 centers. Am J Nephrol 1989; 9: 363–7.
45. Lieberman F, Hidemura R, Peters R, Reynolds T. Pathogenesis and treatment of hydrothorax complicating cirrhosis with ascites. Ann Intern Med 1966; 64: 341–51.
46. Johnston R, Loo R. Hepatic hydrothorax. Studies to determine the source of fluid and report of thirteen cases. Ann Intern Med 1964; 61: 385–401.
47. Grefberg N, Danielson B, Benson L et al. Right-sided hydrothorax complicating peritoneal dialysis. Nephron 1983; 34: 130–4.
48. Boeschoten EW, Krediet RT, Roos CM, Kloek JJ, Schipper MEI, Arisz L. Leakage of dialysate across the diaphragm: an important complication of continuous ambulatory peritoneal dialysis. Neth J Med 1986; 29: 242–6.
49. Bjerke HS, Adkins ES, Foglia RP. Surgical correction of hydrothorax from diaphragmatic eventration in children on peritoneal dialysis. Surgery 1991; 109: 550–4.
50. Trust A, Rossoff LJ. Tension hydrothorax in a patient with renal failure. Chest 1990; 97: 1254–5.
51. Benz R, Schleifer CR. Hydrothorax in CAPD. Successful treatment with intrapleural tetracycline and a review of the literature. Am J Kidney Dis 1985; 2: 136–40.
52. Adam W, Arkies L, Gill G, Meagher E, Thomas G. Hydrothorax with peritoneal dialysis: radionuclide detection of a pleuro-peritoneal connection. Austr NZ J Med 1980; 10: 330–2.
53. Gibbons G, Baumert J. Unilateral hydrothorax complicating peritoneal dialysis. Use of radionuclide imaging. Clin Nucl Med 1983; 3: 83–4.
54. Kennedy J. Procedures used to demonstrate a pleuroperitoneal communication: a review. Perit Dial Bull 1985; 5: 168–70.
55. Mestas D, Wauquier JP, Escande G, Baquet JC, Veyr A. Diagnosis of hydrothorax complicating CAPD and demonstration of successful therapy by scintigraphy (letter). Perit Dial Int 1991; 11: 283–285.
56. Walker F, McAllister C, McKee P, McNulty J. Intraperitoneal Iopamidol, a new radiocontrast agent in the diagnosis of a pleuroperitoneal communication (letter). Perit Dial Int 1986; 6: 108–9.
57. Green A, Logan M, Medawar W et al. The management of hydrothorax in continuous ambulatory peritoneal dialysis (CAPD). Perit Dial Int 1990; 10: 271–4.
58. Vezina D, Winchester JF, Rakowski TA. Spontaneous resolution of massive hydrothorax in

a CAPD patient (letter). Perit Dial Bull 1987; 7: 212–3.
59. Ing A, Rutland J, Kalowski S. Spontaneous resolution of hydrothorax in continuous ambulatory peritoneal dialysis (letter). Nephron 1992; 61: 247–8.
60. Townsend R, Fragola JA. Hydrothorax in a patient receiving continuous ambulatory peritoneal dialysis – successful treatment with intermittent peritoneal dialysis. Arch Int Med 1982; 142: 1571–2.
61. Chow CC, Sung JY, Cheung CK, Hamilton-Wood C, Lai KN. Massive hydrothorax in continuous ambulatory peritoneal dialysis: Diagnosis, management and review of the literature. New Zealand Med J 1988; 101: 475–7.
62. Posen G, Sachs H. Treatment of recurrent pleural effusions in dialysis patients by talc insufflation (Abstract). Am Soc Artif Intern Organs, 25th Annual Meeting, New York 1979; pp 75.
63. Hidai H, Takatsu S, Chiba T. Intrathoracic instillation of autologous blood in treating massive hydrothorax following CAPD (letter). Perit Dial Int 1989; 9: 221–2.
64. Catizone L, Zuchelli A, Zuchelli P. Hydrothorax in a PD patient: successful treatment with intrapleural autologous blood instillation. In: Khanna R, Nolph KD, Prowant BF, Twardowski ZJ, Oreopoulos DG (eds), Advances in Peritoneal Dialysis. University of Toronto Press, Toronto 1991; pp 86–90.
65. Vlachojannis J, Boettcher I, Brandt L, Schoeppe W. A new treatment for unilateral recurrent hydrothorax during CAPD. Perit Dial Bull 1985; 5: 180–1.
66. Pattison C, Rodger R, Adu D et al. Surgical treatment of hydrothorax complicating CAPD. Clin Nephrol 1984; 21: 191–3.
67. Allen SM, Matthews HR. Surgical treatment of massive hydrothorax complicating continuous ambulatory peritoneal dialysis. Clin Nephrol 1991; 36: 299–301.
68. Berlyne G, Lee H, Ralston A, Woolcock JA. Pulmonary complications of peritoneal dialysis. Lancet 1966; 2: 75–8.
69. Ahluwalia M, Ishikawa S, Gellman M et al. Pulmonary functions during peritoneal dialysis. Clin Nephrol 1982; 18: 251–6.
70. Gomez-Fernandez P, Sanchez Agudo L, Calatrava J et al. Respiratory muscle weakness in uremic patients under continuous ambulatory peritoneal dialysis. Nephron 1984; 36: 219–23.
71. Singh S, Dale A, Morgan B, Sahebjami H. Serial studies of pulmonary function in continuous ambulatory peritoneal dialysis. Chest 1984; 86: 874–7.
72. Taveira da Silva A, Davis W, Winchester J, Coleman DE, Weir CW. Peritonitis, dialysate infusion and lung function in continuous ambulatory peritoneal dialysis (CAPD). Clin Nephrol 1985; 24: 79–83.
73. O'Brien AA, Power J, O'Brien L, Clancy L, Keogh JA. The effect of peritoneal dialysate on pulmonary function and blood gasses in CAPD patients. Irish Journal of Medical Science 1990; 159: 215–6.
74. Freedman S, Maberly D. Gas exchange in renal failure (letter). Br Med J 1971; 3: 48.
75. Blumberg A, Keller R, Marti H. Oxygen affinity of erythrocytes and pulmonary gas exchange in patients on continuous ambulatory peritoneal dialysis. Nephron 1984; 38: 248–52.
76. Oreopoulos D, Rebuck A. Risks and benefits of peritoneal dialysis. Chest 1985; 88: 6742.
77. Rebuck A. Peritoneal dialysis and the mechanics of the diaphragm (editorial). Perit Dial Bull 1982; 2: 109–10.
78. Bush A, Gabriel R. Pulmonary function in chronic renal failure: effects of dialysis and transplantation. Thorax 1991; 46: 6, 424–8.
79. Smith S, Goldberg M. Pulmonary insufficiency as a result of chronic aspiration secondary to CAPD therapy (Abstract). Am J, Kid Dis 1985; 6: A19.
80. Eiser A. Pulmonary gas exchange during hemodialysis and peritoneal dialysis: interaction between respiration and metabolism. Am J Kid Dis 1985; 6: 131–42.
81. Fabris A, Biasioli S, Chiaramonte C et al. Buffer metabolism in continuous ambulatory peritoneal dialysis (CAPD): relationship with respiratory dynamics. Trans Am Soc Artif Intern Organs 1982; 28: 270–5.
82. Cohn J, Balk RA, Bone RC. Dialysis-induced respiratory acidosis. Chest 1990; 98: 1285–8.
83. Ahearn DJ, Nolph KD. Controlled sodium removal with peritoneal dialysis. Trans Am Soc Artif Organs 1972; 18: 423–8.
84. Lindholm B, Alvestrand A, Hultman E, Bergstrom J. Muscle water and electrolytes in patients undergoing continuous ambulatory peritoneal dialysis. Acta Med Scand 1986; 219: 323–30.
85. Paulson WD, Bock GH, Nelson AP, Moxey-Mims MM, Crim LM. Hyponatremia in the very young chronic peritoneal dialysis patient. Am J Kid Dis 1989; 14: 196–9.
86. Tzamaloukas A and Avasthi P. Effect of hyperglycemia on serum sodium concentration and tonicity in outpatients on chronic dialysis. Am J Kidney Dis 1986; 7: 477–82.
87. Spital A, Sterns R. Potassium supplementation via the dialysate in continuous ambulatory peritoneal dialysis. Am J Kidney Dis 1985; 6: 173–6.
88. Oreopoulos D, Khanna R, Williams P, Vas S. Continuous ambulatory peritoneal dialysis – 1981. Nephron 1982; 30: 293–303.
89. Rostand S. Profound hypokalemia in continuous ambulatory peritoneal dialysis. Arch Intern Med 1983; 143: 377–8.
90. Bargman J, Jamison R. Disorders of potassium homeostasis. In: Sutton R, Dirks J (eds), Diuretics: Physiology, Pharmacology and Clinical Use. W. B. Saunders Co 1986; pp 296–319.
91. Boen S. Peritoneal dialysis in clinical medicine. Charles C. Thomas: Springfield Illinois 1974.
92. Vaamonde C, Michael V, Metzger R et al.

Complications of acute peritoneal dialysis. J Chron Dis 1975; 28: 637–59.
93. Pedersen F, Ryttov N, Deleuran P, Dragsholt C, Kildeberg P. Acetate versus lactate in peritoneal dialysis solutions. Nephron 1985; 39: 55–8.
94. Ahlmen J, Stelin G. Abdominal pains during CAPD with acetate buffered dialysate (letter). Lancet 1983; 2: 1247.
95. LaGreca G, Biasioli S, Chiaramonte S et al. Acid-base balance on peritoneal dialysis. Clin Nephrol 1981; 16: 1–7.
96. Nissenson A. Acid-base homeostasis in peritoneal dialysis patients. Int J Artif Organs 1984; 7: 175–6.
97. Richardson R, Roscoe J. Bicarbonate, L-Lactate and D-Lactate balance in intermittent peritoneal dialysis. Perit Dial Bull 1986; 6: 178–85.
98. Rubin J, Adair C, Johnson B, Bower JD. Stereospecific lactate absorption during peritoneal dialysis. Nephron 1982; 31: 224–8.
99. Veech R, Fowler R. Cerebral dysfunction and respiratory alkalosis during peritoneal dialysis with D-lactate-containing dialysis fluids (letter). Am J Med 1987; 82: 572–3.
100. Singh S, Hong C, Dale A, Morgan B. Comparison of buffering capacity in patients on hemodialysis and continuous ambulatory peritoneal dialysis. Nephron 1986; 42: 29–33.
101. Naparstek Y, Friedlaender M, Rubinger D, Popovtzer MM. Lactic acidosis and peritoneal dialysis. Isr J Med Sci 1982; 18: 513–4.
102. Conte F, Tommasi A, Battini G et al. Lactic acidosis coma in continuous ambulatory peritoneal dialysis (letter). Nephron 1986; 43: 148.
103. Foulks C, Wright L. Successful repletion of bicarbonate stores in ongoing lactic acidosis: a role for bicarbonate-buffered peritoneal dialysis. Southern Med J 1981; 74: 1162–3.
104. Feriani M, Biasioli S, Borin D et al. Bicarbonate buffer for CAPD solution. Trans Am Soc Artif Intern Organs 1985; 31: 668–72.
105. Lee H, Hill L, Hewill V et al. Lactic acidemia in peritoneal dialysis. Proc Eur Dial Transpl Assoc 1967; 4: 150–5.
106. Tzamaloukas A. 'Contraction' alkalosis during treatment of hyperglycemia in CAPD patients. Perit dial Bull 1983; 3: 196–9.
107. Garella S. Contraction alkalosis in patients on CAPD (letter). Perit Dial Bull 1984; 4: 187–8.
108. Gault M, Ferguson E, Sidhu J et al. Fluid and electrolyte complications of peritoneal dialysis. Ann Intern Med 1971; 75: 253–62.
109. Kenamond T, Graves J, Lempert K, Moss A, Whittier F. Severe recurrent alkalemia in a patient undergoing continuous cyclic peritoneal dialysis. Am J Med 1986; 81: 548–50.
110. Posner J, Plum F. Spinal fluid pH and neurological symptoms in systemic acidosis. N Engl J Med 1967; 277: 605–13.
111. Levy D, Anderson K, Savage D, Balkus S, Kannel W, Castelli W. Echocardiographically detected left ventricular hypertrophy: Prevalence and risk factors. The Framingham Heart Study. Ann Intern Med 1988; 108: 7–13.
112. Silberberg DS, Barre P, Prichard S, Sniderman AD. Left ventricular hypertrophy: An independent determinant of survival in end-stage renal failure. Kidney Int 1989; 36: 286–90.
113. Wizemann V, Timio M, Alpert MA, Kramer W. Options in dialysis therapy: Significance of cardiovascular findings. Kidney Int Suppl 1993; 43: S85–91.
114. Mall G, Huther W, Schneider J, Lundin P, Ritz E. Diffuse intermyocardiocytic fibrosis in uremic patients. Nephrol Dial Transplant 1990; 5: 39–44.
115. Leenen F, Smith D, Khanna R, Oreopoulos DG. Changes in left ventricular anatomy and function on CAPD. Perit Dial Bull Supp 1983; 3: S26–8.
116. Brown P, Johnston K, Fenton S, Cattran DC. Symptomatic exacerbation of peripheral vascular disease with chronic ambulatory peritoneal dialysis. Clin Nephrol 1981; 16: 258–61.
117. Feldman AM, Fivush B, Zahka KG, Ouyang P, Baughman KL. Congestive cardiomyopathy in patients on continuous ambulatory peritoneal dialysis. Am J Kid Dis 1988; 11: 76–9.
118. Guazzi M, Polese A, Magrini F, Fiorentini C, Olivari M. Negative influences of ascites on cardiac function of cirrhotic patients. Am J Med 1975; 59: 165–70.
119. Schurig R, Gahl G, Schartl M et al. Central and peripheral hemodynamics in long term peritoneal dialysis patients. Proc Eur Dial Transpl Assoc 1979; 16: 165–9.
120. Swartz C, Onesti G, Mailloux L et al. The acute hemodynamic and pulmonary perfusion effects of peritoneal dialysis. Trans Am Soc Artif Intern Organs 1969; 15: 367–72.
121. Acquatella H, Perez-Rozas M, Burger B et al. Left ventricular function in uremia: A hemodynamic and echocardiographic study. Nephron 1978; 22: 160–74.
122. Franklin JO, Alpert MA, Twardowski ZJ et al. Effect of increasing intra-abdominal pressure and volume on left ventricular function in continuous ambulatory peritoneal dialysis (CAPD). Am J Kid Dis 1988; 12: 291–8.
123. Rab ST, Alazraki NP, Guertler-Krawczynska E. Peritoneal fluid causing inferior attenuation on SPECT thallium-201 myocardial imaging in women. J Nucl Med 1988; 29: 1860–4.
124. Avram MM. High prevalence of pancreatic disease in chronic renal failure. Nephron 1977; 18: 68–71.
125. Kaysen GA, Majamdar APN, Dubick MA et al. Biochemical changes in the pancreas of rats with chronic renal failure. Am J Physiol 1985; 249: F518–23.
126. Vaziri ND, Dure-Smith B, Miller R, Mirahmadi M. Pancreatic pathology in chronic dialysis patients – an autopsy study of 78 cases. Nephron 1987; 46: 347–9.
127. Sombolos K, McNamee P, Mitwali A, Rabinovich S, Oreopoulos DG. Autopsy findings in patients

treated by continuous ambulatory peritoneal dialysis. Perit Dial Bull 1986; 6: 130–5.
128. Caruana R, Wolfman N, Karstaedt N, Wilson D. Pancreatitis: an important cause of abdominal symptoms in patients on peritoneal dialysis. Am J Kid Dis 1986; 7: 135–40.
129. Rutsky E, Robards M, Van Dyke J, Rostand S. Acute pancreatitis in patients with end-stage renal disease without transplantation. Arch Intern Med 1986; 146: 1741–5.
130. Singh S, Wadhwa N. Peritonitis, pancreatitis and infected pseudocyst in a continuous ambulatory peritoneal dialysis patient. Am J Kid Dis 1987; 9: 84–6.
131. Flynn C, Chandran P, Shadur C. Recurrent pancreatitis in a patient on CAPD (letter). Perit Dial Bull 1986; 6: 106.
132. Donnelly S, Levy M, Prichard S. Acute pancreatitis in continuous ambulatory peritoneal dialysis. Perit Dial Int 1988; 8: 187–90.
133. Gupta A, Yuan ZY, Balaskas EV, Khanna R, Oreopoulos DG. CAPD and pancreatitis: No connection. Perit Dial Int 1992; 12: 309–16.
134. Pitrone F, Pellegrino E, Mileto G, Consolo F. May pancreatitis represent a CAPD complication? Report of two cases with a rapid evolution to death (letter). Int J Artif Organs 1985; 8: 235–6.
135. Royse VL, Jensen DM, Corwin HL. Pancreatic enzymes in chronic renal failure. Arch Int Med 1987; 147: 537–9.
136. Burkart J, Haigler S, Caruana R, Hylander B. Usefulness of peritoneal fluid amylase levels in the differential diagnosis of peritonitis in peritoneal dialysis patients. J Am Soc Nephrol 1991; 1: 1186–91.
137. Luciani L, Gentile M, Scarduelli B, Sinico R, D'Amico G, Samori G. Multiple hepatic abscesses complicating continuous ambulatory peritoneal dialysis. Br Med J 1982; 285: 543.
138. Wanless IR, Bargman JM, Oreopoulos DG, Vas SI. Subcapsular steatonecrosis in response to peritoneal insulin delivery: a clue to the pathogenesis of steatonecrosis in obesity. Modern Pathology 1989; 2: 69–74.
139. Hylander BI, Dalton CB, Castel DO, Burkart J, Rossner S. Effect of intraperitoneal fluid volume changes on esophageal pressures: studies in patients on continuous ambulatory peritoneal dialysis. Am J Kid Dis 1991; 17: 307–10.
140. Korzets Z, Golan E, Ben-Dahan J, Neufeld D, Bernheim J. Decubitus small-bowel perforation in ongoing continuous ambulatory peritoneal dialysis. Nephrol Dial Transplant 1992; 7: 79–81.
141. Rottembourg J, Gahl G, Poignet J et al. Severe abdominal complications in patients undergoing continuous ambulatory peritoneal dialysis. Eur Dial Transpl Assoc Proc 1983; 20: 236–42.
142. Koren G, Aladjem M, Militiano J, Seegal B, Jonash A, Boichis H. Ischemic colitis in chronic intermittent peritoneal dialysis. Nephron 1984; 36: 272–4.
143. Wehling M, Jenni R, Steurer J, Buhler H, Siegenthaler W, Kuhlmann U. Ischemic colitis in a patient undergoing continuous ambulatory peritoneal dialysis. Perit Dial Bull 1982; 2: 123–4.
144. Tomson C, Morgan A. Bleeding from small intestinal telangiectases complicating CAPD (letter), Perit Dial Bull 1985; 5: 258.
145. Faller B, Marichal J. Loss of ultrafiltration in continuous ambulatory peritoneal dialysis: clinical data. In: Gahl G, Kessel M, Nolph K (eds), Advances in Peritoneal Dialysis. Excerpta Medica 1981: pp 227–232.
146. Mactier RA, Khanna R, Twardowski Z, Moore H, Nolph KD. Contribution of lymphatic absorption to loss of ultrafiltration and solute clearances in continuous ambulatory peritoneal dialysis. J Clin Invest 1987; 80: 1311–6.
147. Wu G, Oreopoulos D. Diminished peritoneal ultrafiltration and solute permeability. In: Daugirdas J, Ing T (eds), Handbook of Dialysis. Little, Brown 1988; pp 244-51.
148. Slingeneyer A, Canaud B, Mion C. Permanent loss of ultrafiltration capacity of the peritoneum in long-term peritoneal dialysis: an epidemiological study. Nephron 1983; 33: 133–8.
149. Faller B, Marichal J-F. Loss of ultrafiltration in continuous ambultory peritoneal dialysis: a role for acetate. Perit Dial Bull 1984; 4: 10–3.
150. Krediet R, Boeschoten E, Zuyderhoudt F, Arisz L. Peritoneal transport characteristics of water, low-molecular weight solutes and proteins during long-term continuous ambulatory peritoneal dialysis. Perit Dial Bull 1986; 6: 61–5.
151. Struijk DG, Krediet RT, Koomen GCM et al. Functional characteristics of the peritoneal membrane in long-term continuous ambulatory peritoneal dialysis. Nephron 1991; 59: 213–20.
152. Wideroe T-E, Smeby L, Mjaland S, Dahl K, Berg K, Aas T. Long-term changes in transperitoneal water transport during continuous ambulatory peritoneal dialysis. Nephron 1984; 38: 238–47.
153. Nolph K, Ryan L, Moore H, Legrain M, Mion C, Oreopoulos DG. Factors affecting ultrafiltration in continuous ambulatory peritoneal dialysis. First report of an international cooperative study. Perit Dial Bull 1984; 4: 14–9.
154. Nolph K, Legrain M, Mion C, Oreopoulos DG. Loss of peritoneal ultrafiltration: an international detective story. Perit Dial Bull 1984; 4: 128.
155. Nolph K, Ryan L, Moore H et al. A survey of ultrafiltration in continuous ambulatory peritoneal dialysis. An international cooperative study-second report. Perit Dial Bull 1984; 4: 137–42.
156. Katirtzoglou A, Digenis G, Kontesis P, Karamanos B, Symvoulidis A. Is peritoneal ultrafiltration influenced by acetate or lactate buffers? In: Maher J, Winchester J (eds), Frontiers in Peritoneal Dialysis. Field, Rich and Associates, Inc. 1986; pp 270–3.
157. Ikutaka T, Ishiguro M, Shimabukuro S, Hirano T, Arakawa M. Is peritoneal rest a treatment for ultrafiltration failure during continuous ambulatory peritoneal dialysis? Curr Ther Res 1992; 52: 202–11,

158. DiPaolo N, Buoncristiani U, Gaggiotti E, Capotondo L, DeMia M. Improvement of impaired ultrafiltration after addition of phosphatidylcholine in patients on CAPD (letter). Perit Dial Bull 1986; 6: 44–5.
159. Mactier RA, Khanna R, Moore H et al. Reduction of lymphatic absorption from the peritoneal cavity with intraperitoneal neostigmine, phosphatidylcholine and other drugs. In: Wiching E (ed), Peritoneal dialysis. Editore, Milan 1988: 41–4.
160. Grefberg N, Nilsson P, Andreen T. Sclerosing obstructive peritonitis, beta-blockers, and continuous ambulatory peritoneal dialysis (letter). Lancet 1983; 2: 733–4.
161. Bradley J, McWhinnie D, Hamilton D et al. Sclerosing obstructive peritonitis after continuous ambulatory peritoneal dialysis (letter). Lancet 1983; 2: 113–4.
162. Hauglustaine D, Monballyu J, Van Meerbeek J, Goddeeris P, Lauwarijns J, Pichielsen P. Sclerosing obstructive peritonitis, beta-blockers, and continuous ambulatory peritoneal dialysis (letter). Lancet 1983; 2: 734.
163. Verger C, Celicout B, Larpent L, Goupil A. Sclerosing encapsulating peritonitis during continuous ambulatory peritoneal dialysis. La Presse Medicale 1986; 15: 1311–4.
164. Slingeneyer A, Mion C, Mourad G, Canaud B, Faller B, Beraud JJ. Progressive sclerosing peritonitis: a late and severe complication of maintenance peritoneal dialysis. Trans Am Soc Artif Intern Organs 1983; 29: 633–40.
165. Pusateri R, Ross R, Marshall R, Meredith J, Hamilton RW. Sclerosing encapsulating peritonitis: report of a case with small bowel obstruction managed by long-term home parenteral hyperalimentation, and a review of the literature. Am J Kid Dis 1986; 8: 56–60.
166. Ing T, Daugirdas J, Gandhi V: Peritoneal sclerosis in peritoneal dialysis patients. Am J Nephrol 1984; 4: 173–6.
167. Hauglustaine D, Van Meerbeek J, Monballyu J, Goddeeris P, Lauwerijns J, Michielsen P. Sclerosing peritonitis with mural bowel fibrosis in a patient on long-term CAPD. Clin Nephrol 1984; 22: 158–62.
168. Oreopoulos D. Khanna R, Wu G. Sclerosing obstructive peritonitis after CAPD (letter). Lancet 1983; 2: 409.
169. Dobbie JW. Pathogenesis of peritoneal fibrosing syndromes (sclerosing peritonitis) in peritoneal dialysis. Perit Dial Int 1992; 12: 14–27.
170. Daugirdas J, Gandhi V, McShane A et al. Peritoneal sclerosis in continuous ambulatory peritoneal dialysis patients dialyzed exclusively with lactate-buffered dialysate. Int J Artif Organs 1986; 9: 413–6.
171. Junor B, Briggs J, Forwell M, Dobbie J, Henderson I. Sclerosing peritonitis – The contribution of chlorhexidine in alcohol. Perit Dial Bull 1985; 5: 101–4.
172. Ing T, Daugirdas J, Gandhi V, Leehey D. Sclerosing peritonitis after peritoneal dialysis (letter). Lancet 1983; 2: 1080.
173. Shaldon S, Koch K, Quellhorst E, Dinarello CA. Pathogenesis of sclerosing peritonitis in CAPD. Trans Am Soc Artif Intern Organs 1984; 30: 193–4.
174. Joffe P, Jensen LT. Type I and III procollagens in APD: Markers of peritoneal fibrosis. In: Khanna R, Nolph KD, Prowant BF, Twardowski ZJ, Oreopouls DG (eds), Advances in Peritoneal Dialysis. University of Toronto Press, Toronto 1991; pp 158–60.
175. DeVecchi AF, Castelnovo C, Scalamogna A, Paparella M. Symptomatic accidental introduction of disinfectant electrolytic chlorhexidizer solution into the peritoneal cavity of CAPD patients. Clin Nephrol 1992; 37: 204–8.
176. Greenlee H, Stanley M, Reinhardt G et al. Small bowel obstruction from compression and kinking of intestine by thickened peritoneum in cirrhotics with ascites treated with LeVeen shunt. Gastroenterol 1979; 76: 1282–5.
177. Namasivayam J. Intraperitoneal pseudocyst formation as a complication of continuous ambulatory peritoneal dialysis. Br J Radiol 1991; 64: 463–4.
178. Brown P, Baddeley H, Read A et al. Sclerosing peritonitis, an unusual reaction of a B-adrenergic-blocking drug (practolol). Lancet 1974; 2: 1477–81.
179. Clark C, Terris R. Sclerosing peritonitis associated with metoprolol. Lancet 1983; 1: 937.
180. Hollman AS, McMillan MA, Briggs JD, Junor BJ, Morley P. Ultrasound changes in sclerosing peritonitis following continuous ambulatory peritoneal dialysis. Clin Rad 1991; 43: 176–9.
181. Korzets A, Korzets Z, Peer G et al. Sclerosing peritonitis. Possible early diagnosis by computerized tomography of the abdomen. Am J Nephrol 1988; 8: 143–6.
182. Kittur DS, Korpe SW, Raytch RE, Smith GW. Surgical aspects of sclerosing encapsulating peritonitis. Arch Surg 1990; 125: 1626–8.
183. Lo W-K, Chan K-T, Leung ACT, Pang S-W, Tse C-Y. Sclerosing peritonitis complicating continuous ambulatory peritoneal dialysis with the use of chlorhexidine in alcohol. In: Khanna R, Nolph KD, Prowant BJ, Twardowski ZJ, Oreopoulos DG (eds), Advances in Peritoneal Dialysis. University of Toronto Press, Toronto 1990; 6: 79–84.
184. Slingeneyer A. Preliminary report on a cooperative international study on sclerosing encapsulating peritonitis. Contrib Nephrol 1987; 57: 239–47.
185. Junor BJR, McMillan MA. Immunosuppression in sclerosing peritonitis (Abstract). Perit Dial Int Suppl 1993; 13: S64.
186. Marichal JF, Faller B, Brignon P, Wagner D, Straub P. Progressive calcifying peritonitis: a new complication of CAPD? Nephron 1987; 45: 229–32.
187. Francis DMA, Busmanis I, Becker G. Peritoneal calcification in a peritoneal dialysis patient: A case report. Perit Dial Int 1990; 10: 237–40.

188. Cox SV, Lai J, Suranyi M, Walker N. Sclerosing peritonitis with gross peritoneal calcification: A case report. Am J Kidney Dis 1992; 20: 637–42.
189. Klemm G. Peritoneal calcification and calciphylaxis. Nephron 1989; 51: 124.
190. Seyle H, Gabbiani G, Strebel R. Sensitization to calciphylaxis by endogenous parathyroid hormone. Endocrinology 1962; 71: 554–8.
191. Wakabayashi Y, Kawaguchi Y, Shigematsu T et al. Three cases of extensive peritoneal calcification (ECP) in patients with long-term CAPD (Abstract). Perit Dial Int Suppl 1993; 13: S99.
192. Nace G, George A Jr., Stone W. Hemoperitoneum: a red flag in CAPD. Perit Dial Bull 1985; 5: 42–4.
193. Greenberg A, Bernardini J, Piraino BM, Johnston JR, Perlmutter JA. Hemoperitoneum complicating chronic peritoneal dialysis: single-centre experience and literature review. Am J Kidney Dis 1992; 19: 252–6.
194. Blumenkrantz M, Gallagher N, Bashore R et al. Retrograde menstruation in women undergoing chronic peritoneal dialysis. Obstet Gynecol 1981; 57: 667–70.
195. Harnett J, Gill D, Corbett L, Parfrey PS, Gault H. Recurrent hemoperitoneum in women receiving continuous ambulatory peritoneal dialysis. Ann Intern Med 1987; 107: 341–3.
196. Fraley DS, Johnston JR, Bruns FJ, Adler S, Segel DP. Rupture of ovarian cyst: massive hemoperitoneum in continuous ambulatory peritoneal dialysis patients: diagnosis and treatment. Am J Kidney Dis 1988; 12: 69–71.
197. Coronel F, Maranjo P, Torrente J, Prats D. The risk of retrograde menstruation in CAPD patients (letter). Perit Dial Bull 1984; 4: 190–1.
198. Coward R, Gokal R, Wise M, Mallick NP, Warrell D. Peritonitis associated with vaginal leakage of dialysis fluid in continuous ambulatory peritoneal dialysis. Br Med J 1982; 284: 1529.
199. de los Santos CA, von Eye O, d'Avila D, Mottin CC. Rupture of the spleen: a complication of continuous ambulatory peritoneal dialysis. Perit Dial Bull 1986; 6: 203–4.
200. Williams PF, Beer S. Hemoperitoneum in a patient with idiopathic thrombocytopenic purpura (ITP) and renal failure (letter). Perit Dial Bull 1985; 5: 258–9.
201. Blake P, Abraham G. Bloody effluent during CAPD in a patient with polycystic kidneys (letter). Perit Dial Int 1988; 8: 167.
202. Campisi S, Cavatorta F, DeLucia E. Iliopsoas spontaneous hematoma: an unusual cause of hemoperitoneum in CAPD patients (letter). Perit Dial Int 1992; 12: 78.
203. Huserl F, Tapia N. Peritoneal bleeding in a CAPD patient after extracorporeal lithotripsy (letter). Perit Dial Bull 1987; 7: 262.
204. Hassell L, Moore J Jr., Conklin J. Hemoperitoneum during continuous ambulatory peritoneal dialysis: a possible complication of radiation induced peritoneal injury. Clin Nephrol 1984; 21: 241–3.
205. Modi K, Henderson I. Fatal massive hemoperitoneum after cessation of CAPD (letter). Clin Nephrol 1987; 27: 47.
206. Twardowski ZJ, Schreiber MJ. Peritoneal dialysis case forum: A 55 year old man with hematuria and blood-tinged dialysate. Perit Dial Int 1992; 12: 61–6.
207. Goodkin DA, Benning MG. An outpatient maneuver to treat bloody effluent during continuous ambulatory peritoneal dialysis (CAPD). Perit Dial Int 1990; 10: 227–9.
208. Shohat J, Shapira Z, Yussim A, Boner G. An unusual cause of massive intraperitoneal bleeding in CAPD. Perit Dial Bull 1984; 4: 257–8.
209. Ramon G, Miguel A, Caridad A, Colomer B. Bloody peritoneal fluid in a patient with tuberous sclerosis in a CAPD program (letter). Perit Dial Int 1989; 9: 353.
210. Rambausek M, Waldherr R, Ritz E. Recurrent episodes of bloody dialysate in mesangial IgA-glomerulonephritis (IgA-GN) during upper respiratory tract infections (Abstract). Perit Dial Bull 1987; 7: S62.
211. Ohtomo Y, Higasi Y. A case of MCTD patient with recurrent hemoperitoneum receiving CAPD who had a successful recovery with an increase in steroids. Nippon Jinzo Gakkai Shi 1992; 34: 325–9.
212. Press OW, Press NO, Kaufman SD. Evaluation and management of chylous ascites. Ann Intern Med 1982; 96: 358–64.
213. Vasko J, Tapper R. The surgical significance of chylous ascites. Arch Surg 1967; 95: 355-68.
214. Kelley M Jr., Butt H. Chylous ascites: an analysis of etiology. Gastroenterol 1960; 39: 161–70.
215. Haskim SA, Rohold HB, Babayan JK et al. Treatment of chyluria and chylothorax with medium-chain triglyceride. N Engl J Med 1964; 270: 756–61.
216. Porter J, Wang WH, Oliveria DBG. Chylous ascites and continuous ambulatory peritoneal dialysis. Nephrol Dial Transplant 1991; 6: 659–61.
217. Humayun H, Daugirdas J, Ing T et al. Chylous ascites in a patient treated with intermittent peritoneal dialysis. Artif Organs 1984; 8: 358–60.
218. Pomeranz A, Reichenberg Y, Schurr D, Drukker A. Chyloperitoneum: a rare complication of peritoneal dialysis. Perit Dial Bull 1984; 4: 35–7.
219. Leport J, Devars Du Mayne J-F, Hay J-M, Cerf M. Chylous ascites and encapsulating peritonitis: unusual complications of spontaneous bacterial peritonitis. Am J Gastroenterol 1987; 82: 463–5.
220. Dunnill MS, Millard PR, Oliver D. Acquired cystic disease of the kidneys: a hazard of long-term intermittent maintenance haemodialysis. J Clin Path 1977; 30: 868–77.
221. Crocker JFS, Safe SH. An animal model of hemodialysis induced polycystic kidney disease (PKD) (Abstract). Kidney Int 1984; 25: 183.
222. Bommer J, Waldherr R, VanKaick G, Strauss L, Ritz E. Acquired renal cysts in uremic patients – in vivo demonstration by computed tomography. Clin Nephrol 1980; 14: 299–303.
223. Mickisch O, Bommer J, Bachman S, Waldherr R,

Mann JFE, Ritz E. Multicystic transformation of kidneys in chronic renal failure. Nephron 1984; 38: 93–99.
224. Ishikawa I. Acquired renal cystic disease and its complications in continuous ambulatory peritoneal dialysis patients. Perit Dial Int 1992; 12: 292–7.
225. Miller LR, Soffer O, Nassar VH, Kutner MH. Acquired renal cystic disease in end-stage renal disease: an autopsy study of 155 cases. Am J Nephrol 1989; 9: 322–8.
226. Mallofre C, Almirall J, Campistol JM, Andreu J, Cardesa A, Revert L. Acquired renal cystic disease in HD: a study of 82 nephrectomies in young patients. Clin Nephrol 1992; 7: 297–302.
227. Frifelt JJ, Larsen C, Elle B, Dyreborg U. Multicystic transformation of the kidneys in dialysis patients. Scand J Urol Nephrol 1989; 23: 51–4.
228. Ishikawa I, Shikura N, Nagahara M, Shinoda A, Saito Y. Comparison of severity of acquired renal cysts between CAPD and hemodialysis. In Khanna R, Nolph KD, Prowant BF, Twardowski ZJ, Oreopoulos DG (eds), Advances in Peritoneal Dialysis. University of Tronto Press, Toronto 1991; 7: 91–5.
229. Glicklich D. Acquired cystic kidney disease and renal cell carcinoma: A review. Sem Dial 1991; 4: 273–83.
230. Master U, Cruz C, Schmidt R, Dumler F, Babiarz J. Renal malignancy in peritoneal dialysis patients with acquired cystic kidney disease. In: Khanna R, Nolph KD, Prowant BF, Twardowski ZJ, Oreopoulos DG (eds), Advances in Peritoneal Dialysis. University of Toronto Press, Toronto 1992; 8: 145–9.
231. Spencer SJW and Philips ME. Transitional-cell carcinoma in acquired cystic disease of the kidney in a patient on CAPD. Nephrol Dial Transplant 1990; 464–5.
232. Smith JW, Sallman AL, Williamson MR, Lott CG. Acquired renal cystic disease: two cases of associated adenocarcinoma and a renal ultrasound survey of a peritoneal dialysis population. Am J Kidney Dis 1987; 10: 41–6.
233. Trabucco AF, Johansson SL, Egan JD, Taylor RJ. Neoplasia and acquired renal cystic disease in patients undergoing chronic ambulatory peritoneal dialysis. Urology 1990; 35: 1–4.
234. Cotterell L, Egan JD, Wells IC et al. Significant incidence of ACKD in CAPD patients (Abstract). Perit Dial Bull 1986; 6: S5.
235. Francos GC. Uremic Pruritis. Semin Dial 1988; 1: 209–12.
236. Massry SG, Popovtzer MM, Coburn JW et al. Intractable pruritis as a manifestation of secondary hyperparathyroidism in uremia. Disappearance of itching after subtotal parathyroidectomy. N Engl J Med 1968; 279: 698–700.
237. Balaskas EV, Oreopoulos DG. Uremic pruritis (Part I). Dial Trans 1992; 21: 192–244.
238. Matsumoto M, Ishimaru K, Horie A. Pruritis and mast cell proliferation of the skin in end-stage renal failure. Clin Nephrol 1985; 23: 285–8.
239. Dimkovic N, Djukanovic L, Radmilovic A, Bojic P, Juloski T. Uremic prutiritis and skin mast cells. Nephron 1992; 61: 5–9.
240. Mettang T, Fritz P, Weber J, Machleidt C, Hubel E, Kuhlmann U. Uremic pruritis in patients on hemodialysis or continuous ambulatory peritoneal dialysis (CAPD). The role of plasma histamine and skin mast cells. Clin Nephrol 1990; 34: 136–41.
241. Bencini PL, Montagnino G, Citterio A, Graziani G, Crosti C, Ponticelli C. Cutaneous abnormalities in uremic patients. Nephron 1985; 40: 316–21.
242. Albert C, Michel C, Ikeni A et al. Pruritis in patients on hemodialysis (HD) or peritoneal dialysis (PD) (Abstract). Perit Dial Int Suppl 1, 1991; Abstracts of the XI Annual CAPD Conference, Abstract 5.
243. Tan JKL, Haberman HF, Coldman AJ. Identifying effective treatments for uremic pruritus. J Amer Acad of Derm 1991; 25: 811–8.
244. Balaskas EV, Oreopoulos DG. Uremic pruritis (Part II). Dial Trans 1992; 21: 278–84.
245. Kleinman KS, Coburn JW. Amyloid syndromes associated with hemodialysis (editorial). Kidney Int 1989; 35: 567–75.
246. Gejyo F, Yamada T, Odani S et al. A new form of amyloid protein associated with chronic hemodialysis was identified as beta-2-microglobulin. Biochem Biophys Res Comm 600.
247. Shirahama T, Skinner M, Cohen AS et al. Histochemical and immunohistochemical characterization of amyloid associated with chronic hemodialysis as beta-2-microglobulin. Lab Invest 1985; 53: 705–7.
248. Tielemans C, Dratwa M, Bergmann P et al. Continuous ambulatory peritoneal dialysis vs hemodialysis: A lesser risk of amyloidosis? Nephrol Dial Transplant 1988; 3: 291–4.
249. Sethi D, Gower PE. Dialysis Arthropathy, B2-microglobulin and the effect of dialyser membrane. Nephrol Dial Transplant 1988; 3: 768–72.
250. Miguel Alonso JL, Cruz A, Lopez Revuelta K et al. Continuous ambulatory peritoneal dialysis does not prevent the development of dialysis-associated amyloidosis. Nephron 1989; 53: 389–90.
251. Lysaght MJ, Pollock CA, Moran JE, Ibels LS, Farrell PC. Beta-2 microglobulin removal during continuous ambulatory peritoneal dialysis (CAPD). Perit Dial Int 1989; 9: 29–35.
252. Montenegro J, Martinez I, Saracho R, Gonzalez R. B2 microglobulin in CAPD. In: Khanna R, Nolph KD, Prowant BF, Twardowski ZJ, Oreopoulos DG (eds), Advances in Peritoneal Dialysis. University of Toronto Press, Toronto 1992; 8: 369–72.
253. Benz RL, Siegfried JW, Teehan BP. Carpal tunnel syndrome in dialysis patients: comparison between continuous ambulatory peritoneal dialysis and hemodialysis populations. Am J Kidney Dis 1988; 11: 473–6.
254. Cornelis F, Bardin T, Faller B et al. Rheumatic

254. syndromes and B2-microglobulin amyloidosis in patients receiving long-term peritoneal dialysis. Arthritis Rheum 1989; 32: 785–8.
255. Cruz A, Gonzalez T, Balsa A et al. Destructive spondyloarthropathy in longterm CAPD and hemodialysis (letter). J Rheum 1989; 16: 1169–70.
256. Bicknell JM, Lim AC, Raroque HG, Tzamaloukas A. Carpal tunnel syndrome, subclinical median mononeuropathy, and peripheral polyneuropathy: common early complications of chronic peritoneal dialysis and hemodialysis. Arch Phys Med Rehabil 1991; 72: 378–81.
257. Gagnon RF, Lough JO, Bourgouin PA. Carpal tunnel syndrome and amyloidosis associated with continuous ambulatory peritoneal dialysis. Can Med Assoc J 1988; 139: 753–5.
258. Benhamou CL, Bardin T, Noel LH et al. Beta-2 microglobulin amyloidosis as a complication of peritoneal dialysis treatment (letter). Clin Nephrol 1988; 30: 346.
259. Athanasou NA, Ayers D, Raine AJ, Oliver DO, Duthie RB. Joint and systemic distribution of dialysis amyloid. Quart J Med 1991; 78: 205–14.
260. Jadoul M, Noel H, van Ypersele de Strihou C. B2-microglobulin amyloidosis in a patient treated exclusively by continuous ambulatory peritoneal dialysis. Am J Kidney Dis 1990; 15: 86–8.
261. Colombi A, Wegmann W. Beta-2 microglobulin amyloidosis in a patient on long-term continuous ambulatory peritoneal dialysis (CAPD). Perit Dial Int 1989; 9: 321–4.
262. Allard JC, Artze ME, Porter G, Ghandur-Mnaymneh L, deVelasco R, Perez GO. Fatal destructive cervical spondyloarthropathy in two patients on long-term dialysis. Am J Kid Dis 1992; 19: 81–85.
263. Digenis G, Davidson G, Dombros N, Katz A, Bookman A, Oreopoulos DG. Destructive spondyloarthropathy in a patient on CAPD for 13 years. Perit Dial Int (in press).
264. Ramsay AG. Joint disease in end-stage renal disease. Sem Dial 1988; 1: 21–7.
265. Lustig S, Morduchowicz G, Rosenfeld J, Boner G. Bilateral rupture of the tendon of the long head of the biceps muscle in continuous ambulatory peritoneal dialysis (letter). Perit Dial Bull 1986; 6: 42–3.
266. Baum J, Cestero R, Jain V. Peritoneal-dialysis-spike elbow (letter). N Engl J Med 1983; 308: 1541.
267. Hoffman GS, Schumacher HR, Paul H et al. Calcium oxalate microcrystalline-associated arthritis in end-stage renal disease. Ann Intern Med 1982; 97: 36–42.
268. Cassidy MJD, Owen JP, Ellis HA et al. Renal osteodystrophy and metastatic calcification in long-term continuous ambulatory peritoneal dialysis. Quart J Med 1985; 54: 29–48.
269. Chalmers A, Reynolds WJ, Oreopoulos DG, Meema HE, Meindok H, deVeber GA. The arthropathy of maintenance intermittent peritoneal dialysis. Can Med Assoc J 1980; 123: 635–8.
270. Grinlinton FM, Vuletic JC, Gow PJ. Rapidly progressive calcific periarthritis occurring in a patient with lupus nephritis receiving chronic ambulatory peritoneal dialysis. J Rheum 1990; 17: 1100–3.
271. Hamodraka-Mailis A. Pathogenesis and treatment of back pain in peritoneal dialysis patients. Perit Dial Bull Supp 1983; 3: S41–3.
272. Constable AR, Joekes AM, Kasidas GP et al. Plasma level and renal clearance of oxalate in normal subjects and in patients with primary hyperoxaluria or chronic renal failure or both. Clin Sci 1979; 56: 299–304.
273. Mitwalli A, Oreopoulos D. Hyperoxaluria and hyperoxalemia: one more concern for the nephrologist (editorial). Int J Artif Organs 1985; 8: 71–4.
274. Yamauchi A, Fujii M, Shirai D et al. Plasma concentration and peritoneal clearance of oxalate in patients on continuous ambulatory peritoneal dialysis (CAPD). Clin Nephrol 1986; 25: 181–5.
275. Tomson CRV, Channon SM, Parkinson IS et al. Plasma oxalate in patients receiving continuous ambulatory peritoneal dialysis. Nephrol Dial Transplant 1988; 3: 295–9.
276. Shah GM, Ross EA, Sabo A, Pichon M, Reynolds RD, Bhagavan H. Effects of ascorbic acid and pyridoxine supplementation on oxalate metabolism in peritoneal dialysis patients. Am J Kidney Dis 1992; 20: 42–9.
277. Oren A, Husdan H, Cheng P-T et al. Calcium oxalate kidney stones in patients on continuous ambulatory peritoneal dialysis. Kidney Int 1984; 25: 534–8.
278. Antoniou S, Syreggelas D, Papadopoulos Ch, Dimitriadis A. Intraluminal lithiasis of a peritoneal catheter. Perit Dial Int 1991; 11: 358–60.
279. Schollmeyer P, Bozkurt F. The immune status of the uremic patient: hemodialysis vs CAPD. Clin Nephrol 1988; 30 (suppl 1): S37–40.
280. Goldstein CS, Bomalaski JB, Zurrier RB, Neilson EG, Douglas SD. Analysis of peritoneal macrophages in continuous ambulatory peritoneal dialysis patients. Kidney Int 1984; 26: 733–40.
281. Steinhauer HB, Schollmeyer P. Prostaglandin-mediated loss of proteins during peritonitis in continuous ambulatory peritoneal dialysis. Kidney Int 1986; 29: 584–90.
282. Giacchino F, Alloatti S, Quarello F et al. The influence of peritoneal dialysis on cellular immunity. Perit Dial Bull 1982; 2: 165–8.
283. Giagrande A, Cantu P, Limido A, deFrancesco D, Malacrida V. Continuous ambulatory peritoneal dialysis and cellular immunity. Proc Eur Dial Trans Assoc 1982; 19: 372–9.
284. Webb D, Smith C, Lee G, Wallington TB. Does continuous ambulatory peritoneal dialysis alter immune function? (Abstract). Clin Sci 1984; 66: 14.
285. Shohat B, Boner G, Waller A, Rosenfeld JB. Cell-mediated immunity in uremic patients prior to and after 6 months' treatment with continuous ambu-

latory peritoneal dialysis. Isr J Med Sci 1986; 22: 551–5.
286. Giacchino F, Pozzato M, Formica M et al. Improved cell-mediated immunity in CAPD patients as compared to those on hemodialysis. Perit Dial Bull 1984; 4: 209–12.
287. Collart F, Tielemans C, Schandene L et al. CAPD and cellular immunity: no different than that in hemodialysis patients (letter). Perit Dial Bull 1983; 3: 163–4.
288. Bargman JM, Silverman ED, Klein MH. Effect of in vivo 1,25 dihydroxyvitamin D3 on circulatory lymphocytes. Mineral and Electrolye Metabolism 1989; 15: 359–64.
289. Langhoff E, Ladefoged J. Improved lymphocyte transformation in vitro of patients on continuous ambulatory peritoneal dialysis. Proc Eur Dial Trans Assoc 1983; 20: 230–5.
290. Fivush BA, Case B, May MW, Lederman HM. Hypogammaglobulinemia in children undergoing continuous ambulatory peritoneal dialysis. Ped Nephrol 1989; 3: 186–8.
291. Katz A, Kashtan CE, Greenberg LJ, Shapiro RS, Nevins TE, Kim Y. Hypogammaglobulinemia in uremic infants receiving peritoneal dialysis. J Ped 1990; 117: 258–61.
292. Versluis DJ, Beyer WEP, Masurel N, Diderich PPNM, Kramer P, Weimar W. Intact humoral immune response in patients on continuous ambulatory peritoneal dialysis. Nephron 1988; 49: 16–9.
293. Perez G, Glasson P, Havre H et al. Circulating immune complexes in regularly dialyzed patients with chronic renal failure. Am J Nephrol 1984; 4: 215–21.
294. Wu G, Gelbart D, Hasbargen J et al. Reactivation of systemic lupus in three patients undergoing CAPD. Perit Dial Bull 1982; 6: 6–9.
295. Rodby RA, Korbet SM, Lewis EJ. Persistence of clinical and serological activity in patients with systemic lupus erythematosus undergoing peritoneal dialysis. Am J Med 1987; 83: 613–8.
296. Nossent HC, Swaak TJG, Berden JHM et al. Systemic lupus erythematosus: analysis of disease activity in 55 patients with end-stage renal failure treated with hemodialysis or continuous ambulatory peritoneal dialysis. Am J Med 1990; 89: 169–74.
297. Cardella C. Peritoneal dialysis and renal transplantation (editorial). Perit Dial Bull 1985; 5: 149–51.
298. Winchester JF, Rotellar C, Goggins M et al. Transplantation in peritoneal dialysis and hemodialysis. Kidney Int 1993; 43 (suppl 40): S101–5.
299. Gelfand M, Kois J, Quillin G et al. CAPD yields inferior transplant results compared to hemodialysis (Abstract). Perit Dial Bull 1984; 4: 526.
300. Guillou P, Will E, Davidson A et al. CAPD – a risk factor in renal transplantation? Br J Surg 1984; 71: 878–80.
301. Latta K, Offner G, Hoyer PF, Brodehl J. Reduction of cytotoxic antibodies after continuous ambulatory peritoneal dialysis in highly sensitised patients (letter). Lancet 1988; 2: 847–8.
302. Gokal R, Ramos J, Veitch P et al. Renal transplantation in patients on CAPD. Dial Trans 1982; 11: 125–55.
303. Shapira Z, Shmueli D, Yussim A, Boner G, Haimovitz C, Servadio C. Kidney transplantation in patients on continuous ambulatory peritoneal dialysis. Proc Eur Dial Trans Assoc 1984; 21: 932–5.
304. Evangelista J, Bennett-Jones D, Cameron J et al. Renal transplantation in patients treated with haemodialysis and short term and long term continuous ambulatory peritoneal dialysis. Br Med J 1985; 291: 1004–7.
305. Donnelly P, Lennard T, Proud G et al. Continuous ambulatory peritoneal dialysis and renal transplantation: a five year experience. Br Med J 1985; 291: 1001–4.
306. Tsakiris D, Bramwell S, Briggs J, Junor BJR. Transplantation in patients undergoing CAPD. Perit Dial Bull 1985; 5: 161–4.
307. Diaz-Buxo J, Walker P, Burgess W et al. The influence of peritoneal dialysis on the outcome of transplantation. Int J Artif Organs 1986; 9: 359–62.
308. Glass N, Miller D, Sollinger H, Zimmerman SW, Simpson D, Belzer FO: Renal transplantation in patients on peritoneal dialysis. Perit Dial Bull 1985; 5: 157–60.
309. Rubin J, Kirchner K, Raju S, Krueger RP, Bower JD. CAPD patients as renal transplant patients. Am J Med Sci 1987; 294: 175–80.
310. Cardella C. Renal transplantation in patients on peritoneal dialysis. Perit Dial Bull 1980; 1: 12–4.
311. Fries D, Brocard JF, Plaisant B et al. Continuous ambulatory peritoneal dialysis and renal transplantation. Nephrologie 1989; 10 (suppl): 18–21.
312. O'Donoghue D, Manos J, Pearson R et al. Continuous ambulatory peritoneal dialysis and renal transplantation. A ten-year experience in one center. Perit Dial Int 1992; 12: 242–9.
313. Hurault de Ligny B, Ryckelynck J Ph, Batho JM, Cardineau E, Lavaltier B. Renal transplantation in patients on continuous ambulatory peritoneal dialysis (CAPD) (Abstract). Perit Dial Int 1993; 12 (suppl 1): S22.
314. Rigby R, Petrie J. Transplantation in patients on continuous ambulatory peritoneal dialysis (letter). Transplantation 1984; 37: 533.
315. Ryckelynck J-P, Verger C, Pierre D, Sabatier J-C, Faller B, Beaud J-M. Early post transplantation infections in CAPD patients. Perit Dial Bull 1984; 4: 40–1.
316. Steinmuller D, Novick A, Braun W et al. Renal transplantation of patients on chronic peritoneal dialysis. Am J Kid Dis 1984; 3: 436–9.
317. Stephanidis C, Balfe J, Arbus G, Hardy BE, Churchill BM, Rance CP. Renal transplantation in children treated with continuous ambulatory peritoneal dialysis. Perit Dial Bull 1983; 3: 5–8.
318. Dutton S. Transient post-transplant ascites in

CAPD patients (letter). Perit Dial Bull 1983; 3: 164.
319. Inamoto H, Ozaki R, Matsuzaki T, Wakui M, Saruta T, Osawa A. Incidence and mortality pattern of malignancy and factors affecting the risk of malignancy in dialysis patients. Nephron 1991; 59: 611-7.
320. Digenis G, Pierratos A, Ayiomamitis A, Dombros N, Sombolos K, Oreopoulos DG. Cancer in patients on CAPD. Perit Dial Bull 1986; 6: 122–4.
321. Madden M, Beirne G, Zimmerman S, Sollinger H. Acute bowel obstruction: an unusual complication of chronic peritoneal dialysis. Am J Kid Dis 1982; 1: 219–21.
322. Nassberger L. Enterocele due to continuous ambulatory peritoneal dialysis (CAPD). Acta Obstet Gynecol Scand 1984; 63: 283.
323. Francis D, Schofield I, Veitch P. Abdominal hernias in patients treated with continuous ambulatory peritoneal dialysis. Br J Surg 1982; 69: 409.
324. Lee A, Waffle C, Trebbin W. Clostridial myonecrosis. Origin from an obturator hernia in a dialysis patient. J Am Med Assoc 1983; 246: 1232–3.
325. Lasker N, Burke J, Patchefsky A. Peritoneal reactions to particulate matter in peritoneal dialysis solutions. Trans Am Soc Artif Intern Organs 1975; 21: 342–5.
326. Novello A, Port F. Sclerosing encapsulating peritonitis (editorial). Int J Artif Organs 1986; 9: 393–6.

20 Peritoneal dialysis in children

STEVEN R. ALEXANDER, J. WILLIAMSON BALFE AND ELIZABETH HARVEY

1. Introduction and personal notes — 592
2. Notes on the history of peritoneal dialysis use in children — 592
3. Demographic issues — 594
   3.1. Incidence of ESRD in children — 594
   3.2. Prevalence of ESRD in children — 594
   3.3. Causes of ESRD in children — 595
4. Peritoneal membrane function in children: Physiologic concepts — 595
   4.1. Effective membrane surface area and solute permeability — 596
   4.2. Ultrafiltration — 597
   4.3. Peritoneal lymphatic absorption — 597
   4.4. Peritoneal membrane function in the neonate — 597
   4.5. The peritoneal equilibration test in children — 598
5. Peritoneal dialysis for acute renal failure — 598
   5.1. Indications and contraindications — 598
   5.2. Technical considerations — 599
      5.2.1. Catheters — 599
      5.2.2. Peritoneal dialysis solutions — 600
   5.3. The acute peritoneal dialysis prescription — 600
6. Peritoneal dialysis for ESRD in children — 601
   6.1. Indications and contraindications for chronic peritoneal dialysis — 601
   6.2. Peritoneal dialysis catheters — 601
   6.3. Specialized equipment for pediatric patients — 602
      6.3.1. Small volume bags — 602
      6.3.2. Pediatric cyclers — 603
   6.4. Choosing among commercially available peritoneal dialysis solutions — 603
      6.4.1. Calcium — 603
      6.4.2. Magnesium — 603
      6.4.3. Buffers — 603
      6.4.4. Osmotic agents — 603
   6.5. Dialysis mechanics: The chronic peritoneal dialysis prescription for children — 604
      6.5.1. Chronic intermittent peritoneal dialysis (IPD) — 604
      6.5.2. Continuous ambulatory peritoneal dialysis (CAPD) — 604
      6.5.3. Continuous cycler peritoneal dialysis (CCPD) and nightly intermittent peritoneal dialysis (NIPD) — 604
      6.5.4. Tidal peritoneal dialysis (TPD) — 604
      6.5.5. The CPD prescription — 605
   6.6. Nutritional management of children on CPD — 605
      6.6.1. Nutritional goals — 605
      6.6.2. Controlled enteral nutrition — 607
      6.6.3. Intraperitoneal amino acids — 608
   6.7. A simplified approach to the use of urea kinetic modeling to prescribe and monitor peritoneal dialysis therapy in children — 609
      6.7.1. Kt/V urea — 610
      6.7.2. Practical protein balance in growing children receiving peritoneal dialysis — 610
   6.8. Management of the very young infant: Special considerations — 613
   6.9. Renal anemia and its treatment in children on CPD — 614
      6.9.1. Pre-treatment concerns — 614
      6.9.2. Dosing suggestions — 615
      6.9.3. Monitoring suggestions — 615
      6.9.4. Iron supplementation — 615
   6.10. Renal osteodystrophy — 616
   6.11. Complications — 617
      6.11.1. Peritonitis — 617
      6.11.2. Exit site and tunnel infections — 618
      6.11.3. Hernias, leaks and hydrothorax — 619
      6.11.4. Metabolic abnormalities — 620
      6.11.5. Abdominal catastrophies — 621
      6.11.6. Miscellaneous complications — 621
   6.12. Quality of life and other psychosocial issues — 622
   6.13. Peritoneal dialysis and renal transplantation in children — 623
   6.14. The choice of CPD or hemodialysis as maintenance RRT pending transplantation for children at different ages — 624
   6.15. Training families for home peritoneal dialysis — 625
7. Peritoneal dialysis for intoxications, inborn errors of metabolism and other miscellaneous disorders in children — 626
   7.1. Intoxications — 626
   7.2. Congenital hyperammonemia and other inborn errors of metabolism — 626
   7.3. Miscellaneous pediatric disorders in which treatment with peritoneal dialysis has been attempted — 627
Acknowledgements — 627
References — 627

1. Introduction and personal notes

Like many chapters in this text, the origins of the present chapter can be traced to the 1976 discovery of continuous ambulatory peritoneal dialysis (CAPD) by Moncrief, Popovich and their associates [1]. As pediatric nephrologists trained in the 1970's, the two "senior" authors of this chapter (SRA & JWB) learned the basic techniques of peritoneal dialysis (PD) primarily as a treatment for infants and small children suffering from acute renal failure. Then, as now, PD was widely considered to be the renal replacement therapy (RRT) of choice for acute renal failure in pediatric patients, primarily because PD is intrinsically simple, safe and easily adapted for use in patients of all ages and sizes. However, chronic peritoneal dialysis (CPD) as it was performed in the pre-CAPD era was not very successful in children. During the early 1970's, hemodialysis for children came into vogue, and we learned to use hemodialysis to treat end-stage renal disease (ESRD) in children. The limitations of available hemodialysis techniques for infants and small children soon became painfully apparent. Although separated by 3,000 miles and an international boundary, by 1978 we found ourselves in remarkably similar situations; each of us had become responsible for a group of infants and small children with ESRD who could not be transplanted promptly and for whom the available dialysis treatment options were inadequate. Thus, as with the invention of CAPD itself, the introduction of CAPD into our pediatric ESRD programs was the result of clinical necessity. We suspect that this same process was responsible for the tenacity with which early pediatric CAPD programs struggled to modify original CAPD equipment and techniques (designed exclusively for adults) so that CAPD could be used in children.

Working together to write this chapter has provided us with an opportunity to examine the currently available information on the use of PD in children from a perspective of 15 years of shared experiences and observations. We were pleased and only a little surprised to find that we still have many similar approaches and opinions. However, writing this chapter has also illuminated our differences. As with all complex clinical situations, there is more than one successful way to deal with most problems encountered by a child receiving PD. Throughout this chapter we have attempted to reach consensus whenever possible, and when not, to delineate acceptable alternative approaches. Because pediatric ESRD therapy is an inherently controversial field in which the "definitive" clinical trial is vanishingly rare, writing this chapter together has been a challenge. Fortunately, we were joined in this task by a third author (EH) whose entry into the field of pediatric ESRD care is more recent. The irreverence of youth has been an invaluable addition to the preparation of the more controversial sections of the material that follows. Together the three of us have worked to create a chapter that hopefully provides some practical assistance to those who care for children receiving peritoneal dialysis.

2. Notes on the history of peritoneal dialysis use in children

The peritoneal cavity has been used in the treatment of serious illness in children for at least 75 years. In 1918 Blackfan and Maxcy described the successful use of intraperitoneal injections of saline solution in dehydrated infants [2], a method that is still used in rural areas of some developing countries. The initial reports describing the use of PD to treat children suffering from acute renal failure were published by Bloxsom and Powell in 1948 (in the premier issue of the journal, *Pediatrics*) and by Swan and Gordon in 1949 [3, 4]. These reports appeared at a time when worldwide published clinical experience with PD did not total 100 patients [5].

The experience of Swan and Gordon was the more successful of the two initial pediatric PD reports [4]. The technique ("continuous peritoneal lavage") and apparatus used by these pioneering Denver pediatric surgeons allowed large volumes of dialysate to flow continuously by gravity from 20-liter carboys through a rigid metal catheter that had been surgically implanted into the upper abdomen. Dialysate was constantly drained by water suction through an identical catheter implanted in the pelvis. Fluid balance was maintained by adjusting dialysate dextrose content between 2 gm% and 4 gm%, and excellent solute clearances were achieved by providing an average dialysate delivery of 33 liters per day. Dialysate temperature was regulated by adjusting the number of illuminated 60-watt incandescent light bulbs in a box placed over the dialysate inflow path.

Although two of the three children treated by Swan and Gordon survived after 9 and 12 days of continuous peritoneal lavage, it was more than a decade before the use of PD in children was again reported. During the 1950's the development of disposable nylon catheters and commercially prepared dialysate made PD a practical short-term treatment for acute renal failure [6]. The adaptation of this technique for use in children was described in 1961 by Segar and associates in Indianapolis [7] and in 1962 by Etteldorf and associates in Memphis [8]. Both groups later demonstrated the effectiveness of PD as a treatment for boric acid and salicylate intoxication, two of the most common intoxications in small children during the 1960's [9, 10].

Subsequent reports established PD as the most frequently employed RRT for acute renal failure in pediatric patients [11–17]. PD appeared ideally suited for use in children. As compared to hemodialysis, PD was intrinsically simple, safe, and easily adapted for use in patients of all ages and sizes, from newborn infants to fully grown adolescents. In contrast, hemodialysis at this early stage of development required large extracorporeal blood circuits that were either poorly tolerated or frankly impossible to achieve in many children. The widespread popularity of PD as the acute RRT of choice for children was enhanced by the prevalent notion that the peritoneum was "more efficient" in the child, a concept addressed later in this chapter.

While successful as a treatment for acute renal failure, PD appeared to have much less to offer the child with ESRD. Initial chronic PD techniques required reinsertion of the dialysis catheter for each treatment, making prolonged use in small patients difficult and routinely resulting in inadequate dialysis [18]. The development of a permanent peritoneal catheter, first proposed by Palmer and associates [19, 20] and later refined by Tenckhoff and Schecter [21] made long-term PD an accessible form of RRT for pediatric patients. When Boen [22] and then Tenckhoff [23] devised an automated dialysate delivery system that could be used in the home, chronic intermittent peritoneal dialysis (IPD) became a practical alternative to chronic hemodialysis for children. Largely as a result of the pioneering efforts of the pediatric ESRD treatment team in Seattle [24, 25], pediatric chronic IPD programs were established in a few prominent pediatric dialysis centers [26–29]. However, there was little enthusiasm for chronic IPD among pediatric nephrologists during this period, because it was associated with many of the least desirable features of chronic hemodialysis (e.g., substantial fluid and dietary restrictions, immobility during treatments, and the need for complex machinery), without providing the *efficiency* of hemodialysis.

A new era in the history of PD for children was heralded by the description of CAPD in 1976 by Moncrief, Popovich and associates [1]. CAPD appeared particularly well-suited for use in children. Advantages over hemodialysis of special importance to children included near steady-state biochemical control, no disequilibrium syndrome, greatly reduced fluid and dietary restrictions, and freedom from repeated dialysis needle punctures. CAPD also allowed children of all ages to receive dialysis at home, offering them the opportunity to experience more normal childhoods. Finally, CAPD made possible the routine treatment of very young infants, thereby extending the option of RRT to an entire population of patients previously considered too young for chronic dialysis.

CAPD was first used in a child in 1978 in Toronto [30, 31] and soon became available in other pediatric dialysis programs in North America and Western Europe [32–37]. In Canada, dialysate was available in small volume plastic containers soon after the first pediatric CAPD patients were trained, but in the United States, early efforts to adapt CAPD for pediatric patients were hampered by the commercial availability of dialysate only in 2000 ml containers. Parents were taught to discard surplus fluid from the 2000 ml containers and infuse the remainder [34], or to prepare small volume bags at home by filling blood bank transfer packs [32]. Hospital pharmacies were used to periodically prepare small volume dialysate bags for individual families [33]. These wasteful, expensive, and potentially risky methods became unnecessary in July, 1980, when dialysate in 500 and 1000 ml plastic containers became commercially available in the U.S. [38]. The subsequent addition of 250, 750, and 1500 ml containers completed a range of standardized dialysate containers that accommodated most pediatric CAPD patients.

The next step in the resurgence of chronic peritoneal dialysis (CPD) for children was the reintroduction of the automated cycler. Continuous cycler peritoneal dialysis (CCPD) was first used in a child by Price and Suki in 1981 [39]. Cycler dialysis subsequently became extremely popular among pediatric PD programs in North America [40]. Further modifications of the CCPD regimen focused on elimination of most of the daytime exchange (i.e., nightly intermittent peritoneal dialysis [NIPD]). During the past decade the growth of CAPD, CCPD, NIPD and other CPD variations has been spectacular [40]. Before 1982, fewer than 100 pediatric patients had been treated with CAPD worldwide, and CCPD for children was virtually unknown [39]. By the end of 1989, CPD accounted for 50% of pediatric dialysis patients (<15 years old) in the United States, 65% in Canada, and 75% in Australia and New Zealand [40], and CPD is now the most frequently prescribed chronic dialysis modality for children in many other parts of the world as well.

3. Demographic issues

3.1. Incidence of ESRD in children

ESRD is not a common pediatric disorder. In the United States and Canada there are about 11 new pediatric ESRD cases per million children of similar age reported each year [41, 42]. This contrasts sharply with the incidence of congenital heart disease (8,000 per million) and childhood leukemia (40 per million) [43, 44].

Published information on the incidence of ESRD in pediatric patients reveals marked geographic variability. Reports from single pediatric ESRD treatment centers, national surveys and national and multi-national registries document an incidence ranging from 2.1 to >10 new cases per million children of similar age per year [45]. It is doubtful that such differences reflect actual geographic differences in the prevalence of diseases that result in renal failure. Rather, geographic variability in pediatric ESRD incidence appears to be mainly the result of economic and social conditions. The European Dialysis and Transplant Association reports the mean ESRD incidence for all member countries considered together to be 4.6 new patients per million children per year; however, incidence rates vary from 2 per million in Turkey to 12.5 per million in Finland [45].

ESRD incidence also varies according to age, as shown in Table 1, which provides data from the United States Renal Data System (USRDS) for 1977 and 1987 [46]. Note that ESRD incidence increases dramatically with increasing age. However, even among the oldest pediatric age group (15 to 19 years olds) the incidence of ESRD (21 to 23 per million) is far less than the incidence of ESRD in adults (see Table 1) [46].

Table 1 also shows the differences in ESRD incidence that occur over time. Note that in 1977 only 2 infants per million <1 year of age were reported, compared to 15 per million in 1987. Substantial, though less dramatic increases are also seen for the next two age groups. Above 9 years of age the incidence of ESRD remained essentially unchanged between 1977 and 1987. These data could be interpreted as showing an absolute increase in the disorders leading to ESRD in children <10 yrs of age between 1977 and 1987, but it seems more likely that in 1987 younger children who would not have received RRT in 1977 were no longer being excluded.

The incidence variability seen among different geographic areas, age groups and observation periods serves to emphasize that these are not true disease incidence figures, but rather the incidence of the *decision to treat* children with RRT. That decision is apparently influenced by economic and social conditions, as well as by developing technology.

3.2. Prevalence of ESRD in children

Children account for only a small fraction of the total ESRD patient population. Of the 121,978 registered dialysis patients receiving treatment in the U.S. on December 31, 1990, the USRDS reported that only 1,627 (1.3%) were <20 yrs of age [41]. Table 2 displays USRDS ESRD patient counts for December 31 of 1985 and 1990 by patient age group and treatment modality [41]. Note that absolute pediatric dialysis patient counts are small and increased by only 19% between 1985 and 1990, compared to a 53% increase for adults during the same period. The data in Table 2 clearly demonstrate the importance of transplantation to pediatric ESRD patient management. On December 31, 1990 over 60% of pediatric ESRD patients in the U.S.

Table 1. Pediatric ESRD incidence in the United States in 1977 and 1987 (Adjusted for age, sex and race).

Age group (Years)	New patients PMP per year	
	1977	1987
<1	2	15
1–4	2	4
5–9	4	6
10–14	11	11
15–19	21	23
20–44*	–	79

PMP = Per million population, age-adjusted.
Data from USRDS 1989 (reference [46]).
* Adult data provided for comparison.

were being maintained by a functioning transplant, compared to 26% of adults.

3.3. Causes of ESRD in children

Approximately one-half of children requiring RRT have a congenital or hereditary renal disorder and one-half an acquired renal lesion. This is in contrast to the adult ESRD population in which over 80% of patients have an acquired renal disease. Table 3 lists the primary renal diseases of 762 pediatric dialysis patients reported in 1992 to the Dialysis Patient Data Base of the North American Pediatric Renal Transplant Cooperative Study (NAPRTCS) [47]. The most frequently identified primary renal diseases were aplastic/hypoplastic/dysplastic kidneys (15.7%), focal and segmental glomerulosclerosis (14.6%), obstructive uropathy (14.0%), systemic immunologic disease (7.6%) and the hemolytic uremic syndrome (4.5%).

The frequency with which structural anomalies of the urinary tract occur among children with ESRD has important implications for pediatric PD programs. PD techniques must be made compatible with a wide variety of urinary diversions. Close collaboration with pediatric urologists and surgeons is essential to the successful reconstruction or revision of these urinary tracts prior to transplantation.

4. Peritoneal membrane function in children: Physiologic concepts

It has long been held that the peritoneal membrane of the child is functionally different from that of the adult, and that peritoneal transport kinetics change as a consequence of normal growth and development [15]. This concept can be traced to comparative measurements of peritoneal surface area performed more than 100 years ago. In 1884, in a paper read before the Siberian Branch of the Russian Geographic Society, Putiloff presented comparative data on the peritoneal membrane surface area of infants and adults [48]. Using direct oiled paper tracings of peritoneal contents, Putiloff found that the peritoneal surface area of an infant weighing 2.9 kg was 0.15 m^2, compared to 2.08 m^2 for an adult of unspecified weight. If a weight of 70 kg is assumed for Putiloff's adult subject, the infant's peritoneal surface area is found to be almost twice that of the adult when scaled for body weight (522 cm^2/kg vs 285 cm^2/kg). Earlier studies by Wegner suggested that the peritoneal surface area closely approximated the body surface area in the adult [49]. Because the ratio of body surface area to weight is greater in infants, a greater peritoneal surface area to weight ratio in infants was not surprising.

The clinical implications of these anatomic relationships were explored in 1966 by Esperanca and Collins [50]. Direct measurements of peritoneal surface areas were made during autopsies performed on six neonates and six adults. Mean peritoneal surface area to body weight ratio in the infants was roughly twice that of the adults, confirming Putiloff's measurements made 80 years earlier. Esperanca and Collins assumed that peritoneal surface area and peritoneal membrane function was directly correlated, postulating that "... peritoneal dialysis should be twice as efficient in the infant ..." [50]. Peritoneal urea clearance studies in puppies and adult dogs performed by these same investigators seemed to support their hypothesis. When scaled for body weight, peritoneal urea clearance measured in puppies was two to three times the clearance measured in adult animals. However, these clearance studies were seriously flawed. Widely different dialysate delivery rates were used in the puppies and adult animals (128 vs 42 ml/kg/hour, respectively). In this range, urea clearance is directly proportional to dialysate flow rate, providing ample explanation for the observed differences in urea clearances.

The report by Esperanca and Collins provides an early example of the pitfalls associated with the use of variable dialysis mechanics when studying peritoneal membrane function. These pitfalls can be avoided if peritoneal transport studies are

Table 2. Living U.S. ESRD patients on December 31 of 1985 and 1990 by patient age and treatment modality.

Age group (yrs)	1985 Dialysis	1985 Tx	1990 Dialysis	1990 Tx
0–4	131	111	150	125
5–9	124	251	181	430
10–14	303	468	367	667
15–19	812	980	929	1,188
0–19	1,370	1,810	1,627	2,410
20–85+	78,475	21,308	120,360	43,043
Total	79,845	23,118	121,987	45,453

Tx = Functioning Transplant.
Data from reference [41].

performed in accordance with Gruskin's Rules [51]:

1. Constant inflow, dwell, and outflow times must be used for all study exchanges.
2. Identical dialysate composition must be used in all study subjects.
3. Exchange volumes must be identically scaled per unit body size. (Gruskin allows the use of body weight, height or surface area as the scaling factor, but surface area is probably more reliable).
4. Results must be adjusted and reported according to the body size scaling factor used to determine exchange volume.

Classical studies of peritoneal transport in adults have sought to characterize membrane transport properties in terms of effective membrane surface area and solute permeability, fluid transfer (ultrafiltration), and peritoneal lymphatic absorption [52, 53]. Studies involving pediatric subjects are rare, and available data remain controversial.

4.1. Effective membrane surface area and solute permeability

In an early example of the "peritoneal equilibration test" in pediatric patients, Gruskin and associates examined time-related changes in dialysate-to-blood concentration ratios for seven different solutes in nine children, 4 months to 18.5 years of age [54]. By rigidly controlling dialysis mechanics in these studies, Gruskin demonstrated the distortions created by even minor perturbations in exchange volume and dwell time. Diffusion curves constructed for each solute were found to be fundamentally similar to adult reference curves. Mean peritoneal urea and creatinine clearances were no different in younger compared to older children or adults when scaled to body weight or surface area. Gruskin concluded that apparent age-related differ-

Table 3. Primary renal disease diagnosis in pediatric dialysis patients.

	N	Percent
Diagnosis		
Aplastic/hypoplastic/dysplasic kidneys	119	15.7
Focal segmental glomerulosclerosis	111	14.6
Obstructive uropathy	106	14.0
Systemic immunologic disease	58	7.6
Hemolytic uremic syndrome	34	4.5
Chronic glomerulonephritis	31	4.1
Reflux nephropathy	26	3.4
Polycystic kidney disease	23	3.0
Syndrome of agenesis of abdominal musculature	19	2.5
Medullary cystic disease/juvenile nephronophthisis	18	2.4
Congenital nephrotic syndrome	17	2.2
Pyelonephritis/interstitial nephritis	15	2.0
Membranoproliferative glomerulonephritis Type I	14	1.8
Cystinosis	11	1.4
Familial nephritis	11	1.4
Idiopathic crescentic glomerulonephritis	11	1.4
Membranoproliferative glomerulonephritis Type II	10	1.3
Renal infarct	7	0.9
Drash syndrome	7	0.9
Sickle cell nephropathy	4	0.5
Wilms tumor	3	0.4
Oxalosis	2	0.3
Membranous nephropathy	1	0.1
Other	67	8.8
Unknown	34	4.5

Adapted from reference [47].

ences in peritoneal dialysis "efficiency" described in previous reports were likely the result of differences in dialysis mechanics employed in those studies [51]. Subsequent studies have disputed this conclusion. Analysis of diffusion curves constructed from two studies on separate groups of children suggested that transperitoneal solute movement varied with patient age, not reaching adult values until later childhood [55, 56].

Peritoneal solute transfer in children has also been characterized by measuring the mass-transfer area coefficients (MTAC) for various solutes according to the model of peritoneal membrane transport devised by Pyle and Popovich [57]. Morgenstern and associated found that the MTAC's for urea, creatinine, uric acid, and glucose in eight children, 1.5 to 18 yrs of age were similar to adult reference values when adjusted for body surface area [58]. In contrast, the MTAC for total protein was significantly greater in children than in adults. These results supported earlier clinical observations of increased peritoneal protein losses in younger children treated with CAPD [59, 60]. Subsequent studies by the same investigators supported these observations [61].

In contrast, Geary and associates recently studied peritoneal transport in a large group of children and found that MTAC values for glucose and creatinine were directly related to the age and size of the patients [62]. MTAC values per kilogram body weight were inversely proportional to patient age, suggesting an increased effective peritoneal surface area in younger children.

Attempts to interpret these studies are hindered by the use of different dialysis mechanics in different studies. Geary and associates scaled test exchange volumes by patient weight and used a relatively low standard exchange volume (30 ml/kg). The higher MTAC values per kilogram body weight observed by Geary in younger children could be the result of a relatively greater effective peritoneal surface area *per kilogram body weight* in younger patients.

In summary, no studies have clearly demonstrated an age dependent difference in peritoneal membrane transport function. What has been shown is an anatomically larger and probably functionally larger membrane surface area per kg body weight in younger patients. Proper scaling of test exchange volumes and results to body surface area should eliminate any apparent age related differences in function.

4.2. Ultrafiltration

Early studies and much clinical experience suggested that adequate ultrafiltration could be difficult to achieve in infants and younger children. A more rapid decline in dialysate dextrose concentration and osmolality was observed in younger children, and the inadequate ultrafiltration was attributed to this mechanism [63, 64]. Subsequent studies have failed to find age-related differences in dextrose absorption and intraperitoneal osmolality changes beyond the neonatal period [58, 61, 65].

4.3. Peritoneal lymphatic absorption

Studies of ultrafiltration in children have been hindered by the absence of information on the contribution of lymphatic absorption to net ultrafiltration. Studies by Mactier and associates suggest that children have relatively greater rates of lymphatic absorption than adults [66]. In six children, 2 to 13 years of age, Mactier found that peritoneal lymphatic drainage served to reduce mean ultrafiltration by 27% and mean peritoneal clearances of creatinine and urea by 22% and 24%, respectively. When lymphatic absorption rates were scaled to body weight, higher values were obtained for pediatric patients, compared to adult reference values. However, lymphatic absorption rates were similar to adult reference values when scaled for body surface area [66]. Differences in dialysis mechanics between the adult and pediatric studies and the small number of children studied may explain this discrepancy, but it remains unclear whether lymphatic absorption is an age-related phenomenon.

4.4. Peritoneal membrane function in the neonate

Neonates receiving PD routinely have lower levels of BUN than older children and often have decreased ultrafiltration. A greater membrane solute transport capacity in the young infant is an attractive explanation for these observations. There is evidence to suggest that the peritoneal membrane functions differently during early infancy than at any point later in life. Studies of peritoneal dialysance in puppies demonstrated greater values for all solutes studied compared to adult animals [67]. Studies in human neonates have frequently demonstrated increased peritoneal clearances of small solutes, although most of these studies failed to conform to Gruskin's Rules, confounding interpretation [18, 50, 54, 68]. A more rapid decline in dialysate dextrose concentration due to a relatively greater membrane glucose transport rate may explain the decreased ultrafiltration rates observed in many infants [63, 64], although this has not been demonstrated in controlled studies [56].

There are alternative explanations. Kohaut has shown that ultrafiltration in the neonate is exquisitely dependent on exchange volume [69], suggesting that observed differences in ultrafiltration rates reflect only differences in dialysis mechanics. If Kohaut is correct, proper scaling of exchange volumes and observed ultrafiltration rates to body surface area should resolve any apparent differences between neonates and older subjects. Disappearance rates of glucose from the dialysate and urea from the blood also could be influenced by higher utilization rates of glucose and dietary protein found in the neonate. Growth has been called the "third kidney" of the newborn, because so little dietary protein appears as urea [70]. Glucose utilization by neonates is three times greater than that of adults. These variables must be considered in future studies of peritoneal membrane function in the newborn.

4.5. The peritoneal equilibration test in children

As popularized by Twardowski, the peritoneal equilibration test (PET) has been introduced as a convenient method by which an individual patient's peritoneal membrane transport function may be characterized and compared to population norms [71]. The standardized PET solute curves constructed by Twardowski have been widely used, but are of questionable value as reference standards for pediatric patients. Twardowski reasoned that to be clinically useful the PET should be based on a typical adult CAPD exchange volume of 2,000 ml. Thus, to construct his reference curves, Twardowski used 2,000 ml exchanges in all patients regardless of body size. The importance of scaling test exchange volumes to body size in adults has not been examined, but there is little doubt that pediatric studies must be scaled to body size.

Several investigators have attempted to use the PET to construct solute equilibration curves for pediatric patients [55, 56, 72, 73]. Unfortunately, uniform exchange volumes were not used in these studies, with body weight [55, 56, 73] and body surface area [72] used as scaling factors. Multicenter collaborative studies are currently underway in North America and in Germany to define standardized pediatric PET curves. The ultimate clinical usefulness of such curves has been questioned [74]. Routine PET determinations in individual patients may be helpful in defining the optimum PD prescription and in tracking changes in peritoneal membrane function over time.

5. Peritoneal dialysis for acute renal failure

5.1. Indications and contraindications

The conservative management of acute renal failure in pediatric patients requires meticulous attention to fluid and electrolyte balance. Minor errors can have severe consequences. Dietary restrictions, phosphate binders, diuretics, sodium bicarbonate, calcium salts, antihypertensive medications, and sodium-potassium exchange resins all play important roles in delaying or avoiding dialysis in some children, although such tactics are not likely to be successful in oligo-anuric children. Several factors are at work in the pediatric patient that tend to defeat even the most carefully conceived conservative management plans. Children with acute renal failure are profoundly catabolic, resulting in accumulation of uremic solutes at surprisingly rapid rates. In the oliguric child it is difficult to meet energy requirements while abiding by stringent limitations on allowable fluid intake. As a result, dialysis and hemofiltration tend to be promptly employed in the pediatric patients with acute renal failure.

Widely accepted clinical indications for RRT in children with acute renal failure are listed in Table 4. Such lists may not adequately portray the need to consider the rate at which conditions are deteriorating in the individual child. A marginal clinical situation should not be tolerated in any child when prompt institution of RRT will control fluid and solute derangements and allow adequate nutrition.

The convenience, simplicity and relative safety of PD has allowed the nephrologist to begin dialysis in the child as soon as it is needed, without undue anxiety over potential complications from the procedure itself. The popularity of PD over hemodialysis for critically ill pediatric patients has traditionally rested on two important features: ready access to the peritoneum (vs typically more difficult vascular access), and better tolerance of PD by unstable children. Recent advances in vascular access techniques and equipment along with improvements in hemodialysis (primarily bicarbonate buffers and ultrafiltration control modules) have narrowed the choice between dialysis modalities in many pediatric centers. Moreover, the introduction of continuous hemofiltration techniques for children has begun to challenge the preeminence of peritoneal dialysis for the most critically ill pediatric patients [75–77]. Although vascular access is required, continuous hemofiltration is well tolerated by hemodynamically unstable children. Clear indications for one RRT modality over the others are now rarely present, and often it is the experience of the center that dictates the selection of RRT modality.

There are few contraindications to acute PD. Absolute contraindications all relate to the lack of an adequate peritoneal cavity. Neonates with omphalocele, diaphragmatic hernia or gastroschisis cannot be treated with PD. Recent abdominal surgery is not an absolute contraindication, as long as there are no draining abdominal wounds, but we prefer to treat such patients with continuous venovenous hemofiltration (CVVH) or hemodialysis. Children with vesicostomies and other urinary diversions, polycystic kidneys, colostomies, gastrostomies, prune-belly syndrome and recent bowel anastomoses have been successfully treated with PD in our centers and others. PD can be used to treat acute allograft dysfunction immediately following renal transplantation, as long as the allograft has been placed in an extraperitoneal location. Extensive intra-abdominal adhesions may prevent PD in some patients. Surgical lysis of such adhesions often results in prolonged intra-peritoneal hemorrhage. We now treat such patients acutely with CVVH (if they are unstable) or hemodialysis.

Table 4. Indications[a] for dialysis in children with acute renal failure.

- Hyperkalemia (serum [K+] > 7.0 mEq/L)
- Intractable acidosis
- Fluid overload; often with hypertension, congestive heart failure, or pulmonary edema
- Severe azotemia (BUN > 150 mg/dl)
- Symptomatic uremia (encephalopathy, pericarditis, intractable vomiting, hemorrhage)
- Hyponatremia, hypocalcemia, hyperphosphatemia (severe, symptomatic)
- Fluid removal for optimal nutrition, transfusions, infusions of medications, etc.

[a] These are general guidelines. Each case must be individualized (see text).

5.2. Technical considerations

5.2.1. Catheters

5.2.1.1. Acute catheters: Temporary vs permanent. A reliable catheter is the cornerstone of successful acute PD. The choice between a percutaneously placed temporary catheter and a surgically placed "permanent" catheter is usually somewhat arbitrary, reflecting local practice. An increased incidence of peritonitis has been associated historically with the use of the same temporary catheter for longer than 72 hours [16]. Current practice in our centers is to extend the life of a well-functioning temporary catheter beyond three days, but by the sixth day those catheters usually have been replaced with permanent catheters.

Surgical placement of a cuffed permanent catheter in the setting of acute renal failure has the advantage of assuring good immediate function, but must be weighed against the risks and delays incurred by an operative procedure requiring general anesthesia. Anesthesiologists may be reluctant to administer general anesthesia to a child with the metabolic derangements of acute renal failure. In patients considered high-risk for general anesthesia, initial placement of a percutaneous catheter under local analgesia allows immediate dialysis. A surgical catheter can then be placed once the child is stable and it is clear that more than five days of dialysis will be needed. Surgical catheter placement at the bedside is readily performed in unstable ICU patients [78, 79].

5.2.1.2. Temporary catheters for acute peritoneal dialysis. The familiar pediatric Trocath (McGaw) [80] has been replaced in most pediatric centers by a percutaneously inserted silastic or Teflon catheter that is placed using the Seldinger technique and a peel-away sheath (Cook). The advantages of these catheters were described by Murphy and associates [81]. Poor drainage is a common problem with percutaneous catheters that is usually caused by omental envelopment. When this occurs it is best to avoid repeated abdominal punctures and proceed to surgical catheter placement.

5.2.1.3. Temporary catheters for infants. When treating small infants (e.g. those weighing <1,500 grams) we have frequently resorted to such commonly found ICU items as 14 gauge plastic intravenous catheters (Intracath®, Deseret). In Dallas we have recently had success with a small curled catheter that was designed to drain pleural effusions without a water seal (the Starzl Pleural Catheter®, Cook). This catheter is inserted over a guidewire and can be placed flat just beneath the anterior abdominal wall. Multiple fenestrations in the curled intraperitoneal segment increase drainage and reduce obstructions. In Toronto, a specially designed neonatal acute catheter is used (Cook).

5.2.1.4. Permanent catheters for acute renal failure. Standard, single-cuff Tenckhoff catheters (straight or curled) can be used to treated acute renal failure. In our centers there is no difference in the techniques used to place permanent catheters, whether the patient is to receive acute or chronic PD. Permanent catheters will be discussed later in this chapter in the section on chronic peritoneal dialysis (CPD).

5.2.2. Peritoneal dialysis solutions
Peritoneal Dialysis Solutions (PDS) are commercially available in standard dextrose concentrations of 1.5%, 2.5%, and 4.25%. We usually begin acute dialysis with the 2.5% solution in order to obtain better ultrafiltration at the outset when fluid overload is frequently present and exchange volume must be kept relatively low to avoid leaks from the new catheter insertion site. PDS must be warmed to body temperature before infusion. Adults usually complain of discomfort during the infusion of cool PDS, but infants may respond to unwarmed PDS with a fall in blood pressure. We routinely use either the heater platform of the automated cycler (Baxter PacXtra) or blood transfusion warming devices placed in the PDS inflow path. Alternatively, water-filled heating pads may be wrapped around the hanging bags of fresh PDS.

Some infants do not tolerate the lactate that is absorbed from standard PDS [82]. These babies are often hypoxemic with an ongoing metabolic acidosis. Such infants will do better if they are treated from the outset with a PDS that has been prepared by the hospital pharmacy containing bicarbonate instead of lactate. The bicarbonate PDS formula used in Dallas is shown in Table 5. Note that calcium must be given by an alternate route and serum ionized calcium levels must be closely monitored when bicarbonate dialysis is used.

5.3. The acute peritoneal dialysis prescription

The PD prescription must specify dialysate composition, exchange volume, exchange inflow, dwell and drain times and the number of exchanges to be performed in 24 hours. During the initial 24 hours after catheter placement exchange volume is kept low, usually 15 to 20 ml/kg, to reduce the risk of dialysate leakage. Over the ensuring 3 to 5 days, exchange volume is increased gradually to reach a maximum of 40 to 45 ml/kg. Respiratory embarrassment and hydrothorax have been reported with the use of exchange volumes approaching 50 ml/kg [83, 84].

Initial stabilization on PD requires 24 to 48 hours of frequent exchanges, 40 to 60 minutes each, in order to remove accumulated solutes and excess fluid. This corresponds to a traditional acute intermittent peritoneal dialysis (IPD) regimen. Once stabilized, dialysis can proceed indefinitely. By gradually extending dwell times and increasing exchange volumes toward 40 to 45 ml/kg, a typical maintenance PD regimen can be reached in a few days. Familiarity with CPD regimens used in the treatment of ESRD has led to the popularity of standard CPD regimens for the treatment of acute renal failure [85, 86]. CPD has become the standard approach to acute PD in our centers, once the child has been stabilized with an appropriate period of frequent exchanges to correct fluid and electrolyte disturbances and lower the BUN. There is no need to periodically suspend CPD in order to see if renal function will return; kidneys seem to begin performing again when ready to do so, independent of ongoing CPD. While there have been no systematic studies of this approach to the acute PD prescription, the advantages of the near steady-state biochemical and fluid control achievable with CPD are compelling.

Table 5. Peritoneal dialysis solution containing bicarbonate for use in infants intolerant of lactate dialysate.

NaCl (0.45%)	896.0 ml
NaCl (2.5 mEq/ml)	12.0 ml
NaHCO$_3$ (1.0 mEq/ml)	40.0 ml
MgSO$_4$ (10%)	1.8 ml
D$_{50}$W	50.0 ml

Final composition: Na$^+$ = 139 mEq/L; Cl$^-$ = 99 mEq/L; Mg^{++} = 1.5 mEq/L; SO$_4^=$ = 1.5 mEq/L; HCO$_3^-$ = 40 mEq/L; Hydrous Dextrose = 2.5 g/dl.
Calculated osmolality = 423 mOsm/kg H$_2$O.
Modified from reference [82].

6. Peritoneal dialysis for ESRD in children

6.1. Indications and contraindications for chronic peritoneal dialysis

Most children can be successfully treated at home with chronic peritoneal dialysis (CPD). In the early days of CAPD, we carefully assessed families from the point of view of aptitude, hygiene and motivation to perform home dialysis. Over the years we have been pleasantly surprised that many families who were prejudged as potentially inadequate turned out to be successful CPD families, although some have required extensive home support. In times of limited health care dollars, such support services may not be as readily available.

There are a few situations in which CPD may be considered as being absolutely indicated over chronic hemodialysis: small infants; inadequate vascular access; hypercoagulable states; living a long distance from a pediatric hemodialysis center; and precarious cardiovascular status (Table 6). The preference of the patient and family must be considered a relative indication for CPD, as is the need for better control of hypertension.

As described in the previous section on acute PD, there are a number of conditions that constitute absolute contraindications to CPD, as well as conditions that, while potentially problematic, do not preclude CPD (Table 6). Ureterostomies, pyelostomies, or a vesicostomy have not interfered with CPD in our centers. Bladder augmentation is being employed more frequently for ESRD patients with inadequate bladders in preparation for renal transplantation; even in these children, successful CPD is possible.

6.2. Peritoneal dialysis catheters

Since the outset of CPD, investigators have been attempting to improve on the silastic Tenckhoff catheter. A number of new catheters have been devised, but the ideal catheter is still not available. For most of the available adult catheters there are comparable pediatric models.

The goals of catheter placement include adequate inflow and outflow of dialysate, no fluid leaks, minimal catheter movement at the skin exit site, and placement of the catheter at a site that is both reachable and visible to the patient or caregivers. Pediatric and adult CPD patients differ with respect to body size, underlying diseases and their associated anatomical and surgical features, and the number of alternate caregivers that perform the dialysis procedures. As yet there is no clearly superior catheter for children.

Double-cuff Tenckhoff catheters were originally introduced to overcome the problem of leakage and create a more effective barrier to infection. Early pediatric experience with these catheters was unsatisfactory. The second cuff was large and tended to migrate to the skin exit site, leading to distal cuff erosion. Distal cuff erosion seemed to occur frequently in children, perhaps because most pediatric patients have less abdominal wall adipose tissue than adults. Adoption of single-cuff Tenckhoff catheters resulted in avoidance of distal cuff erosion, but mechanical catheter complications were still common. Subsequently the Toronto Western Hospital catheter was adopted in Toronto, while in Oregon and later in Dallas the short, single-cuff curled Tenckhoff catheter was favored. Both approaches resulted in improved results and have been described in detail [87–90].

The surgical techniques used for catheter place-

Table 6. Indications and contraindications for chronic peritoneal dialysis.

Absolute contraindications for chronic peritoneal dialysis
- omphalocele
- gastroschisis
- diaphragmatic hernia
- obliterated peritoneal cavity
- bladder extrophy
- severe membrane failure

Potentially problematic conditions for chronic peritoneal dialysis
- mentally or physically inadequate patient/parent
- poor hygiene
- lack of motivation
- imminent plans for a living-related-donor transplant, and hemodialysis facility is available
- colostomy
- gastrostomy

Indications for chronic peritoneal dialysis
- small patient
- no vascular access sites
- coagulation disturbances
- blood pressure control
- precarious cardiovascular status
- living a long distance from the pediatric hemodialysis center
- preference of patient/parent

ment in our centers differ in only a few details. For example, a small "porthole" omentectomy is performed routinely in Dallas, whereas in Toronto a partial omentectomy is reserved for catheters being revised for poor outflow. A step-by-step description of the procedure used in Dallas has been published [89, 90]. The catheter placement techniques currently in use in Toronto are reviewed briefly below.

Surgical catheter insertion is performed in children with general anesthesia; muscle relaxation is sometimes required in obese or larger children. At the onset of anesthesia a nasogastric tube is placed to decompress the stomach and an indwelling bladder catheter is placed to insure that the urinary bladder is empty. A 3 to 4 cm transverse incision is made in the skin overlying the middle of the rectus muscle, usually below the level of the umbilicus. The tissues are dissected to the rectus sheath where another transverse incision is made. The muscle fibers are separated bluntly down to the posterior rectus sheath which is then elevated and incised to open the peritoneal cavity. The catheter is inserted into the peritoneal cavity under direct vision, using a stylet to insure that it is positioned in the pelvis. (In Dallas, the short curled catheter is placed just beneath and in the plane of the anterior abdominal wall at the level of insertion [89]). The cuff is sutured in place at the peritoneal edge and the peritoneum closed in a watertight fashion. A trocar is employed to direct the catheter under the rectus muscle a distance of 3 to 5 cm, at which point the trocar is forced through the anterior rectus sheath and subcutaneous tissue to exit the skin at a site well removed from the original skin incision. The rectus muscle and its sheath are closed over the peritoneal entry site of the catheter. Before the skin is closed, 10 to 20 ml/kg of dialysate is instilled and drained to insure adequate inflow and outflow and to confirm that the closure is watertight.

In Toronto a percutaneous insertion technique using the Y-Tec® peritoneoscope (Medigroup, Inc, North Aurora, IL) is being used with increasing frequency. This procedure may be of particular benefit in patients with prune-belly syndrome in whom there is an increased risk of dialysate leakage [91]. The laparoscopic technique requires a smaller (2.5 cm) incision to be made in the same infra-umbilical location over the rectus muscle. The Quill Catheter Guide Assembly® (Medigroup) is inserted and the peritoneal cavity distended with carbon dioxide. The catheter is placed in the quill, which is then peeled away. A purse-string suture closes the rectus sheath around the catheter, which is tunneled subcutaneously as in the open technique.

The catheter break-in period is critical in children, whose thin abdominal walls are prone to leakage and slow to seal around the catheter. The catheter break-in protocol currently used in Toronto is summarized in Table 7.

6.3. Specialized equipment for pediatric patients

6.3.1. Small volume bags

Small volume bags for CAPD have been available for more than a decade. In Canada there are 300, 500 and 750 ml bags, and in the U.S. the volumes are 250, 500, and 750 ml. Because cycler dialysis has nearly replaced CAPD for small patients these small volume products are used less often. For CAPD patients our centers use the spike connection system (System III®, Baxter Healthcare Corp.,

Table 7. Protocol for break-in of a new chronic peritoneal dialysis catheter.

1. Infuse 10 ml/kg body weight 1.5% dialysis fluid (containing heparin 500 IU/L and cefazoline 250 mg/L) with no dwell time until dialysate is clear.

2. When the effluent is clear:
   a) For patients not requiring immediate dialysis or entrance into CPD training:
      – fill the catheter with 3–5 ml (1000 IU/ml) heparin and cap off at the Titanium adapter

      or

      – infuse 10 ml/kg peritoneal dialysis fluid (containing heparin, 500 IU/L), maximum 300 ml, and cap off.
      – irrigate catheter daily for first week.
   b) For patients in need of immediate dialysis, or entrance into CPD training
      – one hour dwell-time for 24 hours
      – two hour dwell-time for 24 hours

3. Gradually increase the exchange volume over a few days to weeks:

	Volume (ml)	
Patient Weight (kg)	INITIAL	FINAL
10	100	400
20	200	600–800
30	300	900–1200
40	400	1200–1500

4. Patients destined to CAPD will get the closest appropriate volume bag; whereas those for CCPD will receive a volume precisely tailored to their size. Prophylactic antibiotic is discontinued once CAPD or CCPD is commenced.

Deerfield, IL) and a disposable disconnect Y-set (Ultraset III®, Baxter) which is compatible with small and standard volume bags. Unfortunately, the integrated disconnect system (Twin Bag) is not available in pediatric sizes, the smallest volume being 1500 ml. The germicidal exchange system (UV-Flash® or UV-XD®, Baxter) is routinely used in our centers, primarily because patients and parents can be confidently trained for CAPD in less time using the germicidal device.

6.3.2. Pediatric cyclers

The first cycler available for pediatric use in North America was the Lasker Cycler (American Medical Products Corporation, Fairfield, NJ) [92]. This simple cycler could be modified to deliver exchange volumes of 200 to 300 ml. The equipment was inexpensive, but commercially purchased dialysate was costly. Cyclers based on the principles of reverse osmosis (Physio-Control Company, Seattle, Washington) were also used to treat pediatric patients during this early period [23]. The reverse osmosis machine was expensive, but operating costs were low and peritonitis was uncommon [23].

Our centers now rely on cyclers manufactured by Baxter Healthcare Corporation, the PAC-X® and the PAC-XTRA®; the latter can deliver exchange volumes as low as 50 ml and offer 10 ml incremental adjustments. There are other excellent pediatric cyclers available: the Impersol Cycler 1000 (Abbott Laboratories); the Microstar VC-1 Cycler (Medionics International Inc.); Peritoneal Dialysis System Fresenius 80/2 or 90/2 (Fresenius). All of these cyclers present problems for small infants for whom the dead space of the tubing greatly reduces dialysis efficiency.

6.4. Choosing among commercially available peritoneal dialysis solutions

Since the advent of CAPD, much investigative effort has been directed toward improving the composition of peritoneal dialysis solutions (PDS). Characteristics of the ideal PDS as proposed by Hutchison and Gokal are: the solution must clear solutes and ultrafilter water in a predictable manner; it must remove uremic toxins; it should provide nutrition to the patient without metabolic complications; it should be isosmotic with a physiological pH using bicarbonate as the buffer; and finally it should have antibacterial and antifungal properties [93].

6.4.1. Calcium

The current trend is toward a PDS with a lower calcium concentration. In North America, PDS was originally available with calcium concentrations of 3.25 or 3.5 mEq/liter (i.e., 1.6 or 1.75 mmol/liter). When oral calcium salts became the preferred phosphate binders in children and adults as a way to avoid aluminum toxicity, a lower calcium dialysate (calcium = 2.5 mEq/liter [1.25 mmol/liter]) became essential for some patients. Use of this lower calcium dialysate in children has had no obvious adverse effects, although systematic studies have not been reported.

6.4.2. Magnesium

It has been shown that children develop hypermagnesemia when treated with CAPD using a PDS containing magnesium at 1.5 mEq/liter (0.75 mmol/liter) [94]. Whether this is harmful is not clear, but most pediatric patients are now treated with a PDS containing less magnesium (i.e., 0.5 mEq/liter [0.25 mmol/liter]).

6.4.3. Buffers

The favored buffer in PDS is lactate. When metabolic acidosis was described in children treated with a PDS containing a lactate concentration of 35 mEq/liter [94], higher lactate concentrations (i.e., 40 to 45 mEq/liter) became the standard for PDS used in children. However, we have observed metabolic alkalosis in some children, even after converting them to the lower lactate solution. This condition may be similar to the contraction alkalosis described in some adult CAPD patients [95].

There are excellent theoretical reasons to prefer sodium bicarbonate as the buffer in PDS used in children. Feriani and associates have described a two-compartment bag separated by a frangible seal [96]. Just prior to fluid instillation the seal is broken, mixing the sodium bicarbonate solution with dialysate containing magnesium and calcium. Yatzidis has experimented with a mixture of glycylglycine and sodium bicarbonate [97]. It seems reasonable to anticipate the availability of a bicarbonate PDS in the near future.

6.4.4. Osmotic agents

Although dextrose (glucose) is the osmotic agent used almost universally in children, it is not ideal. Glucose is readily absorbed and metabolized by pediatric patients, but this may serve as a disadvantage by contributing to a more rapid loss of the osmotic gradient responsible for ultrafiltration [59,

63, 98]. The glucose load from the PDS increases blood sugar, stimulating insulin secretion and leading to hyperlipidemia and obesity.

Of the alternative osmotic agents that have been investigated, the two with the most potential are glucose polymers [99] and amino acids [100]. Glucose polymers are prepared from the fractionation of hydrolyzed corn starch producing oligopolysaccharides of variable size (molecular weight 250 to 20,000 daltons). An ultrafiltrate can be produced through colloid osmosis, even when the solution is isosmolar. However, there is an accumulation of maltose, with unknown metabolic consequences. Glucose polymers have not been studied in pediatric patients.

Amino acid dialysis has been studied in both adults and children [101–104], and will be discussed in detail later in this chapter.

6.5. Dialysis mechanics: The chronic peritoneal dialysis prescription for children

6.5.1. *Chronic intermittent peritoneal dialysis (IPD)*

Published experience with long-term chronic IPD in children is limited [24, 26–29]. When Potter and associates summarized this experience in 1982, they suggested that additional reports were unlikely, because continuous forms of CPD had begun to replace chronic IPD in most pediatric dialysis programs [105]. Compared to continuous forms of peritoneal dialysis, chronic IPD as it is traditionally prescribed is not very attractive. Dialysis consists of only two 20-hour sessions per week (one-hour cycles), resulting in substantially inferior weekly solute clearances. Currently, where it is still used, chronic IPD is only prescribed for short periods for patients who are awaiting CAPD/CCPD training and who have enough residual renal function to maintain acceptable chemistries and fluid balance.

6.5.2. *Continuous ambulatory peritoneal dialysis (CAPD)*

The beauty of CAPD is its simplicity and the fact that there is no need for cumbersome equipment in the home. Prior to automated PD, CAPD was used in children of all ages and sizes. Now CAPD is used primarily in older children and teenagers. For some families the complexity and burden of automated PD is too much. In addition, the sterile disconnect systems available for CAPD make training easier.

Some adolescents with active lives prefer CAPD over cycler dialysis, although most prefer the freedom from daytime exchanges and the improved body image of a near-empty abdomen provided by cycler dialysis (NIPD). The biochemical values reported for children receiving CAPD are similar to those obtained with cycler dialysis. There is a theoretical advantage in middle molecule clearance when CAPD is compared to NIPD [106], but the clinical importance of this observation is unknown. We now train families for CAPD primarily as an adjunct to cycler dialysis for use during travel or at those summer camps at which cyclers are not available. The freedom provided by the portability of CAPD is unmatched by any other currently available dialysis therapy, although the next generation of portable cyclers will challenge this statement.

6.5.3. *Continuous cycler peritoneal dialysis (CCPD) and nightly intermittent peritoneal dialysis (NIPD)*

Cycler dialysis has become the favored mode of peritoneal dialysis in many North American centers. The usual CCPD schedule for older children is five 2-hour exchanges per night with a long daytime exchange using either a full or one-half exchange volume [107, 108]. When the daytime exchange is less than one-half exchange volume the treatment is by convention termed NIPD. There are patients who do not tolerate the daytime exchange. In small children, the daytime exchange may contribute to anorexia. Adolescents frequently complain about the cosmetic effects of the daytime exchange, preferring a near-empty abdomen which they believe allows them to wear more "stylish" clothing.

It is necessary to prescribe more nightly exchanges with NIPD in order to achieve solute clearances equal to those obtained with CCPD. Middle molecule clearance with NIPD will always be inferior to that of CAPD or CCPD, resulting in unknown long-term effects. NIPD is now the most frequently prescribed form of CPD in our centers, largely as a result of patient and family preferences. Systematic studies of NIPD in children have not been reported.

6.5.4. *Tidal peritoneal dialysis (TPD)*

TPD was developed by Twardowski and associates to improve the efficiency of PD [109]. Such an approach could be of particular benefit to children, some of whom, we suspect, continue to be underdialyzed with current CPD techniques. TPD combines the best features of IPD with those of CAPD.

During TPD a constant volume (reserve volume) remains within the peritoneal cavity while the cycler performs rapid smaller exchanges, thus creating an optimal diffusion gradient for solute clearance.

Pediatric experience with TPD is limited [110]. In our two centers we have treated a total of three children with TPD, two with critically decreased ultrafiltration and one who could not achieve an acceptable Kt/V urea using conventional CCPD or NIPD. In all three children, the use of TPD has permitted us to continue CPD for an extended period. The TPD technique was quickly learned by parents already experienced with cycler dialysis. Training can be accomplished in an inpatient or outpatient setting, but initial TPD sessions are best performed in the center to allow adjustment of TPD target parameters. The target ultrafiltration volume is approximated from previous NIPD experience in the individual child, with careful attention directed to fluid balance based on dry weight, home dialysis records and the child's PET. We currently begin with three tidal exchanges each hour during a 10-hour TPD session. Tidal volume is usually 50% of the total exchange volume. To assess the accuracy of the target ultrafiltration volume and prevent accumulation or depletion of dialysate, peritoneal contents can be completely drained hourly or after five hours of TPD. The only problem reported by our patients to date has been minimal drainage pain. Parents have found the work of TPD comparable to that of NIPD. Since we have so far used TPD only in children with membrane dysfunction, we do not know if this technique will be sufficiently beneficial to warrant general use in children with intact peritoneal membranes. TPD should be a practical option for most pediatric CPD patients, in whom smaller total volumes of dialysate would be required, compared to adults.

6.5.5. *The CPD prescription*
The current approach to CPD for children has evolved empirically from early guidelines based on the pediatric adaptation of adult CAPD practices [34, 35, 59]. In general, a CAPD regimen of five exchanges per day has been preferred for small children, using exchange volumes of 35 to 45 ml/kg. The use of 2.5% dextrose solutions is common in oligo-anuric children, yielding up to 40 ml/kg per day in ultrafiltration. This same goal is often achievable with somewhat lower dialysate dextrose concentrations when NIPD regimens are prescribed. Anuric infants require aggressive fortification of formula feedings to achieve nutritional goals within the fluid limits dictated by achievable ultrafiltration and insensible water losses.

In Dallas, we usually begin CPD with a dialysis prescription based on an exchange volume of 40–45 ml/kg. In Toronto, somewhat smaller initial exchange volumes are used in larger children. The individual patient's PET can be used to estimate the dwell time and exchange frequency that will result in optimum small solute clearance. In Dallas, this usually results in a NIPD regimen consisting of 8 to 10 exchanges in 8 to 10 hours each night, 40 to 45 ml/kg per exchange, the dialysate dextrose concentration adjusted to reflect fluid balance requirements. Somewhat fewer exchanges are used in Toronto for larger children. A daytime dwell of 200 to 300 ml is used in most patients.

6.6. Nutritional management of children on CPD

6.6.1. *Nutritional goals*
The goal of nutritional management of children on CPD is to maximize nutrition and normalize growth parameters, while minimizing the metabolic consequences of uremia. This frequently must be accomplished in the face of anorexia, and often necessitates controlled enteral feeding, which may have adverse effects on motor skills and social development. Several reviews of the nutritional approach to pediatric patients on CPD are available, and are summarized below and in Table 8 [112–114]. Recommendations must take into account both losses and absorption of nutrients in the dialysis fluid [98, 115, 116].

Optimal energy requirements have not been established, but consensus recommends that prepubertal children on CPD receive 100% of the recommended daily allowances (RDA's) of the National Academy of Sciences for children of the same height-age and sex [117]. In addition, glucose absorption from dialysate provides up to 12% of the daily caloric intake [118]. Obesity due in part to dialysate glucose absorption is a common problem in adults treated with CPD. Caloric intakes should be adjusted accordingly if obesity develops in children on CPD [115, 119]. Carbohydrates should be complex in nature and provide at least 35% of dietary energy intake.

Protein intake must be carefully controlled to prevent protein-calorie malnutrition while avoiding toxicity from nitrogenous waste products. At least 50% of protein intake should be of high biologic value (e.g., egg, meat, fish and dairy sources) due to the higher percentage of essential amino acids, which may have the beneficial effect of promoting muscle anabolism and decreasing muscle catabolism [120]. If the BUN exceeds 70 mg/dl (30 mmol/l) in a child who is ingesting more than the prescribed dietary protein intake, in the absence of other causative factors, reduction in protein intake should be considered. Alternatively, the amount of dialysis can be increased. Before limiting protein intake in a child on CPD (an infrequent problem in our patients) care should be taken to insure that sufficient dialysis is being provided for the prescribed protein intake and that sufficient non-protein calories are being ingested to prevent protein catabolism. Monitoring of the prescribed protein intake can be accomplished by measuring urea nitrogen appearance in dialysate and urine, as will be discussed later in this chapter. To avoid a progressively negative nitrogen balance, protein supplementation may be necessary in children in whom ad lib dietary intake is unsatisfactory, or in those with recurrent episodes of peritonitis [116, 121, 122].

In infants and young children, approximately 50% of the dietary energy intake should come from fat, with a polyunsaturated-to-saturated fatty acid ratio of 1.5:1.0. Although serum lipid levels are high in patients on CPD, they remain stable on such a regimen [123]. Dietary fat probably should be less in older children, but the age at which fat intake should be curtailed is controversial; inappropriate restriction of fat intake may result in growth impairment [124, 125].

Supplementation of water soluble vitamins is mandatory for children on CPD (Table 8). Provision of the RDA's is sufficient for other vitamins, with the exception of Vitamin D, which must be provided in the activated form either as 1,25 dihydroxy vitamin D3 or 1-alpha hydroxy vitamin D3 (see below). Starting dose for these vitamin D preparations in older children is 0.01 µg/kg per dose given daily, with further titration depending on clinical response. In the erythropoietin era, iron supplementation is necessary in all but those few children on CPD whose iron stores are adequate as a result of prior transfusions (see below). Carnitine levels are frequently low in children who have been on CPD for more than four months, generally reflecting overall nutrition status. Carnitine supplementation is indicated in children who develop signs of myopathy, and may be helpful in other carnitine-deficient patients whose symptomatology is less characteristic [126]. Zinc deficiency has been reported in children on CPD, and routine zinc supplementation has been recommended [127].

In general, fluid, sodium and potassium intake in the child on CPD can be substantially greater than in children treated with hemodialysis. Fluid intake in children on CPD varies widely depending primarily on residual urine output. Restriction of fluid intake is usually only necessary in the small anephric or oligoanuric patient, or those with poor ultrafiltration due to peritoneal membrane failure. Dietary sodium restriction is rarely necessary in children on CPD; only those with severe hypertension despite control of volume status require sodium restriction, and then only to a "no-added salt" diet. Infants routinely require sodium *supplementation* to avoid hyponatremia (see below). Hyperkalemia is not uncommon during the first weeks of CPD. Restrictions of dietary potassium are frequently needed at this time, along with sodium-potassium exchange resins. Constipation must be aggressively avoided and treated, since stool potassium excretion helps to maintain potassium balance in the CPD patient. After the first few weeks of CPD, children can generally be managed

Table 8. Guidelines for nutritional therapy for children receiving chronic peritoneal dialysis.

Nutrient	Infant	Pre-Puberty	Puberty	Post-Puberty
Energy (kcal/kg/day)	110–150	70–100	males-60 females-48	males-60 females-48
Protein (g/kg/day)	2.5-3	2.5	2.0	1.5
Fat		50% dietary intake;		
Pyridoxine B6		5–10 mg/day		
Ascorbic acid		75–100 mg/day		
Folic acid		1 mg/day		

without dietary potassium restriction, although they must be warned against gorging on high potassium foods. Phosphate restriction is an essential, but frequently ignored component of the dietary prescription, resulting in the need for high doses of phosphate binders. Since calcium salts are now used almost exclusively as phosphate binders, additional dietary calcium supplementation is rarely needed.

Monitoring nutritional management requires careful tracking of growth and other anthropometric parameters (e.g., midarm circumference, skinfold thickness), serum protein, albumin and transferrin levels, and three-day dietary intake recalls. Adherence with dietary prescriptions is often a problem, especially for the older child, given the less palatable nature of a phosphate-restricted diet. CPD patients may gain fat and water weight while losing lean body mass, making weights and anthropometric measurements less reliable as determinants of nutritional status [122, 128]. Recent studies with bioelectrical impedance measurements in adult CPD patients have uncovered subtle changes in lean body mass that escape detection by anthropometrics [129]; this technique may also be useful in children.

6.6.2. Controlled enteral nutrition

In the infant and young child on CPD, aggressive feeding is essential to maintain optimal growth rates and neurologic development. Unfortunately, the anorexia associated with ESRD often results in inadequate spontaneous dietary intake. Abdominal fullness from peritoneal fluid, peritoneal dextrose absorption, gastroesophageal reflux, and behavioral problems may also contribute to poor nutrient intake. In addition, when formulas are supplemented with various fat, carbohydrate and protein additives they usually develop the viscosity and palatability of low-grade motor oil, precluding oral acceptance by even the least discriminating infant. These factors, plus the extensive time commitment and negative parent-child interaction that typically accompany attempts to get these children to eat have led to wide-spread reliance on controlled enteral nutrition (tube feeding). Tube feeding can be accomplished using a nasogastric (NG-), gastrostomy (G-) nasojejunal (NJ-), or gastrojejunal (GJ-) tube [130–139]. In patients on NIPD or CCPD, continuous overnight tube feedings have the advantages of delivering fluids and nutrients during the period of most intensive dialysis and consolidating the feeding routine. Nighttime continuous tube feedings also allow the stomach to be empty during the day, which may encourage spontaneous oral intake. In infants it is frequently necessary to combine overnight tube feeds with daytime boluses to achieve caloric intake goals.

While most pediatric centers are quick to employ tube feeding in children unable to meet nutritional goals by spontaneous oral intake, opinions differ regarding the optimum tube feeding technique. In Toronto, gastrostomy tube feedings have been used extensively with good results. In Dallas, similar results have been obtained with nasogastric tube feedings. Neither method is without difficulties.

G-tubes offer convenience and cosmetic advantages and are well-accepted by patients and families who appreciate freedom from the trauma of NG-tube insertion. Complications of G-tube feedings include: nausea, vomiting and diarrhea, which may respond to reduction in the volume and/or nutrient density of the formula; gastritis secondary to an irritant effect of the tube, which may require antacid or histamine-antagonist therapy; displacement of the tube, which is easily replaced at home by a parent; G-tube obstruction, requiring replacement of the tube; G-tube exit site infection; peritoneal dialysis fluid leaks around the G-tube exit site, requiring an alteration in dialysis regimen or switch to hemodialysis; and gastrocutaneous fistula, requiring surgical closure. No increase in peritonitis rate has been seen in patients receiving G-tube feedings [130, 132, 135, 140].

Gastrostomy buttons have also been used successfully in children on CPD. These devices are small and unobtrusive, reducing the stigma of a second abdominal tube. Fungal peritonitis was reported in three patients with gastrostomy buttons, but was probably related to other factors [141]. No cases of fungal peritonitis were seen in another series of 10 children treated with gastrostomy button feedings [139].

NG-tube feedings avoid the trauma of surgical or transabdominal G-tube placement and the risks of dialysate leaks and G-tube exit site infections. Patient acceptance has improved with the development of small (8 Fr), soft silastic tubes that are inserted over a guidewire. However, tube replacement remains an unpleasant experience for even the most adept families. Routine replacement of an NG-tube that has not become spontaneously dislodged is done only once each month, at which time the other nostril is used. The cosmetic effect of the NG-tube in infants is noticed primarily by grandparents, but in school-age children the cosmetic effects become important to the child. Sinusitis and otitis have not been increased in these children, perhaps because the tubes are small and pliable [135, 138].

Both G-tube and NG-tube feedings are associated with vomiting and the risk of aspiration. Despite frequent vomiting, serious aspiration events have been exceedingly rare, perhaps because these children retain an adequate gag reflex and overfeeding is assiduously avoided. The only reported fatality as a result of vomiting and aspiration in a child receiving CPD and tube feedings occurred in a child on G-tube feedings [130]. Children should be evaluated for the presence of gastroesophageal reflux prior to the initiation of either method of tube feeding, and should have a surgical anti-reflux procedure if severe reflux is demonstrated. Medical anti-reflux therapy (e.g., ranitidine, bethanecol, metoclopramide and other similar agents) can be employed in children whose reflux is not severe enough to warrant surgery, but who still vomit. GJ- and NJ-tubes have been used to overcome the problem of vomiting [131, 133]. Maintaining fixation of the tube in the jejunum is difficult, and both GJ- and NJ-tubes are frequently displaced into the stomach.

Both G-tube and NG-tube feedings can interfere with the learning process required to master swallowing. Exclusively tube-fed infants shun solid foods as a consequence of a hyperactive gag reflex [135, 142]. Tube feeding must sometimes be continued for months after successful renal transplantation in these infants while they slowly learn to chew and swallow solids without gagging. Speech development also may be delayed in some NG-tube fed infants [142].

Regardless of the route of enteral feeding, opportunity must be provided for oral stimulation and gratification in order to foster development of oral motor skills and speech production. Pacifier use and gum massage encourage non-nutritive sucking during the tube-feeding sessions and at other times during the day. When possible, oral intake prior to tube feeding should be encouraged, even when the bulk of nutrient intake is via the tube. Reintroduction of oral intake should be a gradual non-aversive process during withdrawal of tube dependence; a multidisciplinary behavioral approach is often useful [120, 122, 124, 142].

Tube feedings can be used as a supplement to voluntary oral intake or as total enteral nutrition. No nutritionally complete commercial formula for children on CPD currently exists. Therapy consists of a basic formula (e.g., Similac PM 60/40 [Ross]; S-29 or S-44 [Wyeth]; Pediasure [Ross]) with added modules of carbohydrate (glucose polymers to avoid hyperosmolality), fat (emulsified fat, or corn or safflower oil), and protein (casein or whey) customized to the needs of the individual child. Whey modules are lower in phosphorus and are more soluble. Emulsified fat is more expensive than vegetable oils, but may be preferable in continuous feedings because of easier mixing and suspension. Aluminum levels must be monitored when using a soy-based formula [136, 140].

6.6.3. *Intraperitoneal amino acids*

While CPD utilizing glucose-based dialysis solutions is effective in controlling uremia and fluid balance, glucose absorption from the dialysis solution with consequent hyperglycemia may contribute to obesity and has been implicated in hypertriglyceridemia and anorexia. Additionally, losses of protein and amino acids (AA) into the dialysis solution may contribute to the hypoalbuminemia, protein-calorie malnutrition, and abnormal plasma AA profiles seen in CPD patients. Greater dialysate losses of protein have been seen in younger patients [98, 115, 143]. Thus, AA solutions have been investigated both in adults and children as alternate dialyzing solutions and have been well tolerated and successful in achieving uremia control and ultrafiltration [98, 102, 103, 104, 119, 144–148].

Utilizing one 5-hour dwell of AA dialysate, Hanning and associates demonstrated adequate removal of urea and creatinine in seven uremic children, when compared to glucose solutions of similar osmolality [98]. AA solutions removed 16% less fluid than their glucose counterpart, but absorption of dialysate AA ($77.3 \pm 5.3\%$) exceeded losses of AA and protein in the glucose solutions, with a single exchange of AA dialysate compensating for the daily effluent protein losses of most patients. Fasting plasma glucose levels were maintained with AA solutions, but hyperaminoacidemia occurred with the more concentrated AA solution [98]. Subsequent studies by this group with a modified AA solution demonstrated that AA are absorbed from the peritoneal cavity of children in proportion to their profile within the dialysate. These observations led to the recommendation that AA solutions be modified to avoid hyperaminoacidemia and to correct the abnormal amino acid profiles which occur in uremic children [104]. A similar study in children demonstrated a 66% and 86% absorption of AA after 1 and 4 to 6 hours respectively, with a plasma AA profile similar to that after a protein meal [147]. Plasma levels of methionine, phenylalanine, valine and isoleucine increased and remained elevated after an AA exchange. AA dialysate also significantly reduced the losses of amino acids not contained in the AA dialysis solution when compared to glucose solution.

Honda and associates [103] studied the short-term effect of an essential amino acid-containing dialysate (EAAD). All serum essential amino acid levels peaked at about 200% one hour after treatment and fell to pretreatment levels by 6 hours, with the exception of methionine which peaked at 680% and fell to 390% of pretreatment values by the end of the cycle. The non-essential amino acid tyrosine, which is low in ESRD patients, increased toward normal levels, and most of the abnormally elevated non-essential amino acids decreased, suggesting a beneficial effect of EAAD on protein synthesis.

While short term studies have shown that AA solutions are well tolerated and effective in achieving uremia control and fluid removal, intermediate and long-term studies in adults have shown conflicting efficacy in improving nutritional status. Oren and associates found significant increases in urea, total body nitrogen, and serum transferrin following four weeks of twice daily exchanges of AA solution in six adults [145]. There was no accumulation of AA in the plasma, and a tendency towards lowering of serum triglyceride levels was noted. In longer studies, Young and associates [149] and Dombros and associates [150] did not observe significant nutritional benefits from prolonged administration of AA, while Bruno and associates [151] noted significant decreases in triglyceride and cholesterol levels as well as improvement in nitrogen balance. Dibble and associates [152] also noted a decrease in total and LDL cholesterol, and apolipoprotein B during 12 weeks of one exchange of 1% AA dialysate per day. Differences in outcome may be related to the initial nutritional state of patients (with severely malnourished patients more likely to achieve positive nitrogen balance), the composition of AA solution used, the time of day or frequency of delivery of the solution, or to other, as yet unidentified factors. In patients with normal total body nitrogen and adequate protein intake, use of AA solutions may be associated with anorexia, which limits caloric intake and offsets any beneficial effect of the AA. Anorexia is associated with the frequency and concentration of AA solution and may be related to increased urea levels, or possibly to central nervous system effects [150]. Other investigators have found no adverse effects on appetite or food intake with administration of AA over four weeks [153]. A significant reduction of serum phosphate during eight weeks of 1% AA dialysate was demonstrated in one study [154], but has not been confirmed by others.

Canepa and associates [102] studied the effect of long term administration of AA solutions (6 to 12 months) in eight children in a cross-over study design, utilizing a once daily AA exchange in the morning. There were no adverse effects (with the exception of an increase in blood urea), and fluid removal and uremia control were adequate. No improvement in growth was observed in these children. Plasma AA levels increased close to normal values, but intracellular AA levels remained low. Qamar and associates [148] performed a 3-month crossover study of AA solutions in seven children, utilizing an overnight AA dwell. They also documented no nutritional benefit, but no adverse effects of long-term AA dialysis. They noted higher potassium and urea levels and an improvement in appetite in the AA group. Elevated plasma albumin levels occurred in the AA group. In all patients net AA absorption exceeded protein losses, with a mean net AA absorption of 79.3 ± 60.8 mg/kg. The serum levels of branched chain AA improved with AA dialysis, but did not reach normal levels.

Further studies of AA dialysate in children are necessary before AA solutions can be recommended for widespread use. AA solutions have the definite disadvantage of requiring refrigeration, making them less convenient, and are more expensive than their glucose counterpart. Studies of long term effects of AA on the peritoneum are also necessary.

6.7. A simplified approach to the use of urea kinetic modeling to prescribe and monitor peritoneal dialysis treatment in children

Urea kinetic modeling has been proposed as a means by which PD can be quantitated and thereby adjusted to ensure delivery of "adequate" RRT. The concepts of kinetic modeling as they apply to PD patients remain highly controversial (see Chapter 14) and will not be reviewed here. Suffice it to say that urea kinetic modeling is of unknown importance to pediatric patients at this time. It remains to be seen if kinetic modeling will be a useful adjunct to the care of children on CPD. The present section is offered as an example of current efforts to apply kinetic modeling to routine pediatric patient management.

6.7.1. Kt/V urea

The Kt/V urea is defined as the total daily (t) urea clearance (K) normalized to the body's volume of distribution of urea (V) [155]. K has peritoneal (Kp) and residual renal (Kr) components:

$$K = Kp + Kr$$

where,

Kp = the peritoneal clearance of urea calculated directly from a complete 24-hour collection of pooled, drained dialysate;
Kr = the residual renal urea clearance calculated from a complete 24-hour urine collection.

Kp and Kr should be measured on the same day.

V is the volume of distribution of urea, which is the total body water (TBW). In non-uremic children, the TBW is approximately 600 ml/kg body weight [156]. In uremic children receiving hemodialysis, V can vary widely from patient to patient [157]. Unlike hemodialysis, there is no convenient way to measure V in children receiving PD. In the absence of a method of direct measurement in the individual patient, an estimate of 600 ml/kg body weight is currently used for V in all patients. This introduces an obvious additional source of error when the patient is an infant, a pubertal adolescent or an obese individual.

6.7.2. Practical protein balance in growing children receiving peritoneal dialysis

The concepts of protein balance as they are related to dietary protein intake, urea nitrogen appearance, Kt/V urea and protein nitrogen losses in the adult CPD patient have been clearly described by Teehan and associates [155]. These concepts form the basis for the material that follows.

6.7.2.1. Total protein nitrogen appearance.
Children on CPD are in daily protein balance. Dietary protein intake must be accounted for in the daily total protein nitrogen appearance (PNA) *plus* any protein nitrogen incorporated into new tissues. Total PNA consists of:

- Dialysate PNA as urea
- Dialysate protein losses
- Dialysate amino acid losses
- Urinary PNA as urea
- Urinary protein losses
- Stool and miscellaneous nitrogen losses (e.g., hair, nails, etc.)

6.7.2.2. Dialysate PNA as urea.
Direct measurement of the dialysate urea nitrogen allows estimation of the dialysate protein nitrogen appearance as urea nitrogen by multiplying by 6.25. For every gram of urea nitrogen that appears in the dialysate, the equivalent of 6.25 grams of dietary protein was metabolized. Of course, the actual protein that appears as urea did not come directly from the metabolism of ingested dietary protein, but for the purposes of protein balance estimates this assumption is useful. The dialysate PNA as urea (the dialysate urea nitrogen appearance [UNA]) must be measured directly, which can be done as part of the determination of Kt/V urea (see below). Dialysate also contains nitrogen in other compounds than urea (see below).

6.7.2.3. Dialysate protein losses in children.
Dialysate protein losses have been reported in children receiving CAPD to range from 0.13 to 0.24 gm/kg body weight per day [60, 118]. It is desirable to measure these losses directly in each patient. For the purposes of this review, dialysate protein losses have been arbitrarily assumed to be 0.2 gm/kg body weight per day.

6.7.2.4. Dialysate amino acid losses.
Data from one pediatric [158] and three adult studies [159–161] indicate that dialysate amino acid losses average 0.05 gm/kg body weight per day.

6.7.2.5. Stool and dialysate and other miscellaneous nitrogen losses.
In the absence of comparable pediatric data, studies in adult CAPD patients must be used to provide an estimate of daily stool and miscellaneous nitrogen losses. From three adult studies, average daily miscellaneous nitrogen losses (expressed as protein intake equivalent by multiplying by 6.25) can be estimated at 0.2 gm protein/kg body weight per day [116, 159, 162]. Nitrogen balance studies in children on CPD are needed to assess the accuracy of these and other approximations based on adult data.

6.7.2.6. "Growth protein".
The most uncertain aspect of the efforts to approximate protein balance in children on CPD is the need to account in some way for protein that is incorporated into new tissue as a consequence of growth. The traditional nomenclature which refers to protein incorporated into new tissue as "positive nitrogen balance" does not comfortably reflect the concepts employed in this review. The term "growth protein" was chosen

instead for this purpose. A rough estimate of "growth protein" can be obtained as follows:

- Between the ages of 3 and 11 years, children can be assumed to grow at a relatively steady rate, with an average weight gain of 2 kg/yr, or 5.5 gm/day. (Of course, children do not grow this way. Daily incremental changes in height and weight vary widely from child to child, and in the same child from day to day. Only by averaging growth over an entire year is the appearance of a steady growth rate obtained. However, the estimation of the "growth protein" components of protein balance in children on CPD requires an assumption of a steady growth rate).
- Approximately 18% of new (lean) body mass is normally protein.
- In the growing child, new protein is added at a rate of about 1 gm per day (0.18 × 5.5. gm/day).
- Thus, about 1 gm/day disappears from protein balance estimates as "growth protein" (i.e., this is protein that does not appear as urea nitrogen for clearance by dialysis).

For children 3 to 11 years old, weighing 10 to 50 kg, "growth protein" ranges from 0.02 to 0.1 gm/kg/day. For the purposes of this review, average daily "growth protein" is assumed to be 0.05 gm/kg per day.

6.7.2.7. Summary of non-urea nitrogen losses in children on CPD. The estimates of daily non-urea losses of protein nitrogen can be expressed as protein intake equivalents as follows:

Dialysate protein	0.20 gm/kg/day
+ Dialysate amino acids	0.05 "
+ Stool and misc. losses	0.20 "
+ "Growth protein"	0.05 "
total	0.50 gm/kg/day

This means that the equivalent of a daily protein intake of 0.5 gm/kg will not appear as urea nitrogen for removal by dialysis and residual renal function. If dialysate and urinary urea nitrogen removal is converted to protein equivalents and another 0.5 gm/kg is added, an estimate of daily protein balance can be obtained. This estimate has implications for both the nutritional and dialysis prescriptions, as we shall see below.

6.7.2.8. The protein nitrogen appearance (PNA) and Kt/V. The estimates of non-urea protein losses described above lead to the hypothesis that in growing children 3 to 11 years of age, protein intake greater than 0.5 gm/kg/day will result in the generation of proportional amounts of urea that must be removed by dialysis ± residual renal function. Urea measured in dialysate or urine is termed the urea nitrogen appearance (UNA). When this amount is converted to its protein equivalent by multiplying by 6.25, the result is termed the protein nitrogen appearance (PNA). A measured UNA of 160 mg/kg/d reflects a PNA of 1.0 gm/kg/d (0.160 × 6.25 = 1.0).

The PNA is presumed to be related directly to dietary protein intake (DPI). When the BUN = 70 mg/dl, it can be postulated that a daily urea clearance (K urea = $K_p + K_r$) of about 225 ml/kg is required to remove the urea that results from every 1.0 gm/kg of dietary protein intake above 0.5 gm/kg. This is calculated as follows:

- Urea nitrogen appearance (UNA) from each 1.0 gm/kg protein intake (above 0.5 gm/kg) = 160 mg/kg urea (1,000 mg ÷ 6.25).
- K urea = UNA/BUN (See Reference 156)
- For BUN = 70 mg/dl, or 0.7 mg/ml,
- K urea = 160 mg/kg ÷ 0.7 mg/ml
  = 228.57 ml/kg
  = ~225 ml/kg
- Kt/V urea = 225 ml/kg ÷ 600 ml/kg
  = 0.375/day
  = 2.625/week

6.7.2.9. The PNA, the Kt/V urea, and the dietary protein intake (DPI). The inter-relationships of the BUN, the K urea, the Kt/V urea and the dietary protein intake (DPI) can be expressed in several ways, as is shown below.

When the BUN = 70 mg/dl, the following relationships should be present:

K urea	Kt/V urea	Approximate DPI
(ml/kg/day)	(per week)	(gm/kg/d)
112	1.3	1.0
157	1.8	1.2
225	2.6	1.5
337	3.9	2.0

A further extension of these relationships can be expressed as a single equation:

Approximate DPI (gm/kg/d) = (BUN/70) × (weekly Kt/V urea /2.6) + 0.5

This equation can be used to monitor dialysis therapy and dietary protein intake in the clinical setting. Consider the case of Robyn, a 12 year old prepubertal girl who is anephric and is managed on NIPD. Weight is 51.3 kg, BUN = 59 mg/dl, 24-hour dialysate volume = 18,250 ml, dialysate urea = 25.3 mg/dl:

- K urea = (24-hr dial vol/pt wt) × (dial urea conc/BUN)
  = (18,250 ml/51.3 kg) × (25.3 mg/dl ÷ 59 mg/dl)
  = 152.6 ml/kg/day
- Kt/V urea = 152.6 ml/kg/d ÷ 600 ml/kg
  = 0.25/day
  = 1.75/week
- Dialysate PNA = (24-hr dial vol/pt wt) × (dial urea conc) × (6.25)
  = (18,250 ml/51.3 kg) × (0.253 mg/ml) × (6.25)
  = 0.563 gm/kg/day
- Approximate DPI:
  •• from measured PNA:
  0.563 gm/kg/d (measured PNA)
  + 0.500 gm/kg/d (est. non-urea losses)
  —————————————
  = 1.063 gm/kg/day
  •• from approximate DPI equation:
  Approximate DPI
  = (BUN/70) × (weekly Kt/V urea/2.6) + 0.5
  = (59/70) × (1.75/2.6) + 0.5
  = 1.067 gm/kg/day
  •• from 3-day diet diary: 1.09 gm/kg/day

Dialysis and nutritional therapy can be monitored in the clinical setting by comparing the approximate DPI obtained from the equation using the BUN and the weekly Kt/V urea with the results of the diet diary. Robyn's dietary prescription was for 1.2 gm protein/kg/day, but her intake was closer to 1.0 gm/kg/day. She was receiving sufficient dialysis to yield a weekly Kt/V urea = 1.75, and her BUN was closer to 60 mg/dl than 70 mg/dl.

There is, of course, no particular advantage to a BUN = 70 mg/dl. This is simply the reference value used to develop the relationships between BUN, DPI and Kt/V urea. However according to these relationships, Robyn's dialysis prescription (Kt/V urea = 1.75/week) and her dietary protein intake prescription (1.2 gm/kg/day) would have resulted in a BUN of about 70 mg/dl. Because her protein intake was less than prescribed, her BUN was proportionately lower than 70 mg/dl.

Another example of the usefulness of the Kt/V urea is seen in the case of Keith, a 7 year old anephric boy on NIPD and nightly nasogastric tube feedings designed to ensure a total dietary protein intake (tube feedings plus ad lib intake) of at least 1.5 gm/kg/day. At a recent visit, Keith's weight was 25.8 kg, BUN = 29 mg/dl, 24-hour dialysate volume = 8,750 ml, dialysate urea concentration = 14 mg/dl.

- Kt/V urea
  = (8,750/25.8) × (14/29) ÷ (600) × (7)
  = 1.86/week
- Approximate DPI
  = (BUN/70) × (weekly Kt/V urea/2.6) + 0.5
  = (29/70) × (1.86/2.6) + 0.5
  = 0.8 gm/kg/day
- DPI from 3-day diet history (included tube feedings) = 1.46 gm/kg/d

When shown the discrepancy between the calculated Approximate DPI and that obtained from their diet history, the parents revealed that they had arbitrarily discontinued tube feedings. It can be seen from these calculations that Keith was not receiving sufficient dialysis to allow a protein intake of 1.5 gm/kg/day and still have a BUN $\leq$ 70 mg/dl. To achieve a BUN = 70 mg/dl on a protein intake of 1.5 gm/kg/day, dialysis must provide a Kt/V urea = 2.6/week, as was noted earlier in this section. Thus, adjustments were needed in both nutritional and dialysis therapy for this boy.

Approximate DPI calculations apparently cannot be used for vigorously growing infants. These babies are usually being tube fed, and so their daily protein intake can be closely estimated. Consider the case of Lea, a 6 month old anephric baby on NIPD and nasogastric tube feedings receiving a consistent protein intake of 2.5 gm/kg/day. She was growing at a normal rate for length and weight, after a period of poor growth in early infancy prior to diagnosis and referral for RRT. Weight = 6.0 kg, BUN = 35 mg/dl, 24-hour dialysate volume = 3,500 ml, dialysate urea concentration = 22 mg/dl.

* Kt/V urea
  = (3,500/6) × (22/35) ÷ (675) × (7)
  [note that an arbitrarily larger V = 675 ml/kg is used in this infant]
  = 3.82/week
* Approximate DPI
  = (35/70) × (3.82/2.3) + 0.5
  = 1.3 gm/kg/day
* DPI from tube feedings = 2.5 gm/kg/day

It is tempting to postulate that protein balance in growing infants is unlike protein balance at any other time during childhood [70]. If this is the case, PNA will be much lower in infants on an equivalent protein intake, resulting in the low BUN's typically seen in these babies. Careful nitrogen balance studies in infants on CPD are needed to define these relationships.

6.8. Management of the very young infant: Special considerations

The past 10 years have seen major advances in CPD for infants [163–165]. Single cuff catheters prevent the cuff erosion noted with double cuff catheters. Tubing and dialysate are now available in appropriate sizes, and automated cyclers simplify patient care. However, several problems are unique to infants on CPD. Peritoneal transport rates of solute and glucose are faster in young children than adults, [55, 63] making long dwell CPD inefficient and prone to inadequate ultrafiltration in a population whose caloric intake is primarily in liquid form. Thus, infants are better suited to short dwell CPD utilizing automated cyclers at night.

Hyponatremia is common, especially in infants with high output renal failure, and may contribute to growth failure. Hyponatremia is due to multiple factors, including low sodium intake from infant formulas, high ultrafiltration requirements relative to body weight with obligate sodium losses in the dialysate, renal sodium losses in non-oliguric patients, and inadequate ultrafiltration. Oral sodium supplementation with sodium chloride or bicarbonate, or supplementation in the dialysate may be necessary to achieve normonatremia [163, 164, 166, 167].

Hypophosphatemia is also common, and may be as deleterious as hyperphosphatemia. Hypophosphatemia may occur with the use of phosphate restricted formulas such as Similac PM 60/40® (Ross Laboratories) which are standard in the treatment of infants with renal failure. Hypophosphatemia requires the cessation of phosphate binders if they are being used, and an increase in dietary phosphate content.

The nutritional management of the infant on CPD represents a special challenge as the optimal requirements are even less well defined than in older children. Using the RDA's as a basis, the following recommendations have been made: energy intake: 110–150 kcal/kg/day, with 50% from carbohydrate and 35% from fat; protein intake: 2.5–3.0 gm/kg/day, with protein of high biologic value, to account for both required intake and dialysate protein losses [112, 114]. Vitamin requirements are similar to older children (Table 8). Gastroesophageal reflux may occur in up to 73% of infants with ESRD, especially in those less than 12 months old, and may contribute to failure to thrive due to food refusal secondary to pain or excessive vomiting [168].

Growth failure in infants treated with CPD is well documented. Optimal growth requires aggressive nutrition (usually with tube feedings), careful attention to correction of acidosis and electrolyte imbalance, aggressive treatment of renal osteodystrophy, and tailoring of CPD prescriptions to achieve adequate dialysis [164, 165, 167, 169–173]. Despite this aggressive approach, growth of infants on CPD may remain suboptimal, and growth potential lost during infancy is rarely recovered.

Developmental delay was previously reported as a significant and serious complication of both conservative management and CPD in infants with chronic renal failure [174]. Improved developmental outcome has been seen with aggressive dietary management, early institution of CPD, control of hyperparathyroidism, and avoidance of aluminum phosphate binders [164, 165, 167, 172, 175]. Despite these improvements, gross motor developmental delay is still common and may be related to prolonged hospitalization and abdominal distension from dialysate. Mild hypotonia is also common, and may be due to carnitine deficiency.

Rates of peritonitis may be higher in infants, due to the proximity of the catheter exit site to the diaper area, and in some cases, the presence of a G-tube. In addition, hypogammaglobulinemia has been reported in infants on CPD, and may be associated with increased infection rates [176]. Use of automated cyclers has reduced peritonitis rates in infants [165].

Mean plasma fluoride concentrations are significantly greater than controls in the first 18 months of life in infants on CPD. No fluorosis in deciduous teeth has been reported, but the effect on permanent teeth remains to be described. Infants on CPD are at risk for markedly elevated fluoride levels and should not be fluoride supplemented [177].

The final goal of ESRD management is a functioning transplant in an intact child. Infants may be an ideal group for transplantation as they have a greater capacity for growth and healing, and are less malnourished, growth retarded and chronically ill than older children with a longer period of renal failure. However, controversy exists as to the optimal timing of transplantation. Traditionally, infants were maintained on CPD until they reached a certain size (approximately 10 kg) to optimize surgical outcome, with the major complication being vascular thrombosis [178, 179]. However, several authors have reported patient and graft survival rates similar to older children and improved growth and neurological development in infants transplanted at less than one year of age, some of whom were transplanted without prior dialysis [164, 165, 175, 180–184]. Living-related donor transplantation appears particularly successful in infants, with dramatically superior graft survival compared to cadaveric grafts [165, 173, 180, 182–184].

Transplantation requires an intensive multidisciplinary approach and should be a calculated step undertaken at the optimal time for each patient, taking into account parental wishes, availability of dialysis and donors, nutritional status, growth status, and surgical experience and outcome for the particular institution [183]. Some infants will require time on dialysis to allow necessary surgical intervention or to correct malnutrition, while others may proceed to transplant without dialysis. The risks of transplantation and prolonged immunosuppression must be weighed against the risks and outcome of prolonged CPD in the developing infant.

Despite the major advances in management of ESRD in infants, the mortality remains higher than in older children [164], and a good outcome as measured by growth and mental development cannot be guaranteed. It is still acceptable for parents to elect conservative therapy if the burden of care outweighs the benefits of dialysis and transplantation [185].

6.9. Renal anemia and its treatment in children on CPD

Recombinant human erythropoietin (rHuEPO) corrects the anemia of chronic renal failure in almost all adult dialysis patients and eliminates the need for red blood cell transfusions [186–189]. Improvements in exercise tolerance, cognitive function, work capacity, sexual function, and overall sense of well-being has been consistently described in adult dialysis patients treated with rHuEPO [190, 191]. A dramatic improvement in the quality of life of the adult dialysis patient is a frequent observation during rHuEPO therapy.

Pediatric dialysis patients may enjoy even greater benefits from rHuEPO therapy than adult patients. Compared with the transfusion dependency seen in only 25% to 60% of adult dialysis patients [192], virtually all children treated with hemodialysis require transfusions from the earliest months of dialytic therapy, and over 75% of children treated with CPD for more than 12 months also become transfusion-dependent [35, 105].

Children with ESRD have problems unique to pediatric patients that might be benefited by rHuEPO treatment. Poor growth is a consistent feature of uremia in children to which anemia may contribute [193, 194]. Cognitive function is diminished in uremic children, a problem that is not improved by dialysis, but does improve with successful renal transplantation [195]. The limited energy and exercise capacity of uremic children are closely related to the degree of renal anemia [196] and adversely affect the capacity of these children to study and play normally with other children. It is a critical task of childhood to develop adequate self-esteem for psychosocial independence in adult life; thus, although difficult to measure, the harmful effects of renal anemia during childhood may be felt for a lifetime.

The initial report describing rHuEPO therapy in pediatric dialysis patients was published in 1989 by Sinai-Trieman and associates [197]. The response seen in five transfusion-dependent adolescents on CCPD was encouraging. Subsequent reports have documented the effectiveness of rHuEPO in pediatric dialysis patients [198–205]. While observations and recommendations must be considered preliminary at this stage in the development of rHuEPO therapy for children [206], the following comments reflect current approaches used in our centers.

6.9.1. Pre-treatment concerns

Treatment with rHuEPO should be considered when a child on CPD has a hematocrit <30%. Before initiating rHuEPO therapy, the child with a borderline hematocrit should be stable on CPD for up to six weeks. Some children will have an increase in hematocrit as they begin CPD that can delay the need for rHuEPO. However, when initial hematocrit is <27% we begin rHuEPO right away.

Hypertension occurs or worsens in one-fourth to one-third of children treated with rHuEPO. It seems prudent to insist on superbly controlled hypertension as a prerequisite for initiating therapy. Particular attention should be paid to maintaining children at their dry weights during initiation of rHuEPO therapy. Blood pressure must be carefully monitored in all treated patients, but especially those not receiving antihypertensive therapy when rHuEPO is begun.

Iron deficiency will inhibit rHuEPO effectiveness. Prior to treatment, iron status should be assessed by measuring serum iron, total iron binding capacity (TIBC), and serum ferritin levels. Transferrin saturation (TS) ≥20%

$$TS(\%) = (serum\ iron/TIBC) \times 100$$

and serum ferritin level >100 ng/ml are reliable indicators of adequate available iron stores. Intravenous iron dextran may be necessary if iron-deficient patients are unable or unwilling to comply with oral iron supplements (see below).

Early concerns about an increased risk of seizures in treated patients have not been substantiated [188, 207]. Early reports of seizures may have described hypertensive encephalopathy rather than a primary neuroelectric event. We do not withhold rHuEPO from children with well-controlled seizure disorders.

6.9.2. Dosing suggestions

The optimum rHuEPO dosing regimen in children on CPD has yet to be defined. rHuEPO may be more effective when administered by the subcutaneous (SC) route [208, 209]. Most children can be maintained on one dose/week when given SC rHuEPO. In Dallas patients begin at 100 units/kg given once/week. The starting dose in Toronto is 50 units/kg given 3 times per week. Target hematocrit in our centers is 36% ± 3%. Dosage adjustments are often necessary before a stable maintenance dose is determined for the individual child.

Subcutaneous rHuEPO can be painful. We teach patients and parents to draw up the prescribed rHuEPO dose in a 1 ml, 27 gauge syringe, and then draw up an equal volume of bacteriostatic saline in the same syringe. The saline contains 10% benzyl alcohol, which acts as a local analgesic when mixed with and administered with rHuEPO. Children are never pleased by the prospect of regular injections of any kind, but the use of bacteriostatic saline has improved acceptability of SC rHuEPO in our centers.

Intra-peritoneal (IP) administration of rHuEPO has been proposed as another method for improving compliance [210]. Early concerns about an increased incidence of peritonitis have not been substantiated. rHuEPO is effective when infused into a dry abdomen for a prolonged period. Until more information is available, IP therapy should probably remain an alternative to SC therapy for those children who are violently intolerant of SC injections.

In the U.S., rHuEPO is sold in single-use vials of various concentrations. In Dallas we have elected to use the highest practical concentration of rHuEPO that will deliver two doses from each vial. Thus, for a child weighing 20 kg, receiving 2000 units SC, once/week, we prescribe the 4000 unit/ml vial. Each 0.5 ml dose of rHuEPO is mixed with 0.5 ml of bacteriostatic saline, and each 1 ml vial is used for two doses, one week apart. The vials are refrigerated between uses. We have systematically cultured vials used twice at home and have had no positive cultures. However, the bioavailability of rHuEPO kept refrigerated for one week after the vial has been entered has not been confirmed.

6.9.3. Monitoring suggestions

During the first 12 weeks of therapy and for a similar period after a change in dose is made, hematocrit should be measured weekly. Once a stable hematocrit and dose are reached, monthly hematocrit measurements are sufficient. Serum iron, TIBC and ferritin are measured monthly for the duration of rHuEPO treatment.

6.9.4. Iron supplementation

Functional iron deficiency must be anticipated and hopefully avoided [211]. Children with high serum ferritin levels need not receive iron supplements as long as transferrin saturation exceeds 20%. However, as available iron stores are used up, transferrin saturation may reach critically low levels before the ferritin level falls below 100 ng/dl. We begin oral iron supplements at a dose of 2 to 3 mg elemental iron/kg per day as soon as the transferrin saturation falls below 50%. When transferrin saturation approaches 20%, iron supplements are increased to 6 mg/kg/day.

Ferrous sulfate is the iron salt most often prescribed in our centers. While this iron salt has the best absorption, it is also associated with the most gastrointestinal side effects [212]. Absorption of oral iron salts is best if given at least two hours away from doses of phosphate binders. A small dose of vitamin C (50 to 100 mg) taken with oral iron preparations will increase absorption. We prescribe iron supplements to be taken with 2 to 4 oz of a vitamin C-containing fruit drink.

When oral iron supplements are inadequate to

maintain transferrin saturation <20%, intravenous iron dextran is indicated [213, 214]. Iron dextran can be given in the outpatient setting. Iron dextran has been used with increasing frequency in children treated with rHuEPO, with few complications. The protocol for iron dextran therapy used in the U.S. pediatric multi-center rHuEPO trial is given in Table 9 (Jabs [Boston], personal communication).

6.10. Renal osteodystrophy

Renal osteodystrophy can contribute significantly to the morbidity and growth failure of children with ESRD [215]. Bone disease can develop rapidly in younger patients, and the probability of bone deformity is greater in this younger age group. It was anticipated at the outset that CAPD would present fewer problems with respect to renal osteodystrophy than had been seen in children treated with hemodialysis, because CAPD provided steady-state biochemical control and permitted a less restrictive diet. In Toronto, early experience showed that these expectations were unduly optimistic [216]. Despite treatment with 1,25 dihydroxy vitamin D3 (calcitriol) and the phosphate binder aluminum hydroxide, nearly all patients had elevated levels of parathyroid hormone (PTH). Gokal and associates reported that in adults treated with CAPD, though not receiving supplemental vitamin D, plasma levels of vitamin D tended to fall after six months of dialysis [217]. Active metabolites of vitamin D have also been shown to be lost in the dialysate [218, 219]. From these early observations it was concluded that supplemental vitamin D was essential in children receiving CPD.

The optimum vitamin D preparation for children is less clear. In a prospective comparison of 1-alpha hydroxy vitamin D3 (10–20 ng/kg/day) and vitamin D3 (400 Units/day), children who received only vitamin D3 developed renal osteodystrophy, whereas those who received 1-alpha hydroxy D3 were protected [220]. Serial bone biopsies showed disappearance of aluminum staining after only six months without aluminum-containing phosphate binders. Others have reported successful treatment for renal bone disease using 1,25 dihydroxy vitamin D3 in pediatric CPD patients [221]. Either of these active metabolites appears capable of controlling hyperparathyroidism; however, when calcium-containing phosphate binders are used, episodic hypercalcemia is a frequent complication.

The optimum route of administration of vitamin D preparations is also incompletely defined. In Toronto, intraperitoneal administration of 1,25 dihydroxy vitamin D3 was compared to the same drug given orally [222]. Identical plasma dose response curves were obtained with the IP and oral routes. While as much as 60% of IP administered drug binds to the dialysis tubing [223], this is apparently offset by a similar amount of drug that is metabolized by enzymes in the gastrointestinal mucosa [224]. Similar studies in adults have been reported by Delmez and associates [225]. There were no adverse effects seen with IP administration.

The potential value of IP administration was recently observed in two Toronto infants who were refractory to large doses of 1,25 dihydroxy vitamin D3 given by gastric tube. A dramatic improvement in bone disease and control of hyperparathyroidism was seen when the infants were switched to IP

Table 9. Iron dextran administration in pediatric peritoneal dialysis patiients.

Indication
Parenteral iron is indicated for patients with low iron stores (transferrin saturation <20%). A trial of oral iron may be attempted before initiation of parenteral iron in those patients with borderline iron stores who are able to tolerate oral iron.

Risks
Side effects are uncommon and include fever, urticaria, headache, malaise, and arthralgias. Anaphylaxis has been reported in <1% of patients given i.v. iron dextran. Recent experience in centers treating adult dialysis patients has shown a much lower incidence if smaller doses are given over a prolonged treatment course. Due to the risk of anaphylaxis each patient is given a test dose prior to initiation of treatment.

Administration of test dose
The test dose is 0.5 ml (25 mg) in patients >20 kg
             0.3 ml (15 mg) in patients 10–20 kg
             0.2 ml (10 mg) in patients <10 kg

Administer dose iv over 1 min. Adverse effects should occur within a few minutes. Observe for 1 hour before giving therapeutic dose or discharging patient from unit.

Administration of dose
Iron dextran will be diluted in normal saline and administered as an intravenous infusion over 2 hours. The patient's Fe and TIBC will be repeated 2 weeks after the dose. If the patient's iron stores are still low the dose will be repeated.

Dose
The dose is adjusted for patient weight.

Weight	Dose	Volume of NS infusion
>20 kg	500 mg	250 ml
10–20 kg	250 mg	125 ml
<10 kg	125 mg	75 ml

administration of the same drug, even though the dose and resulting plasma levels of 1,25 dihydroxy vitamin D3 were lower than when the oral route was used. The reason(s) for this excellent response to IP therapy when oral therapy had failed are unclear. While PTH secretion is down-regulated by raising the plasma calcium level, there is also a well-described direct effect of 1,25 dihydroxy vitamin D3 on the parathyroid gland that reduces PTH secretion independent of changes in calcium concentration [226]. These observations have led Salusky and others to investigate the use of IP, IV, and high-dose oral pulse therapy for refractory cases [227]. Newer vitamin D analogues, which lack a calcemic effect and yet are able to inhibit PTH secretion directly are currently in clinical trails [228].

The role of surgical sub-total parathyroidectomy in pediatrics has greatly diminished in recent years, probably as a result of early and aggressive therapy to control hyperparathyroidism and prevent renal bone disease. Classical tertiary hyperparathyroidism has virtually disappeared from pediatric dialysis programs.

More recently, a newer form of renal osteodystrophy, aplastic bone lesion, has been described in adult and pediatric CPD patients [229, 230]. Aplastic bone lesion may be related in part to overly zealous attempts to lower the plasma PTH level. Unfortunately, aplastic bone lesion can only be diagnosed by bone biopsy, a traumatic procedure that requires heavy sedation to be successful in pediatric patients. Our centers and many others have been reluctant so far to subject our pediatric CPD patients to routine bone biopsies, so the true incidence of aplastic bone lesion is not known. Studies are underway in Los Angeles to better define the role of the bone biopsy and the importance of aplastic bone lesion in pediatric patients (Salusky, [Los Angeles] personal communication).

The use of aluminum-containing phosphate binders has been all but eliminated in most pediatric centers in an effort to avoid chronic aluminum toxicity [231]. Fortunately, for most children, hyperphosphatemia can be controlled using calcium salts. Occasionally, noncompliant adolescents will require a short course of aluminum hydroxide to bring a severely elevated serum phosphate level into line, but for the most part we rely on calcium carbonate or calcium acetate preparations. In some children, relatively high calcium intake results from compliance with prescribed doses of calcium-containing phosphate binders, leading to episodes of hypercalcemia. Hypercalcemia in these children can frequently be avoided with the use of low-calcium dialysate.

6.11. Complications

6.11.1. Peritonitis

Comparative data from the NIH National CAPD Registry have shown that children have a significantly greater peritonitis rate compared to adults, and a greater probability of experiencing an episode of peritonitis during the first year of CPD treatment [232]. Striking reductions in observed peritonitis rates have been reported in adults and children in correlation with recent technical developments in "connectology", the methods by which the patient/peritoneal dialysis system interface is designed [233]. Peritonitis in pediatric CPD patients has been reviewed by several authors [234–237].

Diagnosis of peritonitis in children is based on the same basic clinical criteria as are used in adults: cloudy fluid containing >100 wbc's per cu mm, >50% of which are PMN's [236]. Children may have abdominal pain and fever for a short period before the first cloudy dialysate appears [234]. Causitive organisms are similar to those seen in adult patients. A meta-analysis of several pediatric series totaling 646 episodes of peritonitis found 44% of cases due to gram positive organisms, 21% due to gram negatives, 2% had fungal peritonitis, 8% had a variety of unusual organisms and 25% were culture negative [238].

Current approaches to treatment rely on intraperitoneal administration of antibiotics, following guidelines similar to those developed for adult patients [239] (see Chapter 16). Because exchange volume is based on body size in pediatric patients, it is possible to follow adult dosing guidelines for IP antibiotics when treating children. Newer guidelines based on single weekly IP or IV doses of vancomycin and once daily doses of aminoglycosides [240] have not been evaluated in children and cannot be recommended for pediatric patients at this time.

Although uncommon, fungal peritonitis remains a serious problem in pediatric CPD programs [141]. Following an episode of fungal peritonitis the majority of children suffer peritoneal membrane failure and must be transferred to hemodialysis. Treatment remains highly controversial, a sure sign that no reliably effective, peritoneum-sparing treatment strategy has yet been devised. We rely on gram stains of centrifuged cloudy dialysate for the first evidence of fungal (usually Candida) infections, and begin treatment accordingly. Gram stains rarely provide helpful information for bacterial peritonitis, but a diagnostic gram stain can precede a positive fugal culture by several days. Amphotericin B remains the mainstay of therapy for fungal peritonitis in our programs. In Dallas, Amphotericin B is given at a dose of 1 mg/kg in a single daily IV infusion, after one dose at 0.25 mg/kg to look for adverse reactions. After the third day of therapy the catheter is removed and the child is treated for a short period (3 to 5 days) with hemodialysis. At this point a new peritoneal dialysis catheter is inserted and treatment with Amphotericin B continued for a total of 18 to 21 days. The short period of hemodialysis is intended to allow sterilization of the peritoneal cavity in the absence of a foreign body before placement of the new catheter, while limiting the opportunity for adhesion formation. Alternative approaches to treatment using additional or alternative anti-fungal agents have been reported (see Chapter 16).

The outcome of peritonitis in children is generally favorable. A meta-analysis of 439 episodes of peritonitis in pediatric CPD patients reported that 13% of episodes resulted in catheter removal, 6% led to membrane failure, and only a single episode (0.4%) resulted in death from peritonitis [238].

6.11.2. *Exit site and tunnel infections*
Exit site and tunnel infections continue to plague pediatric CPD programs. The NIH National CAPD Registry has reported an increased incidence of exit site/tunnel infections in children compared to adults (0.8 vs 0.6 episodes/year, respectively), and an increased probability of experiencing a first infection during the initial 12 months of dialysis (0.40[95% CI = 0.34, 0.46] vs 0.30[0.29, 0.32], respectively) [232].

Exit site infections (ESI) in children may present with slight erythema around the catheter to a purulent, ulcerated erosion. The pathogenesis of ESI is uncertain; many potential contributing factors have been proposed, including mechanical irritation, hypersensitivity to silicone rubber, excessive perspiration, and local granulation tissue formation [241]. Levy and associates recently retrospectively reviewed their experience with 157 episodes of ESI occurring in 50 children treated with CPD at a single center during a total of 950 patient-months of dialysis [242]. The ESI was characterized as purulent in 39 and non-purulent in 71 episodes. Staphylococcus aureus was the most frequently cultured organism (46.2%) in both purulent and non-purulent infections. Pseudomonas aeruginosa, the most common gram-negative organism, was cultured from 10.6% of the cases. Patient age, gender and primary renal disease were not correlated with ESI incidence nor did the presence of gastrostomy-tube exit sites, diapers or pyelostomies favor development of ESI in these children. Surprisingly, ESI in diapered infants were more often due to gram-positive organisms than typical enteric bacteria. Thirty-eight of 132 ESI episodes (28.7%) in 28 patients were complicated by peritonitis. The catheter was removed in 13 of 28 patients because of recurrent or pseudomonas peritonitis. ESI incidence was unaffected by catheter removal. Four episodes of ESI were associated with overt tunnel infections; in three cases, the single, deep cuff had migrated to a superficial position [242].

The care of the catheter exit site is thought to hold the key to prevention of ESI [243]. The routine management of the exit site has undergone many changes in our centers, reflecting the failure so far to find a completely satisfactory approach. At times these changes appear more cyclical than evolutionary. In Toronto, until 1982 patients were taught a meticulous sterile dressing technique using an occlusive bandage. Subsequently, sterile gauze dressings changed at least once/week have been used for only the first month after catheter insertion. After the first month, patients were taught to scrub the exit site with povidone iodine when they showered (at least every two days). After 1985 the scrub was discontinued because it caused skin irritation; patients are now taught to shower with plain soap and water, dry with a clean towel, paint a circle of povidone iodine around the exit site and allow it to dry. Any crusting is removed with 3% hydrogen peroxide before applying the iodine paint. The importance of catheter fixation is also stressed. Most patients prefer a small gauze dressing over the exit site applied after the iodine paint is dry. Infants are bathed in a tub in shallow water to avoid soaking the exit site. The gauze dressing is left on during the bath and changed afterwards when the exit site is gently cleaned with a povidone iodine swab.

ESI have traditionally been treated with oral and IP antibiotics, usually given for prolonged periods. In Dallas we have had good results with the early application of Mupirocin ointment (Bactroban®) at the first signs of inflammation at the exit site. The ointment is applied BID for 14 to 21 days. Only if improvement is not seen promptly are IP antibiotics added, based on ESI culture results. In both Dallas and Toronto we have had little success with medical management of ESI due to pseudomonas organisms without catheter replacement.

ESI is a frequent complication of CPD in children [244]. While improved catheter exit site care techniques and more effective ESI treatment strategies may be helpful, the incidence of ESI will only be substantially reduced by advances in CPD technology, such as more biocompatible catheter and cuff materials.

6.11.3. *Hernias, leaks and hydrothorax*

6.11.3.1. *Hernias.* Abdominal wall hernias are common in children treated with CPD, occurring in 22% to 40% of pediatric patients [245, 246]. Multiple hernias are frequently seen. Khoury and associates described 28 hernias in 18 children on CPD [245]. There were 18 inguinal hernias (64%) that occurred in 12 children, 11 of whom were males, whose average age was 5.2 years. The raised intra-abdominal pressure associated with CPD has the potential of converting an asymptomatic patent processus vaginalis into a clinically significant inguinal hernia. The processus vaginalis is patent in 90% of newborns, compared to only 15% of adult males [247]. The incidence of indirect inguinal hernias in CPD patients is 100 times that of the general population. von Lillien and associates reported 60 hernias in 37 children treated with CPD [246]. In contrast to Khoury's experience, the majority of these hernias (60%) were ventral. Incarceration was uncommon, occurring in only one patient in each series.

Prevention and management of hernias varies among pediatric centers. Hernias are likely to occur early in the course of CPD. Poor nutrition, prior abdominal surgery, and recent or concurrent corticosteroid therapy probably place children at increased risk. Young males appear to be at greatest risk for inguinal hernias. In these infants demonstration of a patent processus vaginalis by peritoneography [90] or ultrasound at the time of catheter placement allows pre-emptive repair and thus prevention of subsequent hernia development. The use of NIPD with minimal daytime volumes should be considered for patients felt to be at increased risk for hernia development.

Most hernias can be repaired electively; incarceration is uncommon, especially when the defect is large. Patients should be monitored closely for development of inguinal, umbilical or incisional hernias both before catheter placement and throughout the course of CPD treatment. If a hernia is diagnosed, elective repair is scheduled promptly, avoiding prolonged delays. Parents are instructed to observe carefully for signs of incarceration while awaiting surgery. In most cases of inguinal hernias, especially in males <2 years of age, bilateral repair is recommended.

6.11.3.2. *Leaks.* Dialysate leakage from the catheter exit site has been discussed in the section on catheter placement. Dialysate can also leak from the peritoneal cavity into various tissue planes, most often into the subcutaneous tissue around a previous surgical incision or into the genital area. Subcutaneous leaks usually begin as the dissection of very small amounts of dialysate into a tissue plane that begins at the site of an old or recent surgical incision, often after an episode of coughing or vomiting. The subcutaneous fluid collection enlarges as a consequence of the osmotic pressure of the hypertonic dialysate. Conservative management, occasionally including temporary suspension of CPD, is usually sufficient to allow these leaks to resolve. Aspiration or drainage of subcutaneous fluid collections should be avoided.

A leak into the genital area can be difficult to distinguish from an inguinal hernia. Both CT scan [248] and scintilography [249] have been used for this purpose. Most of these patients can be managed conservatively by reducing exchange volume and prescribing bedrest, or switching from CAPD to NIPD with lower exchange volumes. If a patent processus vaginalis is present it may require ligation to prevent recurrence of a genital leak.

6.11.3.3. *Hydrothorax.* Hydrothorax is an uncommon complication of CPD seen in children [250] and adults [251–253]. It is usually right-sided. The prevalence of pleuroperitoneal connections in the general population is unknown, since hydrothorax only occurs when a patient has a large volume of free intra-peritoneal fluid. It has been suggested that the leak arises because of the effect of raised intra-peritoneal pressure on small defects in the pleuroperitoneum covering the diaphragm [254]. In this scenario, a tiny bleb arises on the superior surface of the diaphragm and then ruptures, forming a one-way valve that can lead to a tension hydrothorax. Alternatively, the potential pleuroperitoneal connection is present as a congenital defect in the diaphragm.

It is important to consider the other causes of pleural effusions in CPD patients, including congestive heart failure, fluid overload and hypoalbuminemia. In many patients without an obvious explanation, tests are necessary to prove the presence of a pleuroperitoneal connection. Various techniques have been described, including thoracentesis to measure pleural fluid dextrose concentration or to detect the presence of intraperitoneally infused dye by colorimetric testing (indigocarmin [255]) or direct visualization (methylene blue), chest fluoroscopy after infusing dilute ratio-opaque contrast media into the peritoneum, and pleural scintilography after infusion of radio-isotope into the peritoneal cavity [256]. We prefer the isotopic technique for children because thoracentesis is not required and radiation exposure is less than with fluoroscopy.

In our programs a total of five children have developed hydrothoraces during CPD, four spontaneously without known antecedent events and the fifth following a percutaneous liver biopsy. The latter child was able to resume CPD without recurrence following 72 hours off dialysis. The four children with spontaneous hydrothorax were transferred to hemodialysis. No attempt was made to seal the pleuroperitoneal communication with intrathoracic sclerosing agents, autologous hemoglobin or surgical patch-grafting as has been reported in adults [252, 255, 257, 258].

6.11.4. Metabolic abnormalities

6.11.4.1. *Glucose and lipids.* Glucose is the best and safest osmotic agent available for peritoneal dialysis. A large fraction of the glucose in peritoneal dialysate is absorbed, providing an added source of energy substrate. While advantageous for many children, these extra carbohydrate calories can contribute to obesity. In Toronto, two children requiring excessive use of high-dextrose dialysate became extremely obese and were transferred to hemodialysis as a consequence However, obesity generally is not considered a contraindication to continued CPD in pediatric patients.

Absorption of dextrose from the peritoneal dialysate induces insulin secretion, resulting in disturbed lipid metabolism. Elevated serum cholesterol and triglyceride levels are seen in a large percentage of pediatric CPD patients [123, 259, 260]. While atherosclerosis is not a clinically visible problem in the pediatric dialysis patient population, hyperlipidemia must be addressed in these children, because they ultimately will receive a renal transplant, thereby incurring additional atherosclerosis risk factors (e.g., anti-rejection medications, hypertension). Although it seems clear that optimum management of the pediatric CPD patient should include efforts to normalize lipid metabolism, available strategies to address hyperlipidemia in these children are limited. Restriction of dietary fat is frequently attempted. However, it is often impossible to achieve adequate energy intake with diets limited in fat. This is particularly true for some oliguric infants, in whom only the inclusion of up to 50% of total calories as high caloric density fats allows energy intake targets to be met within allowable fluid limits. Alternatively, lipid-lowering medications could be used. At this time, experience with these drugs in children is too limited to recommend general use.

The glucose load from peritoneal dialysate does not induce diabetes mellitus, but exposure to intraperitoneal glucose can cause increased glycosylation of protein [261]. ESRD as a result of diabetic nephropathy is vanishingly rare in children (see Table 3), which simplifies the issue of peritoneal glucose absorption for the pediatric CPD patient.

6.11.4.2. *Protein.* Children receiving CPD lose substantial quantities of albumin into the dialysate, with proportionately greater losses occurring in younger patients [59, 60, 262]. Despite aggressive nutritional therapy, including tube feeding, a disturbingly large percentage of pediatric CPD patients have hypoalbuminemia, a well-described mortality risk factor in adult dialysis patients [263]. Coagulation disturbances similar to those seen in the nephrotic syndrome are present in children on CPD [264]. In theory, such children may have an increased risk for graft thrombosis at the time of renal transplantation, although this has yet to be described.

Hypogammaglobulinemia has been reported in infants and younger children on CPD [176, 265]. Mortality rates are highest in this age-group of pediatric CPD patients [232], and the majority of these deaths are due to infectious causes. The possible role of hypogammaglobulinemia in infants on CPD requires further investigation, since it is possible to treat these babies with monthly IV gammaglobulin preparations, an approach currently used in some pediatric centers (Fivush, [Baltimore] personal communication).

Children also experience substantial losses of amino acids into the dialysate, which could contribute to protein-malnutrition. Dietary protein prescriptions in children are routinely adjusted upward to account for intraperitoneal losses of both albumin and amino acids. Unfortunately, many children are unwilling or unable to comply with prescribed protein intake, leading to the risk of chronic malnutrition. The addition of amino acids to the dialysate has been proposed as an alternative to dietary protein supplementation in malnourished children [104].

6.11.5. Abdominal catastrophies

Compared to adult CPD patients, children rarely experience dialysis-related abdominal catastrophies; however, such events have been reported in children and must be considered potential complications in CPD patients of all ages.

6.11.5.1. Encapsulating sclerosing peritonitis.
Encapsulating sclerosing peritonitis is uncommon in children [266]. Gastrointestinal complications of this condition may be fatal. The use of acetate as a dialysate buffer has been implicated in a large percentage of cases reported from Europe [267].

6.11.5.2. Other major disorders of the gastrointestinal tract.
Diverticulitis is a frequent source of bowel perforation and fecal peritonitis in adults which does not occur in children. However, appendicitis must be considered in all children on CPD who present with fever and abdominal pain, which is to say in many children with presenting symptoms suggestive of peritonitis. We have yet to encounter a case of acute appendicitis in a CPD patient in our centers. In such cases, CPD should probably be suspended after appendectomy to allow healing of the appendix stump.

Pancreatitis has been described in adult CPD patients [268]. Early concerns that CPD in some way predisposed patients to the development of pancreatitis have been disputed [269]. Pancreatitis is a rare disorder in children that can be lethal. We have observed pancreatitis in a total of three children in our two programs. Transfer to hemodialysis was included in the management of all three patients.

6.11.5.3. Neoplasia.
Wilms' tumor is a common pediatric malignancy with a known association with ESRD (i.e., the Denys-Drash Syndrome: Wilm's tumor, pseudohermaphroditism, nephropathy) [270]. Wilms' tumors rapidly increase in size and are most often diagnosed by palpation of an abdominal mass.

Children on CPD must be examined regularly with the abdomen empty of dialysate to ensure the absence of an abdominal mass. Rarely, suspicious cells in the dialysate effluent may be identified as malignant using special cytologic techniques.

6.11.6. Miscellaneous complications

It is not possible to address all the complications which may occur in children on CPD. In addition to the major complications discussed above, we will complete this section with a brief review of several of the more important or uniquely pediatric complications.

6.11.6.1. Prune-Belly Syndrome.
Children with Prune-Belly Syndrome can be treated with CPD, despite severely deficient abdominal musculature [91]. In Toronto, percutaneous catheter insertion is preferred as a means of obtaining a more water-tight seal at the thin abdominal wall. In Dallas we prefer to suture the deep cuff to the peritoneal membrane, incorporating the bottom of the cuff in the peritoneal purse-string suture. Both methods have been successful. Although CAPD is possible in these boys, we now treat them with NIPD, limiting daytime volumes to increase patient comfort. Typical exchange volumes are well-tolerated and drain completely if the catheter is unobstructed. Although huge volumes can be infused in these children, this should be avoided.

6.11.6.2. Hydrocephalus.
Children with myelomeningocele typically have neurogenic bladders which may lead to ESRD as a consequence of reflux nephropathy. In addition, these children often have obstructive hydrocephalus requiring shunting of cerebrospinal fluid. Ventriculo-peritoneal (V-P) shunts are preferred due to fewer complications. When children with V-P shunts require dialysis, the choice of CPD raises serious concerns. The risk of peritonitis is sufficiently great in all children treated with CPD that the potential for extension of a simple peritonitis episode to involve the V-P shunt has led some to consider the presence of a V-P shunt an absolute or relative contraindication to CPD. Experience with CPD in children with V-P shunts is limited. At present we would recommend hemodialysis for such children. If hemodialysis is not an option, the V-P shunt could be converted to a ventriculo-atrial or ventriculo-pleural location prior to starting CPD. If these alternatives are not available, CPD in the presence of a V-P shunt is clearly preferable to death from uremia.

6.11.6.3. *Genitourinary surgery*. Children with inadequate urinary bladders are now typically treated with a bladder augmentation procedure using small bowel, large bowel, stomach or dilated ureter [271]. Creation of the augmented bladder requires extensive surgery with attendant risks for development of adhesions. In addition, the augmented bladder segment is attached to a vascular pedicle which resides within the peritoneal cavity. Despite the magnitude of the surgery involved and the potential for complications, we have found these children do well on CPD. In our centers successful CPD has been reliably achieved in children with augmented bladders with no major complications.

Many children on CPD require elective nephrectomies, usually for nephrogenic hypertension or to remove a potential focus for infection (e.g., hydronephrosis or severe vesico-ureteric reflux) prior to transplantation. If it is only necessary to remove the kidneys, the use of a posterior lumbotomy approach avoids invasion of the peritoneal cavity and allows CPD to continue postoperatively, albeit with reduced exchange volumes. For patients requiring nephroureterectomy via a transperitoneal approach CPD often must be suspended for a brief period, during which we treat such children with hemodialysis.

CPD can be offered to children who require a vesicostomy or pyeloureterostomy. We have found no dialysis complications related to these forms of urinary diversion.

6.11.6.4. *Bloody dialysate*. Children on CPD will occasionally experience bloody dialysate following minor abdominal trauma. The bleeding is probably due to catheter trauma in most cases. Mild bleeding can mimic the cloudy fluid of peritonitis. Conservative management has been successful in all such cases seen in our centers. The peritoneal cavity is flushed with dialysate that contains a small amount of heparin (250 Units/liter) to reduce the risk of thrombi obstructing the catheter. Some centers do not use heparin routinely. We do not routinely add antibiotics. Patients, parents, teachers and coaches often need reassurance that such episodes are of little consequence and should not interfere with normal physical activity or participation in sports.

Bloody dialysate can occur in post-menarchal girls secondary to retrograde menstruation. Conservative management is again all that is needed.

6.11.6.5. *Oxalosis*. Oxalosis is a heritable disease of oxalate metabolism that is associated with ESRD in infants and young children [272]. Experience with CPD in infants with oxalosis has generally been dismal [273], although short-term success has been reported. At present we believe such children should be considered early for combined liver-kidney transplantation. Short-term management with hemodialysis or CPD while awaiting transplantation may be successful.

6.12. Quality of life and other psychosocial issues

It is claimed by some authors that survival of patients with ESRD depends on factors other than mode of treatment. Thus, determination of quality of life for ESRD patients is important for clinical decision making and also for allocation of resources. Methodologically sound studies in adults using time trade-off measurements show that successful transplantation is the preferred treatment, providing the best quality of life, with no difference between the various dialysis modalities [274, 275]. This lack of difference in quality of life between hemodialysis and CPD has been confirmed by other authors [276].

One study of 73 children and adolescents compared psychosocial adjustment to ESRD for hemodialysis, CPD and transplantation [277]. Significant advantages of transplantation over dialysis, and of CPD over in-center hemodialysis were found. Children with transplants exhibited less social impairment, less functional impairment, and fewer treatment-associated practical difficulties. Parents of transplanted children also reported fewer practical difficulties. Children on CPD had less social impairment, lower depression scores, better adjustment, and less behavioral disturbance, and reported fewer practical problems related to treatment than their hemodialysis counterparts. Mean depression and anxiety scores were lower in parents of children on CPD. While this study suggests better adjustment of parents whose children are on CPD, possibly due to greater personal control and involvement in their child's care, the potential for parental "burn-out" still exists with prolonged CPD. It is difficult for parents to meet the medical, psychological and social needs of the child on CPD and still have sufficient time and emotional resources to meet the needs of other family members. Parents may also find it difficult to encourage appropriate independence of an ill child [278].

The ultimate success of advances in transplantation and dialysis therapy must be judged by the patient's rehabilitation. Children with ESRD differ from those with many chronic disorders by the persistent manifestations of disease, the continued reliance on medical technology despite successful transplantation, and the 30 times higher incidence of one or more disabilities as compared to the general population. A multicenter study of 479 children and adolescents with ESRD noted that school attendance was well maintained during the first years, but subsequent education was frequently disrupted and inadequate [279]. Attendance in schools providing opportunity for a university career was low, and only 52% of eligible patients attended vocational school. Only 14% of adolescents over 18 years of age achieved independent living. Factors which may contribute to this poor outcome include delays in social maturation, retardation of growth and sexual maturation, and psychological and behavioral disturbances such as depression, anxiety, withdrawal, denial and aggressive behavioral, which have their roots in chronic illness during childhood.

While the outcome of children with chronic renal insufficiency since infancy remains less than optimal, adolescents with later onset of ESRD show great potential for rehabilitation, as demonstrated in a study of 118 patients with onset of renal failure at 12 to 20 years of age [280]. The cumulative survival rate of transplanted patients was 80.1% after 18 years. Functional status was good or excellent in 73.5% of transplant patients, but in only 45% of dialysis patients, with hemodialysis patients functioning poorly compared to CPD patients. Most patients achieved an appropriate level of formal education, but more slowly than their unaffected counterparts. Twenty nine per cent were living independently or with a spouse and four patients had become parents. Significant linear growth retardation (<3rd percentile) was seen in 35.6% of patients, primarily in those with initial growth retardation prior to transplant.

Short stature, as well as alterations in body image related to the need for CPD catheters, central venous lines, feeding tubes or fistulas may contribute to psychosocial maladjustment in children and adolescents with ESRD. While parents can ensure the compliance of younger children for dialysis and medications, adolescents present a particular problem with compliance. Peer pressure often results in dietary non-compliance, and fear of being labelled different may cause a child to forego dialysis exchanges at school, a problem which is helped by using NIPD. Embarrassment over catheters or fatigue related to anemia or underdialysis may result in failure to participate in physical fitness classes, which may result in poor levels of physical activity as adults, with attendant health risks. Ultimately, the child's premorbid personality and the level of parental involvement appear to determine adaptation to ESRD treatment [281].

6.13. Peritoneal dialysis and renal transplantation in children

Pediatric nephrologists agree that the ultimate goal for children with ESRD is a functioning renal transplant. Thus, the effect of pre-transplant dialysis on transplant outcome is vitally important. Following the advent of CPD as widespread treatment for ESRD, Cardella [282] reported no significant difference in graft or patient survival post-transplant in adults regardless of the mode of dialysis pre-transplant. This was confirmed by numerous authors [283–287], with only a few reporting contrary results [288–290]. The major CPD-related complication post-transplant was a 10% incidence of peritonitis which was possibly related to the need for dialysis post-transplant and responded to treatment with antibiotics and sometimes catheter removal [285, 291]. With retroperitoneal graft positioning the peritoneum could be successfully used for dialysis post-transplant if necessary.

In 1983, Stefanidis and associates [292] reported on 23 children transplanted following treatment with CPD. They found no difference in actuarial graft survival in children treated with hemodialysis, CPD or no dialysis. Subsequently, Nevins and Danielson reviewed the outcome of 70 children post-transplantation to determine the effect of prior dialysis therapy [293]. All patients had received prior transfusions allowing the impact of dialysis to be examined separately. They found no difference in patient or allograft survival regardless of the mode of dialysis or absence of prior dialysis.

Reported post-transplant complications in the PD population include fungal peritonitis, and a 10 to 42% (mean 30%) incidence of ascites [292, 294–297]. Numerous reports have confirmed the suitability of children on CPD for transplantation, with no increased risk of rejection and a 5 to 11% incidence of post-transplant peritonitis, which responds readily to antibiotics [294–299]. If left in situ, the catheter can be used for dialysis in the post-transplant period with good catheter patency.

6.14. The choice of CPD or hemodialysis as maintenance RRT pending transplantation for children at different ages

En route to the ultimate goal of renal transplantation, management options for children with ESRD include hemodialysis, CPD or conservative treatment with pre-emptive transplantation. The latter offers the advantage of avoiding the expense and complications of dialysis without influencing the outcome of transplantation. While living-related transplantation may be planned to avoid the need for dialysis, patients awaiting cadaveric transplantation often require dialysis before a kidney becomes available. When dialysis is deemed necessary, the modality chosen should be determined by factors other than the outcome post-transplant, since prior dialysis does not influence transplant outcomes [293]. Since both hemodialysis and CPD are equally effective, the choice of dialysis modality depends on a multitude of factors including availability of services (e.g., proximity to a pediatric hemodialysis center), psychosocial/family considerations, patient factors (e.g., need for or recent intraabdominal surgery) and ESRD treatment program philosophy. Decisions regarding mode of dialysis require objective discussion with the family and child regarding the pros and cons and expected outcome of each modality, regardless of the child's or the family's preconceived notions, as changes in therapy may be necessary for medical or social reasons. Ideally, such discussions should take place prior to the patient's actual need for dialysis to allow time to consider the options and respond appropriately [300, 301]. Social workers and nurses have been found more influential than nephrologists in helping patients to choose a dialysis modality [302].

CPD is generally encouraged for children in our centers. Advantages of CPD which are particularly beneficial to the pediatric age group include: increased attendance at school; less disruption of parents' work schedule; and more flexibility for family activities such as vacations. In particular, nocturnal dialysis modalities (CCPD, NIPD) alleviate the need for dialysis exchanges at school, cause minimal disruption in parental work schedules, and allow consolidation of dialysis and nocturnal tube feedings to decrease the parental work load. In addition, CPD affords better control of blood pressure and fluid balance in anephric or very oliguric patients, allows more liberal food and water intake, and is more readily available than hemodialysis. The primary disadvantage of CPD is infection, namely peritonitis, and to a lesser extent, exit site infections. Other complications include protein malnutrition, obesity, hernias, and membrane failure. Peritoneal access is sometimes unsuccessful, and CPD catheters may need replacement in conjunction with an omentectomy if catheter failure occurs. Parental stress and burn-out may occur. The potential for non-compliance in teenagers is greater on CPD if they are responsible for their dialysis. Non-medical considerations in instituting CPD include the space requirements necessary for dialysis supplies and cycler machines, and hygienic standards within the household.

Hemodialysis is less often recommended for children in our centers because it is technically more demanding in the small child, requires creation of vascular access, may entail the need for repeated venipuncture, and results in significant loss of time from school. It may however, be indicated for patients with a contraindication to CPD or in families who are not motivated or are incapable of performing CPD. The major attraction of hemodialysis is the reduced parental burden of care, though significant time commitments are necessary to transport patients to hemodialysis and for the treatment itself. Disadvantages include more severe fluid and diet restrictions, the relative paucity of pediatric hemodialysis facilities, recurrent bacteremia and sepsis where hemodialysis is performed through an indwelling central venous line, and vascular thromboses related to vascular access. The major contraindications to hemodialysis are lack of an adequate access, and sensitivity to heparin. More severe anemia in hemodialysis patients was once a consideration, but is less relevant in the erythropoietin era.

Another factor which may influence choice of dialysis modality is the anticipated length of time on dialysis prior to transplantation, with hemodialysis favored for short periods of dialysis. In times of fiscal restraint, cost is important. Start up costs are greatest with CPD, but maintenance costs with CPD are much cheaper. Transplantation is cheapest after 18 months of graft survival. Treatment failures maximize costs, so a patient's choice of therapy should be carefully considered for likelihood of success [303]. While some patients have a clear indication or contraindication for one or the other dialysis modality, most patients have a choice. In one study in adults, peritonitis ranked as the most important factor in determining treatment modality, and in general, lifestyles ranked higher than medical consequences for a specific therapy [304]. All forms of ESRD treatment should be viewed as interactive, rather than mutually exclusive. Patients may be required to switch types of dialysis when complications ensue or need for surgery intervenes, or when patients return to dialysis following loss of a renal transplant.

6.15. Training families for home peritoneal dialysis

The goal of a dialysis program is to provide medical and psychosocial management of the child with ESRD until transplantation is achieved. A successful pediatric CPD program requires a multidisciplinary approach, with integral members being the child and family, primary CPD nurse, pediatric nephrologist, renal dietician, social worker, pediatric surgeon and/or pediatric urologist, child life worker, psychiatrist, teacher, financial counselor, and transplant coordinator. Mandatory support systems include Home Care, community visiting nurses and facilities for respite care. Critical to the success of a program are the assumptions that CPD is a successful treatment modality for ESRD, but that complications will occur. Parents maintain the ultimate responsibility for their child, and the dialysis regimen must be fitted into the lives of the child and family, and not the reverse [59, 305].

The initial step in training involves selection of appropriate patients, which will reduce the incidence of treatment failures. Children must have a functional peritoneum, a motivated family, and a primary dialysis caregiver for young children or a backup caregiver for older children. Secondly, the intellectual and functional level of the primary caregiver and child must be evaluated and the training regimen adjusted accordingly. Choices for CPD regimen depend on the needs of the child and the educational limitations of the learner. Factors such as vision and manual dexterity must be considered. We have successfully trained parents with borderline mental retardation to perform limited CPD at home with extensive outpatient nursing support and hospital support for complications such as peritonitis. We have also trained illiterate and non-English speaking parents to perform home dialysis, utilizing pictorial instructions and interpreters. Children older than 12 years of age, unless developmentally or physically handicapped, generally have the cognitive ability and manual dexterity to be taught CPD.

The content of the training program should be outlined to ensure consistency in teaching, and should include the following elements: normal kidney function; complications of chronic renal failure; anatomy and physiology of the peritoneum; the mechanics of CPD (e.g., bag changes, cycler operations, tube change, exit site care etc.); complications (e.g., peritonitis, contamination, exit site infection, fluid overload) and their treatment; monitoring of weights and blood pressure and maintenance of home dialysis records; medications, including intraperitoneal administration of drugs; explanation of laboratory tests, clinic and diagnostic routines, as well as means of contacting the dialysis team; and adaptation of home, school and activity routines to accommodate dialysis [305]. Parents are provided with a home teaching manual that contains the information and protocols covered during the training session and that is used both for initial instruction and for later reference at home. It also includes important phone numbers for contacting the home dialysis team. Another essential teaching aid is a doll with a functioning CPD catheter which allows parents to conceptualize CPD and to practice the procedures until a comfort level is reached prior to applying their newly acquired skills to their child. The doll is also used with age-appropriate children for play therapy pre- and post-operatively.

Preparation for home training involves the establishment of a functioning CPD catheter, family preparations for the training course which involves arranging time off work, and babysitting for siblings, and delivery of supplies to the home. Outcome is considered successful when the child or parent can perform exchanges and/or operate the cycler safely and accurately, can record and interpret weights and blood pressures, and can identify the need for medical consultation or treatment. As well, a parent should be able to establish and maintain age-appropriate patterns of parenting, taking into account the child's developmental status and needs. Training usually lasts for 7 to 10 days, but must be individualized to each family's needs and skills.

Psychosocial support is essential for families of technology-dependent children and can be initiated during the post-training home visit, when suggestions to improve efficiency can also be implemented and provided on an ongoing basis through outpatient clinics. In addition, medical and psychosocial issues are addressed during regular telephone contact with the patient's primary CPD nurse. Many pediatric programs make extensive use of visiting nurse respite care at home and in-center respite care of longer duration in a local rehabilitation facility to prevent parental burn-out and to decrease hospitalization.

The ultimate goal is a well dialyzed, biochemically stable, infection-free child who is growing and developing normally, is attending school, participating in age-appropriate personal and family activities, and is not hospitalized.

7. Peritoneal dialysis for intoxications, inborn errors of metabolism and other miscellaneous disorders in children

7.1. Intoxications

Treatment of intoxications in small children remains an important if infrequently tested area of expertise for the nephrologist who is likely to be consulted regarding the advisability of dialysis in these situations. For many years PD played an important role in the treatment of small children who had been poisoned with substances removable by dialysis [306]. The use of PD in the treatment of poisoning is reviewed in detail in Chapter 26. For information regarding specific intoxications in children the reader in urgent need of this information is advised to contact the nearest Poison Control Center or to call the Rocky Mountain Poison Control Center in Denver, Colorado (303-629-1123).

The use of PD to treat intoxications in children has almost disappeared in our centers. Several factors seem to be responsible for this phenomenon. Improvements in acute hemodialysis techniques and equipment specifically developed for use in small children have made hemodialysis our first choice for intoxications [307–309]. Hemoperfusion techniques and devices are also readily adapted for use in children of almost any size [310]. Reliable percutaneous vascular access procedures and catheters designed for use in small children have become widely available [311, 312]. As a result of these and other developments, emergency hemodialysis is available for infants and children in pediatric dialysis centers throughout North America and Europe. Regardless of a patient's size, hemodialysis is many times more effective than PD at removing dialyzable drugs and poisons [313, 314]. When a child has ingested a potentially harmful amount of dialyzable poison, hemodialysis should be used whenever possible. PD is an acceptable alternative only for those children too small to receive hemodialysis at the facility at which they are being treated and too unstable to be safely transported to a pediatric dialysis center for emergency hemodialysis.

7.2. Congenital hyperammonemia and other inborn errors of metabolism

Congenital urea cycle enzymopathies are characterized by a reduced capacity to synthesize urea, which leads to accumulation of ammonium and other nitrogenous urea precursors [315]. Severely affected neonates develop vomiting, lethargy, seizures and coma within the first few days of life. The central nervous system symptomatology is thought to be primarily due to the effects of increased blood ammonium concentration. Emergency treatment is aimed at rapid and sustained removal of accumulated ammonium.

In our centers PD is still the treatment of choice for infants with congenital hyperammonemia. The superiority of PD over exchange transfusion in this setting has been demonstrated [316]. In studies performed in 53 episodes of hyperammonemic coma, ammonium was removed more rapidly with PD than with exchange transfusion, and the rebound hyperammonemia that often follows treatment with exchange transfusion did not occur in babies treated with PD. Hemodialysis is the most efficient method for removal of ammonium [317], but treatment with hemodialysis must be limited to several hours, whereas endogenous ammonium production in these babies is persistent early in the course of treatment [316]. PD can be continued indefinitely, providing time during which the diagnosis of the specific urea cycle defect can be made and appropriate therapy instituted. PD removes ten times more nitrogen as glutamine than as ammonium; it has been suggested that the effectiveness of PD in hyperammonemic infants may be due in part to the continuous removal of both ammonium and its precursors: glutamine, glutamate, and alanine [316].

PD has also been useful in the acute management of several other congenital metabolic defects: maple syrup urine disease [318], proprionic acidemia [319], and other congenital organic acidemias [320].

7.3. Miscellaneous pediatric disorders in which treatment with peritoneal dialysis has been attempted

Many of the serious afflictions of infants and children have been treated at one time or another with PD. In 1966 Nora and associates demonstrated the effectiveness with which PD removed fluid from children in intractable congestive heart failure [321]. Today such children would be treated with one or more powerful diuretics unknown 25 years ago, or, that failing, with CVVH in our centers.

PD has not been shown to be of sufficient benefit in the treatment of children with the following disorders to warrant further use: hyaline membrane disease [322], neonatal hyperbilirubinemia [323], Reye Syndrome [324], and hepatic coma [325].

Acknowledgements

The authors thank Stanly Lee, MD (Nashville), Denis Geary, MD (Toronto) and Kathy Jabs, MD (Boston) for assistance with portions of the manuscript, Jeanette Kennedy, RN, Mary Blanchett, Janell McQuinn, and Judith McNicoll for technical and clerical assistance, and Johnnie Fairman, RN, Julia Nickles, RN, Jennifer Snell, RN, Becky Nolde-Hurlburt, RN, Margaret Scott, RN and Yolanda Goodman, RN for their expert care of the peritoneal dialysis patients in our programs.

References

1. Popovich RP, Moncrief JW, Decherd JW et al. The definition of a novel wearable/portable equilibrium dialysis technique. (Abstract) Trans Am Soc Artif Intern Organs 1976; 5: 64.
2. Blackfan KD, Maxcy KF. The intraperitoneal injection of saline solution. Am J Dis Child 1918; 15: 19–28.
3. Bloxsum A, Powell N. The treatment of acute temporary dysfunction of the kidneys by peritoneal irrigation. Pediatrics 1948; 1: 52–7.
4. Swan H, Gordon HH. Peritoneal lavage in the treatment of anuria in children. Pediatrics 1949; 4: 586-95.
5. Odel HM, Ferris DO, Power MH. Peritoneal lavage as an effective means of extra-renal excretion. Am J Med 1950; 9: 63–77.
6. Maxwell MH, Rockney RB, Kleeman CR et al. Peritoneal dialysis: I. technique and applications. JAMA 1959; 170: 917–24.
7. Segar WE, Gibson RK, Rhamy R. Peritoneal dialysis in infants and small children. Pediatrics 1961; 27: 603–13.
8. Etteldorf JN, Dobbins WT, Sweeney MJ et al. Intermittent peritoneal dialysis in the management of acute renal failure in children. J Pediatr 1962; 60: 327–39.
9. Segar WE. Peritoneal dialysis in the treatment of boric acid poisoning. NEJM 1960; 262: 798–800.
10. Etteldorf JN, Dobbins WT, Summitt RL et al. Intermittent peritoneal dialysis using 5 per cent albumin in the treatment of salicylate intoxication in children. J Pediatr 1961; 58: 226–36.
11. Lloyd-Still JD, Atwell JD. Renal failure in infancy, with special reference to the use of peritoneal dialysis. J Pediatr Surg 1966; 1: 466–75.
12. Manley GL, Collip PJ. Renal failure in the newborn: treatment with peritoneal dialysis. Am J Dis Child 1968; 115: 107–10.
13. Lugo G, Ceballos R, Brown W et al. Acute renal failure in the neonate managed by peritoneal dialysis. Am J Dis Child 1969; 118: 655–9.
14. Gianantonio CA, Vitacco M, Mendelbarzee J et al. Acute renal failure in infancy and childhood. J Pediatr 1962; 61: 660–78.
15. Wiggelinkhuizen J. Peritoneal dialysis in children. S Afr Med J 1971; 45: 1047–54.
16. Day RE, White RHR. Peritoneal dialysis in children: review of 8 years' experience. Arch Dis Child 1977; 52: 56–61.
17. Chan JCM. Peritoneal dialysis for renal failure in childhood. Clin Pediatr 1978; 17: 349–54.
18. Feldman W, Baliah T, Drummond KN. Intermittent peritoneal dialysis in the management of chronic renal failure in children. Am J Dis Child 1968; 116: 30–6.
19. Palmer RA, Quinton WE, Gray JF et al. Prolonged peritoneal dialysis for chronic renal failure. Lancet 1964; 1: 700–2.
20. Palmer RA, Newell, JE, Gray JF et al. Treatment of chronic renal failure by prolonged peritoneal dialysis. NEJM 1966; 274: 248–54.
21. Tenckhoff H, Schecter H. A bacteriologically safe peritoneal access device. Trans Am Soc Artif Intern Organs 1966; 14: 181–6.
22. Boen ST, Mion CM, Curtis FK et al. Periodic peritoneal dialysis using the repeated puncture technique and an automated cycling machine. Trans Am Soc Artif Intern Organs 1964; 10: 409–14.
23. Tenckhoff H, Meston B, Shilipetar G. A simplified automatic peritoneal dialysis system. Trans Am Soc Artif Intern Organs 1972; 18: 436–40.
24. Counts S, Hickman R, Garbaccio A, Tenckhoff H. Chronic home peritoneal dialysis in children. Trans Am Soc Artif Intern Organs 1973; 19: 157–67.
25. Hickman RO. Nine years' experience with chronic peritoneal dialysis in childhood. Dial Transplant 1978; 7: 803.
26. Brouhard BH, Berger M, Cunningham RJ et al. Home peritoneal dialysis in children. Trans Am Soc Artif Intern Organs 1979; 25: 90–4.
27. Baluarte HJ, Grossman MS, Polinsky MD et al. Experience with intermittent home peritoneal dialysis (IHPD) in children. (Abstract) Pediatr Res 1980; 14: 994.
28. Lorentz WB, Hamilton RW, Disher B et al. Home peritoneal dialysis during infancy. Clin Nephrol 1981; 15: 194–7.

29. Potter DE, McDaid TK, Ramirez JA et al. Peritoneal dialysis in children. In: Atkins RC, Thomson NM, Farrell PC (eds), Peritoneal Dialysis. Churchill-Livingstone, New York 1981; pp 356–61.
30. Oreopoulos DG, Katirtzoglou A, Arbus G, Cordy P. Dialysis and transplantation in young children. (Letter) Brit Med J 1979; 1: 1628–9.
31. Balfe JW, Irwin MA. Continuous ambulatory peritoneal dialysis in children. In: Legrain, M (ed), Continuous Ambulatory Peritoneal Dialysis. Excerpta Medica, Amsterdam 1980; pp 131–6.
32. Alexander SR, Tseng CH, Maksym KA et al. Clinical parameters in continuous ambulatory peritoneal dialysis for infants and young children. In: Moncrief JW, Popovich RP (eds), CAPD Update. Masson Publishing, New York 1981; pp 195–209.
33. Kohaut EC. Continuous ambulatory peritoneal dialysis: a preliminary pediatric experience. Am J Dis Child 1981; 135: 270–1.
34. Potter DE, McDaid TK, McHenry K et al. Continuous ambulatory peritoneal dialysis (CAPD) in children. Trans Am Soc Artif Intern Organs 1981; 27: 64–7.
35. Salusky IB, Lucullo L, Nelson P, Fine RN. Continuous ambulatory peritoneal dialysis in children. Pediatr Clin N Am 1982; 29: 1005–12.
36. Guillot M, Clermont M-J, Gagnadoux M-F, Broyer M. Nineteen months' experience with continuous ambulatory peritoneal dialysis in children: main clinical and biological results. In: Gahl GM, Kessel M, Nolph KD (eds), Advances in Peritoneal Dialysis. Excerpta Medica, Amsterdam 1981; pp 203–7.
37. Eastham EJ, Kirplani H, Francis D et al. Pediatric continuous ambulatory peritoneal dialysis. Arch Dis Child 1982; 57: 677–80.
38. Alexander SR. Pediatric CAPD update – 1983. Perit Dial Bull 1983; 3 (Suppl): S15–22.
39. Price CG, Suki WN. Newer modifications of peritoneal dialysis: options in the treatment of patients with renal failure. Am J Nephrol 1981; 1: 97–104.
40. Alexander SR, Honda M. Continuous peritoneal dialysis for children: a decade of worldwide growth and development. Kidney Int 1993; 43 (Suppl 40): S65–74.
41. U.S. Renal Data System. USRDS 1993 Annual Data Report, The National Institutes of Health, National Institute of Diabetes and Digestive and Kidney Disease, Bethesda, MD., March 1993; B-8, C.2 (Tables).
42. Arbus GS. Pediatric patients in 1989. In: Canadian Organ Replacement Register, 1989 Annual Report. Hospital Medical Records Institute, Ontario, Don Mills, March 1991; pp 71–100.
43. Hoffman JIE. Congenital heart disease. Pediatr Clin N Am 1990; 37: 25–44.
44. Poplack DG. Acute lymphoblastic leukemia. In: Pizzo PA, Poplack DG (eds), Principles and Practice of Pediatric Oncology. Lippincott, New York 1989; p 323.
45. Gusmano R, Perfumo F. Worldwide demographic aspects of chronic renal failure in children. Kidney Int 1993; 43 (Suppl 41): S31–5.
46. U.S. Renal Data System. USRDS 1989 Annual Data Report, The National Institutes of Health, National Institute of Diabetes and Digestive Kidney Diseases, Bethesda, MD, August, 1989.
47. Alexander SR, Sullivan EK, Harmon WE, Stablein DM, Tejani A. Maintenance dialysis in North American children and adolescents: a preliminary report of the North American Pediatric Renal Transplant Cooperative Study (NAPRTCS). Kidney Int 1993; 44 (Suppl 43): S104–9.
48. Putiloff PV. Materials for the study of the laws of growth of the human body in relation to the surface areas of different systems: the trial on Russian subjects of planigraphic anatomy as a means for exact anthropometry – one of the problems of anthropology. Report of Dr. P. V. Putiloff at the meeting of the Siberian Branch of the Russian Geographic Society, 1884 (summarized in ref. 50).
49. Wegner G. Chirurgische Bemerkungen uber die peritoneal Hohle, mit besonder Berucksichtigung der Ovariotomie. Arch Klin Chir 1887; 20: 51.
50. Esperanca MJ, Collins DL. Peritoneal dialysis efficiency in relation to body weight. J Pediatr Surg 1966; 1: 162–9.
51. Gruskin AB, Lerner GR, Fleischman LE. Developmental aspects of peritoneal dialysis kinetics. In: Fine RN (ed), Chronic Ambulatory Peritoneal Dialysis (CAPD) and Chronic Cycling Peritoneal Dialysis (CCPD) in Children. Martinus Nijhoff, Boston 1987; pp 33–46.
52. Nolph KD. Peritoneal anatomy and transport physiology. In: Drukker W, Parsons FM, Maher JF (eds), Replacement of Renal Function by Dialysis, 2nd ed. Martinus Nijhoff, Boston 1983 pp 440–56.
53. Mactier RA, Khanna R, Twardowski Z, Nolph KD. Role of peritoneal cavity lymphatic absorption in peritoneal dialysis. Kidney Int 1987; 32: 65–172.
54. Gruskin AB, Cote ML, Baluarte HJ. Peritoneal diffusion curves. peritoneal clearances, and scaling factors in children of differing age. Int J Pediatr Nephrol 1982; 3: 271–8.
55. Geary DF, Harvey EA, MacMillan JH et al. The peritoneal equilibration test in children. Kidney Int 1992; 42: 102–5.
56. Schroeder CH, Dreumel MJ, Reddingius R et al. Peritoneal transport kinetics of glucose urea and creatinine during infancy and childhood. Perit Dial Int 1991; 11: 322–5.
57. Pyle WK. Mass transfer in peritoneal dialysis. PhD dissertation, University of Texas in Austin, 1981. (Described in: Morgenstern BZ, Baluarte HJ. Peritoneal dialysis kinetics in children. In: Fine RN (ed), Chronic Ambulatory Peritoneal Dialysis (CAPD) and Chronic Cycling Peritoneal Dialysis (CCPD) in Children. Martinus Nijhoff, Boston 1978; pp 47–62.
58. Morgenstern BZ, Pyle WK, Gruskin AB et al. Transport characteristics of the pediatric peritoneal membrane. Kidney Int 1984; 25: 259–64.

59. Balfe JW, Vigneaux A, Williamson J et al. The use of CAPD in the treatment of children with end-stage renal disease. Perit Dial Bull 1981; 1: 35–8.
60. Drachman R, Niaudet P, Dartois A-M, Broyer M. Protein losses during peritoneal dialysis in children. In: Fine RN, Scharer K, Mehls O (eds), CAPD in Children. Springer-Verlag, New York 1985; pp 78–83.
61. Morgenstern BZ, Pyle WK, Gruskin AB et al. Convective characteristics of pediatric peritoneal dialysis. Perit Dial Bull 1984; 4: S155–8.
62. Geary DF, Harvey EA, Balfe JW. Mass transfer area coefficients in children. Perit Dial Int 1994; 14: 30–3.
63. Kohaut EC, Alexander SR. Ultrafiltration in the young patient on CAPD. In: Moncrief JW, Popovich RP (eds), CAPD Update. Masson Publ, New York 1981; pp 221–6.
64. Balfe JW, Hanning RM, Vigneaux A, Watson AR. A comparison of peritoneal water and solute movement in young and older children on CAPD. In: Fine RN, Scharer K, Mehls O (eds), CAPD in Children. Springer-Verlag, New York 1985; pp 14–9.
65. Popovich RP, Pyle WK, Rosenthal DA et al. Kinetics of peritoneal dialysis in children. In: Moncrief JW, Popovich RP (eds), CAPD Update. Masson Publ, New York; pp 227–42.
66. Mactier RA, Khanna R, Moore H, Russ J, Nolph KD, Groshong T. Kinetics of peritoneal dialysis in children: role of lymphatics. Kidney Int 1988; 34: 82–8.
67. Elzouki AY, Gruskin AB, Baluarte JH et al. Developmental aspects of peritoneal dialysis kinetics in dogs. Pediatr. Res 1981; 15: 863–85.
68. Siegel NJ, Brown RS. Peritoneal clearance of ammonia and creatinine in a neonate. J Pediatr 1973; 82: 1044.
69. Kohaut EC. Effect of dialysate volume on ultrafiltration in young patients treated with CAPD. Int J Pediatr Nephrol 1986; 7: 13–6.
70. McCance RA. The maintenance of chemical stability in the newborn in chemical exchange. Arch Dis Child 1959; 34: 361–9.
71. Twardowski ZJ, Nolph KD, Khanna R et al. Peritoneal equilibration test. Perit Dial Bull 1986; 7: 138–47.
72. Schaefer F, Langenbeck D, Heckert KH et al. Evaluation of peritoneal solute transfer by the peritoneal equilibration test in children. Adv Perit Dial 1992; 8: 410–5.
73. Mendley SR, Umans JG, Majkowski NL. Measurement of peritoneal dialysis delivery in children. Pediatr Nephrol 1993; 7: 284–9.
74. Morgenstern BZ. Equilibration testing: close but not quite right. Pediatr Nephrol 1993; 7: 290–1.
75. Leone MR, Jenkins RD, Golper TA, Alexander SR. Early experience with continuous arteriovenous hemofiltration in critically ill pediatric patients. Crit Care Med 1986; 14: 1058–63.
76. Ronco C, Brendolan A, Bragantini L et al. Treatment of acute renal failure in newborns by continuous arteriovenous hemofiltration. Kidney Int 1986; 29: 908–15.
77. Alexander SR. Continuous arteriovenous hemofiltration. In: Levin DL, Morris FC (eds), Essentials of Pediatric Intensive Care. Quality Medical Publishing, St. Louis 1990; pp 1022–48.
78. Leumann EP, Knecht B, Dangel P et al. Peritoneal dialysis in newborns: technical improvements. In: Bulla M (ed), Renal Insufficiency in Children. Springer-Verlag, New York 1982; pp 147–50.
79. Borzotta A, Harrison HL, Groff DB. Technique of peritoneal dialysis cannulation in neonates. Surg Gynecol Obstet 1983; 157: 73–4.
80. Alexander SR. Peritoneal dialysis in children. In: Nolph KD (ed), Peritoneal Dialysis. 3rd ed. Kluwer, Boston 1989; pp 343–64.
81. Murphy JLM, Reznik VM, Mendoza SA, Peterson B et al. Use of a guidewire inserted catheter for acute peritoneal dialysis. Int J Pediatr Nephrol 1987; 8: 199–202.
82. Nash MA, Russo JC. Neonatal lactic acidosis and renal failure: the role of peritoneal dialysis. J Pediatr 1977; 91: 101–5.
83. Lorentz WB. Acute hydrothorax during peritoneal dialysis. J Pediatr 1979; 94: 417–9.
84. Groshong T. Dialysis in infants and children. In: Van Stone JC (ed), Dialysis in the Treatment of Renal Insufficiency. Grune & Stratton, New York 1983; pp 234–6.
85. Posen GA, Luisello J. Continuous equilibration peritoneal dialysis in treatment of acute renal failure. Perit Dial Bull 1980; 1: 6–7.
86. Abbad FCB, Ploos van Amstel SLB. Continuous ambulatory peritoneal dialysis in small children with acute renal failure. Proc EDTA 1982; 19; 607–13.
87. Watson AR, Vigneaux A, Hardy BE, Balfe JW. Six-year experience with CAPD catheters in children. Perit Dial Bull 1985; 5: 119–22.
88. Watson AR, Vigneaux A, Balfe JW, McLorie G, Churchill B. Chronic peritoneal catheters in a pediatric population. In: Khanna R, Nolph KD, Prowant B, Twardowski ZJ, Oreopoulos DG (eds), Advances in Continuous Ambulatory Peritoneal Dialysis 1986. Peritoneal Dialysis Bulletin, Toronto 1986; pp 41–4.
89. Alexander SR, Tank ES, Corneil AT. Five years' experience with CAPD/CCPD catheters in infants and children. In: Fine RN, Scharer K, Mehls O (eds), CAPD in Children. Springer-Verlag, New York 1985; pp 174–89.
90. Alexander SR, Tank ES. Surgical aspects of continuous ambulatory peritoneal dialysis in infants, children and adolescents. J Urol 1982; 127: 501–4.
91. Crompton CH, Balfe JW, Khoury AO. Peritoneal dialysis in the Prune-Belly Syndrome. Perit Dial Int 1994; 14: 17–21.
92. Lasker N. Chronic peritoneal dialysis. PA Med 1971; 74: 67.
93. Hutchison AJ, Gokal R. Peritoneal dialysis fluids for the future: do we have the solution? Dial Transplant 1992; 21: 57–63.

94. Kohaut EC, Balfe JW, Potter D, Alexander SR, Lum G. Hypermagnesemia and mild hypocarbia in pediatric patients on continuous ambulatory peritoneal dialysis. (Letter) Perit Dial Bull 1983; 31: 41–2.
95. Tzamaloukas AH. "Contraction" alkalosis during treatment of hyperglycemia in CAPD patients. Perit Dial Bull 1983; 3: 196–9.
96. Feriani M, Biasioli S, Borin D et al. Bicarbonate buffer for CAPD solution. ASAIO Trans 1985; 31: 668–72.
97. Yatzidis H. A new single bicarbonate CAPD solutions. In: La Greca G, Ronco C, Feriani FM (eds), Fourth International Course on Peritoneal Dialysis. Wichtig Editore, Vincenza 1991; pp 151–7.
98. Hanning RH, Balfe JW, Zlotkin SH. Effectiveness and nutritional consequences of amino acid-based vs glucose-based dialysis solutions in infants and children receiving CAPD. Am J Clin Nutr 1987; 46: 22–30.
99. de Fijiter CWH, Verburugh HA, Liem PO, Heezius E, Donker AJM, Verhoef J et al. Bicompatibility of a glucose polymer-containing peritoneal dialysis fluid. Am J Kid Dis 1993; 21: 411–8.
100. Oreopoulos DG, Crassweler P, Katirzoglou A. Amino acids as an osmotic agent (instead of glucose) in continuous ambulatory peritoneal dialysis. In: Legrain M (ed), International Symposium on CAPD. Excerpta Medica, Amsterdam 1970; pp 335–40.
101. Oreopoulos DG, Marliss E, Anderson GH, Oren A, Dombros N, Williams P, Khanna R, Rodella H, Brandes L. Nutritional aspects of CAPD and the potential use of amino acid containing dialysis solutions. Perit Dial Bull 1983; (Suppl 3): S10–2.
102. Canepa A, Perfumo F, Carrea A, Giallongo F, Verrina E, Cantaluppi A, Gusmano R. Long-term effect of amino-acid dialysis solution in children on continuous ambulatory peritoneal dialysis. Pediatr. Nephrol 1991; 5: 215–9.
103. Honda M. Kamiyama Y, Hasegawa O, Hoshinaga K, Ogawa O, Kawamura T, Ito H. Effects of short-term essential amino acid-containing dialysate in young children on CAPD. Perit Dial Int 1991; 11: 76–80.
104. Hanning RH, Balfe JW, Zlotkin SH. Effect of amino acid-containing dialysis solutions on plasma amino acid profiles in children with chronic renal failure. J Pediatr Gastroenterol Nutr 1987; 6: 942–7.
105. Baum M, Powell D, Calvin S et al. Continuous ambulatory peritoneal dialysis in children: comparison with hemodialysis. NEJM 1982; 307: 1537–42.
106. Bergstrom J, Asaba H, Furst P, Lindholm B. Middle molecules in chronic uremic patients treated with peritoneal dialysis. In: Ghal GM, Kessel M, Nolph KD (eds), Advances in Peritoneal Dialysis: Proceedings of the Second International Symposium on Peritoneal Dialysis, Berlin June 1981. Excerpta Medica, Amsterdam 1981; p. 47.
107. Von Lilien T, Salusky IB, Boechat I et al. Five years' experience with continuous ambulatory or continuous cycling peritoneal dialysis in children. J Pediatr 1987; 111: 513–8.
108. Southwest Pediatric Nephrology Study Group. Continuous ambulatory and continuous cycling peritoneal dialysis in children. Kidney Int 1985; 27: 558–64.
109. Twardowski ZJ. Nightly peritoneal dialysis: why, who, how, and when? ASAIO Trans 1990; 36: 8–16.
110. Flanigan MJ, Doyle C, Lim VS, Ullrich G. Tidal peritoneal dialysis: preliminary experience. Perit Dial Int 1992; 12: 304–8.
111. Alexander SR, Lubischer JT. Continuous ambulatory peritoneal dialysis in pediatrics: 3 years' experience at one center. Nefrologia (Madrid) 1982; 11(Suppl 2): 53–62.
112. Nelson P, Stover J. Principles of nutritional assessment and management of the child with ESRD. In: Fine RN, Gruskin AB (eds), End Stage Renal Disease in Children. W B Saunders Company, Philadelphia 1984; pp 209–26.
113. Hellerstein S, Holliday MA, Grupe WE et al. Nutritional management of children with chronic renal failure. Summary of the task force on nutritional management of children with chronic renal failure. Pediatr Nephrol 1987; 1: 195–211.
114. Salusky IB. The nutritional approach for pediatric patients undergoing CAPD/CCPD. Adv Perit Dial 1990; 6: 245–51.
115. Blumenkrantz MJ, Schmidt RW. Nutritional management of the CAPD patient. Perit Dial Bull 1981; 1: 22–4.
116. Schilling H, Wu G, Pettit J et al. Nutritional status of patients on long-term CAPD. Perit Dial Bull 1985; 5: 12–8.
117. National Research Council. Recommended Dietary Allowances (10th ed). National Academy Press, Washington DC 1989; pp 1–284.
118. Salusky IB, Fine RN, Nelson P, Blumenkrantz MJ, Kopple JD. Nutritional status of children undergoing continuous peritoneal dialysis. Am J Clin Nutr 1983; 38: 599–611.
119. Williams PF, Marliss EB, Anderson GH et al. Amino acid absorption following intraperitoneal administration in CAPD patients. Perit Dial Bull 1982; 2: 124–30.
120. Wassner SJ, Abitbol C, Alexander S et al. Nutritional requirements for infants with renal failure. Am J Kidney Dis 1986; 7: 300–5.
121. Elias RA, McArdle AH, Gagnon RF. The effectiveness of protein supplementation on the nutritional management of patients on CAPD. Adv Perit Dial 1989; 5: 177–80.
122. Buchwald R, Pena JC. Evaluation of nutritional status in patients on continuous ambulatory peritoneal dialysis (CAPD). Perit Dial Int 1989; 9: 295–301.
123. Querfeld U, Salusky IB, Nelson P, Foley J, Fine RN. Hyperlipidemia in pediatric patients undergoing peritoneal dialysis. Pediatr Nephrol 1988; 2; 447–52.
124. Lifshitz F, Moses N. A complication of dietary

treatment of hypercholesterolemia. Am J Dis Child 1989; 143: 537–42.
125. Workshop Proceedings. An evaluation of the 1990 Canadian Nutrition Recommendations for total fat/saturated fat intake for children between the ages of 12 and 18 years. In: Kubow S (ed), Workshop Proceedings, An Evaluation of the 1990 Canadian Nutrition Recommendation for Total Fat/Saturated Fat Intake for Children Between the Ages of 2 and 18 Years. Kush Medical Communications, McGill University 1990; pp 1–52.
126. Murakami R, Momota T, Yoshiya K et al. Serum carnitine and nutritional status in children treated with continuous ambulatory peritoneal dialysis. J Pediatr Gastroenterol Nutr 1990; 11: 371–4.
127. Tamura T, Vaughn WH, Waldo FB, Kohaut EC. Zinc and copper balance in children on continuous ambulatory peritoneal dialysis. Pediatr Nephrol 1989; 3: 309–13.
128. Lindholm B, Bergstrom J. Nutritional aspects on peritoneal dialysis. Kidney Int Suppl 1992; 42(38): S165–71.
129. Schmidt R, Dumler F, Cruz C, Lubkowski T, Kilates C. Improved nutritional follow-up of peritoneal dialysis patients with bioelectrical impedance. Adv Perit Dial 1992; 8: 157–9.
130. Levin L. Balfe JW, Geary D, Wesson D, Steele B. Gastrostomy tube feeding in children on CAPD. Perit Dial Bull 1987; 7: 223–6.
131. Garel L, O'Regan S. Percutaneous gastrojejunostomy for enteral alimentation in children on chronic cycler peritoneal dialysis. Adv Perit Dial 1988; 4: 79–83.
132. Balfe JW, Secker DJ, Coulter PE, Balfe J, Geary DF. Tubing feeding in children on chronic peritoneal dialysis. Adv Perit Dial 1990; 6: 257–61.
133. O'Regan S, Garel L. Percutaneous gastrojejunostomy for caloric supplementation in children on peritoneal dialysis. Adv Perit Dial 1990; 6: 273–5.
134. Warady BA, Kriley M, Belden B, Helerstein S, Alan U. Nutritional and behavioural aspects of nasogastric tube feedings in infants receiving chronic peritoneal dialysis. Adv Perit Dial 1990; 6: 265–8.
135. Wood EG, Bunchman TE, Khurana R, Fleming SS, Lynch RE. Complications of nasogastric and gastrostomy tube feeding in infants receiving chronic peritoneal dialysis. Adv Perit Dial 1990; 6: 262–4.
136. Cunningham C. Tube feeding in the real world: formulas, equipment, finances, and feeding problems. Adv Perit Dial 1990; 6: 255–6.
137. Geary DF, Haka Ikse K, Coulter P, Secker D. The role of nutrition in neurologic health and development of infants with chronic renal failure. Adv Perit Dial 1990; 6: 252–4.
138. Brewer ED. Growth of small children managed with chronic peritoneal dialysis and nasogastric tube feedings: 203-months experience in 14 patients. Adv Perit Dial 1990; 6: 269–72.
139. Watson AR, Coleman JE, Taylor EA. Gastrostomy buttons for feeding children on continuous cycling peritoneal dialysis. Adv Perit Dial 1992; 8: 391–5.
140. Mobarhan S, Trumbore LS. Enteral tube feeding: a clinical perspective on recent advances. Nutrition Rev 1991; 49: 129–40.
141. Murugasu B, Conley SB, Lemire JM, Portman RJ. Fungal peritonitis in children treated with peritoneal dialysis and gastrostomy feeding. Pediatr Nephrol 1991; 5: 620–1.
142. Kamen RS. Impaired development of oral-motor functions required for normal oral feeding as a consequence of tube feeding during infancy Adv Perit Dial 1990; 6: 276–8.
143. Dombros N, Oren A, Marliss E et al. Plasma amino acid profiles and amino acid losses in patients undergoing CAPD. Perit Dial Bull 1982; 2: 27–32.
144. Oreopoulos DG, Marliss E, Anderson GH et al. Nutritional aspects of CAPD and the potential use of amino acid containing dialysis solutions. Perit Dial Bull 1983; (Suppl 3): S10–2.
145. Oren A, Wu G, Anderson GH et al. Effective use of amino acid dialysate over four weeks in CAPD patients. Perit Dial Bull 1983; 3: 66–73.
146. Pederson FB, Dragsholt C, Laier E et al. Alternate use of amino acid and glucose solutions in CAPD. Perit Dial Bull 1985; 5: 215–8.
147. Canepa A, Perfumo F, Carrea A et al. Continuous ambulatory peritoneal dialysis (CAPD) of children with amino acid solutions: technical and metabolic aspects. Perit Dial Int 1990; 10: 215–20.
148. Qamar IU, Levin L, Balfe JW, Balfe JA, Secker D, Zlotkin S. Effects of three month amino acid dialysis compared to dextrose dialysis in children on CAPD. Perit Dial Int 1994; 14: 34–41.
149. Young GA, Dibble JB, Hobson SM et al. The use of an amino-acid-based CAPD fluid over 12 weeks. Nephrol Dial Transplant 1989; 4: 285–92.
150. Dombros N, Prutis K, Tong N et al. Six-month overnight intraperitoneal amino-acid infusion in continuous ambulatory peritoneal dialysis (CAPD) patients – no effect on nutritional status. Perit Dial Int 1990; 10: 79–84.
151. Bruno M, Bagnis C, Marangella M, Rovera L, Cantaluppi A, Linari F. CAPD with an amino acid dialysis solution: a long-term, cross-over study. Kidney Int 1989; 35: 1189–94.
152. Dibble JB, Young GA, Hobson SM, Brownjohn AM. Amino-acid-based continuous ambulatory peritoneal dialysis (CAPD) fluid over twelve weeks: effects on carbohydrate and lipid metabolism. Perit Dial Int 1990; 10: 71–7.
153. Musk M, Anderson H, Oreopoulos D et al. Effects of amino acid dialysate on appetite in CAPD patients. Adv Perit Dial 1988; 4: 153–6.
154. Arfeen S, Kirkwood A, Goodship THJ, Ward MK. Hypophosphatemic effect of 1% amino acid dialysis solution. Adv Perit Dial 1989; 5: 167–70.
155. Teehan BP, Brown JM, Schleifer CR. Kinetic modeling in peritoneal dialysis. In: Nissensen AR, Fine RN, Gentile DE (eds), Clinical Dialysis, 2nd Edition. Appleton & Lange, Norwalk 1990; pp 319–29.

156. Friis-Hansen B. Body water compartments in children: changes during growth and related changes in body composition. Pediatrics 1961; 28: 169–82.
157. Harmon WE, Grupe WE. Urea kinetics in the clinical management of children on chronic hemodialysis. In: Nissenson AR, Fine RN, Gentile DE (eds), Clinical Dialysis 2nd Edition. Appleton & Lange, Norwalk 1990; pp 54–66.
158. DeSanto NG, Capodicasa G, Pluvio M, Gilli G, Girodano C. Nitrogen balance and growth in children on CAPD. In: Gahl GM, Kessel M, Nolph KD (eds), Advances in Peritoneal Dialysis: Proceedings of the Second International Symposium on Peritoneal Dialysis, Berlin June 1981. Excerpta Medica, Amsterdam 1981; pp 397–404.
159. Blumendrantz MJ, Kopple JD, Moran JK et al. Metabolic balances studies and dietary protein requirements in patients undergoing continuous ambulatory peritoneal dialysis. Kidney Int 1982; 21: 849–96.
160. Kopple JD, Blumenkrantz MJ. Nutritional requirements for patients undergoing continuous ambulatory peritoneal dialysis. Kidney Int 1983; 24: S295–302.
161. Maroni BJ, Steinman TI, Walser M et al. Effects of varying protein intake on nitrogen metabolism in chronic renal failure. (Abstract) Am Soc Nephrol 1984; 112A.
162. Walzer M. Determinants of ureagenesis, with particular reference to renal failure. Kidney Int 1980; 17: 709–21.
163. Kohaut EC, Alexander SR, Mehls O. The management of the infant on CAPD. In: Fine RN, Scharer K, Mehls O (eds), CAPD in Children. Springer-Verlag, New York 1985; pp 97–105.
164. Kohaut EC, Welchel J, Waldo FB, Diethelm AG. Aggressive therapy of infants with renal failure. Pediatr Nephrol 1987; 1: 150–3.
165. Tapper D, Watkins S, Burns M, Hickman RO, Avner E. Comprehensive management of renal failure in infants. Arch Surg 1990; 125: 1276–81.
166. Paulson WD, Bock GH, Nelson AP, Moxey-Mims MM, Crim LM. Hyponatremia in the very young chronic peritoneal dialysis patient. Am J Kidney Dis 1989; 14: 196–9.
167. Qamar IU, Balfe JW. Experience with chronic peritoneal dialysis in infants. Child Nephrol Urol 1991; 11: 159–64.
168. Ruley EJ, Bock GH, Kerzner B, Abbott AW, Majad M, Chatoor I. Feeding disorders and gastroesophageal reflux in infants with chronic renal failure. Pediatr Nephrol 1989; 3: 424–9.
169. Alexander SR. CAPD in infants less than one year of age. In: Fine RN, Gruskin AB (ed), End Stage Renal Disease in Children. W B Saunders Company, Philadelphia 1984; pp 149–71.
170. Kohaut EC. Growth in children with end-stage renal disease treated with continuous ambulatory peritoneal dialysis for at least one year. Perit Dial Bull 1982; 2: 159–61.
171. Watson AR, Taylor J, Balfe JW. Growth in children on CAPD; a reappraisal. Adv Perit Dial 1985; 1: 171–7.
172. Warady BA, Kriley M, Lovell H, Farrell SE, Hellerstein S. Growth and development of infants with end-stage renal disease receiving long-term peritoneal dialysis. J Pediatr 1988; 112: 714–9.
173. Fine RN. Renal transplantation of the infant and young child and the use of pediatric cadaver kidneys for transplantation in pediatric and adult populations. Am J Kidney Dis 1988; 12: 1–10.
174. Polinsky MS, Kaiser BA, Stover JB, Frankenfield M, Baluarte HJ. Neurologic development of children with severe chronic renal failure from infancy. Pediatr Nephrol 1987; 1: 157–65.
175. Tagge EP, Campbell DAJ, Dafoe DC et al. Pediatric renal transplantation with an emphasis on the prognosis of patients with chronic renal insufficiency since infancy. Surgery 1987; 102: 692–8.
176. Katz A, Kashtan CE, Greenberg IJ, Shapiro RS, Nevins TE, Kim Y. Hypogammaglobulinemia in uremic infants receiving peritoneal dialysis. J Pediatr 1990; 117: 258–61.
177. Warady BA, Koch M, O'Neal DW, Higginbotham M, Harris DJ, Hellerstein S. Plasma fluoride concentration in infants receiving long-term peritoneal dialysis. J Pediatr 1989; 115: 436–9.
178. Brodehl J, Offner G, Pichlmayr R, Ringe B. Kidney transplantation in infants and young children. Transpl Proc 1986; 18 (4 Suppl 3): 8–11.
179. Koffman CG, Rigden SPA, Bewick M, Chantler C, Haycock GB. Renal transplantation in children less than five years of age. Transpl Proc 1989; 21: 2001–2.
180. Nevins TE. Transplantation in infants less than 1 year of age. Pediatr Nephrol 1987; 1: 154–6.
181. Kalia A, Brouhard BH, Travis LB, Gifford RRM, Winsett OE. Renal transplantation in the infant and young child. Am J Dis Child 1988; 142: 47–50.
182. McMahon Y, MacDonell RCJ, Richie RE et al. Is kidney transplantation in the very small child (<10 kg) worth it? Transpl Proc 1989; 21: 2003–5.
183. Nevins T. Treatment of very young infants with ESRD-renal transplantation as soon as possible (<1 year of age): controversy. Adv Perit Dial 1990; 6: 283–5.
184. Najarian JS, Frey DJ, Matas AJ et al. Successful kidney transplantation in infants. Transpl Proc 1991; 23: 1382–3.
185. Cohen C. Ethical and legal considerations in the care of the infant with end-stage renal disease whose parents elect conservative therapy. An American perspective. Pediatr Nephrol 1987; 1: 166–71.
186. Winearls CG, Oliver DO, Pippard MJ et al. Effect of human erythropoietin derived from recombination DNA on the anemia of patients maintained by chronic haemodialysis. Lancet 1986; 2: 1175–8.
187. Eshbach JW, Egrie JC, Downing MR et al. Correction of the anemia of end-stage renal disease with recombinant human erythorpoietin: results of

a combined phase I and II clinical trial NEJM 1987; 316: 73–8.
188. Eschbach JW, Abdulhadi MH, Brown JK et al. Recombinant human erythropoietin in anemic patients with end-stage renal disease: results of a phase III multicenter clinical trail. Ann Intern Med 1989; 111: 992–1000.
189. Bennett W. A multicenter clinical trial of Epoetin beta for anemia of end-stage renal disease. J Am Soc Nephrol 1991; 1: 990–8.
190. Evans RW, Rader B, Manninen DL. The quality of life of hemodialysis recipients treated with recombinant human erythropoietin. JAMA 1990; 263: 825–30.
191. Canadian Erythropoietin Study Group. Association between recombinant human erythropoietin and quality of life and exercise capacity of patients receiving hemodialysis. Br Med J 1990; 300: 573–8.
192. Eschbach JW. The anemia of chronic renal failure: pathophysiology and the effects of recombinant erythropoietin. Kidney Int 1989; 35: 134–48.
193. Rizzoni G, Broyer M, Guest G et al. Growth retardation in children with chronic renal disease: scope of the problem. Am J Kidney Dis 1986; 7: 256–61.
194. French CB, Genei M. Pathophysiology of growth failure in chronic renal insufficiency. Kidney Int 1984; 30: S59–64.
195. Fennel RS, Rasbury WC, Fennell EB et al. Effects of kidney transplantation on cognitive performance in a pediatric population. Pediatrics 1984; 74: 273–8.
196. Ulmer HE, Greiner H, Schüller HW et al. Cardiovascular impairment and physical working capacity in children with chronic renal failure. Acta Pediatr Scand 1987; 67: 43–9.
197. Sinai-Trieman L, Salusky IB, Fine RN. Use of subcutaneous recombinant human erythropoietin in children undergoing continuous cycling peritoneal dialysis. J Pediatr 1989; 114: 550–4.
198. Scigalla P, Bonzel KE, Bulla M et al. Therapy of renal anemia with recombinant human erythropoietin in children with end-stage renal disease. Contrib Nephrol 1989; 6: 227–40.
199. Offner G, Hoyer PF, Latta K et al. One year's experience with recombinant erythropoietin in children undergoing continuous ambulatory or cycling peritoneal dialysis. Pediatr Nephrol 1990; 4: 498–500.
200. Montini G, Zacchello G, Baraldi E et al. Benefits and risks of anemia correction with recombinant human erythropoietin in children maintained by hemodialysis. J Pediatr 1990; 117: 556–60.
201. Fabris F, Cordinao I, Randi ML et al. Effect of human recombinant erythropoietin on bleeding time, platelet number and function in children with end-stage renal disease maintained by haemodialysis. Pediatr Nephrol 1991; 5: 225–8.
202. Jabs K, Harmon W. Double-blind, placebo-controlled study of the use of epoetin alfa (EPO) in pediatric hemodialysis patients. (Abstract) J Amer Soc Nephr 1990; 1: 400.
203. Rigden SP, Montini G, Morris M et al. Recombinant human erythropoietin therapy in children maintained by haemodialysis. Pediatr Nephrol 1990; 4: 618–22.
204. Campos A, Garin EH. Therapy of renal anemia in children and adolescents with recombinant human erythropoietin (rHuEPO). Clin Pediatr 1992; 31: 94–9.
205. Grimm PC, Sinai-Treiman L, Sekiya NM et al. Effects of recombinant human erythropoietin on HLA sensitization and cell mediated immunity. Kidney Int 1990; 38: 12–8.
206. Alexander SR. Pediatric uses of recombinant human erythropoietin: the outlook in 1991. Am J Kidney Dis 1991; 18(Suppl 1): 42–53.
207. Edmunds ME, Walls J, Tucker B et al. Seizures in haemodialysis patients treated with recombinant human erythropoietin. Nephrol Dial Transplant 1989; 4: 1065–9.
208. Granolleras C, Branger B, Beau MC, Deschodt G, Alsabadani B, Shaldon S. Experience with daily self-administered subcutaneous erythropoietin. Contrib Nephrol 1989; 76: 143–8.
209. Evans JH, Brocklbank JT, Bowmer CJ, Ng PC. Pharmacokinetic of recombinant human erythropoietin in children with renal failure. Nephrol Dial Transplant 1991; 6: 709–14.
210. Reddingius RE, Schroder CH, Monnens LAH. Intraperitoneal administration of recombinant human erythropoietin in children on continuous ambulatory peritoneal dialysis. Eur J Pediatr 1992; 151: 540–2.
211. Van Wyck DB. Iron management during recombinant human erythropoietin therapy. Am J Kidney Dis 1989; 14(2 Suppl 1): 9–13.
212. Crosby WH. The rationale for treating iron deficiency anemia. Arch Intern Med 1984; 144: 471–2.
213. Reed MD, Bertino JS Jr, Halpin TC Jr. Use of intravenous iron dextran injection in children receiving total parenteral nutrition. Am J Dis Child 1981; 135: 829–31.
214. Auerbach M, Witt D, Toler W, Fierstein M, Lerner RG, Ballard H. Clinical use of the total dose intravenous infusion of iron dextran. J Lab Clin Med 1988; 111: 566–70.
215. Hsu AC, Kooh SW, Fraser D et al. Renal osteodystrophy in children with chronic renal failure: an unexpectedly common and incapacitating complication. Pediatrics 1982; 70: 742–50.
216. Hewitt IK, Stefanidis C, Reilly BJ et al. Renal osteodystrophy in children undergoing continuous ambulatory peritoneal dialysis. Pediatrics 1983; 103: 729–34.
217. Gokal R, Ramos J, Ellis HS et al. Histological renal osteodystrophy and 25-hydroxycholecalciferol and aluminum levels in patients on continuous ambulatory peritoneal dialysis. Kidney Int 1983; 23: 15–21.
218. Aloni Y, Shany S, Chaimovitz C. Losses of 25-hydroxyvitamin D in peritoneal fluid: possible mechanism for bone disease in uremic patients treated with chronic ambulatory peritoneal dialysis. Miner Electrolyte Metab 1983; 9: 82–6.

219. Shany S, Rapoport J, Goligorsky M et al. Losses of 1,25- and 24,25-dihydroxycholecalciferol in the peritoneal fluid of patients treated with continuous ambulatory peritoneal dialysis. Nephron 1984; 36: 111–3.

220. Watson AR, Kooh SW, Tam CS, Reilly BJ, Balfe JW, Vieth R. Renal osteodystrophy in children on CAPD: a prospective trail of 1-Alpha-hydroxycholecalciferol therapy. Child Nephrol Urol 1988–89; 9: 220–7.

221. Salusky IB, Fine RN, Kangarloo H et al. "High dose" calcitriol for control of renal osteodystrophy in children undergoing continuous ambulatory peritoneal dialysis. Kidney Int 1987; 32: 89–95.

222. Jones CL, Vieth R, Spino M, Ledermann S, Kooh SW, Balfe JA, Balfe JW. Parenteral 1,25(OH)2D3 therapy in children with chronic renal failure. Clin Nephrol 1994 (in press).

223. Vieth R, Ledermann SE, Kooh SW, Balfe JW. Losses of calcitriol to peritoneal dialysis bags and tubing. Perit Dial Int 1989; 9: 277–80.

224. Vieth R. Presystemic 24-hydoxylation of oral 25-hydroxyvitamin D3 in rats. J Bone Mineral Res 1990; 5: 1177–82.

225. Delmez JA, Dougan CS, Gearing BK, Rothstein M, Windus DW, Rapp N, Slatopolsky E. The effects of intraperitoneal calcitriol on calcium and parathyroid hormone. Kidney Int 1987; 31: 795–9.

226. Slatopolsky E, Weerts C, Thielan J, Horst R, Harter H, Martin KJ. Marked suppression of secondary hyperparathyroidism by intravenous administration of 1,25-dihydroxycholecalciferol in uremic patients. J Clin Invest 1984; 14: 2136–43.

227. Salusky IB, Gooderman WG, Norris KC, Horst R, Fine RN, Coburn JW. Bioavailability of calcitriol after oral intravenous and intraperitoneal doses in dialysis patients. In: Norman AW, Schaefer K, Grigoleit H-G, Herrath D (eds), Vitamin D, Molecular Cellular and Clinical Endocrinology. W de-Gruyter, Berlin 1988; pp 783–4.

228. Finch JL, Brown AJ, Kobodera N, Nishii Y, Slatopolsky E. Differential effect of 1,25(OH)2D3 and 22-oxacalcitriol on phosphate and calcium metabolism. Kidney Int 1993; 43: 561–6.

229. Hutchison AJ, Freemont AJ, Lumb GA, Gokal R. Renal osteodystrophy in CAPD. Adv Perit Dial 1991; 7: 237–9.

230. Salusky IB, Goodman WG. Renal osteodystrophy in dialyzed children. Miner Electrolyte Metab 1991; 17: 273–80.

231. Salusky IB, Coburn JW, Foley J et al. Effects of oral calcium carbonate on control of serum phosphorous and changes in plasma aluminum levels after discontinuation of aluminum-containing gels in children receiving dialysis. J Pediatr 1986; 108: 767–70.

232. Alexander SR, Linblad AS, Nolph KD, Novak JS. Pediatric CAPD/CCPD in the United States: a review of the National CAPD Registry's pediatric population for period January 1, 1981 through August 31, 1986. In: Twardowski ZJ, Nolph KD, Khanna R (eds), Peritoneal Dialysis, New Concepts and Applications. Volume 22 in the series: Contemporary Issues in Nephrology (JH Stein series ed). Churchill-Livingstone, New York 1990; pp 231–55.

233. Port FK, Held PJ, Nolph KD et al. Risk of peritonitis and technique failure by CAPD connection technique: a national study. Kidney Int 1992; 42: 967–74.

234. Fine RN, Salusky IB, Hall T et al. Peritonitis in children undergoing continuous ambulatory peritoneal dialysis. Pediatrics 1983; 71: 806–9.

235. Powell D, San Luis E, Calvin S et al. Peritonitis in children undergoing continuous ambulatory peritoneal dialysis. Am J Dis Child 1985; 139: 29–32.

236. Warady BA, Campoy SF, Gross SP et al. Peritonitis with CAPD and CCPD. J Pediatr 1984; 105: 726–30.

237. Watson AR, Vigneaux A, Bannatyne RM, Balfe JW. Peritonitis during continuous ambulatory peritoneal dialysis in children. Can Med Assoc J 1986; 134: 1019–22.

238. Chesney RW, Zelikovic, I. Peritonitis in childhood renal disease. Am J Nephrol 1988; 8: 147–60.

239. Keane WF, Everett ED, Fine RN et al. Continuous ambulatory peritoneal dialysis (CAPD) peritonitis treatment recommendations: 1989 update. Perit Dial Int 1989; 9: 247–56.

240. Keane WF, Everett ED, Golper TA, Gokal R, Halstenson CH, Kawaguchi Y, Riella M, Vas S, Verbrugh HA. Peritoneal dialysis-related peritonitis treatment recommendations: 1993 update. Perit Dial Int 1993; 13: 14–28.

241. Vas SI. Questions, answers. Perit Dial Bull 1981; 1: 145–6.

242. Levy M, Balfe JW, Geary D, Fryer-Keene S, Bannantye R. Exit-site infection during continuous and cycling peritoneal dialysis in children. Perit Dial Int 1990; 10: 31–5.

243. Schmidt L, Prowant B. The role of the CAPD nurse in decreasing exit site infection. (Abstract) Perit Dial Bull 1984; 4: S57.

244. Warady BA, Jackson MA, Millspaugh J et al. Prevention and treatment of catheter-related infections in children. Perit Dial Bull 1987; 7: 34–40.

245. Khoury AE, Charendoff J, Balfe JW, McLorie GA, Churchill BM. Hernias associated with CAPD in children. Adv Perit Dial 1991; 7: 279–82.

246. Von-Lilien T, Salusky IB, Yab HK et al. Hernias: a frequent complication in children treated with continuous peritoneal dialysis. Am J Kidney Dis 1987; 10: 356–60.

247. White JJ, Haller JA. Groin hernia in infants and children. In: Nyphus LM, Condon RD (eds), Hernia. B Lippincott, Philadelphia 1978; p. 106.

248. Robson WLM, Leung AKC, Putnins RE, Boag GS. Genital edema in children on continuous ambulatory peritoneal dialysis. Child Nephrol Urol 1990; 10: 205–10.

249. Ducassou D, Vuillemin L, Wone C et al. Intraperitoneal injection of technetium-99m sulfur colloid in visualization of a peritoneo-vaginalis connection. J Nucl Med 1984; 25: 68–9.

250. Bunchman TE, Wood EG, Lynch RE. Hydrothorax

as a complication of pediatric peritoneal dialysis. Perit Dial Bull 1987; 7: 237–9.
251. Kuehnal E. Massive pleural effusion secondary to CAPD. (Abstract) Kidney Int 1981; 19: 152.
252. Townsend R, Fragula J. Hydrothorax in a patient receiving CAPD. Arch Intern Med 1982; 142: 1571–2.
253. Scheldewaert R, Rogaerts Y, Pauvels R, Strateon M, Ringor S, Lamiere N. Management of massive hydrothorax in a CAPD patient. A case report and review of the literature. Perit Dial Bull 1987; 2: 69–72.
254. LeVeen HH, Piccone VA, Hutto RB. Management of ascites with hydrothorax. Am J Surg 1984; 148: 210–3.
255. Hidai H, Takatsu S, Chiba T. Intrathoracic instillation of autologous blood in treating massive hydrothorax following CAPD. Perit Dial Int 1989; 9: 221–2.
256 Mestas D, Wanquier JP, Escande G, Baquet JC, Veyr A. Diagnosis of hydrothorax-complicated CAPD and demonstration of successful therapy by scintography. (Letter) Perit Dial Int 1991; 11: 283–4.
257. Benz RL, Schleifer CR. Hydrothorax in continuous ambulatory peritoneal dialysis: successful treatment with intrapleural tetracycline and a review of the literature. Am J Kidney Dis 1985; 5: 136–40.
258. Simmons LE, Rauf Mir A. A review of management of pleuroperitoneal communication in five CAPD patients. Adv Perit Dial 1989; 5: 81–3.
259. Querfeld UWE, LeBouef RC, Isidro B et al. Lipoproteins in children treated with continuous peritoneal dialysis. Pediatr Res 1991; 29; 155–9.
260. Scolnik D, Balfe JW. Initial hypoalbuminemia and hyperlipidemia persist during chronic peritoneal dialysis in children. Perit Dial Int 1993; 13: 136–9.
261. Korbet S, Matika Z, Firanek C, Vlassara H. Advanced glycosylation endproducts (AGE) in CAPD patients. Perit Dial Int 1993; 13: S80.
262. Hanning RH, Balfe JW, Zlotkin S. Dialysate protein and amino acid losses in children receiving continuous ambulatory peritoneal dialysis (CAPD): benefit of a single daily cycle with amino acid dialysis solution. Nutrition Res 1986; 6: 1264–74.
263. Lowrie EG, Lew NL. Death risk in hemodialysis patients. The predictive value of commonly measured variables and an evaluation of death rate differences between facilities. Am J Kidney Dis 1990; 15: 458–82.
264. Jones CL, Andrew M, Eddy A, O'Neil M, Ish Shalom N, Balfe JW. Coagulation abnormalities in chronic peritoneal dialysis. Pediatr Nephrol 1990; 4: 152–5.
265. Fivush BA, Case B, May MW, Lederman HM. Hypogammaglobulinemia in children undergoing continuous ambulatory peritoneal dialysis. Pediatr Nephrol 1989; 3: 186–8.
266. Niaudet P. Loss of ultrafiltration and sclerosing encapsulating peritonitis in children undergoing CAPD/CCPD. In: Fine RN (ed), Chronic Ambulatory Peritoneal Dialysis (CAPD) and Chronic Cycling Peritoneal Dialysis (CCPD) in Children. Martinus Nijhoff, Boston 1987; pp 201–19.
267. Slingeneyer A. Preliminary report on cooperative international study in sclerosing peritonitis. Contrib Nephrol 1987; 57; 239–47.
268. Pitrone F, Pellegrino E, Mileto G, Consolo F. May pancreatitis represent a CAPD complication? Report of two cases with a rapid evolution to death. Int J Artif Organs 1985; 8: 235.
269. Gupta A, Yuan ZY, Balaskas EV, Khanna R, Oreopoulos DG. CAPD and pancreatitis: no connection. Perit Dial Int 1992; 12: 309–16.
270. Drash A, Sherman F, Hartmann W, Blizzard RM. A syndrome of pseudohermaphroditism, Wilm's tumor, hypertension, and degenerative renal disease. J Pediatr 1970; 76: 585–93.
271. Hendren WH, Hendren RB. Bladder agumentation: experience with 129 children and young adults. J Urol 1990; 144: 445.
272. Boquist L, Lindquist B, Ostberg Y et al. Primary oxalosis. Am J Med 1973; 54: 173.
273. Gilboa N, Largent JA, Urizar RE. Primary oxalosis presenting as anuric renal failure in infancy: diagnosis by x-ray diffraction of kidney tissue. J Pediatr 1983; 103: 88–90.
274. Churchill DN, Morgan J, Torrance G. Quality of life in end-stage renal disease. Perit Dial Bull 1984; 4: 20–3.
275. Churchill DN. The effect of treatment modality on the quality of life for patients with end-stage renal disease (ESRD). Adv Perit Dial 1988; 4: 63–5.
276. Tucker CM, Ziller RC, Smith WR, Mars DR, Coons MP. Quality of life of patients on in-center hemodialysis versus continuous ambulatory peritoneal dialysis and transplantation. Perit Dial Int 1991; 11: 341–6.
277. Brownbridge G, Fielding DM. Psychosocial adjustment to end-stage renal failure: comparing haemodialysis, continuous ambulatory peritoneal dialysis and transplantation. Pediatr Nephrol 1991; 5: 612–62.
278. LePontois J, Moel DI, Cohn RA. Family adjustment to pediatric ambulatory dialysis. Amer J Orthopsychiat 1987; 57: 78–83.
279. Rosenkranz J, Bonzel K-E, Bulla M et al. Psychosocial adaptation of children and adolescents with chronic renal failure. Pediatr. Nephrol 1992; 6: 459–63.
280. Roscoe JM, Smith LF, Williams EA et al. Medical and social outcome in adolescents with end-stage renal failure. Kidney Int 1991; 40: 948–53.
281. Fine RN, Salusky IB, Ettenger RB. The therapeutic approach to the infant, child, and adolescent with end-stage renal disease. Pediatr Clin North Am 1987; 34: 789–801.
282. Cardella CJ. Renal transplantation in patients on peritoneal dialysis. Perit Dial Bull 1980; 1: 12–4.
283. Gokal R, Ramos JM, Veitch P et al. Renal transplantation in patients on continuous ambulatory peritoneal dialysis. Proc EDTA 1981; 18: 222–7.
284. Glass NR, Miller DT, Sollinger HW, Zimmerman

SW, Simpson D, Belzer FO. Renal transplantation in patients on peritoneal dialysis. Perit Dial Bull 1985; 5: 157–60.
285. Tsakiris D, Bramwell SP, Briggs JD, Junor BJR. Transplantation in patients undergoing CAPD. Perit Dial Bull 1985; 5: 161–4.
286. Cardella C. Peritoneal dialysis and renal transplantation. Perit Dial Bull 1985; 5: 149–51.
287. Heyka R, Schreiber MJ, Steinmuller DR et al. Renal transplantation in patients on CAPD. Adv Perit Dial 1987; 3: 49–55.
288. Gelfand M, Kois J, Quillin B et al. CAPD yields inferior transplant results compared to hemodialysis. (Abstract) Perit Dial Bull 1984; 4: S26.
289. Cramer SO, Adams MB, Kauffman HMJ. Posttransplant peritonitis in a CAPD patient. Transplantation 1983; 36: 340–1.
290. Guillou PJ, Will EJ, Davison AM, Giles GR. CAPD – a risk factor in renal transplantation? Br J Surg 1984; 71: 878–80.
291. Patel S, Rosenthal JT, Hakala TR. Management of the peritoneal dialysis catheter after transplantation. Transplantation 1983; 36: 589–90.
292. Stefanidis CJ, Balfe JW, Arbus GS, Hardy BE, Churchill BM, Rance CP. Renal transplantation in children treated with continuous ambulatory peritoneal dialysis. Perit Dial Bull 1883; 3: 5–8.
293. Nevins TE, Danielson G. Prior dialysis does not affect the outcome of pediatric renal transplantation. Pediatr Nephrol 1991; 5: 211–4.
294. Leichter HE, Salusky IB, Ettenger RB et al. Experience with renal transplantation in children undergoing peritoneal dialysis (CAPD/CCPD). Am J Kid Dis 1986; 8: 181–5.
295. Malagon M, Hogg RJ. Renal transplantation after prolonged dwell peritoneal dialysis in children. Kidney Int 1987; 31: 981–5.
296. Watson A, Vigneux A, Balfe J. Renal transplantation in children on CAPD and post-transplant ascites. (Letter) Perit Dial Bull 1984; 4: 189.
297. Ogawa O, Hosinaga K, Hasegawa A et al. Successful renal transplantation in children treated with CAPD. Transplant Proc 1989; 21: 1997–2000.
298. Leichter HE, Salusky IB, Ettenger RB et al. Complications after renal transplantation in children undergoing CAPD and CCPD. Adv Perit Dial 1985; 1: 145–8.
299. Hymes LC, Warshaw BL. Renal transplantation in children undergoing peritoneal dialysis. Perit Dial Bull 1986; 6: 74–6.
300. Campbell A. Strategies for improving dialysis decision making. Perit Dial Int 1991; 11: 173–8.
301. Barré PE. Selecting dialysis for chronic renal failure. Diagnosis 1987; 7: 49–55.
302. Holley JL, Barrington K, Kohn J, Hayes I. Patient factors and the influence of nephrologists, social workers, and nurses on patient decision to choose continuous peritoneal dialysis. Adv Perit Dial 1991; 7: 108–10.
303. Prichard SS. The cost of dialysis. Adv Perit Dial 1988; 4: 66–9.
304. Groome PA, Hutchison TA, Prichard SS, ESRD treatment modality selection: which factors are important in the decision? Adv Perit Dial 1991; 7: 54–6.
305. Hall TL, Ann MJ. Nursing management of the child undergoing CAPD. In: Fin RN, Gruskin AB (eds), End Stage Renal Disease in Children. W B Saunders Company, Philadelphia 1984; pp 172–89.
306. Chan JCM, Campbell RA. Peritoneal dialysis in children: a survey of its indications and applications. Clin Pediatr 1973; 12: 131–9.
307. Peterson RG, Peterson LN. Cleansing the blood: hemodialysis, peritoneal dialysis, exchange transfusion, charcoal hemoperfusion, forced diuresis. Pediatr Clin N Am 1986; 33: 675–89.
308. Rothamn A, Normann SA, Manoguerra AS et al. Short-term hemodialysis in childhood ethylene glycol poisoning. J Pediatr 1986; 108: 153–5.
309. Jacobson D, Wirk-Larsen EE, Bredesen JE. Hemodialysis or hemoperfusion in severe salicylate poisoning? Human Toxicol 1988; 7: 161–3.
310. Papadopoulos ZL, Novello AC. The use of hemoperfusion in children, past, present, and future. Pediatr Clin N Am 1982; 29: 1039–52.
311. Moss AH, McLaughlin MM, Lempert KD et al. Use of a silicone catheter with a dacron cuff for dialysis short-term vascular access. Am J Kidney Dis 1988; 12: 492–8.
312. Mahan JD, Mauer SM, Nevins TE. The Hickman catheter, a new hemodialysis access device for infants and small children. Kidney Int 1983; 24: 694–7.
313. Van Stone JC. Hemodialysis. In: Gonick HC (ed), Current Nephrology, Vol. 7. John Wiley & Sons, New York 1984; pp 87–105.
314. Rubin J. Comments on dialysis solution composition, antibiotic transport, poisoning and novel uses of peritoneal dialysis. In: Nolph KD (ed), Peritoneal Dialysis. Martinus Nijhoff, The Hague 1985: p. 253 (Table).
315. Shih VE. Congenital hyperammonemic syndromes. Clin Perinatol 1976; 3: 3–4.
316. Batshaw ML, Brusilow SW. Treatment of hyperammonemic coma caused by inborn errors of urea synthesis. J Pediatr 1980; 97: 893–900.
317. Donn SM, Swartz RD, Thoene JG. Comparison of exchange transfusion, peritoneal dialysis and hemodialysis for the treatment of hyperammonemia in an anuric newborn infant. J Pediatr 1979; 95: 67–70.
318. Sallan SE, Cottom D. Peritoneal dialysis in maple syrup urine disease. Lancet 1969; 2: 1423.
319. Russill G, Thom H, Tarlow JM et al. Reduction of plasma proprionate by peritoneal dialysis. Pediatrics 1974; 53: 281–3.
320. Mahoney MJ. Organic acidemias. Clin Perinatol 1976; 3: 61–78.
321. Nora JJ, Trygstad CW, Mangos JA. Peritoneal dialysis in the treatment of intractable congestive heart failure of infancy and childhood. J Pediatr 1966; 68: 693.
322. Boda D, Muranyi L, Altorjay I, Veress I. Peritoneal

dialysis in treatment of hyaline membrane disease in newborn premature infants. Acta Paediatr Scand 1971; 69; 90–2.
323. Hobolth N, Devantier M. Removal of indirect reacting bilirubin by albumin binding during intermittent peritoneal dialysis in the newborn. Acta Paediatr Scand 1969; 58: 171.
324. Pross DC, Bradford WD, Krueger RP. Reye's syndrome treated by peritoneal dialysis. Pediatrics 1970; 45: 845.
325. Krebs R, Flynn M. Treatment of hepatic coma with exchange transfusion and peritoneal dialysis. JAMA 1967; 199: 430.

21 Peritoneal dialysis in diabetic end-stage renal disease

RAMESH KHANNA

1. Introduction 639
2. The proposed benefits of CAPD/CCPD 640
3. Drawbacks of CAPD 640
4. When is the ideal time to initiate dialysis in diabetics? 640
5. Peritoneal access 640
6. Dialysis schedules 641
   6.1. Intermittent peritoneal dialysis (IPD) 641
   6.2. Automated peritoneal dialysis (APD) 641
   6.3. Tidal peritoneal dialysis 642
   6.4. Continuous cyclic peritoneal dialysis (CCPD) 642
   6.5 Continuous ambulatory peritoneal dialysis (CAPD) 643
7. Glucose as an osmotic agent 643
8. Blood sugar control during peritoneal dialysis 644
   8.1 Kinetics of intraperitoneal insulin 644
   8.2. Benefits of intraperitoneal insulin 644
   8.3. Problems of intraperitoneal insulin therapy 645
   8.4. The steps of blood sugar control in a new CAPD patient using IP route 646
   8.5. Site of intraperitoneal delivery 647
8.6. Blood sugar control during NIPD 647
9. Clinical results 647
   9.1. Blood-pressure control 647
   9.2. Benefits of slow and continuous ultrafiltration during CAPD 648
   9.3. Residual-renal function 648
   9.4. Visual problems 649
   9.5. Cardiac and vascular diseases 649
   9.6 Foot ulceration and care in diabetic patients 649
   9.7. Metabolic and nutritional problems 650
   9.8. Peritonitis 651
   9.9. Patient and technique survival on CAPD 651
   9.10. Technique-related complications 652
   9.11. Hospitalization rates 652
10. Can peritoneal dialysis be a long-term therapy for ESRD patients? 652
11. Can CAPD/CCPD be recommended over hemodialysis for diabetic patients? 653
12. Summary 653
References 653

Introduction

The management of the diabetic patients with end-stage renal disease (ESRD) has undergone significant change over the past 20 years. In countries with adequate socioeconomic conditions, even diabetics with extensive co-morbid diseases denied renal transplantation easily get accepted for chronic dialysis despite the inevitable poor long-term prognosis [1–4]. As a result, diabetes has become the most prevalent cause of ESRD in the USA; on average, about one-third of the new dialysis patients have diabetes as the cause of renal disease [5]. Renal transplantation is the generally preferred treatment for diabetic patients with end-stage renal failure because it leads to better quality of life than any form of dialysis [6]. Although improved compared to a decade ago, the outcome of dialysis therapies (hemodialysis or peritoneal dialysis) for diabetics is still disappointing compared to renal transplantation and dialysis for non-diabetics; nearly half the diabetic patients, who begin dialysis do not survive beyond two years [7] and less than one in five diabetic patients undergoing maintenance dialysis is capable of any activity beyond personal care. In such a setting, choosing a dialytic mode which has a better potential for survival and which promotes better quality of life is extremely important. However, choosing a dialysis therapy at present is subject to strong personal biases of both physician and patient. This is because there is no clear difference between the outcomes of diabetic patients on hemodialysis and peritoneal dialysis. In the 1960's and early 1970's, intermittent peritoneal dialysis (IPD) performed on diabetic ESRD patients either in hospital or at home with a cycler over 30–40 hours/week, showed a promising decline or even arrest of uremic neuropathy and retinopathy. However, the possibilities for patient survival beyond two to three years were dismal [8–12]. On hindsight, it appears that with the loss of residual-renal function, which takes about two-to-three years in PD patients, the amount of dialysis provided with IPD was not adequate, and the majority of patients were dying from either electrolytic abnormalities or progressive uremia. The introduction of continuous ambulatory and continuous cyclic peritoneal dialysis (CAPD/CCPD) during the late 1970's allowed both diabetic and non-diabetic patients to be treated adequately, and was quickly established as a viable alternate renal replacement therapy to hemodialysis [13–21].

2. The proposed benefits of CAPD/CCPD

There are both medical and social benefits of CAPD/CCPD [22]. Since it is essentially a home therapy and allows flexibility in treatment, CAPD/CCPD has several social benefits: it allows home dialysis, permits long distance travel, permits uninterrupted job-related activity, etc. However, in choosing a dialysis therapy both medical and social benefits need to be taken into consideration. The proposed medical benefits of CAPD/CCPD that make it a preferred therapy over hemodialysis are listed in Table 1. During the course of this chapter, I will attempt to examine these issues in more detail to see if there is sufficient evidence to make such claims.

3. Drawbacks of CAPD

Despite the many attractive advantages of CAPD, some of its drawbacks may limit its widespread application. CAPD peritonitis, although less frequent with the use of assist devices remains a major cause of morbidity and therapy failures, its incidence equals that in non-diabetics. Continuous loss of protein through the dialysate may aggravate nutritional problems of some of the chronically ill patients. Long term integrity of the peritoneum, a biological membrane, has not been unequivocally established. Some of the social problems related to CAPD such as distorted body image and burnout due to continuous therapy may also limit its long-term use. Normalization of blood pressure in some

Table 1. Proposed benefits of CAPD.

1. Slow and sustained ultrafiltration and a relative lack of rapid fluid and electrolyte changes compared to hemodialysis
2. Ease of blood pressure control
3. Preservation of residual renal function for a period longer than hemodialysis
4. Access for dialysis is easier
5. Blood sugar control is possible through intraperitoneal route
6. Steady state biochemical parameters.

diabetic patients with autonomic dysfunction and orthostatic hypotension may pose problems with maintaining fluid balance and aggravate ischemic complications. Excessive weight gain and hyperlipidemia as a consequence of continuous glucose absorption in some patients can be causes for concern. During the past few years, advances in the field have enabled us to address some of these concerns and propose remedial measures to improve the risk-benefit ratio of this therapy. These aspects will be discussed more in detail later in this chapter.

4. When is the ideal time to initiate dialysis in diabetics?

Nearly every diabetic patient approaching end-stage renal failure has hypertension [23]. Additionally, the relative or absolute lack of insulin causes hyperglycemia, ketosis and changes in transmembrane electrical potential in diabetics [24]. These problems lead to fluid retention, electrolyte and acid-base disturbances in diabetics at a GFR higher than non-diabetics. Therefore, it has been a practice to initiate dialysis in diabetics when the creatinine clearance is about 8 to 10 ml/min, levels slightly higher than the recommended 5 ml/min for non-diabetics. Although there is no strong opposition to such an approach, the real benefit of early dialysis to the patient remains unsubstantiated. The cost of such an approach is substantial and needs to be taken into account when balancing the benefit-risk ratio.

5. Peritoneal access

One of the advantages of peritoneal dialysis is the ease with which the peritoneum can be accessed. It is possible to use the catheter for supine peritoneal dialysis immediately after its insertion. This avoids the need for temporary access or preplanned-access surgery that is so often necessary in hemodialysis. Access to the peritoneal cavity is obtained through the use of either a Tenckhoff catheter or one of its newer modifications [25, 26]. The technique of catheter insertion, break-in procedure, and post-operative catheter care in diabetics is similar to that used in nondiabetic patients and described in detail in Chapter 10.

The common catheter complications are exit/tunnel infection, catheter-cuff extrusion, poor dialysate flow, dialysate solution leak, pain in association with fluid flow, and peritonitis.

Experience with CAPD over the last 10 years has

confirmed the earlier observations that catheter survival rates, infectious and non-infectious complications of peritoneal access are no different for diabetic patients than non-diabetic patients on peritoneal dialysis [27]. The spectrum of microorganisms causing peritonitis in diabetics is no different; the earlier feared predilection for fungal infection in diabetics has turned out to be ill founded. Although a cause-and-effect relationship is not established, the route of insulin delivery seems to influence the incidence of exit-site and/or tunnel infection; in an exhaustive survey of CAPD/CCPD patients with ESRD attributed to diabetes mellitus done by the USA NIH CAPD Registry [27], exit-site and/or tunnel infection rates per patient year by route of insulin administration were calculated. Although differences in rates were small, diabetics never using insulin had the lowest rate of exit-site/tunnel infection per patient year (0.47), while patients using subcutaneous insulin reported the highest rate (0.65). The exit-site/tunnel infection rate per patient year for patients using intraperitoneally administered insulin (0.60) was similar to the rate reported for patients using a combination of subcutaneous and intraperitoneal insulin (0.54). Blind patients using subcutaneously administered versus blind patients using intraperitoneal insulin reported similar rates per patient year of exit site/tunnel infection. Catheter replacement rates per patient year were similar for all patient groups (0.16 to 0.20).

6. Dialysis schedules

6.1. Intermittent peritoneal dialysis (IPD)

During the 1970's, the recommended scheme of peritoneal dialysis was intermittent peritoneal dialysis with an automated peritoneal dialysis cycler providing 40 hours of dialysis a week, divided into one-to-four sessions [8]. Blood sugar control while on IPD was achieved with insulin administered both subcutaneously and intraperitoneally. The amount of insulin administered was adjusted to individual requirements. On dialysis days, the patients were given the usual daily dose of insulin by subcutaneous injection; an additional amount of regular insulin was added to the dialysis solution until the last five exchanges of dialysis to compensate for the glucose absorbed from the peritoneal cavity during the dialysis solution exchanges. Insulin was omitted from the last few exchanges to prevent post-dialysis hypoglycemia. Insulin requirements were determined at the initiation of each patient's first few treatments. The amount of insulin required was directly proportional to the amount of glucose load instilled during dialysis to achieve ultrafiltration. It took up to two weeks after initiation of dialysis to determine the exact amount of insulin required by an individual patient. Once established, the insulin requirements did not generally change unless new complications were encountered. In these patients, retinopathy and neuropathy seemed to stabilize during the course of IPD treatment. Hemoglobin and hematocrit were maintained at satisfactory levels without blood transfusions. Compared to non-diabetics on IPD, these patients experienced a higher incidence of fibrin-clot formation in dialysis effluent and a higher incidence of peritonitis. The patients also experienced higher rates of arterial calcification and hypertension. The majority of the patients died from cardiac and cerebrovascular complications. Significant percentages of patients died suddenly at home presumably due to a coronary event or from an electrolyte abnormality. The probability of patient survival at one and two years was 44 and 20 percent respectively [8]. Outcome of IPD in other centers with smaller numbers of patients were similar [9–12]. The main reason for the low survival rate may have related to inadequate dialysis since this IPD scheme as advocated in the past provided under the best circumstances a dialysis creatinine clearance of 20 liters/week or less. Presumably, most patients were under dialyzed and became more uremic with the gradual loss of renal function. Since the advent of CAPD, the use of such a scheme of IPD has declined. In any case, due to its inadequacies, such a low prescription is neither recommended nor acceptable as an effective renal replacement therapy.

6.2. Automated peritoneal dialysis (APD)

A variant of IPD, which incorporates longer dialysis times and larger total dialysate volume, daily night time IPD (NIPD), is now used for home treatment in patients who are unsuitable for CAPD [28–31]. The indications for NIPD include those patients having high peritoneal membrane solute transport characteristics and those who develop complications as a result of increased intra-abdominal pressure during CAPD. The rise in intra-abdominal pressure in the supine position is considerably lower than in the upright position [32]. During NIPD treatment at home the patient is bed confined, and sleeps during the most of the therapy time. In order to provide the recommended amount of dialysis of 50 liters/week of creatinine clearance or 2.2 of KT/V urea, NIPD needs to be carried out, depending on the peritoneal solute transport rate, 8 to 12 hours a day using high-dialysis solution volumes ranging from 10–25 liters. A typical NIPD prescription is 1.5 to 2.5 liter fill volume and one hour cycle for an 8 to 10 hour treatment time. In patients with low peritoneal transport characteristics, additional dialysis may be provided by the last bag fill option and leaving the solution dwelling in the peritoneal cavity during the day. Like IPD, the major benefit of NIPD is the lower incidence of complications related to high intra-abdominal pressure compared to CAPD. Importantly, the peritonitis rate is considerably lower probably due to a reduced number of connections and improved host-defence mechanisms [33].

6.3. Tidal peritoneal dialysis

Tidal peritoneal dialysis (TPD) is a modification of the IPD technique whereby after the initial filling of the peritoneal cavity only a portion of dialysate is drained and replaced by fresh solution each cycle, so that there is continuous dialysis solution contact with the peritoneal membrane until the end of the dialysate session when all the fluid is drained out as completely as possible [33, 34]. Preliminary studies indicate that TPD is approximately 20 percent more efficient than NIPD at a dialysis solution flow rate of 3.25–3.5 liter/hour. During an 8 hour session of TPD, ultrafiltration generation is higher, protein losses are similar, and phosphate clearances are lower than 24-hour CAPD for an equivalent glucose load [34]. It has been observed that an eight-to-ten hour daily TPD regimen may provide adequate dialysis (urea clearances and creatinine clearances per day similar to CAPD) to an anuric patient with average to low-average peritoneal membrane transport characteristics. Some of the drawbacks of this technique are the high costs of solution and machine for dialysis. This technique is still in an early stage.

6.4. Continuous cyclic peritoneal dialysis (CCPD)

CCPD is a reversal of the CAPD schedule [35]. It uses multiple short cycles during the night with an automated cycler and a long day time exchange while the patient is ambulatory. With this technique, variable volumes of dialysis solution are delivered for a prescribed dwell time with the aid of an automated cycler during the night (three or four two-liter commercial dialysis solution infusions are generally administered during the night, each dwelling for 2–3 hours) and then are drained by gravity at the end of the dwell. An additional two liters of dialysis solution is infused in the morning and is allowed to dwell intraperitoneally for the next 14 to 15 hours with the catheter capped. Hypertonic dialysis solution containing 2.5 to 4.25 percent dextrose is recommended for the daytime exchange in order to prevent significant absorption of the solution. Diaz-Buxo [35] observed that it is difficult to design a uniform method for intraperitoneal insulin administration for the blood glucose control in CCPD patients due to the fact that during the day, when most of the dietary caloric load is consumed, they carry out only one peritoneal dialysis exchange for 12 to 14 hours and essentially no food is eaten during the night when several dialysis exchanges are carried out.

Diaz-Buxo claims excellent glycemic control can be obtained in the majority of patients if time is spent to calculate the precise dose of insulin required, and if a regular and predictable caloric intake is maintained with little day-to-day variation. He recommends that the insulin dose be appropriately divided among all the dialysis solution bags depending upon the caloric load. Such a distribution avoids sudden and massive infusions of insulin and consequent hypoglycemia or hyperglycemia. The average intraperitoneal insulin dose required for good control of glycemia has been about three times the pre-dialysis total subcutaneous dose. In most cases, 50 percent of the intraperitoneal dose is used for the long-dwell daytime exchange, with the remaining 50 percent equally divided among the nocturnal exchanges. For more detailed instructions, the readers are advised to refer to the protocol recommended by Diaz-Buxo [35].

The one-year patient survival for diabetic patients on CCPD is reported to be 76 percent [35]. The main indications for CCPD in diabetics include: patient preference, young diabetics awaiting cadaver or living-related renal transplantations, and older, blind and dependent diabetics requiring partner support for the dialysis technique. The medical circumstances under which CCPD is recommended over CAPD are when complications occur due to increased intra-abdominal pressure, and chronic low-back pain on CAPD.

6.5. Continuous ambulatory peritoneal dialysis (CAPD)

The standard CAPD technique has been previously reported [13]. In short, the technique consists of exchanging four two-liter dialysis solution bags/day using appropriate glucose concentrations from the range available (0.5, 1.5, 2.5, 42.5 gms percent) to achieve adequate ultrafiltration. The patients are taught to add insulin into the dialysis solution according to the protocol to be discussed later. The technique of CAPD is usually modified to accommodate the handicapped diabetic patient's desire to self-perform dialysis at home. Visual impairment, peripheral vascular disease with amputation of a part or entire limb, and peripheral neuropathy with sensory and/or motor function impairment are some of the physical disabilities observed in these diabetic populations. Devices such as the Ultraviolet box [36], Splicer [37], Oreopoulos-Zellerman connector [38], Y-system [39], and Injecta aid [40] are used with success in many. These devices have enabled a number of blind diabetics to self-perform CAPD. Although the published reports of usage of such devices are scarce, the anecdotal experiences of their usefulness is encouraging. In our center the training period averages five working days while a complex patient may take as much as 20 working days. The recommended dialysis dose (dialysis and residual-renal function) is: a total creatinine clearance by dialysis and GFR of 50 liters per week/$1.73M^2$ BSA or a weekly KT/V urea of 1.7 with a PCR of 0.9 gms/Kg standard body wt [41–43].

7. Glucose as an osmotic agent

Several years of experience with peritoneal dialysis has indicated that glucose has proved to be an effective osmotic agent for inducing ultrafiltration during peritoneal dialysis. However, the use of glucose has been identified with numerous undesirable metabolic effects, which has necessitated a search for alternative osmotic agents. An average CAPD patient typically absorbs 100–150 grams of glucose per day during the course of CAPD therapy. This high carbohydrate absorption leads to unwanted metabolic problems such as obesity, hypertriglyceridemia, and premature atherosclerosis [44]. In addition, higher doses of insulin required to maintain the blood sugar at normal levels may cause hyperinsulinemia which in healthy persons has been shown to be a risk factor for atherosclerotic heart disease [45, 46]. To obviate the unacceptable metabolic consequences of glucose absorption, efforts have been made to substitute glucose with xylitol [47], amino acids [48], gelatin [49], polyglucose [50], or glycerol [51], or polypeptide [52]. Although every agent tried has been found to be an effective osmotic agent and also prevented or minimized some of the unwanted metabolic effects of glucose, none has been utilised long term for peritoneal dialysis because of unacceptable toxicity or metabolic profiles or prohibitively higher cost, compared to glucose.

One-to-two percent amino acid mixtures in the dialysis solution have been used effectively to induce ultrafiltration in nondiabetic CAPD patients [48]. The absorbed amino-acids lead to an increase in the total body nitrogen and transferrin, reduce the inevitable glucose load and lower serum triglyceride levels. Use of such mixtures in diabetic CAPD patients has the potential to reduce many of the undesirable effects of glucose. However, their effectiveness over long periods has not been established. Furthermore, the high cost of amino-acid mixtures could be a major limiting factor in its general use.

Glycerol-containing dialysis solution has been used successfully in diabetic CAPD patients. This agent was well tolerated by the patients, was nontoxic to the peritoneal membrane, did not cause hepatotoxicity, and did not increase protein losses in the dialysate [51, 53]. Blood sugar was easily controlled with insulin. Some patients did develop signs and symptoms of hyperosmolality. However, glycerol showed no benefits over glucose because it delivered similar total caloric load and hyperlipidemia persisted.

Larger molecular-weight poly-glucose appears to be a safe and effective osmotic agent providing sustained ultrafiltration by a mechanism resembling "colloid" osmosis [54]. If long-term studies confirm the safety of moderately elevated maltose levels in the uremic patients, glucose polymer would have a significant role as an osmotic agent in diabetic CAPD patients. A recently completed large multicenter study of polyglucose over 6 months has shown it to be safe and efficacious even in diabetic patients [169].

Polypeptides have been found to be safe in CAPD patients during an acute study [52]. However, long term studies are needed to evaluate its usefulness especially to assess any nutritional value. Currently glucose still remains the best osmotic agent for peritoneal dialysis.

8. Blood sugar control during peritoneal dialysis

The aim of blood sugar control during peritoneal dialysis is to maintain a state of euglycemia throughout the dwell time, control post-meal glycemia, and avoid morning hypoglycemia. Uremia alters the insulin responsiveness and hence the amount required to control blood sugar in a dialysis patient becomes unpredictable [55]. Several methods have been used for blood glucose control during PD especially during CAPD. The survey of the USA NIH CAPD Registry [27] in patients with ESRD attributed to diabetic nephropathy among 499 surveyed patients found five different treatment regimens for blood sugar control during CAPD therapy; eighty-six percent of the patients were taking insulin only, two percent took insulin with an oral hypoglycemic agent, four percent were on an oral agent only, six percent were on diet therapy alone and the remaining two percent were on no specific therapy at all. Of the 434 patients taking insulin, 36 percent received it through subcutaneous injections only, 54 percent through intraperitoneal delivery only, and ten percent through a combination of subcutaneous injections and intraperitoneal delivery. Although there are no studies that show one regimen of insulin administration clearly superior to others for CAPD patients, for reasons discussed below, if insulin is required to control blood sugar, attempts should be made to administer it intraperitoneally.

8.1. Kinetics of intraperitoneal insulin

There is evidence to suggest that intraperitoneal insulin delivery allows more rapid and consistent absorption of insulin; when absorbed, insulin preferentially enters the hepatic portal venous circulation and this hepatic delivery may beneficially affect lipid metabolism and peripheral insulin levels.

There are several similarities between the absorption kinetics of intraperitoneally administered insulin and the normal secretion of insulin by the islet cells. Insulin release in a normal person is a complex coordinated interplay of food absorbed from the gut, gastrointestinal hormones, and other hormonal and neural stimuli. Insulin secreted by the islet cells is taken into the portal vein, and, thereafter, the liver removes 50 to 60 percent of the secreted insulin presented to it [56]. In the basal state, the portal/peripheral ratio of insulin is 3:1. Following bursts of secretion in response to glucose or amino acids, the portal/peripheral ratio may reach a value of 9:1. Insulin administered into the peritoneal cavity is absorbed preferentially by diffusion across the visceral peritoneum into the portal venous circulation. Additionally, direct absorption through the capsule of the liver has also been reported [57]. Once in the liver, a significant fraction of insulin is cleared by the liver during its first pass. Initial delivery of insulin to the liver simulates physiological insulin secretion more closely [58–64]; absorption is continuous until the end of the dwell.

Some of the causes for glycemic lability in diabetic patients taking subcutaneous insulin injections [65, 66] are degradation of insulin in the subcutaneous tissues and variations in absorption due to factors such as depth and location of injection, exercise, or regional blood flow. Peritoneal delivery of insulin alleviates these variables and allows for predictable metabolic management [56, 67, 68].

8.2. Benefits of intraperitoneal insulin

There are benefits when insulin is delivered to the liver during its first pass. Relatively few studies have carefully examined this issue. Studies in dogs show that insulin delivery via the portal route may be necessary to maintain normal levels of hormones and metabolites [69, 70]. However, both portal and peripheral insulin delivery have similar effects on hepatic and extrahepatic carbohydrate metabolism [71].

Excessive basal hepatic glucose output is the principal cause of elevated fasting plasma glucose levels in non-insulin dependent diabetes mellitus (NIDDM) [72, 73]; in normal and NIDDM subjects, hepatic glucose output is much more sensitive to suppression by insulin than is stimulation of peripheral glucose uptake [74]. While reviewing the benefits of intraperitoneal insulin, Duckworth and colleagues argue for treating NIDDM with intraperitoneal insulin because intraperitoneal insulin delivery can selectively inhibit increased hepatic glucose output with a relatively lower degree of hyperinsulinemia in NIDDM compared to subcutaneous insulin injections [75]. Duckworth [56] stresses that, for any given dose of insulin, the amount that reaches the peripheral circulation is considerably less when the insulin is delivered intraperitoneally rather than subcutaneously. This observation is all the more important in view of the increasing evidence suggesting that circulating insulin levels may be directly related to the risk of atherosclerosis [76–78].

In normal subjects, a low basal level of insulin is maintained between meal ingestion [79]. Peritoneal delivery of insulin results in rapid and consistent absorption and allows for maintaining a low basal level between meals. The significance of maintaining a basal level of insulin was clearly shown by studies with programmed insulin-infusion systems which provide insulin in basal as well as pre-meal doses; such systems are far more effective in normalizing blood glucose concentrations in type I diabetes than pre-meal insulin doses alone [80]. Persistent hyperinsulinemia, a rare occurrence in normal subjects, occurs frequently when insulin is subcutaneously injected. One study suggests that intraperitoneal insulin is necessary to normalize lactate levels [81].

A number of studies suggest that intraperitoneal insulin therapy is associated with lipoprotein profiles of lower atherogenic potential [82–84]. These studies demonstrated a reduction in the cholesterol content of high-density lipoprotein in patients treated with intraperitoneal insulin compared with subcutaneous insulin with no change in apolipoproteins A-I and A-II. Moreover, intraperitoneal insulin was associated with lower very-low-density lipoprotein triglycerides, very-low-density lipoprotein apolipoprotein B and near-normal levels of cholesterol ester transfer. The conclusion of these studies was that intraperitoneal insulin was more physiological and corrected a key step in reverse cholesterol transport in patients with IDDM. Hepatic functions, other than carbohydrate and lipid metabolism, that are dependent on insulin may also be improved with intraperitoneal administration [56]. For example, intraperitoneal insulin results in higher levels of plasma hydroxy-vitamin D levels than subcutaneous insulin, even with comparable glucose control [85].

Both intensive subcutaneous insulin therapy and peritoneal insulin delivery can return the blood glucose levels and glycosylated hemoglobin values to normal. But the benefit of peritoneal delivery is fewer glycemic excursions, so that the difference between low and high glucose values during a day are lower compared to subcutaneous insulin [86]. Moreover, the frequency of hypoglycemic episodes is reduced with peritoneal insulin.

A three-step euglycemic clamp in six matched groups (healthy subjects, insulin-dependent diabetics with normal kidney function, nondiabetic uremics, nondialyzed uremic diabetics, and diabetics on hemodialysis and CAPD) showed that the insulin-mediated glucose uptake is closer to normal in CAPD patients taking intraperitoneal insulin that in subjects on hemodialysis taking subcutaneous insulin [87]. In another retrospective study [88], insulin requirements were examined in two groups of dialyzed and non-dialyzed diabetic patients, one treated with subcutaneous insulin and the other with intraperitoneal insulin. The blood glucose levels were significantly lower with the CAPD/IP group compared to both CAPD/subcutaneous and HD/subcutaneous groups at every time interval for as long as 15 months.

Because of the similarities between the effects of intraperitoneally administered insulin and the physiologically secreted insulin, glycemic and metabolic control during CAPD is more physiologic than during hemodialysis. Such an advantage should impact on the overall long-term progression of diabetic complications in patients on dialysis. The effects of intraperitoneal insulin on the progression of target organ diseases in CAPD patients are difficult to ascertain because of the high prevalence of end-stage multi-organ damage at the time of initiation of dialysis; nearly half the patients survive for less than two years on the therapy. Moreover, young patients with early target organ damage, appropriately, are very quickly transplanted and do not stay on the therapy long enough to observe the impact of therapy. Unless observations in diabetic CAPD patients extending over 5 to 10 years are carried out, we will not know the effect of intraperitoneal insulin effect on slowing the progressive end organ damage. For now, it is clear that short-term metabolic control with intraperitoneal insulin is better than that achieved with subcutaneous insulin.

8.3. Problems of intraperitoneal insulin therapy

Some anecdotal experiences suggest increased incidence of peritonitis in patients receiving intraperitoneal insulin [89]. Contrary to this observation, the National CAPD Registry survey of peritonitis revealed that a combination of subcutaneous and intraperitoneal insulin experienced the lowest peritonitis rate (0.93 episodes per patient year) as compared to subcutaneous administered insulin (1.03), and intraperitoneal insulin (1.06). Blind patients using subcutaneously administered versus blind patients using intraperitoneal insulin reported similar rates of peritonitis.

The other problem observed with the use of intraperitoneal insulin is subcapsular liver steatonecrosis [90] and malignant omentum syndrome [91]. Steatosis in a unique subcapsular distribution was observed during autopsy in 10 of 11 CAPD patients treated with intraperitoneal insulin and in none of the 9 control CAPD patients receiving no insulin. More studies are needed to understand the importance of this focal lesion in the livers of CAPD patients receiving IP insulin. In patients with malignant omentum syndrome, insulin is trapped in the omentum, probably in response to foreign protein.

From the above discussion, it is event that there are a number of metabolic and long-term benefits to peritoneal delivery of insulin for diabetic patients. Diabetic dialysis patients, despite the far-advanced target organ-damage, should be given the benefit of peritoneal delivery of insulin for better metabolic control and to derive the anti-atherogenic benefit, however small.

8.4. The steps of blood sugar control in a new CAPD patient using IP route

Several protocols of blood sugar control with IP insulin have been published [15, 19, 92–95]. These protocols are based on the vast experience of the individual centers. There are no studies that compare the effectiveness of different methods, but from a clinical perspective, they all seem effective in achieving the goal of good metabolic control. The method described below is the one practiced at our center.

The goal of therapy is to maintain blood sugar levels at about 150 mg/dl throughout the day. For a week or two after the initiation of CAPD, blood sugar is controlled with daily, multiple subcutaneous injections of regular insulin as per the standard practice of blood sugar control. This interval allows for CAPD to be established and the dialysis dose to be determined. An attempt is made to switch to intraperitoneal route of insulin administration after explaining the practice to the patient. It is not uncommon for patients to refuse the intraperitoneal approach for fear of the unknown. On the first day of the switch, 100 percent of the CAPD daily subcutaneous insulin dose is divided among all four exchanges, with a reduced insulin dose (50 to 70 percent) added to the overnight dwell. Although, many patients may need more than 100 percent of their subcutaneous dose of insulin when switched to the intraperitoneal route, it is recommended to use caution initially to avoid severe hypoglycemia. Although the actual insulin utilized to control blood sugar intraperitoneally is comparatively smaller than by the subcutaneous route (since insulin is only about half absorbed through the peritoneal route during a six-hour dialysis exchange [64]), it is appropriate to initiate the intraperitoneal mode with 100 percent of the subcutaneous dose.

Review of fasting, two-hour post prandial and/or pre-exchange blood glucose results of the previous day allows step wise changes in insulin added to each cycle until desired blood glucose control is achieved. Below are some helpful hints for the use of intraperitoneal insulin. The dialysis exchanges are performed during the day to coincide with the major meals, i.e., breakfast, lunch, and supper. The fourth exchange is made at around 2300 hours, at which time a small snack may be taken. The patient is advised to consume a diet providing 20–25 Kcal/kg body weight/day and containing protein of 1.2 to 1.5 g/kg B.W. During the initial control, blood sugar by finger-stick method is estimated four times a day, pre-exchange. After cleaning the blood port of the dialysis solution bag with a sterilizing solution using a syringe with a long needle, regular insulin is added to each dialysis solution bag. The time of insulin injection into the bag, prior to solution infusion should be standardized. The bag is inverted two or three times to aid mixing. Increments in insulin are required for each additional hypertonic dialysis cycle incorporated into the daily routine. Increments differ among patients. Individual patient requirements are determined during training. Patients are trained to check their blood sugar levels with the finger-prick method. This method, which gives quick results and correlates well with the venous blood sugar levels, helps the patient monitor unexpected fluctuations in blood sugar. The finger-prick test is performed five to ten minutes before each bag exchange and, whenever necessary, the dose of insulin added to the next bag is adjusted according to the guidelines taught to the patient at the time of training.

Intraperitoneal insulin requirements during episodes of peritonitis are believed to be increased, but hypoglycemia has recently been reported when the usual dose of intraperitoneal insulin was continued during peritonitis [97]. Blood glucose levels during peritonitis are determined by the balance between increased insulin absorption and reduced carbohydrate intake due to anorexia versus increased glucose absorption and the infection-related catabolic state. If care is not exercised, severe fatal hypoglycemia may be encountered with intraperitoneal insulin administration.

In diabetic CAPD patients such treatment objectives as maintaining morning-fasting glucose less than 140 mg/dl, post-meal hyperglycemia less than 200 mg/dl, and hemoglobin A_1C levels less than 9 percent is easily achieved with intraperitoneal insulin administration. Insulin injected into the tubing and flushed into the peritoneal cavity with a small volume of dialysis solution reduces the total amount of insulin needed to normalize blood sugar compared to mixing insulin with the dialysis solution prior to infusion [98]. Some type II diabetic patients have difficulty maintaining satisfactory blood sugar levels even with very large doses of insulin. The reason for such refractoriness is not clear but is believed to be due to the trapping of insulin in the mesenteric or omental lymphatics [91].

8.5. Site of intraperitoneal delivery

Most protocols recommend mixing insulin with the dialysis solution before delivery into the peritoneal cavity. This way, insulin is diluted nearly 2000 times and a very low insulin concentration is achieved in the solution. Due to the low concentration gradient, insulin diffusion is slow and continuous. On the other hand, when insulin is injected into the connecting tube through a special injection port, a high concentration of insulin is achieved in the first 50 ml of dialysis solution that gets infused into the peritoneal cavity [92]. This approach reduces the amount of insulin required.

8.6. Blood sugar control during NIPD

Blood-sugar control while on NIPD is achieved with insulin administered either subcutaneously or both subcutaneously and intraperitoneally. The amount of insulin administered is adjusted to individual requirements. During the day, patients are given the daily dose of insulin, usually long acting, by subcutaneous injection, the dose determined both by the patient's dietary-caloric intake and insulin sensitivity. An additional amount of long-acting insulin is given subcutaneously or regular insulin is added intraperitoneally at the initiation of cycler therapy. The amount of insulin needed is dependent on the patient's insulin sensitivity and the amount of glucose absorbed during the dialysis. Type I diabetics typically need considerably less insulin compared to Type II diabetics. During the first few treatments, blood sugar is determined several times and insulin dose is titrated to maintain the desired blood sugar level. It takes several treatment days to determine the exact amount of insulin required by an individual patient. Once stable, blood sugar should be checked periodically during the treatment.

9. Clinical results

9.1. Blood-pressure control

Blood pressure control on CAPD is easy due to continuous sustained ultrafiltration and sodium removal, which maintains patients at their dry body weight [99, 100]. The reduction in blood pressure is most marked during the initial weeks of therapy and additional decreases occur over the next few months [100]. The blood pressure response to CAPD correlates well with the reduction in the fluid body weight, emphasizing the importance of fluid volume in the pathogenesis of hypertension in ESRD. In fact, hypertension can often be controlled without drug therapy, even when plasma renin and aldosterone levels are observed to be increased [101].

During CAPD exchanges, net water as well as sodium is removed. A typical CAPD patient losses about 1 to 1.5 L/day of ultrafiltrate with sodium concentration of about 132 mEq/L since the dialysate equilibrates with serum sodium during a 4 to 6 hour exchange [102, 103]. The total sodium loss during a day can also be readily calculated as the sum of (drain volume × drained dialysate sodium concentration) – (infusion volume × infused dialysate sodium concentration) for each day. Thus, a typical CAPD patient could easily loose up to 132–198 mEq/day of sodium through the ultrafiltrate. A patient accustomed to restricted sodium intake during the course of chronic renal failure often continues his/her low-sodium diet during the CAPD therapy. Consequently, CAPD patients may become sodium depleted over the course of therapy due to the combination of dialysate sodium loss and restricted consumption. Initially, such sodium depletion is beneficial in controlling hypertension. Most CAPD patients, requiring multiple antihypertensive agents for control of hypertension prior to starting CAPD, gradually need fewer and fewer drugs, eventually discontinuing them altogether [100]. If, at this time, dietary sodium intake is not liberalized, severe sodium depletion could lead to hypotension, especially in patients with primary cardiac disease. Total body sodium depletion results in decreased vascular response to infusions of pressor agents such as norepinephrine [104]. Salt repletion in such patients results in restoration of the vascular pressure response, extracellular fluid volume, and blood pressure.

In certain CAPD patients, such as those with diabetic autonomic neuropathy or cardiac dysfunction, hypotension may occur readily and very early after initiating CAPD. Surprisingly, many patients are asymptomatic, despite a severe degree of hypotension. This may possibly be due to the lack of renin response from the kidneys, since most patients are functionally anephric.

On the other hand, during intermittent dialysis therapies, the dialysate sodium concentration decreases due to solute sieving with ultrafiltration, hence sodium loss is considerably diminished [102]. Consequently, hypertension control in patients on intermittent dialysis therapies is not readily achieved. Most patients require fluid and dietary salt restriction and very many need antihypertensive medications. Hypotension, if it occurs in these patients, is generally transient and is a result of rapid ultrafiltration during the treatment. From the above discussion, it is apparent that due to its effect on salt and water balance, CAPD controls blood pressure readily and a significant number of patients do not require medication.

9.2. Benefits of slow and continuous ultrafiltration during CAPD

Rapid ultrafiltration, i.e., three to four liters of fluid removal during a typical three to four hour hemodialysis, three times a week, causes intravascular fluid volume depletion leading to hypotension in many diabetic patients. In most of these patients, this acute transient hypotension is usually managed by infusion of saline or colloid solution to restore intravascular volume and maintain blood pressure. In patients with significant coronary, carotid, or peripheral artery disease, ischemic symptoms or in some instances irreversible ischemic complications such as myocardial infarction or stroke may ensue if hypotension is sustained. Fluid infused to correct hypotension essentially negates the purpose of ultrafiltration and, more importantly, adds to the cost of dialysis. Contrary to hemodialysis, patients on CAPD do not need this rapid rate of ultrafiltration; typically these patients require one to two liters of fluid removal over a 24-hour period. Unless the patient is clearly dehydrated, transient acute hypotension during CAPD is infrequent. There are no data in the literature that compare in a prospective manner the impact of dialysis therapy on the ischemic complications of vascular diseases of similar severity in patients on hemodialysis and CAPD. Nevertheless, analysis of death rates by cause of death for all diabetic ESRD patients on hemodialysis (35,683 patient years at risk) and CAPD (5,254 patient years at risk) during 1987–89 in the USA showed mortality from myocardial infarction and cerebrovascular events were greater among diabetic patients on CAPD/CCPD (151.6 deaths per 1,000 patient years at risk) compared to diabetic patients on hemodialysis (129.7 deaths per 1000 patient years at risk) [7]. This higher death rate from cardiac causes in CAPD diabetic patients may in part be a reflection of selection bias, i.e., preferential use of CAPD/CCPD for patients known to have severe cardiovascular disease.

9.3. Residual-renal function

The importance of residual-renal function in the management of dialysis patients has been under recognized. Residual-renal function contributes to the overall clearance of small and middle molecular weight solutes and fluid removal. In addition, substantial amounts of sodium, potassium, phosphate and acid excretion permit liberal fluid and dietary intake. Due to the contribution of renal function to solute clearance, the dialysis prescription may be modified to reduce the dose of dialysis and, in some, time spent on dialysis per treatment. There are indications that the rate of decline of residual-renal function in patients on hemodialysis and CAPD may be different.

Since the original publication of Rottembourg and colleagues in 1983 [105] which showed a stable residual-renal function (assessed by creatinine clearance) over a period of 18 months in 22 insulin-dependent diabetic patients on CAPD compared to 56 insulin-dependent diabetic patients treated with hemodialysis, several more studies have confirmed the observation that residual-renal function in CAPD patients is preserved for a longer period, in some up to 60 months, compared to hemodialysis patients [106–116]. If, indeed, residual-renal function decays faster in hemodialysis patents than in CAPD patients, several potential mechanisms could be operating simultaneously in hemodialysis.

1. As discussed earlier, patients on hemodialysis

frequently experience rapid changes in extracellular fluid volumes during aggressive ultrafiltration. The result is an acute fall in blood pressure and, most likely, an acute fall in renal blood flow and glomerular capillary pressure, resulting in ischemia of remaining functioning nephrons.

2. There is evidence to suggest that the passage of blood through extracorporeal circulation triggers the secretion of IL-1 and tumor necrosis factor [117]. Levels of tumor-necrosis factor alpha are increased in uremic patients; dialysis further increases their levels. Circulating cytokines may directly or indirectly generate vascular and immune injury in vivo [118]. Alternatively, blood membrane contact may trigger the release of reactive oxygen metabolites into circulation that may damage residual renal tissue [119]. Shah has suggested that reactive oxygen metabolites generated by neutrophils enhance glomerular basement membrane degradation by proteolytic enzymes and may cause a profound constrictive response in the glomerular capillaries [119]. The evidence cited above suggests that hemodialysis could be "nephrotoxic" and, hence, could cause deterioration of residual-renal function at a rate faster than the natural progression of the primary renal disease. Absence of such nephrotoxic effect in patients on CAPD may permit natural progression of renal disease and, in many, preservation of the native kidney function for a longer period.

It is important to point out that the evidence cited above is only suggestive of the trend because many cited studies were retrospective, were not matched for GFR between two therapies at the initiation of dialysis and for frequency of complicating events such as severe hypotension, and were not controlled for administration of other nephrotoxic drugs. Moreover, reliance on creatinine clearance as an estimate of GFR has always been questioned. Several prospective, randomized, comparative studies currently under way, in which inulin clearance is being used as a marker of GFR, should clarify the issue in the near future.

9.4. Visual problems

Most insulin-dependent diabetics have irreversible retinal lesions before they start dialysis, especially during the terminal phase of renal failure when hypertension tends to be severe. In the great majority, by the time they reach the stage of dialysis, ocular lesions are far too advanced to expect any useful recovery. However, attempts should be made to preserve any useful vision the patient has. Specialized eye care is essential for all these patients. Many patients benefit from vitrectomy and panretinal photocoagulation even with advanced retinal lesions [120–122]. The common lesions seen at the time of initiating CAPD are background retinopathy, proliferative retinopathy, and vitreous hemorrhage. Retinal detachment may also be seen in some cases. Therefore, better preservation of ocular function depends on the more aggressive approach to blood pressure and glucose control during the pre-dialysis phase. Retinal ischemia may be made worse by the rapid fluctuations in intravascular volume during the intermittent therapy. CAPD avoids many of the problems inherent in the intermittent forms of dialysis. Stabilization or even improvement of ocular function in diabetic patients maintained on CAPD has been reported by several centers [19, 40, 120, 122].

9.5. Cardiac and vascular diseases

Morbidity and mortality due to atherosclerotic heart disease and microangiopathy remain the main cause of death among diabetics undergoing peritoneal dialysis. Small-vessel disease leading to ischemic gangrene of the extremities is a common complication of type I diabetes. Short-term experience with CAPD in diabetics does not suggest that ischemic complications occur any more frequently in diabetics than in non-diabetics. In the only long-term experience reported by Zimmermann et al. [123], the incidence of ischemic and/or gangrenous complication was extremely low.

9.6. Foot ulceration and care in diabetic patients

Amputation is a distressing complication in patients with end-stage renal disease from diabetes. Studies from Minneapolis report that 17% of patients lost one or both feet during the years following kidney transplantation [163] and in the UK 6.8% of patients receiving dialysis or transplantation had major amputation [164]. Previously these have been thought to be due a macrovascular disease but neuropathic ulceration remains an important preventable contributory factor. True prevalence of these clinical problems, has not been documented although as many as one quarter of patients may have neuropathic ulceration. Foot problems remain a major cause of hospital admissions among diabetic patients. The diabetic foot has tended to be a neglected area because it falls between the specialities of medicine, orthopaedic and vascular surgery. Recent data suggests that doctors are unlikely to examine the patients feet unless their shoes and socks are removed before the patients enters the consulting room and even in the specialist centre only 12% patients attending a Diabetic Clinic had their feet examined [165]. It is estimated that 50–70% of all non traumatic amputations occur in diabetics with an age adjusted major amputation rate 15 times greater than that of the general population.

The major contributory factors in the development of foot ulceration are neuropathy, peripheral vascular disease and abnormal stresses. In the majority of cases the cause of skin breakdown is multifactorial, e.g. ischaemic limb which develops a insensitive ulcer and becomes infected; many become critically ischemic due to increased vascular demand and require amputation. Studies done in Manchester, UK showed that vibration perception threshold was lower in diabetic patients as compared to controls and the mean peak plantar foot pressure (as measured by Pedobiography) was elevated in all diabetic nephropathy patients [166, 167]. These workers conclude that patients at all stages of diabetic nephropathy had increased risk of non vascular foot ulceration.

Prevention of diabetic foot problems entails identifying patients at risk. These are outlined in Table 2 which also show preventative measures in these patients at risk. Of particular interest is the development of the scotch cast boot which is utilised to treat patients with existing diabetic foot ulcers [166]. This consists of a delta light plaster which is weight bearing and has a window cut under the ulcer. This allows redistribution of weight under the foot and avoids any pressure on the ulcer.

A multi disciplinary approach is absolutely crucial [166] and in Manchester a regular combined, joint Diabetic/Renal clinic [167] ensures that the patients are seen by a nephrologist, Diabetologist, Chiropodist and other members of the multi disciplinary team.

9.7. Metabolic and nutritional problems

Losses of proteins, amino acids, polypeptides, and vitamins in the dialysate pose a special problem in those diabetics who may be wasted and malnourished because of poor food intake, vomiting, catabolic stresses, and intercurrent illness. Twenty-four hour amino acid losses in the dialysate average about 2.25 gm/day, with about 8 gm/day of proteins [124]. In uncomplicated cases, daily protein losses in the dialysate correlate with serum-protein concentration and body-surface area. During peritonitis, the protein losses are excessive, and in combination with inadequate food intake may produce severe hypoproteinemia, hypoalbuminemia, and hypo-immunoglobulinemia. Therefore, during the course of a prolonged peritonitis episode, physicians should consider early parenteral nutrition.

Table 2. Prevention of diabetic foot problems in CAPD.

1. *Identification of patients at risk*

    Poor sight
    Elderly
    Previous foot ulcer
    Smokers
    Neuropathy
    Peripheral vascular disease
    Foot deformity
    Limited joint mobility

2. *Regular reinforcement of advice and foot care guidelines*

    DO   Wash feet regularly in warm water check bath water before slipping feet into it.
    Inspect feet daily including sole of feet.
    Avoid dry skin.
    Buying shoes – have feet measured professionally.
    Inspect inside of shoes for foreign bodies.
    Feet examined at each clinic visit.

    DO NOT   Walk barefoot
    Wear new shoes for long periods.
    Smoke
    Use "home remedies to cure foot problems".

3. *Examine feet at each consultation*

    Peripheral Vasc Disease – foot pulses, doppler.
    Neuropathy
    Foot deformity – claw foot, hammer toes, charcot.

4. *Provision of adequate footwear*

    – "Roomey", avoid "crowding of toes" – and pointed shoes.
    – For ulcerated feet – Scotch Cast Boot.
    – Use padded hosiery.

5. *Pre and Post operative care*

    – Feet support with padding.
    – Examine feet daily.

Continuous absorption of glucose during CAPD may aggravate the pre-existing hypertiglyceridemia, a frequent abnormality in uremic patients [19, 125–131]. The prevalence of hypertriglyceridemia in long-term CAPD patients is reported to be about 80 percent [132, 133] and hypercholesterolemia to be about 15–30 percent [132, 134]. Insulin levels correlate directly with the level of serum triglycerides [135]; and since hyperinsulinemia is common, this high prevalence is not surprising. At the start of therapy most patients have either normal or low cholesterol levels. During the initial months after the initiation of therapy, both serum cholesterol and triglycerides increase [44, 127, 136–139]. The increase in cholesterol is predominantly due to the increase in the fractions of VLDL and LDL, and, to a lesser extent, the increase in HDL fraction [44, 134]. The high-density lipoprotein fractions are lost in the dialysate during CAPD [140], but due to increased intake of energy, CAPD patients are reported to have high levels of HDL [141–143]. The lipid disorders are more marked in those with pre-existing lipid abnormalities, especially in the diabetics.

9.8. Peritonitis

CAPD-related peritonitis is one of the major causes of morbidity in CAPD patients. Experiences over ten years have indicated that the spectrum of pathology, clinical manifestations and management of peritonitis in diabetics and non-diabetics are similar. The earlier fears that diabetic-CAPD patients would have a higher frequency of peritonitis with more unusual organisms than non-diabetic patients has been unfounded [144]. About 40 percent of the bacterial peritonitis is due to Staphylococcus epidermidis. While this organism is a weak pathogen, in recent years it has been recognized with increasing frequency as the cause of wound infections and endocarditis. Staphylococcus epidermidis does not produce toxins and pathogenicity depends entirely on its ability to initiate a pyogenic process. The clinical illness is usually mild, and the disease responds well to antibiotic treatment. Other organisms isolated during episodes of peritonitis include Staph. aureus, Strep. viridans, gram-negative enteric organisms, and, very rarely, anaerobic organisms. A very small fraction of peritonitis is caused by fungi.

Insulin administration into the dialysis solution bag breaks the sterility of the system and could potentially contaminate the peritoneal cavity and cause peritonitis. However, clinical experience has shown this not to be a significant problem. The incidence of peritonitis in diabetics is no higher than that in non-diabetics on CAPD [145]. The national CAPD Registry surveyed peritonitis rates per patient year by route of insulin administration and type of diabetes management [27]. Although the differences in the rates were not large, diabetics never using insulin had the highest rate of peritonitis per patient year (1.31), while patients using a combination of subcutaneous and intraperitoneal insulin experienced the lowest rate (0.93). The peritonitis rate per patient year for patients using subcutaneously administered insulin (1.03) was similar to the rate reported for patients using intraperitoneal insulin (1.06). Blind patients using either subcutaneous or intra-peritoneal insulin reported similar rates of peritonitis. The reason for such a protective effect in patients using insulin is unclear.

The recent trend to use devices to facilitate exchange procedures or protect against peritoneal contamination (especially the Y-set system) has significantly reduced the incidence of peritonitis [146].

Treatment of CAPD-related peritonitis is similar for diabetic and non-diabetic patients and has been reported extensively elsewhere [144]. Due to the enhanced absorption of glucose during peritonitis, hyperglycemia is observed frequently in diabetics and insulin requirements may increase. However, some patients may experience hypoglycemia if they are unable to eat and insulin administration is continued at the same dosage as that prior to peritonitis. Close monitoring of blood glucose during episodes of peritonitis is essential to prevent either hypoglycemia or hyperglycemia. Due to increased protein losses during peritonitis, the patient's nutrition must be watched closely during the acute phase and, in some, parenteral nutrition should be considered. Generally, the outcome of peritonitis treatment is good. Most patients continue on CAPD after the peritonitis is cured. A small percentage (2 to 5 percent) will drop out of the CAPD program for a variety of reasons, including membrane failure.

9.9. Patient and technique survival on CAPD

The three-year cumulative patient survival rates on CAPD are significantly better than those achieved with intermittent peritoneal dialysis [13]. However, the actuarial survival and technique success rates for diabetics are lower than non-diabetics of comparable age on CAPD. The reported three-year survival rates for diabetics range from 40 to 60 percent, depending on the age of patients [147–149]. The USRDS Annual report of 1991 compared the one-year survival rate, adjusted for age, sex and race, for diabetics on hemodialysis and CAPD/CCPD from day 90 of dialysis [150]. The one-year survival for the hemodialysis group was slightly better than for CAPD/CCPD (69.6 vs. 65.7 percent). Interestingly, one-year survival for non-diabetic patients was almost identical in the two groups. However, these results are unadjusted for co-morbid conditions such as coronary artery and cerebrovascular diseases. However, when the mortality was analyzed according to the age of the patient, mortality rates tended to be higher for hemodialysis patients than for CAPD patients among younger patients (age 40 years or below), while the opposite was the case among older patients (age over 40 years). The Michigan Kidney Registry [151] using Cox's proportional hazards analysis showed that diabetic patients aged 20 to 59 had a 38 percent lower relative risk of death on CAPD ($p = 0.01$) compared to hemodialysis. Diabetics aged 60 years and older had a 19 percent higher risk on CAPD, but this was not significant ($p = 0.08$). By showing a better survival rate on CAPD compared to hemodialysis, younger patients, who as a group tended to be relatively free from cardiac disease compared to older patients, may be displaying the beneficial effects of CAPD, i.e., better blood-pressure control, use of intraperitoneal insulin. On the other hand, the higher mortality rate for older patients on CAPD is probably a reflection of selection bias; older diabetic patients with severe cardiac and peripheral vascular diseases are preferentially chosen for CAPD/CCPD treatment.

The poorer technique survival rate for CAPD as compared to hemodialysis is a reflection of the CAPD technique related problems of which peritonitis remains the major one [7]. Since the introduction of the Y-set system, the peritonitis rate has improved significantly [152] to about one episode every 16–24 patient months from one episode every 12 patient months before the introduction of the system. This improvement is likely to have a favorable impact on the dropout rate from CAPD. Moreover, during the last few years, adequacy standards for CAPD patients have been proposed [41–43, 153]. Implementation of these will also favorably influence the dropout rates due to inadequate dialysis, which account for nearly 15 to 20 percent of CAPD dropouts.

9.10. Technique-related complications

Complications which are a direct result of increased intra-abdominal pressures, such as dialysate leaks, hernia, hemorrhoids, and a compromised cardiac pulmonary status, occur with the same frequency in diabetics as in non-diabetics. As discussed earlier, peritoneal membrane function as assessed by the serum chemistries and peritoneal equilibration test [154] remains stable in the absence of peritonitis. Transient loss of ultrafiltration during an episode of peritonitis is frequent, but full recovery occurs. Irreversible loss of ultrafiltration may occur as a result of severe peritonitis, repeated episodes of which can lead to sclerosing peritonitis [155–157].

9.11. Hospitalization rates

Because of the numerous complications associated with diabetes, diabetic patients on CAPD tend to have increased morbidity and require more frequent hospitalization than nondiabetic patients. For type I and type II diabetics, the rate of hospitalization (33 days per patient year of treatment) appears to be similar. Hospitalization due to causes directly related to CAPD technique accounting for about a third of the total rate, are progressively decreasing. The rate of hospitalization for diabetics on CAPD is comparable to diabetics on hemodialysis.

10. Can peritoneal dialysis be a long-term therapy for ESRD patient?

During the early years of CAPD, it was feared that long-term CAPD in diabetics may not have been feasible because of extensive microvascular disease. Lower solute and water clearances were predicted for diabetics compared to non-diabetics [158]. In addition, concerns of membrane injury from peritonitis led most to believe there would be a short life for the peritoneal membrane and a high dropout from the therapy after a short period. However, contrary to earlier expectations, a recent study in a group of 130 CAPD patients reported similar peritoneal transport characteristics for both diabetics and non-diabetics [160], and, peritoneal membrane function for solute and water transfer remained stable for up to 60 months [160, 161].

Although experience with long-term survival of diabetics on CAPD is very limited, there are now reports of diabetic patients who have been successfully managed on CAPD for longer than five years [123, 162]. Characteristically, the patients who survive long tend to be free from associated cardiac disease and are non-smokers. The actuarial survival was 44 percent at five years (26 patients at risk) in one of the series [123]. The NIH CAPD registry reported that, of the 7161 CAPD patients surveyed, 19 percent were on treatment for three years or more [27]. These long-term patients included a smaller percentage (18 percent) of patients with diabetes than the short-term cohorts (26 percent).

11. Can CAPD/CCPD be recommended over hemodialysis for diabetic patients?

Diabetes is an exceedingly complex disease and the management of these patients is exceptionally challenging. While acknowledging that both dialysis modalities, CAPD and hemodialysis, have unique advantages and disadvantages for managing diabetic ESRD patients, there is a need to individualize dialysis therapy to derive maximum benefit from a therapy. Based on the available evidence, it is clear that there are some unique features of CAPD that are conducive to better long-term outcomes in some diabetic patients and there are certain features that make diabetic complications more symptomatic. For example, maintenance of residual-renal function for five years or more after initiating dialysis should have great impact on patient management. Residual-renal function allows for liberal diet intake including fluid. Also, the presence of significant residual-renal function gives one the flexibility to modify the dialysis prescription to better adjust to a patient's needs. Lastly, the benefits of intraperitoneal insulin have not been emphasized enough. Besides being convenient, peritoneal delivery of insulin during CAPD achieves better metabolic control compared to subcutaneous injections and, in the long run, produces several effects which are antiatherogenic. Indeed, this is an added advantage in the management of a diabetic patient. Besides these medical benefits, patients with severe coronary or carotid artery diseases and those with diastolic dysfunction may find slow but continuous peritoneal dialysis more tolerable than intermittent hemodialysis. On the other hand, diabetic patients with gastroparesis, CAPD may aggravate their symptoms. This problem may exacerbate nutritional problems of diabetics during CAPD. Similarly, those with diabetic autonomic dysfunction are prone to severe orthostatism because of continuous and sustained sodium loss. Orthostatic hypotension and upper GI symptoms in such patients could be quite crippling. Despite all the technological advances, CAPD can only be done by patients who are highly motivated and has good visual function. Advanced diabetic retinopathy with legal blindness is fairly common in these patients making it extremely difficult for an average patient to self perform CAPD. In conclusion, there are several reasons to recommend CAPD/CCPD over hemodialysis for the many diabetic ESRD patients who choose dialysis as the mode of renal replacement therapy. Similarly, there are several reasons why CAPD should not be recommended for certain diabetic patients. These patients might find hemodialysis more suitable for their medical problems.

12. Summary

It is becoming apparent that with proper selection of patients, diabetic patients can survive for a long period on CAPD. The morbidity and mortality observed on CAPD therapy, like hemodialysis, is primarily related to associated-risk factors such as cardiovascular disease, atherosclerotic complications, and infection. Ability to administer intraperitoneal insulin during CAPD enables simulation of normal insulin secretion by the islet cells. CAPD patients tend to retain residual-renal function for a longer period of time. The incidence of peritonitis is decreasing and is expected to affect the CAPD drop-out rate. Certain features of CAPD make it a suitable therapy for diabetics whereas, other features may negate its use in diabetics.

References

1. Friedman EA. Clinical imperatives in diabetic nephropathy. Kidney Int 1982; 23 (suppl): S16–9.
2. Friedman EA. Overview of diabetic nephropathy. In: Keen H, Legrain M (eds), Prevention and Treatment of Diabetic Nephropathy. MTP, Lancaster 1983; pp 3–19.
3. Friedman EA. Clinical strategy in diabetic nephropathy. In: Friedman E, L'Esperance F (eds), Diabetic Renal-Retinal Syndrome 3. Grune and Stratton, New York 1986; pp 331–7.
4. Legrain M. Diabetics with end-stage renal disease:

the best buy. Editorial. Diabetic Nephropathy 2: 1–3.
5. Markell MS, Friedman EA. Care of the diabetic patient with end-stage renal disease. Semin Nephrology 1990; 10: 274–86.
6. Friedman EA. How can the case of diabetic ESRD patients be improved? Seminars in Dialysis 1991; 4: 13–4.
7. U.S. Renal Data Systems. USRDS 1989 Annual Data Report. The National Institute of Health, National Institute of Diabetes and Digestive and Kidney Diseases, Bethesda, MD, August 1989.
8. Katirtzoglou A, Izatt S, Oreopoulos DG. Chronic peritoneal dialysis in diabetics with end-stage renal failure. In: Friedman EA (ed), Diabetic Renal-Retinal Syndrome. Grune & Stratton, Orlando 1982; pp 317–32.
9. Blumenkrantz MJ, Shapiro DJ, Minura N, Oreopoulos DG, Friedler RM, Levin S, Tenckhoff H, Coburn JW. Maintenance peritoneal dialysis as an alternative in the patients with diabetes mellitus and end-stage uremia. Kidney International 1974; 6 (suppl 1): S108.
10. Quelhorst E, Schuenemann B, Mietzsch G, Jacob I. Hemo and peritoneal dialysis treatment of patient with diabetic nephropathy. A comparative study. Proceedings of the European Dialysis and Transplant Association 1978; 15: 205.
11. Mion C, Slingeneyer A, Salem JL, Oules R, Mirouze J. Home peritoneal dialysis in end-stage diabetic nephropathy. Journal of Dialysis 1978; 2: 426–7.
12. Warden GS, Maxwell JG, Stephen RL. The use of reciprocating peritoneal dialysis with a subcutaneous peritoneal dialysis in end-stage renal failure in diabetes mellitus. Journal of Surgical Research 1978; 24: 495–500.
13. Amair P, Khanna R, Leibel B, Peirratos A, Vas S, Meema G, Chisholm L, Vas M, Zingg W, Digenis G, Oreopoulos DG. Continuous ambulatory peritoneal dialysis in diabetics with end-stage renal disease. N Eng J of Med 1982; 306: 625–30.
14. Legrain M, Rottembourg J, Bentchikou A, Poignet JL, Issad B, Barthelemy A, Strippoli P. Dialysis treatment of insulin dependent diabetic patients. A ten year experience. Clinical Nephrology 1984; 21: 72–81.
15. Lameire N, Dhaene M, Matthys E, de Paepe M, Vereerstraeten P, Drawtwa M, Ringoir S. Experience with CAPD in diabetic patients. In: Keen H, Legrain M (eds), Prevention and Treatment of Diabetic Nephropathy. MTP Ltd, Lancaster 1983; pp 289–97.
16. Polla-Imhoof B, Pirson Y, Lafontaine JJ, Vandenbrouche JM, Cosyns JP, Squifflet JP, Alexandre G, van Ypersele de Strihou C. Resultats de l'hémodialyse chronique et de la transplantation rénale dans le traitement de l'urémie terminale du diabétique. Néphrologie 1982; 3: 80–4.
17. Thompson NW, Simpson RW, Hooke D, Atkins RC. Peritoneal dialysis in the treatment of diabetic end-stage renal failure. In: Atkins R, Thomson NM, Farell PC (eds), Peritoneal Dialysis. Churchill Livingstone, New York 1981; pp 345–55.
18. Khanna R, Wu G, Chisholm L, Oreopoulos DG. Update: further experience with CAPD in diabetics with end-stage disease. Diabetic Nephropathy 1983; 2: 8–12.
19. Khanna R, Wu G, Prowant B, Jastrzebska J, Nolph KD, Oreopoulos DG. Continuous ambulatory peritoneal dialysis in diabetics with end-stage renal disease: a combined experience of two North American centers. In: Friedman E, l'Esperance F (eds), Diabetic Renal Retinal Syndrome 3. Grune and Stratton, New York 1986; pp 363–81.
20. Rottembourg J. Le traitement de l'insuffisance rénale du diabétique. La Presse Med 1987; 46: 437–40.
21. Shapiro FL. Haemodialysis in diabetic patients. In: Keen H, Legrain M (eds), Prevention and treatment of Diabetic Nephropathy. MTP Ltd, Lancaster 1983; pp 247–359.
22. Khanna R, Oreopoulos DG. Continuous ambulatory peritoneal dialysis in diabetics. In: Brenner BM, Stein JH (eds), Diabetes Mellitus. Churchill Livingstone, New York 1989; pp 185–202.
23. Mauer SM, Morgensen CE, Kjellstrand CM. Diabetic nephropathy. In: Schrier RW, Gottschalk CW (eds), Diseases of the Kidney. Little, Brown and Company, Boston 1993; pp 2153–88.
24. Narins RG, Krishna GG, Kopyt NP. Fluid-electrolyte and acid-base disorders complicating diabetes mellitus. In: Schrier RW, Gottschalk GW (eds), Diseases of the Kidney. Little, Brown and Company, Boston 1993; pp 2563–97.
25. Tenckhoff H, Schechter H. A bacteriologically safe peritoneal access device. Transactions of the American Society of Artificial Internal Organs 1968; 14: 181.
26. Khanna R, Twardowski ZJ. Peritoneal access. In: Nolph KD (ed), Peritoneal Dialysis. Kluwer Academic Publishers, Dordrecht 1989; pp 319–43.
27. Lindblad AS, Novak JW, Nolph KD, Stablein DM, Cutler SJ, Steinberg SM, Vena DA. In: Continuous Ambulatory Peritoneal Dialysis in the USA. Kluwer Academic Publishers, Dordrecht 1989; pp 63–74.
28. Twardowski ZJ, Nolph KD, Khanna R, Gluck Z, Prowant BF, Ryan LP. Daily clearances with continuous ambulatory peritoneal dialysis and nightly peritoneal dialysis. Trans Am Soc Artif Intern Organs 1986; 12: 575–80.
29. Khanna R, Twardowski ZJ, Gluck Z, Ryan LP, Nolph KD. Is nightly peritoneal dialysis (NPD) an effective peritoneal dialysis schedule? (Abstracts) American Society of Nephrology-Kidney Int 1986; 29: 233.
30. Nolph KD, Twardowski ZJ, Khanna R. Clinical pathology conference: peritoneal dialysis. Trans Am Soc Artif Intern Organs 1986; 32: 11–16.
31. Scribner BH. Forward to second edition. In: Nolph KD (ed), Peritoneal Dialysis, second edition. Martinus Nijhoff Publishers, Boston/Dordrecht/Lancaster 1985; pp XI–XII.
32. Twardowski ZJ, Khanna R, Nolph KD,

Scalamogna A, Metzler MH, Schneider TW, Prowant BF, Ryan LP. Intraabdominal pressure during natural activities in patients treated with continuous ambulatory peritoneal dialysis. Nephron 1986; 44: 129–35.
33. Twardowski ZJ. New approaches to intermittent peritoneal dialysis therapies. In: Nolph KD (ed), Peritoneal Dialysis. Kluwer Academic Publishers, Dordrecht 1988; pp 133–51.
34. Twardowski ZJ, Nolph KD, Khanna R, Prowant BF, Frock J, Dobbie J, Serkes K, Kenley R, Witsoe D, Barber J. Tidal peritoneal dialysis. Proceedings of the IVth Congress of the International Society for Peritoneal Dialysis, Venice, Italy, June 29–July 2, 1987.
35. Diaz-Buxo JA. Continuous cyclic peritoneal dialysis. In: Nolph KD (ed), Peritoneal Dialysis. Kluwer Academic Publishers, Dordrecht 1989; pp 169–83.
36. Perras ST, Zappacosta AR. Reduction of peritonitis with patients education and Travenol CAPD germicidal exchange system. American Nephrology Nurses Association 1986; 13: 219.
37. Hamilton RW. The sterile connection device: a review of its development and status report – 1986. In: Khanna R, Nolph KD, Prowant BF et al. (eds), Advances in Continuous Ambulatory Peritoneal Dialysis. Peritoneal Dialysis Bulletin Inc, Toronto 1986; pp 186–9.
38. Fenton SSA, Wu G, Bowman C, Cattran DC, Manuel A, Khanna R, Vas S, Oreopoulos DG. The reduction in the peritonitis rate among high-risk CAPD patients with the use of the Oreopoulos-Zellerman connector. Transactions of the American Society for Artificial Internal Organs 1985; 31: 560.
39. Buoncristiani U, Quintaliani G, Cozzari M, Carobia C. Current status of the Y-set. In: Khanna R et al. (eds), Advances in Continuous Ambulatory Peritoneal Dialysis. Peritoneal Dialysis Bulletin Inc, Toronto 1986; pp 165–71.
40. Flynn CT. The diabetics on CAPD. In: Friedman EA (ed), Diabetic Renal-Retinal Syndrome. Grune & Stratton, Orlando 1982; pp 321–30.
41. Keshaviah P. Adequacy of CAPD: a quantitative approach. Kidney Int 1992; 42 (suppl 38): S160–4.
42. Keshaviah P, Nolph KD. The peak concentration hypothesis: a urea kinetic approach to comparing the adequacy of continuous ambulatory peritoneal dialysis (CAPD) and hemodialysis. Perit Dial Int 1989; 9: 257–60.
43. Keshaviah P, Nolph KD, Prowant BF. Defining adequacy of CAPD with urea kinetics. Adv Perit Dial 1990; 6: 173–7.
44. Lindholm B, Bergström J. Nutritional management of patients undergoing peritoneal dialysis. In: Nolph KD (ed), Peritoneal Dialysis. Kluwer Academic Publishers, Dordrecht 1988; pp 230–60.
45. Stout RW. Diabetes and atherosclerosis – the role of insulin. Diabetologia 1979; 16: 141.
46. Zavaroni A, Bonora E, Pagliara M, Dall'Aglio E, Luchetti L, Buonanno G, Bonati PA, Bergonzani M, Gnudi L, Passeri M, Reaven G. Risk factor for coronary artery disease in healthy persons with hyperinsulinemia and normal glucose tolerance. New England Journal of Medicine 1989; 320: 702–6.
47. Bazzato G, Coli U, Landini S. Xylitol and low doses of insulin: new perspectives for diabetic uremic patients on CAPD. Peritoneal Dialysis Bulletin 1982; 2: 161.
48. Williams FP, Marliss EB, Anderson GH et al. Amino acids absorption following intraperitoneal administration in CAPD patients. Peritoneal Dialysis Bulletin 1982; 2: 124.
49. Twardowski ZJ, Khanna R, Nolph KD. Osmotic agents and ultrafiltration in peritoneal dialysis. Nephron 1986; 42: 93.
50. Mistry CD, Mallick NP, Gokal R. The use of large molecular weight glucose polymer as an osmotic agent in CAPD. In: Khanna R, Nolph KD, Prowant BF et al. (eds), Advances in Continuous Ambulatory Peritoneal Dialysis. Peritoneal Dialysis Bulletin Inc, Toronto 1986; pp 7–11.
51. Matthys E, Dolkart R, Lameire N. Extended use of a glycerol containing dialysate in the treatment of diabetic CAPD patients. Peritoneal Dialysis Bulletin 1987; 7: 10.
52. Imholz ALT, Lameire N, Faict D, Koomen GCM, Krediet RT, Martis L. Evaluation of short-chain polypeptides as an osmotic agent in CAPD patients. Peritoneal Dialysis International 1993; 13: S62.
53. Goodship THJ, Heaton A, Wilkinson R, Ward MK. The use of glycerol as an osmotic agent in continuous ambulatory peritoneal dialysis. In: Ota K, Maher J, Winchester J, Hirszel P (eds), Current Concepts in Peritoneal Dialysis. Excerpta Medica, Amsterdam 1992; pp 143–47.
54. Mistry CD, Gokal R. The use of glucose polymer in CAPD: essential physiological and clinical conclusions. In: (Ota K, Maher J, Winchester J, Hirszel P (eds.) Current Concepts in Peritoneal Dialysis. Excerpta Medica, Amsterdam 1992; pp 138–42.
55. Avram MM, Paik SK, Okanya D, Rajpal K. The natural history of diabetic nephropathy: unpredictable insulin requirements. A further clue. Clin Nephrol 1984; 21: 36–8.
56. Duckworth WC. Insulin degradation: mechanisms, products and significance. Endocrine Rev 1988; 9: 319–45.
57. Zingg W, Shirriff JM, Liebel B. Experimental routes of insulin administration. Perit Dial Bull 1982; 2: S24–7.
58. Felig P, Wahren J. The liver as site of insulin and glucagon action in normal, diabetic and obese human. Israel Journal of Medical Sciences 1975; 11: 528.
59. Rubin J, Reed V, Adir C, Bower J, Klein E. Effect of intraperitoneal insulin on solute kinetics in CAPD: insulin kinetics in CAPD. American Journal of Medical Sciences 1986; 291: 81.
60. Rubin J, Bell AH, Andrews M, Jones Q, Planch A. Intraperitoneal insulin – a dose response curve. Transactions of American Society for Artificial Internal Organs 1989; 35: 17–21.

61. Micossi P, Crostallo M, Librenti MC, Petrella G, Galimberti G, Melandri M, Monti L, Spotti D, Scavini M, deCarlo D, Pozza G. Free-insulin profiles after intraperitoneal, intramuscular and subcutaneous insulin administration. Diabetes Care 1986; 9: 575–8.
62. Schade DS, Eaton RP. The peritoneum – a potential insulin delivery route for a mechanical pancreas. Diabetes Care 1980; 3: 229.
63. Shapiro DJ, Blumenkrantz MJ, Levin SR, Coburn W. Absorption and action of insulin added to peritoneal dialysate in dogs. Nephron 1979; 23: 174.
64. Wideroe T, Smeby LC, Berg KJ, Jorstad S, Svartas IM. Intraperitoneal insulin absorption during intermittent and continuous peritoneal dialysis. Kidney International 1983; 23: 22.
65. Paulsen EP, Courtney JW III, Duckworth WC. Insulin resistance caused by massive degradation of subcutaneous insulin. Diabetes 1979; 28: 640–5.
66. Schade DS, Duckworth WC. In search of the subcutaneous insulin degradation syndrome. N Engl J Med 1986; 315: 147–53.
67. Campbell IC, Kritz H, Najemnic C, Hagmueller G, Irsigler K. Treatment of Type I diabetic with subcutaneous insulin resistance by a totally implantable insulin infusion device ("Infusaid"). Diabetes Res 1984; 1: 83–8.
68. Wood DF, Goodchild K, Guillou P, Thomas DJ, Johnston DG. Management of "brittle diabetes" with a preprogrammable implanted insulin pump delivering intraperitoneal insulin. Br Med J 1990; 301: 1143–4.
69. Albisser AM, Normura M, Greenberg GR, Mcphedran NT. Metabolic control in diabetic dogs treated with pancreatic autotransplants and insulin pumps. Diabetes 1986; 35: 97.
70. Ishida T, Chap Z, Chou J, Lewis RM, Hartley CJ, Entman Mark L, Field JB. Effects of portal and peripheral venous insulin infusion on glucose production and utilization in depancreatized conscious dogs. Diabetes 1984; 33: 984–90.
71. Kryshak EJ, Butler PD, March C, Miller A, Barr D, Polonsky K, Perkins JD, Rizza RA. Pattern of postprandial carbohydrate metabolism and effects of portal and peripheral insulin delivery. Diabetes 1990; 39: 142.
72. Olefsky J. Pathogenesis of insulin resistance and hyperglycemia in non-insulin dependent diabetes mellitus. Am J Med 1985; 75: 1–7.
73. DeFronzo RA. Lilly lecture 1987: the triumvirate: B-cell, muscle, liver: a collusion responsible for NIDDM. Diabetes 1988; 3; 667–87.
74. Campbell PJ, Mandarino LJ, Gerich JE. Quantification of the relative impairment in actions of insulin on hepatic glucose production and peripheral glucose uptake in non-insulin dependent diabetes mellitus. Metabolism 1988; 37: 15–21.
75. Duckworth WC, Saudek CD, Henry RR. Why intraperitoneal delivery of insulin with implantable pump in NIDDM? Diabetes 1992; 41: 657–61.
76. Cullen K, Steinhouse NS, Wearne KL, Welborn TA. Multiple regression analysis of risk factors for cardiovascular and cancer mortality in Busselton, Western Australia: thirteen year study. J chronic Dis 1983; 36: 371–7.
77. Fuller JH, Shipley MJ, Rose G, Jarrett RJ, Heen H. Coronary-heart disease risk and impaired glucose tolerance: the White-Hall study. Lancet 1983; 1: 1372–6.
78. Pyorala K. Relationship of glucose tolerance and plasma insulin to the incidence of coronary heart disease: results from two population studies in Finland. Diabetes Care 1979; 2: 131–41.
79. Shafrir E, Bergman M, Felig P. The endocrine pancreas; diabetes mellitus. In: Felig P, Baxter JD, Broadus AE, Forahman LA (eds), Endocrinology and Metabolism. McGraw-Hill Book Company, New York 1987; pp. 1043–178.
80. Tamborlane WV, Sherwin RS, Genel M, Felig P. Reduction to normal of plasma glucose in juvenile diabetes by subcutaneous administration of insulin with a portable pump. New England Journal of Medicine 1979; 300: 573.
81. Selam JL, Kashyap M, Alberti KGM, Lozano J, Hanna M, Turner D, Jean-Didier N, Chan Eve, Charles MA. Comparison of intraperitoneal and subcutaneous insulin administration on lipids apolipoproteins, fuel metabolites, and hormones in Type I diabetes mellitus. Metabolism 1989; 30: 908–12.
82. Kashyap ML, Gupta AK, Selam JL, Turner D, Wuceitich K, White D, Lozano J, Charles MA. Improvement in reverse cholesterol transport associated with programmable implantable intraperitoneal insulin delivery. (Abstract) Diabetes 1991; 40 (suppl 1): 3A.
83. Ruotolo G, Micossi P, Galimberti G, Librenti, MC, Petrella G, Marcovina S, Pozza G, Howard BV. Effects of intraperitoneal versus subcutaneous insulin administration on lipoprotein metabolism in Type I diabetes. Metabolism 1990; 38: 598.
84. Bagdade JD, Subbaiah PV, Ritter M, Dunn FL. Intraperitoneal insulin delivery normalizes cholesteryl ester transfer in IDDM. (Abstract) Diabetes 1991; 40 (suppl): 269A.
85. Colette C, Pares-Herbute N, Monnier L, Swlam JL, Thomas N, Mirouze J. Effect of different insulin administration modalities on vitamin D metabolism of IDDM patients. Horm Metab Res 1989; 21: 37–41.
86. Saudek CD, Salem JL, Pitt HA, Waxman K, Rubio M, Jean Didier N, Turner D, Fischell RE, Charles MA. A preliminary trial of the programmable implantable medication system for insulin delivery. N Eng J Med 1989; 321: 574–9.
87. Schmitz O. Insulin-mediated glucose uptake in nondialyzed and dialyzed uremic insulin-dependent diabetic subjects. Diabetes 1985; 34: 1152–9.
88. Grefberg N, Danielson BG, Nilsson P, Berne C. Decreasing insulin requirements in CAPD patients given intraperitoneal insulin. The Journal of Diabetic Complications 1987; 1: 16–9.
89. Scalamogna A, Castelnova C, Crepaldi M, Guerra L, Graziani G, Cantaluppi A, Ponticelli C. Incidence of peritonitis in diabetic patients on

CAPD: intraperitoneal vs. subcutaneous insulin therapy. In: Khanna R, Nolph KD, Prowant BF, Twardowski ZJ, Oreopoulos DG (eds), Advances in CAPD. University of Toronto Press 1987; pp 166–70.
90. Wanless IR, Bargman JM, Oreopoulos DG, Vas SI. Subcapsular steatonecrosis in response to peritoneal insulin delivery: a clue to the pathogenesis of steatonecrosis in obesity. Modern Pathol 1989; 2: 69–74.
91. Harrison NA, Rainford DJ. Intraperitoneal insulin and the malignant omentum syndrome. Nephrology Dialysis and Transplantation 1988; 3: 103.
92. Rottembourg J. Peritoneal dialysis in diabetics. In: Nolph KD (ed), Peritoneal Dialysis. Kluwer Academic Publishers, Dordrecht 1988; pp 365–79.
93. Khanna R, Oreopoulos DG. CAPD in patients with diabetes mellitus. In: Gokal R (ed), Continuous Ambulatory Peritoneal Dialysis. Churchill Livingstone, Edinburgh 1986; pp 291–305.
94. Carta Q, Monge L, Triolo G, Dani F, Salomone M, Vercellone A, Vitelli A. Continuous insulin infusion in the management of uremic diabetic patients on dialysis: clinical experience with subcutaneous and intraperitoneal delivery. Diabetic Nephropathy 1987; 4: 83–7.
95. Groop LC, van Bonsdorff MC. Intraperitoneal insulin administration does not promote insulin antibody production in insulin dependent patients on dialysis. Diabetic Nephropathy 1985; 4: 80–2.
97. Henderson IS, Patterson KR, Leung ACT. Decreased intraperitoneal insulin requirements during peritonitis on continuous ambulatory peritoneal dialysis. British Medical Journal 1985; 290: 474.
98. Rottembourg J, El Shahat Y, Agrafiotis A, Thuillier Y, de Groc F, Jacobs C, Legrain M. Continuous ambulatory peritoneal dialysis in insulin dependent diabetics: a 40 months experiment. Kidney International 1983; 23: 40.
99. Nolph KD, Sorkin M, Rubin J, Arfania D, Prowant BF, Fruto L, Kennedy D. Continuous ambulatory peritoneal dialysis: three-year experience at one center. Ann Intern Med 1983; 92: 609–13.
100. Young MA, Nolph KD, Dutton S, Prowant BF. Anti-hypertensive drug requirements in continuous ambulatory peritoneal dialysis. Perit Dial Bull 1984; 5: 85–8.
101. Glasson PH, Favre H, Valloton MB. Response of blood pressure and the renin-angiotensin-aldosterone system to chronic ambulatory peritoneal dialysis in hypertensive end-stage renal failure. Clin Sci 1982; 63: S207–9.
102. Nolph KD, Hano JE, Teschan PE. Peritoneal sodium transport during hypertonic peritoneal dialysis: physiologic mechanisms and clinical implications. Ann Intern Med 1969; 70: 931–41.
103. Nolph KD, Sorkin M, Moore H. Autoregulation of sodium and potassium removal during continuous ambulatory peritoneal dialysis. ASAIO Trans 1980; 6: 334–7.
104. Leenen FHH, Shah P, Boer WH, Khanna R, Oreopoulos DG. Hypotension on CAPD: an approach to treatment. Perit Dial Bull 1983; 3: S33–5.
105. Rottembourg J, Issad B, Poignet JL, Stripoli P, Balducci A, Slama G, Gahl GM. Residual renal function and control of blood glucose levels in insulin-dependent diabetic patients treated by CAPD. In: Keen H, Legrain M (eds), Prevention and Treatment of Diabetic Nephropathy. MTP Press Ltd., Lancaster, Boston 1983; pp 339–359.
106. Cancarini GC, Brunori G, Camerini C, Brasa S, Manili L, Maiorca R. Renal function recovery and maintenance of residual diuresis in CAPD and hemodialysis. Perit Dial Bull 1986; 6: 77–9.
107. Lysaght M, Vonesh E, Ibels L, Lindholm B, Nolph KD, Pollock C, Prowant B, Farrell P. Decline of residual renal function in hemodialysis and CAPD patients; a risk adjusted growth function analysis. (Abstract) Nephrol Dial Transplant 1989; 4: 499.
108. Lysaght M, Pollock C, Schindaglm K, Ibeles L, Farrell P. The relevance of urea kinetic modeling to CAPD. (Abstract) ASAIO Trans 1988; 34: 84.
109. Slingeneyer A, Mion C. Five year follow-up of 155 patients treated by CAPD in European-French speaking countries. (Abstract) Perit Dial Int 1989; 7 (suppl 1): 176.
110. Rottembourg J, Issad B, Allouache M, Jacobs C. Recovery of renal function in patients treated by CAPD. In: Khanna R, Nolph KD, Prowant BF, Twardowski ZJ, Oreopoulos DG (eds), Advances in Peritoneal Dialysis. University of Toronto Press, Toronto 1989; pp 63–6.
111. Michael C, Bindi P, Kareche M, Mignon F. Renal function on recovery on chronic dialysis: what is best, CAPD or hemodialysis? (Abstract) Nephrol Dial Transplant 1989; 4: 499–500.
112. Nunan To, Wing AJ, Brunner FB, Selwood NH. Native kidneys sometimes recover after prolonged dialysis and transplantation. In: Giovanetti C (ed), Proceedings of the Vth International Capri Conference on Uremia. Capri 1986; pp 132–49.
113. Nolph KD. Is residual renal failure preserved better with CAPD than hemodialysis? AKF Nephrology Letter 1990; 7: 1–4.
114. Shekkarie MA, Port FK, Wolfe RA, Guire K, Humphrys R, Van Amburg G, Gerguson CW. Recovery from end-stage renal disease. AM J Kidney Dis 1990; 15: 61–5.
115. Mourad G, Mimran A, Mion C. Recovery of renal function in patients with accelerated malignant nephrosclerosis on maintenance dialysis with management of blood pressure by captopril. Nephron 1985; 41: 166–9.
116. Wauters JP, Brunner HR. Discontinuation of chronic hemodialysis after control of arterial hypertension: long-term follow-up. Proc Eur Dial Transplant Assoc 1982; 19: 182–6.
117. Herbelin A, Nguyen AT, Zingraft J, Urena P, Descamps-Latscha B. Influence of uremia and hemodialysis on circulating interleukin-1 and tumor necrosis factor alpha. Kidney Int 1990; 37: 116–25.
118. Cotran RS, Pober JS. Effects of cytokines on

vascular endothelium; their role in vascular and immune injury. Kidney Int 1989; 35: 969–75.
119. Shah AH. Role of reactive oxygen metabolites in experimental glomerular disease. Kidney Int 1989; 35: 1093–106.
120. Rottembourg J, Bellio P, Maiga K, Remaoun M, Rousselie F, Legrain M. Visual function, blood pressure and blood glucose in diabetic patients undergoing continuous ambulatory peritoneal dialysis. Proc Europ Dial Transpl Ass 1984; 21: 330–4.
121. Kohner E, Chahal P. Retinopathy in diabetic nephropathy. In: Prevention and Treatment of Diabetic Nephropathy. MTP Ltd, Lancaster, pp 191–196.
122. Diaz-Buxo JA, Burgess WP, Greenman M, Chandler JT, Farmer CD, Walker PJ. Visual function in diabetic patients undergoing dialysis: comparison of peritoneal and hemodialysis. Int J Artif Organs 1984; 7: 257–62.
123. Zimmerman SW, Johnson CA, O'Brien M. Survival of diabetic patients on continuous ambulatory peritoneal dialysis for over five years. Peritoneal Dialysis Bulletin 1987; 7: 26.
124. Dombros N Oren A, Marliss EB, Anserson GH, Stern AN, Khanna R, Pehl J, Brades L, Roddell H, Libeil BS, Oreopoulos DG. Plasma amino acids profiles and amino acid losses in patients undergoing CAPD. Perit Dial Bull 1982; 2: 37–42.
125. Norbeck H. Lipid abnormalities in continuous ambulatory peritoneal dialysis patients. In: Legrain M (ed), Continuous Ambulatory Peritoneal Dialysis. Excerpta Medica, Amsterdam 1979; pp 298–301.
126. Khanna R, Brechenridge C, Roncari D, Digenis G, Oreopoulos DG. Lipid abnormalities in patients undergoing continuous ambulatory peritoneal dialysis. Peritoneal Dialysis Bulletin 1983; 3: 13–6.
127. Gokal R, Ramos JM, McGurk JG, Ward MK, Kerr DNS. Hyperlipidemia in patient on continuous ambulatory peritoneal dialysis. In: Gahl G, Kessel M, Nolph KD (eds), Advances in Peritoneal Dialysis. Excerpta Medica, Amsterdam 1981; pp 430–3.
128. Moncrief JW, Pyle WK, Simon P, Popovich RP. Hypertriglyceridemia, diabetes mellitus and insulin administration in patient undergoing continuous ambulatory peritoneal dialysis. In: Moncrief J, Popovich R (eds), CAPD Update. Masson, New York 1981; pp 143–65.
129. Sorge F, Castro LA, Nagel A, Kessel M. Serum glucose, insulin, growth hormone, free fatty acids and lipids responses to high carbohydrate and to high fat isocaloric diets in patients with chronic, non-nephrotic renal failure. Horm Metab Res 1975; 7: 118–27.
130. Sanfelippo ML, Swenson RS, Reavan GM. Response of plasma triglycerides to dietary change in patients on hemodialysis. Kidney Int 1978; 14: 180–6.
131. Cattran DC, Steiner GS, Fenton SSA, Ampil M. Dialysis hyperlipemia: response to dietary manipulations. Clin Nephrol 1980; 13: 177–82.

132. Ramos JM, Heaton A, McGurk GJ, Ward MK, Kerr DNS. Sequential changes in serum lipids and their subfractions in patients receiving continuous ambulatory peritoneal dialysis. Nephron 1983; 353: 20–3.
133. Nolph KD, Ryan KL, Prowant B, Twardowski Z. A cross sectional assessment of serum vitamin D and triglyceride concentrations in a CAPD population. Perit Dial Bull 1984; 4: 232–37.
134. Lindholm B, Norbeck HE. Serum lipids and lipoproteins during continuous ambulatory peritoneal dialysis. Acta Med Scan 1986; 220: 143–51.
135. Heaton A, Johnston DG, Haigh JW, Ward MK, Alberti KGMM, Kerr DNS. Twenty-four hour hormonal and metabolic profiles in uraemic patients before and during treatment with continuous ambulatory peritoneal dialysis. Clin Sci 1985; 69: 449–57.
136. Keusch G, Bammatter F, Mordasini R, Binswanger U. Serum lipoprotein concentrations during continuous ambulatory peritoneal dialysis (CAPD). In: Gahl GM, Kessel M, Nolph KD (eds), Advances in Peritoneal Dialysis. Excerpta Medica, Amsterdam 1981; pp 427–9.
137. Lindholm B, Karlander SG, Norbeck HE, Fürst P, Bergström J. Carbohydrate and lipid metabolism in CAPD patients. In: Atkins R, Thomson N, Farrell P (eds), Peritoneal Dialysis. Churchill Livingstone, Edinburgh 1981; pp 198–210.
138. Lindholm B, Alvestrand A, Fürst P, Karlander SSG, Norbeck HE, Ahlberg M, Tranaeus A, Bergrström J. Metabolic effects of continuous ambulatory peritoneal dialysis. Proc EDTA 1980; 17: 283–9.
139. Lindholm B, Karlander SG, Norbeck HE, Bergström J. Glucose and lipid metabolism in peritoneal dialysis. In: La Greca G, Biasoli S, Ronco C (eds), Peritoneal Dialysis. Wichtig Editore 1982; pp 219–230.
140. Kagan A, Barkhayim Y, Schafer Z, Fainaru M. Low level of plasma HDL in CAPD patients may be due to HDL loss in dialysate. (Abstract) Peritoneal Dialysis International 1988; A: 79.
141. Roncari DAK, Breckenridge WC, Khanna R, Oreopoulos DG. Rise in high-density lipoprotein-cholesterol in some patients treated with CAPD. Perit Dial Bull 1987; 1: 136–37.
142. Breckenridge WC, Roncari DAK, Khanna R, Oreopoulos DG. The influence of continuous ambulatory peritoneal dialysis on plasma lipoproteins. Atherosclerosis 1982; 45: 249–58.
143. Tuskamoto Y, Okubo M, Yoneda T, Marumo F, Nakamura H. Effects of a polyunsaturated fatty acid-rich diet on serum lipids in patients with chronic renal failure. Nephrol 1982; 31: 236–41.
144. Vas SI. Peritonitis. In: Nolph KD (ed), Peritoneal Dialysis. Kluwer Academic Publishers, Dordrecht 1989; pp 261–88.
145. Nolph KD, Cutler SJ, Steinberg SM, Novak JW. Special studies from the NIH USA CAPD Registry. Peritoneal Dialysis Bulletin 1986; 6: 28–35.
146. Rottembourg J, Brouard R, Issad B, Allouache M, Jacobs C. Prospective randomized study about Y

146. [...] connectors in CAPD patients. In: Khanna R, Nolph KD, Prowant BF, Twardowski ZJ, Oreopoulos DG (eds), Advances in Continuous Ambulatory Peritoneal Dialysis. Peritoneal Dialysis Bulletin Inc, Toronto 1987; pp 107–13.
147. Madden MA, Zimmerman SW, Simpson DP. CAPD in diabetes mellitus – the risks and benefits of intraperitoneal insulin. (Abstract) Am J Nephrol 1982; 2: 133.
148. Wing AF, Broyer M, Brunner FP, Brynger H, Challah S, Donckerwolcke RA, Gretz N, Jacobs C, Kramer P, Selwood NH. Combined report on regular dialysis and transplantation in Europe 1982. Proc Eur Dial Transplant Assoc-ERA 1983; 20: 5–75.
149. Williams C, University of Toronto Collaborative Dialysis Group. CAPD in Toronto – an overview. Peritoneal Dialysis Bulletin 1983; 35: 2.
150. U.S. Renal Data System. USRDS 1990 Annual Data Report, The National Institute of Health, National Institute of Diabetes and Digestive and Kidney Diseases, Bethesda, MD, August 1991.
151. Nelson CB, Port FK, Wolfe RA, Guire KE. Dialysis patient survival: evaluation of CAPD vs. HD using 3 techniques. (Abstract) Perit Dial Int 1992; 12 (suppl 1): 144.
152. Port KF, Held PJ, Nolph KD, Turenne MN, Wolfe RA. Risk of peritonitis and technique failure by CAPD technique: a national study. Kidney Int: (in press).
153. Keshaviah P, Nolph KD, Prowant BF, Moore H, Ponferrada L, Van Stone J, Twardowski ZJ, Khanna R. Defining adequacy of CAPD with urea kinetics. In: Khanna R, Nolph KD, Prowant BF, Twardowski ZJ, Oreopoulos DG (eds), Advance in Peritoneal Dialysis. University of Toronto Press, Toronto 1990; pp 173–7.
154. Lameire N (Personal communication).
155. Faller B, Marichal JD. Loss of ultrafiltration in CAPD. Clinical data. In: Gahl G, Kessel M, Nolph KD (eds), Advances in Peritoneal Dialysis. Excerpta Medica, Amsterdam 1981; pp 227–32.
156. Slingeneyer A, Mion C, Mourad G, Canaud B, Faller B, Beraud JJ. Progressive sclerosing peritonitis: a late and severe complication of maintenance peritoneal dialysis. Transactions of the American Society of Artificial Internal Organs 1983; 29: 633.
157. Rottembourg J, Brouard R, Issad B, Allouache M, Ghali B, Bourjemaa A. Role of acetate in loss of ultrafiltration during CAPD. In: Berlyne GM, Giovannetti S (eds), Contribution to Nephrology. S. Karger AG, Switzerland 1987; p 197.
158. Nolph KD, Stolta M, Maher JF. Altered peritoneal permeability in patients with systematic vasculitis. Annals of Internal Medicine 1973; 78: 891.
159. Twardowski ZJ, Nolph KD, Khanna R, Prowant BF, Ryan LP, Moore HL, Neilsen P. Peritoneal equilibration test. Peritoneal Dialysis Bulletin 1987; 7: 138.
160. Hallett MD, Kush RD, Lysaght MJ, Farrell PC. The stability and kinetics of peritoneal mass transfer. In: Nolph KD (ed), Peritoneal Dialysis. Kluwer Academic Publishers, Dordrecht 1989; pp 380–8.
161. Struijk DG, Krediet RT, Koomen GCM, Hoek FJ, Boeschoten EW, Reijden HJ, Arisz L. Functional characteristics of the peritoneal membrane in long-term continuous ambulatory peritoneal dialysis. Nephron 1991; 59: 213–20.
162. Gilmore J, Wu G, Khanna R, Oreopoulos DG. Long term CAPD. Peritoneal Dialysis Bulletin 1985; 5: 112.
163. Peters C, Sutherland D, Simmon R, Fryd DS, Najarian JS. Patients and graft survival in amputated vs non-amputated diabetic primary renal allograft recipients. Transplantation 1981; 32: 498–503.
164. Joint Working Party. Renal failure in diabetes in UK: deficient provision of care in 1985. Diabetic Med 1988; 5: 79–84.
165. Bailey TS, Yu H, Royfield E. Patterns of test examination in a Diabetic clinic. Am J Med 1985; 78: 371–4.
166. Thomson FJ, Veves A, Ashe H et al. A team approach to diabetes foot-care – the Manchester experience. The Foot 1991; 2: 75–82.
167. Fernando D, Hutchison A, Veves A, Gokal R, Boulton A. Risk factors for non-ischaemic foot ulceration in Diabetic Nephropathy. Diabetic Med 1991; 8; 1–4.
168. Boulton AJM, Gokal R, Marion EA. The formation of a diabetic nephropathy clinic. Report of the first six months. Postgrad Med J 1988; 64: 84–6.
169. Mistry CD, Gokal R, Peers E, MIDAS Study Group. Multicentre trial of Dextrin 20 in CAPD patients. Kidney Int: 1994 (in press).

22 Peritoneal dialysis in the elderly patient

ALLEN R. NISSENSON

1. Introduction 661
2. Demographics of ESRD in the elderly 661
3. ESRD modality selection in the elderly 663
4. Medical advantages of CPD 665
5. Psychosocial advantages of CPD 666
6. Disadvantages of CPD in the elderly 666
7. CPD in the elderly: current practice and outcome 667
   7.1. Mortality 667
   7.2. Morbidity 670
8. Adequacy of dialysis in the elderly 671
9. Quality of life 671
10. Alternative approaches to CPD in the elderly 674
11. Ethical considerations 675
    11.1. Withdrawal from dialysis 675
References 675

1. Introduction

Although many view *"elderly"* as *". . . being past middle age . . ."* or *". . . characteristic of later life . . ."* [1, 2], this lack of precision has made it difficult to assess the current literature on peritoneal dialysis, as well as other medical procedures, in older patients. It has become traditional in most studies to call patients 65 years old and older "elderly", but this approach is neither uniform nor entirely rational [2]. The "young-old" are likely to be functional mentally and physically, to live at home, to have family or friend support, and to have less medical co-morbidity than the "old-old". The latter often live in institutional settings, may be demented, malnourished, and suffer from serious non-renal medical conditions. Clearly the approach to these two groups, when end-stage-renal disease (ESRD) develops, would be vastly different. If one focuses on the over-75 year old group it is clear that this population is expected to grow dramatically-worldwide into the next century [3]. With this caveat regarding the definition of *"elderly"*, the available data on the use of peritoneal dialysis in older patients will be reviewed.

2. Demographics of ESRD in the elderly

The general population in the United States and in many other parts of the world is aging, placing increasing demands on physicians to understand the special needs of this patient group [4]. It is projected that 21% of the U.S. population will be 65 years old or older by the year 2030. In addition, the incidence of ESRD in the United States is increasing most rapidly in the oldest patients, where the annualized change in incidence from 1985–87 to 1988–90 was 14% for patients over 75 years old and 9.9% for those 65 to 74 [5] (See Figs. 1, 2). Similar trends have been noted worldwide (Table 1, Fig. 3). The prevalence of peritoneal dialysis utilization worldwide is 17%, similar to the prevalence in the U.S. [6]. In the elderly patient, however, chronic peritoneal dialysis (CPD) is used less frequently in the U.S., with only 9% of patients receiving this form of ESRD treatment. This is in marked contrast to other countries where CPD is utilized more frequently than hemodialysis (CHD) is in older patients. This underutilization of CPD in the elderly in the U.S. is particularly ironic considering the results of two recent studies. Mattern *et al.* surveyed physicians in North Carolina, Southern California, and Australia and New Zealand to determine physician attitudes toward various ESRD modalities [7]. Participants were presented with case scenarios and asked to choose which of two ESRD modalities would be preferable for the given clinical situation. The questions were repeated with the same cases and permutations of pairs of all available ESRD modalities including the various forms of dialysis and transplantation. In all three areas of the world physicians chose home CPD as the dialytic treatment of choice for patients over 60 years old (Fig. 4).

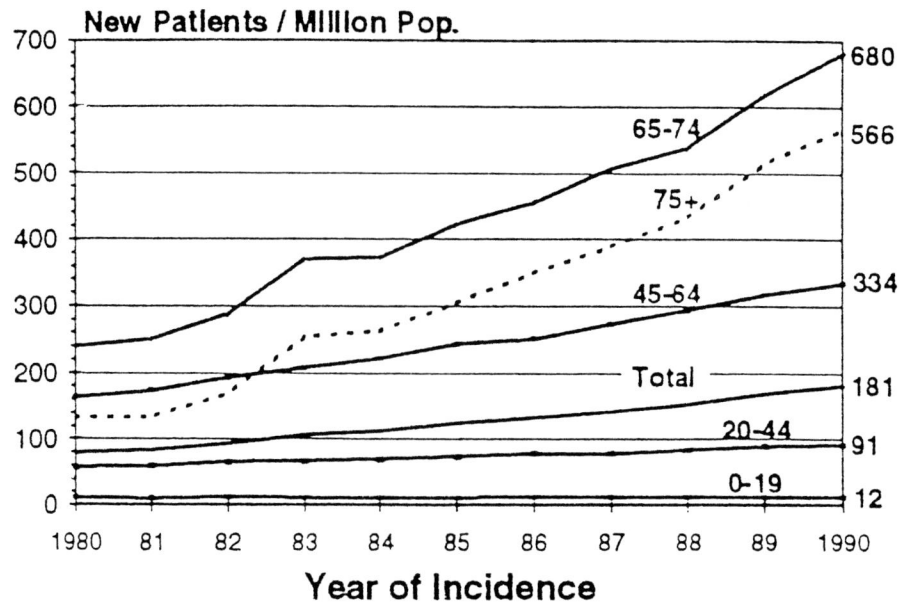

Figure 1. Incidence per million population of treated ESRD by age group, 1980–1990 in the United States.

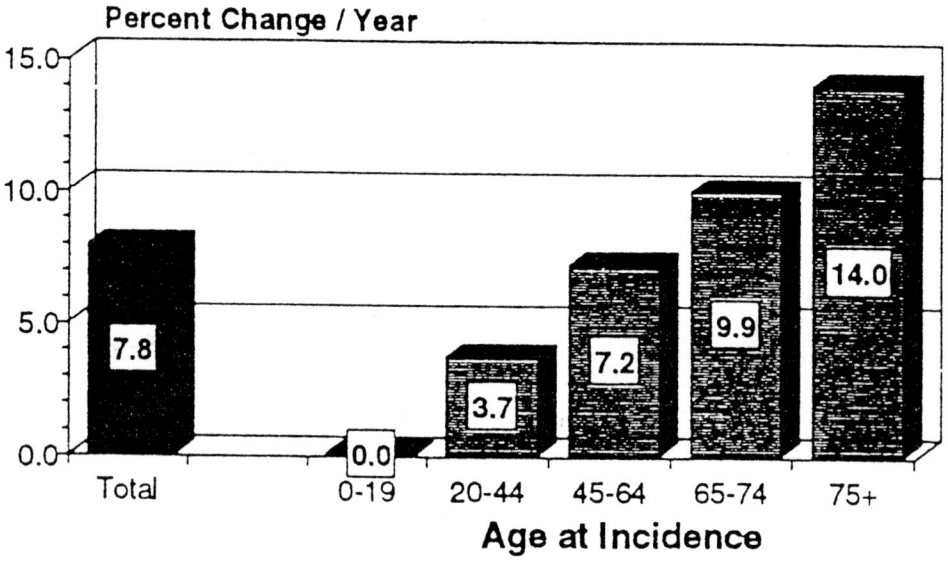

Figure 2. Annualized change in treated ESRD incidence by age (adjusted for sex and race), 1985–1987 to 1988–1990 in the United States.

Despite this, most patients in these areas received in-center hemodialysis (Table 2). A recent survey by Gentile *et al.* of physicians from 11 dialysis centers that utilized CPD in an average of 35% of patients noted that CPD offered better cardiovascular stability than CHD, avoided vascular access concerns, was well tolerated because of slow solute removal, and permitted an independent life style [8].

Again, at these centers, only 27.9% of elderly patients were placed on CPD. Although clearly some "old-old" patients are incapable of performing peritoneal dialysis at home, or have no helper, thus precluding this modality, the current utilization rate seems lower than can be explained on this basis. The role of non-medical factors in modality selection has been studied recently including reim-

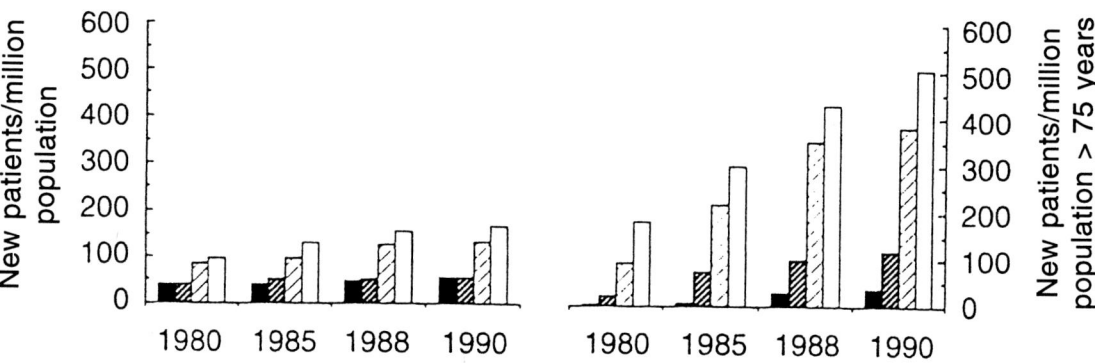

Figure 3. Incidence rates per million population of treated ESRD, 1980–1990. Left hand panel shows data for all new patients and right hand panel data for patients over 75 years old. Reprinted from reference [3], with permission. Symbols are: (■) Australia – New Zealand; (▨) France; (▱) Japan; (□) USA.

bursement, physician bias, educational deficits (physician, nurses, patient), resource availability, social mores, and cultural habits [9]. Clearly these factors in part determine modality selection worldwide, but how they apply specifically to the elderly patient remains to be clarified.

An important question to consider in the treatment of elderly ESRD patients is: What is the life expectancy of such individuals and how is this impacted by ESRD? Data from the USRDS suggests a life expectancy of three and one half years for patients age 65 who started dialysis in 1987, roughly one fifth of that anticipated for a 65 year old without ESRD [10]. The impact of ESRD on life expectancy decreases with increasing age, however, and is small for the older age groups. Of greater importance than life expectancy, however, is the fact that quality of life can be satisfying in these patients, thus supporting the continued offering of ESRD care to this group. Rationing dialysis on the basis of age alone is not supportable based on the currently available outcome and quality of life data.

3. ESRD modality selection in the elderly (see Table 3)

When choosing a dialysis modality for an elderly patient several factors must be considered including the physiologic changes that occur with aging, specific medical conditions that are common in the elderly, and medical and psychosocial advantages and disadvantages of the modality chosen [11, 12]. There are a number of physiologic changes that occur with aging that might impact on the choice of

Table 1. Forecast and relative increase (%) in the number of inhabitants in four industrialized countries.

	1990		2000		2020	
	Total	>75 y/o	Total	>75 y/o	Total	>75 y/o
Australia/ N. Zealand	20.3	0.8	22.5 (10.8%)	1.1 (37.5%)	26.4 (30.0%)	1.6 (100%)
Japan	123.5	5.6	128.5 (4.0%)	7.6 (35.7%)	129.0 (4.0%)	14.0 (150%)
US	249.2	13.1	266.1 (6.7%)	16.1 (22.9%)	294.7 (18.2%)	20.4 (55.7%)
Western Europe	156.9	10.5	159.4 (1.6%)	11.0 (4.7%)	157.6 (0.4%)	14.1 (34.3%)

Total population and population >75 y/o per million.
* Modified from reference [3], with permission.

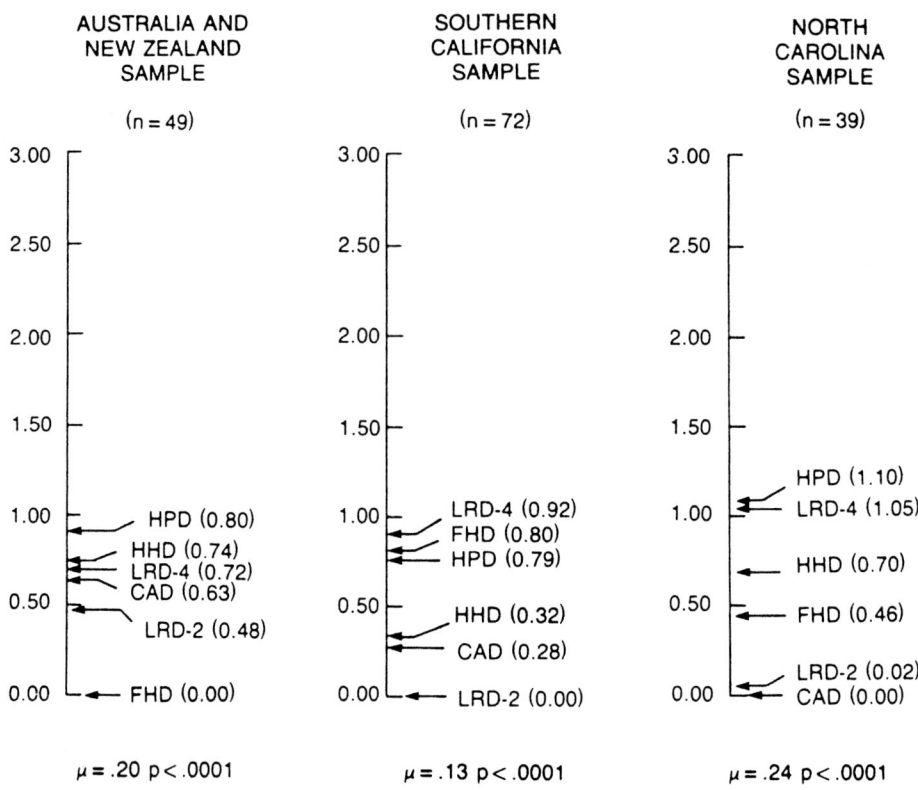

Figure 4. Treatment preferences of nephrologists from three regions of the world for patients over age 60. HPD = home peritoneal dialysis; HHD = home hemodialysis; LRD = living related donor transplantation; CAD = cadaver donor transplantation; FHD = facility hemodialysis. The higher the score on the analog scale, the more often this modality was chosen. Reprinted from reference [7], with permission.

Table 2. Distribution of patients over the age of 60 on the three dialysis modalities in 1985*.

		Aust-NZ		S CA		NC	
		All patients	60+	All patients	60+	All patients	60+
FHD	N	1,098	321	5,457	2,482	1,714	714
	%	43	46	92	95	74	79
HPD	N	762	255	426	112	478	157
	%	30	36	7	4	20	17
HHD	N	692	125	82	12	138	37
	%	27	18	1	<1	6	4
Total		2,552	701	5,965	2,606	2,330	908

* Modified from reference 7, with permission. Aust-NZ = Australian/New Zealand; S CA = Southern California; NC = North Carolina; FHD = facility hemodialysis; HPD = home peritoneal dialysis; HHD = home hemodialysis.

an ESRD modality for an elderly patient [12]. Diminished cardiovascular reserve, clinical or subclinical, is common in this population [13]. Both atherosclerosis and the "normal" impaired baroceptor function of aging may contribute to this phenomenon. Thus, orthostatic hypotension and poor compensatory response to fluid removal with dialysis may occur [14]. Although the use of bicarbonate HD solutions and ultrafiltration-controlled delivery machines have lessened this concern, it is still significant [15]. In addition, cardiac arrhythmias frequently occur during or shortly after HD with its rapid fluid and electrolyte shifts [16]. The frequency of arrhythmias is much less with CPD [17]. Second, there may be a slow deterioration of pulmonary function with aging. Underlying pulmonary disease may preclude a form of ESRD therapy that compromises oxygenation further. Third, the elderly may have impaired delayed hypersensitivity, aggravated by uremia, which may increase their susceptibility to infection. Fourth, the elderly have a number of metabolic characteristics that might impact on modality selection. These include chronic bone loss from osteoporosis, altered protein metabolism, a high rate of malnutrition, a tendency to carbohydrate intolerance and altered metabolism of a variety of drugs. Clearly some of these physiologic characteristics favor CHD, while others favor CPD. Additional benefits of CPD over HD for this group include better correction of brain electrophysiological and cognitive function abnormalities [18], avoidance of vascular access (the gretest source of morbidity in this group when on HD), and an overall superior quality of life [19]. All need to be considered and asessed when choosing a dialytic modality for an elderly patient.

There are a number of health concerns that are common in the elderly that might interfere with the success of CPD. The elderly may be unable, because of dementia, depression or poor social support systems, to perform CPD themselves. To provide this modality, therefore, would require a family member or helper, either of which might be problematic. The elderly are prone to constipation and have a high incidence of chronic diverticulitis. Constipation may prevent adequate catheter drainage, while diverticulitis may be difficult to detect in patients on CPD and confound the diagnosis of peritonitis. Finally, the generally poor tissue turgor and impaired wound healing seen in the elderly may lead to a higher rate of dialysate leaks and hernia formation in this group.

4. Medical advantages of CPD (see Table 4)

There are a number of putative medical advantages of CPD in the elderly patient [11]. First, for those patients with cardiovascular instability, fluid balance is well maintained with few complications with CPD. The continuous slow ultrafiltration that accompanies CPD is generally well tolerated except in the occasional patient with chronic hypotension. Secondly, the anemia of chronic remal failure is often minimal in patients on CPD [20]. This is particularly important in the elderly with underlying

Table 3. Characteristics of the elderly that impact on ESRD modality selection.*

	Favors HD	Favors PD
MEDICAL		
Diminished cardiovascular reserve		+++
Cardiac arrhythmias		++
Decreased pulmonary function	+	
Immunodeficiency		
Bone loss	+	
Carbohydrate intolerance		
Malnutrition	++	+
Bowel dysfunction	+	
Poor wound healing	+	
Access complications		+++
Impaired cognitive function		++
PSYCHOSOCIAL		
Inability to perform self-dialysis	+++	
Impaired quality of life		++
Isolation	++	
Depression	+	
Impaired functional capacity	++	
Lack of self-esteem		++

* Reprinted from reference [1], with permission.

Table 4. Potential medical advantages of CPD in the elderly*.

- Maintenance of hemodynamic stability during dialysis
- Improvement of anemia with low EPO doses (if any)**
- Control of hypertension with few medications (if any)**
- Avoidance of cardiac arrhythmias
- Improvement of nutritional status
- Preservation of renal function**
- Ability to use intraperitoneal insulin in diabetics**
- Enhanced B-2 microglobulin removal**
- Lack of need for vascular access**

* Modified from reference [2], with permission.
** Advantages for younger as well as elderly patients.

atherosclerotic heart disease. In addition, for those patients who are anemic, low dose rhu-Epo therapy compared to hemodialysis, is generally effective, minimizing the cost of this expensive substance [21]. Third, CPD may control hypertension with few anti-hypertensive medications required in the majority of patients [22, 23]. This would be particularly useful in the elderly where hypertension is poorly tolerated and anti-hypertensive medications may have unacceptable side effects. Recent data specifically targeting the elderly population suggest that this benefit of CPD may be overstated [24]. Maiorca studied 15 elderly patients on CPD and compared them to 15 on HD using continuous 24-hour blood pressure monitoring, in the latter during a short-interval interdialytic day [24]. No differences in systolic or diastolic blood pressure were found. In addition, in a larger group of elderly patients followed from 1986–1991, there were no differences in the percentages who become normotensive nor in the number of antihypertensives needed in those on such medications between CPD and HD patients. At least in the elderly, this advantage of CPD is questionable.

The elderly, many of whom have underlying cardiovascular disease, are more susceptible than younger patients to the effects of cardiac arrhythmias, as mentioned above. The detrimental cardiovascular impact of individual hemodialysis treatments in the elderly, for the reasons described, is clear. Controversy continues, however, on the long term cardiovascular effects of these two modalities. Some studies have shown a decrease in intraventricular septum and posterior wall mass and in left ventricular mass index and dilatation in patients on CPD [25, 26]. Others, however, have been unable to confirm these findings. On the other hand, there is little controversy concerning the relative frequency of arrhythmias in patients on HD compared to those on CPD. Using continuous 48 hour Holter monitoring, Timio *et al.* detected supraventricular as well as ventricular arrhythmias (including bigeminy), more frequently in patients on HD and correlated the arrhythmias in both groups with blood norepinephrine levels [27]. Ventricular tachycardia was only seen in patients on HD.

Finally, in the malnourished patient, the absorption of intraperitoneal glucose may be an important source of calories [28]. The prevalence and severity of malnutrition in elderly CPD patients is still undergoing intensive study [24, 29]. A recent cross-sectional study in 8 centers in Italy showed that in patients over the age of 67.4, the percentage with malnutrition was greater for those on HD compared to those on CPD [24]. In a longitudinal study of 11 HD and 22 CPD patients evaluated over 14 months, the percentage with malnutrition decreased in both groups over time and NPCR and serum albumin remained unchanged and similar in both groups [24]. These findings are in contrast to others that have shown a progressive worsening of nutritional status over time in CPD patients [30, 31].

Additional medical advantages of CPD are important in elderly and younger patients alike. These include preservation of residual renal function [32], ability to use intraperitoneal insulin in diabetics [33], enhanced B-2 microglobulin removal compared to CHD [34, 35], and lack of need for vascular access.

5. Psychosocial advantages of CPD

There have been a number of studies of psychosocial adaptation in patients undergoing dialysis. When matched pairs of patients are studied, those on CPD have a higher quality of life, lower illness and modality related stress and lesser mood disturbances than those on CHD [36, 37]. Dialysis modality, therefore, seems to be an independent factor in determining the quality of life of ESRD patients. The elderly, however, have poorer psychosocial adaptation than younger patients on either CHD or CPD [38]. Despite this, the elderly on dialysis often have a high level of life satisfaction, and psychosocial functioning [39, 40]. Some have suggested that long-term success of CPD in this group is dependent on a patient's psychosocial adaptation [41]. In addition, the likelihood of dropout from CPD might be predictable based on pre-CPD psychosocial characteristics [41].

6. Disadvantages of CPD in the elderly

There are contraindications to CPD which apply to elderly as well as younger patients [42, 43]. These include inadequate peritoneal membrane function, hernias that cannot be repaired, and inability to insert a chronic peritoneal access. Relative contraindications include chronic ostomies, recurrent pancreatitis, chronic back pain, recent aortic prosthesis placement, severe peripheral vascular disease and recurrent diverticulitis. In reality, very few patients are excluded from CPD for these reasons.

There are potential disadvantages of CPD in the elderly which should be considered. If a patient is not mentally or physically capable of performing CPD, a family member or helper may be required which adds an additional burden to the technique. Secondly, if peritonitis occurs, the pain, malnutrition and associated in-hospital time may be less well tolerated in the elderly than in younger patients. Thirdly, in the malnourished patient CPD may exacerbate, rather than improve this situation [44, 45]. Anorexia and nausea as well as protein loss in dialysate may contribute to this. Fourth, a higher frequency of hernias and fluid leaks might occur in this population and clearly would be undesirable [46]. Finally, if chronic hypotension occurs, because of poor salt and fluid intake and ongoing ultrafiltration, vascular ischemic syndromes, particularly of the lower extremities, might develop [47].

In summary, there are patient and age specific medical and psychosocial concerns which must be considered when placing an elderly patient on CPD which will impact on the success of this modality.

7. CPD in the elderly: current practice and outcome

7.1. Mortality

CPD has been widely applied to elderly patients throughout the world. Considerable experience with this modality has been published from the United States, the United Kingdom, Italy, Canada, Germany and elsewhere [15, 48–63]. The total experience exceeds 8000 patients in these series (Table 5). There is a predominance of men in this group but this is not different from that seen in younger CPD patients. Outcome of CPD is remarkably similar around the world despite the varying patient selection criteria, management strategies for complications, connector technology used, and availability of alternative ESRD modalities (Table 6). Age is clearly an important risk factor for mortality. Five-year survival (by actuarial analysis) of the elderly on CPD exceeded 35% in only one series [53]. The cause of death was usually cardiovascular or cerebrovascular in younger and older patients, although cachexia and malnutrition may be more common contributing factors in the elderly [64].

There is very little variation in outcome of elderly patients on CPD compared to HD in different parts of the world, although survival is somewhat less on both modalities in older series. Very few of these studies comparing modalities,

Table 5. CPD in the elderly – demographics*.

Reference	No. of patients	Males (%)	Females (%)	Etiology of renal disease (%)**		
				DM	NS	GN
Nolph et al. [48]	7791	55	45	–	–	
Gokal [49]	192	–	–			
Segolino et al. [51]	514	57	43	11	19	9
Posen et al. [50]	1218	–	–	19	29	15
Nissenson et al. [52]	492	57	43	19	31	25
Nebel and Finke [53]	26	–	–	42	12	19
Diaz-Buxo et al. [85]	37	42	58	35	29	13
Benevent et al. [54]	39	64	36	8	15	31
Piccoli et al. [15]	134	–	–	?	31	5
Walls [55]	113	–	–	5	16	11
Garcia-Fontan [59]	20	45	55	10	10	–
Suh [61]	30	60	40	20	7	20
Acchiardo [60]	36	50	50	25	42	14
Issad [62]	109	66	34	12	12	28
Verbeelen [63]	20	NA	NA	40	25	15

* Modified from reference [2], with permission.
** DM = Diabetic nephropathy; NS = Nephrosclerosis (includes hypertensive nephrosclerosis and angiosclerosis); GN = Chronic glomerulonephritis.

however, have considered co-morbid factors and their impact on survival. For example, Benevent et al. reported on 70 patients treated in Lemoges, France from 1980–1988 [54]. CPD patients had twice the number of co-morbid conditions as those on HD, but survival was the same in both groups. Similarly, Walls [55] reported equivalent survival in HD and CPD patients despite a "greater number of patients with a "poor prognosis" condition ... in the CAPD group." More recently, Garcia-Fontan et al. described their experiences with 59 elderly patients (CAPD, N = 20; HD, N = 39) dialyzed in Spain [59]. Survival was not statistically different in the two groups although CAPD patients had more associated risk factors, worse lipid profiles, and better control of anemia and neuropathy compared to those on HD. Acchiardo et al. reported on 50 HD and 36 CAPD over the age of 65 dialyzed between

Table 6. Outcome of dialysis in the elderly**.

Reference	Type of dialysis	Patient survival (%) 3 YR	5 YR	Technique survival (%) 3 YR	5 YR	Comments
Nolph et al. [48]	CPD	–	–	–	–	Risk of death 3.23 times greater than those <60 y/o
Gokal [49]	CPD	–	25	–	34	6 year results
Segoloni et al. [51]	CPD	50	16	75	65	
Posen et al. [50]	CPD	38	15	60	52	
	HD	38	15	80	78	
Nissenson et al. [52]	CPD	52	35	47	27	
Nebel & Fink [53]	CPD	40	40*	–	–	*42 month results
Benevent et al. [54]	CPD	35	–	–	–	
	HD	35	–	–	–	
Piccoli et al. [15]	CPD	43	28	68.7	–	24 month results (Patients aged 65–74)
	HD (Bicarbonate)	56	–	65.3	–	
	HD (Acetate)	43	30*	25.6	–	*48 month results
Walls [55]	CPD	49	35*	–	–	*4 year results
	HD	49	–	–	–	
Tapson et al. [56]	CPD and HD Combined	57	53	–	–	
Jogler & Saade [58]	CPD	70	–	–	–	
	HD	30	–	–	–	
Garcia-Fontan [59]	CPD	30	–	75	–	
	HD	50	–	78	–	
Suh [61]	CPD	50	17*	–	–	*4 year results
Acchiardo [60]	CPD	68*	28	–	–	*2 year results
	HD	59*	29	–	–	
Issad [62]	PD	–	–	22	9	
Verbeelen [63]	CPD	20	12*	–	–	*4 year results
	HD	52	28	–	–	

** Modified from reference [1], with permission.

1983 and 1990 in Tennessee [60]. Similar patient survival was noted at three, five and seven years. Joglar and Saade reported on 50 patients 65 years or older treated with CPD or HD in Puerto Rico [58]. Survival at 36 months was better for patients on CPD compared to those on HD, although the latter patients had more "complicating factors" that might have affected outcome. None of these studies or several others (64–68) used statistical techniques to adjust for these differences in patient characteristics. While suggesting that survival on CPD and HD are similar, these studies are difficult to interpret since patient selection factors or comorbidities do have an impact on the results.

Several studies are now available comparing survival on HD and CPD using the Cox proportional hazards model to adjust the results for patient characteristics [57, 63, 69–71]. Maiorca et al., in a single center study, showed that patient age, and presence of diabetes, malignancy and peripheral vascular disease all impacted on ESRD survival [69]. After adjustment for these factors there was no difference in survival for patients aged 30–66. On the other hand, significantly better survival was found for patients over 66 years old placed on CPD (Fig. 5). This study was expanded to include six centers in Italy [70]. In this larger study, using the Cox model, age, cardiovascular, cerebrovascular, and peripheral vascular disease, presence of diabetes or malignancy, and underlying multisystem disease all impacted on survival. After adjusting for these factors, the rate at which the relative risk of death increased with increasing age was greater for those on HD compared to those on CPD (Fig. 6) [56a]. Finally, Lunde et al. [57] studied elderly patients in Michigan who began dialysis between 1980–1987. Modality was defined as the one being utilized on day 120 of treatment. The relative risk of death was higher in older patients, whites, and those with diabetes or hypertension as a cause of renal failure. Dialysis modality did not impact on the likelihood of death.

On the other hand, data from the USRDS, Michigan Kidney Registry and Belgium conflict with these findings [10, 63, 71]. The most common causes of death in elderly dialysis patients in the United States are cardiac other than myocardial infarction (M.I.), withdrawal from dialysis, and sepsis respectively for patients on HD and CPD. When a 1987–1989 cohort population in the USRDS was examined, the death rate per 1000 patient years at risk from these causes was greater for CPD compared to HD patients. This was particularly true for diabetics (Table 7) [10]. In addition, recent data from the Michigan Registry showed that death rates for elderly non-diabetics were the same for CPD and HD patients, while for diabetics, the increased risk of death seen in the USRDS data persisted (Table 8) [71]. More detailed analyses are ongoing to determine whether the outcome differences by modality are related to patient selection biases, differences in co-morbid conditions, or to some aspect of the treatment itself. Preliminary data shows that peripheral vascular

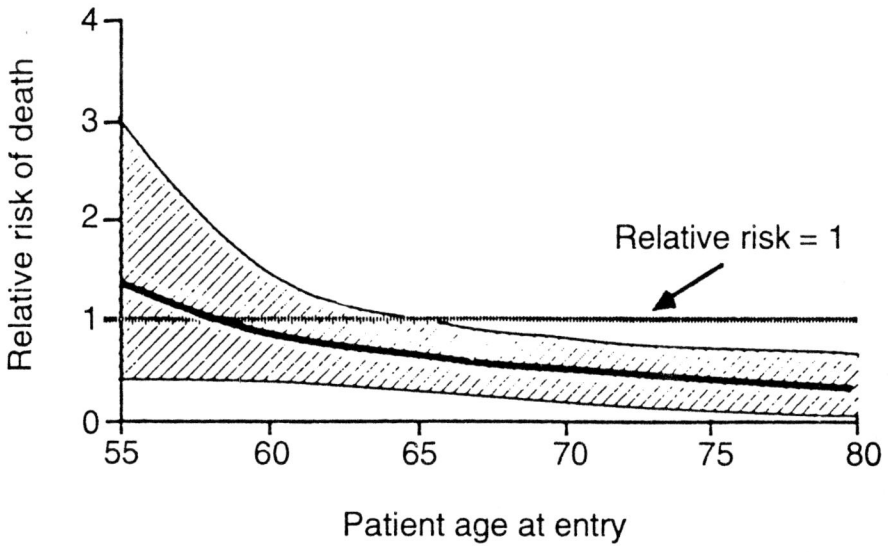

Figure 5. Relative risk of death of patients on CAPD compared to hemodialysis at any given age. ■ = 95% confidence limit. Reproduced from reference [69], with permission.

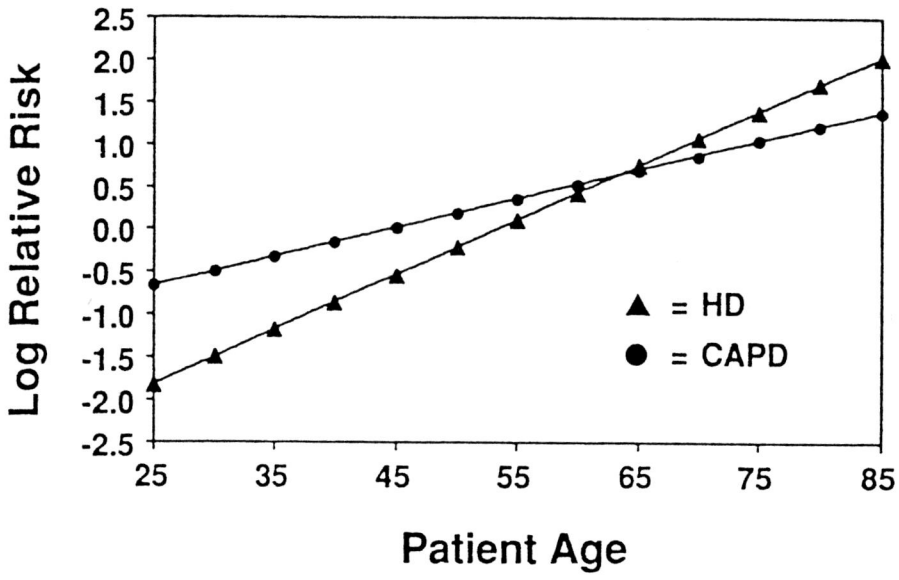

Figure 6. Log of relative risk of death among CAPD and HD patients with increasing age. Reproduced from reference [56a], with permission.

disease is more commonly present in CPD compared to HD patients in the USRDS and may in part account for the differences in survival seen (P. Held, personal communication). In a series from Belgium, on the other hand, median survival for elderly CPD patients was 19 months compared to 47 months for patients on HD [63]. When the Cox analysis was applied, treatment modality as well as functional performance score impacted on survival. More careful statistical analyses of co-morbidity matched patients are needed before firm conclusions can be drawn about the comparative mortality of HD and CPD in the elderly. For non-diabetics this seems less of an issue than for elderly diabetics.

7.2. Morbidity

Many complications of CPD occur no more frequently in elderly CPD patients than in younger ones including peritonitis and exit site infection [48–53]. Recent studies by Piraino, however, have shown that older patients had a higher rate of *S. epidermidis* peritonitis than younger patients, perhaps because touch contamination is more likely in older, less dexterous patients, particularly when spike connection systems are used [72]. On the other hand, older patients had fewer exit site and tunnel infections. Hospitalizations occur more frequently in elderly CPD patients and more days are spent in hospital for the elderly compared to the younger patients [50, 52, 69, 70]. Most of these excess days are related to vascular disease, though longer

Table 7. Death rate in elderly (>65 y/o) ESRD patients (1988–1990) by cause of death*.

Cause of Death	Diabetics		Non-Diabetics	
	HD	CPD	HD	CPD
Cardiac (Other than M.I.)	112.9	173.9	95.5	107.0
M.I.	51.2	89.3	39.2	46.9
Withdrawal from dialysis	48.6	62.8	39.6	47.4
Sepsis	38.6	57.5	25.8	32.4

* Adapted from the USRDS 1993 Annual Data Report for patients on dialysis and not transplanted. Expressed as deaths per 1000 patient years at risk.

Table 8. Dialysis patient survival: evaluation of CAPD vs. HD*.

Age	Diabetics		Non-Diabetics	
	HD	CAPD	HD	CAPD
20–59 (n = 4288)	1.0	0.62	1.0	1.0
60+ (n = 3453)	1.0	1.19	1.0	1.0

* Adapted from reference [71], with permission. Survival is expressed as the relative rate for an incident population beginning dialysis in 1989 (see text for explanation).

hospitalizations for peritonitis are often seen as well. A comparison of complication rates by age groups from the NIH Registry is given in Table 9. When actuarial analysis is performed, the outcome of younger and older patients is again similar, except for a higher mortality in the elderly, as reported by Nissenson et al. [52] (Figs. 7–9). This data is characteristic of that reported in other parts of the world. In addition, intra-abdominal- pressure-related complications of peritoneal dialysis (e.g. hernia, fluid leak, hydrothorax) are more common in older patients and may be a significant source of morbidity [46]. Finally, the need for catheter replacements is lower in the elderly [19, 52].

The likelihood of remaining on CPD over time is less for older compared to younger patients, but this is accounted for almost entirely by the higher mortality rate. Technique success is as low as 9% at five years when all causes of dropout are considered, but is similar in younger and older patients and as high as 78% at five years when death and renal transplantation are considered "lost-to-follow-up" in the analysis.

8. Adequacy of dialysis in the elderly

Increasing emphasis is being placed on quantification of solute removal as a method of assessing adequacy of peritoneal dialysis [73–75]. Urea removal normalized to urea volume of distribution (KT/V urea) as well as weekly creatinine clearance have been proposed to best predict outcomes in CPD patients. Not all investigators agree on the utility of these measures, but increasing data suggest that they may be of use clinically.

Nolph et al. studied indices of adequacy of dialysis and nutrition in young and old CPD patients [76]. They found that creatinine production declines significantly in older CPD patients, emphasizing the fact that serum creatinine is a poor measure of level of renal function or dialysis adequacy. In addition, the relationship of PCR to KT/V seen in younger CPD patients was also seen in older ones. This suggests that increasing dialysis dose in older CPD patients should be reflected in concomitant increases in PCR, as occurs in younger patients [77].

9. Quality of life

There are many psychosocial issues that must be considered when caring for elderly dialysis patients [12]. Many elderly are quite isolated, may live alone, and benefit greatly from the socialization provided at an in-center hemodialysis facility. In addition, an increase in the likelihood of depression has been noted in elderly dialysis patients compared to their peers. Finally, physical limitations or early dementia may impair quality of life. Husebye et al. prospectively studied 78 patients over the age of 70 on long-term dialysis in Minnesota, three years after retrospective analysis of the same group [78]. Over the three year period 54% of the patients had died. The important predictors of survival were all psychosocial in nature and included the score on the Karnofsky scale (functional capacity); weight gain between dialyses (compliance); use of home dialysis (more independent); less often wished for

Table 9. Complication rates for CPD patients per patient year by age**.

Age (yrs)		Peritonitis observed	Ex/tunnel infection	Cath. replace.	All hosp. days	No. of patients
<15		1.64	0.65	0.47	25.0	74
	Partner	1.54	0.78	0.56	26.7	58
	No Part.	1.89	0.35	0.26	21.1	16
15–59		1.34	0.55	0.25	17.7	1,445
	Partner	1.35	0.37	0.28	35.6	166
	No Part.	1.34	0.57	0.25	15.7	1,279
>60		1.26	0.43	0.25	23.1	792
	Partner	1.12	0.34	0.24	26.8	264
	No. Part.	1.32	0.47	0.25	21.6	528

** Adapted from reference [48], with permission.

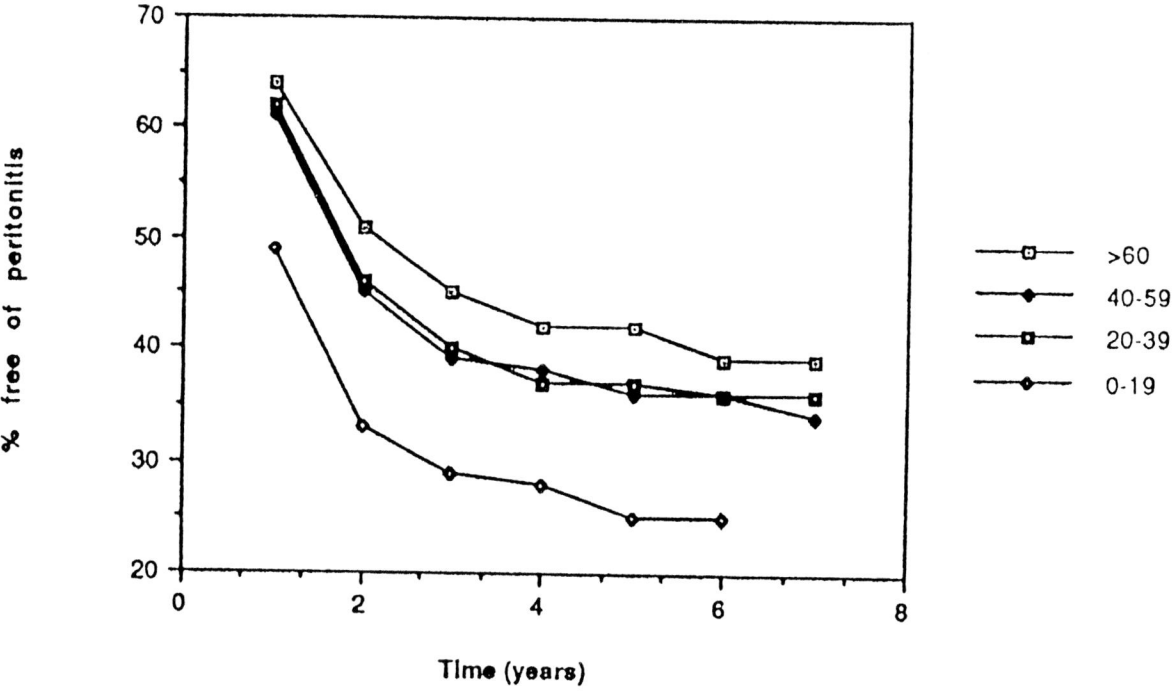

Figure 7. Percent of patients in Southern California and Southern Nevada free of peritonitis over time by age group. Reprinted from reference [52], with permission.

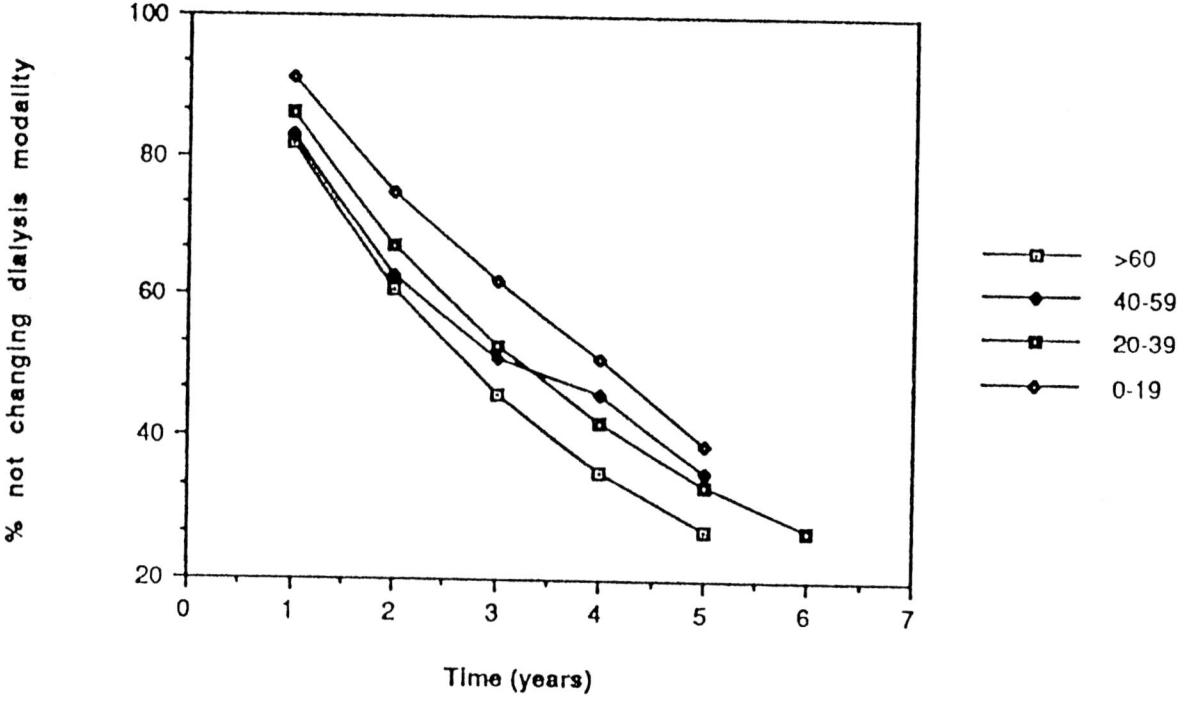

Figure 8. Percent of patients in Southern California and Southern Nevada not changing dialysis modality by age group. Reprinted from reference [52], with permission.

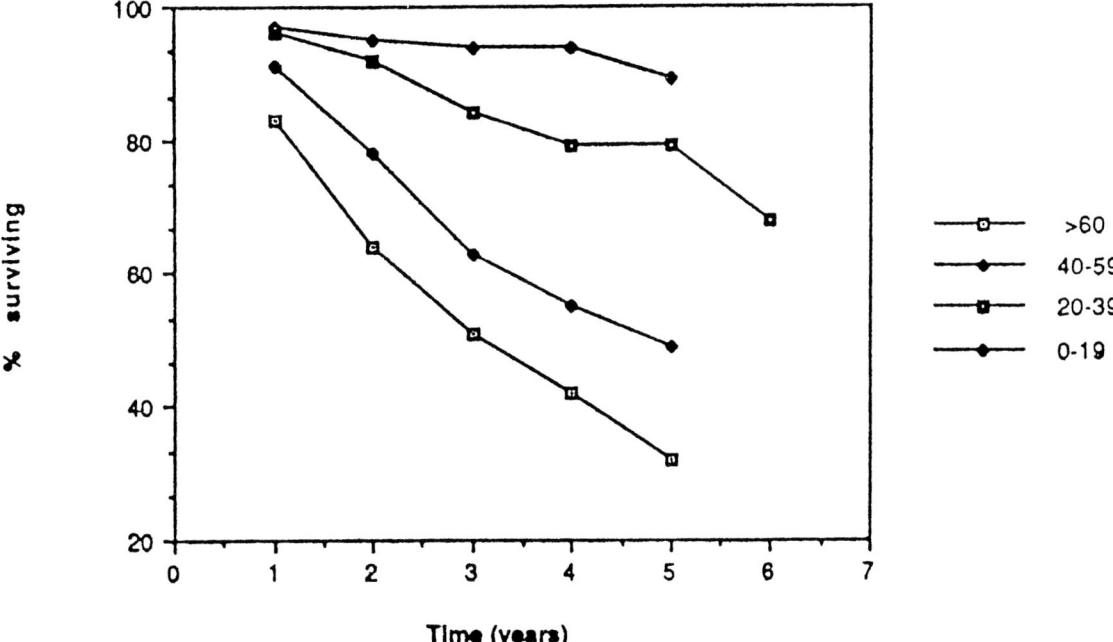

Figure 9. Overall survival of CPD patients in Southern California and Southern Nevada by age group. Reprinted from reference [52], with permission.

a transplant. In the large retrospective study (N = 157), overall quality of life was high compared to patients' impression of the quality of life of their peers [39]. Only 15–30% related their health somewhat worse or worse than others their age without renal failure. A more recent study by McKewitt *et al.* provides a less optimistic view [79]. These investigators studied 60 patients 60–78 years old on chronic dialysis in order to evaluate physical and psychosocial functioning. There was a high degree of disability as indicated by Karnofsky scores (only 32% of patients scored 70 or above). In addition, 33% of patients had mild to severe intellectual impairment on the Pfeiffer Short Portable Mental Status Questionnaire, while 62% demonstrated depressive symptomatology on the Beck Depression Inventory. Finally, this group had many physical limitations to activity that impaired their ability to function. Compared to younger dialysis patients all of these problems were more severe in the elderly.

In contrast, Stout *et al.*, studied 55 patients over the age of 60 on CPD and HD in the U.K. and compared them with 104 younger patients [40]. The older patients perceived life stresses similarly to age matched controls, and as significantly less than younger dialysis patients. In addition, there was no difference between elderly HD and CPD patients, although the number of patients studied in these groups was small.

Additional studies by Marsh *et al.* [18], Wolcott and Nissenson [19] and Wolcott *et al.* [80], suggest an overall better quality of life, cognitive function and brain electrophysiology in CPD compared to HD patients. The elderly on both modalities, however, fared worse on cognitive tests compared to younger patients [38].

Psychosocial evaluation may also be important for optimal initial modality selection in the elderly. Holley and Foulks retrospectively studied 34 elderly dialysis patients and compared them to 61 younger ones [81]. Nurses and social workers assessed patients in 10 categories for their suitability to do CAPD or CCPD. The categories studied included visual acuity, manual dexterity, personal hygiene, family support, adaptability to change, learning ability, motivation, compliance, preference for home dialysis and rehabilitation potential. Failure on CPD could be accurately predicted if the scores were low in these categories. Similarly, Carey *et al.* used the Beavers-Timberlawn Family Evaluation Scale to rate families of CAPD patients in five areas: power structure, individualization/autonomy, separation/loss issues, reality perception, and affect [82]. Patients with low functioning families were twice as likely to transfer from home dialysis for psychosocial reasons. Of those with low functioning families, 67% of elderly CPD patients had transferred to HD by one year compared to only 16% of those with high functioning families. The prospective use of such tools may help assure that patients are placed on the most appropriate modality from the outset of ESRD.

Much additional research is needed in the area of quality of life of elderly dialysis patients. Recent work with the MOS Short-Form Health Survey (SF-36) suggests that this may be a valuable tool in this area, particularly if the existing instrument can be modified to include disease specific information [83].

10. Alternative approaches to CPD in the elderly

The elderly may be more prone to complications of CPD that relate to the high intraperitoneal pressures that develop with an abdomen filled with dialysate. This is a particular problem when patients are ambulatory, since intra-abdominal pressure is greatest with the patient sitting or standing and least when the patient is supine [84]. In such circumstances, CCPD, with exchanges performed at night, might be an ideal alternative. The experience with this modality in the elderly is not extensive, but outcomes seem similar to those seen with CAPD [48, 85, 86]. In addition, for those patients who require assistance to perform CPD, CCPD might be preferable, thus minimizing the time required of an assistant to perform the treatment.

A large number of elderly patients seem excellent candidates for CPD but are not placed on this modality, primarily for logistic or psychosocial reasons. The use of CCPD is one approach to resolving this problem, but three others are worthy of consideration [87–90]. First, about 2%–5% of current ESRD patients live in nursing homes, somewhat less than the rate for non-renal patients of the same age [87]. Most of these patients receive CHD and are transported, at great expense, 2 or 3 times per week to a dialysis facility for treatment. The development of nursing homes capable of carrying out CPD or willing to establish cooperative relationships with CPD centers might permit performance of CPD in this setting, to the benefit of the patient and at a substantial cost saving. The reasons for the reluctance of nursing homes to accept ESRD patients are shown in Fig. 10. Many

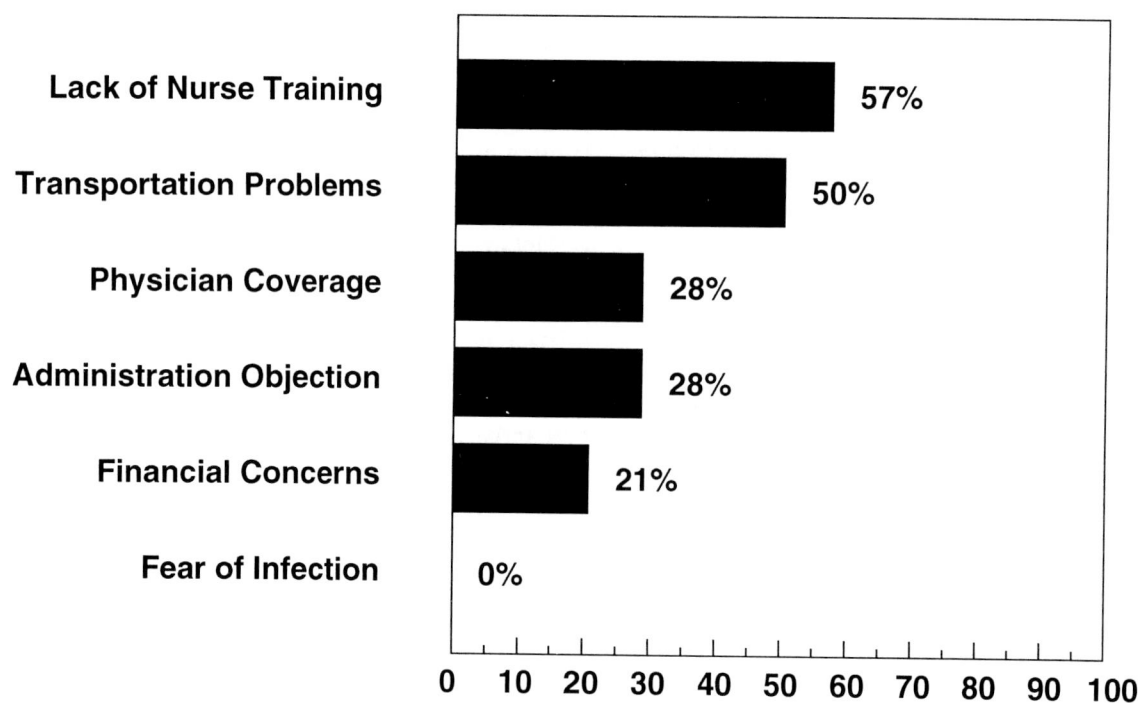

Figure 10. Reasons nursing homes do not accept ESRD patients. Reprinted from reference [87], with permission.

of these concerns might be addressed by a nursing home and dialysis facility working together to establish a CPD program [87, 88]. Even with an excellent cooperative arrangement, however, mortality is high particularly for older patients [88].

Second, adult day care centers (ADC) might be utilized to assist in the care of elderly ESRD patients on CPD [89]. The ADC center could provide a range of services from retraining, performance of exchanges, social services, physical therapy and so on. It could also provide an opportunity for socialization of often lonely and solitary elderly patients. In addition, it could provide an occasional "vacation" for family members from doing dialysis exchanges. Such a program could be integrated into an existing ADC facility, or a dedicated dialysis ADC center could be developed.

Thirdly, some elderly patients need a helper for CPD, but live alone and have no one to assist them. A program of paid home helpers, nurses or technicians, could fill this role [90]. For example, two visits a day could be made for setting up a cycling machine, connecting and disconnecting the patient. The cost of such a program would need to be assessed, but the benefits to the patient could be tremendous.

These concepts are clearly worthy of further exploration so that those elderly who would benefit medically from CPD are able to get it.

11. Ethical considerations

11.1. Withdrawal from dialysis

Withdrawal from dialysis accounts for 9% of deaths in Canadian and U.S. dialysis patients [91, 92]. For patients over 70 years old this is the most common cause of death in U.S. patients [5]. Kjellstrand *et al.* have found that withdrawal is more common in diabetics, whites and home dialysis patients as well [93]. The latter has not been confirmed by other investigators [85].

Elderly patients were not placed on dialysis in the United States or elsewhere in the early years of the ESRD program, a policy that extended into the 1980's [94]. The availability of CPD, permitting less costly and labor intensive treatment to take place in the home was primarily responsible for a change in this practice. The increasing numbers of elderly, debilitated ESRD patients, some of whom are demented and/or nursing home residents has raised a number of ethical concerns about the appropriateness of utilizing scarce technical resources and money on a population with a limited life expectancy. This applies not only to CPD, but to many newer, expensive technologies. Rothenberg suggests the following five points be considered in this regard [95]:

(1) It is inappropriate to make "policy" decisions regarding dialysis for an elderly individual when no such policies in fact exist.
(2) The beneficial effects of dialysis in the elderly are clear and should be kept in mind when considering providing or withholding treatment.
(3) It is important for patients and families to understand the benefits and the burdens of ESRD treatment.
(4) It may be useful to initiate a "trial" of ESRD therapy to better assess the benefits and burdens of the treatment.
(5) It is crucial to support the patient, family and staff, if a decision to withdraw dialysis is made.

In summary, substantial evidence now exists showing the medical success of CPD in the elderly. In a more limited series of studies quality of life has also been reported to be good to excellent in many elderly CPD patients. There appears to be no justification at the present time for systematically excluding the elderly from CPD therapy. Their medical and psychosocial outcomes are similar to those of younger patients and many patients lead productive, satisfying lives.

References

1. Nissenson AR. Dialysis therapy in the elderly patient. Kidney Int 1993; 43 (suppl 40): S51–7.
2. Nissenson AR. Chronic peritoneal dialysis in the elderly. Ger Nephrol Urol 1991; 1: 3–12.
3. Mignon F, Michel C, Mentre F, Viron B. Worldwide demographics and future trends of the management of renal failure in the elderly. Kidney Int 1993; 43 (suppl. 41): S18–26.
4. Schleifer CR. Peritoneal dialysis in the nursing-home patient. In: Oreopoulos DG, Michelis MF, Herschorn S (eds), Nephrology and Urology in the Aged Patient, Kluwer Academic Publishers, Netherland 1993; pp 225–32.
5. US Renal Data System. USRDS 1993 Annual Report, The National Institutes of Health, National Institute of Diabetes and Digestive and Kidney Diseases, Bethesda 1993.
6. Nolph KD. What's new in peritoneal dialysis – An overview. Kidney Int 1992; 42 (suppl 38): S148–52.
7. Mattern WD, McGaghie WC, Rigby RJ, Nissenson AR, et al. Selection of ESRD treatment: An international study. Am J Kidney Dis 1989; 13: 457–64.

8. Gentile DE and the Geruiatric Advisory Committee. Peritoneal dialysis in geriatric patients: a survey of clinical practices. In: Nissenson AR (ed), Adv Perit Dial (Peritoneal Dialysis in the Geriatric Patient). 1990; 6 (suppl): 29–32.
9. Nissenson AR, Prichard SS, Cheng IKP, Gokal R, Kubota M, Maiorca R, et al. Non-medical factors that impact on ESRD modality selection. Kidney Int 1993; 43(40): S120–7.
10. US Renal Data System, USRDS 1989 Annual Report, The National Institutes of Health, National Institute of Diabetes and Digestive and Kidney Diseases Bethesda, MD 1989 August: 17–20.
11. Maiorca R, Cancarini GC, Camerini C, Manili L, Brunori G: Modality selection for the elderly. Medical factors. In: Nissenson AR (ed), Adv Perit Dia (Peritoneal Dialysis in the Geriatric Patient) 1990; 6 (suppl): 18–26.
12. Ross CJ, Rutsky EA. Dialysis modality selection in the elderly patient with ESRD: Advantages and disadvantages of peritoneal dialysis. In: Nissenson AR (ed), Adv Perit Dial (Peritoneal Dialysis in the Geriatric Patient), 1990; 6 (suppl): 11–8.
13. Vlachojannis J, Kerry P, Hoppe D. CAPD in elderly patients with cardiovascular risk factors. Clin Nephrol 1988; 30 (suppl 1): S13–7.
14. Wizemann V, Timio M, Martin AA, Kramer W. Options in dialysis therapy: Significance of cardiovascular findings. Kidney Int 1993; 43 (suppl 40): S85–92.
15. Piccoli G, Quarello F, Salomone M, Bonello F, Pacitti A, Beltrame G, Piccoli Gb, Vercellone A. Dialysis in the elderly: Comparison of different dialytic modalities. In: Nissenson AR (ed), Adv Perit Dial (Peritoneal Dialysis in the Geriatric Patient) 1990; 6 (suppl): 72–81.
16. Epstein AE, Kay GN, Plurab VJ. Considerations in the diagnosis and treatment of arrhythmias in patients with ESRD. Semin Dial 1989; 2: 31–7.
17. Peer G, Korzets A, Hochhauzer E, Eschchar Y, Blum M, Aviram A. Cardian arrhythmias during CAPD. Naphron 1987; 45: 192–5.
18. Marsh JT, Brown WS, Wolcott D, Landverk J, Nissenson AR. Electrophysiological indices of CNS function in hemodialysis and CAPD. Kidney Int 1986; 30: 957–63.
19. Wolcott DL, Nissenson AR. Quality of life in chronic dialysis patients: A critical comparison of CAPD and hemodialysis. Am J Kidney Dis 1988; 11: 402–12.
20. Saltissi D, Coles GA, Napier JAF, Bentley P. The hematological response to CAPD. Clin Nephrol 1984; 22: 21–7.
21. Zimmerman SW, Johnson CA. Erythropoietin use in peritoneal dialysis patients. Am J Kidney Dis 1991; 15(4) (suppl 1): 38–41.
22. Young MA, Nolph KD, Dulton S, Prowant B. Antihypertensive drug requirements in CAPD. Perit Dial Bull 1984; 4: 85–8.
23. Youmbissi J, Sellars L, Shore AC, Poon T. Wilkinson R. Blood pressure on CAPD: relationship to sodium status renin and aldosterone compared with hemodialysis. In Maher JF, Winchester JF, eds. Frontiers in Peritoneal Dialysis, Field, Rich and Assoc., New York 1986; 450–6.
24. Maiorca R, Cancarini G, Brunori G, Vonesh E, Manili L, Camerini R et al. CAPD in elderly. Perit Dial Int (In press 1993).
25. Leehan F, Smith D, Khanna R, Oreopoulos D. Changes in left ventricular hypertrophy and function in hypertensive patients started on CAPD. Am Heart J 1985; 110: 102–6.
26. Alpert MA, Van Stone J, Twardowski Z, Ruder MA, Whiting R, Kelly D, Madsen BR. Comparative cardiac effects of hemodialysis and continuous ambulatory peritoneal dialysis. Clin Cardiol 1986; 9: 52–60.
27. Timio M. Ruolo terapeutico della dialisi peritoneale. In: Timio M (ed), Clinica Cardiologi Nell'Uremia, Wichtig Editore, Milano 1990; p 8.
28. Grodstein GP, Blumenkrantz MJ, Kopple JD, Moran JK, Coburn JW. Glucose absorption during CAPD. Kidney Int 1981; 19: 564–7.
29. Young GA, Kopple JD, Lindholm B, et al. Nutritional assessment of CAPD patients: An international study. Am J Kidney Dis 1991; 17: 462–71.
30. Lindholm B, Bergstrom J. Nutritional aspects on peritoneal dialysis. Kidney Int 1992; 42 (suppl 38): S165–71.
31. Stelin G, Ahlmen J, Morelli B, tylen U. Computed tomography and total body potassium measurements of patients on continuous ambulatory peritoneal dialysis. ASAIO 1985; 8(1): 46–9.
32. Rottembourg J. Residual renal function and recovery of renal function in patients treated by CAPD. Kidney Int 1993; 43 (suppl 40): S106–10.
33. Copley JB, Lindberg JS. Insulin: Its use in patients on peritoneal dialysis. Semin Dial 1988; 1(3): 143–50.
34. Dulanes JT, Hatch FE. Peritoneal dialysis and loss of proteins. Kidney Int 1984; 26: 253–62.
35. Gagnon RF, Somerville P, Kaye M. B-microglobulin serum levels in patients on long term dialysis. Perit Dial Bull 1987; 7: 29–31.
36. Simmons RG, Anderson C, Kamstra L. Comparison of quality of life of patients on continuous ambulatory peritoneal dialysis, hemodialysis, and after transplantation. Am J Kidney Dis 1984; 4(3): 253–5.
37. Gokal R. Quality of life in patients undergoing renal replacement therapy. Kidney Int 1993; 43 (suppl 40): S23–7.
38. Wolcott DL, Nissenson AR, Landsverk J. Quality of life in chronic dialysis patients: factors unrelated to dialysis modality. Gen Hosp Psychiat 10: 267–77.
39. Westlie L, Umen A, Nestrud S, Kjellstrand CM. Mortality and life satisfaction in the very old dialysis patient. Trans Am Soc Artif Intern Organs 1984; 30: 21–30.
40. Stout JP, Gokal R, Hillier VF, Kincey J, Auer J, Oliver D, Simon LG. Quality of life of high risk and elderly dialysis patients in the UK Dial and Transplant 1987; 16: 674–7.
41. Carey H, Finkelstein S, Santacroce s, Brennan N, Raffone D, Rifkin J et al. The impact of psychosocial factors and age on CAPD dropout. In: Nissenson AR (ed), Adv Perit Dial (Peritoneal

Dialysis in the Geriatric Patient) 1990; 6 (suppl): 26–9.
42. Diaz-Buxo JA. Clinical use of peritoneal dialysis. In: Nissenson AR, Fine RN, Gentile DE (eds), Clinical Dialysis, Appleton and Lange, Norwalk 1990: pp 256–300.
43. Moncrief JW, Popovich RP. CAPD. In Nolph KD (ed), Kluwer Academic, The Netherlands 1989; 157–8.
44. Sombolos K, Berkelhammer C, Baker J, Wu G, McNamee P, Oreopoulos DG. Nutritional assessment and skeletal muscle function in patients in CAPD. Perit Dial Bull 1986; 6: 53–8.
45. Dombros NV, Oreopoulos DG. Nutritional aspects of patients on CAPD. In: La Greca G, Chiramonte S, Fabris A, Feriani M, Ronco C (eds), Eichtig Editore, Milano 1988; pp 113–8.
46. Bargman JM. Complications of peritoneal dialysis related to increased intra-abdominal pressure. Kidney Int 1993; 43 (suppl 40): S75–80.
47. Brown PM, Johnston KW, Fenton SSA, Cattran DC. Symptomatic exacerbation of peripheral vascular disease with chronic ambulatory peritoneal dialysis. Clin Nephrol 1981; 16(5): 258–61.
48. Nolph KD, Lindblad AS, Novak JW, Steinberg SM. Experiences with the elderly in the National CAPD Registry. In: Nissenson AR (ed), Adv Perit Dial (Peritoneal Dialysis in the Geriatric Patient) 1990; 6 (suppl): 38–40.
49. Gokal R. CAPD in the elderly-European and UK experience. In: Nissenson AR (ed), Adv Perit Dial (Peritoneal Dialysis in the Geriatric Patient) 1990; 6 (suppl): 56–60.
50. Posen Ga, Fenton SSA, Arbus GS, Churchill DN, Jeffrey JR. The Canadian experience with peritoneal dialysis in the elderly. In: Nissenson AR (ed), Adv Perit Dial (Peritoneal Dialysis in the Geriatric Patient) 1990; 6 (suppl): 38–40.
51. Segoloni GP, Salomone M, Piccoli GB. CAPD in the elderly: Italian multicenter study experience. In Nissenson AR (ed), Adv Perit Dial (Peritoneal Dialysis in the Geriatric Patient) 1990; 6 (suppl): 47–50.
52. Nissenson AR, Gentile DE, Soderblom R. CAPD in the elderly: Southern California/Southern Nevada experience. In: Nissenson AR (ed), Adv Perit Dial (Peritoneal Dialysis in the Geriatric Patient) 1990; 6 (suppl): 51–5.
53. Nebel M, Finke K. CAPD in patients over 60 years of age. In: Nissenson AR (ed), Adv Perit Dial (Peritoneal Dialysis in the Geriatric Patient) 1990; 6 (suppl): 56–60.
54. Benevent D, Benzakour M, Peyronnet P, Lagarde C. comparison of continuous ambulatory peritoneal dialysis and hemodialysis in the elderly. In: Nissenson AR (ed), Adv Perit Dial (Peritoneal Dialysis in the Geriatric Patient) 1990; 6 (suppl): 68–71.
55. Walls J. Dialysis in the elderly: Some UK experience. In: Nissenson AR (ed), Adv Perit Dial (Peritoneal Dialysis in the Geriatric Patient) 1990; 6 (suppl): 82–5.
56. Tapson JS, Rodger RSC, Mansy H, Elliott RW, Ward MK, Wilkinson R. Renal replacement therapy in patients aged over 60 years. Postgrad Med J 1987; 63: 1071–7.
56a. Vonesh EF, Maiorca R. A multicenter, selection-adjusted comparison of patient and technique survival on CAPD and hemodialysis: A classification. Perit Dial Int 1993; 13: 71–2.
57. Lunde NM, Port FK, Wolfe RA, Guire KF. Comparison of mortality risk by choice of CAPD vs. hemodialysis in elderly patients. Adv Perit Dial 1991; 7: 68–73.
58. Jogler F, Saade M. Improved overall survival of elderly patients on peritoneal dialysis. Adv Perit Dial 1991; 7: 68–73.
59. Garcia-Falcon T, Perez-Fontan M, Nogueiro M, Moncalian J, Perez J, Sastre F, Rodriguez-Carmona A. Tratamiento sustitutivo de la insuficiencia renal en el anciano. Es la D.P.C.A. la tecnica de eleccion? In: Nolph KD, Prowant BF, Twardowski ZJ (eds), Adv Perit Dial., Oreopoulos, Multimedia Publishers (In press, 1993).
60. Acchiardo SR, Kraus AP, Kaufman PA, Moore L. Dialysis in the elderly. In: Nolph KD, Prowant BF, Twardowski ZJ (rds), Adv Perit Dial., Oreopoulos, Multimedia Publishers (In press, 1993).
61. Suh H, Wadhwa NK, Cabralda T, Solumbi D, Solomon M. Peritoneal dialysis in elderly end-stage renal disease patients. In: Nolph KD, Prowant BF, Twardowski ZJ (eds), Adv Perit Dial., Oreopoulos, Multimedia Publishers (In press, 1993).
62. Isaad B, Allouache M, Baumelou A, Rottembourg J, Jacobs C. Elderly patients and CAPD riisk factors and withdrawal: A 14 years experience in a single unit. In: Nolph KD, Prowant BF, Twardowski ZJ (eds), Adv Perit Dial., Oreopoulos, Multimedia Publishers (In Press, 1993).
63. Verbeelen D, De Neve W, Van Der P, Sennesael J. Dialysis in patients over 65 years of age. Kidney Int 1993; 43 (suppl 41): S27–30.
64. Piccoli G, Bonello F, Massara C, Salomone M, Maffei S, Iadarola M, et al. Death in conditions of cachexia: The price for the dialysis treatment of the elderly? 1993; 43 (suppl 41): S282–6.
65. Mallinsen WJW, Fleming SJ, Shaw JEH, Baker LRI, Cattell WR. Survival in elderly patients presenting with uraemia. Q J Med (New series) 1984; 53: 301–7.
66. Marai A, Rathaus M, Gibor Y, Bernheim J. Chronic dialysis in the elderly: Intermitent peritoneal dialysis or hemodialysis? Perit Dial Bull 1983; pp 183–6.
67. Taube DH, Winder EA, Ogg C, Bewick M, Cameron JS, Rudge CJ, Williamd DG. Successful treatment of middle aged and elderly patients with ESRD. Brit Med J 1983; 2826: 2018–20.
68. Kaye M, Pajel PA, Somerville PJ. Four years experience with CAPD in the elderly. Perit Dial Bull 1983; 3: 17–9.
69. Maiorca R, Vonesh EF, Cancarini GC, Cantaluppi A, Manili L, Grunori G. A six-year comparison of patient and technique survivals in CAPD and HD. Kidney Int 1988; 34: 518–24.
70. Mairoca R, Vonesh EF, Cavlii P, et al. A multicenter, selection-adjusted comparison of patient and

technique survivals on CAPD and hemodialysis. Perit Dial Int 1991; 11: 118–27.
71. Nelson CB, Port FK, Wolfe RA, Guire KF. Dialysis patient survival: Evaluation of CAPD vs. HD using 3 teniques. (abstract) Perit Dial Int 1992; 12 (suppl): 144.
72. Holley JL, Bernardini J, Perlmutter JA, Piraino B. A comparison of infection rates among older and younger patients on continuous peritoneal dialysis. In: Nolph KD, Prowant BFm Twardowski ZJ (eds), Adv Perit Dial, Oreopoulos, Multimedia Publishers (In press, 1993).
73. Brandes JC, Piering WF, Beres JA, Blumenthal SS, Fritsche C. Clinical outcome of continuous ambulatory peritoneal dialysis predicted by urea and creatinine kinetics. J Am Soc Nephrol 1992; 2: 1430–5.
74. Lameire NH, Vanholder R, Veyt D, Lambert MC, ringoir S. A Longitudinal, five year surveyof urea kinetic parameters in CAPD patients. Kidney Int 1992; 42: 426–32.
75. Gotch FA. Adequacy of peritoneal dialysis. Am J Kidney Dis 1993; 21(1): 96–8.
76. Nolph KD, Moore HL, Prowant B, Meyer M, Twardowski ZJ, Khanna R et al. Age and indices of adequacy and nutrition in CAPD patients. In: Nolph KD, Prowant BF, Twardowski ZJ (eds), Adv Perit Dial., Oreopoulos, Multimedia Publishers (In press, 1993).
77. Bergstrom J, Lindholm B. Nutrition and adequacy of dialysis. How do hemodialysis and CAPD compare? Kidney Int 1993; 43 (supp 40): S39–50.
78. Husebye DG, Westlie L, Styrvoky TJ, Kjellstrand CM. Psychological, social, and somatic prognostic indicators in old patients undergoing long-term dialysis. Arch Inter Med 1987; 147: 1921–4.
79. McKevitt PM, Jones JF, Marion RR. The elderly on dialysis: Physical and psychosocial functioning. Dial Transplant 1986; 15: 130–7.
80. Wolcott DL, Landsverk J, Nissenson AR. Relationship of dialysis modality and other factors to cognitive function in chronic dialysis patients. Am J Kidney Dis 1988; 12: 275–84.
81. Holley JL, Foulks CJ. The utility of a structured evaluation of elderly patients for continuous peritoneal dialysis. Perit Dial Int 1991; 11: 162–5.
82. Carey H, Finkelstein S, Santacroce S, Brenna N, Raffone D, Rifkin J, Loger A, Cooper K, Finkelstein F. The impact of psychosocial factors and age on CAPD droupout. In: Nissenson AR (ed), Adv Perit Dial (Peritoneal Dialysis in the Geriatric Patient) 1990; 6 (suppl): 26–9.
83. Kurtin P, Nissenson AR. Morbidity and mortality of ESRD patients. J Am Soc Neph 1993; 3: 1738–47.
84. Twardowski ZJ, Khanna R, Nolph KD. Intraabdominal pressure during natural activities in patients treated with CAPD. Nephron. 1986; 44: 129–35.
85. Diaz-Buxo JA, Adcock A, Nelms M. Experience with continuous cycle peritoneal dialysis in the geriatric patient. In: Nissenson AR (ed), Adv Perit Dial (Peritoneal Dialysis in the Geriatric Patient) 1990; 6 (suppl): 61–4.
86. Diaz-Buxo JA. The place for cycler-assisted peritoneal dialysis in geriatric patients: comparison with hemodialysis. Ger Nephrol Urol 1993; 3: 7–13.
87. Schleifer CR. Peritoneal dialysis in nursing homes. In: Nissenson AR (ed), Adv Perit Dial (Peritoneal Dialysis in the Geriatric Patient) 1990; 6 (suppl): 92–4.
88. Anderson JE, Kraus J, Sturgeon D. Incidence, prevalence, and outcomes of end-stage renal disease patients placed in ursing homes. Am J Kidney Dis 1993; 21(6): 619–27.
89. Mattern WE. Adult day care centers and peritoneal dialysis. In: Nissenson AR (ed), Adv Perit Dial (Peritoneal Dialysis in the Geriatric Patient) 1990; 6 (suppl): 92–4.
90. Michel C, Bindi P, Viron B. CAPD with private home nurses: An alternative treatment for elderly and disabled patient. In: Nissenson AR (ed), Adv Perit Dial (Peritoneal Dialysis in the Geriatric Patient) 1990; 6 (suppl): 92–4.
91. Mailloux LU, Bellucci AG, Napolitano B, Massey RT, Wilkes BM, Bluestone PA. Death by withdrawal from dialysis: A 20-year clinical experience. J Am Soc Nephrol 1993; 3: 1631–7.
92. Nelson CB, Port FK, Wolfe RA, Guire KE. Comparison of continuous ambulatory peritoneal dialysis and hemodialysis patient survival with evaluation of trends during the 1980's. J Am Soc Nephrol 1992; 3: 1147–55.
93. Kjellstrand CM: Stopping dialysis. In: Nolph KD, Prowant BF, Twardowski ZJ (eds), Adv Perit Dial, Oreopoulos, Multimedia Publishers (In press, 1993).
94. Nicholls AJ, Waldek S, Platts MM, Moorhead PJ, Brown CB. Impact of continuous ambulatory peritoneal dialysis on treatment of renal failure in patients aged over 60. British Med J 1984; 288: 18–9.
95. Rothenberg LS: Ethical concerns for the elderly with ESRD. In: Nissenson AR (ed), Adv Perit Dial (Peritoneal Dialysis in the Geriatric Patient), 1990; 6 (suppl): 6–10.

23 | Quality of life

R. GOKAL

1. Introduction	679
2. Definition	679
3. Dimension and instruments	680
4. Instruments	681
5. Requirements for a measure	681
6. Instruments used in assessments of ESRF patients	682
7. Multi disciplinary team in managing renal failure patients	682
8. Role of social workers in the peritoneal dialysis programme	684
9. Studies on quality of life in ESRF	684
9.1. History	684
9.2. Quality of life in peritoneal dialysis; comparison between PD and HD	686
9.3. Time trade off, sickness impact profile, SK36 and Uraemic Index	689
10. Employment	689
11. Sexual functioning and psychosexual problems	690
12. Psychosocial adjustment and dialysis related stress	691
13. Impact of EPO on quality of life	692
14. Summary of studies on quality of life and future trends	692
15. What do we need to know and how to achieve it	693
16. Summary	694
References	694

1. Introduction

Interest in measuring Quality of Life in relation to healthcare has increased enormously in recent years [1, 2]. This is equally true for end stage renal failure (ESRF), where its importance lies in not only providing for absolute survival but also the quality of that survival. The main purpose, however, is to provide more accurate assessments of individuals or populations health and of the benefits and harms that may result from healthcare. This is even more important in renal failure care where advances are not uncommon and there are alternative therapies available to manage patients; the relative effectiveness of these changes and therapies needs proper evaluation and assessment as regards quality of life [3, 4, 5]. Unquestionably, one of the goals of an end stage renal failure programme (Table 1) is to achieve maximum psychosocial maturation and development, whilst at the same time adapting to the stresses of therapy [6].

2. Definition

The definition of quality of life is difficult as it embraces many dimensions, ranging from physical wellbeing and cognitive competence to the establishment of satisfactory inter-relationships, the occupation of housing which is enjoyed, and possession of sufficient income to explore the world beyond that necessary just for basic biological survival [7].

Before one talks about quality we must define the term. In the dictionary quality is defined as "the degree of excellence of a thing". But how do we know if a thing is excellent or not? Quality is judged by individuals who compare the thing with a standard, which can be a personal one or a consensus one. Quality is also a relative thing that may be perceived differently by different individuals or groups; thus in terms of medical care there is the quality that the doctor perceives, the quality that the patient perceives and the quality that (in a hospital setting) the manager perceives; difficulties can arise because these perceptions may not be the same. From the physicians point of view this perspective may even be somewhat narrower; factors such as

Table 1. Ideal goals for renal replacement programme.

1. Restoration of normal level of biological, psychological and social adaptation and longevity.
2. Minimal adverse effect of treatment as above.
3. Maximum psychological and social maturation.
4. Optimum family function and minimum treatment related stress.
5. Minimal patient care stresses on health professionals and high professional satisfaction.

advancing age, income, and relationships are all outside a physician's control and hence they are principally concerned with measures of health related to quality of life (either measures of health status, e.g. burden of biological disorders or that aspect responsive to therapy – "moveable health status"). In terms of maintaining good health this can be divided into general physical, mental and social aspects [4].

The term quality of life misleadingly suggests an abstract and philosophical approach but indeed should reflect the content and purpose of measures – health related quality of life, subjective health status, functional status [8]. In that respect more specific definitions have emerged. Alexander and Willens [9] state that the fundamental basis of quality of life involves continuously functioning reciprocal interactions between the patient and his environment and encompasses such crucial areas as inter-relationships, physical wellbeing, social activities, personal development, recreation and economic circumstances. Stout and Auer [10] identified several measures which include: mobility, physical performance, employment (objective measures) and ability to lead a satisfactory social life and have sexual and affectionate relationships (subjective measures). Churchill [11] identified a global concept, an estimate of all reciprocal interactions between patients and the environment.

Quality of life measures can be used in may ways in healthcare (Table 2) over and above those stated already [8]. These aspects, especially those related to audit, achievement of standards, quality of patient care and cost effective analysis are assuming greater importance [12]. Indeed the "appropriate healthcare and technology programme" of the World Health Organisation has as target 31: "by 1990 all member states should have built effective mechanisms for ensuring the quality of patient care" and this theme has been taken up by member nations e.g. the United Kingdom in its recent change in health care delivery enshrined in "The Health of the Nation" [13].

Whatever definition of quality of life measures is used or its role in healthcare, consideration of quality of life as well as of survival, always implicit in good clinical practice, has hitherto lacked explicit expression and it is important to do so now. Two important questions come to the fore.

1. Is individual quality of life open to quantitative assessment?
2. Can aggregated indices of quality of individual life be used as a component in deciding health services priorities?

These questions form the basis of a wider debate indirectly addressed here using available publications in the field of renal replacement therapy.

3. Dimension and instruments

Although the concept of quality if life is inherently subjective and definitions vary , the content of the various instruments show some similarity in terms of dimensions which can be subdivided into physical functions (e.g. mobility, self care), emotional functions (wellbeing, life satisfaction, autonomy, depression, anxiety), social function (intimacy, social support, social contact, sexuality), role performance (work, housework), and pain and other symptoms (fatigue and nausea, disease specific symptoms [8]). Hence dimensions of quality of life include not only the physical condition of the patient, important though this is, but also how he feels about life and his relation to it, how he relates to the social environment and his capacity to continue working and achieve contentment. These are, of course, not independent variables and should all be taken into account in assessing quality if life. What is ethically desirable in choosing between all these aspects is difficult to ascertain but Black [14] has set up three possible criteria.

i. Assessments made by sufferers from particular states are to be preferred to vicarious estimates (in the phrase experito credo, the "expert" in the subjective context of the illness is the patient not the doctor or nurse).
ii. A method that takes into account several variables is preferable to uni- or bidimensional methods even at the expense of numerical complexity.
iii. When several variables have been measured,

Table 2. Applications of quality of life measures.

1. Screening and monitoring pyschosocial problems in individual patient care.
2. Medical Audit.
3. Outcome in Health Services.
4. Evaluation Research.
5. Clinical Trials.
6. Population surveys of perceived health problems.
7. Cost-effective analysis.

some weighting should be made in favour of those which can be more rather than less objectively measured. Table 3 shows how fitness for work may be used in comparing the efficacy of different treatments for endstage renal failure [15]. Although fitness for work combines the physical and psychological dimension, it is a simple measure but one not devoid of practicality.

These above concepts thus imply that since quality of life is multi-dimensional it can only be evaluated from multi-dimensional perspective. In addition, a more controversial issue is the need to include multiple items to assess each dimension of quality of life. For conceptual, psychometric and health policy related reasons, multi-item assessments within a given dimension are necessary if one hopes to progress in understanding the dimension and its relationship to patient illnesses, therapies and other life circumstances [5, 16]. However, as is the case in burgeoning research areas, many of the underlying conceptual models and research questions have outstripped the developments and evaluation of suitable measurement instruments.

4. Instruments

There two basic types of instruments, disease specific and generic. The former have been developed for one disease or a narrow range of disease, e.g. arthritis impact measurement scale [17]. Generic instruments are intended to be applicable to a wide range of health problems. Among the commonly used are the Sickness Impact Profile (SIP) [18] and Nottingham Health Profile (NIP) [19]. Though some instruments are administered by clinicians, or intense interviewers, increasingly the emphasis has been on self completed questionnaires for economy of use. The quantitative information provided also varies. Most of these scores with different dimensions of quality of life are not intended to be combined, but others assess dimensions that may be summed to provide a single score e.g. the quality of life (QL index), developed for use in cancer, which consists of five elements (activity, daily living, health, support and outlook) which are summed to provide a single index total [20].

5. Requirements for a measure

a. *Reliability*. All instruments must produce the same results on repeated use under the same conditions. This can be examined by a test, retest of internal reliability (the degree of agreement of items addressing equivalent concepts) -an inter-rater reliability [21].

b. *Validity*. This is more difficult to assess because instruments are measuring an inherently subjective phenomenon. An informal approach is to examine "face validity" – whether instruments cover a full range of relevant topics [22] and the range of patient experiences [23]. A more formal approach is to examine construct validity, which is concerned with the pattern of relations of a quality of life instrument with other more established measures e.g. laboratory vs clinical [24], different health statuses [25]. Above all once validity has been shown for one purpose it cannot be assumed for all possible populations or applications [26].

Table 3.

Method of Treatment	Degree of employment-probability (P)				Relative value
	Full time	Part time	Unemployed		
Hospital HD	0.34	0.25	0.21	0.20	0.54
Home HD	0.64	0.16	0.41	0.06	0.74
Live donor TP	0.75	0.10	0.10	0.05	0.77
Cadaver TP	0.66	0.12	0.13	0.09	0.71
Estimated Utility (U)	0.90	0.60	0.30	0.10	

Fitness for work after Haemodialysis and Transplantation. The horizontal row gives for each modality the probability (P) of the outcome specified at the top of the corresponding column. The final row gives on estimate of the utility (U) of each of the outcomes. The relative value for each modality is the sum of the possibilities of each outcome multiplied by the outcomes probability. Reproduced from reference [14], with permission

c. *Sensitivity of change or responsiveness.* Measures of quality of life that can distinguish between patients at a point in time are not necessarily as sensitive to changes in patients over time when repeated. This aspect is a crucial requirement for longitudinal studies especially clinical trials [27].

d. *Appropriateness.* To ensure that the quality of life measure used is most appropriate, the health problem and likely range of impacts of other treatments need to be carefully considered. Investigators sometimes use a wide range of measures – such "scatter gun" approach has problems and one approach may be to use instruments that let patients select dimensions of most concern which can be assessed over time [28, 29].

e. *Practicality.* This is important and current quality of life measures are most practical for use in clinical trials and formal evaluation studies. For regular use, the more detailed and comprehensive measures are impractical to administer, process, hard to interpret and incorporate into decision making [29].

Overall the design, analysis and interpretation of studies are crucial and are well reviewed by Fletcher *et al.* [30]. More specific to renal diseases Deniston *et al.* [31] assessed quality of life in ESRF using ten different multi-item indices and nine single item measures. Correlations between these measures suggest that these indices tend to represent either functions or feeling with moderate relationships within the two clusters but little between them. These workers concluded that depending on the measures chosen to assess quality of life, different conclusions about the relationship of quality of life to demographic characteristics will be reached. Hence there is the need to think more critically about the nature of the quality of life in arriving at judgements and the relative validity of these different measures.

6. Instruments used in assessments of ESRF patients

Many instruments are available and have been used (Table 4), for assessing quality of life in dialysis and transplant patients. Some of these have not been validated and others have used instruments without controlling for such factors of age, sex, race, ethnicity, educational level, type of job, income and location and associated comorbid conditions. Such considerations make the results reported from such studies questionable. Whatever the instrument that is utilised it is invariably in the form of a questionnaire which solicits a viewpoint, usually that of the patient. It also elicits at a point in time how the patient perceives his overall quality of life or specific measures that are addressed by the actual questionnaire. This is indeed important to understand and bears heavily on some of the requirements addressed previously in choosing the instrument, its validity and reproducibility.

It is at present difficult to advise as to which is the best instruments that would enable an adequate quality of life assessment to be undertaken in dialysis patients. There are only a few specific instruments developed for renal failure (Kidney Disease Questionnaire, and Parfreys Uraemic Index – Table 4). All the others are generic, adapted and to some extent, validated for use in renal replacement therapy patients. For overall objective assessment, Karnofsky performance index, SIP, SF36, NHP (all in Table 4) are good instruments. For those relating to subjective indicators the instruments available are vast in numbers, but those related to wellbeing, life satisfaction and psychological affect are obviously important but may not give specifically detailed nature of aspects of subjective life that is addressed by the more specific measures.

7. Multi disciplinary team in managing renal failure patients

McKevitt [99] defines the Healthcare support system as "Network of Individuals in Groups who provide care and assistance - physical, medical, social, emotional and financial – and who are called on in various degrees, particularly when as individual or family's own resources are insufficient to cope with needs, problems and crisis. Support in the form of care and treatment, information and education, empathy and encouragement and reassurance, guidance and councelling and concrete resources are provided, based on sensitivity and an understanding to the individuals total situation and of their special concerns and needs". It is not surprising, considering the extent to which such supports systems develop that there is a variety of opinions on this elusive question of quality of life. What is well known is that where support systems breakdown or do not exist rehabilitation of the patient can be more difficult [100].

DeNour [101] stresses the importance of staff attitudes and the rehabilitation of haemodialysis

Table 4. Various instruments used in assessing quality of life in renal replacement therapy patients. This is by no means a comprehensive list of instruments but comprise the commonly used ones (as shown in the reference).

OBJECTIVE:	REFERENCES
1. FUNCTIONAL ABILITY:	
Karnofsky Performance Index	[3, 4, 5, 31–36, 39, 40, 41]
Activities of Daily Living (ADL)	[37–38]
Spitzer Quality of Life Index (SQLI)	[31, 36, 50]
2. MEDICAL:	
Chemistry Abnormality Score (CAS)	[39]
Active Clinical Problems Score (ACDS)	[39]
3. Health Status:	
Sickness Impact Profile (SIP)	[38, 42, 43, 45, 46, 51]
Time Trade Off (TTO)	[4, 44, 45, 46, 51]
MOS shortform (SF36)	[47–49, 54, 55]
General Health Questionnaire	[53]
Nottingham Health Profile	[56–58]
*Parfreys Uraemic Index	[59–60]
*Kidney Disease Questionnaire	[46, 51]
EuroQol	[61, 62]

SUBJECTIVE:		REFERENCES
1. GENERAL		
Quality of Life Index (QLI)		[52]
Wellbeing		[3, 4, 5, 34, 35, 63, 65, 69]
Life Satisfaction		[3, 4, 5, 34, 35, 63, 66]
Psychological Affect		[3, 4, 5, 34, 35, 63]
Cantrills Ladder		[67, 68]
Semantic Differential		[66, 67]
Emotional Wellbeing –	Rosenburg selfesteem scale	[65, 70]
	Rosenburg happiness scale	[65, 70]
	Bradburn happiness item	[65, 71]
	Campbells Index of Wellbeing	[65, 72]
	Index of General Affect	[65, 72]
Social Wellbeing –	Vocational rehabilitation	
	Family adjustment	
	Role satisfaction	[65, 72, 73]
	Sexual adjustment and satisfaction	
	Social support satisfaction (SSS)	
	*Dialysis relationship quality (DRQ)	
2. PSYCHOLOGICAL		
Psychological wellbeing		[6, 5, 72]
Self esteem		[39, 74, 75]
Profile of mood states (POMS)		[39, 76, 77, 80]
Simmons Scale		[70, 75, 80]
Multidimensional Health Locus of Control (MHLoc)		[39, 78, 79, 80]
Antonovsky sense of coherence (ASOC)		[80, 81, 82]
Brief Symptom Inventory		[83, 84]
Psychological Adjustment to Physical Illness Scale (PAIS)		[85, 86]
3. STRESSORS AND SATISFACTION WITH THERAPY		
HD Stressor Scale		[91–93]
Stressor Assessment Sacle		[91, 95, 96]
Simmons Multichoice Items		[65, 69, 97]
Dialysis Stress Scale		[67, 87]
General Treatment Stress (GTXS)		[29, 98]
Modality Specific Stress (MSS)		[39, 98]
4. SOCIAL (39, 65, 67, 73)		
Social Support Satisfaction		[39]
Social/Liaison/Activities Index		[39, 98]

* Indicates disease specific for kidney failure – others are generic.

patients, in particular the importance of working as a team to help the patient. Similar arguments would apply equally to CAPD patients. A key factor in the success of treatment is that communication within the healthcare and multidisciplinary team is good and that treatment aims and expectations relayed to the patient and his family are consistent and realistic. Denial in the healthcare team, especially on the part of the physician can lead to conflict and difficulty in adjustment for the patient [101]. Maintaining good communication within such a complex support system can be difficult. The importance of the team developing a consistent and positive philosophy towards treatment is further delineated by McKevitt [102]. Burton et al. [103] found CAPD patients were more satisfied with the support received from household members and from spouses than haemodialysis patients. This could be due to the fact that roles within the family appear less affected with CAPD than with haemodialysis [104].

In the management of patients with ESRF, quality of life has a wide and varied definition, which is undoubtedly connected with the quality and the enthusiasm of the multidisciplinary health care team (nurses, doctors, social workers, physiotherapists, occupational therapists, dietitians, speech therapists, psychologists) who have to liaise closely with other important facets of the patients total environment (family, social groups, community and society – the latter becoming more important especially as it concerns employment, health departments and local authorities) [10].

8. Role of social workers in the peritoneal dialysis programme

Social work with endstage renal failure patients and their families is a specialised branch of this profession demanding not only the general skills taught during professional social work courses but considerable understanding of the medical background. A social worker is indeed a very important and effective member of the multi-disciplinary team and does require special councelling skills, knowledge of group work, handy therapy techniques and an ability to work in difficult social situations and family environments. The role of the social worker in a peritoneal dialysis programme in terms of councelling and support, the role within the multidisciplinary team and the role in the peritoneal dialysis unit are shown in Table 5 [10].

9. Studies on quality of life in ESRF

9.1. History

It is apparent that all the published reports can be classified according to three study periods or eras: these consist of an early period 1966–1972, the middle period 1973–1980, and the contemporary period of 1980 onwards. The types of studies conducted have varied by period with the least amount of empirical work being published during the early periods. This period tended to focus on the "stress" of dialysis and its psychiatric morbidity. It was also related to the maximisation of scarce dialysis and economic resources and patient selection was a primary consideration with rehabilitation used as a selection criteria [105].

The middle period up until 1980 was probably the least exciting. However, it was during this period that the economic issues surrounding dialysis were in large part resolved especially in the United States [106] and in Europe. This by and large, seemed to resolve the inherent patient selection/resource rationing problem and gave rise to a substantial increase in the size of the ESRF patient population. Nevertheless, several studies were published on various aspects of quality of life including psychosocial adaptation and employment and how these varied according to dialysis modality [107, 108].

The contemporary period over the last twelve years or so has proven to be the most exciting. During this time transplantation clearly has come into its own with other interesting innovations including the development of peritoneal dialysis as a major form of renal replacement therapy. It was during this period (in 1981) that Gutman et al. published a landmark study in the New England Journal of Medicine on the physical activity and employment status of maintenenace HD patients [41], and this was accompanied by an editorial in the same issue of the Journal [109]. Considerable doubt about the objective success of dialysis was raised by this survey which showed few ESRF patients were truly rehabilitated; only 25% of hospital haemodialysis patients were capable of doing little more than caring for themselves. Whilst this study may have been "superficial" and suffered form "sampling errors" it reopened a debate on how good these treatments were related to the enormous cost. Rennie [109] argued that there was a need for a national database and debate to better understand this problem. Shortly afterwards the Health Care Financing Administration (HCFA) convened a task force to examine the problem associated with renal patient rehabilitation and at the same time HCFA funded the National Kidney Dialysis and Kidney Transplantation Study [110, 111]. It was not until this contemporary period that a truly comprehensive appreciation of the quality of life of ESRF patients emerged. Many investigations from a wide variety of disciplinary backgrounds embarked upon quality of life assessments. It is also during this time that several innovative features made their mark on renal replacement therapy. These included:

1. Establishment of CAPD and its subsequent growth in the treatment of ESRF.
2. Development of automated peritoneal dialysis and the need to monitor adequacy of peritoneal dialysis.
3. Improving transplantation results with the introduction of Cyclosporin.
4. The introduction of Recombinant human erythropoietin (EPO) for the treatment of anaemia of chronic renal failure. This very significant improvement does question the value of any study completed before the availability of EPO. The numerous and significant improvements in both subjective and objective aspects of quality of life following EPO have now been verified, including those at the energy level, appetite, exercise capability and cognitive function [35, 58, 112–117]. Because previous studies did not usually control for level of anaemia, the results may reflect the adverse effects of anaemia rather than uraemia or its treatment.

Table 5. The role of the social worker in peritoneal dialysis [10].

1. Counselling and Support

1. Creating confidence and rapport with patient and family to facilitate expression of fears, anxieties and problems.
2. Recognition of the patient's right to feel anger and resentment.
3. Helping patient to work through periods of low morale through sympathetic listening.
4. Home visits to mitigate feelings of isolation on leaving hospital.
5. Co-joint sessions with patients and spouse or family to help mutual expression of feelings and improve communication.
6. Sexual counselling where indicated.
7. Encouragement to broaden social contacts/take part in activities where this seems realistic and appropriate.

2. Role within the multi-disciplinary team

1. Input to initial assessment and formulation of the treatment plans including a full social report where requested.
2. Sharing of information (with patient's consent) where circumstances have a bearing on patient's medical condition or treatment.
3. Regular attendance at multi-disciplinary unit meeting to liaise.
4. Liaison with team about practical arrangements, e.g. delivery of supplies, holiday plans, exchanges at work, transport.
5. Referral of patients, e.g. for psychiatric help, genetic counselling.
6. Arranging ward meetings between relatives, doctors, nursing staff, etc., when situations arise that need team discussion.
7. Ensuring that the team understands the social worker's role, so that appropriate referrals can be made by any team member.
8. Assisting in the management of stressful situations confronting the multi-disciplinary team.
9. Educating colleagues in the community about CAPD and the needs of CAPD patients.

3. Role within Dialysis Unit

Social assessment should take into account the following areas:

A. The patient's environment.
   1. The patient's family and support network.
   2. Employment, and prospect for fitting this into the treatment regime.
   3. Accommodation with special reference to (a) problems of space for storage of equipment and performing treatment, (b) need for additional facilities such as handbasin, shower or toilet, (c) the patient's ability to manage stairs (some elderly patients need to have ground floor sleeping, toilet and CAPD exchange facilities).
   4. Financial situation and possible benefits available.
   5. Availability of telephone and transport to mitigate isolation and assist communication.

B. The patient's personality.
   6. The patient's understanding and attitude to his illness and treatment. The family's understanding and attitude to illness and treatment.
   7. Brief assessment of the patient's particular strengths and weaknesses, and an estimation of ability to adjust to treatment.
   8. Evidence of previous ability to cope with setbacks.
   9. Previous interests and hobbies of the patient, especially if these may be affected by the illness or treatment.

Finally, there is the problem about the escalating costs of renal replacement therapy and the desire on the part of governments to ration health care. This has obviously raised a considerable amount of debate, even in countries like the United States where the treatment for patients with ESRF has been financed since 1973 by Medicare's ESRF programme [118–120].

9.2. Quality of life in peritoneal dialysis; comparisons between PD and HD

In 1981 a series of studies began at the Battelle Human Affairs Research Centres in Seattle, USA concerning the Quality of Life of Dialysis and Transplant patients. These studies in chronological order were:

1. The National Kidney Dialysis and Kidney Transplantation Study.
2. The National Heart Transplantation Study.
3. The Kidney Transplant Immunosuppressive Protocol Study.
4. The Amgen Recombinant Human Erythropoeitin Study [5].

These have been referred to as the "Battelle" series. The first of these by Evans et al. [3] was a cross sectional study involving eleven dialysis and transplant centres from which 859 patients were randomly selected to be interviewed. Of these patient 287 were on home HD, 347 on incentre HD, 81 on CAPD, 144 were Transplants. This study looked at objective (functional impairment Karnofsky index, and ability to work) and subjective indicators (life satisfaction, wellbeing and general affect), in the four groups of patients. The overall results are summarised in Table 6 which shows the results for the Karnofsky index. This shows that normal physical activity was present in 79% of transplant patients, 59% home HD and 48% CAPD patients. On the three subjective measures, transplant patients again had a higher quality of life than dialysis patients, who nevertheless compared favourably with the general population. Hence the perceived quality of life of the various groups did not differ significantly. However, the study concluded that objective evidence of successful rehabilitation did not exist except in the case of transplant recipients and some patients undergoing home dialysis. In a similar study, Morris and Jones [53] compared 160 patients with ESRF managed by the same renal replacement modes; they endorsed transplantation as a method of improving the quality of life for the majority of patients with ESRF. This study also showed that for older patients with ESRF, CAPD is well tolerated and shows superiority over in centre HD. However, moderately high levels of psychological distress were noted in all forms of ESRF treatments.

The "Battelle" series of studies, referred to above, address similar subjective and objective measures to assess quality of life; of the three studies that were compiled together for analysis (excluding National Heart Transplantation Study), the subjective quality of life assessment in the various patient groups is summarised in Table 7. This table again highlights the superiority of subjective indicators in the transplant group as well as the improvement in HD patients following EPO therapy. CAPD patients in the Battelle series also demonstrated a better perceived health status, a high index of wellbeing and greater life satisfaction than incentre HD patients.

In the United Kingdom a combined Manchester/Oxford study undertook to review these questions in 159 dialysis patients (78 HD, 81 CAPD) [67]. This study again reported a marked deterioration in the mobility on treatment as compared to that prior to commencement of therapy and the same was also true for items of everyday life (shopping, cooking, travel, social life) [121]. However, subjective measures of quality of life as perceived by the patient showed, no significant difference from a normal population [122]. On Various psychological scales (Cantrill's life satisfaction, semantic differential, life stress, happiness and satisfaction scale), these patients perceived life to be satisfactory and comparable to a normal population. However, one group (males less than 60 years of age with risk factors like diabetes and ischaemic

Table 6. Functional ability according to the Karnofsky index in the four groups of patients studied by Evans et al. [3].

	HHD 287(n)	ICHD 347	CAPD 81 %	TP 144
Normal physical activity	59	44	48	79
Normal p/a part of time	25	25	25	9
Self care only	9	13	12	5
Requires some assistance	7	18	15	7

Abbreviations are: HHD, home haemodialysis; TP, transplant patients; p/a, physical activity ICHD, incentre HD.
[Data are reproduced with permission from reference [4].

heart disease) was consistently less satisfied with life than other groups.

Several comparative studies have subsequently been published which have looked at the issues of quality of life in incentre HD and peritoneal dialysis patients in a controlled manner, looking at various aspects of quality of life and using differing instruments. A well conducted large study done by Simmons et al. [65] assessed 766 patients who experienced one of the renal replacement therapies for at least one year but who in addition were non diabetic and aged between 19 and 56 years. The four groups that were studied were incentre HD (83 patients from eight centres), CAPD (510 patients from 185 centres) current transplants (91 patients, successfully transplanted between 1980 and 1984) and historical transplants (82 performed in the 1970s). Survey questionnaires were administered containing measures of physical, emotional and social wellbeing, vocational rehabilitation, and sexual adjustment. Casemix differences were controlled, in so far as possible, with an analysis of covariance; adjusted means were compared. Findings of the study are shown in Table 8 and again indicate that the quality of life for successful transplant recipients exceeded that of both dialysis groups for almost all variables; however, CAPD patients had a significantly better life and therapy satisfactions as compared to incentre HD patients.

In another comparative study by Walcott and Nissenson 33 matched pairs of CAPD and in centre HD patients were assessed for various measures of quality of life [123]. Here CAPD patients had a higher quality of life, lower illness, lower modality related stress, lower mood disturbances, higher employment, higher community activities and better cognitive function. Similar results were found in the "Batelle" series, who also demonstrated a better perceived health status, higher index of wellbeing and a good life satisfaction than in centre HD patients. In addition Nissenson et al. [80] found that CAPD patients had superior psychosocial adaptation and concluded that patients who had higher levels of stress on in centre HD may benefit from CAPD therapy.

More recent studies of quality of life in ESRF have re-examined these issues. The first of these is by Bremmer et al. [124] which looked at a self administered questionnaire assessing both objective and subjective quality of life in 489 ESRF patients. This study revealed that patients differed in both objective and subjective quality of life when examined as a function of treatment modality. They found that quality of life was similar for successful transplant and home HD patients; these patients appeared to fair better than other treatment groups on both objective and subjective measures. Patients receiving staff assisted incentre HD and CAPD reported markedly diminished quality of life; these differences remained after statistically controlling for non-treatment variables. One of the purposes of the study was to test the representativeness of the results from Evans et al. [3] and indeed Bremmer et al. [124] substantiated the results of Evans and colleagues. The replicability supports the usefulness of these measures for evaluation of different treatment modalities for ESRF and presumably for other

Table 7. Subjective quality of life, by treatment modality.

Treatment	Well-being	Life satisfaction	Psych affect
Home HD	11.12	5.42	5.19
ICHD	10.77	5.15	5.11
CAPD	11.05	5.25	5.30
EPO HD baseline	11.24	5.05	5.63
EPO HD follow up	11.87	5.25	6.02
Conventional TP	11.83	5.66	5.62
CSA nondiabetic TP	11.23	5.17	5.50

Data relating to various renal replacement therapy groups, regarding well-being, life satisfaction and psychological (Psych) affect.
Abbreviations are: EPO human erythropoietin: CsA, Cyclosporin A. [Data quoted from reference [4] with permission]. Psychological affect describes how patients feel about their present life, based on eight bipolar items. The responses are averaged to provide a mean score. The higher the score the better the affect. The index of overall life satisfaction, also based on bipolar responses, ranges from a low of 1 (completely dissatisfied) to a high of 7 (completely satisfied). Index of wellbeing ranges from 2.1 (low level) to 14.7 (high level).

Table 8. Relationships of therapy to quality of life.

Dimension	ICHD	CAPD	Curr TP	Hist TP
Physical wellbeing (4–21)	14.4	14.64	17.55	16.95
Health satis (1–5)	3.24	3.44	3.26	–
Life satisaction (1–7)	4.47	5.07	5.64	–
Therapy satisfaction (1–5)	3.59	4.59	4.85	4.95
Social wellbeing (4–16)	10.12	10.48	11.93	12.89

Figures in parenthesis reflect the range with higher scores reflecting a better level of Quality of Life. Current transplant (Curr TP) are those followed between 1980 to 1984. Historical transplants (Hist TP) from 1970–1973. [Adapted from reference [65] and reproduced from reference [4] with permission].

chronic diseases. The other purpose of the study [124] was to re-examine the impact of transplant failure by defining the three outcomes of transplant (initial success, failure followed by successful retransplant and failure followed by return to dialysis treatment). The results demonstrated that the transplant patients who returned to dialysis treatment suffered substantial impairment of quality of life and that this impairment was masked if these patients were analysed with successfully retransplanted patients in an evaluation of "transplant failure" used as a covariant.

Tucker et al. [125] again compared in centre haemodialysis and CAPD patients on several quality of life variables: dietary adherence, self esteem, hope, wellbeing, marital happiness, perceived control of life, marital status, number of emotional support persons and participation in social recreation and work activities. There were no statistically significant differences in the quality of life variables due to treatment modality or demographic variables. However, CAPD patients did engage in significantly more social and recreational activity, though not more work activity than did incentre HD patients. An interesting point was the skewed racial distribution in this US population in that 73% of the CAPD patients were caucasian whilst 72% of the incentre HD patients were of black origin. This skewed racial composition, also noted in previous research publications, suggests that a choice of treatment is occurring on the basis of some set of patient characteristics or perhaps systematic assignment is occurring on the basis of race, sex and/or education.

Finally a study by Muthny and Koch [126] also confirmed the favourable outcome of renal transplantation in terms of medical and vocational rehabilitation but also with respect to emotional wellbeing, complaints and satisfaction of different life areas (satisfaction with physical performance, intellectual functioning, partnership, family life, sex life and leisure time activities). This study also confirmed the findings of Evans et al. [3] but were in conflict with those of Kalman et al. [127] who did not find differences between treatment groups especially in terms of psychiatric morbidity. For example, using the global anxiety score, in this group of patients from Germany [126], there was no discrimination between the three groups of incentre HD, CAPD and renal transplantation patients.

A recent quality of life study in the UK in ESRF patients undergoing dialysis and transplant treatments shows interesting results. Patients were comprised of incentre HD (95), home HD (59), CAPD (93) and transplant groups (367). A patient questionnaire had been developed to assess quality of life data which could also be converted into the Rosser states of illness [128, 129, 130]. The questionnaire and data analysis took into account comorbidity, severity, an overall disability level and an overall distress level. With respective to comparability and comorbidity the response in this study differed from those involved in Bremer et al. [124] and Evans et al. [3]. This may simply reflect national difference in experience of illness but may also be due to age differences (CAPD and transplant patients in this study were older than their counterparts in the other two studies). In this UK study [128], 35% of the dialysis respondents needed a walking aid or help to get outdoors, or were bedridden, 32% had a problem with some aspect of self care, 30% reported that their usually activity was either severely affected or unable to be carried out, 84% had a problem with some aspect of personal and social relationships. Social life, hobbies, leisure and sex life were affected in 75% of dialysis respondents. However, there were few differences between dialysis groups, and in addition, those with a functioning transplant had a much better quality of life than those on dialysis. When one looked at the overall quality of life score, coded into the Rosser categories of disability and distress, the same trend continued. Two additional comments of concern relating to the design of the research come to mind from this study. Firstly, age was clearly an important factor and in this study there were several areas where significant differences were due to age differences rather than the treatment modes themselves. The second point relates to the questionnaires; quality of life questionnaires can vary considerably depending on the aim and emphasis of the authors. The questionnaire used in the study was designed so that it could be sent out to respondents by mail; whilst they were fairly short, they still aimed to be comprehensive. A disadvantage of this method is a potential loss of data either through non completion or through misunderstandings arising from ambiguous or difficult questions. A alternative design is an interview based questionnaire such as that developed by Parfry [59, 60].

9.3. Time trade off, sickness impact profile, SK36 and Uraemic Index

These new instruments have recently been used to asses quality of life in patients undergoing renal replacement therapy. Timetrade off (TTO) score looks at the ratio between years of full health which the patient would consider equivalent to a lifetime with ESRF [44]. TTO is the ratio of the two where zero equals death, one equals full health. These workers found that scores in various groups were: incentre HD-0.43, home HD-0.49, CAPD-0.56, transplantation 0.84. This instrument has also been used to assess the impact of change from dialysis to transplantation [45]. Sickness Impact Profile (SIP) [18] has now come to be recognised as a very strong instrument for quality of life assessment. 136 questions are put into 12 categories and scores are expressed on a scale of 1–100 with higher scores denoting worse states. Normal individuals have scores between 2 and 3 and terminally ill patients around 35. Hart and Evans [43] looked at this index in 859 renal replacement therapy patients. Scores for the transplant groups were 5.5, home HD 10, CAPD 12.2, and incentre HD 13.9. The "Battelle" series reported by Evans [5] relates this SIP scores by treatment modality breaking down the scores into the physical and psychosocial dimensions (Table 9). Again the superiority of transplantation is obvious while there is little in the way to choose between incentre HD and CAPD.

The MOS shortform health survey – SF36 (Table 4) has been used in assessing the health and functional status of chronic dialysis patients and to compare their health to well subjects and patients with other chronic diseases. Quality of life studies have also been reported in children [131, 132] and the elderly [36, 122, 133–135].

Table 9. Sickness impact profile, by treatment modality.

Treatment	Dimension %		
	Physical	Psychosocial	Total
HHD	6.1	6.4	9.5
ICHD	10.3	9.7	13.9
CAPD	11.3	8.2	13.7
CONV TP	3.3	4.1	5.5
CsA TP	3.8	7.1	6.3

Data are adapted from the Battelle Dialysis and Transplant series [5] and reproduced with permission from reference [4]. For details of the scores, see text. CONV – conventional, CsA – cyclosporin.

Parfrey and colleagues [60] have assessed a health questionnaire specific for ESRF in 107 dialysis and 119 transplant recipients. They looked at the prevalence of 24 physical symptoms and a questionnaire was devised using two new indices (a symptom scale using 12 symptoms and an affect scale comprising 12 emotions) and 6 indices previously used in other chronic illnesses. Constructive validity for the questionnaire was shown by interviewing 97 dialysis and 82 transplant patients in whom the authors hypothesised that physical wellbeing would be better in transplant patients. After each initial matching the transplant were more active with a higher objective quality of life and free of physical symptoms than the dialysis group. Subsequently, 63 stable dialysis and 67 stable transplant patients, 15 dialysis patients successfully transplanted in the intervening year and 5 failed transplant patients were reinterviewed one year later to assess the responsiveness of the questionnaire. In the group who had recently been successfully transplanted both physical affect and quality of life scores showed a major improvement following transplant. The authors conclude that this questionnaire is specific for ESRF, examines physical, psychological and social wellbeing, the instrument is brief, easily administered and reproducible. It also has construct validity and is responsive to changes in therapy. This instrument obviously needs to be utilised further to validate these claims.

10. Employment

Whilst this is an objective parameter of quality of life it is a more difficult parameter to assess because it is related to social circumstances, reimbursement for employment, "employability" in view of employer related bias against dialysis and transplant patients and placing housewives in an unemployed category. Nevertheless, what data are available seem to support better employability of successfully transplanted patients (Table 10). For CAPD patients Fragola et al. [40] found a similar percentage employed after commencement of CAPD; this study was undertaken when the therapy was still in its infancy in the early eighties. Simmons et al. [65], found sharp differences in vocational rehabilitation in the four groups (male patients: historic transplants-75%; current transplant 64%; CAPD 35%; incentre HD 19%. Female patients: 36%, 31%, 15%, 11% respectively). Julius et al. [136] evaluated 742 patients form Michegan reporting CAPD patients were 2.6 times more likely to work than incentre HD patients.

Employment prospects are known to be related to the functional ability of patients. Form the "Battelle" series it is apparent that diabetics were less able initially than non diabetics to work although the outlook for all patients improved with time. Even 15 months after transplantation, 50% of the non-diabetics had returned to work compared to 25% of diabetics. Seedat et al. [137] also reported a decline in employment in both CAPD and incentre HD groups but none in the transplant groups. 32% of the CAPD and 42% of the incentre HD patients were employed in this series from South Africa. Simmons et al. [138] noted that vocational rehabilitation is a particular area of concern. Overall transplant patients are the most likely to be working full time, but pointed out that regulations concerning disability payments under the ESRF programme operate as disincentives for employment. In this study 51% of CAPD patients agreed that they did not work because they were worried losing social security disability payments. Walcott and Nissenson [123] found that 88% of the incentre HD subjects reported no current participation in school, work or household activities as compared with 55% of CAPD subject who reported absence of these vocational activities. These workers felt, therefore, that CAPD is independently associated with higher frequency of maintained vocational function in chronic dialysis patients. Whether this differential level of vocational activity resulted from the relatively small differences in educational history in this population, physician bias to selectively encourage more active patients to begin CAPD, or from true modality effects on vocational function is uncertain and needs further assessment. In a study by Julius et al. [136] the subsample of known diabetic patients aged 20–64 years from the Michigan ESRF disease population was analysed. 742 patients were entered into this study and interviews were conducted from 1984–1986. Significantly higher percentage of the patients undergoing stable CAPD were in the labour force than those undergoing incentre HD (27.4% vs 9.6%). Using logistic regression, and adjusted for sex, race, age, education, marital status, primary diagnosis and duration of the ESRF, this stable CAPD group was 2.6 times more likely to be employed than incentre HD groups. Similar data were reported by Bremmer et al. [124] (28% employed full time on CAPD vs 9% on incentre HD). This group showed that incentre HD patients were more likely to be employed part time than CAPD (23% vs 10%). In Europe the situation is not any different.

In the Oxford-Manchester study [67] there was a dramatic decline in the percentage of patients that were employed while on dialysis as compared to those before dialysis therapy (CAPD 44% from 73%; incentre HD 42% from 83%).

Muthny and Koch [126] in Germany found that the transplant group had the highest vocational rehabilitation. Excluding those above the age of 60 years from the analysis, 31% of the transplant patients, 16% of incentre HD and 19% of CAPD patients were working full time. These are lower rates than in other reported studies but is related to about 50% or so of these patients reporting their vocational status as "retired".

11. Sexual functioning and psychosexual problems

This is an area that has been neglected through ignorance and embarrassment on the part of the renal care team. Nevertheless, studies in this area have shown a dramatic decline in sexual activity for patients on both treatments (PD and HD). Relatively few studies exist in this field and are summarised in a recent review [139]. Auer et al. [67] showed a dramatic decline of sexual activity on dialysis compared to 12 months prior to commencement of therapy. This applied equally to peritoneal dialysis and HD patients; only 31% of patients had sexual activity satisfactory as compared to nearly 60% prior to dialysis, whilst the non existent sexual activity category increased form 22% pre-dialysis to nearly 50% on treatment. Furthermore when the

Table 10. Percentage of patients who are actually working or able to work on the various treatment modalities.

Treatment Modality	Working %	Able to work
Home HD	36.2	59.2
ICHD	20.5	37.2
CAPD	16.2	24.7
EPO HD baseline	22.9	38.7
EPO HD follow-up	24.5	35.9
Conventional TP	45.9	74.1
CSA TP	31.2	60.9
CSA diabetic TP	21.5	37.0

(Data are adapted from reference [5] and reproduced with permission from reference [4] abbreviations as in previous tables).

same cohorts in the study were asked about an affectionate relationship, 87% of married couples were satisfied with marriage but only 24% had satisfactory sexual relationships [140]. Simmons and Abress [138] reviewed satisfaction with sexual activity in male transplant, CAPD and incentre HD patients. On a scale of 1 (complete dissatisfaction) to 7 (complete satisfaction), the three groups had scores of 4.87, 3.11 and 3.21. In the study by Gudex et al. [128] relating to patients in the UK, sex life became seriously affected on therapy in roughly 70% of all dialysis patients (home HD, incentre HD and PD), but only 31% of transplant patients. For hobbies and leisure activities and social life being seriously affected, similar percentages of dissatisfaction were reported in the four treatment groups.

In the study by Muthny and Koch [126] relatively high contentness was reported with respect to family life, partnership and role in the family; less than 10% in this German study showed mild dissatisfaction in these areas. In contrast, however, almost 30% reported marked dissatisfaction with sex life. The highest dissatisfied group being 40% of the incentre HD patients, 33% of the renal transplant, 43% of the HD and 56% of CAPD patients reported that they had had no sexual intercourse in the previous four weeks. Bremmer et al. [124] found sexual activity quite markedly down in incentre HD patients compared to CAPD which in turn was worse than in transplanted patients. Days since last orgasm with intercourse was around 180 days in incentre HD patients as opposed to around 28 days in the CAPD patients and 4 in the transplant patients. Finally, Suskolne and Kaplan DeNour [83] showed that in chronic dialysis patients there was markedly diminished participation in social and leisure activities with increased marital and sexual problems.

12. Psychosocial adjustment and dialysis related stress

Serial studies have looked at effective therapy on subjective indicators of quality of life such as physical wellbeing, emotional wellbeing and social wellbeing [65, 75, 97, 138], as well as psychological status and social status [39, 67, 122, 123] (see Table 4). Simmons et al. [65] found that physical, emotional and social wellbeing and satisfaction with therapy as clusters all correlated significantly with therapy type. These findings clearly indicate the existence of differences among therapies along all dimensions of quality of life. Secondly the effect of therapy type on each specific variable within the clusters was also compared. On most variables, most of the transplant cohorts scored more favourably than either the CAPD or the HD group. For most of the 23 variables differences among the four therapy groups was statistically significant. Comparison of the HD and CAPD groups for 22 variables showed significant differences favouring the CAPD group on nine variables (healthier than before therapy, self esteem, happiness, index of wellbeing, overall life satisfaction, social life satisfaction, happiness with therapy and would still be happy to choose the same therapy). One other characteristic in this study related to the differentiation in the groups with regards to the years on therapy. When this is taken into account the results show that whilst current transplant patients continue to exhibit a more favourable adjustment than HD or CAPD patients, CAPD patients no longer demonstrated an advantage over the HD patients. The CAPD patients showed significantly higher health satisfaction, therapy satisfaction, and higher self esteem than the HD patients and rated at least slightly higher on the other seven variables. In summary, therefore, when background characteristics and disease history variables are controlled, the advantages of transplantation clearly persist but the advantages of CAPD over HD do not. In the study of Walcott and Nissenson [123] looking at 33 matched pairs of incentre HD and CAPD patients from the Los Angeles areas, findings were somewhat different in terms of the psychological status. A larger percentage of CAPD patients had higher self esteem, consistently lower profiles of mood states and total mood disturbances, and lower levels of current emotional distress. CAPD subjects also reported lesser amounts of illness and treatment related stresses than the chronic HD group on the various disease and treatment related stresses (GTXS, modality specific stress Table 4). CAPD subjects also reported a higher frequency of participation in community activities and better relationships with dialysis physicians and patients.

Undoubtedly, dialysis does impart stress and several factors have been identified as stressors. Simmons and Abress [138] looked at satisfaction as an indicator of stress and found that incentre HD patients faired worse. Walcott and Nissenson [123] found that CAPD had a lower modality related stress score; this group also found that in males over

51 years of age, lower vocational activity was associated with poor adaptation to dialysis and increased stress. Bihl et al. [92] found that the severity of stressors in CAPD groups was related to uncertainty of the future, limits on vacations and frequent hospitalisation while in the incentre HD group, stresses were found to be fatigue and boredom, limitation of fluid intake and length of treatment. Similar findings are reported by Eichel [93] and Fuchs and Schreiber [96].

These studies suggest that there is some difference between the treatments in relationship to stress. The stresses are different and there are differing anxieties on the various treatment modalities.

13. Impact of EPO on quality of life

Over the last decade there have been several advances technically and therapeutically in renal replacement therapy. The introduction of recombinant human erythropoietin has indeed been a significant advance in this last decade. The impact of EPO has been quite dramatic and several studies have been published which have shown an improvement in quality of life in dialysis patients [46, 58, 112–117]. Various parameters have shown considerable improvement including energy, physical activity, employment and sleep. However, good prospective studies in CAPD patients are limited. One such looking at improvement of quality of life of CAPD patients treated with subcutaneously administered erythropoietin [58] used the Nottingham Health Profile, before and after treatment. The haemoglobin baseline was 7.5 gm/dl and rose to 10.8 g/dl at retest. There were significant improvements in energy, social life, relationships at home, and leisure pursuits. 12 patients who had already completed more than 9 months on EPO treatment were reassessed to determine whether the changes were sustained. Mean haemoglobin at second retest was 12.8 gm/dl. Improvement in energy continued to be significant and emotional wellbeing showed further improvement. Problems with household tasks which had not shown significant improvement were now considerably reduced. The studies showed far reaching benefits similar to those reported with EPO in haemodialysis patients in a CAPD population with a higher mean age and higher coexisting illness or disability than most reported haemodialysis studies.

More recently the effect of EPO has been evaluated in other CAPD populations. In a double blind placebo controlled study [141] involving 89 patients from 12 centres who had been on CAPD for greater than three months, there was an increase in the haematocrit after 12 weeks to 32% in 87% of the patients, whilst this figure was 25% in the placebo group. Patients on EPO felt better and transfusion requirements decreased.

The optimal haematocrit required to provide an enhanced quality of life, and yet avoid some of the potential risk of EPO resulting form an increased haemtocrit would be important to ascertain. Whilst there is no prospective study to address this question, the Canadian erythropoeitin study group [114] compared patients on placebo, with the HD patients on EPO whose mean level of concentration was maintained at 10.2 gm/dl and 11.7 gm/dl after six months on therapy. They found significant improvement scores for fatigue, physical symptoms, relationships and depression on the Kidney Disease questionnaire [46] and in the global and physical scores of the Sickness Impact Profile for patients on EPO as compared to those on placebo. In addition the time walked in the exercise stress test was significantly longer for patients on EPO. There was however, no significant difference in these parameters for patients in the 10.2 g/dl group as compared to the 11.7 g/dl group. Of significance was the fact that the patients in the higher haemoglobin group had a greater incidence of hypertension and vascular access clotting than patients in the lower haemoglobin group. Based on this study it would seem that an optimal haemoglobin level would be somewhere between 10 and 11 g/dl but a proper evaluation is needed in a prospective manner to ascertain this and to see whether maximum quality of life can be achieved and the level of haemoglobin that is necessary to achieve this [114, 142].

14. Summary of studies on quality of life and future trends

Possibly the most critical issue on quality of life studies that compare modalities of dialysis is the fact that patients are not randomly assigned to a given modality. By and large peritoneal dialysis and home HD are greatly under represented and in centre HD is over represented. This applies to most western countries with perhaps the exception of the United Kingdom [143]. Even within an individual country a given modality of treatment would vary from region to region. Many factors seem to play a role in assigning a particular modality of therapy to a patient. Those reasons have been reviewed in an excellent article by Nissenson et al. [143]. This situation is further complicated since patients frequently change their modality of treatment for both medical and non medical reasons [144]. Therefore the timing of a study comparing modalities becomes a critical variable in itself [65, 145]. Because peritoneal dialysis patients have a higher drop out rate compared to incentre HD patients [146, 147] studies later in the course of therapy can be biased in favour of peritoneal dialysis in that "survivors" of the technique are studied [64]. Very few longitudinal studies of the quality of life of dialysis patients have been done and none have adequately addressed the critical issue of selection bias. Modality selection is important as it has an impact on outcome and quality of life and an analysis of medical decision making such as modality selection must include an understanding of the potential costs and benefits of the decision. In addition to this, few if any studies on patients, have been evaluated pre-dialysis, to determine if quality of life patterns truly represent the effect of dialysis or rather are more representative of the pre-dialysis status of the patient [148]. Only a very few studies have evaluated patients early in the course of treatment to determine what if any effect dialysis of any type might have on the patient. Finally, the impact of recombinant human erythropoietin has been such that one must question the validity of studies prior to the EPO era. Newer studies defined in a prospective manner need to be approached, taking into account the level of anaemia.

15. What do we need to know and how to achieve it

Dialysis care, can be divided into three major component parts; structure, process and outcome. The outcome of most interest in patients is currently, mortality. However, other outcomes of therapy, critical to assessing the quality of care will be added to the ongoing evaluation of endstage renal failure programmes. It is important therefore when making assessments of the outcomes of care that specific areas of structure and process of dialytic care must be examined. Patient specific data and casemix are important variables that have an impact on outcome. Information that describes the relative importance and effects of various comorbid conditions, weighted by severity, is essential. These data are needed to adjust and evaluate outcome such as mortality, hospitalisation rates, cost of care, intensity of resource utilisation, quality of life, rehabilitation and patient satisfaction. In addition more information is needed regarding the influence of psychosocial and demographic characteristics on outcomes. The effects of income, job status, family status, education and various psychological factors (such as depression or coping mechanism) need to be examined. Other specific areas that need to be built into the equation related to treatment that the patient receives, are the effect of dose of dialysis prescribed and delivered, time of treatment versus solute clearances, dialyser uses, and changes of modality of dialysis. Finally, how the choice of modality is made and how this decision is controlled by the physician or by other factors is also going to be important.

When all these factors are corrected for, one then has to decide on what instruments are available to assess this quality of life and outcome. Many instruments are available (Table 4) and have been used for assessing the quality of life of dialysis patients. The central theme has always been to arrive at an instrument which is comprehensive enough to include many dimensions of quality of life, short enough to minimise respondent burden, reliable and valid, easily scored, interpreted and inexpensive. Such comprehensive overall instruments are limited and have their drawbacks but the SF36, Sickness Impact Profile, Nottingham Health Profile and a Karnofsky Performance Index (functional ability), are good instruments. It would be important to supplement these with disease specific information which is incorporated in Parfrey's Uraemic Index and the Kidney Disease Questionnaire (Table 4). In terms of assessing patients mental or emotional condition and social wellbeing, various instruments also exist but those that are easy to utilise include POMS, PAIS. The overall scales of wellbeing, life satisfaction and psychological affect are also useful.

One cannot stress enough the urgent need for a core battery to assess quality of life in endstage renal failure patients. Amongst hundreds of published papers one can hardly find half a dozen that are studied by the same methods to ascertain quality of life aspects. This lack of agreement about methods of measurement is at least a partial explanation for the contradictory information that is presented above. There is not general agreement about the quality of life of patients in renal replacement therapy. Some results are very hard to accept (e.g. in the study by Evans [3] American home dialysis and transplant patients were found to be happier than the general American public). The lack of consensus about patients quality of life is not only an academic problem but also a highly practical one. If we do not know patients adjustment how can we study and elucidate the factors that influence adjustment, how can we improve adjustment or how can we suggest to patients which of the available renal replacement therapies is better for them. In this respect it is of interest that the US Renal Data System casemix-adequacy of dialysis study has commenced and because of the size, complexity and cost of these projects it is unlikely to be repeated but is likely to provide useful data relating to risk stratification based upon patient casemix and the impact this has on quality of care provided and the outcome of this care.

16. Summary

Rehabilitation can be achieved by renal replacement therapy. Data to date would indicate that most successfully transplanted patients achieve rehabilitation both on objective and subjective criteria in a cost effective manner; however, unsuccessful transplantation has a poor quality of life outcome. Home dialysis patients achieve this same goal to a certain extent. For incentre haemodialysis and peritoneal dialysis patients, the objective evidence of rehabilitation is lacking; however perceived quality of life on subjective measures shows results comparable to a normal population. Comparisons between incentre haemodialysis and CAPD populations are difficult but different modality related stressors impart differing stresses to the patient. CAPD has marginal advantages over incentre dialysis. What is needed in the future in unravelling the many questions facing the endstage renal dialysis community with respect to outcome appears to be the development of a model of risk stratification based upon patient casemix. Patients can then be characterised in sufficient details to draw practical conclusions. Whilst the effect on patient survival is important, of much greater relevance is the effect of the treatment of renal failure on patient quality of life. Improving this outcome should be the primary goal of endstage renal failure care whether or not life is substantially prolonged. Future studies in this area, addressing the shortcomings of the available ones as outlined in this review, should be given high priority for research funding.

References

1. Spilker B, Molinek F, Johnston K, Simpson RL, Tilson HH. Quality of life bibliography and indexes. Med Care 1990; 28 (suppl): D51–77.
2. Wilkin D, Hallam L, Doggett M. Measure of need and outcome for primary care. Oxford University Press, Oxford 1992.
3. Evans RW, Manninen DL, Garrison LP et al. The quality of life of patients with endstage renal failure. N Engl J Med 1985; 312: 553–9.
4. Gokal R. Quality of Life in patients undergoing renal replacement therapy. Kidney Int 1993; 43 (suppl 40): S23–7.
5. Evans RW. Quality of Life assessment and the treatment of endstage renal disease. Transplant Rev 1990; 4: 28–51.
6. Mathers DF. Beyond survival. Dial Transplantation 1980; 9: 657–61.
7. Hopkins A. How might measures of quality of life be useful to me as a Clinician? In: Hopkins A (ed), Measures of the Quality of Life. Royal College of Physicians of London publications, London 1992; 1–13.
8. Fitzpatrick R, Fletcher A, Gore S, Jones D, Spiegelhalter D, Cox D. Quality of Life measures in healthcare. I: Applications and issues in assessment. Brit Med J 1992; 305: 1074–7.
9. Alexander JL, Willems EP. Quality of Life; some measurement requirements. Arch Phys Med Rehabil 1981; 62: 261–5.
10. Stout J, Auer J. Rehabilitation and Quality of Life on CAPD. In: Gokal R (ed), Continuous Ambulatory Peritoneal Dialysis. Churchill Livingstone, Edinburgh 1986; 327–48.
11. Churchill DN. The effect of treatment modality on the Quality of Life for patients with end stage renal disease. Adv Perit Dial 1988; 8: 63–5.
12. Hopkins A. Measuring the Quality of Medical Care. Royal College of Physicians of London Publications, London 1990.
13. Department of Health. The Health of a Nation. HMSO, London 1991.
14. Black D. Ethical issues arising from measures of the Quality of Life In: Hopkins A (ed), Measures of the Quality of Life. Royal Colege of Physicians of London Publications, London 1992; 121–9.
15. Black D. Paying for Health. J Med Ethics 1991; 17: 117–23.
16. Dew MA, Simmons EG. The advantages of multiple measures of the Quality of Life. Scand J Urol Nephol 1990 (suppl 131): 23–30.
17. Meenan R, Gertman P, Mason J, Dunaif R. The arthritis impact measurement scales: further investigations of a Health Status instrument. Arch Rheum 1982; 19: 1048–53.
18. Bergner M, Bobbett R, Carter W. Gibson B. The sickness impact profile: development and final

revision of a health status measure. Med Care 1981; 19: 787–805.
19. Hunt S, McEwen J, McKenna S. Measuring health status. Croom Helm, London 1986.
20. Spitzer W, Dobson A, Hall J et al. Meauring the Quality of Life of cancer patients: a concise QL-index for use by Physicians. J Chron Dis 1981; 34: 585–97.
21. Cox D, Fitxpatrick R, Fletcher A et al. Quality of Life assessment: can we keep it simple? J Roy Stats Soc Series A 1992; 155: 353–92.
22. Lomas J, Pickard L, Mohide A. Patients versus clinician item generation for Quality of Life measures. Med Care 1987; 25: 764–9.
23. Anderson R, Bury M. Living with Chronic illness: the experience of patients and their families.Unwin. Hyman, London 1988.
24. Guyatt G, Bernan L, Townsend M, Pingsey SO. Chambers LW. A measure of Quality of Life for clinical trials in chronic lung disease. Thorax 1987; 42: 773–8.
25. Stewart A, Greenfield S, Hays R et al. Functional status and wellbeing of patients with chronic conditions. JAMA 1989; 262: 907–13.
26. Jenkinson C, Fitzpatrick R. Measurements of health status in patients with chronic illness: comparison of the Nottingham Health Profile and the general health questionnaire. Fam Pract 1990; 7: 121–4.
27. Patrick D, Deyo R. Generic and disease-specific measures in assessing health status and quality of life. Med Care 1989; 27: S217–32.
28. Guyatt G, Walter S, Norman G. Measuring changes over time: assessing the usefulness of evaluation instruments. J Chron Dis 1987; 40: 171–8.
29. Tugwell P, Bombardier C, Buchanan W et al. Methotrexate in rheumatoid arthritis: impact on Quality of Life assessed by traditional standard item and individual patient preference health status questionnaire. Arch Intern Med 1990; 150: 59–62.
30. Fletcher A, Gore S, Jones D, Fitzpatrick R, Spiegelhalter D, Cox D. Quality of Life measures in Healthcare II: Design analysis and interpretation. Brit Med J 1992; 305: 1145–8.
31. Deniston OL, Carpenter-Alting P, Kneisly J, Hawthorne M, Port FK. Assessment of Quality of Life in endstage renal disease. Health Serv Res 1989; 24: 555–78.
32. Grieco A, Long CJ. Investigation of the Karnofsky Performance Status as a measure of Quality of Life. Health Psychol 1984; 3: 129.
33. Karnofsy DA, Burchenal JH. The clinical evaluation of chemotherapeutic agents in cancer. In: McLeod CM (ed), Evaluation of chemotherapeutic index in Cancer. Columbia University Press, New York 1949, 191–204.
34. Bremer BA, McCauley CR, Wrona RM, Johnson JP. Quality of Life in endstage renal disease: a re-examination. Am J Kid Dis 1989; 13: 200–9.
35. Evans RW. Recombinant Human Erythropoietin and the Quality of Life of endstage renal disease patients: a comparative analysis. Am J Kid Dis 1991; 18 (suppl 1): 62–70.
36. MaClennan WM, Anson C, Birkeli K, Tuttle E. Functional status and Quality of Life. Predictors of early mortality among patients entering treatment for endstage renal disease. J Clin Epidemiol 1991; 44: 83–9.
37. Kutner NG, Brogan DJ. Assisted survival, ageing and rehabilitation needs: comparison of older dialysis patients and age matched peers. Arch Phys Med Rehabil 1992; 73: 309–15.
38. Julius M, Hawthorn JM, Carpenter-Acting P, Kneisley J, Wolfe RA, Port FK. Independence in activities of daily living for endstage renal disease. Am J Kidney Dis 1989; 13: 61–9.
39. Wolcott DL, Nissenson AR, Landiverk J. Quality of Life in Chronic Dialysis Patients. Gen Hosp Psych 1988; 10: 267–77.
40. Fragola JA, Grube S, VanBlock L, Bourke E. Multicentre study of physical activity and employment status of CAPD patients in the United States. Proc EDTA 1983; 20: 243–9.
41. Gutman RA, Stead WW, Robinson RR et al. Physical activity and employment status of patients on maintenance haemodialysis. N Engl J Med 1981; 304: 309–13.
42. Bergner M, Bobbett RA, Carter WV, Gibson BS. The sickness impact profile: development and final revision of a health status measure. Med Care 1981; 19: 787–805.
43. Hart LG, Evans RW. The functional status of ESRD patients as measured by the sickness impact profile. J Chron Dis 1987: 40 (suppl 1): 117S–30S.
44. Churchill DN, Torrance GW, Taylor DE et al. Measurements of Quality of Life in endstage renal failure. The time trade off approach. Clin Invest Med 1987; 10: 14–27.
45. Russell JD, Beecroft ML, Ludwen D, Churchill DN. The Quality of Life measures in renal transplantation – a prospective study. Transplantation 1992; 54: 656–60.
46. Laupacis A, Wong C, Churchill DN. The use of generic and specific Quality of Life measures in haemodialysis patients treated with erythropoeitin. The Canadian EPO study. Cont Clinc Trials 1991; 12 (suppl 4): 168S–79S.
47. Ware JE, Sherbourne CD. The MOS 36-Item Shortform Health Survey (SF36) Med Care 1992; 30: 473–83.
48. Ware J. Measuring patients views; the optimum outcome measures. SF36: Brit Med J 1993; 306: 1429–30.
49. Jenkinson S, Coulter A, Wright L. Shortform 36 (SF36) health survey questionnaire: normative data for adults of working age. BMJ 1993; 306: 1437–40.
50. Fox E, Peace K, Neale TJ, Morrison RB, Hartfield PJ. Quality of Life for patients with ESRF. Ren Fail 1991; 13: 31–5.
51. Laupaces A, Muirhead N, Keown P, Wong C. A disease specific questionnaire for assessing quality of life in patients on haemodialysis. Nephron 1992; 60: 302–6.
52. Ferrans CE, Powers MJ. Pyschmetric assessment

of the Qaulity of Life index. Res Nurs Health 1992; 15: 29–38.
53. Morris PLP, Jones B. Transplantation versus dialysis: a study of Quality of Life. Transpl Proceedings 1988; 20: 23–6.
54. Kurtin PS, Davies AR, Myer KB, De Giacomo JM, Kantx ME. Patient based health status measures in outpatient dialysis. Med Care 1992; 30: MS136–49.
55. Kurten P, Nissenson AR. Variation in ESRD patient outcomes: What we know, what should we know and how do we find it out? J. Am Soc Nephrol 1993; 1738–47.
56. Hunt SM, McKenna SP, McEwen J, Backett EM, Williams J, Papp E. A quantitative approach to perceived health status: A validation study Epidemol Community Health 1980; 34: 281.
57. Hunt SM, McKenna SP, McEwan J et al. The Nottingham Health Profile: Subjective health status and medical consultations. Soc Sci Med 1981; 15: 221–32.
58. Auer J, Simon G, Oliver DO, Anastassiades E, Stephens J, Gokal R. Improvements in quality of life on CAPD patients treated with subcutaneoulsy adminsitered erythropoietin for anaemia. Perit Dial Int 1992; 12: 40–42.
59. Parfrey PS, Vavasour HM, Henry S et al. Clinical features and severity of non specific symptoms in dialysis patients. Nephron 1988; 50: 121–8.
60. Parfrey PS, Vavasour HM, Bullock M et al. Development of a health questionnaire specific for ESRD. Nephron 1989; 52; 20–9.
61. EuroQol Group. EuroQol – a new facility for the measurement of health related quality of life. Health Policy 1990, 16: 199–208.
62. Coyle B. Measuring outcomes in clinical audit: developing a quality of life protocol for regional renal service. Health Service Journal 1993 (in press).
63. Campbell A, Converse PE, Rogers WL. The Quality of American Life: perceptions, evaluations and satisfactions. Russell Sage Foundation, New York 1976.
64. Kutner NG, Brogan D, Kutner MH. Endstage renal disease treatment modality and patients Quality of Life. Am J Nephrol 1986; 6: 396–402.
65. Simmons RG, Anderson CR, Abress LK. Quality of Life and rehabilitation differences among four ESRD therapy groups. Scand J Urol Nephrol 1990; (suppl) 131: 7–22.
66. Johnson JP, McCauley CR, Copley JB. The Quality of Life of haemodialysis and transplant patients. Kidney Int 1982; 22: 286–91.
67. Auer J, Gokal R, Stout JP et al. The Oxford/Manchester Study of dialysis patients. Scand J Urol Nephrol 1990 (suppl) 131: 31–37.
68. Cantril H. The pattern of human concerns. Rutgers Univ Press, New Brunswick 1985.
69. Simmons RG, Anderson C, Kamstra L, Amer NG. Quality of Life and alternate ESRD therapies. Transplant Proc 1985; 17: 1577–8.
70. Rosenburg M. Society and adolescent self image. Princeton. Univ. Press, Princeton 1965.
71. Veroff J, Kulko RA, Douvan E. Mental Health in America: patterns of help seeking from 1957 to 1976. Barrie Books, New York 1981.
72. Campbell A, Converse PE, Rodgers WL. The Quality of American Life. Russell Sage Foundation, New York 1976.
73. Evan RW, Manninen DL, Maier A, Garrison LP, Hart LG. The Quality of Life of Kidney and Heart Transplant recipients. Transplant Proc 1985; 17: 1579–82.
74. Simmons RG. Longterm reactions of renal recipients and donors. In: Levy NB (ed), Psychonephrology 2: Psychological problem in Kidney Failure and their treatment. Plenum, New York 1983: 275–87.
75. Simmons RG, Klein SD, Simmons RL. Gift of Life: The social and psychological impact of organ transplantion. Wiley, New York 1977.
76. McNair DM, Lorr M, Dropplenam LF. Manual for the Profile of mood state. Educational and Industrial Testing Service, San Diego 1981.
77. Wolcott DL, Wellish DK, Fawzy FI, Landsverk J. Psychological adjustment of adults bone marrow transplant donors whose recipient survives. Transplantation 1986; 41: 484–8.
78. Wallston KA, Wallston BS. Health locus of control scales. In: Lefcourt HM (ed), Research with the locus of control Constrict. Vol 1: Assessment methods. Academic, New York 1981: 189–243.
79. Poll B, DeNour AK. Locus of control and adjustment to chronic dialysis. Psychol Med 1980; 10: 153–7.
80. Nissenson AR, Maida CA, Katz AH et al. Psychological adaptation of CAPD and centre haemodialysis patients. Adv Perit Dial 1986; 4: 47–56.
81. Antonovsky A. The sense of coherence: Development of a research instrument. Newsletter and research reports, William S Schwartz Research centre, Tel-Aviv University, Israel 1983; 1: 11–22.
82. Antonovsky A. The sense of coherence as a determinant of health. In: Matarazzo JD, Herd JA, Miller NE, Weiss S (eds), Behavioural Health. J Wiley, New York 1984; pp 114–9.
83. Soskolne V, DeNour AK. Psychological adjustment of Home haemodialysis, CAPD and hospital dialysis patients and their spouses. Nephron 1987; 47: 266–73.
84. Derogatis LR, Melisaratis N. The brief symptom inventory and introductory report. Psychol Med 1983; 13: 595–605.
85. Derogatis LR, Lopez MC. PAIS and PAIS-SR administration survey and procedure manual. Clin Psychometric Res, Baltimore 1983.
86. DeNour AK. Renal replacement therapies. In: Spiker B (ed), Quality of Life assessments on Clinical trials. Raven Press Ltd., New York 1990; 381–9.
87. Conley JA, Burton HJ, DeNour AK et al. Support systems for patients and spouses on home dialysis. Int J Family Psychiatry 1981; 2: 45–54.
88. Chyatte SB. Rehabilitation medicine in Chronic Renal Failure. In: Chyatte SB (ed), Rehabilitation

in chronic renal failure. Williams and Wilkins, Baltimore 1979; pp 28–45.
89. Gray H, Brogan D, Kutner NG. Status of life areas. Congruence/noncongruence in ESRD patients and spouse perceptions. Soc Sci Med 1985; 20: 341–6.
90. Levinson JL, Glocheski S. Psychological factors affecting ESRD. Psychosomatic 1991; 32: 382–389.
91. Balaru K, Murphy S, Powers M. Stress identification and coping patterns in patients on haemodialysis. Nursing Research 1982; 31: 107–112.
92. Bihl MA, Ferrans CE, Powers MJ. Comparing stressors and Quality of Life of Dialysis patients. ANNA J 1988; 15: 27–36.
93. Eichel CJ. Stress and coping in patients on CAPD compared to haemodialysis patients. ANNA J 1986; 13: 9–73.
94. Lindary R. Adaptation to home dialysis: the use of haemodialysis and peritoneal dialysis. ANNA J 1982; 9: 49–51.
95. Luby C. Stressor response identification in CAPD population – Masters Thesis. Kent State University, Kent, Ohio.
96. Fuchs J, Schreiber M. Patients Perceptive of CAPD and Haemodialysis Stressors. ANNA J 1988; 15; 282–300.
97. Simmons RG, Anderson C, Kamstra L. Comparison of Quality of Life of patients on CAPD, haemodialysis and after transplantation. Am J Kidney Dis 1984; 4: 253–5.
98. Lindsay RM, Burton HJ, Kline SA. Quality of Life and psychosocial aspects of chronic peritoneal dialysis. In: Nolph KD (ed), Peritoneal Dialysis. Martinez Nichkoff, Boston 1985; pp 667–84.
99. McKevitt P 1980. Support and support sytems in dialysis. Dial Transplantation 1980; 9: 980–1.
100. Perras SP, Zappacosta AR. Identifying candidates for CAPD. Dial Transplant 1981; 10: 108–112.
101. DeNour AK. Medical Staff's attitude and patient rehabilitation. Proc. EDTA 1980; 17: 520–3.
102. McKevitt P. Support in home and selfcare. Dial Transpl 1980; 9; 1097–100.
103. Burton H, DeNour DK, Cowley JA, Wells CA, Wai L. Comparison of psycholgical adjustment to CAPD and home haemodialysis. Perit Dial Bull 1982; 2: 76–86.
104. Auer J. Quality of Life in CAPD related to sex and age – a comparison with haemodialysis. Proc EDTNA 1981; 9: 204–10.
105. deWardener HE. Some ethical and economic problems associated with intermittent haemodialysis. In: Wolstenholme GEW, O'Conner M (eds), Ethics in Medicine progress. Luth Brown, Boston 1966; pp 104–26.
106. Evans RW, Blagg CR, Bryan FA. Implications for healthcare policy. A social and demographic profile of haemodialysis patients in the United States. JAMA 1981, 245: 487–92.
107. Hagberg B, Malnquist AA. A prospective study of patients on chronic haemodialysis. Pretreatment of psychiatric and psychological variables predicting outcome. J Psychosom Res 1974; 18: 315–22.
108. DeNour AK, Czaczkes JW. Adjustment to chronic haemodialysis. Isr J Med Sci 1974; 10: 498–505.
109. Rennie D. Renal rehabilitation – where are the data? N Engl J Med 1981; 304: 351–3.
110. Evan RW. Manninen DL, Garrison LP et al. Special reports: Fundings from the National Kidney Dialysis and Kidney Transplantation Study. HCFA Pub No 3230. Baltimore, MD Health Care Financing Adminstration 1987.
111. National ESRD Patient Rehabilitation task force: final report of the National ESRD Patient Rehabilitation task force. Transmitted by Guttman RA, June 1980.
112. Deniston OL, Luscombe FA, Buesching DP, Richer RE, Spinowitz BS. Effect of long term erythrpoietin beta therapy on the quality of life of haemodialysis patients. Am Soc Artif Int Organs Trans 1990; 36: M157–60.
113. Wolcott DL, Marsh JT, LaRue A, Carr C, Nissenson AR. Recombinant human eythropoietin treatment may improve quality of life and cognitive function in chronic haemodialysis patients. Am J Kid Dis 1989, 14 (suppl 1): 14–18.
114. Canadian Erythropoietin Study group. Association between recombinant human erythropoietin and quality of life and exercise capacity of patients receiving haemodialysis. BMJ 1990; 300: 573–8.
115. Evans RW. Recombinant human erythropoietin and the quality of life of endstage renal disease patients: a comparative analysis. Am J Kid Dis 1991: 18 (suppl 1); 62–70.
116. Evans RW, Rader B, Manninen DL. The quality of life of haemodialysis recipients treated with recombinant human erythropoietin. Cooperative multicentre EPO clinical trial group. JAMA 1990; 263: 825–30.
117. Nissenson AR. National cooperative rHuEPO study in patients with CRF. a phase IV multicentre study. Am J Kid Dis 1991; 18 (suppl 1): 24–33.
118. Klahr S. Rationing of Health Care and the endstage renal disease programme. Am J Kid Dis 1990; 16: 392–5.
119. Ari D, Held PJ, Pauly MV. The medicare cost of renal dialysis. Med Care 1992; 30: 879–91.
120. Friedman EA. Nephrology and the rationing of Healthcare. Contrib Nephrol Basle Karger 1993; 102: 200–36.
121. Stout J. How does dialysis effect the lifestyle of renal patients? A comparative study between CAPD and HD. EDTNA J 1988; 9: 11–2.
122. Stout J, Gokal R, Hillier V et al. Quality of Life of high risk and elderly dialysis patients in the UK. Dial Transplant 1987; 16: 674–7.
123. Wolcott DL, Nissenson AR. Quality of Life in chronic dialysis patients: a critical comparison of CAPD and HD. Am J Kid Dis 1988; 11: 402–12.
124. Bremmer BA, McCauley CR, Wrona RM, Johnston JP. Quality of life in endstage renal disease: A re-examination. AM J Kid Dis 1989; 13: 200–9.
125. Tucker CM, Ziller RC, Smith WR, Mars DR, Coone MP. Quality of Life of patients on incentre haemodialysis versus CAPD. Perit Dial Int 1991; 11: 341–6.

126. Muthny FA, Koch K. Quality of Life of patients with endstage renal failure. In: La Greca G, Olivares J, Feriani M. Passlick-Deitjen J (eds), In. CAPD – a decade of experience. Contrib Nephrol – Basel Karger 1991; 89; 265–73.
127. Kalman TP, Wilson PG, Kilman CM. Psychiatric morbidity in longterm renal transplant recipients and patients underoing haemodialysis. JAMA 1983; 250: 55–58.
128. Gudex C, deChano F, Feest TG (personal communication).
129. Rosser R, Kind P. A seale of valuations of State of Illness: Is there a social consensus? Int J Epidemiol 1978; 7: 347–58.
130. deCharo FT, Gudex C, Feest TG et al. Stastical projection and Scenario forecasts of the audit ESRF programme. BMJ in press.
131. Doyle CL, Flannigan J, Mabe C. Tidal peritoneal dialysis vs CAPD. Childrens preference. ANNA J 1992; 19: 249–54.
132. Roscoe JM, Smith CF, Williams EA et al. Medical and social outcome in adolescents with end stage renal failure. Kidney Int 1991; 40: 948–53.
133. Sandroni S, Arora N, Vidrene L, Moles K. Feasibility of incentre staff assisted cycler dialysis. Adv Perit Dial 1990; 6: 76–78.
134. Kutner NG, Brogan DJ. Assisted survival, ageing and rehabilitation needs: comparison in older dialysis patients and age matched peers. Arch Phys Med Rehabil 1992; 73: 309–15.
135. Avram MR, Pena C, Burrell D, Antignani A, Avram MM. Haemodialysis and the elderly patients: potential advantages as to quality of life. Urea generation, serum creatinine and less interdialysate weight gain. Am J Kid Dis 1990; 16: 342–5.
136. Julius M, Kneisley J, Carpentier-Alting P, Hawthorne V, Wolfe R, Port K. A comparison of employment rates of patients treated with CAPD vs incentre haemodialysis. Arch Int Med 1989; 149: 839–42.
137. Seedat YK, MacIntosh CG, Subban JV. Quality of Life for patients in an endstage renal disease programme. S Afr Med J 1987; 71: 500–4.
138. Simmons RG, Abbress L. Quality of Life issues for endstage renal disease patients. Am J Kid Dis 1990; 15: 201–8.
139. Gokal R, Uttley L. A collection of problems in CAPD. Adv Perit Dial 1989; 5: 76–80.
140. Stout JP, Auer J, Kincey J et al. Sexual and marital relationships and dialysis patients viewpoint. Perit Dial Bull 1987; 7: 97–101.
141. Nissenson AR, Swartz R, Zimmerman S, Watson A. A double blind placebo controlled study of rHuEPO in peritoneal dialysis patients. J Am Soc Nephrol 1990; 1: 405 (abstract)
142. Korbet SM. Anaemia and erythropoeitin in haemodialysis and CAPD. Kidney Int 1993; 43 (suppl 40): S111–9.
143. Nissenson AR, Prichard SS, Cheng IKP et al. Non medical factors that impact on ESRD modality selection. Kidney Int 1993; 43 (suppl 40): S120–7.
144. Porter GA, Lowson L, Buss J. Bias in selecting treatment for endstage renal disease. Kidney Int 1985; 28 (suppl 17): S34–7.
145. Parfrey PS, Vavasour HM, Gault MH. A prospective study of health status in dialysis and transplant patients. Transplant Proc 1988; 20: 1231–2.
146. Gokal R, Jakubowksi C, King J et al. Outcome in patients in CAPD and haemodialysis: 4 year analysis of a prospective multicentre study. Lancet 1987; 2: 1105–9.
147. Serles KD, Blagg CR, Nolph KD, Vonesh EF, Shapiro F: Comparison of patient and technique survival in CAPD and haemodialysis: a multicentre study. Perit Dial Int 1990; 10: 15–9.
148. Oldenburg B, MacDonald GS, Perkins RJ. Prediction of quality of life in a cohort of endstage renal disease patients. J Clin Epidemiol 1988; 41: 555–64.

24 Outcome of peritoneal dialysis: comparative studies

Rosario Maiorca and Giovanni C. Cancarini

1. Introduction	699
2. Cardiovascular morbidity	700
2.1. Blood pressure control	701
2.2. Arrhythmia	701
2.3. Myocardial ischemia	701
2.4. Hypotensive episodes	701
2.5. Dyslipidemia	702
3. β2-Microglobulin and uremic amyloidosis	702
4. Immunological status	702
5. Nervous system	704
6. Endocrine system	705
6.1. Thyroid function	705
6.2. Pituitary hormones	705
6.3. Sexual function	706
6.4. Growth hormone	706
6.5. ACTH and cortisol	706
7. Uremic osteodystrophy	707
8. Metabolism	708
8.1. Carbohydrates	708
8.2. Lipids	709
8.3. Proteins	709
9. Residual renal function	710
10. Transplantation	710
11. Hospitalization	711
12. Technique failure	713
12.1. Technique survival	714
12.2. Technique success	714
12.3. Causes of technique failure	716
13. Mortality on CAPD	716
13.1. Observed results	717
13.2. Factors affecting patient survival	719
13.2.1. Modality	719
13.2.2. Age	719
13.2.3. Sex	722
13.2.4. Race	722
13.2.5. Cardiac and vascular disease	722
13.2.6. Diabetes	722
13.2.7. Peritonitis	724
13.2.8. Malignancy	724
13.2.9. Other patient-related factors	724
13.2.10 Effects of experience and technical improvement on patient survival	724
13.3. Causes of death	725
14. Conclusion	725
References	726

1. Introduction

Since the introduction of Continuous Ambulatory Peritoneal Dialysis (CAPD) nephrologists have been questioning the ability of the method to achieve the same results as hemodialysis (HD). Unfortunately, clinical and ethical considerations, including the right of patients to select their preferred dialysis treatment, make such an evaluation impossible in prospective, randomized studies. Hence, comparisons can be made only for series with differing case-mix which have been only occasionally and partially corrected for pretreatment differences by sophisticated statistical analysis. Moreover, the results are greatly affected by differences in experience with the two methods: the shorter existence of CAPD pays the price of all limited experiences, in terms of number of patients and duration of treatment. CAPD technique is still insufficiently standardized, with important differences in different centers in incidence of peritonitis and in catheter-related complications that greatly affect results. Moreover, one should not forget the indisputable fact that the comparison must be critical. CAPD treatment, with its basic differences from HD in terms of small and large molecule dialysis profiles, with its continuous 24-hours-a-day blood purification, its cardiovascular and blood chemistry stability, and its better preservation of residual diuresis may be preferentially indicated, but it, like HD, has also contraindications. This renders slightly nonsensical any conclusions based on results obtained with unselected series.

In this chapter we examine several aspects of uremic pathology for which there is enough experience to allow appraisal of their behaviour in the two methods. When evaluating these results the limitations described above must be kept in mind.

2. Cardiovascular morbidity

Cardiovascular disease is the most frequent cause of death in dialysis patients, accounting for about 50% of all deaths. Among the risk factors for cardiovascular disease are uremic cardiomyopathy, with myocardial hypertrophy and intermyocardiocytic fibrosis, coronary artery disease, hypertension and dislipidemia. Theoretically, CAPD has some hemodynamic advantages over HD. The main ones are: no need for an arterio-venous fistula, constant electrolyte and acid-base balance, constant removal of uremic waste products (some of them possible etiological factors in uremic cardiopathy) and the lack of intradialytic or interdialytic changes in cardiac filling, inotropism and oxygen request, all detrimental to long-term cardiac performance. Another favorable effect of CAPD was lesser degree of anemia, but this advantage has now been nullified with the introduction of human recombinant erythropoietin.

Cardiac systolic function is usually normal in CAPD and HD patients but can be subnormal in the elderly or in patients with ischemic cardiomyopathy and can become hyperdynamic on HD in patients with high output-arteriovenous fistulae [1]. Diastolic function is, on the contrary, often altered in both methods, due to uremic cardiomyopathy with left ventricular hypertrophy (LVH) and intermyocardiocytic fibrosis [2–6]. In the uremics, the left ventricle (LV) becomes progressively stiffer and in the early phase of diastole its dilatation becomes progressively difficult and less efficient. LV end-systolic and end-diastolic pressures increase. Ventricular filling will depend more and more on atrial contraction, with consequent atrial hypertrophy and enlargement. During fluid retention, e.g., in the interhemodialytic interval, such patients are at risk of atrial arrhythmia and pulmonary and peripheral congestion. Increased LV pressure and fibrosis are responsible for subendocardial ischemia, which alters propagation of action potentials, and facilitates arrythmias of the reentry type [7].

Alpert et al. [8] did a cross-sectional study of 54 patients on HD and 39 on CAPD. They found a lower incidence, on CAPD, of end-diastolic and end-systolic left ventricular dilatation, higher cardiac output and lower mean velocity of circumferential fiber shortening. The same group obtained concordant results for patients switching from HD to CAPD and vice-versa. Septal and posterior wall thickness were increased by similar percentages in patients on the two methods. Some studies have evaluated the echocardiographic changes in LVH during CAPD and HD. In 18 patients on CAPD for 6–12 months, Leenen and coworkers [9] observed decreases in left ventricular mass, wall thickness and end-diastolic and end-systolic dimensions. In a longitudinal study, Timio and coworkers [10] observed, after six months of treatment, decreases in thickness of the myocardial interventricular septum, posterior wall mass and left ventricular mass index on CAPD, but not on HD. Decreased left ventricular mass and end-diastolic volume on CAPD and increased on HD were seen by Deligiannis et al. [11]. These data are in contrast with those published by Eisenberg et al. [3] who observed worsening of myocardial hypertrophy on CAPD, from normal/mild to moderate in 5 of 10 cases, and from moderate to severe in 2 of 6 cases. These discrepancies between reported series may result from differences in case-mix, diets, dialysis treatment, or control of hypertension and ECV.

LVH has many possible causes in uremia. Most important among them is persistently elevated blood pressure over 24h; other factors are anemia, hyperparathyroidism, renin angiotensin system (local), endothelin, sympathetic overactivity, salt/ouabain-like factor, and pulsatile vs steady LV work load [12]. Its reduction on CAPD and not on HD has been related to the nocturnal blood pressure lessening seen only on CAPD, and to the norepinephrine levels, which are lower on CAPD than on HD [10]. We saw no differences in nocturnal blood pressure between 15 pairs of randomly selected elderly CAPD and HD patients (mean ages 72 ± 5 and 71 ± 5 years on dialysis for 31 ± 18 months and 31 ± 19 months); 24 hour blood pressure readings were taken with an automatic apparatus, choosing the short interval day for HD patients [13].

Intermyocardiocytic fibrosis is an early complication of uremia. In parathyroidectomized and subtotally nephrectomized rats given PTH there is three times more myocardial interstitium and lesser capillary density [14]. There are no comparative studies of changes in intermyocardiocytic fibrosis on HD and CAPD, but evidence exists of its progression in patients on maintainance HD [15, 16]. If high PTH levels really have a detrimental effect, then the differential effect of the two dialysis methods on fibrosis can be understood. There is some evidence for lower PTH levels on CAPD and greater prevalence of the adynamic lesion, which is associated with low PTH levels [134].

2.1. Blood pressure control

Clinical data demonstrate that CAPD is effective in controlling hypertension. The continuous removal of sodium and excess water limits ECV fluctuation, avoiding those hypertensive peaks connected with fluid overfilling that can be seen on HD. Since the large majority of hypertensive states in uremics can be corrected by ultrafiltration, blood pressure control on CAPD depends on accurate maintainance of dry weight. This can be achieved by appropriate use of hypertonic dialysis fluid. In the 1987 Report of the NIH-CAPD Registry, 30% of 400 hypertensive patients reverted to normal by one year and others tended to take less medication [17]. In two other studies [18, 19], CAPD appeared to be as effective as HD, whereas in another one [8] thre was better control of blood pressure on CAPD than on HD. A decreased vascular response to exogenous angiotensin infusion, possibly related to the peritoneal clearance of some still unknown substance(s) enhancing the vascular effect of circulating vasopressive agents, has been observed [20]. Greater reduction of nocturnal blood pressure, close to physiological values, has been observed on CAPD as compared to HD, on continuous 24-hour monitoring of blood pressure, and it has been suggested that this contributes to the lessening of LVH [21]. Such differences were not observed by us in a randomly selected group of elderly patients, referred to earlier [13].

2.2. Arrhythmia

Arrhythmias, due to cardiovascular disease but also to intercompartmental water and electrolyte shifts during dialysis, is frequent in hemodialysis patients. Moreover, as documented in patients with essential hypertension, LV hypertrophy is a strong predictor of ventricular premature beats, cardiac arrhythmia and sudden death. In patients on hemodialysis or hemofiltration, the incidence of premature beats was frequent, 25%, especially in the last two hours of treatment [22]. In a multicenter, cross-sectional study, ventricular arrhythmias were seen in 79% of patients from the third hour of HD to five hours or more after dialysis; 21% of these arrhythmias was Lown class 4A or B. On the contrary, in a Holter study of 21 CAPD patients [23] the incidence of arrhythmia was no different, even in elderly or cardiac patients, during treatment as compared to a day in which the treatment was deliberately withheld. In a comparative study with continuous 48h Holter monitoring, supreventricular, isolated ventricular and bigeminal arrhythmias were seen, more frequently on HD than on CAPD and in both treatments rates of ventricular extrasystoles correlated with blood norepinephrine levels. Ventricular tachycardic episodes were seen only in HD patients, whereas on CAPD hypokinetic arrhythmias prevailed [21].

2.3. Myocardial ischemia

Occurrence of myocardial ischemic episodes is frequent on HD, whereas data for CAPD are lacking. Zuber et al. [22] observed ST depression, indicative of ischemic episodes, predominantly in the last two hours of treatment in 25% of their patients on hemodialysis or on hemofiltration studied with continuous Holter monitoring. ECG changes lasted for 40–90 minutes and half of them were asymptomatic. None of these patients had objective signs of coronary artery pathology.

To our knowledge, no study has compared the appearance rates of de-novo coronary disease on CAPD and HD. In separate studies, this rate was evaluated as 8.8% at one year and 15% at two years on CAPD [24], and as 12 and 18% on HD [25].

2.4. Hypotensive episodes

Hypotensive episodes and other intra- or peridialytic symptoms are rare on CAPD and common on HD. Hypotension, multifactorial in origin, is ultimately a result of an imbalance between ultrafiltration rate and vascular refilling [26], (which is frequent on HD and uncommon on CAPD), and to uremic cardiomyopathy. Frequent hypotensive episodes are seen much more often in patients with LVH than in those without LVH [1].

In a study by Charytan et al. [27], 92 patients on HD and 72 on CAPD on treatment for up to 26 months, there were 15.6 episodes per patient per year on HD versus only 0.46 on CAPD of hypotension or hypertension, significant arrhhythmias, chest pain, seizures, muscle cramps, headaches, twitching, and gastrointestinal troubles; on HD they occurred in 20% of treatments. In HD, hypotension rates, 20 to 50 per cent of dialysis, resulted in hypotension in the past [28–30] but this has improved considerably since the introduction of convective or mixed dialyses techniques, use of bicarbonate buffer and automated ultrafiltration [31–33]. We recently evaluated the incidence of hypotensive episodes (i.e., a drop of systolic blood pressure to 90 mmHg or less, or a drop of 20 mmHg if the initial SBP was 100 mmHg or less) in one year, in 63 patients (34 M, 29 F) mean age 62 ± 15 years, on dialysis for 87 ± 63 months, treated with bicarbonate-HD (59 pts) or acetate-HD (4 pts), all on automated ultrafiltration. In a total of 1034 treatments, hypotensive episodes occurred in 10.8% of dialyses; 30% of the patients had 74% of the hypotensive episodes, and these patients did not differ from the others in age (62 ± 16 versus 62 ± 15 years; $p = 0.95$) or in time on dialysis (92 ± 62 vs 84 ± 63 months; $p = 0.68$) [34].

2.5. Dyslipidemia

Finally, dyslipidemia is also a risk factor for cardiovascular disease and CAPD treatment is associated with a more atherogenic lipoprotein profile than is HD (see below, in Metabolism section).

In conclusion, it seems reasonable to consider CAPD as the method that preserves cardiovascular function better. Myocardial hypertrophy is more progressive on HD, wherease there is regression on CAPD, provided that good control of ECV is obtained. On HD, the progressively increasing impairment of early left ventricular filling can have devastating effects during the sessions, due to the rapid blood ultrafiltration that can dramatically worsen the cardiovascular refilling and can lead to collapse, induce arrhythmias, and cause sudden death [16]. Between the sessions, HD patients are at increased risk of atrial, pulmonary and peripheral congestion and atrial arrhythmia. On CAPD, all these effects are avoided by the continuous ultrafiltration. Moreover, the absence of an arteriovenous fistula, the steady-state level of acid-base balance, the concentrations of sodium, potassium, calcium and the constant removal of uremic waste products are all favorable factors in the control of uremic cardiomyopathy.

On the other hand, CAPD has a more atherogenic lipid profile, the negative effects of which are hard to predict.

3. β2-Microglobulin and uremic amyloidosis

The amount of β2 microglobulin removed by dialysis depends on the characteristics of dialysis membranes but is less than that removed by normal kidneys (1350 mg/week) [35–38]. Dialysis *per se* might stimulate the production of β2-microglobulin. On HD possible causes are acetate, endotoxins, becterial cell fragments in dialysis solution and the use of a cellulose membrane that activates monocytes to produce IL-1 [37, 39]. In CAPD, β2-microglobulin stimulation might arise from biocompatibility of dialysis solution and from immune stimulation during peritonitis [34, 40].

Lower plasma levels of β2-microglobulin in CAPD than in HD patients have been reported, suggesting a reduced risk of renal amyloidosis in patients on peritoneal dialysis [36, 41, 42]. The lower plasma levels of β2-microglobulin on CAPD are due to the greater preservation of residual renal function than in HD [34, 43–51].

However, β2-m plasma levels in all dialysis patients are so elevated that the risk of deposition remains high. Since bone lesions referable to β2-microglobulin deposition have been found in about 16% of pre-dialysis uremic patients (when plasma levels of β2-microglobulin are lower than in dialyzed patients [46]), uremia *per se* also plays a role in the appearance of β2m-related amyloidosis. Whether more permeable membranes and biocompatible solutions are able to reduce plasma β2-m concentrations and renal amyloidosis remains to be seen.

Comparative studies of CAPD and HD patients with similar demographic and dialytic ages [52] show a similar incidence of bone lesion [34], nerve entrapment or surgery for carpal tunnel syndrome (Figs. 1–3) [34, 35, 53].

4. Immunological status

Uremia impairs the immunological status, as demonstrated by lymphopenia, delayed rejection of allografts and leucocyte recruitment at the site of infections, cutaneous anergy, defective chemotaxis and phagocytosis, attenuated humoral responses to vaccine administration and reduced interferon production [54–56] These changes might be the cause of the increased susceptibility to infections and neoplasms in uremics [57]. Dialysis may further impair the immunological status through depletion of useful proteins, trace-metals and vitamins or an immune response through bioincompatibility of dialysis membranes and dialysis fluid or entry into the blood of microorganisms or endotoxins. Entry of microorganisms is frequent on HD and accounts for approximately half of the life-threatening infections of dialysis patients [58]. Endotoxins can more easily enter the blood stream in uremic patients and

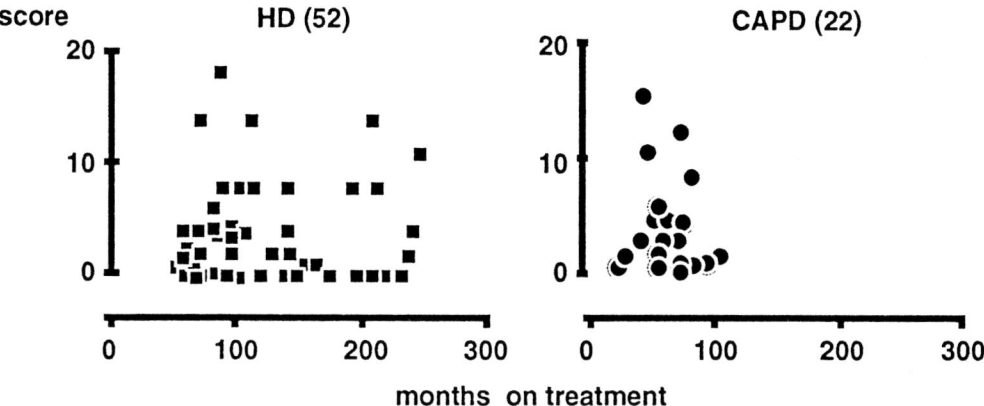

Figure 1. Presence, at last X-ray control, of radiolucent bone lesions referable to uremic amyloidosis. Scored according to number and size of lesions. (Reprinted from reference [34] by permission of Blackwell Scientific Publications, Ind.)

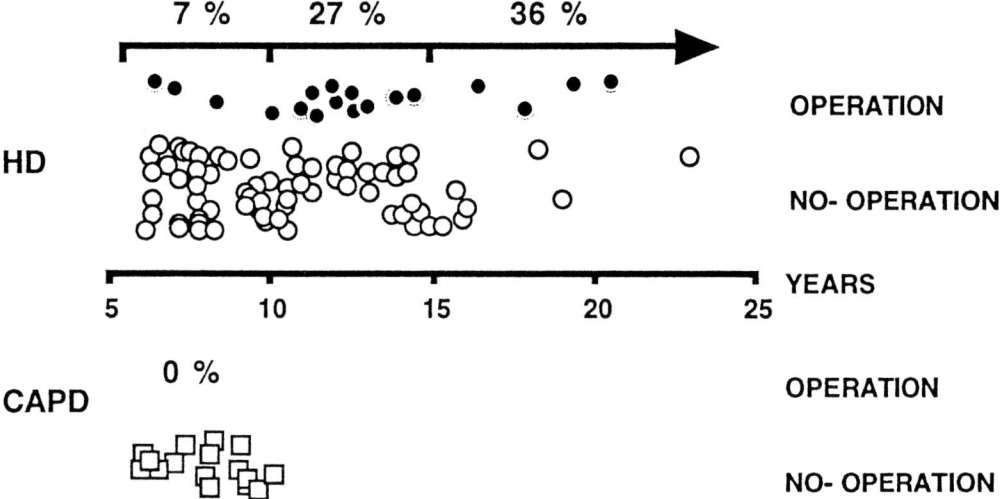

Figure 2. Carpal tunnel operations in HD and CAPD patients on treatment for more than five years. Cross sectional study. Symbols are: (●) HD, operation; (○) HD, no operation; (□) CAPD, no operation. (Reprinted from reference [34] by permission of Blackwell Scientific Publications, Inc.)

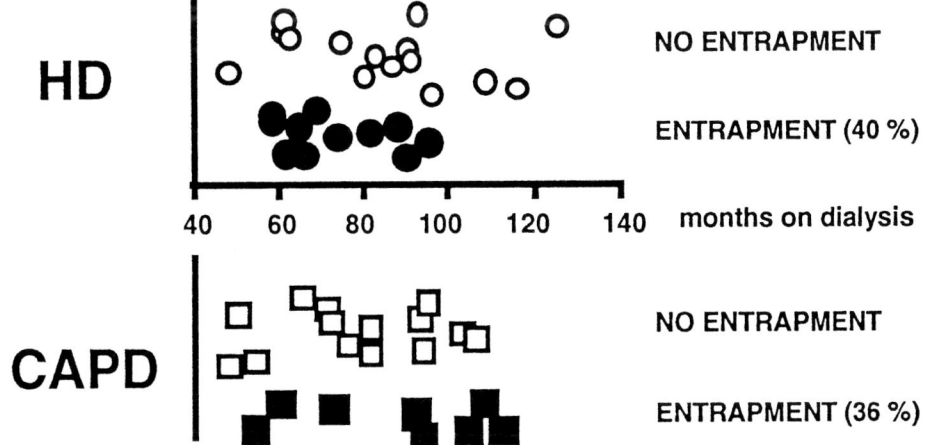

Figure 3. Slowing of median nerve conduction velocity in the carpal tunnel (entrapment). Cross sectional study on CAPD and HD. Symbols are: (●) HD, entrapment; (○) HD, no entrapment; (■) CAPD, entrapment; (□) CAPD, no entrapment. (Reprinted from reference [34] by permission of Blackwell Scientific Publications, Inc.)

important increases of their plasma levels have been found in patients on conservative treatment (17.0 ± 2.09 ng/L), on HD (40.0 ± 4.7 ng/L) and on hemofiltration (19.0 ± 7.5 ng/l). On the contrary, levels were similar to those of healthy controls (7 ± 0.6 ng/L) in patients with transplants and in peritoneal dialysis patients [59].

Serum antibacterial activity is depressed in uremics and further depressed by either HD and CAPD [60]. Sera from HD patients and from non-dialyzed uremics showed non-complement related antibacterial activity that did not appear in normal controls and in CAPD patients; this residual activity might be due to the greater ease of middle molecule removal by peritoneal dialysis (PD) than by HD [60]. Sera from CAPD lost the ability to inhibit E-rosette formation over time while patients on HD did not [61]. Neutrophils from CAPD patients had chemotactic and bactericidal activities similar to those from HD patients, but better phagocytic function [62]. There was significantly less chemiluminescence of stimulated PMN cells from HD patients, while CAPD patients did not differ from controls [56].

CAPD patients showed improvement in cellular immunity (tested by E-rosette count) and in delayed hypersensitivity reactions (tested by DNCB and PPD skin test) in contrast to HD patients in whom no changes were found [61, 63]. Collart et al. [64] found increased OKT4+/OKT8+ ratios on both HD and CAPD due to reduced percentages of OKT8+ cells with normal values of both OKT4+ and OKT3+. In contrast, others [65] observed significant increases in percentages of OKT3+ and OKT4+ cells and a higher OKTA+/OKT8+ ratio in only CAPD patients. The lymphoblastic response in autologous serum was better in CAPD than in HD patients, perhaps due to the removal of some inhibitory factor(s) [56, 66, 67]. T-cell function appeared to be impaired in HD patients, as demonstrated by a complete loss of inducibility of the IL-2 gene and decreased inducibility of gamma-IFN-mRNA, which appears to be normal in PD patients [68]. The proliferative response to mitogens is also similar or better on CAPD than on HD [64, 69, 70].

Sensitization to membrane or tubing or to sterilizing agents has been observed on HD. Similar percentages of patients (12%) with IgE antibodies against ethylene oxide have been found on HD, on bemofiltration and on intermittent peritoneal dialysis [71]. This was not confirmed in another study [72] where positive skin tests were found in 9% of HD patients but not in patients on PD whilst positive RAST tests in 12% of HD patients contrasted with only 2% in PD patients.

In conclusion, in the majority of the studies, CAPD appears to preserve immune function better than HD. However, do these laboratory differences have any clinical significance? In a retrospective clinical study we found that HD patients required more admissions per patient-year than CAPD patients for infections (other than those related to the technique, e.g., infection of access, peritonitis): 0.158 vs. 0.096, but days of hospitalization were the same (1.55/patient-year) [34]. Respiratory tract infections were more than 45% of all causes. No statistically significant difference was found in the incidence of any other infectious diseases. The incidence of malignancy did not significantly differ, 4.2% on HD and 5.9% on CAPD. Follow-up was comparable, but the mean age of patients on CAPD was seven years greater than on HD ($p < 0.001$), and this might have influenced the results. There were no significant differences in the localization of neoplasias. Thus, our clinical results do not support the contention that the improved immunity in CAPD has clinical significance.

5. Nervous system

On CAPD, nerve conduction velocity has been stable or slightly worsened in most of the studies [73–79]. In two groups of 20 patients on CAPD and HD, comparable for age and time on dialysis, we observed similar slight deterioration of the external sciatic popliteal nerve conduction velocity on both CAPD and on HD [45]. Acoustic nerve latency was slightly and similarly increased in both groups, and the internuclear latency was normal in both groups [80]. No differences were found between CAPD and HD patients in Visual Evoked Potentials (VEP) and Somatosensory Evoked Potentials (SEP) [78].

Changes in brain density have been observed with computerized tomography only in patients on HD, probably related to changes in water content during dialysis [78]. Many studies have shown better brain function in CAPD than in HD patients and this might result from the greater stability of water content and of plasma electrolytes and acid-base status in the brain on CAPD [81–83]. Marsh et al. [81] found that the attention and the efficiency of cognitive processing were more similar to normal in CAPD that in HD patients. Similar results were obtained by Wolcott et al. [82] and Garcia-Maldonado et al. [83]. The better brain tolerance to CAPD than to HD is also supported by the lesser risk of dialysis-associated seizures in children and adolescents on CAPD [84].

6. Endocrine system

Many studies have evaluated the effect of dialytic methods on the endocrine abnormalities caused by uremia.

6.1. Thyroid function

Plasma levels of Thyroxine (T4) were reduced either to the same degree in both HD and CAPD [85-88] or more in HD patients [89]. In one study T4 levels were reduced in HD and normal in CAPD patients [90] resulting from the longer treatment of the CAPD group [90]. Discordant results have also been obtained for free thyroxine (FT4): normal in CAPD and reduced in HD [85, 91], normal in HD and increased in CAPD [91], reduced in both HD and CAPD [87, 88, 91]. These discrepancies may reflect different laboratory methods [89]. Triiodothyronine (T3) has been reported to be more reduced on HD than on CAPD [85], reduced to the same degree in both modalities [86-89, 91], reduced on HD and normal on CAPD [90]. Plasma free-T3 levels, normal in some studies [86, 87], reduced in others [88, 91], were not significantly different between CAPD and HD. Plasma levels of thyroid stimulating hormone (TSH) though similar in CAPD and HD, were sometimes normal [85, 87, 89-92], sometimes slightly increased [85, 88], but always inappropriately low with respect to plasma levels of T3 and T4. Impairment of pituitary function is also supported by the reduced and blunted response of plasma TSH levels to the injection of TRH [85, 88, 91-93].

Thyroid hormone status on CAPD (FT3 normal, FT4 and reverse-T3 increased, T3 and T4 decreased) might result from the reduction of peripheral de-iodination of T4 to T3 or of the amounts of hormone-binding proteins, or on a defective hormone-protein bonding [86]. However, plasma TBG levels have been found to be normal [94], since the daily dialysate loss of this protein is only about 1/6 its daily production. The increase in FT4 and decrease in T4 might be due to an inhibitor of the T4 bond to protein [87], as in other metabolic diseases [89, 95-97]. The higher levels of reverse T3 (rT3) on CAPD than on HD might be due to increased inhibitor of peripheral uptake of rT3 on HD. Moreover, direct relationships between rT3 and fasting plasma glucose, or the glucose peak after an oral load, or plasma insulin levels have been demonstrated in HD patients [87]. No relationship to T3 concentrations was found [87]. Thus, the reduced tolerance to glucose appears to play a role in peripheral conversion of T4 to rT3 as demonstrated by the lowest levels of T3 and the highest of rT3 being found in HD and CAPD patients with reduced glucose tolerance, as in diabetics [98], and that fasting increased the plasma levels of rT3 [99]. This might have been important in CAPD patients, who continuously absorb glucose from the peritoneal cavity, but it was not confirmed by clinical studies [100] that have found normal rT3 levels on CAPD and low levels on HD.

The presence of a relative thyroid dysfunction in dialysis is also supported by the observation of anatomical and functional impairments in 11/13 CAPD patients and in 26/33 HD patients by thyroid scintigraphy even in the absence of clinical or laboratory data of hypothyroidism [100]. The reports of these studies do not state whether or not some patients had to be given thyroid hormones to correct the relative reductions of T3 and T4. Walker et al. [101] reported that 14/104 CAPD patients were given T4 before the start of CAPD and that another 7 patients were given T4 during CAPD because of increased plasma levels of TSH and reduced T4 and FT4. To our knowledge, there is no other report that supports the need to treat such a large number of CAPD patients with thyroid hormones. On the other hand, giving T3 to uremics might make the nitrogen balance negative, whereas the low level of thyroid hormone might protect nitrogen metabolism [102]. In any case, uremics rarely show clinical findings suggesting hypothyroidism and need for substitutive therapy.

6.2. Pituitary hormones

Plasma levels of PRL, FSH, LH are reported to be similarly increased in HD compared to CAPD patients [91, 103-105]. More patients on CAPD had hyperprolactinemia than on HD (73% versus 50%) [105] or did not differ [104]. In one study [104], men on HD had significantly higher levels than those on CAPD, whereas the difference in women was not significant. High levels of prolactinemia, due to increased synthesis and to reduced renal clearance [106], might compensate for the low levels of $1,25(OH)_2$-D_3 since PRL stimulates its synthesis [106]. However no relationship between PRL and PTH has been found [104].

6.3. Sexual function

The testosterone levels were higher in CAPD than in HD patients [103], as free hormone. The concentrations of sex hormone binding globulin (SHGB) are similar in both groups. Sexual function appeared to be similarly impaired in men on boh CAPD and HD [103]. Erectile impotence was found in 66% of CAPD males and 60% of HD. 82% of CAPD and 82% of HD had some degree of testicular atrophy [103]. Three of 12 women on HD and six of seven on CAPD had regular menses, but only one patient in each group had ovulatory cycles. Two of three women, amenorrheic on HD, had regular menses some months after being switched to CAPD [107].

6.4. Growth hormone

Increased growth hormone (GH) levels have been found in both CAPD and HD patients [91], as were the plasma cortisol and prolactin responses to insulin-induced hypoglycemia [108], while mean plasma levels of growth hormone were signifantly lower in CAPD patients than in HD patients. This suggests again that there is some degree of anterior pituitary disfunction in dialyzed patients. Bessarione et al. [109] found that GH response to insulin was significantly greater in uremics than in normal children. There was no difference between uremic children on conservative treatment and on CAPD. This suggests that CAPD does not correct the pituitary disfunction due to uremia.

6.5. ACTH and cortisol

Reduced responses of plasma levels of aldosterone and 18-hydroxycortisterone after injection of ACTH were found in HD [110], but not in CAPD patients [111]. Siamopoulos et al. [112] found normal basal levels of ACTH in uremics on conservative management, on HD and on PD. Basal levels of cortisol (normal values: mean ± SEM 4.4 ± 0.8 mcg/dL) were slightly increased on CAPD (8.4 ± 1.1 mcg/dL), higher on HD (13.3 ± 1.6) and much more on conservative therapy (24.5 ± 3.8). After stimulation with CRH (corticotropin-releasing hormone), only CAPD patients showed adequate peaks of ACTH (42.1 ± 8.5 pg/ml). However, the plasma cortisol peak was adequate in all three groups. The relatively low level of cortisol in CAPD is the result of peritoneal loss of the hormone and this might favour the ACTH response to CRH [113].

Administration of ACTH, after inibition of endogenous ACTH with dexamethasone, elicits normal-high values of plasma corticosteroids on CAPD [111, 113], but not on HD [110].

Plasma aldosterone and 18-hydroxycorticosterone were higher in CAPD than in HD patients, while plasma levels of cortisol were similar [115]. The differences in concentration were not due to differences in binding to plasma proteins or to differences in clearance [114]. On the contrary, aldosterone clearance was higher on CAPD than on HD [114]. Renin-angiotension systems might be more activated in CAPD patients than in HD patients, and this might amplify the steroidogenic effect of the greater free potassium intake of CAPD patients [115]. The greater responsiveness of adrenal glands to standing and to ACTH in IPD [111] than in HD anephrics [116] might be due to better metabolic status or to inibition of secretion of aldosterone and 18-hydroxycorticosterone by heparin in HD patients [116].

Kumar et al. [117] studied four patients on HD and after changing to CAPD. Plasma renin activity increased from 0.9 to 14.1 ng/ml/hr and aldosterone from 3.4 to 67.4 ng/dL, whereas mean blood pressure decreased, from 114 to 102. Plasma volume was greater in CAPD patients than in normal controls, 3600 versus 3000 ml. Epinephrine and nor-epinephrine was increased on CAPD [117]. In another study, a reduction in plasma norepinephrine was observed in patients switched from HD to CAPD, with levels going back to the basal levels when CAPD patients were switched to HD. [10]. The increases in DRA and aldosterone, in spite of the normal or large plasma volumes might be due to increased sympathetic stimulation [117]. On this basis PRA and aldosterone concentration would not be useful for evaluation of the extent of volume changes in CAPD [117], whereas it might help to evaluate atrial natriuretic factor (ANF). HD patients have pre-dialysis plasma levels of ANF significantly higher than CAPD patients and controls (271.8 ± 173.4 pg/ml; 81.8 ± 80.5; 31.5 ± 19.8; CAPD vs controls: P: NS), although ANF has similar clearance on HD and CAPD (35.5 ± 12.0 and 3.35 ± 12.0 liters/week) [118]. Plasma levels of ANF were directly related to plasma volumes [118] and during HD and ultrafiltration, ANF levels dropped to 124.4 ± 58.7 pg/ml.

7. Uremic osteodystrophy

This topic is reviewed in depth in Chapter 7. Many papers report the effects of PD on the factors affecting bone disease (calcium, PTH, aluminum, vitamin D, etc.). In CAPD there is peritoneal removal of PTH whereas there is no PTH removal on HD. Urinary removal is present more frequently on CAPD, since residual renal function lasts longer on this method (see section on residual renal function). On CAPD, serum iPTH levels have sometimes been found to decline to normal levels [119], sometimes to increase [120] and sometimes to become significantly lower than to HD [121], these conflicting results possibly depending on the optimal control of calcium and phosphorus balance.

In a cross-sectional study (unpublished data) we recently evaluated serum PTH, calcium and phosphate levels in our new patients, put on their first treatment between 1.1.80 and 31.12.92. Serum samples were taken in the morning, on HD in the short interval, on CAPD before the first bag-exchange (Table 1). There is some evidence of lower PTH levels on CAPD, but the stability of blood chemistries on CAPD and their fluctuations on HD obviously limit the significance of any differences observed.

In the ESRD patients put on dialysis between 1.1.80 and 31.12.92 parathyroidectomy was necessary in 1 CAPD and 7 in HD patients. These data are impressive but misleading. In fact, life table survival of patients with parathyroid glands (that is parathyroid survival, after defining the patients dead or leaving the method as lost to follow-up) shows (Fig. 4) that differences appear only for the group of patients with more than 10 years of treatment, who are limited on CAPD. The difference, if any, will be measurable only after longer follow-ups.

Several studies have evaluated the evolution of uremic osteodystrophy from a histological and

Table 1. Serum levels of PTH, calcium and phosphate in CAPD and HD patients.

	CAPD	HD	P =
Number of patients	72	103	
Age (years)	66 ± 12	62 ± 16	0.085
Follow-up (months)	39 ± 32	56 ± 45	0.006
PTH$_{COOH}$ (pg/ml)	2804 ± 2469	3658 ± 2824	0.042
PTHintact (pg/ml)	153 ± 217	182 ± 215	0.398
Calcium (mg/dl)	9.9 ± 1.2	9.5 ± 0.7	0.015
Phosphate (mg/dl)	4.7 ± 1.0	4.7 ± 1.2	0.959

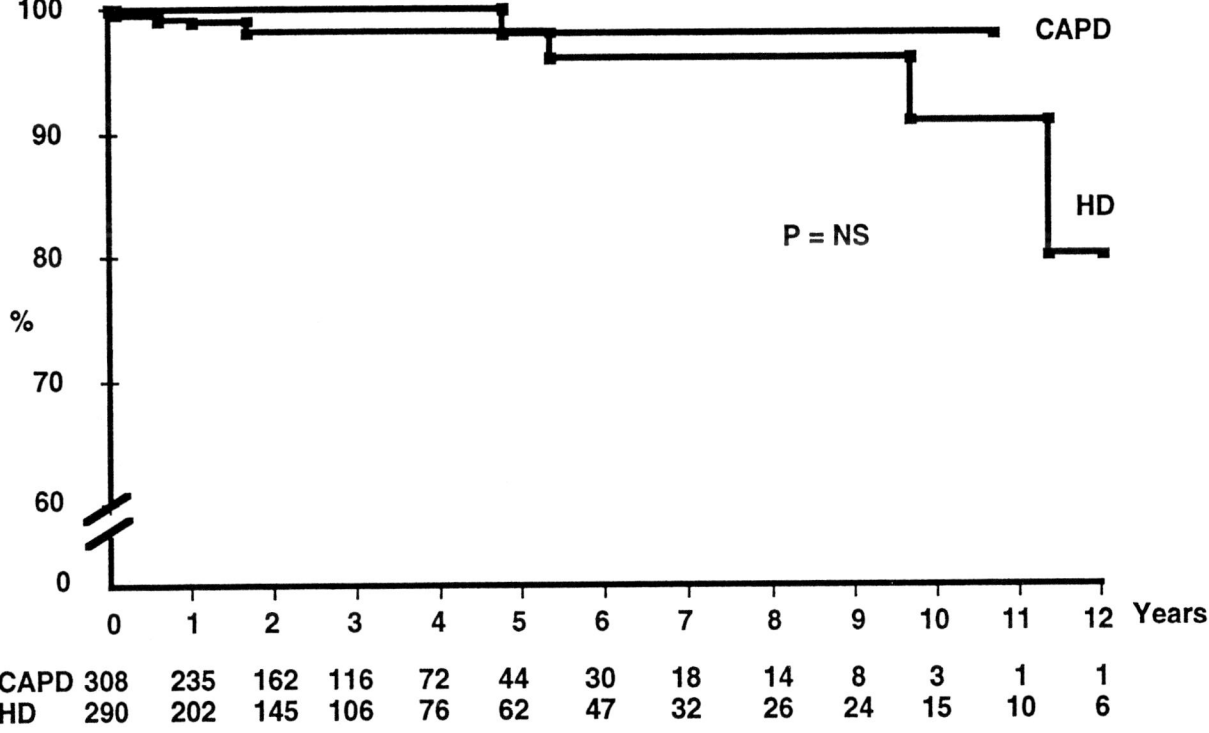

Figure 4. Parathyroidectomy-free patients in CAPD and HD (life table analysis). Numbers at bottom indicate the patients at risk.

radiological point of view [119, 122–135]. Only a few of them have compared the results on CAPD and on HD. Improvement of osteomalacia on CAPD more than on HD is one of the most frequently reported results. Osteitis fibrosa was improved or worsensed in approximately and equal number of papers. However, in the studies done after 1986 [130–133], there seems to be a constant trend toward improvement of both osteomalacia and osteitis fibrosa on CAPD.

In CAPD patients aluminum bone disease is less frequent [135, 136], whereas aplastic bone disease is more frequent. In the Toronto Osteodystrophy Study [134], aplastic bone was present in 48.8% of all patients, being more frequent in CAPD (68%) than in HD patients (35%). This difference was attributed to a greater frequency of hypercalcemic episodes in CAPD, and greater use of calcium carbonate as a phosphate binder. Adynamic bone was not related to the presence of aluminum, but was associated with high values of serum calcium, low/normal PTH and vascular calcification. The greater incidence of adynamic bone disease on CAPD than on HD was also found by Pei *et al.* [136], 48% in 142 PD patients and 16% in 117 HD patients. Hutchison *et al.* [137] found adynamic bone disease in 10/32 CAPD patients; in 7/10 the histological picture was evident at the start of CAPD and in three it developed on a pre-existent osteomalacia.

8. Metabolism

8.1. Carbohydrates

Reduced tolerance to glucose is a characteristic finding in uremia. It appears in spite of higher levels of plasma insulin and is probably due to a defect in the post receptor binding [138]. The continuous peritoneal absorption of glucose, amounting to 120–245 grams/day [139], may further impair carbohydrate metabolism and lead to diabetes. In fact, 3 of 5 patients studies by Armstrong *et al.* [140] showed decreased glucose tolerance on CAPD. Lameire *et al.* [141] reported that 3 of 135 non-diabetic patients developed diabetes but quoted an incidence of diabetes of 5–7.5% in other studies. However, there are still doubts about whether the reported cases had preclinical diabetes before starting CAPD or whether all CAPD patients are at risk of worsening their glucose tolerance or of developing diabetes. Heaton [142] found that uremics have daily profiles of serum glucose higher than normals, but these improve after three months on CAPD in spite of unchanged plasma levels of insulin. Ketone bodies are increased in uremia and revert to normal values on CAPD. Triglycerides increase in uremia and further increase on CAPD [142]. The response to an intravenous glucose load was studied in 9 normals, 16 patients on CAPD, 32 on HD and 31 as yet undialyzed uremics [143]. Basal C-peptide and glucagon were increased in all uremics, whilst plasma insulin levels were increased only in CAPD patients. Conard's "K" values indicating reduced glucose tolerance was found in 50% of non-dialyzed uremics, in 37% of CAPD patients and in only 6% of patients on HD. However the CAPD patients were older than the HD ones and it is well known that age reduces glucose tolerance. When only patients comparable for age were considered, there was no difference between CAPD and HD [143].

Glucose given intraperitoneally causes a more prolonged hyperglycemia and a longer lasting increase of plasma insulin levels than an oral glucose load [144, 145]. In one study, the longer duration of high glucose concentrations and of insulin promoted increased triglyceride and VLDL synthesis in the liver [146]. However, in that study [146], basal plasma insulin was normal and the C-peptide/insulin ratio was higher than in other studies [147, 148]. In Heaton's study [148] of six non-diabetic CAPD patients, basal plasma insulin was twice the normal value and lactate concentration was also increased, probably due to the load of lactate present as buffer in the dialysis solution. Pyruvate levels showed a slight increase after hypertonic glucose solutions and ketone bodies were also reduced, more so with hypertonic solutions.

On the other hand the continuous glucose load during CAPD can lead to spontaneous reduction in carbohydrate consumption as food [149], in spite of stability of the glucose tolerance level. The response to the oral glucose load resembles that of type II diabetes with hyperinsulinemia. In 13 CAPD patients, Lindholm *et al.* [150] found that fasting blood glucose, serum insulin and glucagon levels during an oral glucose tolerance test were not different from those of normals and concluded that glucose intolerance persists during CAPD, but than this therapy does not further impair this metabolic derangement.

In summary, the majority of the studies indicates that the reduced tolerance to glucose does not progress in CAPD. However, the levels of triglycerides and cholesterol appear to increase [146, 149] and this might favour the tendency of uremics to accelerated atherosclerosis [143].

8.2. Lipids

Dialysis patients are hyperlipidemic due to an increased production and a decreased removal of triglycerides on both CAPD and HD, positively correlated to plasma immunoreactive insulin levels [151]. Serum cholesterol is generally normal in HD patients, while it has been found either increased [149, 151] or unchanged [141] in CAPD patients. In these patients, plasma lipid concentrations before dialysis are relevant to their final concentrations during the treatment. In fact, patients on CAPD starting with low plasma levels of triglyceride have the lowest triglyceride [152, 153], and the highest HDL cholesterol levels, and no increase in VLDL [153]. This suggests that lipoprotein response to continuous glucose supply differs from patient to patient according to the efficiency of their lipoprotein metabolism [154].

In a longitudinal assessment, the risk of atherogenesis did not change over 24 months of follow-up; however, when evaluated over six years, in a cross-sectional study, the risk appeared to be greater in patients on CAPD. [155]. This probably indicates that a long time is necessary to develop significant lipid changes. In a comparative study Avram *et al.* [156] found CAPD treatment to be associated with a more atherogenic lipoprotein profile than is HD, but the potential risk associated with hyperlipidemia was far outweighted by the increased overall mortality of patients with hypolipidemia due to malnutrition, which is a more important prognostic factor for patient survival.

8.3. Proteins

In a small series of HD and CAPD patients, an increase in mortality was observed as malnutrition worsened [157].

Hypoalbuminemia is one of the most reliable signs of malnutrition in non-proteinuric and non-enteropathic patients and has often been used to define the nutritional status of dialyzed patients. CAPD does not correct the hypoalbuminemia present before dialysis, whereas HD does [158]. An inverse relationship between albuminemia and mortality in HD patients was also found in CAPD patients [159, 160]. On the other hand, a recent report showed that stable low serum levels of albumin in CAPD patients were not correlated with a worse patient outcome [161].

In an international study of 224 CAPD patients using the "subjective nutritional assessment," based on 21 variables derived from history and clinical examination or anthropometry and biochemistry, 8% of the patients were severely mainourished and 32.6% were mildly or moderately malnourished [162]. In a Italian multicenter study [13], the same method, applied to 256 HD and 204 CAPD patients, showed severe malnutrition in 3% of the HD and 7.8% of the CAPD patients, moderate/mild malnutrition in 27% and 33.8% and good nutritional status in 70% and 58.3%, with differences between treatments statistically not significant. There were no relationships between mortality and subjective global assessment of nutritional status or serum albumin levels. When all malnourished were combined, percentages of malnourished patients increased with age, on both HD and CAPD, and the increase was higher on HD than on CAPD in patients older than 65, suggesting that there is better preservation of the nutritional status in the elderly CAPD patients. Other studies based on anthropometric measurements found no differences in nutritional status between CAPD and HD [163, 164]. In addition, the percentages of deaths due to cachexia were similar for HD and CAPD in a multicenter study [165].

Another approach to the problem is longitudinal study of nutritional parameters in patients on each treatment. In our experience, CAPD patients have lower serum protein levels than HD patients [158]. However, long term CAPD patients, up to 8 years of treatment, maintain unchanged plasma levels of albumin and transferrin (Table 2) [166], indicating that long-term CAPD treatment is not necessarily associated with malnutrition. These data are in agreement with our own which show the stability of the protein catabolic rate and the creatinine appearance rate in patients on long-term CAPD treatment [166]. CAPD patients usually have lower protein intake than that recommended (1.1–1.3 g/Kg BW/day) for nitrogen balance [167, 168] and this should expose them to a greater risk of malnutrition [161, 166]. However, this protein need was assessed in patients 44–48 years old, a range quite different from the older CAPD patients. Studies also including elderly patients, have shown that on both CAPD and HD there is an inverse relationship between normalized protein catabolic rate and age [166, 169]. According to these studies, it seems reasonable to suggest that CAPD patients, the majority of whom are elderly, can have an average lower protein requirement than that usually suggested to maintain nitrogen balance.

9. Residual renal function

After the initial reports [170–172] which suggested that in CAPD residual renal function was maintained for a longer time as compared to HD, several studies have confirmed this in non-diabetics [173–175] and in diabetics [176–178]. Moreover, CAPD is more favourable in terms of recovery of renal function; in several studies [172, 179–181] this has been seen in 1–8% of CAPD patients, compared to 0.86%–1.2% of HD patients. In patients recovering renal function, nephroangiosclerosis, interstitial nephropathy and systemic disease were the more frequent causes of renal failure [179–181]. This is in agreement with data from Cancarini et al. [172], who showed that the mean annual reduction of creatinine clearance was similar on CAPD and HD in patients with primary glomerulonephropathy, whereas it was much smaller on CAPD in patients with nephrangiosclerosis and interstitial nephropathy. The preservation of renal function in dialyzed patients has indisputable advantages as it allows reduction of the dose of dialysis.

10. Transplantation

The suggestion that CAPD is more able than HD to improve the impaired immune status caused by uremia raises the question of whether transplantation in CAPD patients might have a worse outcome. In 1984 Guillou et al. [65] reported inferior graft survival in CAPD as compared to HD patients treated mainly with azathioprine and prednisolone. The patients did not differ in age, time on dialysis, or HLA-A, HLA-B, HLA-DR mismatches. The only difference was a significantly higher OKT4+/OKT8+ ratio in CAPD patients. The investigators suggested that CAPD restored or maintained an immune response sufficient to increase the risk of graft rejection, whereas HD patients, having a lower percentage of OKT4+, were more easily immunosuppressed by conventional therapy, which mainly acts on OKT4+ cells. That modality has an effect was supported by the high incidence of early rejection on CAPD. However, graft survival curves, which different greatly in the first month after transplantation, later became parallel. One year later, Donnelly et al. [70] did not find any difference in plasma suppressive activity and in lymphocyte function between patients coming from CAPD or HD who had the same graft survival. Since then, many groups have compared the outcomes of transplantation in HD and CAPD patients without showing any differences in patient and graft survival [182–194]. These results have also been confirmed for children [195].

Transplanted patients coming from peritoneal dialysis are at risk of development of catheter-related infections. Post-tranplant prevalence of peritonitis varies from 0% to 40% [183, 184, 186, 188–191, 193–197]. Peritonitis developed very rarely in patients not using CAPD after surgery [193, 195]. In any case, post-transplant peritonitis is not a major problem if it is managed aggressively by antibiotic therapy and early catheter removal [191, 193]. Diaz-Buxo et al. [182] suggest removing the catheter one day before transplantation from living-related donors and 1-2 week after surgery for kidneys from cadaveric donors. Wood et al. [193] and Ogawa et al. [196] removed the

Table 2. Serum albumin and serum transferrin over time in 21 CAPD patients (M ± SD). (Reprinted with permission from reference [166]).

Albumin	CAPD start	1	2	3	4	5	6	7	8 years
ALL (n = 21)	3.6 ± 0.2	3.7 ± 0.3	3.7 ± 0.4	3.7 ± 0.4	3.7 ± 0.3				
Subgroup A (n = 13)	3.6 ± 0.2	3.7 ± 0.4	3.7 ± 0.3	3.8 ± 0.3	3.9 ± 0.3*				
Subgroup B (n = 8)	3.7 ± 0.2	3.7 ± 0.3	3.6 ± 0.4	3.6 ± 0.5	3.5 ± 0.3⁰	3.4 ± 0.3⁰	3.5 ± 0.5	3.6 ± 0.3	3.7 ± 0.3

Transferrin	CAPD start	1	2	3	4 years				
ALL (n = 21)	277 ± 73	280 ± 72	261 ± 59	255 ± 46	272 ± 54				
Subgroup A (n = 13)	252 ± 73	275 ± 62	257 ± 55	258 ± 41	263 ± 37				
Subgroup B (n = 8)	319 ± 90	289 ± 90	267 ± 68⁰	250 ± 56*	287 ± 75	264 ± 56⁰	257 ± 64⁰	266 ± 44⁰	264 ± 47

* $p < 0.01$ vs CAPD start   ⁰ = $p < 0.05$ vs CAPD start.

catheter perioperatively, while others 1–26 weeks after transplantation [182, 186, 191, 193, 194].

The percentages of transplanted patients with infections of the wound were sometimes similar in HD and CAPD [193] sometimes greater in CAPD patients: 19% versus 9% [188]; 26% versus 11% [194]. In the last study, the percentage increased to 56% when only patients needing CAPD post-transplantation were taken into account [194]. On the other hand, no wound infection was observed in 20 children by Ogawa et al. [196] who had removed the catheters at the time of tranplants from 16 of them.

Exit site infections have complicated the post-transplant course in 2% to 8% of patients [186, 190, 191, 193, 194] while leakage from the transplant wound occurred in 1.8% to 5% [190, 194, 198]. Ascites developed in 2 of 10 patients reported by Odor-Morales et al. [183] in 2 of 42 patients studied by Evangelista et al. [188] and 1 of 56 of those reported by Glass et al. [198].

Incidences of infections other than peritonitis, wound infection and catheter exit-site infection were similar in CAPD and HD patients [198].

11. Hospitalization

The causes for hospitalization are partially different for PD and HD, and this must be considered in evaluating comparative results.

One interesting study compared similar numbers of patients randomly assigned to home IPD (HIPD) and home hemodialysis (HHD) [199]. The mean days of hospitalization were 16.3 ± 3.2 on HHD and 18.3 ± 2.8 on HIPD in the first 6 months and 24.0 ± 5.8 and 28.4 ± 5.8 in the following 6 months. In the first six months there were 30 admissions of the HIPD and 9 of the HHD group. Surgical revision for dialytic access was less frequent for the HHD group (9.5%) than for the HIPD group (12.8%). Patients on HHD had 12 cardiac accidents (arrhythmia, angina, myocardial infarction, cardiac decompensation, pericarditis), but none of the patients on HIPD. On the other hand, only one patient on HHD had peritonitis which was the reason for 20 of the 58 admissions of the HIPD group.

Several other investigators have evaluated the need for hospitalization on CAPD and on HD (Table 3), but their results are hard to compare because hospitalization incidences may differ according to the center's policy and their availability of out-patient care and social facilities and attention to cost saving. Case mix is another variable, since age and diabetes, do influence the hospitalization rate [202, 206]. The studies cited here compare the incidence of hospitalization in the same center/s, thus overcoming the bias due to center-effect. When comparing home treatment to in-center treatment, it is important, for better comprehension, to separate the first hospitalization from later ones, as the need of training greatly prolongs the first hospitalization much.

The incidence of hospitalization is greater on CAPD than on HD in some studies [34, 201, 204, 206] and similar in others [202–204, 207]. In the study of Serkes et al., the difference was statistically significant although small [202]. Diabetics on CAPD are admitted more often than non-diabetics [202, 203, 206]. Days of hospitalization for diabetics on CAPD have been reported as both more [202] and less [203, 208, 209] than those for diabetics on HD. Unfortunately, not all the studies give the percentage of diabetics and this can influence the results. It is noteworthy that studies that divide the days of hospitalization according to their causes [34, 207] or that report the incidence of hospitalization due to peritonitis [201, 205] show that the difference between CAPD and HD disappears or becomes negative when admissions due to peritonitis are excluded. This supports the hope that progressive reduction in the frequency of peritonitis will be able to reduce the gap between the two modalities. In the study of Kurtz et al. [201], 43% of CAPD patients were not hospitalized during the time of the study versus only 23% of HHD patients; once hospitalized, however, patients on CAPD were hospitalized longer.

Burton and Walls analyzed the hospitalization of dialysis patients in greater depth [206]. They applied a generalized linear model to 227 patients on either CAPD or HD to identify confounding factors, estimate the magnitude of their effects and adjust for any bias influencing hospitalization. Six of 86 variables studied influenced hospitalization, some adversely others beneficially. Diabetes and atherosclerotic disease significantly increased the hospitalization rate, while having a living spouse and the initial presentation via out-patient department reduced it. After correcting for the above, the investigators found a quadratic relationship between patient age and hospitalization rate: the ratio of the estimated rate at a specific age to the rate at 50 years of age increased below the age of 20, and much more above the age of 60 years. When the need for hospitalization was examined according to the date of commencement of dialysis, it remained stable on HD over the course of the study, whereas it markedly diminished on CAPD, so that the annual hospitalization ratio between CAPD and HD fell, with time, from the initial 7.8 to 1.33 days/patient-month. The conclusion of the investigators is that, with growing experience, hospitalization on CAPD can become very close to that on HD. The same conclusion was reached by Khanna et al. [210], who observed a progressive reduction of the incidence of hospitalitazion of CAPD patients from 26.1 days/patient-year (13.1 due to peritonitis) in the period 1977–78 to 16 (5.1 due to peritonitis) in 1982. A similar positive trend was found by Nolph in the US CAPD Registry [211].

We recently reevaluated hospitalization in 254 CAPD and 240 HD patients treated in our center between 1 Jan. 1981 and 31 Dec. 1991 [34]. The two groups had comparable follow-ups (32 ± 29 months on HD vs, 34 ± 26 on CAPD). Hospitalizations were classified into: first hospitalization (diagnosis period, preparation of dialytic access, CAPD training), hospitalization due to technique-related problems (peritonitis, exit-site and tunnel

Table 3. Hospitalization rate in some studies.

Author [reference]	Years studies	Modality	# of pts	Mean age	Diabetics %	All admissions (days/p-y)	First admissions (days)	Following admissions (days/p-y)
Non-diabetics								
Mion et al. [200]	1981	HIPD	17	NA		26.1		
		CAPD	15	NA		22.3		
		ICHD	52	NA		10.6		
		HHD	60	NA		14.9		
Kurtz et al. [201]	1979–83	CAPD	21	49.6		9.9		
		HHD	30	47.8		4.7		
Serkes et al. [202]	1981–85	CAPD	219	NA		10.14		
		ICHD+HHD	261	NA		9.18		
All patients								
Charytan et al. [203]	1980–81	CAPD	72	50.0	12.5	17.2		
		ICHD	92	57.7	14.1	19.0		
Blagg et al. [204]	1982	HIPD	NA	NA	NA	26.28		
		CAPD	NA	NA	NA	19.74		
		ICHD	NA	NA	NA	19.29		
		ICIPD	NA	NA	NA	39.81		
		HHD	NA	NA	NA	9.19		
Frascino et al. [205]	NA	CAPD	10	NA	2	16.4		
	NA	HHD	10	NA	2	14.8		
	NA	ICSCHD	20	NA	NA	6.9		
Burton and Walls [206]	1980–85	CAPD	123	51.2	15	39.0		
		HD	121	44.1	5	14.7		
Gokal et al. [207]	1983–86	CAPD	610	52	16	14.8		
		HD	329	48	4 (?)	12.4		
Maiorca et al. [34]	1981–91	CAPD	254	NA	NA		32.5	20.0
		HD	240	NA	NA		22.1	AcHD: 9.1
								Bic-HD: 12.4
								HF/HDF: 9.5
Diabetics								
Charytan et al. [203]	1980–81	CAPD	9	NA		40.3		
		HD	13	NA		48.4		
Legrain et al. [208]	1978–83	CAPD	38	52.2		42		
	1973–83	HD	67	41.3		46		
Mejia et al. [209]	1978–83	CAPD	33	42.1		84	25	15.6
		HD	33	43.6		90	14	36.0
Serkes et al. [202]	1981–85	CAPD	119	NA		19.4		
		HD	104	NA		13.4		

infection, hernias, problems related to the vascular access, etc.), hospitalizations in some way connected to pathology already present at the beginning of treatment, (cardiovascular disease, diabetes, etc.) all other reasons for hospitalization (diagnostic needs, hemorrhages, infectious diseases, metabolic problems, surgical problems, etc.). First hospitalization, which included training as in-patients, was longer on CAPD than on HD, 32.5 days versus 22.1 The duration of hospitalization for all other admissions was longer on CAPD than on HD: 20.0 days/patient-year on CAPD, 12.4 on bicarbonate-HD, 9.1 on acetate HD and 9.5 on HF/HDF (Fig. 5). The incidence of the days spent in hospital because of complications of the technique was almost twice as great for CAPD as for HD patients, the difference being due to peritonitis. There were no differences in hospitalizations due to pathologies already present at the start of treatment, whereas the length of hospitalization due to other causes was longer on CAPD and on bicarbonate-HD than on other methods.

12. Technique failure

PD technique survival is one of the most widely discussed topics. In its evaluation some investigators also include death of the patients, since death while on one method can be considered a failure of that method. However, it is well known that about 50% of deaths are due to cardiovascular disease and many others (such cause as malignancy) are not strictly relatable to the method. This is why it is preferable to treat dead patients as lost to follow-up. This approach has been followed in many of the published studies. On the other hand, to include deaths among final events in technique survival can be useful evaluating the probability for one patient to live while on that method. This approach, often called "technique success analysis," can be impor-

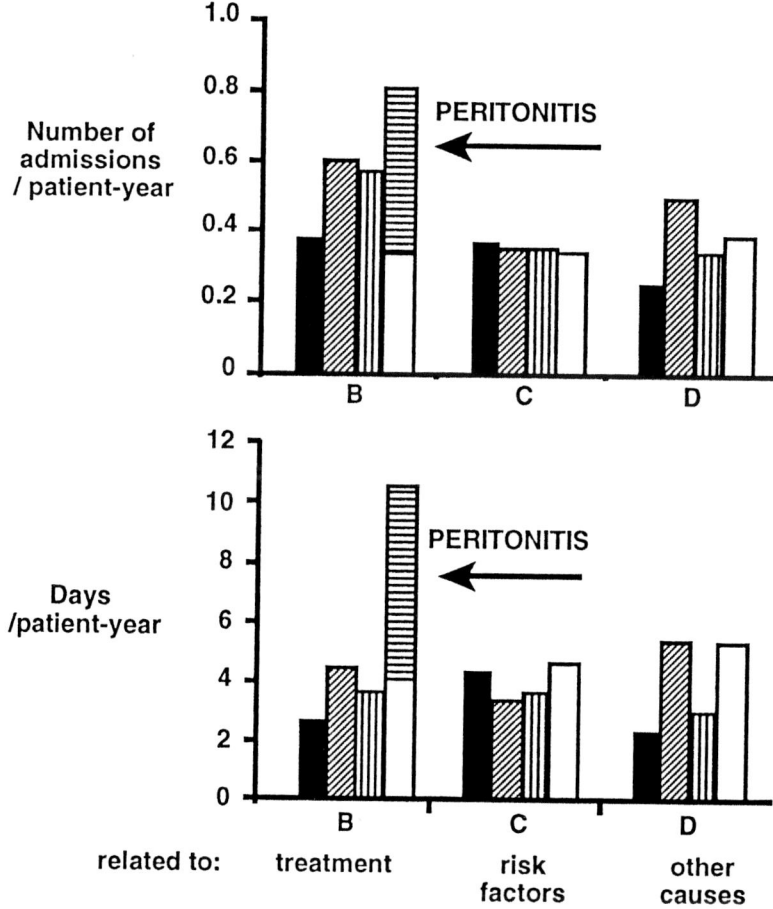

Figure 5. Number of hospitalizations per patient-year (A) and days of hospitalization per patient-year (B) for four dialysis modalities. Symbols are: (■) acetate HD; (□) bicarbonate HD; (□) HF/HDF; (□) CAPD, peritonitis excluded; (□) CAPD, peritonitis. (Reprinted from reference [34] by permission of Blackwell Scientific Publications, Inc.).

tant in forecasting the center's work load and the number of patients who will remain on the method over a certain period of time.

In the following analysis of the published studies, we will discuss the two different approaches in different paragraphs; the first is called technique survival, the second technique success.

12.1. Technique survival

The technique survival of intermittent peritoneal dialysis is worse than that of HD. In one prospective, randomized study [199] 49.2% of the patients were switched from home intermittent peritoneal dialysis (HIPD) to HD versus only 9.1% from HHD to IPD.

More studies have compared technique survivals for CAPD and HD, some reporting worse results on CAPD [165, 207, 212, 213], others with comparable results [214, 215] (Table 4). Two large studies, one Canadian, the second Italian, are not included in the table as they do not include the percentages of survivors on the treatments. In the first [216], data from the Canadian Renal Failure Registry for non-diabetic patients are reported. For the age group 15–44 years, CAPD patients had the same technique survival as HD patients in the first six months, but afterwards the CAPD curve continued to decrease while the HD curve was stable, and after 30 months technique survival was 45% for CAPD and 85% for HD. A similar trend was observed in the age group 45–64, but the final diffences were less than for younger patients (55% on CAPD vs 70% on HD). Finally, in the older age group (65 years or more), treatment survival was better for CAPD in the first 24 months, but at 30 months any difference had disappeared. These data suggest worse technique survival for CAPD in youth, with differences progressively decreasing with age. These conclusions are supported by observations of better CAPD technique survival in the elderly [216] and of decreasing risk of change to HD from CAPD [212].

The second paper [217] cites data from the Dialysis and Transplantation Registry of the Italian Piedmont Region over the period 1981–87. Approximated technique survivals after 42 months were 55% for CAPD (359 patients), 65% for bicarbonate-HD (431 patients), and 30% for acetate-HD (1231 patients). Comparison of the CAPD patients with the 53 hemofiltration patients showed similar results after 24 months of treatment.

Several studies have attempted to identify causes of CAPD technique failure. Peritonitis still stands as the most important cause and its frequency significantly affects technique survival (Fig. 6) [218]. Excellent technique survival data have been obtained [214] since the introduction of the Y-system [219–220]. The influence of peritonitis on technique survival was assessed in a cause-specific analysis [165]. Considering "changes of modality due to peritonitis" as "lost to follow-up" the relative risk for CAPD failure decreased from 1.81 to 1.06, similar to that of HD, put at 1.

Other studies have examined the role of diabetes in CAPD technique survival. Diabetics on CAPD have a higher risk of modality change than either non-diabetics or diabetics on HD [202]. However another study shows the very opposite [212]. The presence of cerebro-cardiovascular disease was associated with both an increased [207] and decreased [212] risk of modality change (from HD to CAPD). In an Italian study [165] no patient related factor was found to significantly affect technique survival. Firanek found a higher relative risk of need to change from CAPD for black patients than for white [221].

Other not patient-related factors influence technique survival. Progressive experience lessens the risk of CAPD failure but not of ICHD. [212]. In a multicenter study, differences were seen among centers [165], probably due to different center policies in patient selection, treatment, training and propensity to change method because of peritonitis or other technique-related complications.

12.2. Technique success

In one of the first studies, Rubin et al. [222] found a higher modality failure rate (mortality and technique failure) on CAPD that on HD, 43% versus 16%. However the two groups were not comparable because there were more diabetics on CAPD (25% versus 5%), more cardiovascular disease (37% versus 8%) and more patients with lower incomes. The mean age was 5 years older for the CAPD, but this was not significantly different. In a study in 1983 [200], the percentages of "standard patients" continuing on their first treatment modality were 90% for HHD, 80% for CHD, 42% for IPD and 50 % for CAPD. Interestingly, the main reason for transferring CAPD patients to another modality was loss of ultrafiltration, with peritonitis the second reason. At that time the buffer used was acetate, which leads to loss of ultrafiltration.

Table 5 reports the results of some other studies. The percentages of success were similar on CAPD

Table 4. Technique survival in some studies.

Author [reference]	Years studied	Modality	Number of patients	Mean age	Percentage of diabetics	1 year	2 years	3 years	4 years	5 years	6 years	Comments
Gokal et al. [207]	1983–86	CAPD	610	52	16				91			
		HD	329	48	4 (?)				61			
Maiorca et al. [213]	1981–86	CAPD	120	58	23	98	89	84	71	71		$P = 0.0457$ vs HD
		HD	139	48	9	96	96	96	96	96		
Maiorca et al. [165]	1981–87	CAPD	480	56.2	20.2	94.7	87.5	81.1	72.8	71.6	71.6	$P = 0.0491$ vs HD
		ICHD	373	50.0	7.2	94.3	90.6	87.0	87.0	87.0	87.0	
Cavalli et al. [214]	1981–88	CAPD	42	61.6	14.3			75				
		HD	48	57.8	7.1			73				
Gentil et al. [212]	1984–88	CAPD	272	NA	28.7	80	64	56				$P < 0.001$ vs ICHD
		ICHD	842	NA	2.3	95	94	94				
Lupo et al. [215]	1985–89	CAPD	660	59.7	13					67		$P = NS$ vs HD
		HD	968	53.6	8					82		

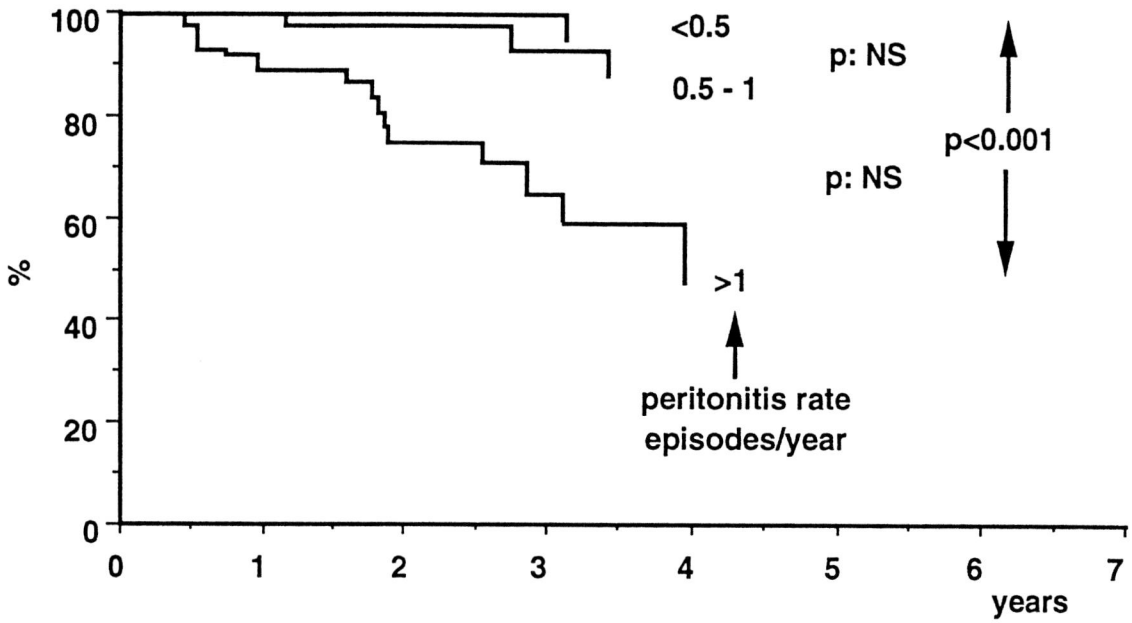

Figure 6. True technique survival (only CAPD failure considered as final event), according to peritonitis rate. (Reprinted from reference [218] by permission of Springer-Verlag).

and HD [203, 233] or worse on CAPD [212], even after adjusting for pretreatment differences [165].

12.3. Causes of technique failure

As for the causes of technique failure, 3 to 78% of HD patients change type of dialysis, as compared with 11 to 15% of the CAPD patients [165, 202, 207, 213]. On CAPD, peritonitis is the main cause (40–47%), loss of peritoneal function accounts for 15–19% and catheter related problems for 9–15%. A very small percentage of drop-outs is due to malnutrition and 4–15% are due to patient preference. On HD, cardiovascular instability, loss of vascular access and other medical reasons are the main causes for abandoning the technique. In the analysis of Registries [224], peritonitis accounted for 27 to 52% of drop-outs, and loss of petitoneal function for 8 to 14%. The loss of peritoneal function was higher (30% after two years) in France [225]. In absolute figures, only 1.7–2.5% of patients at risk leave the treatment due to loss of peritoneal function and 5 to 7.2% due to peritonitis [165, 207, 213].

Table 6 shows that causes for changing modality in two multicenter studies.

13. Mortality on CAPD

Several studies have tried to assess patient survival on CAPD compared to that on HD. Unfortunately, due to objective and ethical limitations, no study

Table 5. Technique success in some studies.

Reference	Years studied	Modality	Number	Mean age	Percentage of diabetics	1 year	2 years	3 years	6 years	Comments
Charytan et al. [203]	1980–81	CAPD	72	50.0	12.5		70*			* = at the 26th month
		ICHD	92	57.7	14.1		70*			* = at the 26th month
Gentil et al. [212]	1984–88	CAPD	272	NA	28.7	71	46	36		$p < 0.001$ vs ICHD
		ICHD	842	NA	2.3	86	80	75		
Marichal et al. [223]	1978–89	CAPD	139	50.5	17.2			49	20	
	1972–89	ICHD	137	50.9	5.1			49	31	

* = Changes to HHD or to Tx treated as lost to follow-up.

has prospectively compared large numbers of unselected, randomly allocated patients. Therefore, it is impossible to establish with absolute scientific rigor whether one method is definitely better than another. Published survival studies are usually retrospective and in many of them no attempt was made to correct for pretreatment differences. These are mentioned below as "observed results." Some studies found differences among subgroups of patients (older, diabetics, etc.) or made comparisons for selected subgroups (such as "standard population").

Some studies have used statistical analysis to find factors that influence survival and to correct results for them. The search for risk factors has sometimes led to different results or has been successful for only one modality. There differences are due to the different numbers of patients considered, to different lengths of follow-up or to the number of fatalities associated with each cause, sometimes insufficient for statistical significance. As a consequence, greater numbers of risk factors have emerged from the largest studies and from those searching for the largest number of risk factors. It follows from this that in many studies the corrections were only partial.

13.1. Observed results

In the only study, to our knowledge, in which patients were randomly allocated to HIPD or HHD [199], there were no differences between groups.

Table 7 shows the patient suvivals seen in different studies. Frequently the results on CAPD and HD were similar [165, 200, 201, 203, 213, 215], even in a study in which CAPD patients were older and burdened by more risk factors than HD patients [165]. Other studies have shown better results on HD [207, 212, 226]. Definitely better survival on HHD was found [226, 227]. The presence of a higher percentage of diabetics sometimes worsens results for CAPD. In studies of standard populations [200] or restricted to non-diabetics of similar age [201], or separating diabetics from non-diabetics [202], or comparing patients without high risk or diabetics [215], patient survival was the same on CAPD and HD. Cavalli et al. [214] observed better results on CAPD in spite of a higher percentage of patients with diabetic nephropathy or aged 70 years or more, but the HD group contained more patients with malignancy and hypertension. The observed differences due to patient selection add further support to the need to correct the case mix. In a study by Capelli et al. [226], the differences in survival observed at three-years (32% on CAPD versus 50% on ICHD) disappeared after adjusting for age and diabetes only.

Other studies of survival do not report percentages and are therefore not included in the table. In the large series of Burton and Walls [228], life-expectancy is better with transplantation than with either form of dialysis ($p < 0.05$), and probably better with hemodialysis than with CAPD. In the Regional Piedmont Dialysis and Transplantation Registry, there were no significant differences between CAPD, acetate-HD and bicarbonate-HD after 60 months. Patients on hemofiltration had significantly worse survival. The similarity of results on CAPD, Bic-HD and Ac-HD was also confirmed for the subgroups of "standard patients'

Table 6. Cause for leaving modality, in percent.

	Gokal et al. [207]		Maiorca et al. [165]	
	CAPD	HD	CAPD	HD
Peritonitis	47		40	
Loss of ultrafiltration	8			
Loss of peritoneal cavity	4		19	
Loss of biochemical control	3			
Catheter related	13		9	
Malnutrition	2			
Patient choice	4	4	11	11
Cardiovascular instability		9	2	37
Loss of vascular access		27		11
Medical (peritonitis excluded)			13	33
Patient unable to cope			5	
Other	17	59	2	7

Table 7. Patient survival in some comparative studies. See text for comments.

Author [reference]	Years studied	Modality	Number of patients	Percentage of diabetics	Mean age	1 year	2 years	3 years	4 years	5 years	6 years	Comments
Capelli et al. [226]	1974–81	CAPD	88	35.2	55.7	86	50	32				
		IPD	26	42.3	53.2	70	20	10				
		ICHD	276	14.9	52.0	85	63	50				
		HHD	64	4.7	44.2	98	85	66				
Charytan et al. [203]	1980–81	CAPD	72	12.5	50.0		≈ 80					Standard population
		ICHD	92	14.1	57.7		≈ 80					Standard population
Mion et al. [200]	1978–82	CAPD	20	0	42.8		90					Standard population
	1976–82	ICHD	91	0	40.9		92					Standard population
	1976–82	HHD	87	0	42.2		98					
	1976–82	HIPD	30	0	39.8		100					
Kurtz et al. [201]	1979–83	CAPD non-diab	21	0	49.6	91	91	78*				* = at 32th month
		HHD non-diab	30	0	47.8	96	96	84*				* = at 32th month
Mailloux et al. [227]	1970–85	CAPD	46	NA	NA					43		
		ICHD	425	NA	NA					35		
		HHD	52	NA	NA					≈ 90		
Gokal et al. [207]	1983–86	CAPD	610	16	52				62			
		HD	329	4 (?)	48				74			
Maiorca et al. [213]	1981–86	CAPD	120	23	50	89	81	73	64	46		P = 0.2694 vs HD
		HD	139	9	48	92	88	80	72	66		
Maiorca et al. [165]	1981–87	CAPD	480	20.2	56.2	91	79	68	60	49	38	P = 0.0725 vs HD
		ICHD	373	7.2	50.0	92	84	79	67	62	54	
Cavalli et al. [214]	1981–88	CAPD	42	14.3	61.6			71				
		HD	48	7.1	57.8			58				
Gentil et al. [212]	1984–88	CAPD	272	28.7	NA	89	73	64				Mantel: P = 0.008
		ICHD	842	2.3	NA	91	85	80				Breslow: P = 0.17
Lupo et al. [215]	1985–89	CAPD	660	13	59.7					45		P = NS vs HD
		HD	968	8	53.6					54		
		CAPD No-HR pts	240	0	NA					65		P = NS vs HD
		HD No-HR pts	527	0	NA					66		
		CAPD diabetics	89	100	NA			45				P = NS vs HD
		HD diabetics	80	100	NA			50				

and "high risk patients" [217]. Posen et al. [216] compared the non-diabetic patients of the Canadian Renal Failure Registry. CAPD patients aged 15–44 had the same survival as compared to HD patients up to 30 months of follow-up. No differences were found for patients aged 45–64 after 42 months. For the age group 65 and older, survival on CAPD was better than that on HD at 6 and 12 months, but the differences narrowed after the 18th month and had disappeared by the 36th month.

13.2. Factors affecting patient survival

13.2.1. Modality

Many studies have tried to measure the risk of death due to modality for CAPD and HD. Results are summarized in Table 8. The only statistically significant differences observed were in the study by Rubin et al. [222] comparing CAPD to home hemodialysis (HHD).

After adjusting data for bias among groups, Burton and Walls [228] estimated that the proportion of patients predicted to survive 10 years were 53% for CAPD, 45% for hemodialysis and 50% for transplantation. However, these figures were projections calculated on the basis of clinical data with a follow-up of 5.5 years for transplantation and less than 2 years for CAPD. In the studies by Maiorca et al. [165, 213], the risk of death on each modality changed with age. In another study [231] patients aged 60 or older had similar patient survival on CAPD and HD but worse on IPD.

The higher drop-out on the CAPD technique might positively influence patient survival figures by dropping the worst patients and leaving the best patients on treatment. If that was true, patients dropping-out from CAPD should be at higher risk of death, e.g., should be older or have more risk factors. This was excluded in one study [34]: the only statistically significant differences between patients leaving the method and the others were incidence of systemic diseases (higher) and mean age (lower) in patients leaving CAPD (Table 9).

13.2.2. Age

Age heavily influences mortality. Shapiro and Umen [232] showed that age had a non-linear effect on patient survival in HD patients, the relative risk of death being 0.21 for patients 1–45 years old, 0.53 for 46–60 and 1.0 over 61. In one of the first studies on patient survival on CAPD [210], age was a powerful negative factor. For the patients in the EDTA-ERA Registry, there were important differences between age groups in primary renal disease, but no differences between CAPD and HD for any of them, with survivals on CAPD no worse, and possibly better, than on other modes of treatment [233]. The relative risks of death due to age in different studies are shown in Table 10.

Only a few studies have compared the effect of age on CAPD and HD patients. In the USRDS Annual Data Report 1991 [235], survival on CAPD was lower than on HD for the elderly, and higher for younger patients. In the elderly, Gokal found a greater risk of death on CAPD than on HD [207] whereas Gentil et al. [212] found that patients on

Table 8. Relative risk of death with different modalities.

	Relative risk of death for					
	HD versus CAPD		CAPD versus HD		Tx versus CAPD	
	RR	P	RR	P	RR	P
Gentil et al. [212]	0.82	= 0.325				
Burton and Walls [206]	1.30	> 0.3			1.09	> 0.3
Maiorca et al. [213]			1.34	= 0.6041		
Rubin et al. [222] HHD			1.30	= 0.020		
LCD			1.03	NS		
Wolfe et al. [229]			0.98	NS		
Maiorca et al. [165]			1.30	= 0.1612		
Serkes et al. [202] (non-diabetics)			0.62	= 0.08		
Lunde et al. [230]			1.025*	NS		
Lupo et al. [215]	1.571	NS				

* Patients ≥ 65 years.

Table 9. Comparison of risk factors in patients leaving CAPD due to method failure vs patients continuing on CAPD (waiting permission to reproduce it from KI).

Factor	Pts shifted from CAPD %	Pts remaining on CAPD %	
Peripheral vasculopathy	28.6	18.0	
Cerebral vasculopathy	14.3	16.4	
Ischemic cardiopathy	17.5	22.8	
Cardiac arrhythmia	7.9	14.0	
Hypertension	61.9	64.0	
Malignant hypertension	1.6	1.2	
Diabetes Type I	6.3	3.2	
Diabetes Type II	20.6	20.4	
Hyperlipemia	23.8	26.0	
Chronic respir. infection	9.5	13.6	
TBC	6.3	4.8	
Systemic disease	1.6	9.2	$p = 0.04$
Cirrhosis	6.3	7.2	
UTI	7.9	10.0	
Malignancy	3.2	6.4	
Average number of risk factors/patient	2.54	2.68	
No risk (%)	6.3	2.8	
Age (years)	56	63	$p < 0.001$

ICHD had higher risk than those on CAPD. Maiorca et al. [213] found that the rates of increase of mortality connected with increasing age were different for the two methods (Fig. 7). After correcting for the risk of death linked to pretreatment risk factors, survival was the same on CAPD and HD for patients aged 30–66, but not for patients 67 and over, who had a significantly lower mortality rate on CAPD than on HD [213]. When the study was extended to five other centers, the statistically significant difference of survival in the elderly disappeared [165], but the risk of death connected with age increased at a greater rate on HD than on CAPD (Fig. 8) [13]. In a larger study, [215] Lupo et al. also found that the impact of age on survival is greater on HD than on CAPD: four-year patient survival was 85% on HD and 70% on CAPD for patients 21–50 years old, 63% and 54% for 51–65 years old and 30% and 40% for patients over 65.

Lunde et al. [230] compared mortality in 1552 elderly patients divided according to the treatment in use on the 120th day. Diabetes, hypertension, white race and age significantly increased the risk of death. They concluded that CAPD had similar outcomes to HD in geriatric non-diabetic patients. These data are questionable since they consider the events that occurred after the 120th day, even if patients changed treatment subsequently. Moreover,

Table 10. Effect of age on patients survival in different studies.

Study	Age groups (years) or increments	Relative risk	P	Comments
Capelli et al. [226]	10-year increment	1.20		
Burton and Walls [206]	10-year increment	1.68	< 0.001	
Gokal et al. [207]	Age ≥ 60	3.28	< 0.001	IN CAPD patients
	Age ≥ 60	2.3	< 0.5	In HD patients
Maiorca et al. [213]	Age − 53.2	1.14	= 0.0003	CAPD + HD pts
Walker et al. [234]	(Age − 51)/10	1.45	= 0.0003	CAPD + HD pts
Rubin et al. [222]	by 20 year difference	1.17	= 0.001	CAPD + HD pts
Wolfe et al. [229]	10 year increment	1.2	< 0.001	CAPD + ICHD patients 20–60 years old
Serkes et al. [202]	Age < 46	0.34	< 0.05	Non-diabetics (Age 46–60 = 1.00)
	Age > 60	2.77	< 0.003	Non-diabetics (Age 46–60 = 1.00)
Gentil et al. [212]	Age > 60	4.10	0.000	CAPD + ICHD
	Age > 60	4.10	< 0.001	ICHD
	Age > 60	3.69	< 0.001	CAPD
Maiorca et al. [165]	Age − 53.5	1.07	0.0001	CAPD + HD
Lupo et al. [215]	Age	1.047	0.000	CAPD + HD
	Age	1.040	0.025	CAPD
	Age	1.055	0.000	HD

OUTCOME OF PERITONEAL DIALYSIS: COMPARATIVE STUDIES

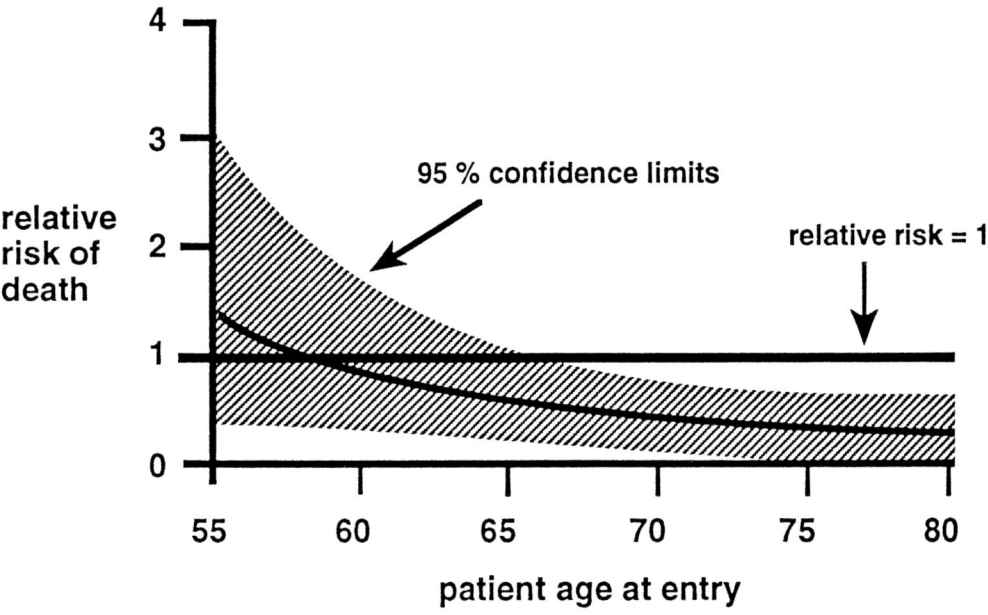

Figure 7. Relative risk of death on CAPD according to age. The risk of death on HD at every age set equal to 1. (Used with permission from Kidney International, volume 34, page 522, 1988).

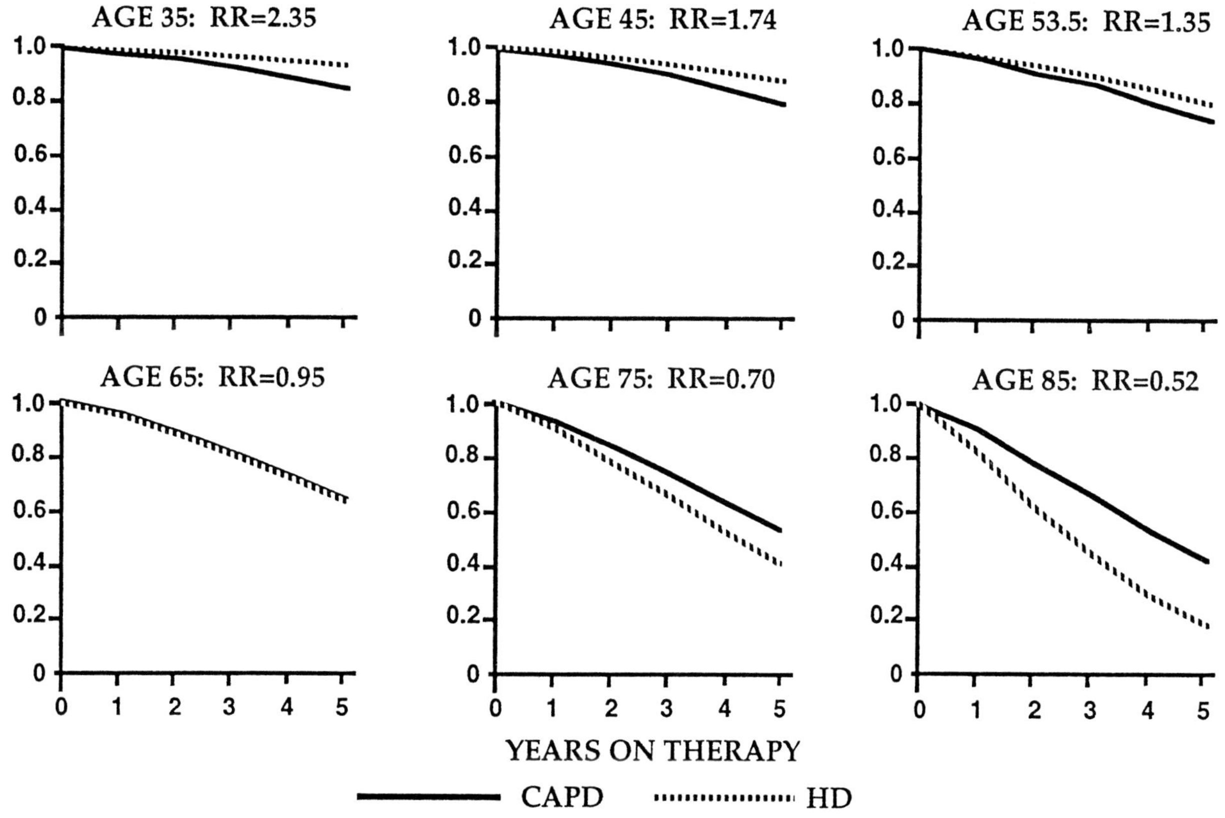

Figure 8. Effect of age on patient survival in CAPD and HD (reprinted from reference [13] by permission of Multimed, Inc).

co-morbid conditions other than primary renal disease were not considered.

13.2.3. Sex
In 672 non-diabetics on HD from 1976 to 1982, Shapiro and Umen found a negative effect of male sex on survival [232]. However, when other risk factors were simultaneously taken into account, the sex influence disappeared. Presumably, the higher mortality in males, not confirmed elsewere, was to be attributed to the higher prevalence of cardiovascular disease in men. Table 11 shows the conflicting data related to the influence of gender on outcomes.

13.2.4. Race
White race has also been charged with having a negative effect on survival. This was true in the study of Wald [229], who also found greater risk for patients with a primary diagnoses of hypertension or diabetes, and that of Lunde [230] which related to white patients aged 65 years or more [230]. However this was not shown in other studies [202, 222].

13.2.5. Cardiac and vascular disease
In a study by Shapiro and Umen, cardiovascular, cerebrovascular and other vascular diseases accounted for 48% of all causes of death in HD patients [232]. The relative risk of death was still high but had decreased when age was taken into account. For CAPD patients, the negative effect of heart disease was confirmed by Khanna et al. [210]: two-year survival was 95% for patients without cardiac abnormalities before dialysis, 51% for patients with previous myocardial infarction and 62% for patients with previous angina. After 42 months, survival was 46% for patients with cardiomegaly compared to 88% for those without cardiac abnormalities. On the other hand, dialysis increases the risk for developing cardiovascular disease. Khanna et al. [210] showed that 40–59 year old CAPD patients had cumulative incidences of de novo ischemic heart disease of 8.8% and 15% one and two years after therapy, similar to the 12% and 18% found for HD patients [236] and greater than the 12.7% at six years in the non-uremic matched population of Framingham [237].

A strong negative effect of cardiovascular disease on patient survival has been assessed by the Cox hazard regression model [238] (Table 12).

13.2.6. Diabetes
Patient survival is worse for diabetics than for non diabetics [202, 213, 217, 233]. The relative risk of death for dialyzed diabetics versus non-diabetics range from 1.71 to 5.71 in different studies [165, 207, 212, 229, 230, 231, 234]. Survival of diabetics after four years was about 60% versus about 99% for non-diabetics, after correcting for the negative effects of other factors [213], and 60% versus 84% after two years in CAPD patients in the study of Khanna et al. [210]. This is contrary to the data of Chandran et al. [239] for CAPD patients, who found the same life-expectancy in diabetics as in non-diabetics, but the two groups were of different ages and this might have affected survival.

The risk of death for diabetics increased with age in the study of Capelli et al. [226] but not in that of Serkes et al. [202] where the risk increased for non-diabetics. According to Walker et al. [234], the greater risk of death on dialysis for diabetics than for non-diabetics has lessened with time: from 5.71 in 1977 to 3.92 in 1980 to 2.69 in 1983.

Different results for diabetic survivals on PD and HD have been reported, for diabetics 20–60 years old. Wolfe found a significantly higher relative risk of death on CAPD than on ICHD [229]. In the USRDS annual data Report 1991 [235], one-year survival was lower on CAPD that on HD (65.7% vs

Table 11. Effect of sex on patients survival in some studies.

Study	Sex	Relative risk	P
Burton and Walls [206]	Male	0.48	<0.001
Maiorca et al. [213]	Female	0.65	= 0.3465; NS
Wolfe et al. [229]	Male (all)	1.09	NS
	Male (diabetics)	1.27	P < 0.01
Serkes et al. [202]	Female Diabetic	0.55	< 0.03
	Female non-diabetic	0.70	NS
Maiorca et al. [165]	Female	1.13	NS
Lunde et al. [230]	Male	1.05	NS

69.6%), but the results were not adjusted for race or for diagnosis other than diabetes. The mean age was 53 for CAPD and 55 years for HD patients [235]. White patients with diabetic or hypertensive ESRD tended to survive better on CAPD up to age 40, and survive better on HD above that age. According to the USRDS study [235], these data represent general trends, because of the small sample size and the substantial random variability in the individual estimates. In a study by Zimmerman et al., CAPD was the best primary modality for patients not for transplantion [240]. Mejia et al. [209] found that survival of diabetics was no different on HD and CAPD for up to 12 months, after which it became higher on CAPD, being 81% vs 40% on HD [209]. In 298 diabetics of the Piedmont Dialysis and Transplantation Registry, Triolo et al. [241] found that one-year survival was 85% for patients younger than 50 years versus 63% for patients older than 60. Survival was better on CAPD, hemofiltration and bicarbonate HD (82%, 81% and 80%) than on acetate HD (66%).

Survival was no different for diabetics on CAPD and HD, in the studies of Maiorca and Serkes [165, 202, 213], after correcting for pretreatment differences.

The most frequent cause of death of diabetics on dialysis is cardiovascular disease: 55.8% of deaths versus 51.1% for non-diabetics in the EDTA report [242]. Infections caused 14.6% and 14.3% of deaths. In the study of Legrain et al. [208], the causes of death for HD and CAPD patients expressed as percentages of patients at risk, were: cerebrovascular + cardiac: 12% versus 15%. Arteritis + sepsis both 10%, Sepsis 9% versus 2%, stopping of treatment 6% versus 2%, other causes 6% vs 2%. Peritonitis was the cause of death in 10% of CAPD patients and hyperkalemia and malnutrition each caused 4% of deaths in the HD group.

The worse results obtained for diabetics are due to several factors, the main one being the presence of complications of diabetes at the start of dialysis. Peripheral vascular disease, hypertension and retinopathy are present in a large majority of diabetics and 10–20% of them are blind at the start of dialysis [209, 243, 244].

Some complications seem to progress differently on CAPD or HD. For example, diabetic retinopathy appeared to improve more frequently in patients on CAPD than in those on HD in the studies of Legrain et al. and Khauli et al. [208, 245], while its progression was the same on CAPD and HD in other studies [244, 246]. In spite of the different results these studies agree that control of hypertension is important for slowing the rate of progression of retinopathy [208, 246]. Legrain et al. reported data supporting better control of hypertension in CAPD than in HD patients and this might explain the better results in progression of retinopathy obtained on CAPD [208]. On the other hand, a major problem in diabetics on both HD and CAPD is hypotension [208], consequent to autonomic nervous system dysfunction due to both diabetes and uremia.

Peripheral vascular disease is one of the more frequent complications in diabetes and, in fact, 4–5% of diabetics on dialysis have amputations

Table 12. Effect of cardiovascular diseases on patients survival in some studies.

Study	Definition	Relative risk	P
Burton and Walls [206]	Ischemic heart disease	1.65	< 0.025
Gokal et al. [207]	Cerebrovascular and cardiovascular disease	3.36	< 0.001
Maiorca et al. [213]	Peripheral vascular	2.21	0.0227
Walker et al. [234]	Previous myocardial infaction (year 1983)	1.21	
Panarello et al. [231]	Heart failure	2.0	0.002
	Peripheral vascular	2.1	0.002
Serkes et al. [202]	Arteriosclerotic heart disease; non-diabetics	1.14	NS
	Arteriosclerotic heart disease; diabetics	1.93	< 0.02
	Peripheral vascular disease; non-diabetics	1.01	NS
	Peripheral vascular disease; diabetics	1.84	< 0.03
Gentil et al. [212]	Cardiovascular (CAPD + ICHD)	1.53	0.038
	Cardiovascular (CAPD)	0.77	NS
	Cardiovascular (ICHD)	2.06	0.003
Maiorca et al. [165]	Ischemic cardiopathy	2.02	0.0001
	Peripheral vascular disease	1.61	0.0103
	Cerebrovascular disease	1.60	0.0184

[240, 244]. Concerns have been raised about the possibility that CAPD worsens the course of peripheral vascular disease in diabetics as well as in non-diabetics [247]. However, the data for diabetics show similar incidences of amputation in both CAPD and HD patients [208, 245]. In HD patients, diabetic vascular disease negatively affects the duration of vascular access [208, 248]. On the other hand, the presence of an arteriovenous fistula was significantly associated with hand gangrene in the same limb [248]. Mejia et al. showed that CAPD and HD diabetics had about the same incidence of complications (4.6 ± 1.2 expisodes/patient-year versus 3.6 ± 0.7), but vascular access required interventions more often than peritoneal access (1.3 ± 0.5 episodes/patient-year versus 0.2 ± 0.1) [209].

13.2.7. Peritonitis

Patients with a higher incidence of peritonitis have worse survival [218]. In a study of 288 CAPD patients we found significant difference in death rates between patients with less than 0.5 and more than one peritonitis episode per year (Fig. 9) [218]. The peritonitis rate was not related to time on CAPD or on the age of patient at start of treatment. The influence of peritonitis rate on mortality was seen both when peritonitis alone was the cause of death and when all the causes of death were included. In the last analysis, the difference appeared even more impressive. In 8 of 9 patients who died from peritonitis, the etiology was fungal.

13.2.8. Malignancy

Malignancy imparts a high relative risk (from 2.06 to 6.09) for survival of uremics ($p < 0.004$ to < 0.0001) [165, 213, 231, 234]. It follows that correction for this factor is of paramount importance when comparing different methods.

13.2.9. Other patient-related factors.

Other factors have been shown in single studies to affect patient survival, some adversely, others favourably. Burton and Walls [228] found a negative effect of amyloidosis (RR = 8.26), acute presentation or "acute on chronic" presentation (RR = 2.73) and convulsions (RR = 3.17). Parenthood (RR = 0.64) had a positive effect. Walker et al. [234] and Wolfe et al. [229] found a significant positive effect of glomerulonephritis. Maiorca et al. [165] has reported a relative risk of 2.58 for multisystem diseases.

13.2.10. Effects of experience and technical improvement on patient survival

In dialysis patients, Walker et al. [234] found a progressive reduction in the relative risk of death over time, irrespective of the modality. For a patient 55 years old the reduction was calculated to be 50% in six years (from 1977 to 1983). The risk of death

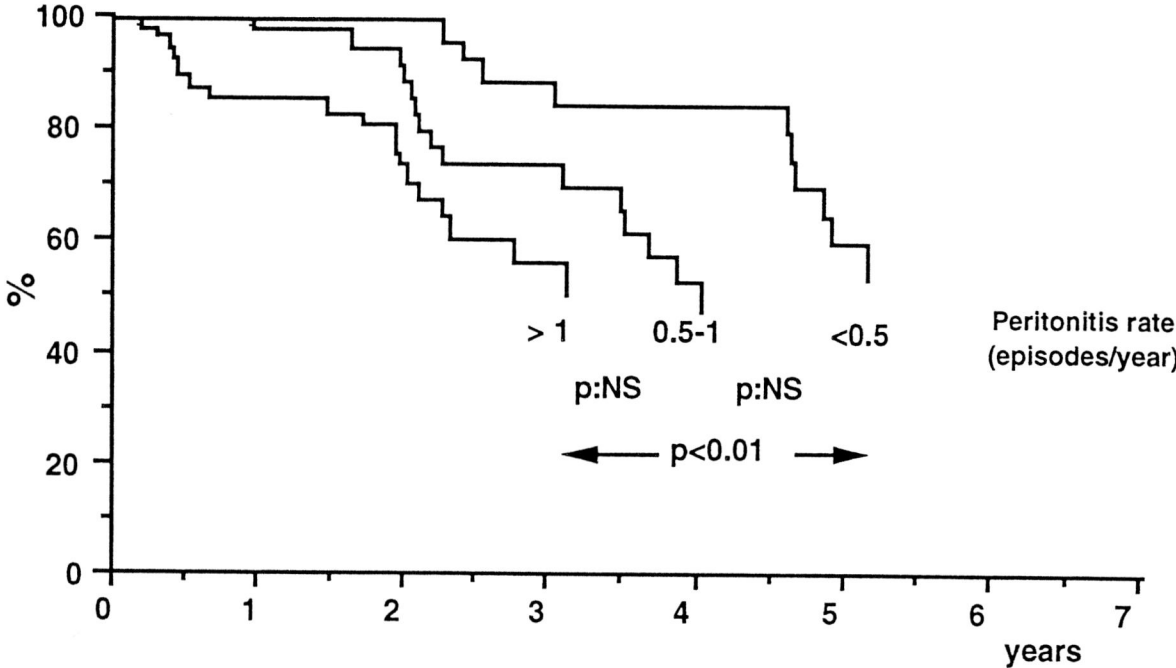

Figure 9. Patient survival according to peritonitis rate. (Reprinted from reference [218] by permission of Springer-Verlag).

related to modality, which was not different for CAPD and HD in 1980, dropped more on CAPD (from 1.00 to 0.27 in 1984) than in HD (from 1.00 to 0.77), after 4 years.

Wolfe et al. found an increase in the risk of dealth on dialysis by a factor of 1.04 per year after 1980 [229]. However, there were important differences between methods, perhaps due to the increased experience with CAPD and a change in patient mix. The risk decreased by 1% per year in the CAPD patients (P = NS) and increased significantly, by 6% per year ($p < 0.001$), in ICHD patients. In spite of these differences, death rates were not different on CAPD and ICHD at the start and at the end of the study.

Gentil et al. [212] found that for CAPD and ICHD considered together the relative risk of death lowered by 0.84 per year after 1984. Separately, the two modalities did not show any significant improvement with time.

13.3. Causes of death (Table 13)

Cardiovascular pathology is the main cause of death being responsible for 27 to 54% of deaths on CAPD and for 29 to 50% on HD [165, 206, 207, 213, 240, 249]. According to the EDTA Registry [250], cardiovascular deaths accounted for 51% of deaths on HD, for 55% of deaths on CAPD and for 36% in patients with transplants in 1990. These data do not take into account differences in age or other pretreatment risk factors. As for specific cardiovascular cause, deaths from myocardial infarction were 14% on HD, 20% on PD and 17% in transplanted patients; cardiac arrests were 13, 12 and 6%, cardiac failures 13, 12, and 6%, and cerebrovascular deaths 11, 11 and 7%. Total and cardiovascular mortality in dialysis was, in the EDTA Registry, higher in Northern than in Southern Europe.

The only unequivocal difference between CAPD and HD is in deaths for peritonitis. Among the causes of death on CAPD, sclerosing encapsulating peritonitis seems to be disappearing since chlorhexidine and acetate buffer were discontinued. In France, there has been a progressive reduction of this complication, with no deaths from this cause recorded since 1985 [250].

Dementia and cachexia have similar incidences in CAPD and HD patients [165]. Peritonitis is directly responsible for 7–10% of deaths on CAPD, i.e., for the death of 1.3–1.9% of all patients on this treatment [165, 206, 207, 213]. However, as said above, peritonitis, worsening the general condition of the patients, might be responsible for more deaths.

14. Conclusion

From the data in the literature, CAPD and on HD do not seem to differ greatly in respect to morbidity or mortality in dialysis patients. CAPD patients have a greater need for hospitalization, mainly due to peritonitis, the "case-mix" and also to lack of

Table 13. Causes of death in percent in some comparative multicenter studies.

	Gokal et al. [207]		Gentil et al. [212]		Maiorca et al. [165]	
	CAPD	HD	CAPD	ICHD	CAPD	HD
Patients at risk	610	329	272	842	480	373
Patients dead	77	44	48	107	119	59
Cause of death in percent						
Cardio/cerebrovascular	48	29	44	42	54	50
Septicaemia/Infections ≠ peritonitis	1	14	8	8	6	3
Peritonitis	10	4	13	1	7	–
Treatment stopped	12	11	–	–	–	–
Malignant disorder	8	18	10	7	7	17
Haemorrhage	6	9	–	–	–	–
Social	–	–	4	10	–	–
Dementia	–	–	–	–	4	2
Cachexia	–	–	–	–	16	13
Bone marrow depression					–	3
Other	14	13			4	10
Undetermined			8	22	2	–

experience. HD has a greater incidence of intra- and peridialytic cardiovascular instability and arrhythmia, and greater ECV espansion in the interdialytic period, which can have adverse effects on cardiovascular function, mainly in cardiac patients and in the elderly. Hypertension is corrected equally well. Hormonal and immunological conditions are not different on CAPD and HD, although they seem to be slightly better preserved by CAPD. As for neuropathy, osteodystrophy, uremic amyloidosis, malnutrition, there are differences between the two methods, but neither of them seems to control these complications better than the other. Diabetes negatively affects survival in both CAPD and HD, and no significant differences in the evolution of diabetes complications have come out, so far.

Method survival is worse for CAPD, due to peritonitis, but there is also an influence of patient selection and a "center" effect. The higher drop-out rate did not artefactually influence the calculation of survival.

On CAPD, the high frequency of peritonitis increases the risk of death, so it is very important to reduce the peritonitis rate, as Y-connectors and double bags have been demonstrated to do. Sclerosing encapsulating peritonitis is now disappearing. All things considered, patient survival does not differ for the two methods, but for older patients it seems to be better on CAPD.

References

1. Wizemann V, Timio M, Alpert M, Kramer W. Options in dialysis therapy: significance of cardiovascular findings. Kidney Int 1993; 43 (suppl 40): S85–91.
2. Levy D, Anderson K, Savage D, Balkus S, Kannel W, Castelli W. Echocardiographically detected left ventricular hypertrophy: prevalence and risk factors. The Framingham Hearth Study. Ann Intern Med 1988; 108: 7–13.
3. Eisenberg M, Prichard S, Barre P, Patton R, Hutchinson T, Sniderman A. Left ventricular hypertrophy in end-stage renal disease on peritoneal dialysis. Am J Cardiol 1987; 60: 418–9.
4. Silberberg DS, Barre P, Prichard S, Sniderman AD. Left ventricular hypertrophy: an independent determinant of survival in end-stage renal failure. Kidney Int 1989; 36: 286–90.
5. Harnett JD, Parfrey PS, Griffiths SM, Gault MH, Barre P, Bultmann RD. Left Ventricular hypertrophy in end-stage renal disease. Nephron 1988; 48: 107–15.
6. Kamer W, Hüting J, Wizemann V. Left ventricular hypertrophy in end-stage renal failure: functional findings and therapeutical implications. In: Timio M, Wizemann V (eds), Cardionephrology. Wichtig Editore, Milano 1991; pp 97–100.
7. Levy D, Anderson KM, Savage DD, Balkus SA, Kannel WB, Castelli WP. Risk of ventricular arrhythmias in left ventricular hypertrophy. The Framingham Heart Study. Am J Cardiol 1987; 60: 560–5.
8. Alpert MA, Van Stone J, Twardwoski ZJ et al. Comparative cardiac effects of hemodialysis and continuous ambulatory peritoneal dialysis. Clin Cardiol 1986; 9: 52–60.
9. Leenen FHH, Smith DL, Khanna R, Oreopoulos DG. Changes in left ventricular hypertrophy and function in hypertensive patients started on continuous ambulatory peritoneal dialysis. Am Heart J 1985; 10: 102–5.
10. Timio M, Ronconi M, Lori G, Venanzi S, Pede S. Effetto differenziato dell'emodialisi e della dialisi peritoneale ambulatoriale continua (CAPD) sull'ipertrofia asimmetrica settale dei pazienti uremici. G Ital Nefrol 1985: 4: 157–60.
11. Deligiannis A, Paschalidou E, Sakellariou G et al. Changes in left ventricular anatomy during haemodialysis, continuous ambulatory peritoneal dialysis and after renal transplantation. Proc Eur Dial Transpl Ass 1984; 21: 185–9.
12. Amann K, Rambausek M, Mall G, Ritz E. Structural causes of cardiac dysfunction in uremia. Contribution to Nephrology 1993. (in press).
13. Maiorca R, Cancarini G, Brunori G et al. CAPD in the elderly. Perit Dial Internat 1993; 13 (suppl 2): S165–71.
14. Malle G, Rambausek M, Neumeister A, Kollmar S, Vetterlein F, Ritz E. Myocardial interstitial fibrosis in experimental uremia. Implications for cardiac compliance. Kidney Int 1988; 33: 804–11.
15. Malle G, Huther W, Schneider J, Lundin P, Ritz E. Diffuse intermyocardiocytic fibrosis in uremic patients. Nephrol Dial Transplant 1990, 5: 39–44.
16. Ritz E, Rambausek M, Mall G, Ruffmann K, Mandelbaum A. Cardiac changes in uremia and their possible relationship to cardiovascular instability on dialysis. Nephrol Dial Transplant 1990; Supplement 1: 93–7.
17. Report of the National CAPD Registry of the National Institutes of Health, 1987.
18. Ramos J, Gokal R, Siampoulos K, Ward MK, Wilkinson R, Kerr DNs. CAPD: three year experience. Q J Med 1983; 52: 165–86.
19. Young MA, Nolph KD, Dulton S, Prowant B. Anti-hypertensive drug requirements in continuous ambulatory peritoneal dialysis. Perit Dial Bull 1974; 4: 85–8.
20. Glasson PH, Favre H, Vallotton MB. Response of blood pressure and the renin-angiotension-aldosterone system to chronic ambulatory peritoneal dialysis in hypertensive end-stage renal failure. Clin Sci 1982; 63: 207s.
21. Timio M. Clinica cardiologica nell'uremia. Ruolo terepeutico della dialisi peritoneale. Wichtig Editore, Milano 1990; pp 73–8.
22. Zuber M, Steinmann E, Huser B, Ritz R, Thiel G,

Brunner F. Incidence of arrhythmias and myocardial ischaemia during haemodialysis and hemofiltration. Nephrol Dial Transplant 1989; 4: 632–4.
23. Peer G, Korzets A, Hochhauzer E, Eschchar Y, Blum M, Aviram A. Cardiac arrhythmia during continuous ambulatory peritoneal dialysis. Nephron 1987; 45: 192–5.
24. Wu G and the University of Toronto Collaborative Dialysis Group. Cardiovascular deaths among CAPD patients. Perit Dial Bull 1983; 3 (suppl): S23–6.
25. Rostand SG, Gretes JC, Kirk KA, Rutsky EA, Andreoli TE. Ischemic heart disease in patients with uremia undergoing maintenance hemodialysis. Kidney Int 1979; 16: 600–11.
26. Maiorca R. Cardiovascular problems in the choice of dialysis therapy for the elderly. Cardionephrological meeting, Assisi 1993. Contribution to Nephrology 1993 (in press).
27. Charytan C, Spinowitz BS, Galler M. A comparative study of continuous ambulatory peritoneal dialysis and center hemodialysis. Arch Intern Med 1986: 146: 1138–43.
28. Henderson LW: Symptomatic hypotension during hemodialysis. Kidney Int 1980: 17: 571–6.
29. Rosa AA, Fryd DS, Kyellstrand CM. Dialysis symptoms and stabilization in long-term dialysis. Arch Intern Med 1980: 140: 804–7.
30. Degoulet P, Reach I, Di Giulio S, De Vries C, Rouby JJ, Aime F, Volanthen M. Epidemiology of dialysis-induced hypotension. Proc Eur Dial Transplant Assoc 1981; 18: 133–8.
31. Ronco C, Fabris A, Chiaramonte S, De Dominicis E et al. Comparison of four different short dialysis techniques. Internat J Artif Organs 1988; 11: 169–74.
32. De Vires PMJM, Othof CG, Solf A et al. Fluid balance during haemodialysis and hemofiltration: the effect of dialysate sodium and a variable ultrafiltration rate. Nephrol Dial Transplant 1991; 6: 257–63.
33. Zucchelli P, Santoro A, Ferrari G, Spongano M. Acetate-free biofiltration: hemodiafiltration with base-free dialysate. Blood Purif 1990; 8: 14–22.
34. Maiorca R, Cancarini GC, Brunori G, Camerini C, Manili L. Morbidity and mortality of CAPD and hemodialysis. Kidney Internat 1993; 43 (suppl. 40): S4–15.
35. Cornélis F, Bardin T, Zingraff J, Drüeke T. Beta-2-microglobulin amyloidosis and peritoneal dialysis. In: Gejyo F, Brancaccio D, Bordin T (eds), Dialysis amyloidosis. Wichtig Editore, Milano 1989; pp 119–22.
36. Tielemans C, Dratwa M, Bergmann P et al. Continuous ambulatory peritoneal dialysis vs hemodialysis: a lesser risk of amyloidosis. Nephrol Dial Transplant 1988: 3: 291–4.
37. La Greca G. L'amiloidosi da β2-microglobulina. In: Saporiti E, Marchini P (eds), Beta2microglobulina: realtà e fantasie. Aula Medica, Roma 1990; 3: 1–6.
38. Catizone L. Cocchi R, Dalla Rovere S, Viglietta G, Fusaroli M, Zucchelli P. Beta-2-microglobulina e dialisi peritoneale ambulatoriale continua. In: Saporiti E, Marchini P (eds), Beta2microglobulina: realtà e fantasie, Aula Medica 1990; 3: 47–56.
39. Shaldon S, Dinarello CA, Wyler DJ. Induction of Interleukin-1 during CAPD. Contrib Nephrol 1987; 57: 207–12.
40. Carozzi S, Nasioni MG, Schelotto C et al. Bacterial peritonitis and beta-2 microglobulin (β2M) production by peritoneal macrophages (PMO) in CAPD patients. Adv Perit Dial 1990; 6: 106–9.
41. Rottembourg J, Allouache M, Musset L, Jacobs C. Beta2 microglobulin kinetics in dialysed patients: haemodialysis vs continuous ambulatory peritoneal dialysis. Nephrol Dial Transplant 1987; 2: 448–9.
42. Di Raimondo CR, McCarley P, Stone WJ. Beta-2 microglobulin in peritoneal dialysis patients: serum levels and peritoneal clearance. Perit Dial Int 1988; 8: 43–7.
43. Mistry CD, O'Donoghue DJ, Nelson S, Gokal R, Ballardie FW. Kinetic and clinical studies of β2-microglobulin in continuous ambulatory peritoneal dialysis: influence of renal and enhanced peritoneal clearance using glucose polymer. Nephrol Dial Transplant 1990; 5: 513–9.
44. Ballardie FW, Ferr DNS, Tennent G, Pepys MB. Haemodialysis versus CAPD: equal risk of amyloidosis? Lancet 1986; 1: 795–6.
45. Maiorca R. Cancarini GC, Camerini C et al. Is CAPD competitive with hemodialysis for long-term treatment of uraemic patients. Nephrol Dial Transplant 1989; 4: 244–53.
46. Catizone L, Cocchi R, Fusaroli M, Zucchelli P. Studio del comportamento della Beta 2-microglobulina in CAPD: confronto con l'emodialisi. In: Passione A, Procaccini DA, Querques M (eds), Dialisi Peritoneale. Wichtig Editore, Milano 1991: pp 489–94.
47. Canaud B, Assounga A, Flarier JL, Slingeneyer A et al. β-2 microglobulin serum levels in maintenance dialysis. What does it mean? ASAIO Trans 1988; 34: 23–9.
48. Scalamogana A, Imbasciati E, De Vecchi A et al. Beta-2 Microglobulin in patients on peritoneal dialysis and hemodialysis. Perit Dial Int 1989; 9: 37–40.
49. Lysaght MJ, Pollock CA, Moran JE, Ibels LS, Farrel PC. Beta-2-microglobulin removal during continuous ambulatory peritoneal dialysis (CAPD). Perit Dial Int 1989; 9: 29–35.
50. Acchiardo S, Kraus AP Jr, Jennings BR. Beta-2 microglobulin levels in patients with renal insufficiency. Am J kidney Dis 1989; 13: 70–4.
51. Blumberg A, Burgi W. Bahaviour of beta 2-microglobulin in patients with chronic renal failure undergoing hemodialysis, hemodiafiltration and continuous ambulatory peritoneal dialysis. Clin Nephrol 1987; 27: 245–9.
52. van Ypersele de Strihou C, Jadul M, Malghemm J, Maldague B, Jamart J, the working party on dialysis amyloidosis. Effect of dialysis membrane and patient's age on signs of dialysis related amyloidosis. Kidney Int 1991; 39: 1012–9.

53. Benz RL, Siegfried JW, Tehen BP. Carpal tunnel syndrome in dialysis patients: comparison between continuous ambulatory peritoneal dialysis and hemodialysis populations. Am J Kidney Dis 1988; 11: 473–6.
54. Keane WF, Raij LR. Host defenses and infectious complications in maintenance hemodialysis patients. In: Drukker W, Parsons FM, Maher JF (eds), Replacement of kidney function by dialysis. 2nd revised edition. Martinus Nijhoff, Boston 1983; pp 646–58.
55. Van der Meer JWM. Defects in host-defense mechanism. In: Rubin RH, Young LS (eds), Clinical approach to infection in the compromised host. 2nd ed. Plenum Medical Book, New York 1988; pp 41–73.
56. Zucchelli P, Perrari G, Catizone L, Beltrandi E. Clinical importance of immunological disturbances in hemodialysis and CAPD patients. In: La Greca G, Chiaramonte S, Fabris A, Feriani M, Ronco C (eds), Peritoneal Dialysis. Wichtig Editore, Milano 1988; pp 101–6.
57. Schollemeyer P, Bozkurt F. The immune status of the uremic patients: hemodialysis versus CAPD. Clin Nephrol 1988; 30 (suppl 1): S37–40.
58. Tolkoff-Rubin NE, Rubin RH. Uremia and host defenses. New Engl J Med 1990; 322: 770–2.
59. Nisbeth U, Hällgren R, Eriksson Ö, Danielson BG. Endotoxemia in chronic renal failure. Nephron 1987; 45: 93–7.
60. Bertazzoni EM, Panzetta G. Effects of different forms of dialytic treatment on serum antibacterial activity in patients with chronic renal failure. Nephron 1984; 36: 224–9.
61. Giacchino F, Quarello F, Pellerey M, Piccoli G. Continuous ambulatory peritoneal dialysis improves immunodeficiency in uremic patients. Nephron 1983; 35: 208–10.
62. Huttenen K, Lampainen E, Silvennoinen-Kassinen S, Tiilikanan A. The neutrophil function of uremic patients treated by hemodialysis or CAPD. Scand J Urol Nephrol 1984; 18: 167–72.
63. Giacchino F, Pozzato M, Piccoli G. Evaluation of the influence of peritoneal dialysis on cellular immunity by the E-rosette inhibition test. Artif Organs 1984; 8: 156–60.
64. Collart F, Tielemans C, Dratwa M, Schandene L, Wybran J, Dupont E. Hemodialysis, continuous ambulatory peritoneal dialysis and cellular immunity. Proc Eur Dial Transplant Ass 1983; 20: 190–4.
65. Guillou PJ, Will EJ, Davison AM, Giles GR. CAPD-a risk factor in renal transplantation? Br J Surg 1984; 71: 878–80.
66. Giacchino F, Alloatti S, Quarello F Coppo R, Pellerey M, Piccoli G. The influence of peritoneal dialysis on cellular immunity. Perit Dial Bull 1982; 2: 165–8.
67. Giangrande A, Cantù P, Limido A, de Francesco D, Malacrida V. Continuous ambulatory peritoneal dialysis and cellular immunity. Proc Eur Dial Transplant Ass 1982; 19: 372–9.
68. Gerez L, Madar L, Shkolnik T, Kristal B et al. Regulation of interleukin-2 and interferon-gamma gene expression in renal failure. Kidney Int 1991; 40: 266–72.
69. Langhof E, Ladefoged J. Improved lymphocyte transformation in vitro of patients on continuous ambulatory peritoneal dialysis. Proc Eur Dial Transplant Ass 1983; 20: 230–5.
70. Donnelly PK, Shenton BK, Lennard TWJ, Proud G, Taylor RMR. CAPD and renal transplantation. Br J Surg 1985; 72: 819–21.
71. Rumpf KW, Seubert S, Seubert A et al. Association of ethylene-oxide-induced IgE antibodies with symptoms in dialysis patients. Lancet 1985; 2: 1385–7.
72. Marshall C, Shimizu A, Smith EKM, Dolovich J. Ethylene oxide allergy in a dialysis center: prevalence in hemodialysis and peritoneal dialysis populations. Clin Nephrol 1984; 21: 346–9.
73. Kim D, Blair G, Wu G, Ayiomamitis A, Oreopoulos DG. Electrophysiological studies of nerve function in patients on CAPD over long periods. Perit Dial Bull 1985; 5: 45–8.
74. Sunderrajan S, Nolph KD. Longitudinal study of nerve conduction velocities during continuous ambulatory peritoneal dialysis. Perit Dial Bull 1985; 5: 48–50.
75. Lindholm B, Tegner R. Deterioration of peripheral nerve function during continuous ambulatory peritoneal dialysis. Perit Dial Bull 1986; 6: 20–7.
76. Lindholm B, Bergstrom J. Nutritional aspects of CAPD. In: Gokal R (ed), Continuous ambulatory peritoneal dialysis. Churchill Livingstone, Edinburgh 1986; pp 228–64.
77. Tegner R, Lindholm B. Uremic polyneuropathy: different effects of hemodialysis and continuous ambulatory peritoneal dialysis. Acta Med Scand 1985; 218: 409–16.
78. Albertazzi A, Di Paolo B, Amoroso L. Central and peripheral nervous system in dialysis patients: CAPD vs HD. In: La Greca G, Chiaramonte S, Fabris A, Feriani M, Ronco C (eds), Peritoneal Dialysis. Wichtig Editore, Milano 1988; pp 281–6.
79. Mallamaci F, Zoccali C, Ciccarelli M, Briggs JD. Autonomic function in uremic patients treated by hemodialysis or CAPD and in transplant patients. Clin Nephrol 1986; 25: 175–80.
80. Camerini C, Bonfioli F, Movilli E et al. Potenziali evocati uditivi del tronco encefalico (ABR: auditory brainstem responses): confronto tra pazienti in emodialisi ed in dialisi peritoneale ambulatoriale continua. Nefrologia Dialisi Trapianto 1988. Milano: Wichtig Editore, 1988: 551–2.
81. Marsh JT, Brown WS, Wolcott D, Landsverk J, Nissenson AR. Electrophysiological indices of CNS function in hemodialysis and CAPD. Kidney Int 1986; 30: 957–63.
82. Wolcott DL, Wellisch DK, Marsh JT, Schaeffer J, Landsverk J, Nissenson AR. Relationship of dialysis modality and other factors to cognitive function in chronic dialysis patients. Am J Kidney Dis 1988; 12: 275–84.
83. Garcia-Maldonado M, Williams C, Smith ZM.

Mental performance in CAPD. Adv Perit Dial 1991; 7: 105–7.
84. Glenn GM, Astley SJ, Watkins SL. Dialysis-associated seizures in children and adolescents. Pediatr Nephrol 1992; 6: 182–6.
85. Semple GC, Beastal GH, Henderson IS, Thomson JA, Kennedy AC. Thyroid funtion and continuous ambularory peritoneal dialysis. Nephron 1982; 32: 239–52.
86. Giordano C, De Santo NG, Carella C et al. Thyroidal status in uremia -Effects of hemodialysis and CAPD. Intern J Artif Org 1982; 5: 339–44.
87. Pagliacci MC, Pelicci G, Grignani F et al. Thyroid function tests in patients undergoing maintenance dialysis: characterization of the 'low-T4 syndrome' in subjects on regular hemodialysis and continuous ambulatory peritoneal dialysis. Nephron 1987; 46: 225–30.
88. Kerr DJ, Singh VK, Tsakiris D, McConnell KN, Junor BJR, Alexander WD. Serum and peritoneal Dialysate Thyroid Hormone levels in patients in Continuous Ambulatory Peritoneal Dialysis. Nephron 1986, 43: 164–8.
89. Thynsen B Gatz M, Freeman M, Alpert BE, Charytan C. Serum thyroid hormone levels in patients on continuous ambulatory peritoneal dialysis and regular hemodialysis. Nephron 1983; 33: 49–52.
90. Verger MF, Verger C, Mercier-Hatt D, Perrone F. Diminution de la triiodothyronine et de sa forme inverse sous l'effet de l'épuration extra-rénale: role de l'apport glucidique. La Presse Médicale 1984; 13: 1613–6.
91. Ross RJ, Goodwin FJ, Houghton BJ, Boucher BJ. Alteration of pituitary-thyroid function in patients with chronic renal failure treated by hemodialysis or continuous ambulatory peritoneal dialysis. Ann Clin Biochem 1985; 22: 156–60.
92. Boero R, Quarello F, Isais GC et al. Valutazione dinamica della funzionalità ipotalamo-ipofisaria nei pazienti in CAPD: confronto con l'emodialisi. In: Giordano D, De Santo NG (eds), Dialisi peritoneale. Atti del I Convegno Nazionale. Wichtig Editore, Milano 1984; pp 259–64.
93. Giordano C, De Santo NG, Carella C et al. TSH response to TRH in hemodialysis and CAPD patients. Int J Artif Org 1984; 7: 7–10.
94. Inaba M, Nishizawa Y, Nishitani H et al. Concentrations of thyroxine-binding globulin in sera and peritoneal dialysates in patients on chronic peritoneal ambulatory dialysis. Nephron 1986; 42: 58–61.
95. Kaptein EM, MacIntyre SS, Weiner JM, Spencer CA, Nicoloff JT. Fre thyroxine estimates in nonthyroidal illness: comparison of eigth methods. J Clin Endoc Metab 1981; 52: 1073–7.
96. Chopra IJ, Van Herle AJ, Chau Teco NG, Nguyen AH. Serum free thyroxine in thyroidal and nonthyroidal illness: a comparison of measurements by radioimmunoassay, equilibrium dialysis, and free thyroxine index. J Clin Endoc Metab 1980; 51: 135–43.
97. Wartofsky L, Burman KD. Alteration in thyroid functin in patients with systemic illness: the 'euthyroid sick syndrome'. Endocr Rev 1982; 3: 164–217.
98. De Marchi S, Cecchin E. Alterations of circulating thyroid homrone levels in dialysis patients: another piece to solve the puzzle. Nephron (letter) 1987; 46: 400–1.
99. Spaulding SW, Chopra IJ, Sherwin RS, Lyall SS. Effect of caloric restriction and dietary composition on serum T3 and rT3 in man. J Clin Endocr Metab 1976; 42: 197–200.
100. Princi P, Pitrone F, Princi P Jr et al. La scintigrafia della tiroide nella insufficienza renale cronica in HD ed in CAPD e IPD. In: Giordano C, De Santo NG (eds), Dialisis Peritoneale. Atti del II Convegno Nazionale. Wichtig Editore, Milano 1984; pp 561–3.
101. Walker F, Form G, Khanna R, Digenis GE, Oreopoulos DG. Study of thyroid function in patients on CAPD. Abstracts of the American Society of Nephrology. Kidney Int 1983; 23: 164.
102. Lim VS, Flanigan MJ, Zavala DC and Freeman RM. Protective adaptation of low serum triiodothyronine in patients with chronic renal failure. Kidney Int 1985; 28: 541–9.
103. Rodger RSE, Letcher K, Genner D, Dewar J, War MK and Kerr DNS. Sexual disfunction in patients treated by CAPD. In: Maher JF, Winchester JF (eds), Frontiers in Peritoneal Dialysis. Field, Rich and Associates, New York 1986; pp 512–5.
104. Biasioli S, Feriani M, Chiaramonte S et al. Hormonal status. In: La Greca G, Chiaramonte S, Fabris A, Feriani M, Ronco C (eds), Peritoneal Dialysis. Wichtig Editore, Milano 1988; pp 247–52.
105. Hou HS, Grossman S, Molitch ME. Hyperprolactinemia in patients with renal insufficiency and chronic renal failure requiring hemodialysis or chronic ambulatory peritoneal dialysis. Am J Kidney Dis 1986; 6: 245–9.
106. Kokot F, Wiecek A. Endocrine changes in chronic dialysis patients. In: Maher JF (ed), Replacement of renal function by dialysis. IIIrd edition. Kluwer Academic publishers, Dordrecht 1989; pp 953–71.
107. Galler M, Spinowitz B, Charytan C, Kabadi M, Freeman R. Reproductive function in dialysis patients: CAPD vs Hemodialysis. Perit Dial Bull 1983; 3: S30–2.
108. Rodger RSC, Dewar JH, Turner SJ, Watson MJ, Ward MK. Anterior pituitary dysfunction in patients with chronic renal failure treated by hemodialysis or continuous ambulatory peritoneal dialysis. Nephron 1986; 43: 169–72.
109. Bessarione D, Perfumo F, Giusti M et al. Growth hormone response to growth hormone-releasing hormone in normal and uraemic children. Comparison with hypoglycaemia following insulin administration. Acta Endocrinologica (Copenh) 1987; 114; 5–11.
110. Williams GH, Bailey GL, Lampers CL et al. Studies on the metabolism of aldosterone in chronic renal failure and anephric man. Kidney Int 1973; 4: 280–5.

111. Mitra S, Genuth SM, Berman LB, Vertes V. Aldosterone secretion in anephric patients. New Engl J Med 1972: 286: 61.
112. Siamopoulos KC, Dardamanis M, Kyriaki D, Pappas M, Sferopoulos G, Alevisou V. Pituitary adrenal responsiveness to corticotropin-releasing hormore in chronic uremic patients. Perit Dial Int 1990; 10: 153–6.
113. Zager PG, Spalding CT, Frey HJ, Brittenhom ME. Low dose adrenocorticotropin infusion in continuous ambulatory peritoneal dialysis patients. J Clin Endocr Metab 1985; 61: 1205–10.
114. Zager PG, Frey HJ, Spalding CT, Nevarez M. Removal of adrenocorticoids during CAPD and hemodialysis. Adv Perit Dial 1986: 70–2.
115. Zager PG, Frey HG, Gerdes BG. Plasma concentrations od 18-hydroxycorticosterone and aldosterone in continuous ambulatory peritoneal dialysis and hemodialysis patients. Am J Kidney Dis 1983; 3: 213–8.
116. Abbott EC, Gornell AG, Sutherland DJA et al. The influence of heparin-like compound on hypertension, electrolytes. Can Med Assoc J 1966; 94: 1155–64.
117. Kumar DN, Zabetakis PM, Gardenswartz MH, Gleim GW, Agrawal M, Michelis MF. Elevated renin activity associated with increased cathecholamines in chronic ambulatory peritoneal dialysis. Abstract of the III International Symposium on Peritoneal Dialysis. Perit Dial Bull 1984; 4: S34.
118. Ryoichi A, Osamu M, Shozo M, Naoki Y. Plasma levels of human natrial natriuretic factor in patients treated by hemodialysis and continuous ambulatory peritoı eal dialysis. Nephron 1988; 50: 225–8.
119. Gokal R, Ramos JM, Ellis HA, Parkinson I et al. Histological renal osteodystrophy, and 25 hydroxycholecalciferol and aluminium levels in patients on continuous ambulatory peritoneal dialysis. Kidney Int 1983; 23: 15–21.
120. Kurtz SB, McCarthy JT, Kumar R. Hypercalcemia in continuous ambulatory peritoneal dialysis (CAPD) patients: observations on parameters of calcium metabolism. In: Gahl GM, Kessel M, Nolph KD (eds), Advances in Peritoneal Dialysis. Excerpta Medica, Amsterdam 1981; pp 467–72.
121. Zucchelli P, Catizone L, Casanova S, Fusaroli M, Fabbri L, Ferrari G. Renal osteodystrophy in CAPD patients. Miner Electrolyte Metab 1984; 10: 326–32.
122. Shusterman NH, Wasserstein AG, Morrison G, Audet P, Fallon MD, Kaplan F. Controlled study of renal osteodystrophy in patients undergoing dialysis. Improved response to continuous ambulatory peritoneal dialyis compared to hemodialysis. Am J Med 1987; 82: 1148–56.
123. Calderaro V, Oreopoulos DG, Meema HE et al. The evolution of renal osteodystrophy in patients undergoing continuous ambulatory peritoneal dialysis. Proc Eur Dial Transplant Ass 1980; 17: 533–41.
124. Tielemans C, Aubry C, Dratwa M. The effects of continuous ambulatory peritoneal dialysis on renal osteodystrophy. In: Gahl GM, Kessel M, Nolph KD (eds), Advances in peritoneal dialysis: proceedings of the 2nd symposium on peritoneal dialysis. Amsterdam: Excerpta Medica, 1981: 455–60.
125. El Shahat Y, Issad B, Jacobs C et al. Evolution of renal osteodystrophy in patients treated with CAPD. Mineral Electrolyte Metab 1981; 6: 265.
126. Teitelbaum S, Fallon MD, Gearing BK, Dougan CS, Delmez JA. The effects of CAPD on bone histomorphology (abstract). Kidney Int 1982; 21: 180.
127. Digenis G, Khanna R, Pierrators A et al. Renal osteodistrophy in patients maintained on CAPD for more than three years. Perit Dial Bull 1983; 3: 81–6.
128. Llach F. Metabolic bone disease in the CAPD patient. Perit Dial Bull 1983; 3 (suppl): S24–7.
129. Buccianti G, Bianchi ML, Valenti G. Progress of renal osteodystrophy during continuous ambulatory peritoneal dialysis. Clin Nephrol 1984; 22: 279–83.
130. Lo Schiavo C, Fabris A, Adami S et al. Effects of continuous ambulatory peritoneal dialysis on renal osteodystrophy. Perit Dial Bull 1985; 5: 53–5.
131. Delmez JA, Fallon MD, Bergfeld MA, Gearing BK, Dougan CS, Teitelbaum SL. Continuos ambulatory peritoneal dialysis and bone. Kidney Internat 1986: 30: 379–84.
132. Rahman R, Heaton A, Goodship THJ. Renal osteodystrophy in patients on continuous ambulatory peritoneal dialysis: a five-year study. Perit Dial Bull 1987: 7: 20–6.
133. Giangrande A, Ballanti P, Castiglioni A et al. L'osteodistrofia renale nel paziente uremico in CAPD. Studio prospettico a 5 anni. In: Passione A, Procaccini DA, Querques M (eds), Dialisi Peritoneale. Atti del VI Congresso nazionale, 1991. Wichtig Editore, Milano 1991: 149–54.
134. Hercz G, Pei Y, Manuel A et al. Aplastic osteodistrophy without aluminium in dialysis patients (abstract). Kidney Int 1990; 37: 449.
135. Joffe P, Podenphant J, Heaf JG. Bone histology in CAPD patients: a comparison with hemodialysis and conservatively treated chronic uremics. Adv Perit Dial 1989; 5: 171–76.
136. Pei Y, Horcz G, Greenwood C et al. Non-invasive prediction of aluminium bone disease in hemo- and peritoneal dialysis patients; Kidney Int 1992; 41: 1374–82.
137. Hutchison AJ, Whitehouse RW, Boulton HF et al. Characteristics and natural history of adynamic bone in CAPD (abstract). Nephrol Dial Transplant 1992; 7: 759–60.
138. Smith D, DeFronzo RA. Insulin resistance in uremia mediated by postbinding defects. Kidney Int 1982; 22: 54–62.
139. Lindholm B, Karlander SG. Glucose tolerance in patients undergoing continuous ambulatory peritoneal dialysis. Acta Medica Scand 1986; 220: 477–83.
140. Armstrong VW, Creutzfeldt W, Ebert R, Fuchs C, Hilgers R, Scheler F. Effect of dialysate glucose

load on plasma glucose and glucoregolatory hormones in CAPD patients. Nephron 1985; 39: 141–5.
141. Lameire N, Matthys D, Matthys E, Beheydt. Effects of long-term CAPD on carbohydrate and lipid metabolism. Clin Nephrol 1988; 30 (suppl 1): S53–8.
142. Heaton A, Johnston DG, Haigh JW, Ward MK, Alberti KGMM, Kerr DNS. Twenty-four hour hormonal and metabolic profiles in uraemic patients before and during treatment with continuous ambulatory peritoneal dialysis. Clin Sci 1985; 69: 449–57.
143. Maiorca R, Panzetta G, Broccoli R, Rigosa C, Valentini U, Sandrini S. Glucose metabolism in CAPD: intravenous glucose load and C-peptide, insulin and glucagone variations. Int J Nephrol Urol Androl 1981; 1 (suppl): 66–8.
144. Wideroe TE, Smeby LC, Myking OL. Plasma concentrations and transperitoneal transport of native insulin and C-peptide in patients on continuous ambulatory peritoneal dialysis. Kidney Int 1984, 25: 82–7.
145. Wideroe Te, Smeby LC, Myking OL, Wessel-Aas T. Glucose, insulin and C-peptide kinetics during continuous ambulatory peritoneal dialysis. Proc Eur Dial Transpl Assoc 1983, 20: 195–200.
146. Crapo PH, Reaven GM, Olefsky JM. Ormonal and substrate responses to a standard meal in normal and hypertriglyceridemic subjects. Metabolism 1981; 30: 231–4.
147. Kajinuma H, Tanabashi S, Ishiwata K et al. Symposium on proinsulin, Insulin and C-peptide. Tokushima, Japan 1978. International Congress Series 486. Excerpta Medica, Amsterdam 1978: 183.
148. Heaton A, Johnston DG, Burrin JM et al. Carbohydrate and lipid metabolism during continuous ambulatory peritoneal dialysis (CAPD): the effect of a sigle dialysis cycle. Clin Sci 1983; 65: 539–45.
149. Von Baeyer H, Gahl GM, Riedinger H et al. Adaptation of CAPD patients to the continuous peritoneal energy uptake. Kidney Int 1983; 23: 29–34.
150. Lindholm B, Karlander SG. Glucose tolerance in patients on continuous ambulatory peritoneal dialysis (CAPD). Trans Am Soc Artif Intern Organs 1981; 27: 58–60.
151. Chanz MK, Varghese Z, Persaud JW, Baillod RA, Moorhead JF. Hyperlipidemia in patients on maintenance hemo- and peritoneal dialysis: the relative pathogenetic role of triglycerides production and triglyceride removal. Clin Nephrol 1982; 17: 183–90.
152. Cancarini GC, Brasa S, Camerini C, Maiorca R. I problemi della CAPD: quali progressi dopo 4 anni di esperienze. In: Giordano C, De Santo NG (eds), Dialisi peritoneale, Atti del II Convegno Nazionale. Wichtig Editore, Milano 1984; pp 77–82.
153. Breckenridge WC, Roncari DAK, Khanna R, Oreopoulos DG. The influence of continuous ambulatory peritoneal dialysis on plasma lipoproteins. Atherosclerosis 1982; 45: 249–58.
154. Lindholm B, Bergstrom J, Norbeck HE. Lipoprotein metabolism in patients on continuous ambulatory peritoneal dialysis. In: Gahl GM, Kessel M, Nolph KD (eds), Advances peritoneal dialysis. Excerpta Medica, Amsterdam 1981; pp 434–6.
155. Tane D, Fein PA, Antignani A, Mittman N, Avram MM. The impact of CAPD treatment on lipid metabolism and cardiovascular risk. Adv Perit Dial 1990; 6: 234–7.
156. Avram MM, Goldwasser P, Burrel DE, Antignani A, Fein PA, Mittman N. The uremic dislipidemia: a cross-sectional study. Am J Kidney Dis 1992; 20: 324–35.
157. Marckmann P. Nutritional status and mortality of patients in regular dialysis therapy. J Intern Med 1989; 266: 429–32.
158. Maiorca R, Cancarini G, Manili L, Brunori G, Camerini C, Strada A, Feller P. CAPD is a first class treatment: results of an eight-year experience with a comparison of patient and method survival in CAPD and hemodialysis. Clin Nephrol 1988; 30 (suppl 1): S3–7.
159. Lowrie EG, Lew NL. Death risk in hemodialysis patients: the predictive value of commonly measured variables and an evaluation of death rate differences between facilities. Am J Kidney Dis 1990; 15: 458–82.
160. Teehan BP, Schleifer CR, Brown JM, Sigler MH, Raimondo J. Urea kinetic analysis and clinical outcome on CAPD. A five year longitudinal study. Adv Perit Dial 1990; 6: 181–5.
161. Fine A, Cox D. Modest reduction of serum albumin in continuous ambulatory peritoneal dialysis is common and of no apparent clinical consequence. Am J Kidney Dis 1992; 20: 50–4.
162. Young GA, Kopple JD, Lindholm B et al. Nutritional assessment of continuous ambulatory peritoneal dialysis patients: an international study. Am J Kidney Dis 1991; 17: 462–71.
163. Nelson EE, Hong CD, Pesce AL et al. Anthropometric norms in the dialysis population. Am J Kidney Dis 1990; 16: 32–7.
164. Marckmann P. Nutritional status of patients on hemodialysis and peritoneal dialysis. Clin. Nephrol 1988; 29: 75–8.
165. Maiorca R, Vonesh EF, Cavalli PL et al. A multicenter selection-adjusted comparison of patient and technique survivals on CAPD and hemodialysis. Perit Dial Int 1991; 11: 118–27.
166. Cancarini GC, Costantino E, Manili L et al. Nutritional staus in long-term CAPD patients. Adv Perit Dial 1992; 8: 84–7.
167. Kopple JD, Blumenkrantz MJ. Nutritional requirements for patients undergoing continuous ambulatory peritoneal dialysis. Kidney Int 1983; 24 (suppl): S295–302.
168. Blumenkrantz MJ, Kopple JD, Moran JK, Coburn JW. Metabolic balance studies and dietary protein requirements in patients undergoing continuous ambulatory peritoneal dialysis. Kidney Int 1982; 21: 849–61.
169. Movilli E, Mombelloni S, Gaggiotti M, Maiorca R.

Effect of age on protein catabolic rate (PCRn), morbidity and mortality in uremic patients with adequate normalized dose od dialysis (Kt/V urea). Nephrol Dial Transplant (in press).
170. Rottembourg J, Issad B, Gallego JL et al. Evolution of residual renal function in patients undergoing maintenance hemodialysis or continuous ambulatory peritoneal dialysis. Proc Eur Dial Tranplant Ass 1982; 19: 397–409.
171. Rottembourg J, Issad B, Poignet JL et al. Residual renal function and control of blood glucose levels in insulin-dependent diabetic patients treated by CAPD. In: Keen H, Legrain M (eds), Prevention and treatment of diabetic nephropathy. MTP Press Limited, Lancaster 1983; pp 339–52.
172. Cancarini GC, Brunori G, Camerini C, Brasa S, Manili L, Maiorca R. Renal function recovery and maintenance of residual diuresis in CAPD and hemodialysis. Perit Dial Bull 1986; 6: 77–9.
173. Lysaght MJ, Vonesh EF, Gotch F et al. The influence of dialysis treatment modality on the decline of remaining renal function. Trans Am Soc Artif Internal Org 1991; 37: 598–604.
174. Hallet M, Owen J, Becker G, Stewart J, Farrel PC. Maintenance of residual renal function: CAPD versus HD. (abstract) Perit Dial Int 1992; 12 (suppl 1): 124.
175. Nolph KD. Is residual renal function preserved better with CAPD than with hemodialysis? Am Kidney Fund Lett 1990; 7: 1–7.
176. Rottembourg J, Issad B, Allouache M, Baumelou A, Deray G, Jacobs C. Clinical aspects of continuous ambulatory and continuous cyclic peritoneal dialysis in diabetic patients. Perit Dial Int 1989; 9: 289–94.
177. Khanna R, Oreopoulos DG. Peritoneal dialysis in diabetic end-stage renal disease. J Diab Complications 1989; 3: 12–7.
178. Coronel F, Hortal L, Naranjo P et al. Analysis of factors in the prognosis of diabetics on continuous ambulatory peritoneal dialysis: long-term experience. Perit Dial Int 1989; 3: 12–7.
179. Lindblad AS, Nolph KD. Recovery of renal function in continuous ambulatory peritoneal dialysis. A study of National CAPD Registry data. Perit Dial Int 1992; 12: 43–7.
180. Michel C, Haddoum F, Viron B, Mignon F. Reprise de la fonction rénale après traitement par dialyse péritonéale continue ambulatoire? Nephrologie 1989; 10 (suppl 2): 53–5.
181. Rottembourg J, Issad B, Allouache M, Jacobs C. Recovery of renal function in patients treated by CAPD. Adv Perit Dial 1989; 5: 63–6.
182. Diaz-Buxo JA, Walker PJ, Burgess WP et al. The influence of peritoneal dialysis on the outcome of transplantation. Intern J Artif Organs 1986; 9: 359–62.
183. Odor-Morales A, Casterona G, Jimeno C et al. Hemodialysis or continuous ambulatory peritoneal dialysis before transplantation: prospective comparison of clinical and hemodynamic outcome. Transplantation Proc 1987; 19: 2197–89.
184. Triolo G, Segoloni GP, Salomone M et al. Comparison between two dialytic populations undergoing renal transplantation. Adv Perit Dial 1990; 6: 72–5.
185. Kyllönen L, Helanterä A, Salmela K, Ahonen J. Dialysis method and kidney graft survival. Transplantation Proc 1992; 24: 354.
186. O' Donoghus D, Manos J, Pearson R et al. Continuous ambulatory peritoneal dialysis and renal transplantation: a ten-year experience in a single center. Perit Dial Int 1992; 12: 242–9.
187. Taylor RMR, Proud G, Donnelly PK. Continuous ambulatory peritoneal dialysis. Br J Surg 1985; 72: 250.
188. Evangelista JB, Bennett-Jones D, Cameron JS et al. Renal transplantation in patients treated with haemodialysis and short term and long term continuous ambulatory peritoneal dialysis. Br Med J 1985; 291: 1004–7.
189. Shapira Z, Shmueli D, Yussim A, Boner G, Haimovitz C, Servadio C. Kidney transplantation in patients on continuous ambulatory peritoneal dialysis. Proc Eur Dial Transpl Ass 1984; 21: 932–5.
190. Rubin J, Kirchner KA, Raju S, Krueger RP, Bower JD. CAPD patients as renal transplant patients. Am J Med Sci 1987; 294: 175–80.
191. Gokal R. Renal transplantation in patients on CAPD. In: La Greca, Chiaramonte S, Fabris A, Feriani M, Ronco C (eds), Peritoneal dialysis. Proc 2nd International Course. Wichtig Editore, Milano 1985; pp 283–8.
192. Poole-Warren LA, Disney APS, Schindhelm K, Farrel PC. Australian renal, transplant experience in CAPD patients. In: La Greca, Chiaramonte S, Fabris A, Feriani M, Ronco C (eds), Peritoneal dialysis. Proc 2nd International Course. Wichtig Editore, Milano 1985; pp 289–90.
193. Wood CJ, Thomson NM, Scott DF, Holdsworth SR, Boyce N, Atkins RC. Renal transplantation in patients on CAPD. In: Maher JF, Winchester JF (eds), Frontiers in peritoneal dialysis, Field and Rich, New York 1986; pp 353–6.
194. Tsakiris D, Brawell SP, Briggs JD, Junor BJR. Transplantation in patients undergoing CAPD. Perit Dial Bull 1985; 5: 161–4.
195. Hymes LC, Warshaw BL. Renal transplantation in children undergoing peritoneal dialysis. Perit Dial Bull 1986; 6: 74–6.
196. Ogawa O, Hoshinaga K, Hasegawa A et al. Successful renal transplantation in children treated with CAPD. Transplantation Proc 1989; 21: 1997–2000.
197. Robinson RJ, Leapman SB, Wetherington GM, Hamburger RJ, Fineberg NS, Filo RS. Surgical considerations of continuous ambulatory peritoneal dialysis. Surgery 1984; 96: 723–9.
198. Glass NR, Miller DT, Sollinger HW, Zimmerman SW, Simpson D, Belzer FO. Renal transplantation in patients on peritoneal dialysis. Perit Dial Bull 1985; 5: 157–60.
199. Gutman RA, Blumenkrantz MJ, Chan YK et al.

Controlled comparison of hemodialysis and peritoneal dialysis: Veterans Administration multicenter study. Kidney Int 1984; 26: 459–70.
200. Mion C, Mourad G, Canaud B et al. Maintenance dialysis: a survey of 17 years' experience in Languedoc-Roussillon with a comparison of methods in a "standard populations". ASAIO J 1983; 6: 205–13.
201. Kurtz SB, Johnson WJ. A four-year comparison of continuous ambulatory peritoneal dialysis and home hemodialysis: a preliminary report. Mayo Clin Proc 1984; 59: 659–62.
202. Serkes KD, Blagg CR, Nolph KD, Vonesh EF, Shapiro F. Comparison of patient and technique survival in continuous ambulatory peritoneal dialysis and hemodialysis: a multicenter study. Perit Dial Int 1990; 10: 15–9.
203. Charytan C, Spinowitz BS, Galler M. A comparative study of continuous ambulatory peritoneal dialysis and center hemodialysis. Arch Intern Med 1986; 146: 1138–43.
204. Blagg CR, Wahl PW, Lamers JY. Treatment of chronic renal failure at the Northwest Kidney Center, Seattle, from 1960 to 1982. ASAIO J 1983; 6: 170–5.
205. Frascino J. A comparison of self-care dialysis modalities. Home hemodialysis, Continuous ambulatory peritoneal dialysis, In-center self-care hemodialysis. Dial Transplant 1985; 14: 13–6.
206. Burton PR, Walls J. A selection adjusted comparison of hospitalization on continuous ambulatory peritoneal dialysis and haemodialysis. J Clin Epidemiol 1989; 42: 531–9.
207. Gokal R, Jakubowski C, King J et al. Outcome in patients on continuous ambulatory peritoneal dialysis and haemodialysis: 4-year analysis of a prospective multicentre study. Lancet 1987; ii: 1105–9.
208. Legrain M, Rottembourg J, Bentchikou A et al. Dialysis treatment of insulin dependent diabetic patients: ten years experience. Clin Nephrol 1984; 21: 72–81.
209. Mejia G, Zimmerman SW. Comparison of continuous ambulatory peritoneal dialysis and hemodialysis for diabetics. Perit Dial Bull 1985; 5: 7–11.
210. Khanna R, Wu G, Vas S, Oreopoulos DG. Mortality and morbidity on continuous ambulatory peritoneal dialysis. ASAIO J 1983; 6: 197–204.
211. Nolph KD. Pyle WK, Hiatt M. Mortality and morbidity in continuous ambulatory peritoneal dialysis: full and selected registry populations. ASAIO J 1983; 6: 220–6.
212. Gentil MA, Cariazzo A, Pavon MI et al. Comparison of survival in Continuous Ambulatory Peritoneal Dialysis: a multicenter study. Nephrol Dial Transplant 1991; 6: 444–51.
213. Maiorca R, Vonesh E, Cancarini GC et al. A six-year comparison of patient and technique survivals in CAPD and HD. Kidney Int 1988; 34: 518–24.
214. Cavalli PL, Viglino G, Goia F, Cottino R, Mariano F, Gandolfo C. CAPD versus Hemodialysis: 7 years of experience. Adv Perit Dial 1989; 5: 52–5.
215. Lupo A, Cancarini G, Catizone L et al. Comparison of survival in CAPD and hemodialysis: a multicenter study. Adv Perit Dial 1992; 8: 136–40.
216. Posen G, Arbus G, Hutchinson T, Jeffery J. Survival comparisonm of adult non-diabetic patients treated with either hemodialysis or CAPD for end-stage renal failure. Perit Dial Bull 1987: 7: 78–9.
217. Quarello F, Bonello F, Boero R et al. CAPD in a large population: a 7-year experience. Adv Perit Dial 1989; 5: 56–62.
218. Maiorca R, Cancarini GC, Camerini C, Manili L, Brunori G. The impact of the Y-system and low peritonitis rate on CAPD results. In: Hatano M (ed), Nephrology. Springer-Verlag, Tokyo 1991; pp 1592–601.
219. Buoncristiani U, Bianchi P, Cozzari M et al. A new safe simple connection system for CAPD. Int J Nephrol Urol Androl 1980; 1: 50–3.
220. Maiorca R, Cantaluppi A, Cancarini GC et al. Prospective controlled trial of a Y-connector and disinfectant to prevent peritonitis in continuous ambulatory peritoneal dialysis. Lancet 1983; 2: 642–4.
221. Firanek CA, Vonesh EF, Korbet SM. Patient and technique survival among an urban population of peritoneal dialysis patients: an 8-year experience. Am J Kidney Dis 1991; 18: 91–6.
222. Rubin J, Barnes T, Burns P et al. Comparison of home hemodialysis to continuous ambulatory peritoneal dialysis. Kidney Int 1983; 23: 51–6.
223. Marichal JF, Cordier B, Faller B, Brignon P. Continuous ambulatory peritoneal dialysis (CAPD) or center hemodialysis? Retrospective evaluation of the success of both methods. Perit Dial Internal 1990; 10: 205–208.
224. Nolph KD. Clinical Results with peritoneal dialysis. Registry experiences. In: Twardowski Z, Nolph KD, Khanna R, Stein JH (eds), Peritoneal dialysis. Contemporary Issues in Nephrology, volume 22. Churchill Livingstone, New York 1991; pp 127–144.
225. Slingeneyer A, Canaud B, Mion C. Permanent loss of ultrafiltration capacity of the peritoneum in long-term peritoneal dialysis: an epidemiological study. Nephron 1983; 33: 133–8.
226. Capelli JP, Camiscioli TC, Vallorani RD. Comparative analysis of survival on home dialysis, in-center hemodialysis and chronic peritoneal dialysis (CAPD-IPD) therapies. Dial Transplant 1985; 14: 38–52.
227. Mailloux LU, Bellucci AG, Mossey RT et al. Productors of survival in patients undergoing dialysis. Am J Med 1988; 84: 855–62.
228. Burton PR, Walls J. Selection-adjusted comparison of life-expectancy of patients on continuous ambulatory peritoneal dialysis, haemodialysis, and renal transplantation. Lancet 1987; 1: 1115–9.
229. Wolfe RA, Port FK, Hawthorne VM, Guire KE. A comparison of survival among dialytic therapies of choice: in-center hemodialysis versus continuous

229. ambulatory peritoneal dialysis at home. Am J Kidney Dis 1990; 15: 433–40.
230. Lunde NM, Port FK, Wolfe RA, Guire KE. Comparison of mortality risk by choice of CAPD varsus hemodialysis among elderly patients. Adv Perit Dial 1991: 68–72.
231. Panarello G, De Baz H, Cecchin E, Tesio F. Dialysis for the elderly: survival and risk factors. Adv Perit Dial 1989; 5: 49–51.
232. Shapiro FL, Umen A. Risk factors in hemodialysis patient survival. ASAIO J 1983; 6: 176–84.
233. Brunner FP, Brynger H, Challah S et al. Renal replacement therapy in patients with diabetic nephropathy, 1980–85. Report from the European Dialysis and Transplantation Association Registry. Nephrol Dial Transplant 1988; 3: 585–95.
234. Walker JV, Grove MA. Survival in a community hospital dialysis center. Am J Nephrol 1988; 8: 40–8.
235. Excerpts from United States Renal Data System. 1991 Annual Data Report. V. Survival probabilities and cause of death. Am J Kidney Dis 1991; 18 (suppl 2): 49–60.
236. Rostand SG, Gretes JC, Kirk KA, Rutsky EA, Andreoli TE. Ischemic heart disease in patients with uremia undergoing maintenance hemodialysis. Kidney Int 1979; 16: 600–11.
237. Kannel WB, Dawber TRE, Kagan A, Revotskie N, Stokes J. Factors of risk in the development of coronary heart disease: Six-year follow-up experience. The Framingham study. Ann Intern Med 1961; 55: 33–50.
238. Cox DR. Regression models and life tables (with discussion). J R Statist Soc 1972; B34: 197–220.
239. Chandran PK. Lane T. Flynn CT. Patient and technique survival for blind and sighted diabetics on continuous ambulatory peritoneal dialysis: a ten-year analysis. Int J Artif Organs 1991; 14: 262–8.
240. Zimmerman SW, Glass N, Sollinger H, Miller D, Belzer F. Treatment of end-stage diabetic nephropathy: over a decade of experience at one institution. Medicine 1984; 63: 311–7.
241. Triolo G, Segoloni GP, Pacitti A et al. The treatment of uremic diabetic patient (UDP) in Piemonte (Dialysis and Transplantation Registry – RPDT): survival analysis. In: Andreucci VE, Dal Canton A (eds), New therapeutic strategies in nephrology. Kluwer Academic Publishers, Boston 1991; pp 440–2.
242. Brunner FP, Broyer M, Brynger H, Challah S, Dykes SR, Fassbinder W, Oulès R, Rizzoni G, Selwood NH, Wing AJ. Survival on renal replacement therapy: data from the EDTA Registry. Nephrol Dial Transplant 1988; 2: 109–22.
243. Rottembourg J, Bellio P, Maiga K, Remaoun M, Rousselie F, Legrain M. Visual function, blood pressure and blood glucose in diabetic patients undergoing continuous ambulatory peritoneal dialysis. Proc Eur Dial Transplant Ass 1985; 21: 330–4.
244. Catalano C, Postorino M, Kelly PJ, Fabrizi F, Enia G, Maggior Q. Diabetes and renal replacement therapy in Italy: mode of treatment and major complications. In: Andreucci VE, Dal Canton A (eds), New therapeutic strategies in nephrology. Kluwer Academic Publishers, Boston 1991; pp 443–5.
245. Khauli RB, Novick AC, Steinmuller DR et al. Comparison of renal transplantation and dialysis in rehabilitation of diabetic end-stage renal disease patients. Urology 1986; 27: 521–5.
246. Diaz-Buxo JA, Burgess WP, Greenman M, Chandler JT, Farme CD, Walker J. Visual function in diabetic patients undergoing dialysis: comparison of peritoneal and hemodialysis. Int J Artif Organs 1984; 7: 257–62.
247. Mion C. Practical use of peritoneal dialysis. In: Maher JF (ed), Replacement of renal function by dialysis. Kluwer Academic Publishers, Dordrecht 1989; pp 537–89.
248. Tzamaloukas AH, Murata GH, Harford AM et al. Hand gangrene in diabetic patients on chronic dialysis. ASAIO Trans 1991; 37: 638–43.
249. Heaton A, Rodger RSC, Sellars L et al. Continuous ambulatory peritoneal dialysis after the honeymoon: review of experience in Newcastle 1979–84. Br Med J 1986; 293: 938–41.
250. Brunner FP, Ehrich JHH, Fassbinder W et al. Combined report on regular dialysis and transplantation in Europe, XXI, 1990. Nephrol Dial Transplant 1991; 6 (suppl 4): 5–29.

25 Registry results

KARL D. NOLPH

1. Introduction — 735
2. The worldwide survey of Baxter Healthcare Inc. — 735
3. United States Renal Data System — 738
4. Michigan Registry — 743
5. European Dialysis and Transplant Association – European Renal Association (EDTA Registry) — 746
6. Canadian Registry — 746
7. The Australia and New Zealand Dialysis and Transplant Registry — 748
8. Missouri Kidney Program — 748
9. General trends — 749
References — 749

1. Introduction

Previous editions of *Peritoneal Dialysis* have included results of the USA NIH CAPD Registry [1]. The USA NIH CAPD Registry activities were assumed by the United States Renal Data System in 1988. The Final Report of the USA NIH National CAPD Registry was published in book form in 1989 [2]. Previous editions of *Peritoneal Dialysis* also contained peritoneal dialysis results from the Registry of the European Dialysis and Transplant Association (EDTA Registry) [3]. The EDTA Registry is still active and still collecting information relative to peritoneal dialysis.

In this chapter, I will focus on registry information that has been collected by active registries throughout the world over more recent years and published mainly from 1991 to 1993. Although some of the findings of these registries are similar, there are other studies and findings which are unique to each source. Therefore, I will review the highlights of registry reports sequentially rather than in an integrated fashion.

2. The worldwide survey of Baxter Healthcare Inc.

For over a decade, Baxter Healthcare Inc. has conducted an annual survey of worldwide chronic peritoneal dialysis activities, the more recent of which has been released in early 1993 [4]. At the close of 1992, there were near 535,100 total patients on chronic dialysis around the world. Of these, near 16% were maintained on some form chronic peritoneal dialysis (85% on CAPD). From the end of 1991 to the end of 1992, the worldwide chronic hemodialysis population had grown 9% while the worldwide chronic peritoneal dialysis population grew by 16%. Figure 1 shows the growth of the worldwide chronic peritoneal dialysis population over recent years to almost 80,000 patients by the end of 1992.

Figure 2 shows the percentage of dialysis populations in different countries maintained on chronic peritoneal dialysis as the end of 1992. Reasons for variations in the proportions of patients on chronic peritoneal dialysis have been recently explored in an international study; reimbursement issues, lifestyle considerations, and geographical factors appear to be more dominant than medical factors in their impact on the utilization of chronic peritoneal dialysis [5].

In the United States in 1992, 28% of 60,200 new ESRD patients went to chronic peritoneal dialysis as their initial therapy. The USA peritoneal dialysis population grew 13.5% while the hemodialysis population grew 33%. At the end of 1992, the number of peritoneal dialysis patients using automated peritoneal dialysis techniques was 5650 compared to 21,072 patients on CAPD.

Figure 3 shows the latest estimate of the worldwide peritoneal dialysis type and system mix. Note that only 20% of chronic peritoneal dialysis patients were using simple straight-line connectology as of 1993. Figure 4 shows the most recently estimated US peritoneal dialysis type and system mix. Note that less than 10% of the patients on chronic peritoneal dialysis were using standard straight-line connectology as of 1993. The disposable and UV

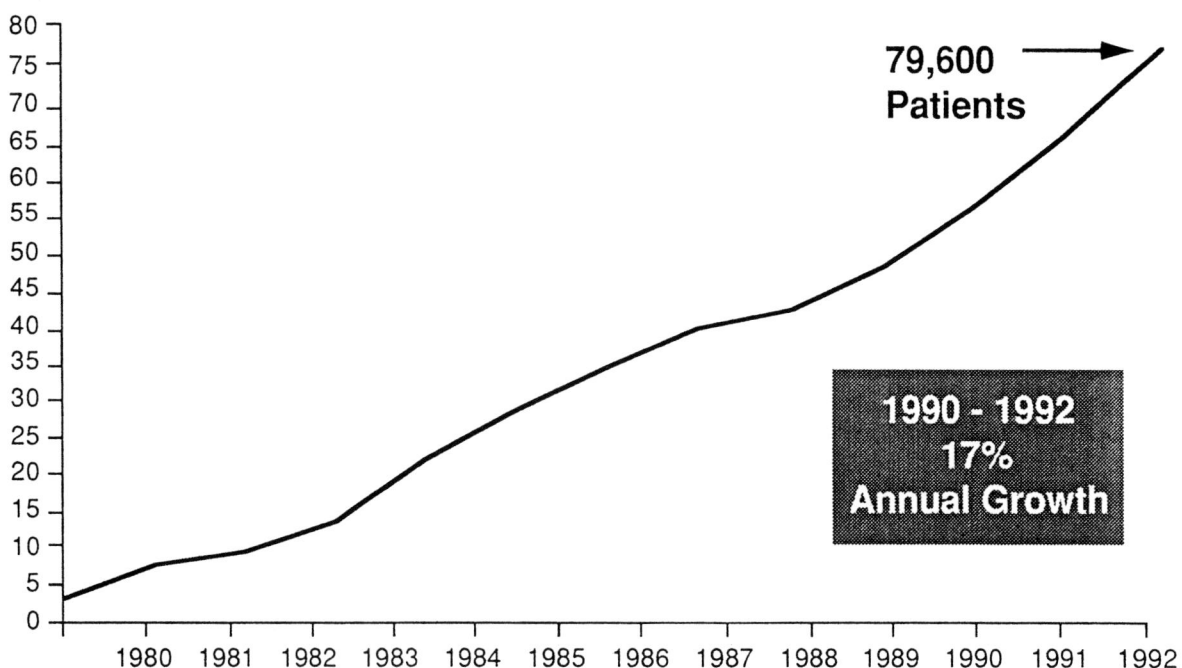

Figure 1. The worldwide population of patients maintained on chronic peritoneal dialysis (vertical axis in thousands) is shown over recent years. With permission – reference [4].

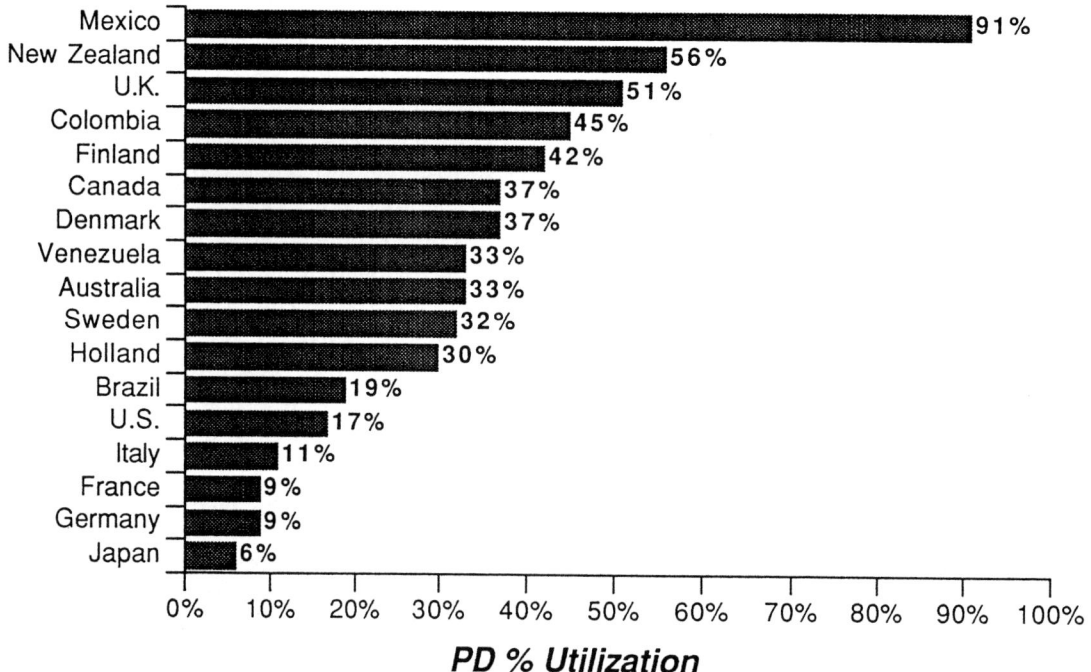

Figure 2. The percentage of national dialysis populations maintained on chronic peritoneal dialysis (horizontal axis) as of the end of 1992. With permission – reference [4].

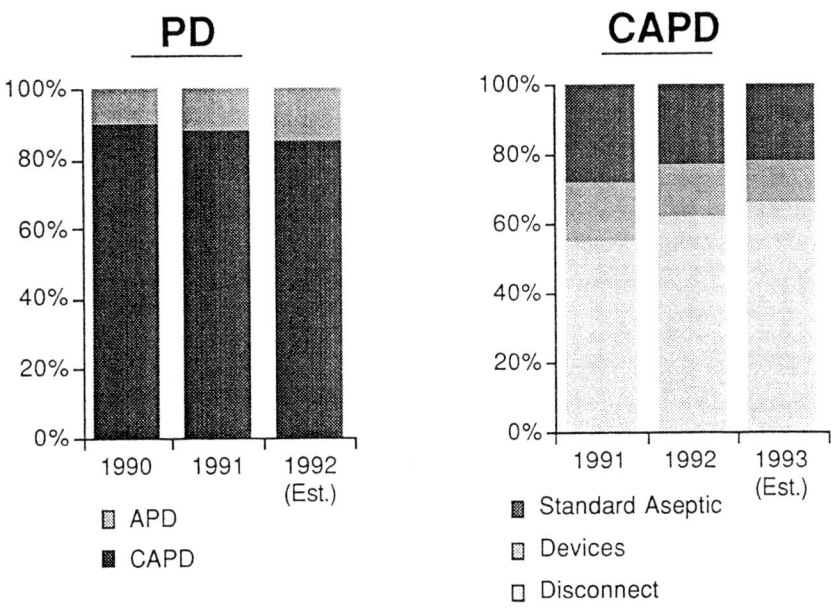

Figure 3. The worldwide distribution of automated peritoneal dialysis (APD) and continuous ambulatory peritoneal dialysis (CAPD) is indicated to the left for 1990, 1991, and 1992. To the right, for 1991, 1992, and 1993 are shown percentages of patients using standard aseptic technique, non-disconnect devices, and disconnect devices for CAPD. with permission – reference [4].

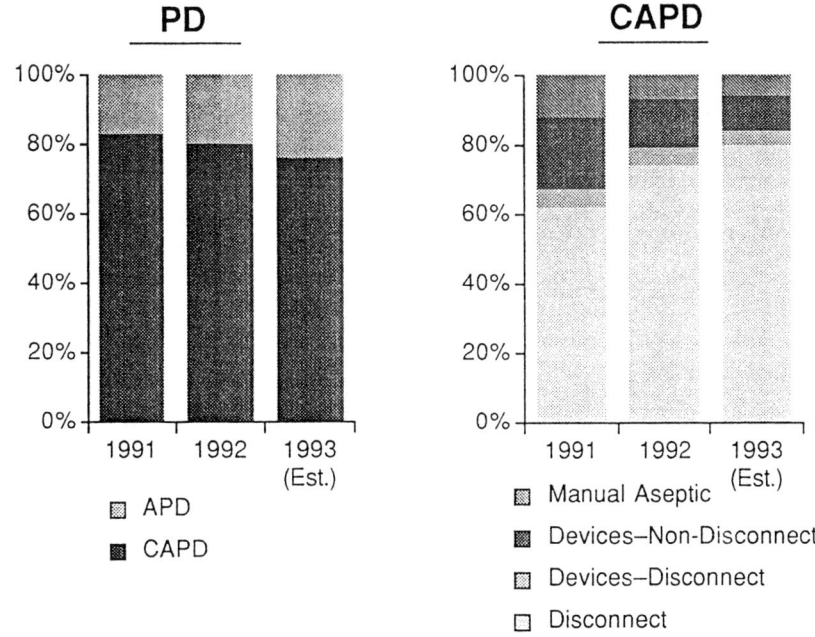

Figure 4. Percentage distributions on APD and CAPD as in Figure 3 are shown to the left for the USA for 1991, 1992, and 1993. To the right, USA percentages of the USA CAPD population using manual aseptic connectology, devices that are non-disconnect, devices coupled with disconnect, and simple disconnect are indicated for 1991, 1992, and 1993. With permission – reference [4].

3. United States Renal Data System

Highlights of the 1991 Annual Data Report of the United States Renal Data System were published in the *American Journal of Kidney Diseases* [6]. Figure 5 shows the one-year age, race, and sex adjusted patient survival for all dialysis patients incident in 1986–88 by diabetic status and modality on day 91 following onset of ESRD. The one-year survivals for hemodialysis and CAPD for the diabetics and nondiabetics are indicated on the respective bars.

Figure 6 shows mortality rate in deaths per thousand patient years at risk by age, race, and dialytic modality. Note the death rate is shown on a log scale. The prevalent cohort is the 1987–89 population. All patients had a primary diagnosis of glomerulonephritis. Although age impacts on mortality, consistent effects of race and modality are not as evident.

Figure 7 shows a similar kind of analysis in patients with diabetic nephropathy. Among white patients with diabetic ESRD, death rates tend to be lower among CAPD patients up to approximately age 40 and death rates tend to be lower among hemodialysis patients above that age. Results in patients with hypertensive ESRD showed no consistent impact of race or modality similar to the results with glomerulonephritis. Even though these figures adjust for age, race, and modality, there may be other differences in the populations represented by each curve that account for differences, if any, that are seen.

The Report contains analyses of modality distribution over time in the cohort of patients starting ESRD therapy in 1985–86. These will not be presented herein since they do not reflect the increasing use of chronic peritoneal dialysis in later cohorts.

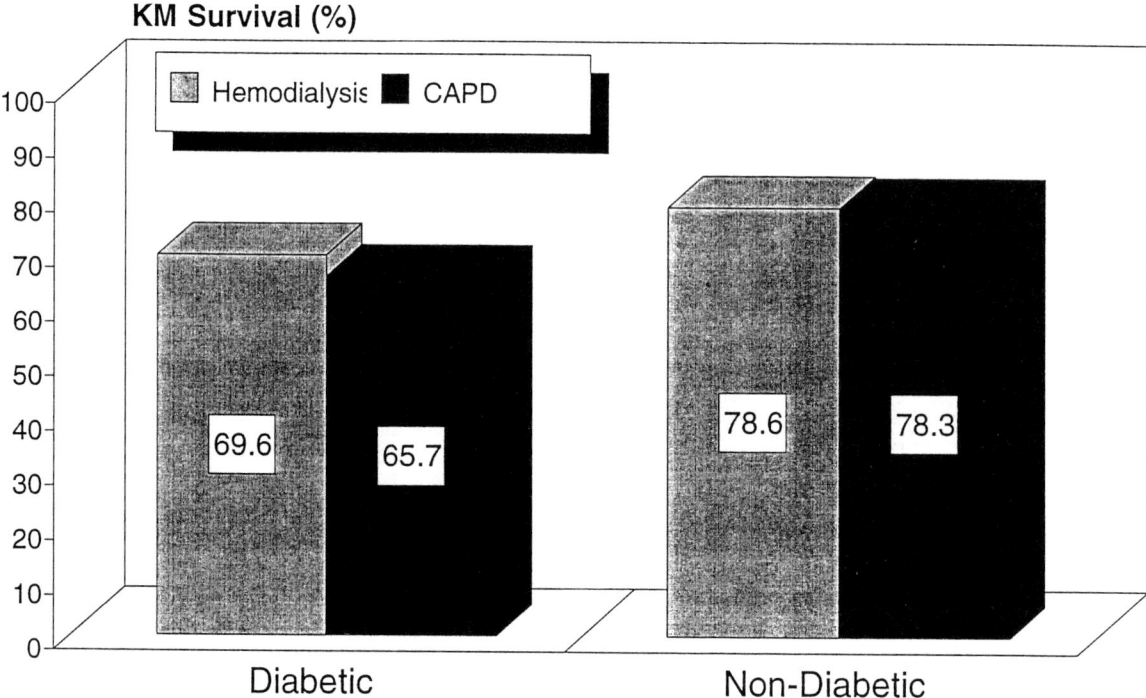

Figure 5. One-year age, race, and sex adjusted patient survival for all dialysis patients incident in 1986–88 by diabetic status and modality on day 91 following onset of ESRD. With permission – reference [4].

Mortality by Age, Race, and Modality - Glomerulonephritis

Mortality Rates for All Prevalent ESRD Patients Receiving Dialysis at the Beginning of the Year by Age, Race, and Dialytic Modality, 1987-89

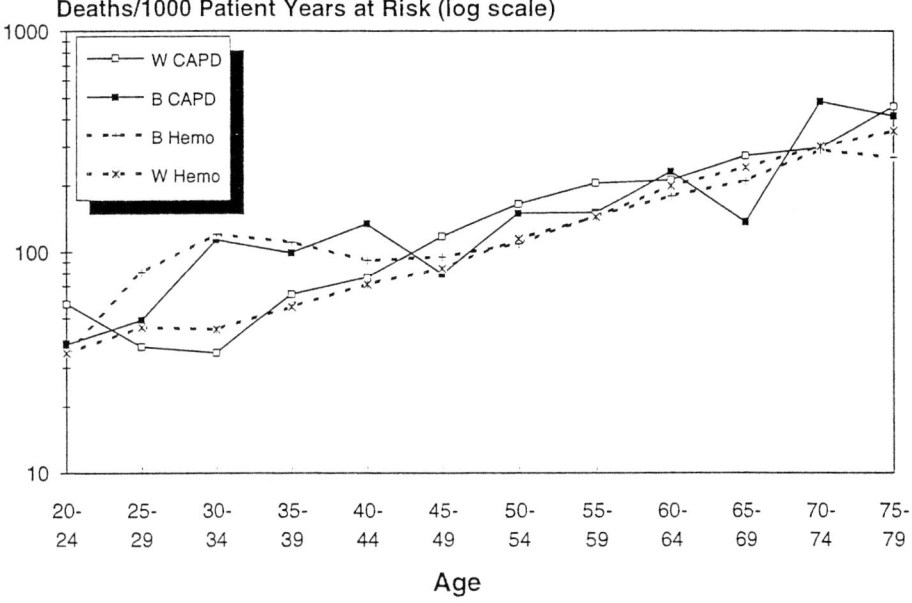

Figure 6. Mortality rate in death per thousand patient years (vertical axis, log scale) are related to age, race, and dialytic modality. All patients had a primary renal diagnosis of glomerulonephritis. W – white; B – black. With permission – reference [4].

Mortality by Age, Race, and Modality - Diabetes

Mortality Rates for All Prevalent ESRD Patients Receiving Dialysis at the Beginning of the Year by Age, Race, and Dialytic Modality, 1987-89

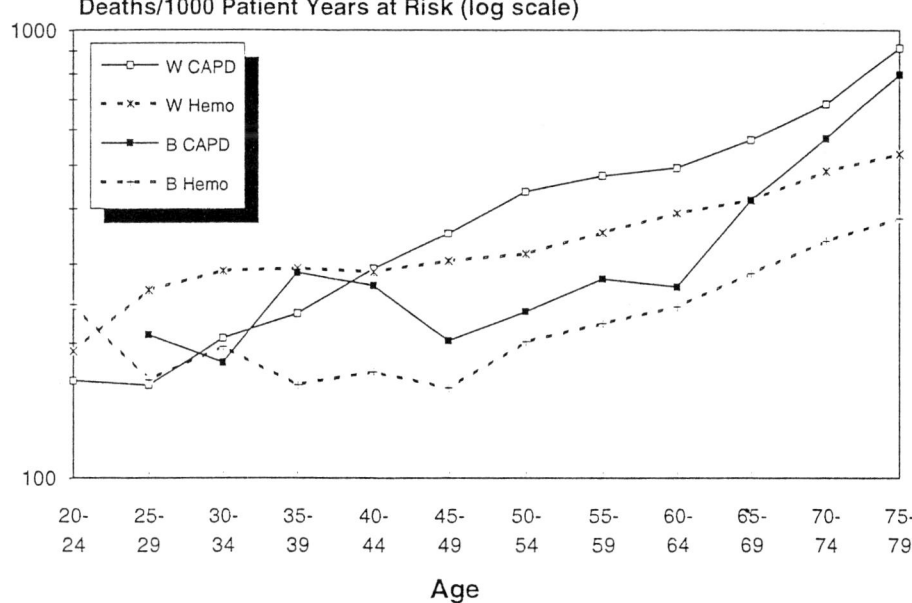

Figure 7. This figure is similar to Figure 6, except that all patients were thought to have diabetic nephropathy. With permission – reference [4].

Excerpts from the USRDS 1992 Annual Data Report were also published in the *American Journal of Kidney Diseases* [7]. One study consisted of an historical prospective sample of 2,420 nondiabetic and 1,738 diabetic patients incident from 1986–87 analyzed according to comorbid factors and their selection to peritoneal dialysis and hemodialysis. Table 1 summarizes selected patient characteristics for peritoneal dialysis vs. hemodialysis in these 1986–87 incident patients. Patients selected for PD were on average younger than those selected for HD (54 vs. 59, respectively). PD patients were less likely to be black (26 vs. 37%). The sex distribution was more similar (46 vs. 48% female). Patients selected to PD were more likely to have a history of diabetes (46 vs. 41%).

Table 2 shows the relative chance of selected comorbid conditions being present at the time of ESRD controlling for age and diabetes and looking at peritoneal vs. hemodialysis patients. For the adjusted count of risk factors hemodialysis patients were considered the reference (1.00). The significance of the difference of the risk of having the comorbid condition in the peritoneal dialysis population was assessed by Cochran-Mantle-Haenszel statistics. PD patients had a higher risk for peripheral vascular disease. The HD patients were more likely to have had a cerebral vascular accident, an amputation, or to be incapable of independent ambulation.

Figure 8 shows a count of comorbid factors by age and diabetes controlling for gender and race in a case mix study of 3,962 patients. Counts are controlled for gender and race looking at diabetic and nondiabetic patients within two age groups (less than 60 and 60 years or older). All adjusted counts of risk factors are expressed relative to the reference group of nondiabetic HD patients 60 years or older for whom the absolute count of risk factors was 3.31. The statistical differences was assessed by the t-test. Among diabetic patients less than 60 years of age, the difference in the relative count of comorbid factors between HD and PD was found to be statistically significant.

Overall, HD patients were more likely to be older, more likely black, less likely diabetic, and had more comorbid conditions at the time of ESRD than did PD patients. The fact that HD patients were older accounts for a substantial portion of the differences in reported comorbid conditions. Controlling for age, race and diabetes, the observed differences in the number of comorbid conditions was greatly reduced, although HD patients still had more comorbid conditions.

The USRDS 1992 Annual Data Report summarized the prescribed liters per exchange in the 1986–87 incident CAPD patients. Figure 9 shows that 77.9% of patients surveyed used 2–2.5 liters per exchange. The prescribed exchanges per day in this same 1986–87 incident CAPD population are depicted in Fig. 10. The figure shows that 86.6% of patients were prescribed 4 exchanges per day. Figure 11 shows the prescribed liters of dialysate per week (which here refers to the instilled volume) in this same incident population. 68.3% of patients

Table 1. Selected patient characteristics of 1986–87 incident patients for peritoneal dialysis vs. hemodialysis.

Patient characteristics	PD	HD
Age at ESRD (mean, years)	53.5	58.7
Race (%):		
White	69.1	56.8
Black	26.2	36.7
Other	4.7	6.5
Gender: Female (%)	46.0	48.0
Diabetes (%):		
Primary cause of ESRD*	36.2	28.1
As cause of ESRD or prior history**	45.6	41.0
Count of cases (n)	759	3,399

* As cause of ESRD from USRDS patient database.
** Database or Case Mix Severity Form. Includes diabetes as primary cause of ESRD (above) and prior history of diabetes as reported to the USRDS.
With permission – reference [7].

Table 2. Relative chance* of selected comorbid conditions being present at the time of ESRD, controlling for age and diabets, peritoneal dialysis vs. hemodialysis (USRDS case mix severity study, 1986–87 incident ases).

Comorbid condition at time of ESRD	Hemodialysis (Reference)	Peritoneal dialysis Relative chance	p
Congestive heart failure	1.00	0.93	0.19
Coronary heart disease**	1.00	0.98	0.75
Cerebrovascular accident	1.00	0.66	0.01
Peripheral vascular disease (PVD)***	1.00	1.20	0.02
Amputation due to PVD	1.00	0.66	0.05
Not capable of independent ambulation	1.00	0.57	0.01

* Cochran-Mantel-Haenszel.
** Coronary heart disease includes coronary heart disease, bypass surgery (CABG), coronary angioplasty, abnormal angiography.
*** Peripheral vascular disease includes PVD, amputation due to PVD, absent foot pulses, claudication.
With permission – reference [7].

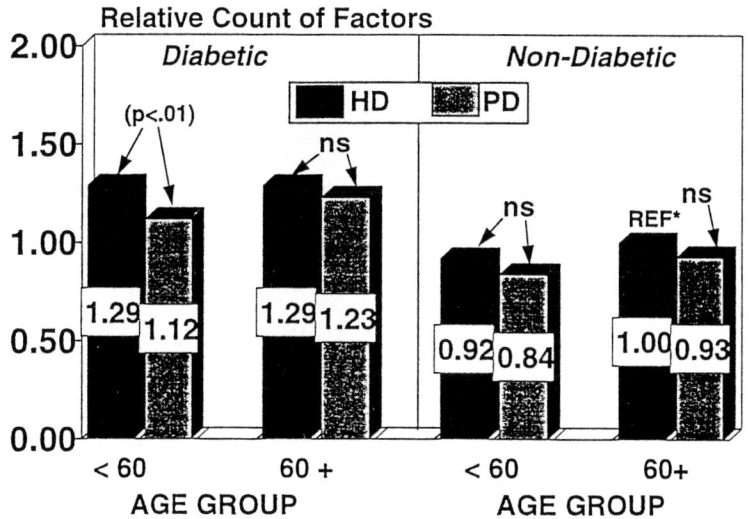

Figure 8. The relative count of comorbid factors controlling for gender and race is shown by age and diabetes from a case mix analysis of 3,962 patients. A relative count of 1.0 implies the presence of 3.31 comorbid factors. With permission – reference [7].

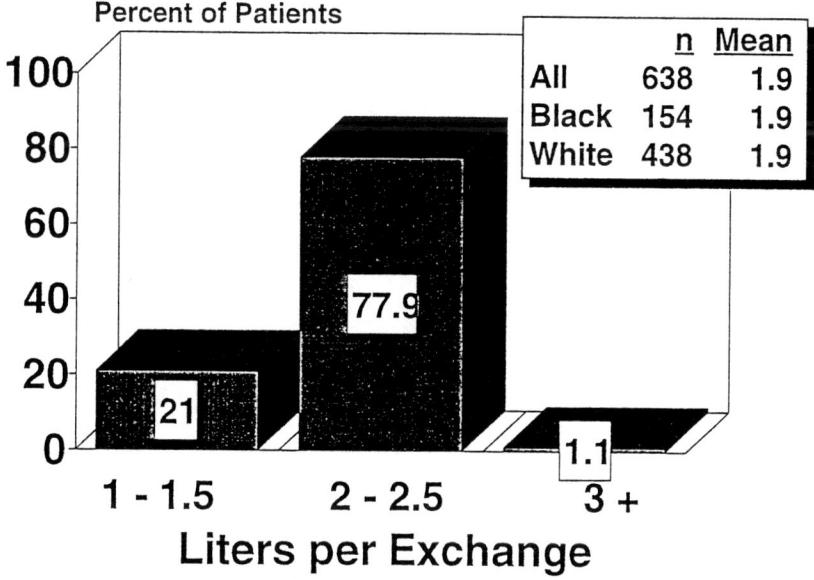

Figure 9. The prescribed liters per exchange in 1986–87 incident USA CAPD patients. Percentages of patients (vertical axis) using different liters pre exchange (horizontal axis) are shown. With permission – reference [7].

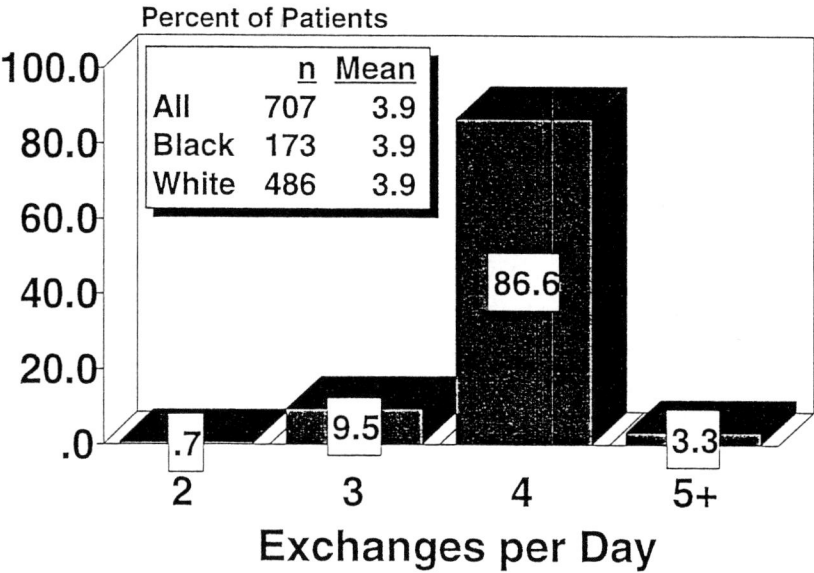

Figure 10. The percentages of patients (vertical axis) using different numbers of exchanges per day (horizontal axis) are shown for 1986–87 USA CAPD incident patients. With permission – reference [7].

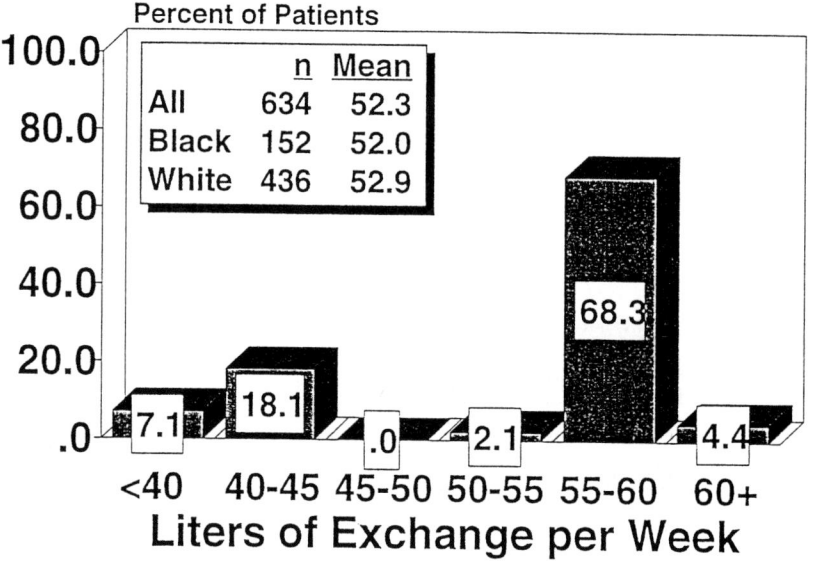

Figure 11. The percentages of patients (vertical axis) prescribed different exchange volumes per week in liters (horizontal axis) are shown for 1986–87 incident USA CAPD patients. With permission – reference [7].

in this same incident population. 68.3% of patients used 55–60 liters per week of dialysis solution.

In a 1989 survey of 2,807 CAPD patients, 44% of patients used straight catheters, 40% curled, 12% catheters with a permanent swan-neck bend, and 4% other types of catheters. 72% used double-cuff catheters. In only 20% were deep cuffs placed in the midline; 33% used paramedian and 14% lateral placement. Surgeons inserted 88% of the catheters in this patient group, using surgical dissection 74% of the time. Only 10% were placed by nephrologists. Alternative insertion techniques used by surgeons or nephrologists were peritoneoscopy in 6% and blind insertion in 8%. 43% of patients received prophylactic antibiotics at the time of catheter insertion. The risk of peritonitis by a Cox analysis was not increased relative to the specialty of the physician placing the catheter, the use of intraperitoneal drugs, the type of insertion technique, or the deep cuff position. The risk of peritonitis was increased with the use of single superficial catheters ($p < 0.02$).

Data forms were analyzed on 3,366 CAPD patients who started CAPD at home for the first time during the first 6 months of 1989 [8]. A total of 706 CAPD units submitted theses data forms. Standard connectology was used in 34%, the Y-set in 32% (with or without UV), standard ultraviolet light in 27%, O-set in 5%, and other forms of connectology in 2%. Figure 12 shows the actuarial percent of patients remaining peritonitis free in days since the start of CAPD at home relative to the connection technique used. Note that the peritonitis free survival was higher with the Y-set and ultraviolet light devices. The relative risks of first peritonitis with the Y-set and standard UV was 0.60 and 0.75 compared to standard connection technique and these values were significantly reduced relative to the standard reference ($p < 0.01$ and $p < 0.01$, respectively). Figure 13 shows the actuarial percent of patients remaining on their initial connection technique (technique survival) in days since the start of CAPD at home (deaths and transplants are censored in this analysis). The relative risk of technique failure was significantly ($p < 0.01$) reduced by the Y-set (relative risk 0.49 compared to standard at 1.0), standard UV (relative risk 0.73) and the O-set (relative risk 0.64). The reductions in time to first peritonitis with the Y-set compared to standard connectology are comparable percentage-wise to those reported by the Canadian CAPD Clinical Trials Group [9] and the report of the Italian CAPD reported by the Canadian CAPD Clinical Trials Group [9] and the report of the Italian CAPD Study Group [10].

4. Michigan Registry

Mortalities for CAPD patients and hemodialysis patients were compared in all Michigan residents 20–59 years of age who initiated therapy for end-stage renal disease during the 1980's (n = 4288)

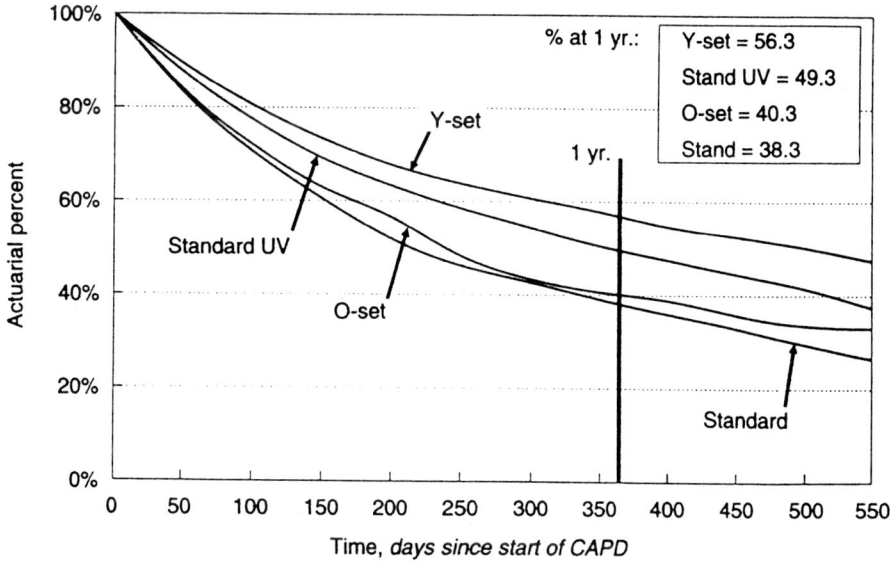

Figure 12. The actuarial percent of patients remaining peritonitis free in days since the start of CAPD at home by connection technique is shown from a survey of USA centers. N:Y-set = 1,067, Standard UV = 916, O-set = 167, Standard = 1,133. With permission – reference [8].

[11]. The study populations were stratified by primary renal diagnosis and analyses were controlled for age, race, sex, and year in which chronic dialysis was initiated using the Cox proportional hazards methods. Using an intention to treat analysis (not censoring data at the time of a modality change), glomerulonephritic and diabetic patients on CAPD experienced mortality rates lower than their hemodialysis counterparts. Figure 14 shows the risk of death and 95% confidence limits for diabetics on CAPD relative to diabetics on HD according to age of onset of ESRD with adjustments for race, sex, and year of ESRD onset. The relative risks of death were significantly lower in the CAPD patients ($p < 0.05$ through the age of 52). For the subgroups 20–29, 30–39, and 40–49, the CAPD relative risks were significantly less to the $p < 0.01$ level. For the 50–59 year old group, the relative risk of death for CAPD was below that of HD to the $p = 0.06$ level.

Older age was associated with an increased mortality rate in all diagnostic groups. Diabetics also showed significant differences in mortality rates for white vs. black patients. There were no significant differences in mortality associated with race and sex for nondiabetic patient groups.

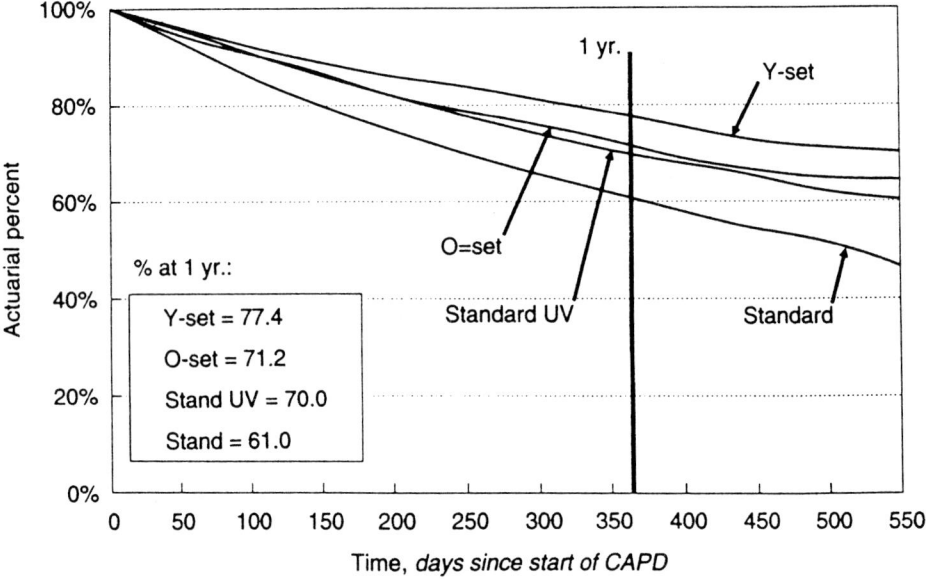

Figure 13. The actuarial percent of patients remaining on the initial connection technique (technique survival) in days since the start of CAPD at home (death and transplants are censored in this analysis). The results are from the USA center survey study. N:Y-set = 1,067, O-set = 167, Standard UV = 916, Standard = 1,133. With permission – reference [8].

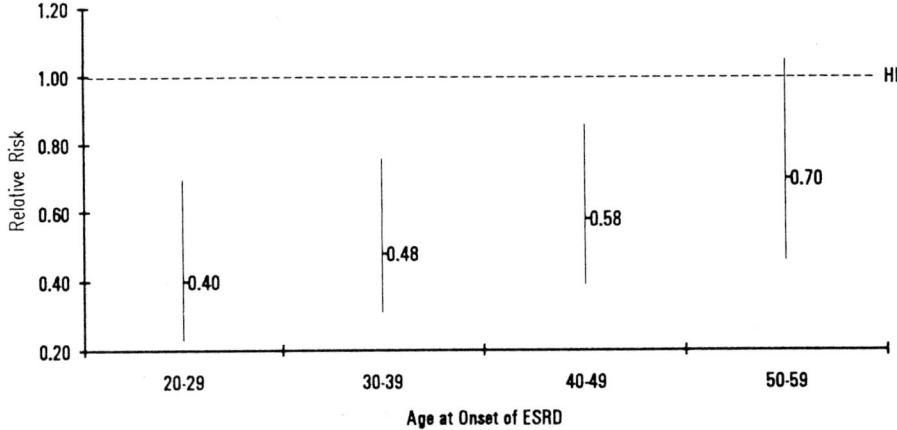

Figure 14. This study represents findings in diabetics in the Michigan Registry. The relative risks of death (and 95% confidence limits) for CAPD relative to HD by age and onset of ESRD are shown. Risks are adjusted for race, sex, and year of ESRD onset. For each age group, the relative risk of death on HD is defined as 1.00. With permission – reference [11].

Mortality trends across the 1980's showed no statistically significant pattern for diagnostic groups other than diabetics. In the diabetic patients, however, the death rates of CAPD cohorts have been decreasing an average of 9% per year while those of HD cohorts appear to be increasing with an overall linear trend of 4% per year. Figure 15 shows the log of the relative risk for CAPD and HD by year of incidence adjusted for age, race, and sex.

Figure 16 shows survival of glomerulonephritic and diabetic patients using CAPD and HD with all curves adjusted for a 45-year-old white man initiating therapy in 1989. The curves were generated by a Cox model with the intention to treat censoring approach. Among diabetics, median survival for HD patients was 23.8 months whereas median survival for CAPD patients was 36.1 months. The 1, 3, and 5 year survival rates for diabetic HD patients were 80, 33, and 12%, while those for CAPD patients were 87, 50, and 27%, respectively. In patients with glomerulonephritis on HD, the 1, 3, and 5 year survival rates were 94, 72, and 57%, respectively, while the corresponding figures for CAPD patients were 95, 79 and 67%.

The authors of the paper stress that the results of the study must be interpreted with caution and do not imply a causal relationship between the use of CAPD and lower mortality rates. There is the

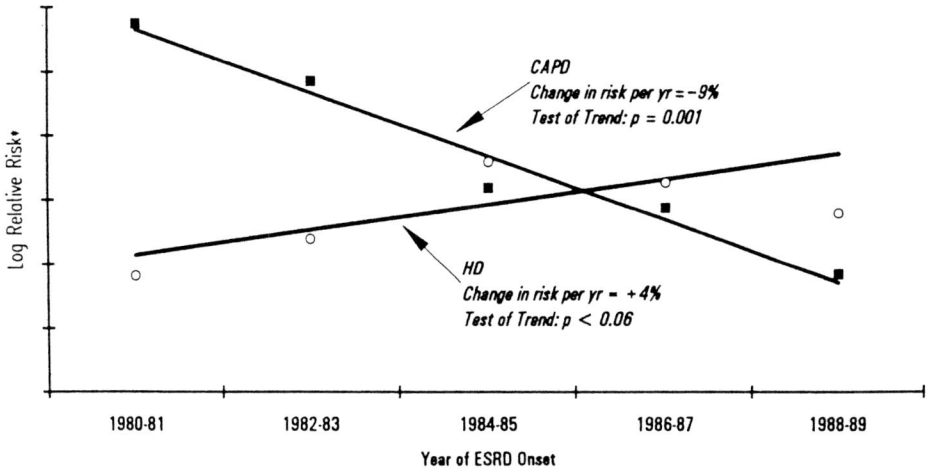

Figure 15. In this study of diabetics in the Michigan Registry, changes in CAPD and HD mortality risk by year of incidence from 1980–89 are shown. The vertical axis represents the log of the relative risk and each marked increment represents a 22% higher risk. With permission – reference [11].

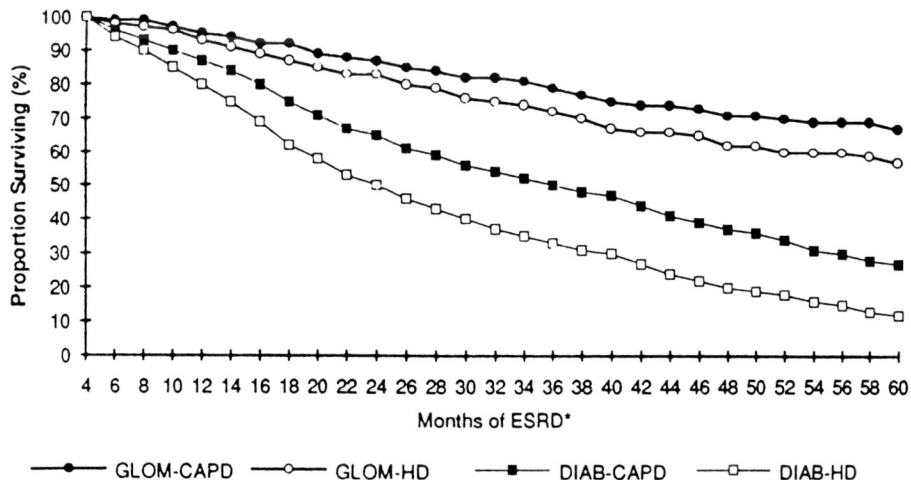

Figure 16. From the Michigan Registry, survival of glomerulonephritic (GLOM) and diabetic (DIAB) patients using CAPD and HD. Curves are for a 45-year-old white man initiating therapy in 1989 and were generated by a Cox model with ITT-sensoring criteria. Follow-up began at day 120 of ESRD. With permission – reference [11].

possibility of a lower count of comorbid conditions among CAPD diabetic patients not considered in this analysis [7]. They also point out, however, that the existence of real difference in therapy efficacy cannot be completely ruled out. There is the question as to whether avoidance of sudden drastic hemodynamic and biochemical changes as well as improved control over glycemia may contribute to lower morality rates among CAPD patients [12]. The rising death rates on hemodialysis may reflect USA trends perhaps resulting in part from delivered small solute clearances on hemodialysis that are less in many centers in the US than in Europe where HD survivals are better than in the USA [7].

5. European Dialysis and Transplant Association – European Renal Association (EDTA Registry)

The most recent report of the EDTA Registry covers the 1991 update of their data [13]. As of December 31, 1991, there were 97,447 patients on hospital/center hemodialysis, 4,568 on home hemodialysis, 1,117 on intermittent peritoneal dialysis, 14,057 on continuous forms of peritoneal dialysis, and 51,738 patients with a functioning transplant graft. 5% or 741 patients were on continuous cyclic peritoneal dialysis (CAPD). There were high percentages of patients using disconnect or Y systems for CAPD; the overall percentage is 67%, with the highest percentages by country in Italy (91%) and the Netherlands (91%). The frequency of peritonitis in CAPD patients expressed as patient months/peritonitis episode in 1990 range from 2.6 in Egypt to 31.3 in Iceland. The overall Registry average was 10.2 patient months/peritonitis episode. In Italy, where the use of the Y-set is extensive, the rate was 19.0 patient months/peritonitis episode overall.

In chronic peritoneal dialysis patients, myocardial infarctions were responsible for 20% of the deaths; myocardial infarctions caused 14% of deaths on chronic HD. Percentage distributions of other cardiovascular events are every similar between the two therapies. The highest percentage of deaths due to infection is seen in transplant patients.

The EDTA Registry analyzed successful pregnancies in women on renal replacement therapy [14]. Over 10 years of data collection since 1977, there have been 490 pregnancies and 500 babies born to mothers on renal replacement therapies in member countries of the EDTA Registry. Mothers with a functioning transplant had 88.4% of these babies, mothers on CHD 11.2%, and mothers on CAPD 0.4%.

The EDTA Registry analyzed the rehabilitation of 617 young adults from different European countries who started dialysis or transplantation before the age of 15 years [15, 16]. The analysis showed that 32% of patients on renal replacement therapies aged 21 and 40 years who started treatment under 15 years had one or more disabilities which affected their rehabilitation, even though they were mild in the majority of patients. Effective vision did not seem to be altered by renal replacement therapies. Motor dysfunctions, however, changed in 76% of patients, improving in 39% and deteriorating in 37%. Patients starting renal replacement therapy with hearing deficiencies had worsening in 2/3 and improvement in 1/3. There were 30% of patients on renal replacement therapies who started secondary school or university but did not complete their training. There were 16% who had to attend a special school for the handicapped. The proportion of patients who were employed was lower among dialyzed patients than among those with a functioning graft. In these studies, the impact of mode of dialysis was not assessed relative to the degree of school attendance or employment. Interestingly, 85.5% of the study population remained unmarried.

The EDTA Registry published a special report analyzing renal replacement therapy for end-stage renal failure before two years of age [17]. During the 1986–88 period, the initial therapy for end-stage renal failure was CAPD in 60%, hemodialysis in 25%, intermittent peritoneal dialysis in 8%, and transplantation prior to dialysis in 7% of these very young patients. Figure 17 shows the proportional distribution methods of treatment in children starting renal replacement therapies under the age of two years during 1983–1987 and who survived three years. CAPD was the most commonly used dialysis therapy initially in these patients and four the first one and a half years after starting dialysis. The percentage on CAPD declines as the percentage with a functioning transplant increases. The percentage of patients on chronic hemodialysis remains relatively constant.

6. Canadian Registry

The 1991 data from the Canadian Organ Replacement Register was presented to the 25th

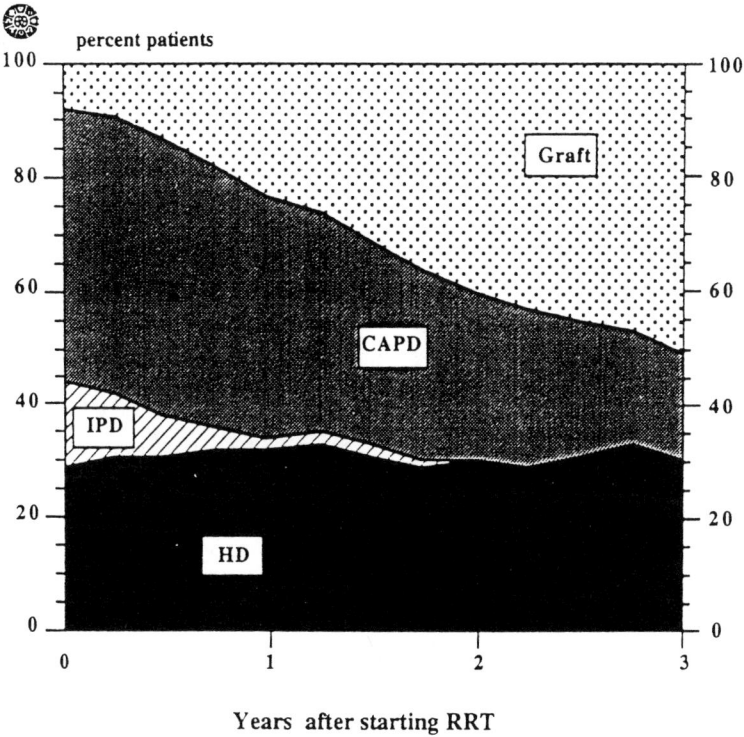

Figure 17. From the European Dialysis and Transplant Association-European Renal Association Registry, the proportional distribution of methods of treatment for ESRD in surviving children starting renal replacement therapy under the age of 2 years in 1983–87. With permission – reference [17].

Annual Meeting of the Canadian Society of Nephrology and the Canadian Transplant Society in September of 1992 [18]. This report added the 1991 experience to the previous 1990 report [19]. There were 2,482 patients who began renal replacement therapies in Canada in 1991. There were 867 of these patients aged 45–64 and 985 greater than 64 years of age. This 1992 population represents an incident rate near 95 per million population. Near 39% started on chronic peritoneal dialysis. By the end of 1991, 941 patients (38% of all who started therapies in 1991 and 44% of all dialysis patients at the end 1991) were on peritoneal dialysis. Reasons for discontinuing CAPD during different treatment years from 1984 through 1991 were compared. There has been a decline in the percentage of CAPD patients discontinuing for reasons of peritonitis, perhaps related to the widespread use of disconnect systems and lower peritonitis rates. Even though the numbers of patients starting dialysis has increased year by year in Canada and the numbers of patient starting CAPD have increased since 1988, the numbers of patients discontinuing CAPD in the first year of treatment have declined from 558 in 1988 to 470 in 1991.

The percentage distribution of the prevalent end-stage renal disease population in Canada at the end of respective years was examined. The overall cumulative percentage of chronic peritoneal dialysis patients in Canada had been running near 20%, including patient with a functioning transplant in the total prevalent end-stage renal disease population. As of the end of 1991, the 2,593 patients on chronic peritoneal dialysis represent 37.7% of the 6,877 total dialysis population; there were 2,593 total patients on chronic peritoneal dialysis. Of these, 2,239 were on CAPD, 165 on incenter intermittent peritoneal dialysis, 163 on CCPD, 16 on home intermittent peritoneal dialysis, and 10 on combined PD/HD.

At year end 1991, there were 50.3% of hemodialysis patients and 32.2% of peritoneal dialysis patients receiving erythropoietin therapy. It is interesting that there 22 chronic peritoneal dialysis patients living in nursing homes and 17 patients on chronic peritoneal dialysis living in chronic care facilities at the end of 1991.

7. The Australia and New Zealand Dialysis and Transplant Registry

The Fifteenth Report of the Australia and New Zealand Dialysis and Transplant Registry was published in October of 1992 [20]. There were 958 patients (55 per million) new to renal replacement therapies in 1991. As of December 31, 1991, the cumulative population was 6,658 total patients (3,546 with a functioning transplant and 3,112 dialysis-dependent). They also note an age profile shift towards the elderly. The median age of their new patient population was 56, 25% were 65 years and over and 29% were age 55–64 years.

In Australia, 60% of CAPD patients used disconnect systems as of March 31, 1992. The risk of developing peritonitis at 6 months of CAPD was 45%. Of patients starting CAPD over the 12 months prior to March 31, 1992, 62% had no reported episodes of peritonitis. Median survival free of infection estimated by actuarial survival methods was 9.3 months.

In Australia, 382 of 891 home CAPD patients were considered able to work (43%). There were 837 home CAPD patients (94%) able to care for themselves with no or occasional assistance.

In Australia, the death rate among CAPD patients for 1991 was 12%. The same gross annual death rate for center hemodialysis was 10% The death rates of hemodialysis and CAPD patients in Australia in 1991 were similar for hemodialysis and CAPD except for age 75–84, where the death rate on CAPD was higher. These differences could be accounted for by differences in risk factors between the two populations.

8. Missouri Kidney Program

The Missouri Kidney Program, sponsored by the state of Missouri, maintains a registry of end-stage renal disease therapies in the state [21]. In 1992, 61% of new dialysis patients were over age 60. Diabetes and hypertension were the two leading causes of the primary renal disease (26.5% and 19.8% of new patients, respectively). Figure 18 shows the distribution by treatment modality of all Missouri dialysis patients as of June 30, 1992. Of these patients, 21.1% were on chronic peritoneal dialysis (17.4% CAPD, 3.7% cycler PD).

Table 3 shows the treatment distribution by patient characteristics as of this same time. Note

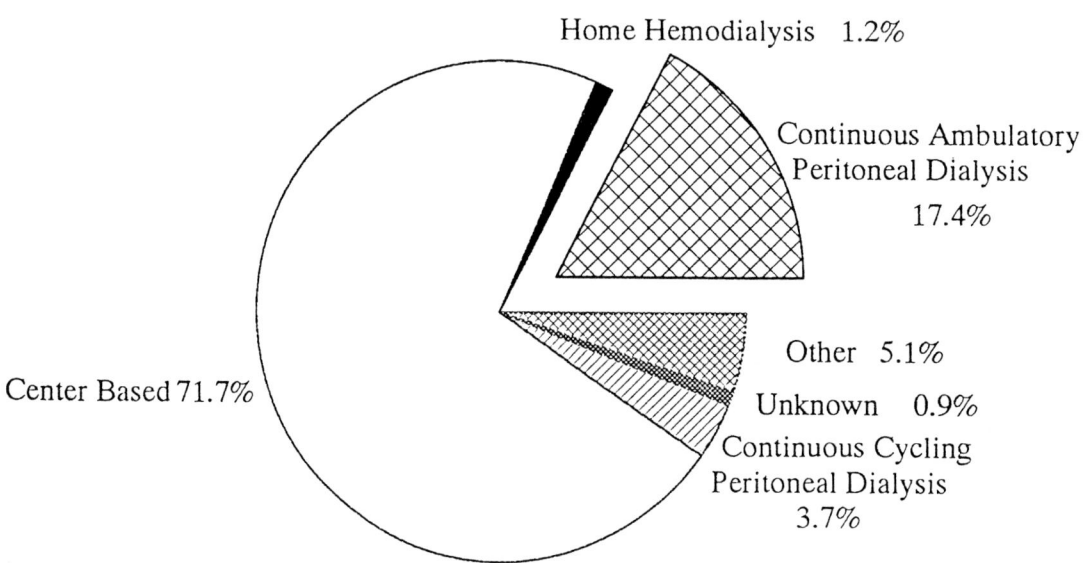

Figure 18. From the Missouri Kidney Program Registry, the distribution by treatment modality is shown for all Missouri dialysis patients as of June 30, 1992. With permission – reference [21].

that the percentage of non-white patients on CAPD is lower than the percentage of white patients on CAPD. This is a typical finding that has been mentioned before.

9. General trends

The chronic peritoneal dialysis population continues to grow, and in many areas of the world, the growth rates are proportionately greater than those seen in the chronic HD population. Most chronic peritoneal dialysis patients are on CAPD, but the use of cycler techniques such as nightly intermittent peritoneal dialysis and continuous cyclic peritoneal dialysis is increasing.

Patient survivals with CAPD and HD are often similar in comparable populations; when differences are seen variations in comorbid risk factors between the populations cannot be excluded. Declining death rates in diabetes on CAPD and increasing death rates in diabetics on HD in Michigan have not been definitively explained.

The age of the dialysis population everywhere in the world seems to be increasing. Presumably the comorbid risk factors of dialysis populations are also increasing. These changing characteristics of the dialysis population must be kept in mind in comparing outcomes from one period to another.

The shift from standard CAPD connectology to disconnect devices has been evident in multiple registry reports. The use of disconnect devices seems to be associated with lower peritonitis rates.

The utilization of chronic peritoneal dialysis varies markedly in different regions. It appears that these differences in the proportion of dialysis patients on chronic peritoneal dialysis mainly reflect geographical, social, and reimbursement issues.

The role and methods of peritoneal dialysis continue to undergo evolution. These changes suggest an ever-increasing role of peritoneal dialysis, hopefully with fewer complications than in the earlier years.

References

1. Lindblad AS, Novak JW, Nolph KD. The USA CAPD Registry. Characteristics of participants and selected outcome measures for the period January 1, 1981 to August 31, 1937. In: Nolph KD (ed), Peritoneal Dialysis. 3rd ed. Kluwer Academic Publishers, Dordrecht 1989; pp 389–413.
2. Lindblad AS, Novak JW, Nolph KD (eds). Continuous ambulatory peritoneal dialysis in the USA: final report of the National CAPD Registry 1981–1988. Kluwer Academic Publishers, Dordrecht 1989.
3. Golper TA, Geerlings W, Selwood NH, Brunner FP, Wing AJ. Peritoneal dialysis results in the EDTA Registry. In: Nolph KD (ed), Peritoneal Dialysis. 3rd ed. Kluwer Academic Publishers, Dordrecht 1989; pp 414–28.
4. Westman J. Worldwide dialysis update. Annual survey by Baxter Healthcare Inc., Deerfield, IL 1993.
5. Nissenson AR, Prichard SS, Cheng IKP et al. Nonmedical factors that impact on ESRD modality selection. Kidney Int 1993; 43 (suppl 40): in press.
6. Excerpts from United States Renal Data System, 1991 Annual Data Report. Am J Kidney Dis 1991; 18 (suppl 2): 1–127.
7. Excerpts from United States Renal Data System, 1992 Annual Data Report. AM J Kidney Dis 1992; 20 (suppl 2): 1–113.
8. Port FK, Held PJ, Nolph KD, Turenne MN, Wolfe RA. Risk of peritonitis and technique failure by CAPD connection technique: a national study. Kidney Int 1992; 42: 967–74.
9. Canadian CAPD Clinical Trials Group. Peritonitis in continuous ambulatory peritoneal dialysis. Randomized clinical trial comparing the Y connector disinfectant system to standard systems. Perit Dial Int 1989; 9: 159–64.
10. Fellin G, Gentile MG, Manna GM, Redaelli L, D'Amico G. Peritonitis prevention: a Y-connector and sodium hypochlorite. Three years' experience. Report of the Italian CAPD Study Group. In: Khanna R, Nolph KD, Prowant B, Twardowski ZJ, Oreopoulos DG (eds), Advances in Continuous Ambulatory Peritoneal Dialysis. Peritoneal Dialysis Bulletin Inc., Toronto 1987; pp 114–8.
11. Nelson CB, Port FK, Wolfe RA, Guire KE. Comparison of continuous ambulatory peritoneal dialysis and hemodialysis patient survival with evaluation of trends during the 1980s. J Am Soc Neph 1992; 3: 1147–55.
12. Diaz-Buxo JA. Continuous ambulatory peritoneal

Table 3. Treatment Distribution by patient characteristics.

Characteristics	Center Hemo (#/%)	Home Hemo (#/%)	CAPD (#/%)
Male	1409/78.8	29/1.6	350/19.6
Female	1369/80.8	20/1.2	306/18.0
White	1566/74.2	27/1.3	517/24.5
Non-white	1199/88.2	22/1.6	139/10.2
New patient	777/80.8	4/0.4	181/18.8
All other patients	2001/79.4	45/1.8	475/18.8
Hypertension	618/84.2	6/0.8	110/15.0
Glomerulonephritis	259/74.4	7/2.0	82/23.6
Diabetes	696/78.1	9/1.0	186/20.9
Hospital days (mean)	12.1	4.7	11.6

With permission – reference [21].

dialysis (CAPD) and hemodialysis: pride and prejudice. Perit Dial Int 1990; 10: 5–7.
13. Raine AEG, Margreiter R, Brunner FP et al. Report on management of renal failure in Europe, XXI, 1991. Nephrol Dial Transplant 1992; 7 (suppl 2): 7–35.
14. Rizzoni G, Ehrich JHH, Broyer M et al. Successful pregnancies in women on renal replacement therapy: report from the EDTA Registry. Nephrol Dial Transplant 1992; 7: 279–87.
15. Rizzoni G, Ehrich JHH, Broyer M et al. Rehabilitation of young adults during renal replacement therapy in Europe: 1. the presence of disabilities. Nephrol Dial Transplant 1992; 7: 573–8.
16. Ehrich JHH, Rizzoni G, Broyer M et al. Rehabilitation of young adults during renal replacement therapy in Europe: 2. schooling, employment, and social situation. Nephrol Dial Transplant 1992; 7: 579–86.
17. Ehrich JHH, Rizzoni G, Brunner FP et al. Renal replacement therapy for end-stage renal failure before 2 years of age. Nephrol Dial Transplant 1992; 7: 1171–7.
18. Fenton SAA, Jeffery JR. 1991 preliminary statistics: Canadian Organ Replacement Register. Hospital Medical Records Institute, Don Mills, Ontario, Canada September 1992.
19. Canadian Organ Replacement Register, 1990 Annual Report. Hospital Medical Records Institute, Don Mills, Ontario, Canada April 1992.
20. Disney APS (ed). Fifteenth report of the Australia and New Zealand Dialysis and Transplant Registry. The Queen Elizabeth Hospital, Woodville, South Australia October 1992.
21. Warady BA, Druse K. Annual report of the Missouri Kidney Program, 1992. Missouri Kidney Program, University of Missouri, Columbia, MO 1992.

26 The use of peritoneal dialysis in special situations

SARAH S. PRICHARD AND JOANNE M. BARGMAN

1. Introduction 751
2. Renal failure: Special situations 751
   2.1. Pregnancy in ESRD 751
   2.2. HIV infected patients 752
      2.2.1. Management of HIV patients on peritoneal dialysis 753
      2.2.2. Disposal of dialysate 753
   2.3. Chronic liver disease 753
   2.4. Acute renal failure 754
   2.5. Hyper and hypocalcemia 754
3. Non-uremic indications for peritoneal dialysis 755
   3.1. Congestive heart failure 755
   3.2. Inborn errors of metabolism 757
      3.2.1. Urea cycle defects and neonatal hyperammonemia 757
      3.2.2. Organic acidemias 757
      3.2.3. Disorders of amino acid metabolism 758
      3.2.4. Disorders of carbohydrate metabolism 758
   3.3. Acute pancreatitis 758
      3.3.1. Other surgical indications 759
   3.4. Psoriasis 760
   3.5. Acute hepatic failure 761
   3.6. Hypothermia and hyperthermia 761
   3.7. Poisoning 761
   3.8. Multiple myeloma 762
   3.9. Experimental uses for the peritoneal cavity: Total peritoneal nutrition and paracorporeal membrane oxygenation 763
      3.9.1. Total peritoneal nutrition 763
      3.9.2. Paracorporeal membrane oxygenation and removal of carbon dioxide 763
References 764

1. Introduction

Peritoneal Dialysis is now widely and successfully used to treat ESRD patients. The continuous nature of the therapy and its home based, self care nature make it particularly advantageous for certain subgroups of patients. Using the peritoneal cavity as access provides additional uses of the therapy in both uremic and non-uremic states. This chapter focuses on the use of peritoneal dialysis in special groups of ESRD patients and in a variety of non-uremic conditions.

2. Renal failure: Special situations

2.1. Pregnancy in ESRD

Pregnancy is a relatively rare event in patients with advanced renal failure. In 1978, a report from the European Dialysis and Transplantation Association (EDTA) reported on 115 pregnancies amongst 13,000 women of child bearing age followed by the registry. [1] Of the pregnancies that were not terminated, 16 live births occurred, representing a 23% success rate. Prematurity and low birth weight almost always occurred. Recent results show a marked improvement. In a survey undertaken in 1990, 1.5% of women of child bearing age on ESRD therapy conceived and the success rate of live births was 52%. Prematurity and low birth weights remain almost the rule.

Early reports of pregnancy with End Stage Renal Disease (ESRD) were exclusively of experience with patients on hemodialysis. With the wide spread use of peritoneal dialysis, there is emerging a series of successful reports of managing pregnant ESRD patients on peritoneal dialysis [2–7]. CAPD offers several theoretical advantages to the pregnant patient; the continuous nature of the therapy avoids the fluid shifts and blood pressure variations seen in hemodialysis, and no heparin is required which should reduce bleeding complications, especially abruptio placentae.

Problems peculiar to CAPD do occur. Peritonitis has been reported in 3 instances and in one episode at 24 weeks gestation, was associated with the onset of premature labour and a stillbirth [7]. As the pregnancy advances, the intraperitoneal volume of fluid tolerated may be reduced, requiring more frequent small volume exchanges in order to achieve the usual targeted plasma urea level of less than 18 mmol/L [5]. Catheter placement can generally be achieved without complication at any stage of pregnancy [6]. One patient was reported to have developed a leak and one had several catheters fail requiring a change to hemodialysis.

The present use of erythropoietin (EPO) has alleviated the high transfusion requirements reported in the ESRD pregnancies prior to 1988. However, hypertension which often complicates pregnancy in dialysis, might be aggravated [8, 11]. Hou reported on 5 cases managed with EPO, and in none was hypertension a difficult management issue. The CAPD patient in that series requires no additional anti-hypertensive medication [8].

Spontaneous hemoperitoneum in the non pregnant young women on CAPD is rarely a cause for concern. In pregnancy, however, it may represent the onset of an abruptio or the rupture of a uterine vessel and should be treated seriously, including observation in hospital and urgent ultrasound assessment.

A potential therapeutic manoeuver for CAPD patients with premature labour is the addition of magnesium to the bath. Careful attention must be paid to serum magnesium levels, particularly when intravenous boluses of magnesium are also used.

In choosing CAPD vs. hemodialysis for a pregnant ESRD patient, there is insufficient experience reported to be conclusive as to which modality is best. There are less than 20 cases of pregnancy in CAPD, and the success rate exceeds 50% which is far superior to the 1978 EDTA report; however present day hemodialysis results also seem to be improved [9]. The use of EPO, bicarbonate baths and more biocompatible membranes, all contribute to better outcomes. Nonetheless, there is no doubt that CAPD can be used safely during pregnancy with minimal inconvenience to the patient and with a high probability of a successful live birth.

2.2. HIV infected patients

Renal disease, including end-stage renal disease, is a frequent complication of HIV infected patients [12, 13]. The prognosis for ESRD patients who are HIV positive is poor, particularly for those with AIDS at the time of starting dialysis.

Both hemodialysis and peritoneal dialysis have been used to manage these patients. There are some reasons to advocate the use of peritoneal dialysis preferentially, including higher hematocrits, caloric supplementation provided by the dialysate glucose, the maintenance of a home environment and reduced risk exposure for the health care providers.

There can also be disadvantages. Dialysate protein losses in these patients, who are often otherwise nutritionally compromised and/or nephrotic, may worsen their nutritional status. Neurologic involvement causing physical and intellectual impairment sometimes contraindicates home peritoneal dialysis as an initial form of therapy, or may require a modality change to hemodialysis after some period of time on home based peritoneal dialysis. Finally, the immunocompromised state common to all HIV positive patients could predispose to an increased incidence of peritonitis or exit site infections with unusual and difficult to treat infecting organisms.

There is somewhat conflicting data in the literature on the incidence and type of peritonitis in HIV infected patients. Cruz reported on his experience with 5 patients in 1989 [14]. Their peritonitis rate was extremely high (1 in every 2.7 patient months). The predominant organism was staphylococcus. Their overall survival after starting CAPD was 7.8 ± 2.4 months.

In 1990, Graham reported on a multi centre trial in which data was collected from 32 CAPD units [15]. Fifty-eight percent of the population were HIV drug abusers. In this study population, 53% were asymptomatic, 37% had AIDS and 10% had ARC. Twenty-five of the 32 centers reported that home peritoneal dialysis was the preference modality for HIV patients. There were 226 episodes of peritonitis in the 79 patients. Over half (55%) of these were gram positive, with staphylococcus being the predominant organism. Gram negative infections were 20% of the reported peritonitis episodes, of which almost 30% were pseudomonas. Fungal organisms were isolated in 6% of the episodes and there was no growth in 18%. There was a substantial rate (29%) of modality change to hemodialysis reported. This high incidence of pseudomonas and fungal peritonitis has also been reported by others [22, 23].

In 1991, Wasser et al. did not report an increased incidence of peritonitis in HIV patients, nor did they report a higher rate of gram negative or fungal peritonitis [16]. However, in 1992, Schloth et al. reported on their experience with HIV positive patients [17]. There was a two fold increase in peritonitis in this population compared to their HIV negative population (1 in 4.6 vs. 1 in 9.9 patient months). Although gram positive organisms were the most frequent infecting organisms, there was a tendency (though not statistically significant) for a higher rate of gram negative and fungal peritonitis. These authors could not correlate infection rates with serum albumin levels in the HIV positive patients.

Most recently, Teblin et al. [18] analyzed their experience with 39 HIV infected patients. The peritonitis rates were more than 2 times higher in their HIV patients, with pseudomonas and fungal infections being notably more frequent. In contrast, Wasser et al. [19] reported on 16 HIV positive patients and found no increase in peritonitis compared to their HIV negative patients (1 in 13.15 vs 1 in 11.04 patient months). In both of the later studies, the peritonitis rates are high for the non HIV groups compared to the experience widely reported with disconnect flush-before-fill systems. Perhaps once these baseline peritonitis rates are reduced, a more consistent difference between HIV positive and negative patients will become apparent.

Retention rates at the end of one year for HIV patients is variably reported from 28% to 45% [14, 15, 18]. Drop out occurs largely because of death. In addition, modality change is frequent, largely to hemodialysis, but also to automated peritoneal dialysis, because of an inability to cope with standard CAPD therapy. Frequent peritonitis may also require a modality change.

2.2.1. *Management of HIV patients on peritoneal dialysis*

Management of the HIV population with the ESRD requires an understanding of and management of their primary disease, its clinical course and therapy. In particular, appropriate adjustment for drug dosages must be made. Commonly administered drugs, including AZT, DDI, Gancyclovir, Acyclovir, intravenous Pentamadine and Foscarnet all require a decrease in dosage with advanced renal failure. The peritoneal clearance of these drugs is minimal. The use of amphotericin at any therapeutic dose may result in loss of residual renal function.

The maintenance of adequate nutrition is essential and difficult because of frequent concurrent diarrhea and esophagitis. A careful record of dietary intake with appropriate supplementation will help maximize general well being.

2.2.2. *Disposal of dialysate*

Peritoneal dialysate drainage contains the HIV antigen and as such is a potential source of contamination. It is recommended that universal precautions, as proposed by Center for Disease Control [20, 21], be followed for these patients. Disposal of the spent dialysate can be in the toilet after treatment with bleach (sodium hypochlorite). The empty dialysate bags should be double bagged prior to disposal and needles used at home should be brought back to the hospital center for disposal. Adherence to these guidelines can minimize any risk of transmission of the virus. Some countries may have more stringent regulations with regard to HIV waste handling.

In summary, peritoneal dialysis can be successfully used to manage HIV positive patients. There are reasons to favour this modality choice but there are some circumstances in which peritoneal dialysis may not be feasible. Peritonitis rates may be higher for this patient population, particularly for pseudomonas and fungus, but this has not precluded the use of peritoneal dialysis. Finally, retention rates are low due to a high mortality rate and a failure to cope with a self care, home based program as their primary disease progresses.

2.3. Chronic liver disease

Peritoneal dialysis offers several advantages over hemodialysis in the management of patients with advanced chronic liver disease, with or without ascites. The avoidance of anticoagulation and intradialytic hypotension and the direct drainage of ascites should facilitate patient care. However, there are surprisingly few reports on the use of peritoneal dialysis in this population.

In 1977, Wilkinson et al. reported on a large series of patients using acute peritoneal dialysis in 20 patients with chronic liver disease, and 50 patients with fulminant acute liver disease [24]. None of the cirrhotic group survived to leave the hospital. Perhaps these early poor results have discouraged the use of peritoneal dialysis in cirrhotic patients. More recent reports have shown much better success using peritoneal dialysis.

In 1992, Marcus reported on a series of 9 patients, all with ESRD and advanced cirrhosis with ascites, managed on peritoneal dialysis [25]. They had survivals of up to 8 years on CAPD with 3 of the patients still being alive and well on peritoneal dialysis after 18 to 24 months at the time of their report. Noted complications included pleural effusions in two, with one of these patients developing an empyema, recurrence of repaired umbilical and other hernias, and a peritonitis rate similar to the overall centre experience. Interestingly, these patients' serum albumin levels remained unchanged while on peritoneal dialysis.

More recently, Durand has reported a series of 4 patients with chronic cirrhosis and tense ascites who have been successfully treated on CAPD for periods of 2 to 11 years [26]. They reported excellent peritoneal clearance and ultrafiltration. Nutritional deficiencies were not a problem. Horie also reported on a single case treated successfully for 30 months on CAPD [27].

Dadone et al. studied the transport characteristics of 10 patients on peritoneal dialysis with chronic hepatic disease (CHD) compared to normals [28]. The duration of CAPD therapy at the time of study for the CHD group exceeded 12 months. This again underlines the usefulness of peritoneal dialysis in managing these patients. With regard to water and solute transport, the CHD patients had higher rates of ultrafiltration and higher small solute transport, but no correlation between dialysate glucose absorption and ultrafiltration. On the basis of these observations, one can presume that the ongoing production of ascites likely contributes to the excess ultrafiltration and that a high rate of lymphatic absorption continues in CHD patients on peritoneal dialysis, just as is found in CHD patients not on dialysis. In spite of this, peritoneal dialysis effectively maintained both fluid balance and adequate solute clearance.

Patients who have hepatitis B or C do shed viral particles into the peritoneal fluid. As such, handling of the patient's blood and spent dialysate should be similar to HIV contaminated fluids and the guidelines recommended by the CDC should be followed [20, 21].

In summary, patients with ESRD and concurrent chronic liver disease can be successfully managed on peritoneal dialysis. Since the peritoneal drainage also manages the ascites, peritoneal dialysis may be the modality of choice if the patient is able to carry out the therapy.

2.4. Acute renal failure

Acute renal failure (ARF) requiring a dialytic intervention can be treated with hemodialysis, continuous arterio-venous hemodialysis (CAVHD) or peritoneal dialysis [29–34]. Peritoneal dialysis offers the advantage of being a continuous therapy, which does not require anticoagulation nor vascular access. Furthermore, it can be performed in hospitals or on wards where hemodialysis nursing expertise does not exist. However, it cannot be utilized in patients with open abdominal wounds or abdominal surgical drains. It can be used in patients with recent abdominal surgery provided the incision site is intact.

Acute renal failure patients are frequently severely catabolic. Therefore, a high dose peritoneal dialysis therapy is required to maintain adequate clearances for both small and larger molecular weight substances [29, 31, 32]. This may involve the use of up to 48 litres of dialysate per 24 hour period. The use of large doses of peritoneal dialysis fluid also gives the patients a substantial caloric load which can help reduce the catabolic state.

Careful attention needs to be paid to the patients' net nitrogen loss in assessing the success of peritoneal dialysis in ARF. Although azotemia can be controlled, the patient may remain in net negative nitrogen balance [29]. Potentially, the addition of amino acids to the dialysate could improve nitrogen balance at the risk of worsening azotemia [35]. If an appropriate balance between azotemia and catabolism cannot be achieved, aggressive daily hemodialysis or CAVHD may be necessary.

Access for acute peritoneal dialyses may be achieved either by a temporary stylet catheter or a chronic PD catheter. If the expertise is easily available for its insertion, the latter is generally preferable because of its longevity. In patients starting ESRD therapy, it has been advocated to have the peritoneal catheter in place for several weeks prior to its use because of the increased risk of leaks when it is used early. This delay is obviously not possible in ARF, but maintaining the patients in the recumbent position in the first few days after catheter insertion can reduce this risk.

In summary, patients with ARF can be managed on peritoneal dialysis provided their peritoneal cavity is intact. In order to obtain adequate solute clearances, high dose peritoneal dialysis must be utilized and additional nutritional support is often necessary even though the peritoneal dialysis itself supplies a large caloric load.

A summary of the potential advantages and disadvantages of peritoneal dialysis for ESRD patients with concurrent pregnancy, HIV infection and chronic liver disease, as well as patients with acute renal failure, is shown in Table 1.

2.5. Hyper and hypocalcemia

Hypercalcemia in non uremic patients can virtually always be treated successfully with rehydration in conjunction with bisphosphonates, calcitonin or mithramycin. Prior to the development of these pharmacologic agents, there were scattered reports of using peritoneal dialysis with low or zero calcium dialysate to treat hypercalcemia [37].

Presently, hypercalcemia has become a frequent complication of patients with ESRD who are managed with calcium containing phosphate binders. The availability of a lower calcium dialysate has somewhat alleviated this problem and is discussed elsewhere in this book. However, there remain a small number of patients on peritoneal dialysis who develop severe hypercalcemia [38, 39]. These cases can be well managed by utilizing a calcium free dialysate solution made up by the local hospital pharmacy using distilled water, 50% dextrose, NaCl and NaHCO3.

Similarly, non uremic hypocalcemic patients can be managed medically with appropriate administration of calcium, vitamin D and magnesium. There is however, a subgroup of ESRD patients who have undergone parathyroidectomy who may benefit from intraperitoneal calcium supplementation. Both Thompson [40] and Benz [41] have reported cases of hungry bone syndrome post parathyroidectomy with prolonged hypocalcemia in whom calcium gluconate was safely added to the peritoneal dialysate for periods of weeks to months. The continuous nature of CAPD gave all 4 of these cases excellent calcium control. Thus, prolonged post parathyroidectomy hypocalcemia in ESRD patients may be an additional indication for peritoneal dialysis.

3. Non-uremic indications for peritoneal dialysis

3.1. Congestive heart failure

In the severest forms of cardiac failure, the salt and water retention which accompanies this condition may become unresponsive to even the most potent diuretics. With pump failure, forward perfusion can become so compromised that renal blood flow is severely reduced and renal insufficiency supervenes. The decrease in peritubular blood flow and tubular fluid flow rate limits the delivery of diuretic to its target sites within the nephron. Furthermore, with limited renal blood flow even if the diuretic were to reach its effector site, the resultant diuresis

Table 1. Peritoneal dialysis in special ESRD populations.

PATIENT GROUP	PERITONEAL DIALYSIS POTENTIAL ADVANTAGES	PERITONEAL DIALYSIS POTENTIAL DISADVANTAGES
PREGNANCY	– No anticoagulation – Stable BP – Minimal blood loss – Stable chemistries – Home based – May add magnesium to dialysate	– May require frequent exchanges – Tolerance of only small I.P. Volumes – Peritonitis precipitating labour
HIV INFECTED PATIENTS	– Reduced Health Care Provider Risk exposure – Caloric loading with glucose – Home based – Minimal blood losses	– Additional protein losses in dialysate – Increased peritonitis esp. Pseudomonas and fungus – Inability to cope requiring modality change
CHRONIC LIVER DISEASE	– No anticoagulation – Stable BP – Direct ascites drainage – Caloric loading with glucose	– Recurrence of hernias – Pleural effusions (Pleural-peritoneal communication) – Large protein losses in dialysate
ACUTE RENAL FAILURE	– No anticoagulation – No vascular access – Stable BP – Continuous solute clearance – Caloric loading with glucose – Can be done in locations where hemodialysis expertise is unavailable	– Requires high dose PD to achieve adequate clearance in catabolic patients – Requires an intact peritoneal cavity – Protein losses contribute to net nitrogen losses

and natriuresis is limited by counter regulatory effects within the renal circulation. The end result is the lack of response to diuretics in the face of severely limited renal blood flow.

In the 1960's intermittent peritoneal dialysis (IPD) was reported to be useful in the treatment of volume overload in patients with cardiac disease. The dialysis effected rapid fluid removal (more than 7 litres on average). Diuretic responsiveness was reported to be restored in the majority of patients, presumably by the subsequent "unloading" of the heart, increased inotropy and hence improved renal blood flow. Because the dialysis ultrafiltrate is hypotonic to plasma, the hyponatremia in these patients was corrected by the removal of water in excess of salt. It was postulate that peritoneal dialysis could be used in the treatment of refractory congestive heart failure in patients with concomitant renal disease, severe hyponatremia, or for the optimization of a patient prior to cardiac surgery [42]. This method was also successful in treating severe cardiac failure in babies and children with congenital heart disease. Although the improvement was transient, it enabled the infants and children with correctable lesions to undergo cardiac surgery [43]. Other reports of the use of IPD confirmed its usefulness in severe heart failure. Dilution studies confirmed that salt and water removal led to an increased cardiac index. The majority of patients treated in this manner entered remission and some were able to undergo corrective cardiac surgery such as valve replacement [44]. IPD was used in the setting of acute myocardial infarction with subsequent severe cardiac failure and was again found to be effective in fluid removal and correction of electrolyte abnormalities. It was suggested that peritoneal dialysis could be used to tide a patient over this period until the myocardium was able to repair itself from the ischemic event [45].

In each of the above reports IPD was used transiently. The patients who had remediable disease were benefitted by the ultrafiltration and had opportunity to recover or undergo corrective surgery. Those without potential for improvement in their cardiac disease succumbed at some point after the dialysis. It became clear that for this kind of patient the only option to extend life in any real way would be to provide repeated dialysis. Subsequently a patient with severe arteriosclerotic heart disease and normal renal function was described who received repeated sessions of IPD every few months and who survived for 21 months after his initial presentation with anasarca and pulmonary edema [46].

A larger cohort of patients with refractory congestive heart failure who received repeated IPD was reported more than a decade later by Shapira et al. [47]. Ten patients with severe cardiac disease and baseline serum creatinine concentrations ranging between 2.7 and 7.1 mg/dL received up to 7 sessions of IPD. Between 4.5 and 15 litres was ultrafiltrated with each dialysis. These patients experienced improvement in their quality of life with relief of pulmonary edema or anasarca and a reduction in the frequency and length of hospitalization. Interestingly, a dramatic increase in urine output was noted after the completion of each dialysis, again presumably related to improve cardiac function and renal perfusion. Unfortunately, despite the implied improvement in overall quality of life (not formally examined), survival remained short because of the severity of the heart disease [47]. Similar results were seen in the patients reported by Weinrauch et al., who also noted that these patients didn't tolerate ultrafiltration by hemodialysis because of hypotension and angina, but were able to tolerate IPD somewhat better [48].

Continuous ambulatory peritoneal dialysis (CAPD) was used in three patients with intractable congestive heart failure. Once again the dialysis effected an almost 10 kilogram weight loss with marked improvement in symptoms. However, recurrent peritonitis precluded continuation of CAPD, and all three patients died shortly after discontinuing dialysis [49].

Despite this disappointing initial report, it was clear that CAPD, given is continuous nature, would be more suitable than IPD for the treatment of heart failure. With IPD there is the opportunity for reaccumulation of salt and water, and hence interdialytic weight gain. Furthermore, the rapid ultrafiltration which must occur during the IPD poses the risk of hypotension and unwanted electrolyte fluxes.

The optimism for CAPD was borne out by the report of a patient with severe ischemic cardiomyopathy, serum creatinine of 2.4 mg/dL and volume overload uncontrolled by diuretics who was placed on CAPD, 2 to 3 exchanges daily, and was maintained successfully on this treatment for two years despite an ejection fraction of just 14% [50]. Subsequent reports demonstrated that CAPD was successful in maintaining euvolemia for months to years in patients with severe cardiac disease with or without renal impairment [51–55]. As a result of controlling hypervolemia, long-term CAPD led to improvement in cardiac function in some patients [51, 52, 55].

Other benefits noted included improved renal function. Shilo *et al.* noted an almost fourfold increase in renal plasma flow as measured by PAH clearance, and doubling of the creatinine and inulin clearance [53]. Presumably the improved renal perfusion was the result of increased left ventricular function. Coincident with correction of hypervolemia there is an appropriate fall in plasma concentration of atrial natriuretic factor (ANF) and, in addition, the increased renal perfusion leads to a dramatic fall in plasma renin concentration and aldosterone levels [55]. (Table 2)

The prognosis for these patients, however, must remain guarded. If the cardiac condition is not operable or self-limited, these patients are at risk for early cardiac death. In one study 16 to 19 patients died of sudden death, probably the result of ventricular arrhythmias [54]. In Rubin's report overall median survival was less than one year, and the patients were hospitalized as often for dialysis-related problems as they had been before dialysis for cardiac-related problems [52].

In summary, CAPD can be useful in the management of intractable congestive heart failure which has become unresponsive to drug therapy. Peritoneal dialysis is very effective in controlling salt and water overload and in correcting the hyponatremia so frequently found in these patients. With the attendant ultrafiltration, there have been reports of improved cardiac function, increased renal perfusion and renewed responsiveness to diuretics. In the occasional patient there has been a remarkable prolongation of life, and in patients with transient cardiac dysfunction intervention with ultrafiltration can be lifesaving. Overall, however, most patients are still left with very severe cardiac disease and have a poor prognosis.

Table 2. The effect of CAPD on patients with congestive heart failure.

Konig et al., Advances in Peritoneal Dialysis, 1991

PARAMETER	BEFORE CAPD	AFTER 1.5–32 MOS CAPD
Systolic BP	82	122
Diastolic BP	55	72
Serum ANF (ng/L)	1253	295
Renin (pg/mL)	12730	3800
Aldosterone (ng/dL)	35	13
Na (mmol/L)	126	136

3.2. Inborn errors of metabolism

The Inborn errors of metabolism comprise a large and diverse group of diseases wherein there is often a missing intermediary step or enzyme abnormality leading to a block in the normal degradative pathways of metabolism. Such a block leads to the accumulation of precursors which can cause toxic manifestation, often in the neonatal period. Current therapy revolves around the recognition of the disorder, the rapid removal of the accumulated toxic metabolites, dietary modification and vitamin supplementation [56].

Given the small molecular weight of the products to be cleared, dialysis has become important in the urgent removal of these toxic metabolites in the neonatal period.

3.2.1. *Urea cycle defects and neonatal hyperammonemia*

In the hepatic urea cycle, several enzymes are involved in the metabolism of ammonia to urea. Deficiency of any of these enzymes can lead to a marked accumulation of ammonia in the blood which manifests as neurologic changes up to and including coma and death [56]. The mainstay of the treatment of this neonatal emergency is the rapid removal of ammonia.

The clearance of ammonia by hemodialysis and peritoneal dialysis has been compared by several investigators, and in each case the clearance by hemodialysis was approximately 10-fold that achieved by peritoneal dialysis [57–59]. Since the goal of treatment is to lower plasma ammonia levels as quickly as possible, it would seem prudent to use hemodialysis, if available, as the first line of therapy. As suggested by Wiegand et al., peritoneal dialysis may be useful adjunctive therapy once the ammonia levels have been lowered and dietary therapy is being introduced [58]. In a baby with deficiency of the urea cycle enzyme ornithine transcarbamylase (OCT), treatment with rapid peritoneal dialysis alone did not lower blood ammonia levels and the baby died [60]. A recent report suggests that the combination of peritoneal dialysis and venovenous hemofiltration can effectively reduce ammonia to safe levels [61].

3.2.2. *Organic acidemias*

Deficiency of a degradative enzyme leads to accumulation of organic acids with a number of deleterious consequences, including metabolic acidosis, elevated ammonia levels, and, clinically, failure to thrive, poor feeding, vomiting, lethargy and coma [56]. Absent proprionyl-CoA-carboxylase activity leads to proprionic acidemia. Clinical outcome appears to be related to the plasma proprionic acid concentration. Russell et al. described acute peritoneal dialysis to reduce plasma levels of proprionic acid; during the first six hours of peritoneal dialysis the blood levels deceased from 5.22 mmol/L to 0.66 mmol/L. Although the patient was being treated for sepsis simultaneously, the finding of proprionic acid in the dialysis fluid suggested that improvement was in large part due to the removal of the acid by dialysis [62]. Subsequent reports have confirmed the effectiveness of peritoneal dialysis in the treatment of proprionic acidemia, with [63] or without [64, 65] accompanying exchange transfusion.

Deficiency of the methylmalonyl-CoA mutase apoenzyme leads to methylmalonic acidemia. The combination of acute peritoneal dialysis and exchange transfusion proved lifesaving in a neonate with this condition, who unfortunately succumbed soon after from sepsis [66]. Another 2 1/2 year old child with methylmalonic acidemia who was failing to thrive was placed on CAPD, 6 exchanges daily, to remove methylmalonate and control metabolic acidosis. The patient experienced a remarkable improvement, both clinically and biochemically, despite a number of dialysis-related complications [67].

3.2.3. *Disorders of amino acid metabolism*
Perhaps the most well-known of these disorders is maple syrup urine disease (MSUD), so named because of the distinct odor of the urine. Infants with this condition present with feeding problems and neurologic deterioration. The mechanism of the toxicity is unknown but an abnormality in myelin formation has been noted [68].

The biochemical defect is a block in the decarboxylation of the ketoacids of branched chain amino acids (BCAA). Because of this block, there is accumulation of the branched chain amino acids (leucine, isoleucine, valine) and their ketoacids. Again the goal of treatment has rested in part in removing the retained metabolites and in inducing anabolism, but with foods deficient in branched chain amino acids.

Sallan et al. [69] reported treating an infant with MSUD with 100 hours of IPD, along with high calorie feeding by the intravenous and nasogastric routes. There was a gratifying reduction in blood and CSF BCAA levels, and the peritoneal clearance of leucine was similar to that of creatinine. The authors concluded that peritoneal dialysis was more effective than repeated exchange transfusions for the urgent treatment of MSUD. Subsequent studies have revealed that hemodialysis results in a 7–10 fold increase in the clearance of BCAA and their ketoanalogues compared to peritoneal dialysis [59].

However, as noted by McMahon and MacDonnell [68], hemodialysis and exchange transfusions are difficult, labor-intensive procedures carrying the risk of septicemia and hypotension. Moreover, feeding, which is a crucial part of treatment, often must be suspended during these procedures. On the other hand, peritoneal dialysis leads to a steady reduction of BCAA levels while allowing for the feeding of the infant. This has been confirmed by reports of rapid reduction in plasma levels of BCAA with PD alone [65, 68]. Followup of patients with MSUD treated with peritoneal dialysis, in addition to parenteral and intestinal alimentation, has revealed normal somatic and intellectual development [70].

3.2.4. *Disorders of carbohydrate metabolism*
A 42 year old woman with glucose-6-phosphatase deficiency (von Gierke disease) and renal failure was treated with CAPD. The use of hypertonic high-glucose solution overnight was able to prevent the nocturnal hypoglycemia seen in this glycogen storage disease [71].

3.3. Acute pancreatitis

Acute inflammation of the pancreas leads to the elaboration of a number of potentially toxic substances from this organ into the peritoneal cavity. It is probable that these compounds are absorbed into the systemic circulation where they contribute to the serious complications seen in severe pancreatitis, such as hypotension and noncardiogenic pulmonary edema. Suggested mediators produced by the inflamed pancreas include histamine, lipase, trypsin, kallikrein, kinins, and prostaglandins [72].

Lavage of the peritoneal cavity with dialysate or some other physiologic fluid would seem to be an effective method to clear the potentially harmful mediators before they are absorbed. In 1965 Wall required that the institution of peritoneal dialysis for renal failure in three patients with acute pancreatitis led to rapid improvement in their overall status [73].

Subsequent animal studies suggested that peritoneal lavage conferred benefit in experimental acute pancreatitis. In dogs with pancreatitis induced by the injection of trypsin and taurocholate into the pancreatic duct, intervention with peritoneal dialysis for 6 hours led to a marked reduction of short term mortality, and histologically, by decreased fat necrosis and pancreatic hemorrhage and necrosis [74]. More than two decades later similar results were obtained in dogs with pancreatitis induced by retrograde injection of bile and trypsin into the pancreatic duct. The survival rate was higher in dogs receiving peritoneal lavage and higher still in dogs lavaged with aprotinin, an inhibitor of trypsin, in the dialysis fluid. As in the first study, a marked reduction in necrotizing and hemorrhagic lesions were seen historically [75]. Subsequent experimental work in rats also gave encouraging results [76, 77, 78].

In 1976, Ranson et al. randomized 10 patients with acute pancreatitis of mixed etiology into 2 groups of equal severity. Five patients received peritoneal dialysis with dialysate containing potassium, heparin and ampicillin for 48 to 96 hours. Five patients received the usual supportive care. In the group receiving peritoneal dialysis, the duration of stay in the intensive care unit was half that of those receiving conventional treatment. In addition, oral intake was resumed more quickly and the duration of hospitalization shorter in the dialyzed group [79]. However, after more experience with peritoneal lavage, they observed that while peritoneal dialysis lead to a striking early improvement, there was no difference in overall mortality between the two groups. The later deaths in the dialyzed patients were due to sepsis, particularly pancreatic abscesses [80]. To address the problem of late sepsis, Ransom and Berman [81] randomized 29 patients presenting with acute pancreatitis to peritoneal lavage for 2 days or for 7 days. Once again ampicillin was added to the dialysate. The longer lavage reduced the frequency of sepsis and death from sepsis. In the subgroup of patients with many signs of poor prognosis, lavage for 7 days was associated with no deaths from sepsis compared to a 54% death rate in those receiving the 2 day lavage. There were small numbers, however, and it is interesting to note that the overall mortality in both groups was similar, with 3 deaths out of 15 patients receiving the short lavage, and 2 deaths (neither due to abscess) out of 14 in those receiving lavage for 7 days. The authors postulated that the longer dialysis is more effective because the inflamed pancreas continues to secrete enzymes and other harmful mediators for many days [81]. A trial of peritoneal dialysis in acute alcoholic pancreatitis by Stone and Fabian noted a greater frequency of early improvement and lower mortality compared to those patients who received supportive care only [82].

Another important study led to a different conclusion. A large multicentre randomized study [83] of 3 days of peritoneal dialysis showed no difference in outcome in the 45 patients who received dialysis compared to the control group of 46 patients who received maximum supportive care. There were 13 deaths (28%) in the control group and 12 deaths (27%) in the lavage group. Furthermore, lavage did not change the length of survival nor the incidence of pseudocyst nor abscesses. (It is interesting to note that the lavage group lost a median of 44 g of protein daily in the dialysate.) Criticism of the study include the fact that the median time to the start of dialysis was too long at 38 hours, longer than the previous studies discussed above. The authors, however, suggest that the transperitoneal route of absorption of pancreatic toxins may not be as important as other routes, such as the lymphatics and pancreatic veins and so peritoneal lavage is not that crucial to treatment [83].

In summary, there is a good physiologic and experimental basis to support using peritoneal dialysis in severe acute pancreatitis. On the other hand, the human data have not convincingly demonstrated reduced overall mortality in those receiving peritoneal lavage. Probably this is related to the multisystem deterioration that accompanies severe acute pancreatitis; these patients are so ill that any one intervention may be unlikely to change overall outcome. Still, the treatment options are so limited in this devastating condition that a recent review on the management of acute pancreatitis still recommends peritoneal dialysis for patients with severe pancreatitis who fail to improve with intensive supportive care during the first 24 to 48 hours [84].

3.3.1. *Other surgical indications*

A patient has been reported with chyloperitoneum associated with alcoholic pancreatitis. In addition to supportive measures, the patient underwent peritoneal dialysis with rapid improvement in abdominal pain and overall condition [85]. Peritoneal dialysis has also been successful in the management of traumatic hemoperitoneum [86] and to temporize in patients with perforated gastroduodenal ulcers [87].

3.4. Psoriasis

The chance observations that psoriasis improved with both hemodialysis [88] and peritoneal dialysis [89] led Twardowski and colleagues to try peritoneal dialysis in non uremic patients with severe forms of this skin disease [90]. Of the three patients, two experienced rapid improvement with almost complete resolution of the skin manifestations. Dialysis did not effect improvement in the third, who had pustular psoriasis. However, as the authors pointed out, the study was uncontrolled and spontaneous remissions are seen in this disease.

Since these original observations, there have been numerous reports on the effects of peritoneal dialysis on the natural history of psoriasis. Given the bias for reporting only positive results, it is perhaps not surprising that the majority of reports are of patients improving on dialysis [91–98]. Moreover, peritoneal dialysis appeared to be more effective than hemodialysis in this respect [91, 97–99].

As emphasized by Kramer *et al.* [94], however, there are pitfalls in the interpretation of these studies. The ability of psychological factors to lead to improvement in psoriasis has been demonstrated [100]. Therefore the institution of dialysis may lead to remission by a "placebo effect" rather than by removal of pro-psoriatic factors in the dialysate. In addition, if the treating physician truly believes the dialysis will be effective, the results could be misinterpreted. Finally, if the followup period is too short the relapse rate may be underestimated.

However, the study by Whittier *et al.* presented cogent evidence that peritoneal dialysis led to real improvement in severe intractable plaque-type psoriasis [95]. In random order, patients received 48 hours of sham or real peritoneal dialysis weekly for four weeks. This was followed by a 2 month observation period after which the patient then received the alternative dialysis (sham or real peritoneal dialysis) for 4 weeks, followed by another 2 month period of observation. Four of the five patients had a striking response to real peritoneal dialysis whereas none of the patients had improvement with the sham procedure. The results strongly suggested that peritoneal dialysis is effective in altering the natural course of psoriatic skin disease. The authors recommended trying peritoneal dialysis in patients with other forms of treatment have failed.

If peritoneal dialysis does lead to improvement of psoriasis, the mechanism of the improvement is far from clear. How could the peritoneal cavity clear a factor(s) that the normally-functioning kidney couldn't? Suggested explanations are that the factors are large molecular weight or extensively protein-bound, and therefore unable to pass through the glomerular capillary bed, but able to enter the peritoneal cavity. In a related fashion, the factors may be rejected by electrostatic forces at the glomerular capillary wall. Finally, perhaps the factors are filtered, but completely reabsorbed by the renal tubules [102].

Glinski and colleagues [103] suggest that the improvement seen with peritoneal dialysis is the result of removing polymorphonuclear leukocytes (PMNL) from the peritoneal cavity. These cells contain higher than normal amounts of proteases capable of inducing destructive changes in the stratum corneum of the skin. In a study of 16 patients with psoriasis, there was a strong correlation between the number of PMNL removed by dialysis and the improvement in the skin disease. Content of the proteases in the PMNL was highest in the first few days of dialysis and fell thereafter. The authors speculated that the "activated" PMNL are replaced over time by nonstimulated PMNL with normal or reduced content of proteolytic enzymes [103] (Interestingly, Whittier *et al.* [95] could not find any correlation between the occurrence of peritonitis, with its high rate of neutrophilic exudation into the peritoneal cavity, and improvement of psoriasis). These investigators also found that leukopheresis had a beneficial effect in psoriasis similar to that of peritoneal dialysis, which is consonant with the hypothesis that the pro-psoriatic factor is contained within the PMNL [104].

Despite the flurry of favorable reports in the 1970's and 1980's, peritoneal dialysis has not found widespread use in the treatment of severe, resistant psoriasis. It is expensive treatment and requires the involvement of nephrologists and nephrology nurses. There is the ever-present risk of peritonitis and other complications. Koebner's phenomenon may occur at the exit site [97] which could predispose to infection. Finally, the results do not appear, for the most part, to be long-lasting, and reactivation of disease may occur soon after discontinuation of dialysis [93, 97]. Therefore, this treatment should be reserved for the very exceptional cases of disabling plaque-type psoriasis where no improvement is effected by the current armamentarium of topical and systemic medications.

3.5. Acute hepatic failure

The liver possesses the capacity to regenerate. Because of this, the goal of treatment of fulminant hepatic failure has been to support the patient and optimize his status until the liver can begin to heal. Unfortunately, the advent of coma as a result of hyperammonemia and other retained metabolites is a poor prognostic sign. Clinicians have attempted to remove the retained toxins by various methods to lessen the encephalopathy. Peritoneal dialysis has been said to be helpful in treating the coma resulting from liver failure.

In 1967, Krebs and Flynn [105] reported on reversal of hepatic coma in a young man with viral hepatitis who received exchange transfusion and peritoneal dialysis. The rationale for the concurrent use of dialysis was to aid in the removal of ammonia, not only that retained with liver failure but also that contained in the massive amount of old blood the patient received by transfusion. The authors were uncertain of the contribution of the dialysis to the patient's recovery. The use of dialysis in four patients (3 peritoneal, 1 hemodialysis) by Pirola et al. did not ameliorate hepatic coma [106].

A more optimistic report came from Mactier et al. [107] who used rapid exchange intermittent peritoneal dialysis in 5 patients with fulminant hepatic failure of diverse etiology. Four of the patients had concomitant renal failure. During the first period of IPD (up to 4 days) hepatic coma improved in 4 patients. Three of the patients recovered completely with normal hepatic and renal function as followup. The authors suggested that because the overall prognosis of combined hepatic and renal function is poor, the recovery seen in 3 of the 5 patients suggests that peritoneal dialysis indeed conferred a true benefit. The authors suggested that the results with IPD are comparable to those seen with hemoperfusion [107].

Perhaps the only real way to discern the effect of peritoneal dialysis would be by means of a controlled clinical trail. This, of course, would be very difficult to carry out, particularly with the advent of successful liver transplantation for fulminant hepatic failure.

However, if the patient is not a transplant candidate, or there are no organs available, peritoneal dialysis can prove helpful, particularly in the setting of associated renal failure. As suggested by Mactier [108], in contrast to charcoal hemoperfusion, peritoneal dialysis can treat the extracellular fluid volume overload and hyponatremia so often seen in this condition, remove uremic and perhaps hepatic toxins, treat hypoglycemia, and obviate the need for anticoagulation of an extracorporeal circuit.

3.6. Hypothermia and hyperthermia

In 1967, Lash et al. reported the use of peritoneal dialysis as a method of core rewarming in patients with accidental hypothermia [109]. The use of external rewarming (blankets, etc.) in the absence of a method of core rewarming is felt to be dangerous. The peripheral vasodilatation can lead to the shunting of cold peripheral blood to the core, producing further chilling of the heart and increasing the risk of serious arrhythmia. The vasodilatation of peripheral vessels with external rewarming can also contribute to hypovolemia by decreasing the circulating volume [110]. Dogs undergoing experimental hypothermia needed larger volumes of fluids and electrolytes when warmed externally compared to those who underwent core rewarming by cardiac bypass or peritoneal dialysis [111]. The setup for core rewarming by peritoneal dialysis is not difficult and should be available in most emergency units. As pointed out by Reuler et al. [110], an added advantage to peritoneal dialysis is the clearance of alcohol and some other drugs in those patients whose hypothermia is associated with an overdose of these substances.

There have been many reports of successful resuscitation from hypothermia with warmed peritoneal dialysis [112–114] even when the original core temperature at presentation has been as low as 16 C [112].

Given the ease of access to the peritoneal cavity as a conduit for alteration of core temperature, it is not surprising that cold peritoneal dialysis has been used in the hyperthermia associated with heat stroke [115] and meningococcal septicemia [116].

3.7. Poisoning

The clearance of small molecular weight substances depends on blood and dialysate flow rates. For the majority of ingested poisons, which are of low molecular weight, clearance of toxins is consistently higher with hemodialysis than peritoneal dialysis [117].

The reports documenting the effectiveness of peritoneal dialysis in the treatment of drug intoxication predate the widespread use of hemodialysis. Peritoneal dialysis proved beneficial in the treatment of salicylate poisoning [118] and barbiturate overdose [119] although the clearance of barbiturate is limited by its large volume of distribution [119]. Interestingly, the effectiveness of peritoneal dialysis reported in Reye's syndrome [120] may have actually been the result of clearing salicylate by dialysis, before the association between salicylates and Reye's syndrome was appreciated [121].

Other intoxications in which peritoneal dialysis has been used to increase clearance of the toxin are listed in Table 3.

There are perhaps some extraordinary circumstances where peritoneal dialysis might be more effective than extracorporeal dialysis. For example, the anticonvulsant phenytoin is highly protein-bound and therefore poorly dialyzable. However, a newborn with phenytoin poisoning was successfully treated by peritoneal dialysis. The authors suggested that the permeability of the newborns' peritoneum is so great that the protein-phenytoin complexes were able to be cleared from the peritoneal cavity [122]. Intraperitoneal EDTA has been reported in the treatment of lead intoxication, but the patient had end stage renal disease [123].

However, except in these unusual circumstances or when hemodialysis is not available, peritoneal dialysis should not be the treatment of choice for the management of poisoning. Hemodialysis affords higher small solute clearances which is important in the urgent treatment of intoxication.

3.8. Multiple myeloma

Although the causes of renal failure in multiple myeloma are diverse, the most frequent association is with "myeloma kidney". Histologically, there is deposition of immunoglobulin light chains in the tubules with surrounding inflammation. With progressive tubular damage, renal failure supervenes.

Immunoglobulin light chains, present in high concentration in plasma cell disorders, are tubulotoxic. What is not clear is whether the removal of large amounts of light chains, by plasmapheresis or peritoneal dialysis, is of benefit in reversing the renal failure of multiple myeloma. Although the total immunoglobulin has a molecular weight in the hundreds of thousands, depending on subtype, the light chain has a molecular weight of 22000 and so may be partially transported across the peritoneum.

Yium et al. [131] reported a 54 year old man with IgG lambda myeloma who responded clinically to IPD. He was uremic at presentation and improvement in his status could have resulted from the coincident treatment of sepsis and uremia. Moreover, he remained in renal failure. However, the first IPD session removed 22 g of IgG, and the second 72 g of IgG. For this quantity to be removed by plasmapheresis instead would have entailed the removal of unacceptably large volumes of plasma [131]. On the other hand, when light chain rather than the whole immunoglobulin was measured, Russell and colleagues found that one 5 litre plasma exchange removed 10 times as much Bence Jones protein as 50 hours' worth of peritoneal dialysis [132]. They concluded that plasma exchange was more efficient to remove light chains than peritoneal dialysis. Moreover, Rosansky and Richards reported that peritoneal dialysis removed just 104 mg of IgG per hour, which would extrapolate to about one tenth as much IgG removed by this method than that reported by Yiu. Plasmapheresis removed over 100 times as much IgG per hour as did peritoneal dialysis [133].

It remains controversial whether plasmapheresis has a role in the treatment of myeloma for reasons other than hyperviscosity, i.e. to remove light chains and so lessen the renal insult. Insofar as peritoneal dialysis may be even less effective in removing significant amounts of Bence Jones protein, it is doubtful that intervening with peritoneal dialysis for reasons other than uremia would benefit the patient with multiple myeloma.

Despite these concerns, there are some reports of patients with myeloma who improved after receiving peritoneal dialysis. In one patient CAPD was commenced to increase the light chain clearance. The patient's renal function improved and repeat renal biopsy showed amelioration of the tubulopathy. Chemotherapy was given concurrently and light chain clearance by peritoneal dialysis was not documented, and so the relationship of the PD to the improved kidney function remains tenuous

Table 3. Intoxications treated by peritoneal dialysis.

Salicylates [118]
Barbiturates [119]
Isopropyl Alcohol [124]
Potassium dichromate [125]
Bromates [126, 127]
Organophosphates [128, 129]
Carp gall bladder [130]
Lead [123]
Phenytoin [122]

[134]. Another patient with lambda light chain myeloma and renal failure was treated with CAPD. She refused chemotherapy but on dialysis alone experienced improvement in the hematologic parameters [135]. Finally, a review by Cosio et al. of their myeloma patients and those in the literature gave perhaps the most intriguing results: If the patients were divided into those who recovered renal function and those who remained on chronic renal replacement therapy, the absence of light chain disease and the use of peritoneal dialysis were both associated with increased recovery of renal function. In other words, patients treated with peritoneal dialysis recovery renal function more often than patients undergoing hemodialysis. As the authors note, however, the number of patients treated by peritoneal dialysis was small, and there may be a bias to reporting successful results [136].

While it is conceivable that peritoneal dialysis could lessen the burden of immunoglobulin light chains presented to the kidney, there is insufficient evidence to recommend its use in non uremic patients. In the patient with renal failure there may be an advantage to peritoneal dialysis over hemodialysis because of the greater clearance of immunoglobulin light and heavy chains with peritoneal dialysis. However, the role of light chain clearance, even by the more effective plasmapheresis, remains controversial, and it is well to remember that patients treated with hemodialysis have shown improved renal function also [137, 138].

3.9. Experimental uses for the peritoneal cavity: Total peritoneal nutrition and paracorporeal membrane oxygenation

3.9.1. *Total peritoneal nutrition*

When the gut is unable to support enteral feedings, total parental nutrition has served as a useful alternative. However, the administration of large amounts of carbohydrates, lipids, and amino acids via the venous system has a number of drawbacks, both from a nutritional/metabolic standpoint and from a mechanical perspective. The latter includes exit site infection, thrombosis and septicemia. Furthermore, these problems may be amplified in the pediatric population, where long term venous access may be troublesome.

Given the transport capabilities of the peritoneal cavity, it became clear that not only intraperitoneal glucose but amino acids [139, 140] and lipids [141] were transported across the peritoneal membrane. Preliminary studies have documented the absorption of amino acids from dialysis fluid. A potentially useful role for the peritoneal cavity would be to absorb all the nutrients necessary for total nutritional support, in the event that oral feedings or intravenous alimentation were not feasible.

Sprague-Dawley rats were given nothing per os but dialyzed for 7 days with a solution containing 10% dextrose and 2% amino acids, electrolytes, vitamins, trace elements, carnitine and choline [142]. They were compared to a cohort who underwent laparotomy and sham peritoneal dialysis setup but who were fed orally with the same amount of nutrients. The intraperitoneal feeding was found to support body weight and positive nitrogen balance. No hepatic steatosis developed in the animals fed intraperitoneally. The absorption of amino acid nitrogen and absorption of glucose from the peritoneal cavity averaged 95%.

The authors concluded that, even without data on lipid absorption, peritoneal dialysis represents an alternative route for nutritional support. The peritoneal cavity might be especially useful in patients with problems with venous access or in patients in whom large fluid loads directly into the vascular tree may pose difficulty, such as the patient with poor cardiac reserve. It remains to be seen if long term nutritional support, with or without lipids, can be maintained in humans by the use of peritoneal nutrition.

3.9.2. *Paracorporeal membrane oxygenation and removal of carbon dioxide*

In acute lung disease, such as noncardiogenic pulmonary edema, the maintenance of tissue oxidation is important for survival. There are a number of extracorporeal bypass-type membrane oxygenators that oxygenate the red cells and return them to the body. The peritoneal cavity has a large surface area with large splanchnic blood flow. If the peritoneal cavity could function as a paracorporeal membrane oxygenator, it would obviate the need for the extracorporeal circuit or the attendant complex technology.

New Zealand white rabbits were intubated and ventilated with a high nitrous oxide, low oxygen-containing gas to simulate severe hypoxia [143]. Two peritoneal catheters were inserted. Dialysate was bubbled with 100% O_2 and dialysis was carried out in this manner. The peritoneal oxygenation resulted in augmentation of PO_2 to very satisfactory levels. No gas trapping or surgical emphysema was noted. In addition, CO_2 was adequately removed by the dialysate. The authors concluded that peritoneal oxygenation is capable of augmenting oxygenation and carbon dioxide removal in the critically ill patient with acute respiratory failure [143].

In a different model, the peritoneal cavity was simulated by a bubble oxygenator into which 10% CO_2 was added. The rate of CO_2 removal was a linear function of dialysate flow rate, gas flow rate, and concentration of bicarbonate. This model removed 60 ml/min of CO_2, which represents 30% of CO_2 production, a rate predicted to be able to treat hypercapnea associated with acute respiratory failure [144]. It is hoped that further animal studies will be forthcoming on the potential cavity as a gas exchange organ.

References

1. Registration Committee of the European Dialysis and Transplant Association. Successful pregnancies in women treated by dialysis and kidney transplantation. Br Journal Obstet Gynecol 1990; 87: 839–45.
2. Hou S. Peritoneal dialysis and hemodialysis in pregnancy. Baillieres Clin Obstet and Gynecol 1987; 1: 1009–25.
3. Hou S. Pregnancy in women requiring dialysis for renal failure. Am J Kid Dis 1987; 9(4): 368–73.
4. Lavoie SD, Jonson-Whittaker L, Huard PJ et al. Two successful pregnancies on CAPD. Advances Perit Dial 1988; 4: 90–5.
5. Hou S. Pregnancy in Continuous Ambulatory Peritoneal Dialysis (CAPD) patients. Perit Dial Int 1990; 10: 201–4.
6. Redav M, Cherem L, Eliot J et al. Dialysis in the management of pregnant patients with renal insufficiency. Medicine 1988; 67: 199.
7. Gadallah MF, Ahmad B, Karubian F et al. Pregnancy in patients on chronic ambulatory peritoneal dialysis. Am J Dis 1992; 20(4): 407–10.
8. Hou S, Orlowski J, Pahl M et al. Pregnancy in women with end-stage renal disease: treatment of anemia and premature labor. Am J Kid Dis 1993; 21(1): 16–22.
9. Nagiotte MP, Grundg HO. Pregnancy outcome in women requiring chronic hemodialysis. Obstet Gynecol 1988; 72: 456–9.
10. Barri YM, Al Furayh O, Quinibi WY et al. Pregnancy in women on regular hemodialysis. Dial Transplant 1991; 20: 652–6.
11. Fujimi S, Hori K, Mujemd C et al. Successful pregnancy and delivery in a patient following rHuEPO therapy and on long-term dialysis. J Am Soc Nephro (abstract) 1990; 1: 397.
12. Rao TK, Friedman EA, Nicastri AD. The types of renal disease in the acquired immunodeficiency syndrome. N Eng J Med 1987; 316: 1062–8.
13. Gardenswartz MH, Lerau CW, Seligson AR et al. Renal disease in patients with AIDS: a clinicopathological study. Clin Nephro 1984; 21: 197–204.
14. Cruz C, Kaul R, Markowitz N. Dialysis options for HIV infected patients. Perit Dial Int 1989; 9 (suppl 1): 89.
15. Graham MM, Bonini LA, Verdi MM. A multicenter study: clinical practices of HIV infected patients on CAPD/CCPD. Advances Perit Dial 1990; 6: 88–91.
16. Wasser WG, Beryl MJ, Brandons et al. HIV positively does not predispose peritoneal dialysis patients to peritonitis. J Am Soc Neph 1991; 2: 369–73.
17. Schloth T, Genabe I, Pilgrim W et al. Peritonitis and the patient with human immunodeficiency virus (HIV). Advances Perit Dial 1992; 8: 250–2.
18. Teblin JA, Rigsby M, Kliger A et al. Outcome of HIV infected patients on continuous peritoneal dialysis. (Abstract) Perit Dial Int 1993; 13 (suppl 1): S35.
19. Wasser WG, Bajl MJ, Brandon S et al. HIV positively does not predispose peritoneal dialysis patients to peritonitis. Perit Dial Int (abstract) 1993; 13 (suppl 1): S88.
20. Centre for Disease Control. Recommendations for providing dialysis treatment for patients infected with Human-T-Lymphotrophics Virus Type III/Lymphadenopathy related virus. Ann Int Med 1986; 106: 558–9.
21. MMWR. Recommendations for Prevention of HIV Transmission in Health Care Settings. Aug 21 1987; 36(25): 25–185.
22. Lewis M, Gorban-Brennan NL, Kliger A et al. Incidence and spectrum of organisms causing peritonitis in HIV positive patients on CAPD. Adv in CAPD 1990; 6: 136–8.
23. Drissler R, Peters AT, Lynn RI. Pseudomonal and candidal peritonitis as a complication of continuous ambulatory peritoneal dialysis in human immunodeficiency virus-infected patients. Am J Med 1989; 86: 787–90.
24. Wilkinson SP, Weston MJ, Parsons V et al. Dialysis in the treatment of renal failure in patients with liver disease. Clin Neph 1977; 8: 287–92.
25. Marcus RG, Messana J, Swartz R. Peritoneal dialysis in end-stage renal disease patients with preexisting chronic liver disease and ascites. Am J Med 1992; 93: 35–40.
26. Durand PY, Friedd P, Chanleau J et al. Long term follow up in cirrhotic patients with chronic renal failure undergoing CAPD. Perit Dial Int (abstract) 1993; 13 (suppl 1): S47.
27. Horie M, Kobayashi S, Nezassa S et al. A case report of hepatic cirrhosis with ascites and uremia treated by CAPD. Perit Dial Int (abstract) 1993; 13 (suppl 1): S73.
28. Dadone C, Pincella G, Bonoldi G et al. Transport of water and solutes in uremic patients with chronic hepatic disease in CAPD. Advances Perit Dial 1990; 6: 23–5.

29. Steiner RW. Continuous equilibration peritoneal dialysis in acute renal failure. Perit Dial Int 1989; 9: 5–7.
30. Cameron JS, Ogg CH, Trounce JR. Peritoneal dialysis in hypercatabolic acute renal failure. Lancet 1967; 1: 1188–91.
31. Posen GA, Luisello J. Continuous equilibration peritoneal dialysis in the treatment of acute renal failure. Perit Dial Bull 1981; 1: 6.
32. Katirtzoglous A, Kontesis P, Myopoulou-Symvoulidis D et al. Continuous equilibration peritoneal dialysis (CEPD) in hypercatabolic renal failure. Perit Dial Bull 1983; 3: 178–80.
33. Trevino-Becerra A, Munoz P, Avilez C et al. Equilibrium peritoneal dialysis (EPD) in acute renal failure (ARF) secondary to rhabdomyolysis (sic). Perit Dial Bull 1987; 7: 244–6.
34. Siemons L, van den Heuvel P, Parizel G et al. Peritoneal dialysis in acute renal failure due to cholesterol embolization: two cases of recovery of renal function and extended survival. Clin Nephrol 1987; 28: 205–8.
35. Nolph KD. Peritoneal dialysis for acute renal failure. Trans Am Soc Artif Intern Organs 1988; 34: 54–5.
36. Oreopoulos DR, Marliss E, Anderson GH et al. Nutritional aspects of CAPD and the potential use of amino acid containing dialysis solutions. Perit Dial Bull 1983; 3: S10–2.
37. Hamilton JW, Lasrich M, Hergil P. Peritoneal dialysis in the treatment of severe hypercalcemia. J Dial 1980; 4: 129–35.
38. Heyburn PJ, Selby PL, Peacock M et al. Peritoneal dialysis in the management of severe hypercalcemia. Br Med J 1980; 280: 525–6.
39. Querfel U, Salusky IB, Fine RN. Treatment of severe hypercalcemia with peritoneal dialysis in an infant with end-stage renal disease. Pediatr Nephrol 1988; 2: 323–5.
40. Thompson TJ, Neale TI. Intraperitoneal calcium for resistant symptomatic hypocalcaemia after parathyroidectomy in chronic renal failure. Br Med J 1988; 296: 896–7.
41. Benz RL, Schleifer CR, Teehan BP et al. Successful treatment of postparathyroidectomy hypocalcemia using continuous ambulatory intraperitoneal calcium (CAIC) therapy. Perit Dial Int 1989; 9: 285–8.
42. Mailloux LU, Swartz CD, Onesti G et al. Peritoneal dialysis for refractory congestive heart failure. JAMA 1967; 199(12): 873–8.
43. Nora JJ, Trygstad CW, Mangos JA et al. Peritoneal dialysis in the treatment of intractable congestive heart failure of infancy and childhood. J Pediatr 1966; 68(5): 693–8.
44. Cairns KB, Porter GA, Kloster FE et al. Clinical and hemodynamic results of peritoneal dialysis for severe cardiac failure. Am Heart J 1968; 76(2): 227–34.
45. Malach M. Peritoneal dialysis for intractable heart failure in acute myocardial infarction. Am J Cardiol 1972; 29: 61–3.
46. Raja RM, Kransoff SO, Moros JG et al. Repeated peritoneal dialysis in treatment of heart failure. JAMA 1970; 213(13): 2268–9.
47. Shapira J, Lang R, Jutrin I et al. Peritoneal dialysis in refractory congestive heart failure. Part I: intermittent peritoneal dialysis (IPD). Perit Dial Bull 1983: 130–2.
48. Weinrauch LA, Kaldany A, Miller DG et al. Cardiorenal failure: treatment of refractory biventricular failure by peritoneal dialysis. Uremia Invest 1984; 8(1): 1–8.
49. Robson M, Biro A, Knobel B et al. Peritoneal dialysis in refractory congestive heart failure. Part II: continuous ambulatory peritoneal dialysis (CAPD). Perit Dial Bull 1983: 133–4.
50. McKinnie JJ, Bourgeois RJ, Husserl FE. Long-term therapy for heart failure with continuous ambulatory peritoneal dialysis. Arch Intern Med 1985; 145: 1128–9.
51. Kim D, Khanna R, Wu G et al. Successful use of continuous ambulatory peritoneal dialysis in refractory heart failure. Perit Dial Bull 1985: 127–30.
52. Rubin J, Ball R. Continuous ambulatory peritoneal dialysis as treatment of severe congestive heart failure in the face of chronic renal failure. Arch Intern Med 1986; 146: 1533–5.
53. Shilo S, Slotki IN, Iaina A. Improved renal function following acute peritoneal dialysis in patients with intractable congestive heart failure. Isr J Med Sci 1987; 23(7): 821–4.
54. Mousson C, Tanter Y, Chalopin JM et al. Treatment of refractory congestive cardiac insufficiency by continuous ambulatory peritoneal dialysis. Long-term course. Presse Med 1988; 17(32): 1617–20.
55. Konig PS, Lhotta K, Kronenberg F et al. CAPD: a successful treatment in patients suffering from therapy-resistant congestive heart failure. In: Khanna R, Nolph KD, Prowant BF, Twardowski ZJ, Oreopoulos DG (eds), Advances in Peritoneal Dialysis. Perit Dial Bull Inc, Toronto 1991; 7: 97–101.
56. Burton BK. Inborn errors of metabolism: the clinical diagnosis in early infancy. Pediatr 1987; 79(3): 359–69.
57. Donn SM, Swartz RD, Thoene JG. Comparison of exchange transfusion, peritoneal dialysis and hemodialysis for the treatment of hyperammonemia in an anuric newborn infant. J Pediatr 1979; 95(1): 67–70.
58. Wiegand C, Thompson T, Bock GH et al. The management of life-threatening hyperammonemia: a comparison of several therapeutic modalities. J Pediatr 1980; 96(1): 142–4.
59. Rutledge SL, Havens PL, Haymond MW et al. Neonatal hemodialysis: effective therapy for the encephalopathy of inborn errors of metabolism. J Pediatr 1990; 116(1): 125–8.
60. Siegel NJ, Brown RS. Peritoneal clearance of ammonia and creatinine in a neonate. J Pediatr 1973; 82(6): 1044–6.
61. Lettgen B, Bonzel KE, Colombo JP et al. Therapy of hyperammonemia in carbamyl phosphate synthase deficiency with peritoneal dialysis and

venovenous hemofiltration. Monatsschr Kinderheilkd 1991; 139(9): 612–7.
62. Russell G, Thom H, Tarlow MJ et al. Reduction of plasma propionate by peritoneal dialysis. Pediatr 1974; 53(2): 281–3.
63. Hsu WC, Lin SP, Huang FY et al. Propionic acidemia: report of a case that is successfully managed by peritoneal dialysis and sodium benzoate therapy. Chin Med J 1990; 46(5): 306–10.
64. Robert MF, Schultz DJ, Wolf B et al. Treatment of a neonate with propionic acidemia and severe hyperammonemia by peritoneal dialysis. Arch Dis Child 1979; 54(12): 962–5.
65. Gortner L, Leupold D, Pohlandt F et al. Peritoneal dialysis in the treatment of metabolic crises caused by inherited disorders of organic and amino acid metabolism. Acta Paed Scand 1989; 78(5): 706–11.
66. Sanjurjo P, Jaquotot C, Vallo A et al. Combined exchange transfusion and peritoneal dialysis treatment in a neonatal case of methylmalonic acidemia with severe hyperammonemia. An Esp Pediatr 1982; 17(4): 317–20.
67. Moreno-Vega A, Govantes JM. Methylmalonic acidemia treated by continuous ambulatory peritoneal dialysis. (Letter) N Engl J Med 1985; 312(25): 1641–2.
68. McMahon Y, MacDonnell RC Jr. Clearance of branched chain amino acids by peritoneal dialysis in maple syrup urine disease. In: Khanna R, Nolph KD, Prowant BF, Twardowski ZJ, Oreopoulos DG (eds), Advances in Peritoneal Dialysis. Perit Dial Bull Inc, Toronto 1990; 6: 31–4.
69. Sallan SE, Cottom D. Peritoneal dialysis in maple syrup urine disease. Lancet 1969; 635(2): 1423–4.
70. Clow CL, Reade TM, Scriver CR. Outcome of early and long-term management of classical maple syrup urine disease. Pediatr 1981; 68(6): 856–62.
71. Vandepitte K, Lins RL, Daelemans R et al. Continuous ambulatory peritoneal dialysis (CAPD) in a patient with glucose-6-phosphatase deficiency. Perit Dial Int 1989; 9(2): 111–4.
72. Lankisch PG, Koop H, Winckler K et al. Continuous peritoneal dialysis as treatment of acute experimental pancreatitis in the rat. II: analysis of its beneficial effect. Dig Dis Sci 1979; 24(2): 117–22.
73. Wall AJ. Peritoneal dialysis in the treatment of severe acute pancreatitis. Med J Aust 1965; 2(7): 281–3.
74. Rasmussen BL. Hypothermic peritoneal dialysis in the treatment of acute experimental hemorrhagic pancreatitis. Am J Surg 1967; 114(5): 716–21.
75. Bassi C, Briani G, Vesentini S et al. Continuous peritoneal dialysis in acute experimental pancreatitis in dogs. Effect of aprotinin in the dialysate medium. Int J Pancreatol 1989; 5(1): 69–75.
76. Lankisch PG, Koop H, Winckler K et al. Continuous peritoneal dialysis as treatment of acute experimental pancreatitis in the rat. I: effect on length and rate of survival. Dig Dis Sci 1979; 24(2): 111–6.
77. Tilquin BM, O'Connor TC, Hancotte-LaHaye CM et al. The effect of peritoneal dialysis with and without aprotinin on acute experimental pancreatitis in rats. Int Surg 1990; 75(3): 174–8.
78. Fric P, Slaby J, Kosafirek E et al. Effective peritoneal therapy of acute pancreatitis in the rat with glutaryl-trialanin-ethylamide: a novel inhibitor of pancreatic elastase. Gut 1992; 33: 701–6.
79. Ranson JHC, Rifkind KM, Turner JW. Prognostic signs and nonoperative peritoneal lavage in acute pancreatitis. Surg Gynecol Obstet 1976; 143: 209–19.
80. Ranson JHC, Spencer FC. The role of peritoneal lavage in severe acute pancreatitis. Ann Surg 1978; 187: 565–75.
81. Ranson JHC, Berman RS. Long peritoneal lavage decreases sepsis in acute pancreatitis. Ann Surg 1990; 211(6): 708–18.
82. Stone HH, Fabian TC. Peritoneal dialysis in the treatment of acute alcoholic pancreatitis. Surg Gynecol Obstet 1980; 150(6): 878–82.
83. Mayer AD, McMahon MJ, Corfield AP et al. Controlled clinical trial of peritoneal lavage for the treatment of severe acute pancreatitis. NEJM 1985; 312(7): 399–404.
84. Crist DW, Cameron JL. The current management of acute pancreatitis. Adv Surg 1987; 20: 69–123.
85. Goldfarb JP. Chylous effusions secondary to pancreatitis: case report and review of the literature. Am J Gastroenterol 1984; 79(2): 133–5.
86. Moncade F, Fortier A, Guyon P et al. Peritoneal puncture dialysis in the monitoring and treatment of hemoperitoneum of traumatic origin? J Chir 1991; 128(6–7): 285–9.
87. Delaitre B, Attailia A, Chihaoui M. Perforated gastroduodenal ulcers. Treatment by peritoneal dialysis. 72 cases. Presse Med 1988; 17(25): 1297–300.
88. McEvoy J, Kelly AMT. Psoriatic clearance during hemodialysis. Ulster Med J 1976; 45: 76–8.
89. Twardowski ZJ. Abatement of psoriasis and repeated dialysis. Ann Intern Med (letter) 1977; 86: 509–10.
90. Twardowski ZJ, Nolph KD, Rubin J et al. Peritoneal dialysis for psoriasis. An uncontrolled study. Ann Intern Med 1978; 88(3): 345–51.
91. Hanicki Z, Cichocki T, Klein A et al. Dialysis for psoriasis-preliminary remarks concerning mode of action. Arch Dermatol Res 1981; 271(4): 401–5.
92. Goring HD, Thieler H, Guldner G et al. Peritoneal dialysis therapy in psoriasis. Hautarzt 1981; 32(4): 173–8.
93. Halevy S, Halevy J, Boner G et al. Dialysis therapy for psoriasis. Report of three cases and review of the literature. Arch Dermatol 1981; 117(2): 69–72.
94. Kramer P, Brunner FP, Brynger H et al. Dialysis treatment and psoriasis in Europe. Clin Neph 1982; 18(2): 62–8.
95. Whittier FC, Evans DH, Anderson PC et al. Peritoneal dialysis for psoriasis: a controlled study. Ann Intern Med 1983; 99(2): 165–8.
96. Glinski W, Jablonska S, Imiela J et al. Peritoneal

dialysis and leukopheresis in psoriasis: indications and contraindications. Hautarzt 1985; 36(1): 16–9.
97. Twardowski ZJ, Lempert KD, Lankhorst BJ et al. Continuous ambulatory peritoneal dialysis for psoriasis. A report of four cases. Arch Inter Med 1986; 146(6): 1177–9.
98. Sobh MA, Abdel Rasik MM, Moustafa FE et al. Dialysis therapy of severe psoriasis: a random study of forty cases. Nephrol Dial Transplant 1987; 2(5): 351–8.
99. Nissenson AR, Rapaport M, Gordon A et al. Hemodialysis in the treatment of psoriasis: a controlled trial. Ann Intern M ed 1979; 91: 218–20.
100. Goldsmith LA, Fisher M, Wacks J. Psychological characteristics of psoriasis: implications for management. Arch Dermatol 1969; 100: 674.
101. Anderson PC. Dialysis treatment of psoriasis. (Editorial) Arch Dermatol 1981; 117: 67–8.
102. Chen WT, Hu CH, Schiltz JR et al. In search of "psoriasis factor(s)": a new approach by extracorporeal treatment. Artif Organs 1978; 2(2): 203–5.
103. Glinski W, Zarebska Z, Jablonska S et al. The activity of polymorphonuclear leukocyte neutral proteinases and their inhibitors in patients with psoriasis treated with a continuous peritoneal dialysis. J Invest Dermatol 1980; 75(6): 481–7.
104. Glinski W, Jablonska, Imiela J et al. Peritoneal dialysis and leukopheresis in psoriasis: indications and contraindications. Hautarzt 1985; 36(1): 16–9.
105. Krebs R, Flynn M. Treatment of hepatic coma with exchange transfusion and peritoneal dialysis. JAMA 1967; 199(6): 430–2.
106. Pirola RC, Ham JC, Elmslie RG. Management of hepatic coma complicating viral hepatitis. Gut 1969; 10(11): 898–903.
107. Mactier RA, Dobbie JW, Khanna R. Peritoneal dialysis in fulminant hepatic failure. Perit Dial bull 1986; 6(4): 199–202.
108. Mactier R. Non-renal indications for peritoneal dialysis. In: Khanna R, Nolph KD, Prowant BF, Twardowski ZJ, Oreopoulos DG (eds), Advances in Peritoneal Dialysis. Perit Dial Bull Inc, Toronto 1992; (in press).
109. Lash RF, Burdette JA, Ozdil T. Accidental profound hypothermia and barbiturate intoxication: a report of rapid "core" rewarming by peritoneal dialysis. JAMA 1967; 201: 269–70.
110. Reuler JB, Parker RA. Peritoneal dialysis in the management of hypothermia. JAMA 1978; 240(21): 2289–90.
111. Moss JF, Haklin M, Southwick HW et al. A model for the treatment of accidental severe hypothermia. J Trauma 1986; 26(1): 68–74.
112. DaVee TS, Reineberg EJ. Extreme hypothermia and ventricular fibrillation. Ann Emerg Med 1980; 9(2): 100–2.
113. Davis FM, Judson JA. Warm peritoneal dialysis in the management of accidental hypothermia: report of five cases. New Zeal Med J 1981; 94(692): 207–9.
114. Troelsen S, Rybro L, Knudsen F. Profound accidental hypothermia treated with peritoneal dialysis. Scand J Urol & Nephrol 1986; 20(3): 221–4.
115. Horowitz BZ. The golden hour in heat stroke. Use of iced peritoneal lavage. Am J Emerg Med 1989; 7: 616–9.
116. Khan IH, Henderson IS Mactier RA. Hyperpyrexia due to meningococcal septicaemia treated with cold peritoneal lavage. Postgrad Med J 1992; 68: 129–31.
117. Blye E, Lorch J, Cortell S. Extracorporeal therapy in the treatment of intoxication. Am J Kid Dis 1984; 3(5): 321–38.
118. Schlegel RJ, Altstatt LB, Canales L et al. Peritoneal dialysis for severe salicylism: an evaluation of indications and results. J Pediatr 1966; 69(4): 553–62.
119. Arieff AI, Friedman EA. Coma following non-narcotic drug overdosage: management of 208 adult patients. Am J Med Sci 1973; 266(6): 405–26.
120. Pross DC, Bradford WD, Krueger RP. Reye's syndrome treated by peritoneal dialysis. Pediatr 1970; 45: 845.
121. Shaw EB. Reye's syndrome and salicylate intoxication. Pediatr 1970; 46(6): 976–7.
122. Narcy P, Zorza G, Taburet AM et al. Severe poisoning with intravenous phenytoin in the newborn. Value of peritoneal dialysis. Arch Fran Pediatr 1990; 47(8): 591–3.
123. Roger SD, Crimmins D, Yiannikas C et al. Lead intoxication in an anuric patient: management by intraperitoneal EDTA. Aust & New Zeal J Med 1990; 20(6): 814–7.
124. Dua SL. Letter: peritoneal dialysis for isopropyl alcohol poisoning. JAMA 1974; 230(1): 35.
125. Kaufman DB, DiNicola W, McIntosh R. Acute potassium dichromate poisoning. Treated by peritoneal dialysis. Am J Dis Child 1970; 119(4): 374–6.
126. Lichtenberg R, Zeller WP, Gatson R et al. Bromate poisoning. J Pediatr 1989; 114(5): 891–4.
127. Warshaw BL. Treatment of bromate poisoning. J Pediatr 1989; 115(4): 660–1.
128. Duo LJ, Zhi ZG, Ji LY. Peritoneal dialysis in the treatment of severe poisoning with organophosphorous pesticides: experience with twenty-two patients. Perit Dial Int 1990; 10(3): 242–3.
129. Kassa J. Use of peritoneal dialysis as a therapeutic method in poisoning by Neguvon. Ceskoslovenska Farmacie 1990; 39(1): 7–10.
130. Yamamoto Y, Wakisaka O, Fujimoto S et al. Acute renal failure caused by ingestion of the carp gall bladder-a report of 3 cases, with special reference to the reported cases in Japan. J Jap Soc Intern Med 1988; 77(8): 1268–73.
131. Yium J, Martinez-Maldonado M, Eknoyan G et al. Peritoneal dialysis in the treatment of renal failure in multiple myeloma. South Med J 1971; 64(11): 1403–5.
132. Russell JA, Fitzharris BM, Corringham R et al. Plasma exchange versus peritoneal dialysis for removing Bence Jones protein. BMJ 1978; 2(6149): 1397.
133. Rosansky SJ, Richards FW. Use of peritoneal dialysis in the treatment of patients with renal

failure and paraproteinemia. Am J Nephrol 1985; 5: 361–5.
134. Rose PE, McGonigle R, Michael J et al. Renal failure and the histopathological features of myeloma kidney reversed by intensive chemotherapy and peritoneal dialysis. BMJ 1987; 294(6569): 411–2.
135. Boyce NW, Holdsworth SR, Thomson NM et al. "Long-term" survival in light-chain myeloma with dialysis therapy alone. Aust & N Zeal J Med 1984; 14(5): 676–7.
136. Cosio FG, Pence RV, Shapiro FL et al. Severe renal failure in multiple myeloma. Clin Neph 1981: 15(4): 206–10.
137. Brown WW, Hebert LA, Piering WF et al. Reversal of chronic end-stage renal failure due to myeloma kidney. Ann Intern Med 1979; 90(5): 793–4.
138. Johnson WJ, Kyle RA, Dahlberg PJ. Dialysis in the treatment of multiple myeloma. Mayo Clin Proc 1980; 55: 65–72.
139. Goodship THJ, Lloyd S, McKenzie PW et al. Short-term studies on the use of amino acids as an osmotic agent in continuous ambulatory peritoneal dialysis. Clin Sci 1987; 73: 471–8.
140. Oreopoulos DG, Marliss EB, Anderson GH et al. Nutritional aspects of CAPD and the potential use of amino acid containing dialysis solutions. Perit Dial Bull 1983; 3(1)(Suppl): 510–2.
141. Mitwalli A, Rodella H, Brandes L et al. Is fat absorbed through the peritoneum? Perit Dial Bull 1985; 5(2): 165–8.
142. Pessa ME, Sitren HS, Copeland EM III et al. Nutritional support by intraperitoneal dialysis in the rat: maintenance of body weight with normal liver and plasma chemistries. J Parenteral and Enteral Nutrition 1988; 12(1): 63–7.
143. Siriwardhana SA, Newfield AM, Lipton JM et al. Oxygen delivery by the peritoneal route. Can J Anesthesia 1990; 37 (4 pt 2): S159.
144. Shah BS. An in vitro model for chemical extraction of carbon dioxide via modified peritoneal dialysis. ASAIO Transactions 1988; 34(2): 112–5.

27 Intraperitoneal chemotherapy

MICHAEL F. FLESSNER AND ROBERT L. DEDRICK

1. Introduction 769
2. Model concept 771
3. Model implementation 772
   3.1. Estimation of solute-independent parameters 772
   3.2. Peritoneal transport of small molecules: Theory 774
   3.3. Estimation of parameters dependent on molecular weight 775
      3.3.1. Variation of PA with molecular weight 775
      3.3.2. Variation of PA with body size 775
      3.3.3. Areas for transport 778
      3.3.4. Role of capillary permeability 778
      3.3.5. Regional permeabilities 778
   3.4. Lipid solubility 778
   3.5. Blood flow 778
4. Pharmacokinetic advantage: Theory 779
5. Application of model to evaluation of the pharmacokinetic advantage 780
   5.1. Antineoplastic agents 780
      5.1.1. Cisplatin 780
      5.1.2. 5-fluorouracil 781
   5.2. Antibiotics: Vancomycin 782
   5.3. Intraperitoneal insulin 783
   5.4. I.P. antibody therapy 784
6. Summary 785
References 785

1. Introduction

A wide variety of therapeutic drugs are administered into the peritoneal cavity as a portal of entry to the body and as a localized treatment. Because of intravenous access problems in neonates, transfusion of packed red blood cells was one of the earliest uses of intraperitoneal (i.p.) therapy [1, 2]. Insulin is often placed in the dialysate in order to treat glucose intolerance during peritoneal dialysis [3], and i.p. insulin delivery is currently undergoing investigation as a means of long-term therapy in diabetes [4]. Erythropoietin, prescribed as replacement therapy for the anemia related to end-stage renal disease (ESRD), has recently been administered intraperitoneally [5]. In contrast to these forms of i.p. therapy which are designed to treat systemic illnesses, antibacterial agents are injected intraperitoneally in order to treat peritonitis [6, 7]. And in the last 20 years, i.p. chemotherapy has been evaluated extensively for treatment of malignancies localized to the peritoneal cavity [8–16].

Prior to prescribing i.p. therapy, the critical point which the clinician must determine is the usefulness of such an approach. Is there a pharmacokinetic advantage of administering the drug regionally (i.p.) versus systemically (intravenously or i.v.)? In other words: does the drug approach therapeutic concentration in the region of interest, while maintaining a relatively low, non-toxic level in the general circulation?

A good example of a drug with a significant therapeutic advantage is cisplatin, which is therapeutic for metastatic ovarian carcinoma and which is toxic to the kidney when administered systemically. Drug levels within the peritoneal cavity can be maintained at levels 10–25 times plasma levels [17] by i.p. administration with the simultaneous i.v. infusion of thiosulfate to block the systemic action of cisplatin.

On the other hand, the i.p. administration of a drug such as erythropoietin, which has a site of action in the bone marrow and not the peritoneal cavity, may not be an appropriate use of this route. Because of a slow rate of systemic absorption, very large concentrations of erythropoietin must be injected with the peritoneal dialysate to attain levels in the blood which are equivalent to those attained with i.v. or subcutaneous (s.c.) dosing. Much of this expensive agent must be wasted, since the solution must be drained from the patient before the drug is fully absorbed [5].

What follows is an analytical approach to the evaluation of the i.p. route of administration with respect to the i.v. route. The approach assumes that the target of the therapy is either a cellular component in the peritoneal cavity (bacteria or tumor ascites cells) or the tissues surrounding the peritoneal cavity.

At steady state the quantitative formula for pharmacokinetic advantage (R_d) in its simplest form is [18]:

$$R_d = \frac{\left(\frac{C_P}{C_B}\right)_{ip}}{\left(\frac{C_P}{C_B}\right)_{iv}} \quad (1)$$

where: C_P = concentration in the peritoneal cavity, C_B = concentration in the systemic circulation, and the subscripts indicate the route of administration. In planning a therapeutic strategy, the physician would like to predict R_d prior to administration of the drug in humans. The pharmacokinetics of a particular drug are based on the transport physiology of the region in which it is administered as well as pharmacokinetic processes in the rest of the body.

Physiologic characteristics of the peritoneal cavity which cause it to be advantageous for removal of waste metabolites and poisons from the body also provide an excellent portal of entry into the body for many drugs. The tissue space surrounding the cavity is capable of absorbing almost any agent, including cell-sized materials, placed in the cavity. As illustrated in Fig. 1, blood and lymphatic capillary networks are contained within the tissue space. The density of these networks depends on the specific organ tissue. As drugs transport into the tissue from the cavity, they will be taken up by these networks and returned to the general circulation. The rate of a drug's transfer to the blood is governed by its effective diffusivity and convection (solvent drag) within the tissue space, the permeability-surface area of the blood and lymphatic capillaries for a given volume of tissue, and the blood perfusion. The process of drug uptake from the peritoneal cavity includes the same physiologic mechanisms responsible for transport during dialysis except that their direction has been reversed.

Our goal in this chapter is to illustrate how the

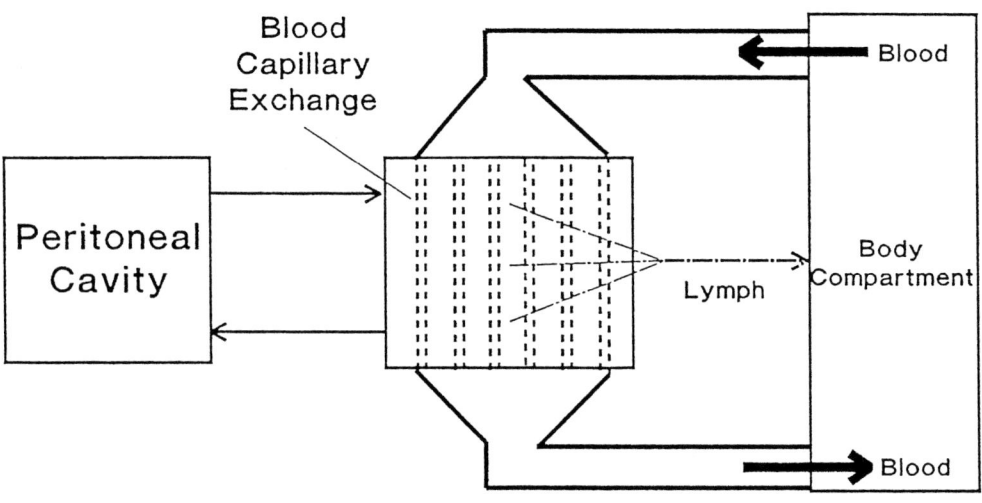

Figure 1. *Distributed Model* concept in which blood flows through exchange capillaries which are distributed uniformly in the tissue surrounding the peritoneal cavity. Drugs introduced into the peritoneal cavity transport into the surrounding tissue interstitium. From the tissue interstitium, the solutes transfer into either blood capillaries (small molecules) or lymphatic capillaries (the pathway for macromolecules).

INTRAPERITONEAL CHEMOTHERAPY

physician can implement the above equation to estimate the pharmacokinetic advantage in a proposed therapy which utilizes the peritoneal cavity as a drug delivery system. We will first present a detailed conceptual model of peritoneal transport, followed by a brief explanation of the mathematical consequences of this conceptual model over a range of molecular weights. Then we will give a number of examples in which the theory is applied.

2. Model concept

Although the simplicity of the concept presented in Fig. 1 is appealing, the anatomy and physiology of the peritoneal cavity are far more complex. Figure 2 illustrates a conceptual model which attempts to include some of the diversity of organ physiology which exists in the tissue surrounding the peritoneal cavity [19].

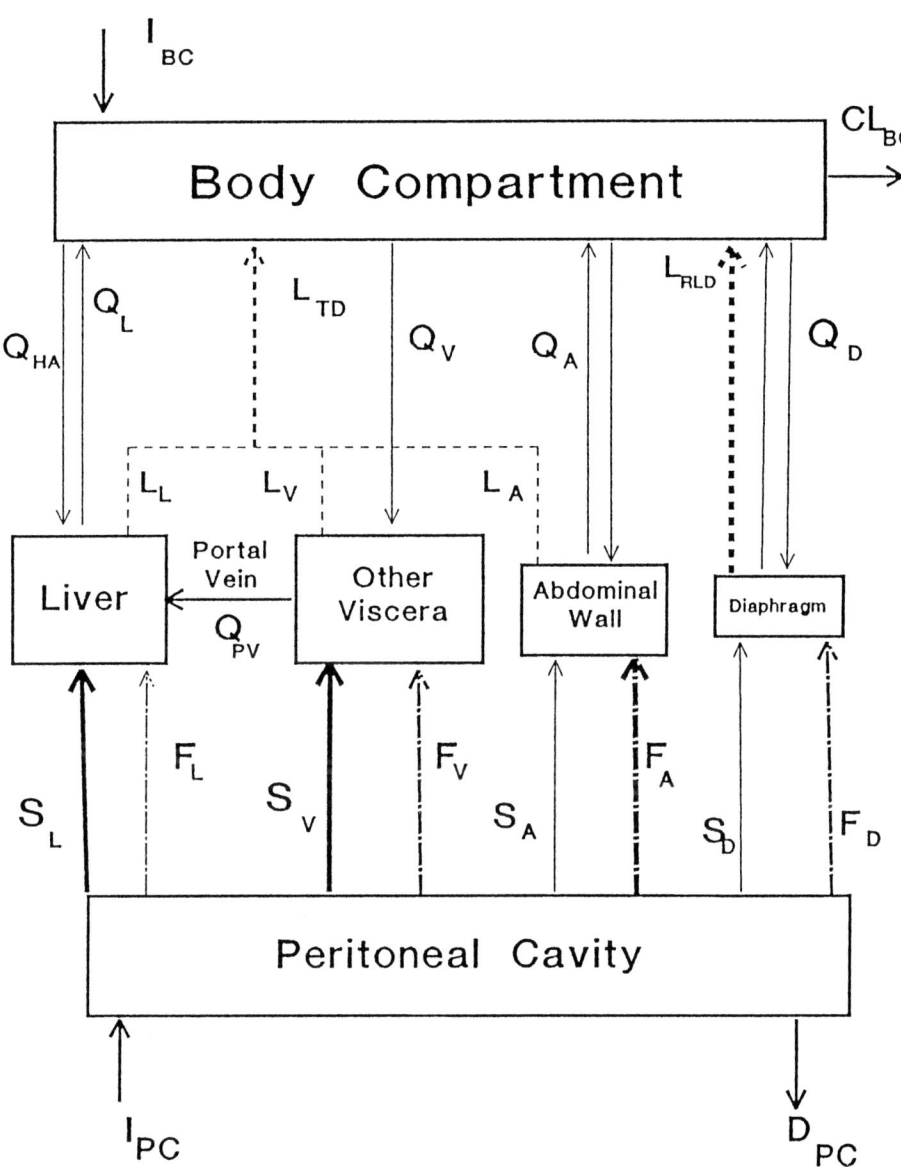

Figure 2. Compartmental model concept of intraperitoneal drug delivery in which transport occurs between the cavity and specific tissues surrounding the cavity. *Symbols:* I = infusion; CL = clearance; D = drainage from the cavity; Q = blood flow through organ or vessel; L = lymph flow from tissue to body compartment; F = rate of convection from the cavity to tissue; S = rate of solute transfer from the cavity to tissue. *Subscripts:* A = abdominal wall and psoas; BC = body compartment; D = diaphragm; HA = hepatic artery; L = liver; PC = peritoneal cavity; PV = portal vein; RLD = right lymph duct; TD = thoracic duct; V = other viscera including the intestines, stomach, pancreas, and spleen. See text for a full description.

The body is shown as a single compartment in Fig. 2, but could be represented by multiple compartments, if the pharmacokinetic characteristics of the drug demand it. The volume of the Body Compartment equals the volume of distribution of the drug in the total body excluding the tissues surrounding the peritoneal cavity. Its concentration is assumed to equal the mixed venous concentration. The drug is cleared at some rate CL_{BC} and there may exist some rate of input into the compartment (I_{BC}). Blood flows from the Body Compartment through each peritoneal compartment with rate Q_i. Lymph flows from each organ system (L_i) through two major systems into the body compartment: the thoracic duct (L_{TD}) and the right lymph duct (L_{RLD}).

The single "Peritoneal Tissue" compartment has been divided into four major compartments. Each of these compartments receives blood originating in the Body Compartment. The blood flows through capillary exchange vessels distributed throughout the tissue (as illustrated in Fig. 1 but left out of Fig. 2 for clarity) and returns to the body compartment. Lymph flows from each tissue space to the body compartment as illustrated in Figs. 1 and 2. Each tissue compartment receives solutes from the peritoneal cavity with a solute mass transfer rate of S and fluid at rate F (S and F are illustrated as positive from the cavity into the tissue).

The diaphragm is included as a separate compartment because of the specialized sub-diaphragmatic lymphatic system [20, 21] which accepts cell sizes to 25 µm in diameter [22] and which accounts for 70–80% of the total lymph flow from the cavity [23–25]. The diaphragm also experiences relatively large but variable hydrostatic pressure gradients during respiration, because of its position between the thoracic and abdominal cavities. Expiration facilitates direct fluid movement into the diaphragmatic interstitium and into the lacunae of the subdiaphragmatic lymphatic apparatus [20–21].

The abdominal wall is shown as a separate compartment because it is the single largest recipient of fluid transfer from the cavity. In animal experiments, this amounts to 25–30% of the total fluid movement out of the cavity [24–26]. The reason for this fluid movement has been attributed to the hydrostatic pressure gradient across the abdominal wall. In addition, the lymphatics are not well developed in this tissue and therefore do not provide the safety valve that they do in intestinal tissue [27]. Proteins or other macromolecular drugs which are carried into the tissue as a result of the hydrostatic pressure-driven convection will circulate to the Body Compartment very slowly [26, 28].

The liver is separated from the other visceral tissues because of the unique architecture of its microcirculation (very large pores) and its possible role in protein losses into the cavity. The "other viscera" include the spleen, stomach, intestines, and the pancreas. These have been found to have similar transport characteristics and are therefore lumped together in a single tissue compartment.

The peritoneal cavity compartment is assumed to be well-mixed; i.e., the concentration is the same throughout the cavity. The cavity may have a solute input rate of I_{PC} and a drainage rate of D_{PC}. The cavity does not exchange directly with the body compartment; transport occurs only with the tissue compartments.

3. Model implementation

In order to use equation (1), C_P must be estimated. In order to do this, the mathematical model corresponding to the conceptual model of Fig. 2 must be solved. This consists of: (a) a series of mass and volume balances on each compartment, (b) rate equations (defining each S and CL), and (c) boundary conditions (defining initial concentrations, volumes, and inputs (I) and outputs (D)). Critical to the solution of these equations are a large number of parameters which describe the system.

3.1. Estimation of solute-independent parameters

A necessary step in the solution is the determination of the parameters in Fig. 2: Q_i, L_i and F_i. Each of these numbers does not depend on solute characteristics but upon the underlying physiology of the tissue. Table 1 is a listing of these parameters. Because many of these numbers had to be estimated from incomplete information or scaled from animal experiments, they should be considered order-of-magnitude.

The first two columns concern peritoneal surface area. The first column specifies the percent of the total peritoneal surface area, while the second tabulated the total surface area in cm^2. We chose Rubin et al. [29] because the measurements were more conservative than Esperanca and Collins [30], since the mesentery was not included. The areas have been scaled to a 70 kg body weight by the factor (body weight)$^{0.7}$ [18].

The tissue weights were estimated as follows. The liver weight was taken directly from a table in Ludwig [31]. The "other viscera" weight was computed from the sum of the spleen (0.14 kg) and intestines. The weight of the intestines was estimated from the product of the total surface area [29], the average thickness of 2.5 mm [32], and the specific gravity of these tissues, which was assumed to equal 1 g/cm^3. The thickness of the abdominal wall and diaphragm were estimated to be 2 cm and 0.3 cm [33, 34], respectively, and the tissue weight was calculated in the same fashion as in the case of the hollow viscera.

There have been a number of estimates of the rate of perfusion (q_i) of the abdominal tissues. We used Rubin *et al.*'s [35] measurement in the control animals for the parietal wall (0.06 ml/min/g tissue) and diaphragm (0.31). Other estimates [36] for the parietal wall tended to be much higher, because of the specific preparation and use of vasodilators. The perfusion rates in the "other viscera" and the liver (includes both hepatic artery and portal flow) were estimated from total organ blood flows [37–38] and divided by the weight of each system. The estimates for the g.i. tract agree with several other measurements made in a variety of tissues from other species [39–41]. The total blood flows for the diaphragm and abdominal wall (Q_i) can be calculated from the product of the organ weight and q_i.

Thoracic duct lymph flow has been measured in man and typically has a flow rate of 1–1.6 ml/hr/kg body weight [42–43]. Non-ruminant animals have flow rates on the order of 2–3 ml/hr/kg body weight [24, 44–46]. Morris [46] estimates that the contributions of the liver and gastrointestinal tract amount to 30% and 64%, respectively, of the thoracic duct flow. The remaining 6% of the total flow is from all the skeletal muscle below the diaphragm, including the psoas, the abdominal wall, and the lower limbs. In order to estimate the lymph flow for humans, the mean value for the thoracic duct (1.3 ml/hr/kg body weight) was multiplied by the percentages obtained by Morris for each organ system: 30% for liver and 64% for other viscera. One third of the remaining 6% was arbitrarily assumed to be the contribution of the abdominal wall. Total lymph flows were then calculated by multiplying each tissue specific lymph flow rate times the body weight (70 kg) and converting to ml/min.

Seventy to eighty percent of the lymph which exclusively leaves the peritoneal cavity flows through the subdiaphragmatic system [47]. It is a major site for transport of fluids, macromolecules, and cellular materials from the cavity to the blood. Values for flow range from 0.6–1.8 ml/hr/kg body weight in the anesthetized rat [24] to 0.1 ml/hr/kg in anesthetized sheep and 0.50 ml/hr/kg in awake sheep [48]. Flow rates in awake, healthy CAPD patients vary from 0.14–0.28 ml/hr/kg body weight [49–50]. The rates appear to increase in cirrhosis to 0.43 ml/hr/kg [51]. We have chosen the mean rate of 0.23 ml/hr/kg and multiplied it by 70 kg to find the diaphragmatic lymph flow rate of 16.1 ml/hr.

The next to last column in Table 1 lists estimated total flow rates of fluid in ml/min to each organ system. The total flow from the cavity has been estimated from the average of three studies in healthy CAPD patients [49–50, 52] to be 1.33 ml/min. This flow is thought to be due to the hydrostatic pressure in the cavity [24, 53] and occurs in the face of hyperosmolar solutions which draw fluid into the cavity [26, 28, 54–55]. These studies have shown that protein acts as a marker for fluid movement. The total hourly flow rate has been partitioned to each set of tissues on the basis of the

Table 1. Adult human parameters which are independent of solute size (scaled to 70 Kg body weight).

Tissue	% total surface area	A_i (cm^2)	Weight (g)	q_i (ml/min/g)	Q_{tot} (ml/min)	L (ml/min)	F (ml/min)	L/F
Liver	13.2	1056	1800	0.83	1500	0.46	0.07	6.83
Other viscera (intestines, spleen, stomach)	67.9	5432	1700	0.65	1100	0.97	0.33	2.91
Abdominal wall	11	880	1960	0.06	118	0.04	0.67	0.05
Diaphragm	7.9	632	190	0.3	57	0.27	0.27	1.01

fraction of protein deposition from the cavity [26] with corrections for the rates of lymph flow from each tissue.

3.2. Peritoneal transport of small molecules: Theory

The next step in the implementation of our model concept is the definition of the appropriate rate equations. This has been rigorously performed only for small molecules.

Transfer of small molecules from the peritoneal cavity can be viewed as a process of diffusion from the fluid in the cavity into the adjacent tissues followed by absorption from the tissue extracellular space into blood in the exchange vessels (Fig. 1). Convection generally does not play a quantitatively significant role for small solutes, and lymphatic uptake is negligible compared with removal from the tissue by the flowing blood. The result is that a concentration profile is established within the tissue. At steady state, the rate of diffusion down the profile at any location is exactly balanced by the combination of irreversible chemical reaction in the tissue and removal by flowing blood. For a non-reactive solute and a uniformly distributed capillary network, it is easily shown that the rate of uptake into blood perfusing the viscera may be calculated from the equation [56]:

$$S_V = \sqrt{D_V(p_V a_V)} \, A_V(C_P - C_B) \qquad (2)$$

where S_V = net rate of uptake of the solute (µg/min), D_V = the effective diffusivity of the solute in the viscera (cm²/min), p_V = the intrinsic permeability of the blood capillaries in the viscera (cm/min), a_V = the capillary surface area per unit tissue volume (cm²/cm³), A_V = the superficial surface area of the viscera exposed to peritoneal fluid (cm²), C = the free solute concentration (µg/cm³), and the subscripts P and B refer to peritoneal fluid and blood, respectively. The effective diffusivity is equal to the diffusivity in the tissue interstitial space multiplied by the tissue fractional interstitial space which is available to the solute.

A number of observations may be made about Equation (2). First, the effective diffusivity, capillary permeability and capillary surface area enter as their square root so that doubling of the capillary permeability, e.g., would be expected to be associated with only a 41 percent increase in mass transfer ($2^{1/2}$ = 1.41). Second, the net transport rate is proportional to the superficial area of the tissue.

And, third, the rate of transport is proportional to the difference in the free concentration of solute between the peritoneal fluid and blood.

Equation (2) serves as the basis for the definition of an equivalent "permeability" P_V of the tissue. If there were a thin membrane separating the peritoneal fluid from the blood, the rate of uptake would be given by

$$S_V = P_V A_V \, (C_P - C_B). \qquad (3)$$

Comparison of Equations (2) and (3) shows that the equivalent tissue permeability can be calculated from:

$$P_V = \sqrt{D_V(p_V a_V)} \, . \qquad (4)$$

Either Equation (2) or (3) can be used to calculate the rate of absorption of a drug from the peritoneal cavity into the blood as they are exactly equivalent. The spatially distributed view of the tissue offers certain advantages because it provides some insight into the underlying transport mechanisms and how these might be altered by pathologic processes or pharmacologic manipulations. It also serves as a natural link to the very large body of literature on capillary physiology and provides a natural framework to incorporate this into descriptions and predictions of peritoneal transport rates. Further, it explicitly predicts that a concentration profile extends a finite depth into the tissue, and tissue penetration is an important consideration if the goal of intraperitoneal therapy is to treat disease in the tissue or disease of finite thickness such as peritoneal carcinomatosis on serosal surfaces. Explicitly, the concentration profile is given by:

$$\frac{C - C_B}{C_P - C_B} = \exp - \sqrt{\frac{p_V a_V}{D_V}} \, x \qquad (5)$$

where x is the distance from the serosal surface.

Equations similar to (2) and (3) can be written for as many types of peritoneal tissue as desirable. Since uptake rates into the various tissue types are parallel processes, they may be summed to provide:

$$S = [(P_L A_L) + (P_V A_V) + (P_A A_A) + (P_D A_D)] \, (C_P - C_B) \qquad (6)$$

with the subscripts defined in Fig. 2.

Equation (6) is usually given simply as:

$$S = (PA) \, (C_P - C_B) \qquad (7)$$

where (PA) is the mass transfer-area coefficient which incorporates all absorbing structures in contact with peritoneal fluid. The PA product is a single parameter defined as the sum of the individual tissue PA's as indicated by comparison of Equations (6) and (7).

The "A" of equation (7) should not, in general, be equated to the topological surface area of the peritoneum; "A" would be equal to the sum of the individual tissue areas only if all tissue permeabilities were equal. The data below do not support that equality.

It is instructive to examine the magnitudes of some of the parameters that have been discussed above in order to place them in quantitative perspective.

3.3. Estimation of parameters dependent on molecular weight

In order to calculate the rates S_i of solutes with low lipid solubility in Fig. 2, transport parameters such as the mass transfer-area coefficient (P_iA_i) for each solute and each organ system must be determined. To illustrate parameters over a wide range of molecular weights, we have estimated values for P_iA_i in Tables 2–4 for sucrose (mwt 342), inulin (mwt 5250), and IgG (mwt 160,000), respectively. The values for A_i are taken from Table 1. P_i can be estimated from equation (4), the expression for a diffusion-limited solute transporting in a distributed system.

Values for p_i and a_i for the liver in Tables 2 and 3 have been taken from Crone [57]. Since the "other viscera" are chiefly the stomach and intestines and since the serosal side of these viscera is made up of layers of muscle, their capillary transport characteristics are assumed to be equal to those of the hind limb. These same values are used for the diaphragm and abdominal wall. The p_ia_i for IgG (Table 4) are taken from values from Carter *et al.* [58] for skeletal muscle (viscera, abdominal wall, and diaphragm) and scaled by data of Mayerson [59] to the liver.

Values for D_e, the diffusivity in the interstitial space, are estimated from a variety of sources. For sucrose and inulin, the diffusivity was taken from Schultz and Armstrong [60] and Flessner *et al.* [61]. Since macromolecular diffusion through tissue is markedly restricted [62], D_e is roughly only 5% of the diffusivity in water [63]. The value in Table 4 is derived from Clauss and Jain [64] for normal (granulation) tissue.

The interstitial fractions (Θ_i) for sucrose have been obtained from values for EDTA, which has an equivalent molecular size to sucrose [65]. Values for the liver and viscera were taken directly from the paper. Values for the abdominal wall and diaphragm have been equated to those for skeletal muscle. In Table 3 and 4, the values for liver have been obtained from Goresky [66]. The remainder of the fractional interstitial spaces have been compiled for inulin from work of Rippe [67] and for IgG, from Bill [68].

3.3.1. Variation of PA with molecular weight

The value of PA has been studied extensively because of its importance to peritoneal dialysis. Therefore, our best data exist for the common indicators of azotemia and physiologic markers that have been measured in this context. Fig. 3 shows some values of PA plotted against molecular weight [69]. The data vary approximately as the inverse of the square root of molecular weight. This would be expected from the penetration model if the capillary permeability varies with the –0.63 power of molecular weight (Fig. 4) and the diffusivity in tissue varies with the –0.45 power of molecular weight observed for diffusion in water [56]. From this correlation, PA for sucrose would equal 8.5 cm/min; the PA for inulin would be 2.8 ml/min. These compare favorably with our estimates of 5.0 and 1.6 cm/min in Tables 2 and 3, respectively.

Rubin measured a mass-transfer-area coefficient (MTAC) for inulin to be 3.3 ml/min in humans. However, the convective component of transport has likely been included in Rubin's calculation [3]. It is interesting to note that the sum of the PA_{tot} and F_{tot} in Table 3 equals 2.9 ml/min, nearly the same as the MTAC calculated by Rubin.

Values for the IgG PA, the mass transfer-area coefficient for transport of protein from the blood to the cavity, have been calculated and listed in Table 4. The overall value of 0.03 ml/min compares favorably with those measured by Rippe [70], who found 0.05 ml/min, and Krediet *et al.* [71], who measured rates on the order of 0.04 ml/min.

3.3.2. Variation of PA with body size

Figure 5 shows the PA product for urea and inulin for the rat, rabbit, dog and human; these species cover a body-weight range from 200 g to 70 kg [18]. The parameter increases as the 0.62 to 0.74 power of body weight for inulin and urea, respectively. The average of these two values is very close to the 2/3 expected for body-surface-area scaling.

Table 2. Adult human parameters for sucrose.

Tissue	a_i (cm²/cm³)	p_i (cm/min × 10⁵)	D_e (cm²/min × 10⁵)	Θ_i	P_i (cm/min × 10⁴)	A_i (cm²)	P_iA_i (cm³/min)	F_i (ml/min)	PA/F	q_i (ml/min/g)	pa/q
Liver	250	396	3.3	0.14	21.7	1056	2.28	0.07	34.18	0.83	1.19
Other viscera (intestines, spleen, stomach)	70	32.4	3.3	0.21	4.0	5432	2.17	0.33	6.52	0.65	0.03
Abdominal wall	70	32.4	3.3	0.12	3.0	880	0.27	0.67	0.40	0.06	0.38
Diaphragm	70	32.4	3.3	0.12	3.0	632	0.30	0.27	1.13	0.30	0.08

Overall parameters: PA = 5.02 ml/min; F = 1.34 ml/min; PA/F = 3.75.

Table 3. Adult human parameters for inulin.

Tissue	a_i (cm²/cm³)	p_i (cm/min × 10⁵)	D_e (cm²/min × 10⁵)	Θ_i	P_i (cm/min × 10⁴)	A_i (cm²)	P_iA_i (cm³/min)	F_i (ml/min)	PA/F	q_i (ml/min/g)	pa/q
Liver	250	174	1.2	0.078	6.43	1056	0.68	0.07	10.19	0.83	0.52
Other viscera (intestines, spleen, stomach)	70	15.6	1.2	0.13	1.31	5432	0.71	0.33	2.14	0.65	0.02
Abdominal wall	70	15.6	1.2	0.1	1.15	880	0.10	0.67	0.15	0.06	0.18
Diaphragm	70	15.6	1.2	0.1	1.15	632	0.07	0.27	0.27	0.30	0.04

Overall parameters: PA = 1.56 ml/min; F = 1.34 ml/min; PA/F = 1.16.

Table 4. Adult human parameters for IgG.

Tissue	p_ia_i (cc/g/min)	D_e (cm/min × 10⁷)	Θ_i (cm²)	P_i (cm/min × 10⁷)	A_i (cm²)	P_iA_i (cc/min)	q_i (ml/min/g)	pa/q
Liver	0.07	1.44	0.06	24.6	1056	0.026	0.83	0.08
Other viscera (intestines, spleen, stomach)	0.00014	1.44	0.08	1.3	5432	0.007	0.65	0.00
Abdominal wall	0.00014	1.44	0.015	0.55	880	0.0005	0.06	0.00
Diaphragm	0.00014	1.44	0.015	0.55	632	0.0003	0.30	0.00

Overall parameters: PA = 0.034 ml/min.

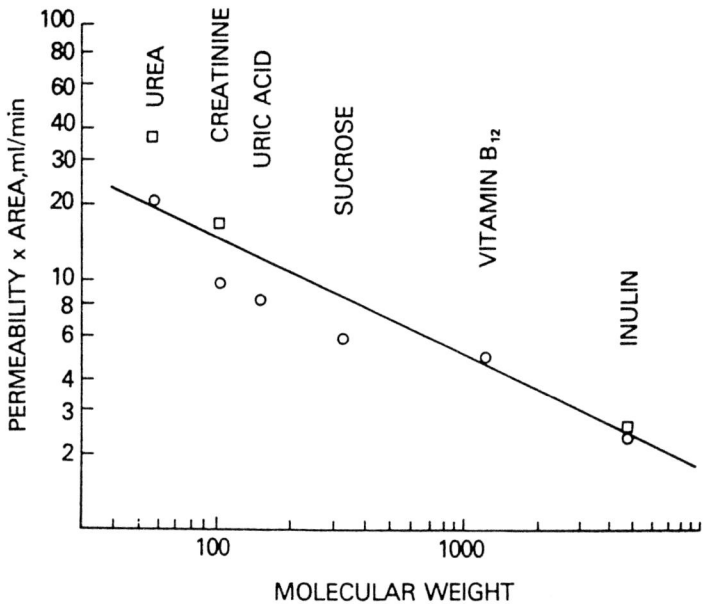

Figure 3. Peritoneal permeability times area (or mass transfer-area coefficient) versus molecular weight. See text for a complete discussion. From reference [69].

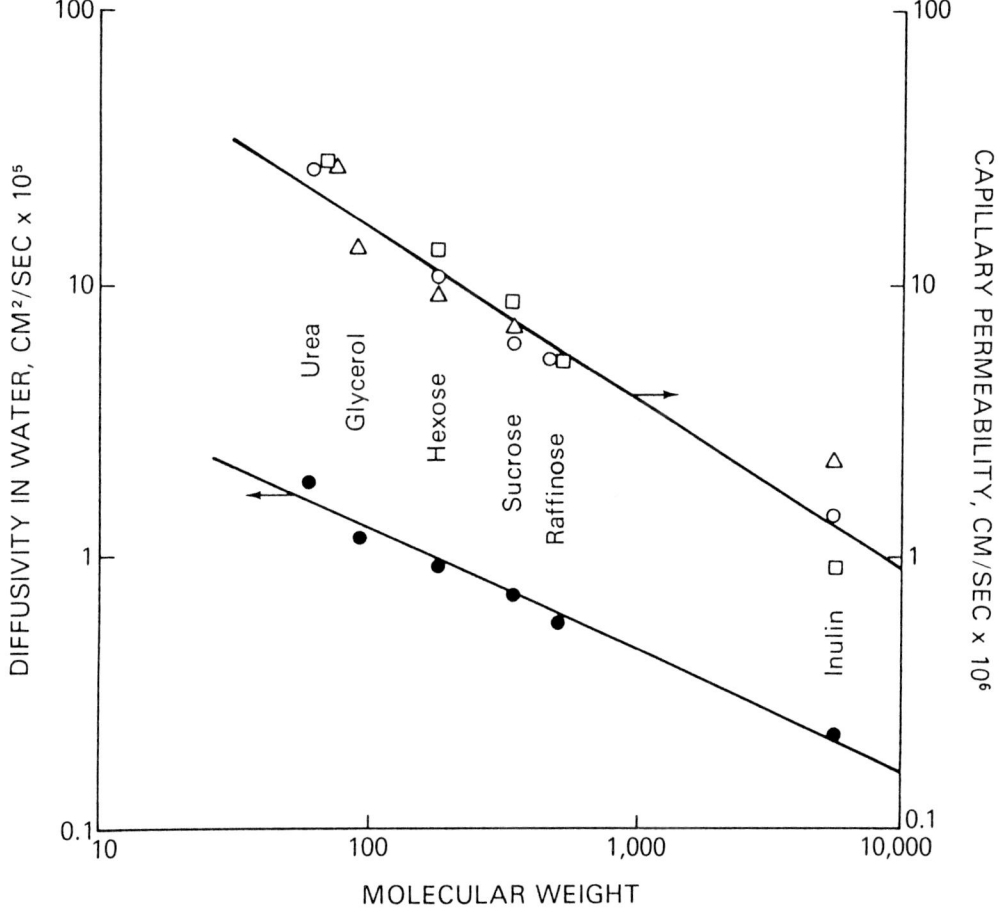

Figure 4. Capillary permeability versus molecular weight (right axis) and diffusivity in water versus molecular weight (left axis). Adapted from reference [56].

Since the characteristic time for absorption from the peritoneal cavity is equal to V_p/PA, similar time scales can be achieved in humans and experimental animals if the volume is scaled as the 2/3 power of the body weight. For example, 2 liters in the peritoneal cavity of a 70-kg human patient (29 ml/kg) would be equivalent to 40 ml in a 200-g rat (200 ml/kg) because $(200/70,000)^{2/3} (2000) = 40$.

3.3.3. Areas for transport

The peritoneal surface area of the adult human has been estimated to be of the order of 8000 to 10,000 cm² [29–30]. Of this value, the surface of the liver constitutes about 6–13% (range of averages from the two references), the diaphragm 4–8%, the peritoneal walls 11% (anterior abdominal wall 7%). Corresponding percentages for the 595 cm² surface area of the adult rat were: liver, 16%; diaphragm, 3%; peritoneal walls, 19% [29].

3.3.4. Role of capillary permeability

Figure 3 shows that the PA product for a 250-dalton hydrophilic drug in a human would be expected to be about 10 ml/min. If the peritoneal surface area is approximately 8,000 cm² as discussed above, then the average equivalent peritoneal permeability would be 1.3×10^{-3} cm/min. Figure 4 shows that the intrinsic permeability, p, of mammalian muscle capillaries is 10^{-5} cm/sec or 0.6×10^{-3} cm/min. This remarkable similarity is probably fortuitous. Peritoneal transport appears to derive its selectivity partly from the properties of the capillaries; however, the quantitative contribution of the capillaries must be interpreted in conjunction with diffusion into the tissues as shown in Equation (4).

3.3.5. Regional permeabilities

In Tables 2 and 3, the lumped coefficients of diffusive transfer for each tissue (P_iA_i) suggest that the liver is roughly equal to all other viscera in terms of relative importance to mass transfer. The ratios of PA/F demonstrate that, over most of the peritoneal surface, diffusive transport dominates in the transfer of small solutes from the cavity to the tissue during the typical dialysis.

The transport of large proteins, such as IgG, is dominated chiefly by convection or solvent drag from the cavity [26, 28]. Once in the tissue, they are removed by lymphatic flow. Table 1, therefore, lists values for L/F for each tissue. These suggest that the transport of protein from the cavity to the blood may be limited by its transport from the cavity to the tissue space in the diaphragm, viscera, and the liver, which contain extensive lymphatic systems. On the other hand, transport of protein from the cavity via the abdominal wall interstitium is limited by the lymphatic flow.

3.4. Lipid solubility

Increasing lipid solubility increases the rate of transfer of a drug from the cavity into the surrounding tissue and the blood. Torres et al. [72] measured the absorption of model compounds dissolved in 50 ml of saline in the rat. They found that as the heptane-water partition coefficient (K_{hep}) increased above 0.001, the rate of absorption increased significantly. Barbital with a K_{hep} of 0.001 was found to have an absorption of 57% at the end of one hour. On the other hand, thiopental, with a K_{hep} of 3.3, had an absorption of 96% at the end of one hour. Subsequent studies with the lipid soluble drugs hexamethylmelamine in the mouse [73] and thioTEPA in human subjects [74] have shown peritoneal clearances about an order of magnitude greater than would be expected for hydrophilic drugs. Unfortunately, capillary permeabilities and tissue diffusivities are not available for these compounds. Therefore, a table similar to Table 2 or 3 cannot be constructed.

3.5. Blood flow

Estimates of the effective blood flow surrounding the peritoneal cavity suggest that transport between the blood and the cavity is not limited by the supply of blood. Physiologists have attempted to estimate the "effective" blood flow by measuring the clearances of various gases from the peritoneal cavity, assuming that these were limited by blood flow only. Gas clearances of hydrogen [75–76] and CO_2 [77], have been determined in small mammals and found to be equal to 4–7% of the cardiac output. However, this method of determining the effective peritoneal blood flow may actually underestimate the true blood flow. Collins [78], who studied absorption of several inert gases from peritoneal gas pockets in pigs, found almost a three-fold range in clearance which correlated with the gas diffusivity in water. If the transport of these gases was limited by blood flow, the clearance of each gas would have been the same. The results imply that the transport of these gases is not limited by blood flow but by resistance to diffusion in the tissue. Gas clearance data therefore underestimates the true peritoneal blood flow, and the conclusion, based on lumped clearance data, would be that blood flow limitation in the peritoneal cavity is unlikely.

The lumped clearance argument does not rule out specific limitations in a portion of the peritoneal cavity, which may be offset by another set of tissues. In Tables 2–4, the ratios $p_i a_i / q_i$ are compiled for our three solutes for each tissue. The blood flow does exceed the transendothelial permeability-area product by a factor of 3 or more in all tissues except for the liver. Since our numbers are not precise measurements but order-of-magnitude estimates, conclusions concerning blood flow limitations in the liver cannot be drawn from Tables 2 and 3. However, its possibility should be further investigated.

4. Pharmacokinetic advantage: Theory

If a drug is infused at a constant rate into a fixed volume of fluid in the peritoneal cavity until steady state is achieved, then a regional advantage will be observed:

$$R_{ip} = (C_P/C_B)_{ip}. \quad (8)$$

Similarly, if the drug is infused at a constant rate intravenously with the same fixed intraperitoneal volume of fluid, then the corresponding concentration ratio may be defined

$$R_{iv} = (C_P/C_B)_{iv}. \quad (9)$$

The pharmacokinetic advantage R_d is defined as the ratio:

$$R_d = R_{ip}/R_{iv}. \quad (10)$$

Conceptually, R_d expresses the relative advantage that may be achieved by administration of a drug directly into the peritoneal cavity compared with intravenous administration. It has been shown [18] that the pharmacokinetic advantage may be expressed as a remarkably simple equation if there is no elimination of the drug from the peritoneal region:

$$R_d = 1 + CL_{TB}/PA \quad (11)$$

where CL_{TB} = total body clearance (cm³/min). The same equation may be used for drug that is not administered by continuous infusion to steady state if the exposure terms are defined as the areas under the peritoneal and plasma concentration curves (AUC_p and AUC_B) following any schedule of administration. The system must be linear in the sense that none of the relevant parameters changes with drug concentration or time.

Equation 11 indicates a large pharmacokinetic advantage for most hydrophilic drugs administered to the peritoneal cavity. For example, a typical antibiotic would be expected to have a PA of the order of 10 ml/min (Fig. 3). If the drug is cleared from the body by glomerular filtration at the rate of inulin, 125 ml/min [79], then the expected value of R_d is approximately 14.

Many drugs are eliminated by tissues within the peritoneal cavity, particularly the liver. This provides a first-pass effect which has the effect of increasing the natural pharmacokinetic advantage given by Equation (11). The regional advantage expected in the presence of some extraction of the drug by liver may be obtained from Dedrick [18]:

$$R_{ip} = \frac{1 + \dfrac{CL_{TB}}{PA}}{1 - fE} \quad (12)$$

where f = the fraction of the absorbed drug that enters the liver through the portal system or by direct absorption into its surface, and E = the fraction of that drug which is removed by the liver on a single pass. The quantity (1 – fE) is the fraction of the absorbed drug that reaches the systemic circulation. If this fraction is small, then the natural advantage to regional administration can be considerably enhanced.

We do not have adequate information on the value of f. It is generally thought that small molecular weight compounds are absorbed primarily through the portal system [80]; however, there is evidence that some significant fraction of the absorbed drug can bypass the liver [10]. In the Speyer study, concentrations of 5-fluorouracil were observed to be higher in a peripheral artery than in the hepatic vein in three of four patients. Calculation of f was not reliable because analysis of the data depended upon knowledge of the blood flows in the portal vein and drug metabolism by gastrointestinal tissues, and these were not measured. The fact that about 15–20 percent of the peritoneal surface area covers tissues which are not portal to the liver is consistent with the transport observations.

5. Application of model to evaluation of the pharmacokinetic advantage

5.1. Antineoplastic agents

The pharmacokinetic rationale for the intraperitoneal administration of drugs in the treatment of microscopic residual ovarian cancer was described in 1978 [69]. The procedure has been the subject of numerous preclinical and clinical studies during the subsequent years, and these have been reviewed periodically [81–83]. The pharmacokinetic theory has been consistently validated, and there is clear evidence of response in terms of surgically staged complete remissions in a number of studies. Markman et al. [16] reviewed several of these and concluded that there may be an advantage to regional drug delivery of cisplatin-based therapy for small-volume refractory residual ovarian cancer. Subsequently, Markman et al. [84] concluded that attainment of a surgically staged complete remission may have a favorable impact on survival. However, the role of intraperitoneal drug therapy in the management of abdominal cancer remains controversial [85], and there have not yet been properly controlled clinical trials to define what patient populations might benefit from intraperitoneal chemotherapy.

While the place of intraperitoneal drug administration in cancer chemotherapy has not been adequately defined, some important pharmacologic principles have been explored during the investigation of antineoplastic agents. Some of these principles are illustrated by a discussion of two specific drugs: cis-diamminedichloroplatinum (II) (cisplatin) and 5-fluorouracil (5-FU). At issue are both the pharmacology of intracavitary administration and the depth of penetration of drug into both normal and neoplastic tissues.

5.1.1. Cisplatin

Cisplatin is among the most active agents used in the treatment of ovarian cancer. Its pharmacokinetics have been studied extensively, and a physiological model has been developed and applied to several species [86–88]. Briefly, the drug reacts with both small and large molecular weight nucleophiles in plasma and tissue compartments. The tissue-specific rate constants vary among the tissues but are relatively constant across species. Release of (presumably inactive) platinum from macromolecules is dominated by their catabolism.

Goel et al. [89] studied the intraperitoneal administration of cisplatin in combination with etoposide and examined the effect of concurrent administration of sodium thiosulfate to protect the kidney against platinum toxicity. They administered the drug combination in 2 L of normal saline and observed a cisplatin clearance from the peritoneal cavity of 15 ml/min and a clearance from the plasma of 329 ml/min. These clearances resulted in a regional advantage (AUC_p/AUC_B) of 26 in those patients who did not receive sodium thiosulfate. This advantage is similar to the value of 16 obtained by Piccart et al. [90] for cisplatin administered in combination with melphalan.

Los et al. [91] conducted pharmacokinetic studies of cisplatin in rats bearing CC531 colonic adenocarcinoma on serosal surfaces of the peritoneal cavity in order to determine the effect of route of administration on tumor and normal tissue levels of platinum. The AUC_B was approximately the same following both i.v. and i.p. administration while the regional advantage was 7.6 based on ultrafiltered plasma and peritoneal fluid. Clearance from the peritoneal cavity may be calculated from their data to be 0.42 ml/min for a 200-g rat. The rat clearance is thus predictive of the human values on the basis of body weight to the 2/3 power in general agreement with the allometric variation in Fig. 5.

Average tumor levels of platinum in the i.p. group were twice those in the i.v. group; however, the excess platinum was confined to the periphery of the tumor. Measurements of platinum concentrations by proton-induced X-ray emission (PIXE) showed substantially higher levels in the outer 1.0 mm of the tumor; concentrations at 1.5 and 2.2 mm from the surface were independent of route of administration of the drug. This limited penetration is consistent with theoretical calculations for hexose [56] and experimental data for [^{14}C] EDTA [92] in normal tissues. It is instructive to apply a penetration model to cisplatin. As a rough approximation, let us assume that the diffusivity in tissue, D, is 1.9×10^{-6} cm^2/sec based on transport in brain [93]; that the capillary pa product is of the order of 1.4×10^{-3} sec^{-1} based on hexose in jejunum; and that the tissue specific reaction rate, k, is 8×10^{-5} sec^{-1} based on muscle [87]. Then the nominal diffusion distance $[D/(pa + k)]^{1/2}$ is 0.4 mm which would imply that 9/10 of the gradient would be confined to the first millimeter from the surface of the tissue. While these calculations are provided for illustrative purposes and are very approximate, they

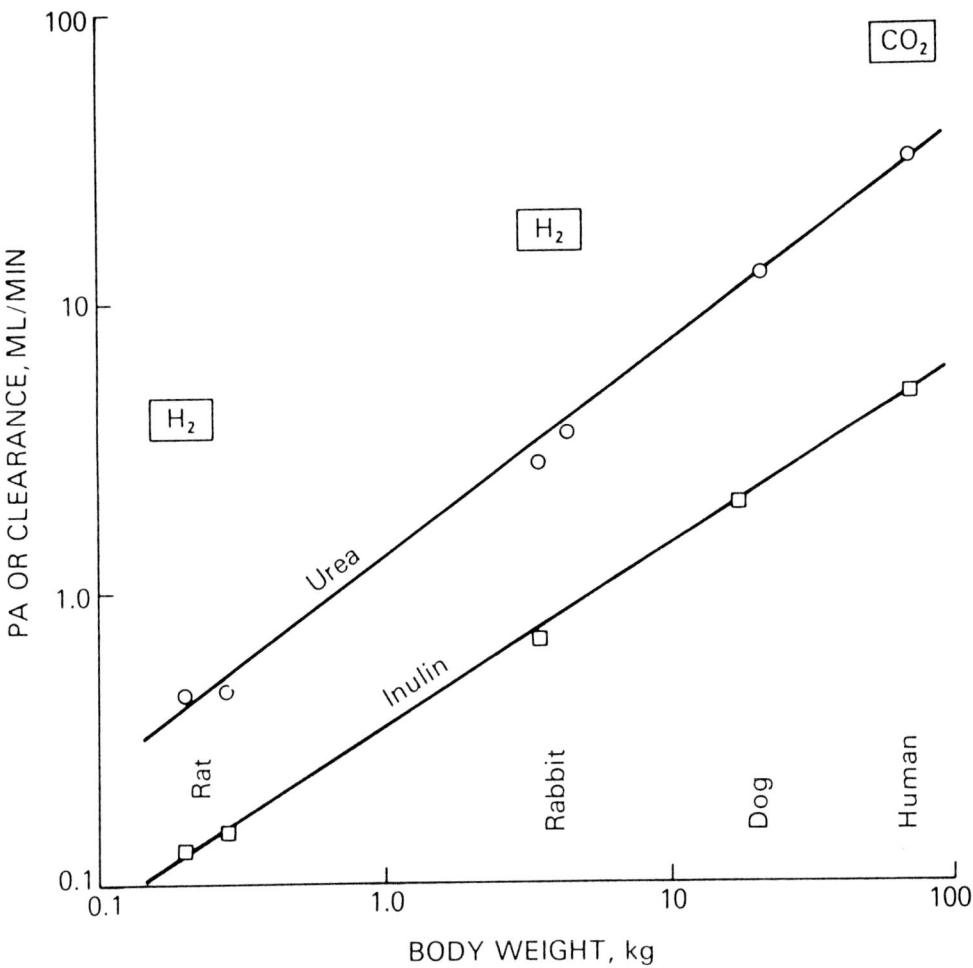

Figure 5. Peritoneal permeability times area (or mass transfer-area coefficient) for the indicated gases, urea, and inulin versus body weight. From reference [56].

are almost certainly much better that order-of-magnitude. They support the idea that direct diffusion of cisplatin into tissue is very limited in extent.

The above reaction ($k = 8 \times 10^{-5}$ sec^{-1}) and permeability (1.4×10^{-3} sec^{-1}) parameters predict that $[1.4 \times 10^{-3}/(1.4 \times 10^{-3} + 8 \times 10^{-5})] (100) = 95\%$ of the drug would be expected to be absorbed into the systemic circulation. This large bioavailability is consistent with the observations of Los *et al.* [91] in the tumor bearing rat and of Pretorius *et al.* [94] in the dog as well as with considerable human experience.

5.1.2. 5-fluorouracil

As discussed by Chabner [95], phosphorylation of 5-FU to nucleotide analogs appears necessary for its subsequent biological effects. Elimination from the body is primarily by metabolism believed to require reduction of the pyrimidine ring by dihydrouracil dehydrogenase. This enzyme is present in both the liver and other tissues such as the gastrointestinal mucosa. 5-FU exhibits strongly nonlinear elimination in humans subjects with a half-saturating concentration of 15 µM as reviewed and discussed in the development of a physiologic pharmacokinetic model [96]. Further, the observation of total body clearances at low infusion rates that considerably exceed expected hepatic blood flow suggests the presence of extensive extrahepatic metabolism.

5-FU has pharmacologic properties which commended it to intraperitoneal trials in the treatment of intra-abdominal cancer. It is a hydrophilic drug with a molecular weight of 130 daltons which would be expected to have a relatively slow clearance from the peritoneal cavity (Fig. 3) and a total body clearance ranging from 0.94 l/min at an infusion rate of 134 mg/kg/day to as high as

4–7 l/min at infusion rates of 10–30 mg/kg/day [96]. In addition to the high ratio of CL_{TB} to predicted PA, significant removal of the drug by peritoneal tissues would be expected to further limit systemic exposure.

The prediction of a high regional advantage has been shown in a number of clinical trials. Values of the AUC ratio between peritoneal cavity and plasma have been reported to be strongly dose dependent, ranging form 124 at a dose of 3.5 mM to 461 at a dose of 2.0 mM [14]. These are in general agreement with the observations of Speyer et al. [9], who observed peritoneal-to-plasma concentration ratios of 298 at four hours and of Sugarbaker et al. [97] who reported a mean AUC ratio of 200 in patients administered 5-FU in the immediate postoperative period. Clearance from the peritoneal cavity has been in good agreement with the predictions from Fig. 3: 14 ml/min [9] and 24 ml/min [14]. Nonlinearity in systemic exposure deriving from the saturable metabolism (and possible saturable first-pass effect) of the agent was associated with an extraordinarily steep dose-response curve [9].

There has been considerable interest in the detailed mechanism of absorption of 5-FU from the peritoneal cavity because of the possibility of using this route as a way to perfuse the liver through the portal vein. Speyer et al. [10] placed catheters in the portal vein, hepatic vein, peripheral artery and peripheral vein of human patients. The hepatic extraction was calculated to decrease slightly from about 0.7 to 0.6 from the first to the 7th exchange. The estimated value of the fraction, f, of the absorbed drug entering the portal system was strongly dependent on assumptions relating to the blood flow rate in the portal vein and metabolism by tissues draining into the portal system, neither of which was directly assessed. Estimated values of f ranged from 0.3 to 1 depending on the assumptions made. There was direct evidence of drug bypassing the portal system in three of the four patients in whom the AUC in the peripheral artery actually exceeded the AUC in the hepatic vein. Also, in studies in rats, Archer et al. [98] observed that systemic 5-FU levels were significantly lower during mesenteric vein infusion (0.9 ± 0.2 μM) compared with i.p. infusion at the same rate (2.1 ± 0.3 μM).

Indirect evidence of a pharmacologic first-pass effect is provided by the observations of Gianola et al. [99], who were able to administer a mean of 1.5 g per treatment cycle i.p. but only 1.0 g i.v.; the i.p route was actually accompanied by less hematological toxicity.

Penetration of 5-FU into tissues surrounding the peritoneal cavity has not been studied experimentally. Collins et al. [100] observed a strongly concentration-dependent rate of 5-FU disappearance from the peritoneal cavity of the rat. The peritoneal clearance increased from 0.20 ml/min, consistent with its molecular weight, to 10 times that value as the peritoneal concentration was decreased from 10 mM to 20 μM. This was explained by assuming that the drug is metabolized in tissues adjacent to the peritoneal cavity. A one-dimensional diffusion model with saturable intratissue metabolism (V_{max} = 36 nmol/min/g, K_m = 5 μM) simulated the peritoneal concentrations reasonably well. The model predicted that the concentration in the tissue would be 10% of its value at the tissue surface at a depth of 0.6 mm following a 12 mM dose; the corresponding 10% level would be reached at only 0.13 mm following a 24 μM dose. Observations that the toxicity profile associated with intraperitoneal administration is similar to that observed following i.v. administration [9, 99] seem to confirm limited tissue penetration. If the drug reached the gastrointestinal crypt cells in high concentration, one would expect substantial toxicity there.

5.2. Antibiotics: Vancomycin

Intraperitoneal antibiotic therapy is used to treat localized peritonitis. The goal of such therapy is the same as that of antineoplastic agents: to maximize the concentration in the cavity in order to target the superficial tissues in the peritoneal cavity. Since the subject of i.p. antibiotic therapy has been covered thoroughly in another chapter of this text, we will illustrate the general approach to calculation of the regional pharmacokinetic advantage by application of the theory to vancomycin, a drug which is currently one of the recommended "first-line" therapies [101].

Vancomycin has molecular weight of 1500. 55% of the drug is bound to serum protein [102–104]. Its volume of distribution is variable and is cited over a range of 0.64 L/kg in normal young humans [102] to 0.93 L/kg in the elderly [102–103]. Patients with renal failure (creatinine clearance less than 10 ml/min) have volumes of distribution averaging 0.9 L/kg [104]. The serum half-life of vancomycin is typically 6 hours. However, since 90% of the injected dose is excreted by the kidneys [105–106], the normal half life of 6 hours becomes markedly prolonged in renal failure. Clearance of the drug in normal (70 kg) patients is 100–140 ml/min. In the patient with renal failure, the clearance is correlated with iothalamate, a marker for glomerular filtration rate [105]. Typical clearance rates for patients with creatinine clearance less than 10 ml/min average approximately 5 ml/min [104, 107].

Table 5 lists model parameters which can be used to calculate the pharmacokinetic advantage. We have estimated the capillary permeabilities from our range of values in Tables 2 and 3 and Figure 4. D_e has been equated to the value derived from experiments performed with polyethylene glycol (MW = 900 daltons) [61]. The interstitial fractions have been set equal to those of sucrose. The calculated overall PA equals 3.2 ml/min, which is slightly lower than the value given by Fig. 3: 4.0 ml/min. For the purpose of illustration, let us assume that the overall clearance from the body of our patient on peritoneal dialysis is 5 ml/min and that the drug is given by continuous infusion. Under these circumstances, the relative advantage of i.p. administration relative to i.v. administration is calculated from equation (11) modified to account for protein binding: $R_d = 1 + 5/(3.2 \times 0.45) = 4.5$.

Because of the long half-life and the toxicity of high serum levels which might result if continuous infusion were performed [103], the drug is usually given in either a single i.p. dialysate dwell every 24 hours of as an i.v. infusion approximately once a week. Bunke et al. [108] studied vancomycin pharmacokinetics by dosing patients with either 10 mg/kg i.v. in a saline solution over 30 min or 10 mg/kg diluted in 2 liters of 1.5% dextrose dialysate, which was allowed to dwell over 4 hours. By computing the AUC_P/AUC_B for i.p. delivery during the first 24 hours, the regional advantage (R_{ip}) is 429/109 = 3.9. Repeating the same for i.v. delivery, the AUC_P/AUC_B (R_{iv}) is 78.4/297 = 0.26.

The pharmacokinetic advantage would then be $R_{ip}/R_{iv} = 3.9/.26 = 15$. This provides a strong theoretical and experimental argument for i.p. vancomycin in appropriate cases of peritonitis.

5.3. Intraperitoneal insulin

Human insulin is a small protein with a molecular weight of 5808, which is secreted by the beta cells of the pancreatic islets of Langerhans in response to a glucose load in the plasma [109]. The secretion occurs directly into blood which circulates via the portal vein to the liver. The bulk of the hormone in the blood is in the unbound form [110]. Extraction of the hormone by the liver is receptor-mediated, saturable, and typically amounts to 40–60% of the drug delivered in the portal system [111]. After entering the general circulation, insulin distributes to the entire extracellular space [110]. In particular insulin circulates to the kidney and muscle, which, aside from the liver, are its other major targets. Under normal conditions, there is a portal-to-peripheral insulin concentration gradient, with the highest concentrations in the liver [112]. In an effort to control diabetic hyperglycemia in a more physiological way, replacement insulin is increasingly being administered intraperitoneally in order to mimic the normal physiology.

Insulin is often administered dissolved in the dialysate to diabetic patients who suffer from ESRD and are treated with CAPD [113]. This results in the simultaneous transfer of insulin and dextrose from the cavity into the body. Because of the extensive extraction by the liver, equation (12) must be used in order to predict the regional advantage of i.p. insulin therapy. Rubin [3] has shown that the transport properties of insulin (Mass-Transfer-Area Coefficient or MTAC = 2.9 m./min) are nearly identical to those of inulin (MTAC = 3.3 ml/min).

Table 5. Adult human parameters for vancomycin.

Tisue	a_i (cm²/cm³)	p_i (cm/min × 10⁵)	D_e (cm²/min × 10⁵)	Θ_i	P_i (cm/min × 10⁴)	A_i (cm²)	P_iA_i (cm³/min)	F (ml/min)	PA/F	q_i (ml/min/g)	pa/q
Liver	250	300	1.7	0.14	13.4	1056	1.41	0.07	21.2	0.83	0.90
Other viscera (intestines, spleen, stomach)	70	30	1.7	0.21	2.7	5432	1.49	0.33	4.5	0.65	0.03
Abdominal wall	70	30	1.7	0.12	2.1	880	0.18	0.67	0.3	0.06	0.35
Diaphragm	70	30	1.7	0.12	2.1	632	0.13	0.27	0.5	0.30	0.07

Overall parameters: PA = 3.21 ml/min; F = 1.34 ml/min; PA/F = 2.4.

Table 3 contains estimates of transport parameters for inulin and these will be used as parameters for insulin. PA is highest for the liver and the "other viscera", both of which account for nearly 90% of the total diffusive transfer of insulin from the cavity. F, the convective flow rate from the cavity to the tissue, does not enter directly into the calculation. In equation (12), f = 0.9 and E = 0.5. PA_{tot} from Table 3 = 1.57 ml/min. While the normal total body clearance of insulin is typically 650–750 ml/min (referenced to 1.73 m^2), the clearance of ^{125}I-insulin is approximately half or 350 ml/min in chronic renal failure [114–115]. The regional advantage can be calculated from equation (12): R_R = [1 + 350/1.57]/(1 – 0.9 (0.5)) = 407. The measured ratio of intraperitoneally-administered ^{125}I-insulin (AUC_p/AUC_B) was approximately 500 in dogs [113] while the value was 200–300 in humans [116].

Recent efforts in insulin replacement therapy for patients, who suffer from diabetes mellitus but who are not on dialysis, have tested i.p. administration as a more physiological method of drug delivery [112]. In a study which compared free insulin peaks after i.m., s.c., and i.p. injections, intraperitoneal insulin produced serum insulin peaks at 15 min, while i.m and s.c. insulin resulted in a much slower increase with peaks at 60 and 90 min respectively [117]. The rapid rise in serum insulin, produced by i.p. administration, followed by a gradual fall in concentration more closely mimics the true pancreas. The same study demonstrated that insulin delivered to the upper part of the peritoneal cavity was more quickly absorbed than insulin introduced into the lower part of the cavity. This is likely due to the rapid transfer into tissues of the gastrointestinal tract and direct diffusion into the liver. Delivery into the cavity by a pump has also led to more consistent serum levels than with administration into subcutaneous tissue, which produces variability in absorption rates [118].

In contrast to the relatively steady delivery of i.p. insulin in CAPD, this therapy is typically given episodically in small volumes in the upper part of the cavity. The ratio of portal to systemic venous levels of insulin (AUC_{portal}/AUC_B) can give us a rough estimate of the utility of the delivery technique. It should be pointed out that the concentration in the portal vein probably reflects only a portion of the insulin delivered to the liver, since direct absorption across the surface of the liver is known to occur [119]. Selam *et al.* [120] the demonstrated in dogs that the ratio of i.p. insulin delivery to the portal vein over the amount appearing in the plasma is 17. Although this regional advantage is not as dramatically high as in the case of CAPD patients, it nonetheless supports the concept of i.p. delivery of insulin in order to reestablish the normal portal-to-peripheral insulin concentration gradient.

5.4. I.P. antibody therapy

A relatively new concept in cancer therapy is the use of i.p.-administered monoclonal antibodies in the treatment of intra-abdominal cancers. These antibodies, which are typically linked to some toxic agent, react specifically with antigens on the tumor cell and bind strongly, with subsequent killing of the cell [121]. As outlined in Dedrick and Flessner [122] the general equation for the calculation of the pharmacokinetic advantage is the same as that for small substances (see equation (11)). From Table 4, PA_{tot} = 0.03 ml/min, which is in agreement with Rippe's recent estimate [70] of 0.05 ml/min. The total body clearance of IgG has been estimated to be 0.5–1.0 ml/min [122]. Inserting this into equation (11), one may calculate a R_d of 17–33. This suggests a considerable pharmacokinetic advantage in i.p. administration of monoclonal antibody.

The usefulness of this therapy must also be assessed in terms of the ultimate goal. Free ascites cells are readily accessible to MAbs [123]; in this case the R_d would be the number calculated by equation (11). Unlike smaller molecules, however, large proteins do not penetrate tissues readily. Because of their large size (molecular radius = 52 Å), the effective diffusivity in tissue is on the order of 10^{-9} cm^2/s [64]. Since this is 100–1000 times less than the diffusivity of small molecules, the diffusive transport of macromolecules such as IgG within normal or neoplastic tissue is very slow. Recent mathematical analyses have also shown that MAbs with high affinity to their antigens are even more severely retarded by the "binding-site barrier" [124–126]. The transport of these molecules is typically dominated by convection, both within the interstitial space [127] and across capillary endothelium [128]. Tissue penetration studies of antibodies administered i.p. in animals [28] have shown that most of the IgG is contained in the initial 300–400 μM of tissue during the first 3 hours. These studies also demonstrated that diffusion likely plays only a minor role in the transport of the protein. Studies in tumor-bearing animals confirm these findings and have not demonstrated large advantages of i.p. MAb administration over i.v. administration [123]. This means that there may be limitations in the treatment of solid tumors and metastases with MAbs or other macromolecules.

6. Summary

Intraperitoneal chemotherapy should be considered as an alternative to intravenous therapy when the target is contained within the peritoneal cavity or within the adjacent tissue. The distributed model concept has been used to formulate a calculational scheme in order to evaluate the solute transport to specific tissue groups surrounding the cavity. With parameters derived from the literature, the model can be used to solve for the steady-state concentrations in the peritoneal cavity and the plasma. The ratio of these two concentrations defines the regional advantage of intraperitoneal therapy. Several applications of the theory are presented in order to illustrate the method in which a new i.p. therapy may be evaluated prior to use in patients.

References

1. Cole WCC, Montgomery JC. Intraperitoneal blood transfusion. Amer J Dis Child 1929; 37: 497–510.
2. Clausen J. Studies on the effects of intraperitoneal blood transfusion. Acta Paediatr, Stockholm. 1940; 27: 24–31.
3. Rubin JA, Reed V, Adair C, Bower J, Klein E. Effect of intraperitoneal insulin on solute kinetics in CAPD: insulin kinetics in CAPD. Am J Med Sci 1986; 291: 81–7.
4. Pitt HA, Saudek CD, Zacur HA. Long-term intraperitoneal insulin delivery. Ann Surg 1992; 216: 483–92.
5. Bargman JM, Jones JE, Petro JM. The pharmacokinetics of intraperitoneal erythropoietin administered undiluted and diluted in dialysate. Perit Dial Intl 1992; 12: 369–72.
6. Lamiere N, Bogaert M, Belpaire L. Peritoneal pharmacokinetics and pharmacological manipulation of peritoneal transport. In: Gokal R (ed), Continuous Ambulatory Peritoneal Dialysis. Churchill Livingstone, New York 1986; pp 56–93.
7. Hirszel P, Maher JF. Pharmacologic alteration of peritoneal transport rates. In: Nolph K (ed), Peritoneal Dialysis, 3rd Ed 1990; pp 184–95.
8. Jones RB, Myers CE, Guarino AM, Dedrick RL, Hubbard SM, DeVita VT. High volume intraperitoneal chemotherapy ("Belly Bath") for ovarian cancer. Cancer Chemother Pharm 1978; 1: 161–6.
9. Speyer JL, Collins JM, Dedrick RL, Brennan MF, Buckpitt AR, Londer H, DeVita VT, Myers CE. Phase I and pharmacological studies of 5-fluorouracil administered intraperitoneally. Canc Res 1980; 40: 567–72.
10. Speyer JL, Sugarbaker PH, Collins JM, Dedrick RL, Klecker RW, Jr, Myers CE. Portal levels and hepatic clearance of 5-Fluorouracil after intraperitoneal administration in humans. Cancer Res 1981; 41: 1916–22.
11. Jones RB, Collins JC, Myers CE, Brooks AE, Hubbard SM, Balow JE, Brennan MF, Dedrick RL, DeVita VT. High-volume intraperitoneal chemotherapy with methotrexate in patients with cancer. Cancer Res 1981; 41: 55–9.
12. Ozols RF, Young RC, Speyer JL, Sugarbaker PH, Greene R, Jenkins J, Myers CE. Phase I and pharmacological studies of adriamycin administered intraperitoneally to patients with ovarian cancer. Cancer Res 1982; 42: 4265–9.
13. Gianni L, Jenkins JF, Greene RF, Lichter AS, Myers CE, Collins JM. Pharmacokinetics of the hypoxic radiosensitizers misonidazole and demethylmisonidazole after intraperitoneal administration in humans. Cancer Res 1983; 43: 913–6.
14. Arbuck SG, Trave F, Douglas Jr HO, Nava H, Zakrzewski S, Rustum MY. Phase I and pharmacologic studies of intraperitoneal leucovorin and 5-fluorouracil in patients with advanced cancer. J Clin Oncol 1986; 4: 1510–7.
15. Urba WJ, Clark JW, Steis RG, Bookman MA, Smith II JW, Beckner S, Maluish AE, Rossio AL, Rager H, Ortaldo AR, Longo DL. Intraperitoneal lymphokine-activated killer cell/interleukin-2 therapy in patients with intra-abdominal cancer: immunologic considerations. J Natl Canc Inst 1989; 81: 602–11.
16. Markman M, Hakes T, Reichmann B, Hoskins W, Rubin S, Lewis Jr JL. Intraperitoneal versus intravenous cisplatin-based therapy in small-volume residual refractory ovarian cancer: evidence supporting an advantage for local drug delivery. Regional Canc Treatment. 1990; 3: 10–2.
17. Howell SB, Pfeifle CE, Wung WE, Olshen RA. Intraperitoneal cis-diamminedichloroplatinum with systemic thiosulfate protection. Cancer Res 1983; 43; 1426–31.
18. Dedrick RL. Interspecies scaling of regional drug delivery. J Pharm Sci 1986; 75: 1047–52.
19. Crafts RC: A Textbook of Human Anatomy. 2nd Ed. New York: John Wiley and Sons. 1979: 213–345.
20. Leak LB, Rahil K. Permeability of the diaphragmatic mesothelium: the ultrastructural basis for "stomata". Am J Anat 1978; 151: 557–94.
21. Bettendorf U. Lymph flow mechanism of the subperitoneal diaphragmatic lymphatics. Lymphology 1978; 11: 111–6.
22. Allen L. On the penetrability of the lymphatics of the diaphragm. Anat Rec 1956; 124: 639–58.
23. Yoffey JM, Courtice FC. Lymphatics, Lymph, and the Lymphomyeloid Complex. Academic Press, New York 1970
24. Flessner MF, Parker RJ, Sieber SM. Peritoneal

25. Abernathy NJ, Chin W, Hay JB, Rodela H, Oreopoulos, Johnston MG. Lymphatic drainage of the peritoneal cavity in sheep. Am J Physiol 1991; 260: F353–8.
26. Flessner MF, Dedrick RL, Reynolds JC. Bidirectional peritoneal transport of immunoglobulin in rats: compartmental kinetics. Am J Physiol 1992; 262: F275–87.
27. Pearson CM. Circulation in skeletal muscle. In: Abramson DI (ed), Blood Vessels and Lymphatics. Academic Press, New York 1862; pp 520–1.
28. Flessner MF, Dedrick RL, Reynolds JC. Bidirectional peritoneal transport of immunoglobulin in rats: tissues concentration profiles. Am J Physiol 1992; 263: F15–23.
29. Rubin J, Clawson M, Planch A, Jones Q. Measurements of peritoneal surface area in man and rat. Amer J Med Sci 1988; 295: 453–8.
30. Esperanca MJ, Collins DL. Peritoneal dialysis efficiency in relation to body weight. J Pediatr Surg 1966; 1: 162–9.
31. Ludwig J. Current Methods of Autopsy Practice. Philadelphia: WB Saunders, 1972.
32. Rhodin JAG. Histology: A Text and Atlas. New York: Oxford University Press, 1974.
33. Richardson KC. Illustrations of Light Microscopical Preparations from Various Tissues and Organs. Baltimore: University of Maryland School of Medicine, 1976.
34. diFiore MSH. Atlas of Human Histology. Lea and Fegiger, Philadelphia 1981.
35. Rubin J, Jones Q, Planch A, Stanek K. Systems of membranes involved in peritoneal dialysis. J Lab Clin Med 1987; 110: 448–53.
36. Vetterlein F, Schmidt G. Functional capillary density in skeletal muscle during vasodilation induced by isoprenaline and muscular exercise. Microvas Res 1980; 20: 156–64.
37. Guyton AC. Textbook of Medical Physiology, 6th Ed. WB Saunders Co, Philadelphia 1981; pp 349.
38. Mapleson WW. An electric analogue for uptake and exchange of inert gases and other agents. J Appl Physiol 1963; 18: 197–204.
39. Bonaccorsi A, Dejana E, Quintana A. Organ blood flow measured with microspheres in the unanesthetized rat: effects of three room temperatures. J Pharmacol Meth 1978; 1: 321–28.
40. Grim E. The flow of blood in the mesenteric vessels. In: Hamilton WF, Dow P (eds), Handbook of Physiology, Vol II Sect 2. American Physiological Society, Washington 1963; pp 1443–56.
41. Chow CC, Grassmick B. Motility and blood flow distribution within the wall of the gastrointestinal tract. Am J Physiol 1978; 235: H34–9.
42. Crandall LA Jr, Barker SB, Graham DG. A study of the lymph flow from a patient with thoracic duct fistula. Gastroent 1943; 1: 1040.
43. Courtice FC, Simonds WJ, Steinbeck AW. Some investigations on lymph from a thoracic duct fistula in man. Austral J Exptl Biol Med Sci 1951; 29: 201.
44. O'Morchoe CCC, O'Morchoe DJ, Holmes MJ, Jarosz HM. Flow of renal hilar lymph during volume expansion and saline diuresis. Lymphology 1978; 11: 27–31.
45. Shad H, Brechtelsbauer H. Thoracic duct lymph in conscious dog at rest and during changes of physical activity. Pfluegers Arch 1978; 367: 235–40.
46. Morris B. The exchange of protein between the plasma and the liver and intestinal lymph. Quart J Exptl Physiol 1956; 41: 326.
47. Yoffey JM, Courtice FC. Lymphatics, Lymph, and Lymphoid Tissue. Harvard University Press, Cambridge 1956; pp 121–219.
48. Tran L, Rodela H, Abernethy NJ, Yuan Z-Y, Hay JB, Oreopoulous D, Johnston MG. Lymphatic drainage of hypertonic solution from peritoneal cavity of anesthetized and conscious sheep. J Appl Physiol 1993; 74: 859–67.
49. Daugirdas JT, Ing TS, Gandhi VC, Hano JE, Chen WT, Yuan L. Kinetics of peritoneal fluid absorption in patients with chronic renal failure. J Lab Clin Med 1980; 85: 351–61.
50. Rippe B, Stelin G, Ahlmen J. Lymph flow from the peritoneal cavity in CAPD patients. In: Maher JF, Winchester JF (eds), Frontiers in Peritoneal Dialysis. Field, Rich, New York 1986; pp 24–30.
51. Dykes PW, Jones JH. Albumin exchange between plasma and ascites fluid. Clin Sci 1964; 34: 185–97.
52. Mactier RA, Khanna R, Twardowski Z, Nolph KD. Role of peritoneal cavity lymphatic absorption in peritoneal dialysis. Kidney Int 1987; 32: 165–74.
53. Zink J, Greenway CV. Control of ascites absorption in anesthetized cats: effects of intraperitoneal pressure, protein, and furosemide diuresis. Gastroent 1974; 73: 1119–24.
54. Nolph KD, Mactier R, Khanna R, Twardowski ZJ, Moore H, McGary T. The kinetics of ultrafiltration during peritoneal dialysis: the role of lymphatics. Kidney Int 1987; 32: 219–26.
55. Flessner MF. Net ultrafiltration in peritoneal dialysis: role of direct fluid absorption into peritoneal tissue. Blood Purif 1992; 10: 136–47.
56. Dedrick RL, Flessner MF, Collins JM, Schultz JS. Is the peritoneum a membrane? ASAIO J 1982: 5: 1–8.
57. Crone C. The permeability of capillaries in various organs as determined by use of the 'indicator diffusion' method. Acta Physiol Scand 1963; 58: 292–305.
58. Carter RD, Joyner WL, Renkin EM. Effects of histamine and some other substances on molecular selectivity of the capillary wall to plasma proteins and dextran. Microvas Res 1974; 7: 31–8.
59. Mayerson HS, Wolfram GC, Shirley HH, Wasserman K. Regional differences in capillary permeability. Am J Physiol 1960; 198: 155–60.
60. Schultz JS, Armstrong W. Permeability of inter-

stitial space of muscle (rat diaphragm) to solutes of different molecular weights. J Pharm Sci 1978; 67: 696–700.
61. Flessner MF, Dedrick RL, Schultz JS. A distributed model of peritoneal-plasma transport: analysis of experimental data in the rat. Am J Physiol 1985; 248: F413–24.
62. Watson PD, Grodins FS. An analysis of the effects of the interstitial matrix on plasma-lymph transport. Microvas Res 1978; 16: 19–41.
63. Flessner MF, Dedrick RL, Schultz JS. Exchange of macromolecules between peritoneal cavity and plasma. Am J Physiol 1985; 248: H15–25.
64. Clauss MA, Jain RK. Interstitial transport of rabbit and sheep antibodies in normal and neoplastic tissues. Cancer Res 1990; 50: 3487–92.
65. Larsson M, Johnson L, Nylander G, Ohman U. Plasma water and ^{51}Cr EDTA equilibration volumes of different tissues in the rat. Acta Physiol Scand 1980; 110: 53–7.
66. Goresky CA. The interstitial space in the liver: its partitioning effects. In: Crone C, Lassen NA (eds), Capillary permeability. Alfred Benzon Symposium III. Academic Press, New York 1970; pp 415–33.
67. Rippe B. Personal Communication.
68. Bill A. Plasma protein dynamics: albumin and IgG capillary permeability, extravascular movement and regional blood flow in unanesthetized rabbits. Acta Physiol Scand 1977; 101: 28–42.
69. Dedrick RL, Myers CE, Bungay PM, DeVita VT. Pharmacokinetic rationale for peritoneal drug administration in the treatment of ovarian cancer. Cancer Treatment Rep 1978; 61: 1–11.
70. Rippe B, Stelin G, Ahlmen J. Basal permeability of the peritoneal membrane during continuous ambulatory peritoneal dialysis (CAPD). In: Maher J (ed), Advances in Peritoneal Dialysis, 1981. Excerpta Medica, Amsterdam 1981; pp 5–9.
71. Krediet RT, Struijk DG, Koomen GCM, Zemel D, Boeschoten EW, Hoek FJ, Arisz L. Peritoneal transport of macromolecules in patients on CAPD. Contrib Nephrol 1991; 89: 161–74.
72. Torres IJ, Litterst Cl, Guarino AM. Transport of model compounds across the peritoneal membrane in the rat. Pharmacol 1978; 17: 330–40.
73. Lewis C, Lawson N, Rankin EM, et al. Phase I and pharmacokinetic study of intraperitoneal thioTEPA in patients with ovarian cancer. Cancer Chemother Pharmacol 1990; 26: 283–7.
74. Wikes AD, Howell SB. Pharmacokinetics of hexamethylmelamine administered via the ip route in an oil emulsion vehicle. Cancer Treatment Rep 1985; 69: 657–62.
75. Aune S. Transperitoneal exchange. II Peritoneal blood flow estimated by hydrogen gas clearance. Scand J Gastroent 1970; 5: 99–104.
76. Flessner MF. Transport of water soluble solutes between the peritoneal cavity and the plasma in the rat. [Dissertation]. Ann Arbor, Mich: Department of Chemical Engineering, University of Michigan, 1981.
77. Grzegorzewska AE, Moore HL, Nolph KD, Chen TW. Ultrafiltration and effective peritoneal blood flow during peritoneal dialysis in the rat. Kidney Int 1991; 39: 608–17.
78. Collins JM. Inert gas exchange of subcutaneous and intraperitoneal gas pockets in piglets. Resp Phys 1981; 46: 391–404.
79. Pitts RF. Physiology of the kidney and body fluids. Year Book Medical Publishers, Chicago 1963; p 63.
80. Lukas G. Brindle SD, Greengard P. The route of absorption of intraperitoneally administered compounds. J Pharmacol Exptl Therap 1971; 178: 562–6.
81. Myers CE, Collins JM. Pharmacology of intraperitoneal chemotherapy. Cancer Investigation 1983; 1: 395–407.
82. Brenner DE. Intraperitoneal chemotherapy: a review. J Clin Oncol 1986; 4: 1135–47.
83. Los G, McVie JG. Experimental and clinical status of intraperitoneal chemotherapy. Eur J Cancer 1990; 26: 755–62.
84. Markman M, Reichman B, Hakes T et al. Impact on survival of surgically defined favorable responses to salvage intraperitoneal chemotherapy in small-volume residual ovarian cancer. J Clin Oncol 1992; 10: 1479–84.
85. Ozols RF. Intraperitoneal chemotherapy. Current Prob Cancer 1992; 16: 99–101.
86. Farris FF, King FG, Dedrick RL, Litterst CL. Physiological model for the pharmacokinetics of cis-dichlorodiammineplatinum(II) (DDP) in the tumored rat. J Pharmacokin Biopharm 1985; 13: 13–39.
87. King FG, Dedrick RL, Farris FF. Physiological pharmacokinetic modeling of cis-dichlorodiammineplatinum(II) (DDP) in several species. J Pharmacokin Biopharm 1986; 14: 131–55.
88. King FG, Dedrick RL. Physiological pharmacokinetic parameters for cis-dichlorodiammineplatinum(II) (DDP) in the mouse. J Pharmacokin Biopharm 1992; 20: 95–9.
89. Goel R, Cleary SM, Horton C et al. Effect of sodium thiosulfate on the pharmacokinetics and toxicity of cisplatin. J Nat Cancer Inst 1989; 81: 1552–60.
90. Piccart MJ, Abrams J, Dodian PF et al. Intraperitoneal chemotherapy with cisplatin and melphalan. J Nat Cancer Inst 1988; 80: 1118–24.
91. Los G, Mutsaers PHA, van der Vigh WJG, Baldew GS, de Graaf PW, McVie JG. Direct diffusion of cis-diamminedichloroplatinum(II) in intraperitoneal rat tumors after intraperitoneal chemotherapy: a comparison with systemic chemotherapy. Cancer Res 1989; 49: 3380–4.
92. Flessner MF, Fenstermacher JD, Dedrick RL, Blasberg RG. A distributed model of peritoneal-plasma transport: tissue concentration gradients. Am J Physiol 1985; 248: F425–35.
93. Morrison PF, Dedrick RL. Transport of cisplatin in rat brain following microinfusion: an analysis. J Pharm Sci 1986; 75: 120–8.
94. Pretorius RG, Petrilli ES, Kean C, Ford LC,

Hoeschele JD, Lagasse LD. Comparison of the iv and ip routes of cisplatin in dogs. Cancer Treatment Rep 1981; 65: 1055–62.
95. Chabner BA. Fluorinated pyrimidines. In: Chabner B (ed), Pharmacologic principles of cancer treatment. W B Saunders, Philadelphia 1982; pp 183–212.
96. Collins JM, Dedrick RL, King FG, Speyer JL, Myers CE. Nonlinear pharmacokinetic models for 5-fluorouracil in man: intravenous and intraperitoneal routes. Clin Pharmacol Therap 1980; 28: 235–46.
97. Sugarbaker PH, Graves T, DeBruijn EA et al. Early postoperative intraperitoneal chemotherapy as an adjuvant therapy to surgery for peritoneal carcinomatosis from gastrointestinal cancer: pharmacological studies. Cancer Rest 1990; 50: 5790–4.
98. Archer SG, McCulloch RK, Gray BN. A comparative study of the pharmacokinetics of continuous portal vein infusion versus intraperitoneal infusion of 5-fluorouracil. Reg Cancer Treat 1989; 2: 105–11.
99. Gianola FJ, Sugarbaker PH, Barofsky I, White DE, Meyers CE. Toxicity studies of adjuvant intravenous versus intraperitoneal 5-FU in patients with advanced primary colon or rectal cancer. Am J Clin Oncol 1986; 9: 403–10.
100. Collins JM, Dedrick RL, Flessner MF, Guarino AM. Concentration-dependent disappearance of fluorouracil from peritoneal fluid in the rat: experimental observations and distributed modeling. J Pharm Sci 1982; 71: 735–8.
101. Peritoneal dialysis-related peritonitis treatment recommendations, 1993 update. Perit Dial Intl 1993; 13: 14–28.
102. Cutler NR, Narang PK, Lesko LJ, Ninos M, Power M. Vancomycin disposition: the importance of age. Clin Pharmacol Ther 1984; 36: 803–10.
103. Moellering RC. Pharmacokinetics of vancomycin. J Antimicr Chemother 1984; 14 (suppl): D43–52.
104. Matzke GR, McGory RW, Halstenson CE, Keane WF. Pharmacokinetics of vancomycin in patients with various degrees of renal function. Antimicrob Agents Chemother 1984; 25: 433–7.
105. Rotschafer JC, Crossley K, Zaske DE, Mead K, Sawchuk RJ, Solem LD. Pharmacokinetics of vancomycin: observations in 28 patients and dosage recommendations. Antimicrob Agents Chemother 1982; 22: 392–4.
106. Nielsen HE, Hansen HE, Korsager B, Skov PE. Renal excretion of vancomycin in kidney disease. Acta Med Scand 1975; 197: 261–4.
107. Cunha BA, Ristuccia AM. Clinical usefulness of vancomycin. Clin Pharmacol 1983; 2: 417–24.
108. Bunke CM, Aronoff GR, Brier ME, Sloan RS, Luft FC. Vancomycin kinetics during continuous ambulatory peritoneal dialysis. Clin Pharmacol Ther 1983; 34: 621–37.
109. Guyton AC. Textbook of Medical Physiology, 6th Ed. WB Saunders Co, Philadelphia 1981; p 959.
110. Larner J. Insulin and oral hypoglycemic drugs and glucagon. In: Gilman AG, Goodman LS, Rall TW, Murad F (eds), Goodman and Gilman's The Pharmacological Basis of Therapeutics. 7th ed. Macmillan Publishing Co, New York 1985; pp 1490–503.
111. Duckworth WC. Insulin degradation: mechanisms, products, and significance. Endocrine Rev 1988; 9: 319–45.
112. Duckworth WC, Saudek CD, Henry RR. Why intraperitoneal delivery of insulin with implantable pumps in NIDDM? Diabetes 1992; 41: 657–61.
113. Shapiro DJ, Blumenkrantz MJ, Levin SR, Coburn JW. Absorption and action of insulin added to peritoneal dialysate in dogs. Nephron 1979; 23: 174–80.
114. Fuss M, Bergans A, Brauman H, Toussaint C, Vereerstraeten P, Franckson M, Corvilain J. ^{125}I-insulin metabolism in chronic renal failure treated by renal transplantation. Kidney Int 1974; 5: 372–7.
115. Navalesi R, Pilo A, Lenzi S, Donato L. Insulin metabolism in chronic uremia and in the anephric state: effect of the dialytic treatment. J Clin Endocrinol Metab 1975; 40: 70–85.
116. Wideroe T-E, Smeby LC, Berg KJ, Jorstad S, Svart TM. Intraperitoneal (^{125}I) insulin absorption during intermittent and continuous peritoneal dialysis. Kidney I 1983; 23: 22–8.
117. Micossi P, Cristallo M, Librenti MC, Petrella G, Galimberti G, Melandri M, Monti L, Spotti D, Scavini M, Di Carlo V, Pozza G. Free-insulin profiles after intraperitoneal, intramuscular, and subcutaneous insulin administration. Diabetes Care 1986; 9: 575–8.
118. Williams G, Pickup J, Clark A, Bowcock S, Cooke E, Keen H. Changes in blood flow close to subcutaneous insulin injection site in stable and brittle diabetics. Diabetes 1983; 32: 466–73.
119. Zingg W, Rappaport AM, Leibel BS: Studies on transhepatic absorption. Can J Physiol Pharmacol 1986; 64: 231–4.
120. Selam J-L, Bergman RN, Raccah D, Jean-Didier N, Lozano J, Charles MA. Determination of portal insulin absorption from peritoneum via novel nonisotopic method. Diabetes 1990; 39: 1361–5.
121. Ward BG, Mather SJ, Hawkins LR, Crowther ME, Shepherd JH, Granowska M, Britton KE, Slevin ML. Localization of radioiodine conjugated to the monoclonal antibody HMFG2 in human ovarian carcinoma: assessment of intravenous and intraperitoneal routes of administration. Cancer Res 1987; 47: 4719–23.
122. Dedrick RL, Flessner MF. Pharmacokinetic considerations on monoclonal antibodies. Immunity to Cancer. II. Alan R. Liss, Inc, New York 1989; pp 429–38.
123. Griffin TW, Collins J, Bokhari F, Stochl M, Brill AB, Ito T, Emond G, Sands H. Intraperitoneal immunoconjugates. Cancer Res 1990; 50: S1031–8.
124. Fujimori K, Covell DG, Fletcher JE, Weinstein JN. Modeling analysis of the global and microscopic

125. Fujimori K, Covell DB, Fletcher JE, Weinstein JN. A modeling analysis of monoclonal antibody percolation through tumors: a binding-site barrier. J Nucl Med 1990; 31: 1191–8.
126. van Osdol W, Fujimori K, Weinstein JN. An analysis of monoclonal antibody distribution in microscopic tumor nodules: consequences of a "binding site barrier". Cancer Res 1991; 51: 4776–84.
127. Flessner MF. Peritoneal transport physiology: insights from basic research. JASN 1991; 2: 122–35.
128. Rippe B, Haraldsson B. Fluid and protein fluxes across small and large pores in the microvasculature. Application of two-pore equations. Acta Physiol Scand 1987; 131: 411–28.

distribution of immunoglobulin G, F(ab')$_2$, and Fab in tumors. Cancer Res 1989; 49: 5656–63.

Index

abdominal
    bloating 565
    catastrophies 621
    events 369
    pain 292, 366
    pores (peritoneal canals) 27
    reflux 565
    viscera 478
    wall 370, 478
acetate 249
acetazolamide 540
acid base balance 562
acidemias, organic 757
acidosis 245, 451, 535, 540
acquired renal cystic disease (ARCD) 572
ACTH 706
acute renal failure (ARF) 754
adequate dialysis 10, 419
adhesion 490
    molecule, intercellular 518
    molecule, vascular cell 518
adsorbents 168
adult day care centers 675
advanced glycosylation end products (AGE) 36
adynamic bone
    disease 377
    lesion 531
age 719
agents 238
    high molecular weight 238
    low molecular weight 238
AIDS 482, 752
albumin 80, 86, 96, 129, 144, 245
    concentrations 447
    flux 82
    loss of 620
aldosterone 98, 706
alkalosis, respiratory 563
allergic reactions 302
aluminium 535
    related bone diseases 535
    toxicity 237
amino acids 95, 242, 452
    beneficial effects 245
    clinical efficacy 245
    ineffectiveness of 244
    intraperitoneal 375
    loss of 452, 608
aminoglycoside antibiotics 205
    stability of 204
amphotericin B 175

amputation 649
amyloidosis 100, 574
    related disorders 378
anaerobic organisms 483
anatomical resistance sites 119
anemia 376, 461
angiopathy 35
angiotensin II 98
anionic sites 176
anionic solutes 50
anorexia 453
antibiotic prophylaxis 492
antibiotics 298, 323, 485, 782
    sensitivities 480
antineoplastic agents 780
appendicitis 491
appetite
    loss of 453
arachidonic acid metabolite leukotrine B4 61
arrhythmias 701
arteriosclerotic cardiovascular disease 459
ascites 121
    lymphatic absorption in 120
    peritoneal lymphatic absorption rate in 120
ascitic protein 141
asepsis 319
antherosclerosis 381
ATP formation 163
Australia and New Zealand Dialysis and Transplant Registry 748
automated peritoneal dialysis (APD) 8, 9, 399, 641
    adequacy of 407, 429
    advantages 399
    compared to CAPD 403
    efficiency of 405
    history 399
    physiological considerations 403
    selection of 407
    technique 400
aztreonam 205

B lymphocytes 578
backfiltration 126
    consequences of 126
    decreasing 128
back pain 372, 576
bacteraemia 516
bacteria 482, 511
bacterial
    colonization 278
    penetration 475

bacteria to cell ratio 478
barbiturates 175
    removal of 175
basic fibroblast growth factor (β-FGF) 42
Battelle series 686
Baxter Healthcare Inc. 735
Best Demonstrated Practices database 427
beta-2-microglobulin (B_2M) 86, 378, 702
beta-lactam antibiotics 191
bicarbonate 250
    solution 252
bidirectional transfer 183
biochemical monitoring 545
biocompatible membrane 452
biofilm 477, 515
biopsy 19
    histopathological feature 33
    registration 20
bladder augmentation procedure 622
blind insertion
    of catheters 322
blood
    time dependence of 149
blood capillary 69
blood flow 52, 778
    capillary 53
    clearance 53
    hydrostatic pressure 164
    in the peritoneal capillary bed 53
    splanchnic 97
    regulation 97
blood pressure 98, 376, 410, 563
blood sugar control 644
    while on NIPD 647
    with IP-insulin 646
blood-to-lymph transport 50
blood urea nitrogen clearance 360
bloody dialysate 622
bloody effluent 366
bloody fluid 485
body clearance 179
bone
    deformity 616
    diseases 530, 616, 707
    lesion
        aplastic 617
        idiopathic adynamic 543
    mineral stores 540
branched chain amino acids (BCAA) 758
breathing 560
buffer 562, 603
BUN 365
    clearance 360
    profile 425
burnout syndrome 340

C3 511
calcific periarthritis
calcifications 569
calcifying peritonitis 570
calcitonin 535
calcitriol 542

calcium 237, 409, 461, 529, 603
    balance 237, 537
    carbonate precipitation 252
    channel blockers 171
    dialysis fluid 539
    fluids 238
    metabolism 532
    salts 538
    uptake 237
Canadian Organ Replacement Registry 746
cancer 579
    intra-abdominal 784
CAPD 5, 37, 162, 357, 444, 604, 699
    associated fibrosis 37
    benefits 640, 648
    blood pressure control 647
    causes of death 383, 669
    cessation of 40
    clinical results 647
    compared to hemodialysis 361, 379, 454, 668
    compared to IPD/CCPD 360
    complications 373
    concepts 358
    contraindications to 11
    diabetics on 653
    discontinuing 383
    drawbacks 640
    future developments 383
    growth 6
    hospitalization rates 652
    hyperlipidemic effect 240, 459
    history 357
    in children 592
    inception 17
    indications 11
    management program 364
    mass transfer area coefficient in 78
    metabolic complications 372
    nutritional complications 372, 444
    patient and technique survival 651
    peritoneal cavity 504
    peritoneum in 31
    portability 362
    principles 358
    psychosocial aspects 381
    results 8
    solutions 250
    systems 6, 252
        connection methods 253
        connectology 256
        connector designs 253
        disconnect systems 259
        double bag 256
        sterile connection device (SCD) 258
        ultraviolet devices 258
        'Y' shape 254
    technique 6, 362
    therapy 19
        circumstances during 19
    visual problems 649
capillary 47, 57
    basement membrane 51

bed 26
- blood flow in the peritoneal 53
- blood 69
- blood flow 53
  - peritoneal 50
- continuous 70
- endothelium 51, 70, 163
- filtration coefficient 54
- hydrostatic pressure 50, 141
  - gradient 136
- intestinal 50
- lumen 51
- lymphatic 115
- perfused 92
- peritoneal 48, 49
- permeability 778
- surface area 50, 70
- venules 70

captopril 171
carbohydrates 708
carbohydrate metabolism 373, 758
carbon dioxide
- removal of 763

cardiac
- disease 722
- failure 755
- output 52

cardiovascular
- complications 376, 563
- disease 700
- drugs 191
- morbidity 700

care 295
- late 296
- outcomes 693

carnitine depletion 460
catecholamines 98, 170
- dialysate level 98

catheters 3, 271, 315, 515, 599
- break-in techniques 326, 346
- column disc 303
- complications 272, 290, 302, 366, 412, 640
- designs 274
- dislodgement 367
- exit site 272
- failure 305
- fixation device 323
- for infants 599
- hernias 330
- historical perspective 272
- implantation techniques 274, 288, 294
  - stencils 288
  - stilette 288
- indwelling silicone rubber 4
- leaks 330
- luer-locking titanium peritoneal 7
- malfunction 367
- mechanical stress 295
- migration 274, 297
- obstruction 282, 297, 300, 367
- performance 306
- placement 315
- preparation 293
- relocation 297
- removal 302, 315
- repair 315
- replacement 411
- resilience force 282
- rigid 290
- skin-exit direction 279
- soft 293
- surgical insertion in children 602
- survival 368
- Swan neck 284, 305
- Tenckhoff 7, 272, 303
- Toronto Western Hospital 283
- tunnel infections 272
- tunnel morphology 276
- viscus perforation 297

caudal exit direction 279
cell-cell interaction 517
cell count 480
cell proliferation 515
cellular
- defenses 504
- desert 40
- response 477

charge 93
chelating agents 168
chemical mediators 60
chemotherapy 769
children
- disorders 626
- ESRD 594
- management 613
- membrane function 595
- peritoneal dialysis 591
- transplantation 623
- treatment 414, 591

chylomicrons, triglyceride-rich 572
chlorpromazine 175
cholecystitis 491
cholecystokinin 54
cholesterol 460
chronic peritoneal dialysis (CPD)
- alternative approaches 674
- choice as maintenance RRT pending transplantation 624
- comparison to CHD 662, 667, 686
- complications 322
- design 315
- disadvantages 666
- extraperitoneal designs 315
- insertion 322
- intraperitoneal designs 315
- materials 318
- medical advantages 665
- placement techniques 319
- position 317
- prescription for children 604
- problems 318
- psychosocial advantages of 666
- survival on 669

chronic liver disease 753
chyloperitoneum 572

cisplatin 769, 780
cleansing agents 278
clearance 50, 55
clinical
   concerns 243
   features 536
   implications 595
   studies 432
      large patient population 432
      longitudinal 432
      multicenter 433
      single center 432
clinic visits 344
coelomic cavity 26
   history 27
cognitive function 614
collagen attachment 281
colloid 144
   mass transfer rates
      from the peritoneal cavity 123
      intraperitoneal 123
   radio 120
   radio-labelled 123
   tracer 120
color flow-Doppler ultrasound (CFDU) 406
column disk catheter 304
combined peritoneal dialysis 9
communication within healthcare 684
complications
   respiratory 560
computer model 125
conditions
   optimal experimental 149
conductivity
   hydraulic 136
congenital hyperammonemia 626
connections 491
constipation 491
containers 364
contamination
   infectious 517
   microbial 516
   noninfectious 516
continuous ambulatory peritoneal dialysis (CAPD) see CAPD
continuous arterio-venous hemodialysis (CAVHD) 754
continuous cyclic peritoneal dialysis (CCPD) 8, 163, 191, 360, 399, 430, 604, 642
   benefits 640
   biochemical parameters 408
   clinicial experience 408
   complications 410
   growth 9
   hematologic parameters 408
   protocol 404
   renal transplantation 414
   treatment of acute renal failure 413
   treatment of children 413
   treatment of diabetics 413
continuous venovenous hemofiltration (CVVH) 599
controlled enteral nutrition 607
convection 76, 96
   diffusion ratio 96
   free 80

convective transport 77, 164
cortisterone 706
creatinine 85, 96, 147, 153, 163
   clearance 422, 437, 671
   efficacy number (EN) 423
Cruz 317
cryptogenic peritonitis 484
crystalloid 140, 144
cuffs 280, 315
   catheters 280
   Dacron 315
   external 281
   extrusion 281, 299, 369
   number of 280
cycle duration 403
cycles 404
cyclers 401, 603
cyclic adenosine monophosphate (cAMP) 533
cyclooxygenase products 518
cytochalasins 173
cytokeratin 41
cytokines 98, 511, 518
cytological inclusion disorder 29
cytoplasm 76

Dacron cuffs 330
death
   causes 380, 383, 725
Denys-Drash Syndrome 621
desferrioxamine 211
developmental delay 613
devices
   for CAPD systems 251
dextrans (DEAE Dextran) 81, 93, 97, 163
   neutral 94
   polydispersed neutral 147
diabetes mellitus 100, 348, 413, 446, 543, 639, 722
   treatment of 413
diabetic 11
   angiopathy 35
   foot 650
   hyperglycemia 36
diabetiform
   basement membrane pathology 35
   stromal pathology 36
diagnostic problems 490
dialysate
   acid 99
   amino acid containing 99
   calcium 237
   concentration 95, 149
   glucose
      based 140
      rapid absorption of 127
   hypertonic 99
   intraperitoneal
      volume profile 140
      reabsorption 141
   leaks 282, 346, 366, 369
   pathological consequences 17
   return 296
   solute concentration 149
   tonicity 363

INDEX

    to plasma concentration ratio (D/P) 82, 421
    volume 155, 405
dialysis 8
    adequacy 419
        nutrition 438
    dose 420, 643
        clinical outcome 434
    ethical considerations 675
    fluids 3, 233
        based on amino acids 456
    containers 252
    hypertonic solution 145, 155
    in children 598
    index 423
    initiate in diabetics 640
    modality 663
    performance 19
        deterioration in 19
    related stress 691
    schedules 641
    solutions 233
        choosing among 603
        composition 233
        leak localization 300
        leaks 292, 300
    therapy 8
        intermittent 8
        nutrional effects 443
    withdrawal from 675
dialytic
    procedure 451
    sodium balance 234
Dianeal 56
dietary protein intake (DPI) 611
diatrizoate 557
diazoxide 170
diffusion 76, 96, 162
    free 80
    pharmalogically influenced 162
diffusive transport 76
diltiazem 56
dilute solutions 137
dipyridamole 169
disaster plans 353
disconnect systems 8
dissective placements 294
dissective techniques 319
distributed exchange model 76
diurnal cycles 404
diurnal Vip 405
diverticulitis 490
dopamine 170
D/P ratio 82, 421
drainage 292
drainage volumes
    decreased 101
driving force 136
dropouts 381
drugs 161
    absorption 183
        adverse effects 185
        degradation 184
        electric charge 183

        peritoneal lymphatic absorption 184
        peritonitis 184
    abusers 752
    affecting peritoneal bloodflow 173
    antiviral 205
    antifungal 205
    binding 180
    chronic administration 179
    class of 186
    dialysate concentrations 182
    distribution 179
    dose adaptation 182
    fate 180
    half-life 178
    infusion 779
    intoxication 761
    intraperitoneal administration 183
    pharmacokinetics 181
    protein binding 185
    renal clearence 180
    therapeutic 769
    therapeutic effects 177
    toxic effects 177
    transfer to the blood 770
    used in gastroenterology 208
drug-protein binding 182
dual-cuff catheter 329
dual-energy X-ray absorptiometry (DEXA) 546
dual photon absorptiometry (DPA) 546
dyslipidemia 702

effective peritoneal blood flow (EPBF) 53
effusions
    pericardial 100
    pleural 100
elderly patients 349, 661
    adequacy of dialysis 671
    CPD 667
    morbidity 670
    poor nutrition 349
    quality of life 671
elective nephrectomies 622
electric charge 81
electrochemical concentration coefficient 163
electrolyte balance 234
employment 689
encapsulating sclerosing peritonitis 621
endocrine abnormalities 705
endogenous infections 477
endosteal fibrosis 530
end-stage chronic renal disease (ESRD) 186
    demographics 661
    in children 592, 594
    life expectancy 663
    pregnancy 751
end stage renal failure (ESRF) 679
energy
    intake 448, 464
    malnutrition 445
    requirements 449
enteritis, necrotizing 565
environmental infections 477
eosinophils 479

epidermal cells 275
epidermis 276
epinephrine 54, 98
epithelialization 278
epithelium 41, 277
Epo 348
    impact 692
erythema 369
    treatment of 369
erythropoietin 208, 461, 769
    administration of 208, 348
    recombinant human 692
essential amino acid-containing dialysate (EAAD) 609
European Dialysis and Transplant Association Registry (EDTA Registry) 532, 746
exchange
    fluids 46
    hypertonic 146
    isotonic dependence 155
    time dependence 155
exit direction 278
exit site care 369
exit site appearances 298
    classification of 298
    placement 319
exit site infection 274, 297, 347, 368, 411, 480, 618
    treatment 299
exit trocar 288
exogenous toxins 162
extraperitoneal space 292
    penetration of 292
extraskeletal 536
exuberant granulation tissue 299

failure 40
family 625
fenestrated 70
fibrin 477
    exudation 40
    insudation of 39
fibroconnective tissue
    excess 41
    growth of 41
fibrogenesis
    uncontrolled serosal 41
fibronectin 477, 513
fibroneogenesis 40
fibrosis 37
    CAPD-associated 37
    mural 37, 38
    pathogenesis of peritoneal 39
        in CAPD 39
    schistosomal hepatic 121
fibrosing syndromes
    categorization of 37
Fick's first law of diffusion 76
flow
    bulk 126
fluids 135
    absorption 57
        transcapillary 141
    biological 477

    loss 126
    movement 119, 135
    overload 101
    transperitoneal 135
        mathematical models describing 155
    transport of 69
5-fluorouracil (5-FU) 780
fluoroquinolones 191
fructose 242
fungi 481, 484

gastrointestinal
    absorption of calcium 537
    complications 377, 564
gastrostomy buttons 607
genital edema 370, 556
genitourinary surgery 622
glucagon 172
glucose 36, 80, 85, 96, 157, 239, 363, 452, 620, 643
    absorption 457
    based dialysate 140
    concentration 364
    free diffusion coefficient of 93
    intolerance 457
    metabolism 457
    polymer (GP) 246
    rapid absorption of dialysate 127
    reduced tolerance 708
    transport 363
glucagon 54
    intravenous 99
glycerol 95, 241
glycopeptides 191
glycoproteins 60
glycosylation 42
glycylglycine-bicarbonate solution 252
gram negative organisms 369, 483
gram positive organisms 482
gram stain 479
gross ultrafiltration rate 166
growth hormone (GH) levels 706
growth failure in infants 613, 616
growth protein 610
G-tubes 607

haematogenous infections 476
haemodialysis 2, 336
    programme 4
haemoglobin
    autologous 97
        intraperitoneally administered 96
healing process 277
    mechanical factors 277
    systemic factors 278
heart disease 376
heart failure 755
    treatment of 168
hematocrit 692
hematological parameters 408
hemodialysis (HD) 19, 161, 361, 559, 606, 624, 699
hemoglobin
    autologous 140
hemoperitoneum 371, 570

hemorrhage 168
heparin 211, 489
hepatic
    complications 565
    failure 761
hepatitis 482
hernia 370, 412, 555, 619
heteroporous 84
heteroporosity 88
high clearance intermittent therapies 361
high molecular weight agents 238, 245
histamine 54, 171
histological classification 20
histopathological
    changes 18
    feature of biopsies 33
HIV infected patients 752
home
    dialysis 364
    intermittent peritoneal dialysis (HIPD) 714
    nursing 341
    patients 341
    visits 344
homoporous membrane 79
hospitalization 711
host defense 10, 503
    contribution to the 118
    effect of dialysate on 513
host nutrition 521
humoral
    defences 511
    immune factors 512
hydraulic conductance 88
hydralazine 170
hydrocephalus 621
hydrothorax 292, 371, 557, 619
    diagnosis of 558
    treatment of 559
hypercalcaemia 539, 754
hypercalcemic patients 755
hypercatabolic patients 162
hypercholesterolemia 460
hyperglycemic damage 34
hyperkalemia 36, 236, 562
hyperkalemic patients 162
hyperlipidemia 376, 459, 709
hypermagnesemia 236
hyperosmolar solutions 56
hyperparathyroidism 461
hyperphosphatemia 617
hypersensitive reactions 489
hypertension 100, 376, 701
    infrahepatic portal 121
hyperthermia 761
hypertonic
dialysate 99
    dialysis solution 145, 155
    exchange 146
    peritoneal dialysis 122
hypertriglyceridemia 459
hypertrophy 381
hyperventilation 119
hypoalbuminemia 709

hypocalcemia, persistent 563
hypogammaglobulinemia 620
hypokalemia 365, 562
hyponatremia 613
hypophosphatemia 613
hypotensive episodes 701
hypothermia 761

IgG 88, 511
IgM 88
immune
    alterations 447
    response 451, 511
    status, impaired 710
immunocompetence 577
immunologic defense mechanisms 62
immunological status 702
immunoglobulins 148, 478
inadequate dialysis 419
infants
    management of 613
infections 276, 347, 381, 447, 475, 489, 515
infectious organisms 475
inflammatory
    cells 504
    response 517
inflammation 298, 477
    mediators 477
    peritoneal response 62
    the role of microcirculation 58
infusion pain 301
instillation volumes
    to increase 9
instruments
    disease specific 681
    generic 681
insulin 208
    administration 651
    diffusion 647
    intraperitoneal 644
    metabolism 457
    release 644
integrins 60
interleukin-1 568
intermittent peritoneal dialysis (IPD) 186, 360, 399, 443, 604, 641, 714
intermittent
    procedures 360
    therapy 485
internal organs 292
    perforation 292
International Peritoneal Biopsy Registry 18, 19, 20
interstitial 50, 74
    diffusion resistances 90
        series-coupled 90
    gel matrix 50
    oncotic pressure 141
    resistance 93
    space 74
    tissue 157
        connective 163
interstitium 70, 74
intestinal perforation 490

intoxications, treatment in children 626
intra-abdominal pathology 38
intra-abdominal pressure (IAP) 346, 404, 412, 555, 652
intracristal swelling 33
intraluminal 516
   infections 476
intraperitoneal (IP)
   administration 95, 348, 615, 769, 780
      antibiotic therapy 782
         antibody therapy 784
      bacteria 128
   chemotherapy 769
      colloids
         mass transfer rates to the blood 123
      dialysate volume profile 140
      fluid
         accumulation 120
      infusion of isotonic saline 141
      insulin 644, 783
         benefits 644
         problems 645
      isosmotic fluid 119
      pressure 126, 674
      prolonged dwell 162
      prostaglandin levels 518
      reabsorption of dialysate 141
      therapy 769
      volume 406
intravenous
   administration 95
   glucagon 99
inulin 96, 163
   free diffusion coefficient 93
iopamidol 557
iron supplementation 615
ischemic colitis 565
isoporous membrane 84
isoproterenol 55, 93, 169
   enhancement 169
isosmolar 122
   bimodal formulation 145
isotonic saline
   intraperitoneal infusion 141
isovolemia 85

kidney
   extracorporeal artificial treatment 135
   stones 576
   transplant 11
kinetics
   of osmotic pressure 137
   parameter
      reliably estimate 152
   role of lymphatic absorption 121
KT/V urea index 10, 423, 610, 671
KT/V values 437

laboratory evaluation 365
lactate 85, 249
   absorption 95
   buffering effect 249
   dissapearance rate 249
   infusion 249
      metabolic side effects 251
   safety 252
   toxicity 251
lamellar
   bodies 23, 25
   structure 25
Laplace's law 555
large pore system 73
L-carnate 460
leakage, dialysate 619
left ventricular hypertrophy (LVH) 563
leukocyte
   endothelial interactions 62
   interaction 58
licenced practical nurses 339
licenced vocational nurses 339
Lifecath catheter 319
limitations 125
limited energy and exercice capacity 614
lipids 165, 620
   abnormalities 373
   levels 459
   metabolism 458
      disturbances in 458
   solubility 778
lipoprotein profiles 645
liver 115, 761
   cirrhosis 475
   compression 118
   disease 115
low molecular weight agents 238
lubricants 28
lymphatics 166
   absorption 166
   flow rate in CAPD patients 166
lymphatic 46, 75, 118, 141
   absorption 117, 121, 127
      estimating 122, 125
      factors controlling 119
      in ascites 120
      rate 119, 122, 124
      role in kinetics 121
   cannulation 125
   capillaries 115
   circulation 46
   drainage 115
      rate 126
   flow 119
   openings 115
   peritoneal 115
      absorption 119
   rate in ascites 120
      drainage 119
      function of cavity 118, 121
   system 75
lymphocytes 508
lymphopenia, peripheral 508
lymphoscintigram 121
lymphoscintigraphy
   mediastinal 121

macrophages 504

INDEX

macromolecules 96
  charged 174
  dilution of a marker 154
  disappearance rate 97
  tracer 129
  transport 69
magnesium 236, 461, 603
  intake 237
  metabolism 535
  removal 237
  solution 236
magnitude of therapy 429
maintenance dialysis therapy 446
malate 163
malignancy 115, 491, 724
malnutrition 10, 374, 443, 709
  causes 445
  prevalence 446
  prevention 375, 455
  signs 445
  treatment 375, 455
malonate 163
maple syrup urine disease (MSUD) 758
mass transfer 31, 77
  area coefficient (MTAC) 77, 78, 151, 360, 597, 775
  in CAPD 78
material breakdown 302
mechanical accidents 302
medications 366
mediators, release of 518
membrane
  biocompatible 452
  capillary basement 51
  effects
    drugs that have specific 162
  homoporous 79
  isoporous 84
  models of exchange 76
  pathology
    diabetiform basement 35
  peritoneal 2, 70
    determining the solute reflection coefficient 155
    osmosis 157
    surface area 92
    sieving coefficients for the human 146
    ultrafiltration properties 156
  permeability 137, 138
  semipermeable
    ideal 138
    partially permeable 138
  solute-permeable
  surface-active agents 173
  three-pore 90
mesenchymal stem cells
  proliferation 41
mesenteric
  blood flow 163
  circulation
    topography 46
mesentery 45, 163
mesothelial
  cell 20, 510
    cell junctions 20

cell monolayers 62
cell nuclei 20
cytoskeleton 21
  immunocytochemical staining 21
denudation 36
stem cells 42
  entrapment 42
sub-cellular organisation 28
mesothelium 17, 18, 22, 31, 163
  changes in response 31
  changes in surface topography 32
  defoliation 29
  electron micrographs 17
  function 28
  morphological alterations 35
  parietal 25
  similarities of 23
    and type II pneumocytes 23
  visceral 25
metabolic abnormalities 443, 620
metabolic acidosis 10, 450
  correction 248
metabolic changes 243
metabolic problems 651
metabolism 457, 708
  amino acid 758
  inborn errors 626, 757
  oxalate 576
  oxidative 163
metabolites 212
metabolizing renal tissue 451
Michigan Kidney Registry 652, 669
Michigan Registry Study 379, 743
microbiological
  culturing 479
  environment 475
microcirculation
  inflammation 58
  physiologic principles 50
microporous bacterial filter 257
microorganisms 277
microvascular
  exchange 54
  permeability 50
microvasculature 47
  hemodynamic pressure profiles 47
  transport 51
microvilli 20, 75
mid-arm muscle circumference (MAMC) 446
mineral metabolism 461
minerals 464
minimal effective concentration (MEC) 179
Missouri coiled catheter 323
Missouri Kidney Program 748
mitochondria 20
  degenerative changes 33
mitochondrial pyknosis 33
modality 719
  selection 673
model
  implementation 772
  multicompartmental 152
  multiexponential 152

molecular
  large 144
  size 93
  weight 86, 771, 775
  weight toxins 423
molecules 362
  removal 362
Moncrief technique 294, 326
monitoring suggestions 615
monocytes 504
morbidity 381, 412, 447, 616, 649, 670
  cardiovascular 381
mortality 412, 447, 490, 649, 667, 693, 709
MTAC 77, 78
  of creatinine 95
multi-disciplinary team 682
multiple myeloma 762
mycobacteria 483
myeloma kidney 762
myocardial ischemic episodes 701
myofibroblasts 41
myoglobin 86

National Academy of Sciences for children 605
National CAPD Registry of the National Institute of Health 304
National Cooperative Dialysis Study (NCDS) 10, 426, 453
necrotizing enteritis 565
neonatal hyperammonemia 757
neonates 597
neoplasia 621
neoplastic transformation 573
neostigmine 128, 175
neovascularization 102
nephrology nursing 337
nephrostomes 27
nerve conduction velocity 704
net catabolism of protein 451
net ultrafiltration rate (NUFR) 53
neutrophil 60, 507
neurotension 50
NG-tubes 607
nightly intermittent peritoneal dialysis (NIPD) 9, 399, 430, 604
nightly peritoneal dialysis (NPD) 9
nitrogenous waste-products 409
nitroprusside 55, 93, 169
noncompliance 352
non-dialyzed chronic renal failure 447
non-insulin dependent diabetes mellitus (NIDDM) 644
non-urea nitrogen losses 611
norepinephrine 98, 171
Nottingham Health Profile 692
nuclear
  fibrous lamina 20
  profile 32
    alteration in 32
nursing 335
  at home 341
  back up support 341
  care 339
  cost effectiveness 341
  homes 674
  job enrichment 340
  legal complications 341
  licenced 339
  methods 340
  practice 341
  procedures 347
  qualifications 337
  quality improvement 342
  research 353
  staffing levels 338
  stress 340
  teaching 342
nutrition 438, 443
  and dialysis adequacy 438
nutritional
  abnormalities 443
  efficacy 243
  intake 463
  management of children on CPD 605
  problems 650
  status 409, 445

omenta 45
omental attachment 330
oncotic
  pressure 141
    interstitial 141
  transcapillary reabsorption 143
operative repair 559
opsonic
  activity 513
  capacity of the dialysate 519
oral pulse therapy 542
organ erosion 302
orthostatic systolic pressure 235
osmolality 238
osmolality gradient 138
osmolar concentration 137
osmosis 79
osmotic 137
  agent 129, 144, 238, 456, 603, 643
    alternative 143
  conductance 156
  efficacy 242
  flow with a hyposmolar solution 144
  fluid flow 90
  forces 137
  peritoneal membrane 157
  pressure 137
    equilibrium 122
    gradient 136
    kinetics 137
  reflection coefficient 47, 81, 138, 157
  solute 157
  ultrafiltration 135
osteitis fibrosa cystica 530
osteoblasts 532
osteoclasts 530
osteocytes 532
osteodystrophy 544
osteomalacia 530

INDEX

outflow failure 330
outflow obstruction 303
oxalate metabolism 576

PA
   values 151
   variation 775
pain 283, 615
Palmer catheter 273
p-aminohippurate (PAH) 147
pancreatitis 491, 564, 758
Pappenheimer theory 165
paracorporeal membrane oxygenation 763
paracrystalline intracytoplasmic inclusions 28
   formation 29
parallel pathway model 76
paraproteinemia 100
parathyroid glands 533
parathyroid hormone (PTH) 461, 532, 616, 617
parathyroidectomy 541
particles 128
pathogenesis
   of hydrothorax 557
   of renal osteodystrophy 531
   of SEP 568
pathognomic 35
patients
   body image 352
   care 295, 337, 344
   drop-outs 381
   elderly 349
   environment 365
   high risk 338
   holiday arrangements 351
   hospitalized 346
   infection rate of 347
   management 365
   personal hygiene 351
   preparation 293
   selection 10, 492, 625
   sex life 352
   situation 353
   size 422
   survival 379, 716, 719
   training of 335, 342, 364
   transport rates 349
Patlak equation 77
PCR 437
peak concentration hypothesis 437
pediatric patients 602
peptides 248
perforated ulcer 491
pericatheter hernias 330
pericatheter leaks 282, 300, 330
perichromatin granules 32
periluminal 516
   infections 476
peripheral
   lymphopenia 508
   monocyte function 505
   neuropathy 424
   oedema 3

peritoneal
   access 4, 272, 640
   anatomy 1
   barrier 125
      exchange characteristics 90
   biopsy 19
      opportunity for 19
   bleeding 371
   canals 27
   capillary 48, 49
      blood flow 50
   catheter tunnels 276
   cavity 45, 51, 69, 128, 504, 763
      access to 272
      as a drug delivery system 771
      complications related to 370
      experimental uses for 763
      function of lymphatics 118, 121
      homeostasis 477
      in CAPD patients 516, 517
      mass transfer rates of colloids 123
      physiologic characteristics 770
   cells 503
   clearance 83
   dialysis
      access care 271
      adequacy 419, 671
      automated (APD) 8, 9
      clinical studies 432
      combined 9
      comparative studies 699
      complications 617
      continuous ambulatory (CAPD) 5, 37
      continuous cyclic (CCPD) 8
      cyclers 401
      efficiency 102, 169
      exit site care 271
      fluid 249
      hypertonic 122
      history 592
      in children 591, 601
      in elderly patients 661
      intermittent 4, 85, 140, 248
      long-duration 102
      luer-locking titanium 7
      nightly intermittent (NIPD) 9
      noninfectious complications of 555
      nursing 335
      nutritional requirements 443
      patients 443
      program 335
      pump-driven systems 402
      rabbit model of 154
      special situations 751
      surface area 778
      solutions 233, 403, 600
      tidal (TPD) 9, 642
   disappearance rate of tracer 126
   drainage 516
   drug clearence 181
   effective blood flow (EPBF) 53
   equilibration test (PET) 82, 349, 361, 421, 598

exchange 46, 76
   contribution 46
   membrane models 76
fibrosis 34
   pathogenesis in CAPD 39
fluid
   biocompatibility 241
   mathematical model 148
flux 539
gas clearance 53
inflammation 33
International Biopsy Registry 18, 19, 20
lavage 1, 489
lymphatic 115
   absorption 119, 597
   drainage 119
lymphocytes 508
macrophage 518
   function 505
mass transport 169
membrane 2, 70, 510
   characteristic 349
   determining the solute reflection coefficient 155
   function in children 595
   osmotic 157
   surface area 92
   sieving coefficients 146
   ultrafiltration properties 156
mesothelial cells 518
microcirculation 45
microvascular architecture of the parietal 47
microvasculature in transport 51
morphology 10
nutrition 763
opacification 37
permeability 31
   area coefficient 162
   inter-patient variability 31
   intrinsic clinical measurement 94
reaction 20
response to inflammation 62
solute transfer in children 597
solute transport 101
   effect of posture 406
   rate 407
surface area 70, 430
   effective 94, 101
transport 51, 169
   accelerating 166
   drugs 177
   in children 597
   kinetics 170
   mathematical description 51
   model 771
   pharmalogical manipulations 161
   physiological manipulations 161
   rate 163
   small molecules 774
   three-pore model 157
ultrafiltration 56
volume 430
peritoneoscopic equipment 289, 294
peritoneoscopic technique 322, 330

peritoneum 17, 18, 26
   anatomical surface area 136
   blood circulation 46
   catheter adherence 296
   defense mechanisms 478
   denuded 33
   endothelioid covering 17
   human 151
   in CAPD 31
   parietal 18, 45
   subdiaphragmatic 75, 116
   surface area 46
   'tanned' 37
   visceral 45
peritonitis 4, 18, 36, 92, 101, 301, 347, 410, 451, 473, 617, 651, 724, 782
   aseptic 484
   bacterial 555
   based on connectology 257
   CAPD-related 651
   causative organisms 481
   clinical course 480
   complications 490
   definition 480
   diagnosis 479
   diagnostic problems 490
   encapsulating sclerosing 621
   eosinophilic 484
   episodes 492
   history 473
   incidence 505
   incubation period 480
   indicators 18
   inflammation 92
   neutrophilic 484
   pathogenesis 473
   prevention 491
   rate 8, 492
   evaluation 7, 492
   sclerosing 34, 102, 127, 490
   sclerosing encapsulating (SEP) 38, 670
   symptoms 480
   treatment 485
      side effects 489
permeability 77
   area product (PA) 145
   membrane 137
   regional 778
   surface area product 77
   to inulin 81
permselectivity 49
PGE_2 518
phagocytes 513
pharmacokinetics 177
pharmacokinetic advantage 779
pharmacokinetic alterations 180
pharmacokinetic concepts 177
pharmacokinetic theory 780
pharmacologic manipulations 164
phentolamine 171
phosphate 529
   metabolism 534
phosphatidylcholine (PC) 22, 165, 175

phospholipids 120, 128
phosphorus 409, 461
    balance in CAPD 537
physiological state 407
physiology of tissue 772
pituitary hormones 705
plasma
    clearance 179
    concentration 178
    fluoride concentrations 613
    levels of Thyroxine 705
    lipoprotein (a) levels 460
    renin activity 98
    solute concentration 85
    substitutes 246
platelet activating factor (PAF) 60
pleural effusions 371
pleurodesis 559
plexus
    subperitoneal 115
PMN 507
PMØ 504
pneumocytes 22
    similarities of mesothelium and type II 23
Poiseuille's law 88
poisoning 761
polycystic kidney disease 571
polyethylene plastic tubes 3
polypeptides 163
    gastrointestinal hormones 172
polyurethane catheter 319
polyvinylchloride 3
Popovich technique 294, 326
pore 49
    radius 82
    small 88
postcapillary venules 47, 70
potassium 153, 461, 562
    balance 236
    removal 236
povidine-iodine 296
practical protein balance in growing children 610
pregnant patients 751
preserve immune function 704
pressure, intra-abdominal 563
prophylactic antibiotics 323, 492
prostacyclin 102, 518
prostaglandin 98, 171
    inhibitors 172
    levels 511
    synthase stimulators 172
protamine sulphate 81
protein 163, 511, 620, 709
    breakdown 449
    catabolic rate (PCR) 448
    catabolism 449
    intake 447, 463
    loss of 101, 176, 452, 608
    malnutrition 445
    nitrogen appearance (PNA) 611
    oxidation rate 449
    requirements 448
    total 153
    transport 778
Prune-Belly Syndrome 621
pruritis 573
psoriasis 760
psychosexual problems 690
psychosocial adjustment 691
psychosocial issues 622, 671
pulmonary oedema 3
purulent drainage 369
pyeloureterostomy 622
Pyle-Popovich model 83

quality of life 622, 671, 679
    as a function of treatment modality 687
    assessing 682
    definition of 679
    dimensions 680
    employment 689
    future trends 692
    in relation to healthcare 679
    instruments 680
    sexual functioning 690
    stress 691
    studies 684
quantitative computed tomography (QCT) 546
QL index 681

race 722
radio-colloids 120
radio-labelled colloid 123
radio-labelled serum albumin (RISA) 75
radiological monitoring 546
reactive oxygen metabolites 61
recombinant human erythropoietin (rHuEPO) 208, 348, 461, 614
    optimum dosing regimen
recurrence 481
recurrent peritonitis 451
redox dye 163
reflex ileus 366
Registry of the European Dialysis and Transplant Association (EDTA Registry) 736
registry results 736
regression
    linear 149
    nonlinear 149
rehabilitation
    medical 688
    vocational 688
reinfection 481
relaps 481
remesothelialization 40
renal
    anemia 614
    cancer 573
    failure 29
        children with acute 598
        chronic 161, 447
        end-stage 135
        uremic manifestations 29
    function 177, 710
    impairment 531
    malignancy 573

osteodystrophy 409, 529, 531, 537, 616
replacement therapy (RRT) 1, 592, 624
tissue 451
transplantation 19, 623
RER 29
degenerative changes 33
hyperplasia 32
residual-renal function 437, 648
resilient lining cell
role as a 28
respiration 561
respiratory
alkalosis 563
burst activation 514
complications 560
dysfunction 372
restricted diffusion 80, 165
rHuEPO see: Recombinant human erythropoietin
rigid catheters 290
complications 291
loss of 292
risk factor analysis 433, 447
rough endoplasmic reticulum (RER) 20

Scanlan tunneler 288
sclerosing encapsulating peritonitis (SEP) 38, 372, 567
sclerosing peritonitis 34, 102
sclerotic tissue 39
secretin 54, 172
Seldinger guide wire 289, 294, 322
selectins 60
septicemia 447
sex 722
sexual functioning 690, 706
serine depletion 451
serositis
etiology of uremic 29
initiation of the exudative 29
serotonin 54
serum albumin 460
serum antibacterial activity 704
serum lipid concentrations 460
serum magnesium 540
serum potassium 365
serum proteins 94, 104
shape 93
sickness impact 689
sieving coefficient 146, 147, 148
for the human peritoneal membrane 146
silicone catheter 319
single cuff catheter 329
single photon absorptiometry (SPA) 546
sinus tract 279
sinus tract length 279
SK36 689
skeletal manifestations 536
skeletal scintigraphy 546
skeletoarticular complications 377, 381
small solute indices 421
social workers 684
sodium 153, 234
anions 157
balance 234

bicarbonate 251
chloride 92
intake 234
side effects 234
removal 234
solution 235
transfer 92
soft catheters 293
complications 296
solute
characteristics 772
clearance 421
independent parameters 772
permeability 596
removal 403, 425, 671
solutions 85, 456
dialysate concentration 149
large 128
lipid soluble 163
low molecular weight
disappearance rate 95
mass transfer 127, 167
MTAC 85
permeable membrane 138
reflection coefficient 146, 148
accuracy from computer experiments 151
of the peritoneal membrane 155
removal 145
transfer 76
transport 48, 76, 87, 135, 148
of small molecules 69
peritoneal 101
ultrafiltration 155
volume 430
warming 351
water soluble 163
sorbitol 242
splanchnic perfusion 166
splanchnic vascular bed 164
spontaneous bacterial peritonitis 475
staff
attitudes 682
level 337
orientation 339
recruitment 339
stress 340
staff-patient ratio 339
staphylococcus aureus nasal carriage 279
staphylococcus epidermidis 42
staphylococci 510
Starling
equation 57
forces 141
stem cells 41
sterile connections 491
stomata 115, 116, 117
stromal diabetiform lesions 34
studies 432
subcutaneous
administration 348
cuff 326
removal of 326
dosing 769

INDEX

submersion in water 296
submesothelial stroma 26
surgical wound infections 366
sutures 319
Swan neck catheter 284, 305, 318
    complications 284
    survival probability 305
Swan neck presternal 294
synthetic polymers 246
systemic administration 181
systemic antibiotics 298
succinate 163
superimmunoglobulins 60
surface area
    effective filtering 136
    regulations 97
surgical peritonitis 474
synoviocytes 41
systemic
    circulation 118
    disease 101
    lupus erythematosus (SLE) 100
    sclerosis 100
    vasculature 45

T lymphocytes 577
technique
    failure 716
    success 714
    survival 380, 713
Tenckhoff catheters 272, 283, 303, 515, 600
    complications 303
Tenckhoff trocar method 288, 322
tendonitis 575
tendon rupture 575
terminal arterioles 47
testosterone levels 706
TGF-β-1 41
therapy adequacy requirements 421
theophylline 170
theoretical concerns 148
thermoclave 257
thoracentesis 559
thoracic duct 116
three-pore membrane 90
three-pore model 86, 93
three-stream method 251
Thyroxine 705
tidal
    dialysis 350
    peritoneal dialysis (TPD) 9, 350, 604
    ultrafiltration volume 350
time trade off (TTO) 689
tissue
    perfusion 277
    reaction 275
    solute concentration profiles 74
    weights 773
topographical alterations 32
Toronto Western Hospital catheters 282, 304, 319, 601
    complications 282
toxicity 427
    to mesothelial cells 515

trace elements 463
tracer colloid 120
training program 335, 625
transcapillary
    fluid absorption 141
    oncotic reabsorption 143
    ultrafiltration 121, 136
transcellular ultrafiltration 49
transcutaneous catheter 322
transcytosis 86
transiliac bone biopsy 546
transmembrane fluid transport 28
transmittance coefficient 148
transmural infections 476
transperitoneal 74, 79
    absorption 119
    fluid 135
        mathematical models describing 155
    transfer
        bidirectional 118
    transport 74
    ultrafiltration 79, 155
        hydraulically induced 148
        model of 156
        osmotically induced 148
        rate 136, 147
transplantation 335, 578, 613, 710
transport
    augmented 162
    mechanisms 162
    of fatty acids 165
    of lipids 165
    parameters
        accurate calculations of 85
    resistance 163
    size independent 96
    velocity 93
Travasol-base AA solutions 456
triglyceride 709
triglyceride-rich chylomicrons 572
Trocath 599
tube feeding 607
    continuous 607
    technique 607
tunnel infections 347, 368, 480, 618
tunneling devices 288
two-pore model 87
two-stream method 251
tyton ties 290

ultrafiltration 50, 77, 403, 597
    coefficient decrease 175
    cumulative net transcapillary 121, 124
    failure 372, 566
    high transmembrane 146
    importance on transperitoneal solute transport 155
    loss of 126, 127
        net 102
    net transcapillary 127
    osmotic 135
    rate 174, 363
        pharmacological alteration 174
    transcapillary 136

transperitoneal 79, 155
   model of 155
      hydraulically induced 148
      osmotically induced 148
      rate 136, 147
under dialysis 10, 425
United States Renal Data System (USRDS) 280, 306, 412, 669, 735
uraemia 3
urea 85, 92, 153, 157, 163
   clearances 53
   cycle effects 757
   free diffusion coefficient 93
   kinetic indices 436
   kinetic modeling (UKM) 407, 609
uremia 100, 577
uremic
   index 689
   osteodystrophy 707
   pathology 699
   pruritus 378
   serositis 29
      etiology 29
   state 29
ureteric ligation 2
urinary stones 378
USA NIH CAPD Registry 735

vancomycin 782
van 't Hoff's law 79, 138
vascular
   bed 26, 164
   calcification 544
   diseases 168, 722
   endothelium 58, 60
   surface area
      recruitment 92
vasoactive
   agents 54
   effects 162
vasoconstrictor response 164
vasopressin 98
ventricular ectopy 376
ventriculo-peritoneal (V-P) shunts 621
verapamil 56
vesicostomy 622
vimentin 41
   synthesis 21
viruses 481
visceral trauma 366
vitamins 212, 376, 464
   deficiencies 462
   fat-soluble 462
   intake 465
   losses 212
   status 212
   water-soluble 462, 606
vitamin C 577
vitamin D
   metabolites 212
   metabolism 533, 541
   preparation for children 616
von Recklinghausen's stomata 75

water
   metabolism 561
   movement 136
   soluble vitamins 606
WBC yields 504
Weibel-Palade body 76
Wilm's tumor 621
wound hematoma 367

xylitol 242

yeasts 484
Y-set system 652
Y-TEC system 322